APA Handbook of
Psychopharmacology

APA Handbooks in Psychology® Series

APA Addiction Syndrome Handbook—two volumes
    Howard J. Shaffer, Editor-in-Chief

APA Educational Psychology Handbook—three volumes
    Karen R. Harris, Steve Graham, and Tim Urdan, Editors-in-Chief

APA Handbook of Behavior Analysis—two volumes
    Gregory J. Madden, Editor-in-Chief

APA Handbook of Career Intervention—two volumes
    Paul J. Hartung, Mark L. Savickas, and W. Bruce Walsh, Editors-in-Chief

APA Handbook of Clinical Geropsychology—two volumes
    Peter A. Lichtenberg and Benjamin T. Mast, Editors-in-Chief

APA Handbook of Clinical Psychology—five volumes
    John C. Norcross, Gary R. VandenBos, and Donald K. Freedheim, Editors-in-Chief

APA Handbook of Community Psychology—two volumes
    Meg A. Bond, Irma Serrano-García, and Christopher B. Keys, Editor-in Chief

APA Handbook of Comparative Psychology—two volumes
    Josep Call, Editor-in-Chief

APA Handbook of Contemporary Family Psychology—three volumes
    Barbara H. Fiese, Editor-in-Chief

APA Handbook of Counseling Psychology—two volumes
    Nadya A. Fouad, Editor-in-Chief

APA Handbook of Dementia—one volume
    Glenn E. Smith, Editor-in-Chief

APA Handbook of Ethics in Psychology—two volumes
    Samuel J. Knapp, Editor-in-Chief

APA Handbook of Forensic Neuropsychology—one volume
    Shane S. Bush, Editor-in-Chief

APA Handbook of Forensic Psychology—two volumes
    Brian L. Cutler and Patricia A. Zapf, Editors-in-Chief

APA Handbook of Giftedness and Talent—one volume
    Steven I. Pfeiffer, Editor-in-Chief

APA Handbook of Human Systems Integration—one volume
    Deborah A. Boehm-Davis, Francis T. Durso, and John D. Lee, Editors-in-Chief

APA Handbook of Industrial and Organizational Psychology—three volumes
    Sheldon Zedeck, Editor-in-Chief

APA Handbook of Men and Masculinities—one volume
    Y. Joel Wong and Stephen R. Wester, Editors-in-Chief

APA Handbook of Multicultural Psychology—two volumes
    Frederick T. L. Leong, Editor-in-Chief

APA Handbook of Nonverbal Communication—one volume
    David Matsumoto, Hyisung Hwang, and Mark Frank, Editors-in-Chief

APA Handbook of Personality and Social Psychology—four volumes
    Mario Mikulincer and Phillip R. Shaver, Editors-in-Chief

APA Handbook of Psychology and Juvenile Justice—one volume
    Kirk Heilbrun, *Editor*-in-Chief

APA Handbooks in Psychology

APA Handbook of
Psychopharmacology

Suzette M. Evans, *Editor-in-Chief*

Kenneth M. Carpenter, *Associate Editor*

AMERICAN PSYCHOLOGICAL ASSOCIATION
Washington, DC

Chapter 29 was coauthored by employees of the United States government as part of official duty and is considered to be in the public domain.

The opinions and statements published are the responsibility of the authors, and such opinions and statements do not necessarily represent the policies of the American Psychological Association.

Published by
American Psychological Association
750 First Street, NE
Washington, DC 20002
https://www.apa.org

Order Department
https://www.apa.org/pubs/books
order@apa.org

In the U.K., Europe, Africa, and the Middle East, copies may be ordered from Eurospan
https://www.eurospanbookstore.com/apa
info@eurospangroup.com

AMERICAN PSYCHOLOGICAL ASSOCIATION STAFF
Jasper Simons, *Chief Publishing Officer*
Brenda Carter, *Publisher, APA Books*
Kristen Knight, *Senior Reference Editor, APA Books*

Typeset in Berkeley by Circle Graphics, Inc., Reisterstown, MD

Printer: Sheridan Books, Chelsea, MI
Cover Designer: Naylor Design, Washington, DC

Library of Congress Cataloging-in-Publication Data

Names: Evans, Suzette M., editor. | American Psychological Association, issuing body.
Title: APA handbook of psychopharmacology / editor-in-chief, Suzette M. Evans.
Other titles: Handbook of psychopharmacology | American Psychological Association handbook of psychopharmacology
Description: Washington, DC : American Psychological Association, [2019] | Series: APA handbooks in psychology series | Includes bibliographical references and index.
Identifiers: LCCN 2018043964 (print) | LCCN 2018044895 (ebook) | ISBN 9781433830761 (eBook) | ISBN 1433830760 (eBook) | ISBN 9781433830754 (hardcover) | ISBN 1433830752 (hardcover)
Subjects: | MESH: Mental Disorders—drug therapy | Psychotropic Drugs
Classification: LCC RC483 (ebook) | LCC RC483 (print) | NLM WM 402 | DDC 616.89/18—dc23
LC record available at https://lccn.loc.gov/2018043964

http://dx.doi.org/10.1037/0000133-000

Printed in the United States of America

10 9 8 7 6 5 4 3 2 1

Contents

Editorial Board

About the Editor-in-Chief

Suzette M. Evans, PhD, is a psychologist trained in biopsychology at The University of Chicago and in behavioral pharmacology at the Johns Hopkins University School of Medicine. She is currently a professor of clinical neurobiology (in psychiatry) at the Columbia University Vagelos College of Physicians and Surgeons and research scientist VI at the New York State Psychiatric Institute. She has been a member of the American Psychological Association (APA) and Division 28 (Psychopharmacology and Substance Abuse) since 1992. She served as president of Division 28 in 2007 and served as a member of the APA Board of Convention Affairs from 2011 to 2014. She is also a recent past editor of the APA journal *Experimental and Clinical Psychopharmacology* (2011–2017).

Dr. Evans has more than 100 publications and 30 years of research experience that span preclinical research with laboratory animals, human laboratory research, and clinical treatment research in substance abuse. Over the past 25 years Dr. Evans has received continuous research funding, primarily from the National Institute on Drug Abuse. Much of her research has used controlled laboratory procedures in humans to examine the acute behavioral and reinforcing effects of drugs of abuse, including alcohol, cannabis, and cocaine. Her focus is identifying potential behavioral and neurobiological markers of vulnerability to identify high-risk individuals before they transition from casual recreational use to problematic drug use. Several of these factors include stress, impulsivity, and decision making. Moreover, she has been at the forefront of exploring the role of sex as a biological variable. Much of her past and current research focuses on examining potential differences between males and females, including hormonal influences across the menstrual cycle.

Contributors

Alfredo Carlo Altamura, MD, Department of Neurosciences and Mental Health, Psychiatry Unit, Fondazione IRCCS Cà Granda Ospedale Maggiore Policlinico, University of Milan, Milan, Italy

Andrea Arighi, MD, Department of Pathophysiology and Transplantation, Neurodegenerative Disease Unit, Dino Ferrari Center, Fondazione IRCCS Cà Granda Ospedale Maggiore Policlinico, University of Milan, Milan, Italy

Amit Bhaduri, MBChB, BSc (Hons), MRCPsych, Orygen, The National Centre of Excellence in Youth Mental Health, Parkville, Victoria, Australia

Paolo Brambilla, MD, PhD, Department of Neurosciences and Mental Health, Psychiatry Unit, Fondazione IRCCS Cà Granda Ospedale Maggiore Policlinico, University of Milan, Milan, Italy, and Department of Psychiatry and Behavioural Neurosciences, UT Houston Medical School, Houston, TX

Ana J. Bridges, PhD, Department of Psychological Science, University of Arkansas, Fayetteville

Claire O. Burns, MA, Department of Psychology, Louisiana State University, Baton Rouge

Andrew Chanen, MBBS(Hons), BMedSci(Hons), MPM, PhD, FRANZCP, Clinical Services, Orygen, The National Centre of Excellence in Youth Mental Health, Parkville, Victoria, Australia, and Centre for Youth Mental Health, University of Melbourne, Melbourne, Victoria, Australia

Emil F. Coccaro, MD, Department of Psychiatry and Behavioral Neuroscience, Pritzker School of Medicine, University of Chicago, Chicago, IL

Hilary S. Connery, MD, PhD, Division of Alcohol and Drug Abuse, McLean Hospital, Belmont, MA, and Department of Psychiatry, Harvard Medical School, Boston, MA

Jan Copeland, PhD, Faculty of Medicine, University of New South Wales, Sydney, Australia, and Cannabis Information and Support, St. Ives, New South Wales, Australia

Marc L. Copersino, PhD, ABPP-CP, Division of Alcohol and Drug Abuse, McLean Hospital, Belmont, MA, and Department of Psychiatry, Harvard Medical School, Boston, MA

Patrick H. DeLeon, PhD, JD, MPH, Daniel K. Inouye Graduate School of Nursing and the F. Edward Hebert School of Medicine, Uniformed Services University of the Health Sciences, Bethesda, MD

Fernanda P. De Oliveira, Doctoral Candidate, Department of Medical and Clinical Psychology, Uniformed Services University of the Health Sciences, Bethesda, MD

David J. Drobes, PhD, Department of Health Outcomes and Behavior, Moffitt Cancer Center, Tampa, FL

Emmanuel H. During, MD, The Stanford Center for Sleep Sciences and Medicine, and Department of Psychiatry and Behavioral Sciences, Stanford Sleep Medicine Center, Stanford University School of Medicine, Redwood City, CA

Meredith K. Ginley, PhD, Department of Psychology, East Tennessee State University, Johnson City, and The Pat and Jim Calhoun Cardiology Center, UConn Health, Farmington

Jon E. Grant, MD, Department of Psychiatry and Behavioral Neuroscience, Pritzker School of Medicine, University of Chicago, Chicago, IL

Amie Hall, PharmD, 96th Medical Group Hospital, U.S. Air Force, Eglin Air Force Base, FL

Liisa Hantsoo, PhD, Department of Psychiatry, Perelman School of Medicine at the University of Pennsylvania, Philadelphia

Angela M. Heads, PhD, Department of Psychiatry and Behavioral Sciences, Center for Neurobehavioral Research on Addiction, McGovern Medical School at The University of Texas Health Science Center at Houston

Jack E. Henningfield, PhD, PinneyAssociates, Bethesda, MD

Denise A. Hien, PhD, Center of Alcohol Studies, Graduate School of Applied and Professional Psychology, Rutgers The State University of New Jersey, New Brunswick

Tom Hildebrandt, PsyD, Department of Psychiatry, Icahn School of Medicine at Mount Sinai, New York, NY

Maree Hunt, PhD, School of Psychology, Victoria University of Wellington, Wellington, New Zealand

Kyle K. Kampman, MD, Department of Psychiatry and Center for Studies of Addiction, Perelman School of Medicine, University of Pennsylvania, Philadelphia

Therese K. Killeen, PhD, Medical University of South Carolina, Charleston

Bethea A. Kleykamp, PhD, Analgesic, Anesthetic, and Addiction Clinical Trial Translations, Innovations, Opportunities, and Networks, and University of Rochester School of Medicine and Dentistry, Rochester, NY

F. Scott Kraly, PhD, Department of Psychological and Brain Sciences, Colgate University, Hamilton, NY

Clete A. Kushida, MD, PhD, The Stanford Center for Sleep Sciences and Medicine, and Department of Psychiatry and Behavioral Sciences, Stanford Sleep Medicine Center, Stanford University School of Medicine, Redwood City, CA

Scott D. Lane, PhD, Department of Psychiatry and Behavioral Sciences, Center for Neurobehavioral Research on Addiction, McGovern Medical School at The University of Texas Health Science Center at Houston

Matteo Lazzaretti, MD, PhD, Department of Neurosciences and Mental Health, Psychiatry Unit, Fondazione IRCCS Cà Granda Ospedale Maggiore Policlinico, University of Milan, Milan, Italy

Paula Lopez-Gamundi, BS, Department of Psychiatry and Behavioral Sciences, Center for Neurobehavioral Research on Addiction, McGovern Medical School at The University of Texas Health Science Center at Houston

Anne Macaskill, PhD, School of Psychology, Victoria University of Wellington, Wellington, New Zealand

Barbara J. Mason, PhD, Department of Neuroscience, The Scripps Research Institute, La Jolla, CA

Sarah Mathews, MD, Department of Psychiatry, Perelman School of Medicine, University of Pennsylvania, and the Penn Center for Women's Behavioral Wellness, and the Penn Center for the Study of Sex and Gender in Behavioral Health, Philadelphia

Johnny L. Matson, PhD, Department of Psychology, Louisiana State University, Baton Rouge

Robert E. McGrath, PhD, School of Psychology, Fairleigh Dickinson University, Teaneck, NJ

R. Kathryn McHugh, PhD, Division of Alcohol and Drug Abuse, McLean Hospital, Belmont, MA, and Department of Psychiatry, Harvard Medical School, Boston, MA

Roger S. McIntyre, MD, FRCPC, Mood Disorders Psychopharmacology Unit, University Health Network, and Department of Psychiatry and Pharmacology, University of Toronto, Toronto, Ontario, Canada

Dean McKay, PhD, ABPP, Department of Psychology, Fordham University, Bronx, NY

Robert Miranda, Jr., PhD, Department of Psychiatry and Human Behavior, Center for Alcohol and Addiction Studies, Brown University, Providence, RI

Bret A. Moore, PsyD, ABPP, U.S. Army Regional Health Command-Central, San Antonio, TX

Lisa Namerow, MD, Departments of Psychiatry and Pediatrics, University of Connecticut School of Medicine; Consultation Service to Pediatrics, Connecticut Children's Hospital; and Child and Adolescent Psychiatry, Institute of Living/ Hartford Hospital, Hartford

Lorenz S. Neuwirth, PhD, Department of Psychology and SUNY Neuroscience Research Institute, SUNY College at Old Westbury, Old Westbury, NY

Stephanie S. O'Malley, PhD, Department of Psychiatry, Yale School of Medicine, New Haven, CT

Nancy M. Petry, PhD, (deceased) The Pat and Jim Calhoun Cardiology Center, UConn Health, Farmington

Michaela Pettie, BSc(Hons), School of Psychology, Victoria University of Wellington, Wellington, New Zealand

Alessandro Pigoni, MD, Department of Neurosciences and Mental Health, Psychiatry Unit, Fondazione IRCCS Cà Granda Ospedale Maggiore Policlinico, University of Milan, Milan, Italy

Julie R. Price, PsyD, MSCP, RYT200, Department of Anesthesiology/Pain Medicine, 96th Medical Group Hospital, U.S. Air Force, Eglin Air Force Base, FL, and Sacred Integrative Healing, Shalimar, FL

Micah J. Price, PsyD, Department of Anesthesiology/Pain Medicine, Naval Hospital Pensacola, Pensacola, FL, and Sacred Integrative Healing, Shalimar, FL

Antonio E. Puente, PhD, Department of Psychology, University of North Carolina Wilmington

Lynette A. Pujol, PhD, U.S. Army Regional Health Command-Central, San Antonio, TX

Carla J. Rash, PhD, The Pat and Jim Calhoun Cardiology Center, Behavioral Health, UConn Health, Farmington

Lara A. Ray, PhD, Department of Psychology, University of California, Los Angeles

Erin K. Reid, Doctoral Candidate, Department of Psychological, Health, and Learning Sciences, College of Education, University of Houston, Houston, TX

Joshua D. Rosenblat, MD, Mood Disorders Psychopharmacology Unit, University Health Network, Department of Psychiatry and Pharmacology, University of Toronto, Toronto, Ontario, Canada

Lesia M. Ruglass, PhD, Department of Psychology, City College of New York, City University of New York, New York

Patrick Sajovec, Doctoral Candidate, Department of Psychological, Health, and Learning Sciences, College of Education, University of Houston, Houston, TX

Elio Scarpini, MD, Department of Pathophysiology and Transplantation, Neurodegenerative Disease Unit, Dino Ferrari Center, Fondazione IRCCS Cà Granda Ospedale Maggiore Policlinico, University of Milan, Milan, Italy

Susan Schenk, PhD, School of Psychology, Victoria University of Wellington, Wellington, New Zealand

Joy M. Schmitz, PhD, Department of Psychiatry and Behavioral Sciences, Center for Neurobehavioral Research on Addiction, McGovern Medical School at The University of Texas Health Science Center at Houston

Mark R. Serper, PhD, Department of Psychology, Hofstra University, Hempstead, NY, and Department of Psychiatry, Icahn School of Medicine at Mount Sinai, New York, NY

Bradley H. Smith, PhD, Department of Psychological, Health, and Learning Sciences, College of Education, University of Houston, Houston, TX

Kathryn Z. Smith, PhD, Columbia University Medical Center/New York State Psychiatric Institute, New York

Dan J. Stein, MD, PhD, Department of Psychiatry and Mental Health, University of Cape Town, Cape Town, South Africa

Robyn Sysko, PhD, Department of Psychiatry, Icahn School of Medicine at Mount Sinai, New York, NY

Katherine Thompson, PhD, Orygen, The National Centre of Excellence in Youth Mental Health, Parkville, Victoria, Australia, and Centre for Youth Mental Health, University of Melbourne, Melbourne, Victoria, Australia

Keith A. Trujillo, PhD, Department of Psychology and Office for Training, Research, and Education in the Sciences, California State University San Marcos

B. Timothy Walsh, MD, Department of Psychiatry, Columbia University College of Physicians and Surgeons, and New York State Psychiatric Institute, New York

Karin Tong Wang, Doctoral Candidate, Department of Psychology, Hofstra University, Hempstead, NY

Margaret C. Wardle, PhD, Department of Psychology, University of Illinois at Chicago

Michael F. Weaver, MD, Department of Psychiatry and Behavioral Sciences, Center for Neurobehavioral Research on Addiction, McGovern Medical School at The University of Texas Health Science Center at Houston

Allanah J. Wilson, MBChB, Department of Psychiatry and Mental Health, University of Cape Town, Cape Town, South Africa

Jin H. Yoon, PhD, Department of Psychiatry and Behavioral Sciences, Center for Neurobehavioral Research on Addiction, McGovern Medical School at The University of Texas Health Science Center at Houston

Kristyn Zajac, PhD, The Pat and Jim Calhoun Cardiology Center, Behavioral Health, UConn Health, Farmington

A Note From the Publisher

The *APA Handbook of Psychopharmacology* is the 31st publication to be released in the American Psychological Association's *APA Handbooks in Psychology®* series, instituted in 2010. The series comprises both single volumes and multivolume sets focused on core subfields or on highly focused content areas and emerging subfields. A complete listing of the series titles to date can be found on pp. ii–iii.

Each publication in the series is primarily formulated to address the reference interests and needs of researchers, clinicians, and practitioners in psychology. Each also addresses the needs of graduate students for well-organized and highly detailed supplementary texts, whether to "fill in" their own specialty areas or to acquire solid familiarity with other specialties and emerging trends across the breadth of psychology. Many of the sets additionally bear strong interest for professionals in pertinent complementary fields (i.e., depending on content area), be they corporate executives and human resources personnel; psychiatrists; doctors, nurses, and other health personnel; teachers and school administrators; counselors; legal professionals; and so forth.

Under the direction of small and select editorial boards consisting of top scholars in the field, with chapters authored by both senior and rising researchers and practitioners, each reference commits to a steady focus on best science and best practice. Coverage converges on what is currently known in the particular topical area (including basic historical reviews) and the identification of the most pertinent sources of information in both the core and evolving literature. Volumes and chapters alike pinpoint practical issues; probe unresolved and controversial topics; and highlight future theoretical, research, and practice trends. The editors provide guidance to the "dialogue" among chapters through internal cross-referencing that demonstrates a robust integration of topics. Readers are thus offered a clear understanding of the complex interrelationships within each field.

With the imprimatur of the largest scientific and professional organization representing psychology in the United States and the largest association of psychologists in the world, and with content edited and authored by some of its most respected members, the *APA Handbooks in Psychology* series is an indispensable and authoritative reference resource for researchers, instructors, practitioners, and field leaders alike.

Introduction

The field of psychology has played a significant role in furthering an understanding of the joys as well as the trials and tribulations of the human condition. Psychology's scope includes developing experimental methods and procedures to identify and study the processes affecting an individual's emotional and behavioral functioning, utilizing this knowledge to develop programs and treatments that can help mitigate the suffering associated with emotional and behavioral dysregulation, and contributing to awareness of the "bigger picture": the larger contextual factors that influence and circumscribe this important work.

Psychopharmacology is a branch of pharmacology that focuses on the study and development of psychoactive drugs (i.e., drugs that affect the brain). These drugs typically interact with specific target sites in the central nervous system, which results in temporary changes in biology, mood, and behavior. One of the primary goals of psychopharmacology is to develop medications and evaluate their effectiveness and safety for the treatment of mental health conditions. While physicians and other medical professionals are the primary prescribers of medications for mental health disorders, there is a growing intersection between psychology and medicine. Thus, all psychologists and other mental health professionals would benefit from having a basic understanding of psychopharmacological methods and procedures, their application to address human suffering, and the key contextual factors involved.

The *APA Handbook of Psychopharmacology* is designed to provide a working knowledge of basic pharmacology and psychopharmacology, to illustrate the utility of pharmacotherapy for addressing different dimensions of human suffering, and to highlight the broader professional and social issues involved in this work in a language suitable for a broad readership. We envision this handbook as being helpful in several ways: by providing a library reference that captures the most current research to date on pharmacotherapy strategies for addressing emotional and behavioral conditions, as an informative guide for educators and students to strengthen their understanding of the scientific and professional issues associated with the field of psychopharmacology, and as an invaluable desk reference for both researchers and practicing clinicians. Psychopharmacology is constantly changing, particularly as new medications emerge, and thus the primary goal of this handbook is to summarize the current and emerging research and clinical evidence related to the pharmacologic treatment of mental health disorders. Many treatment approaches incorporate pharmacological interventions, and although currently few psychologists prescribe medications to their patients, this may change in the future. Regardless, it is likely that psychologists and other mental health professionals will be working with patients who either are taking psychotropic medications or have questions concerning their utility. Thus, a more in-depth understanding of the literature and issues surrounding pharmacotherapy can help facilitate the types of clinical conversations many practitioners will have with their clients. Further, as the health care system changes—we hope to become more integrated—and psychologists become more informed on the role of psychopharmacology for mental health disorders, the more helpful they will be to their patients and society as important members of multidimensional treatment communities.

Distinction in the field was the primary criterion we used when selecting chapter contributors for this handbook. Another important consideration was that contributors (particularly contributors to Part II of the handbook) had to be amenable to writing their chapters according to our structured thematic framework. This framework was employed to provide readers with a more consistent experience across chapters. Our hope was that the parallel structure of chapters also would allow the handbook to be used as a go-to desk reference for specific information (e.g., evidence for pharmacotherapy across the lifespan).

Upon undertaking the task of identifying potential contributors, based on the breadth of mental health disorders covered in the handbook, it became clear that this was beyond the scope of our personal expertise. This forced us, as editors, to reach out far beyond our normal circle of colleagues. We are extremely pleased with the positive response we received from our colleagues and from experts in their respective fields, many of whom we interacted with for the first time. While we anticipated that many seasoned individuals would contribute to the handbook, we also encouraged joint contributions with more junior individuals. Consequently, this handbook has a broad and diverse range of contributors, including researchers working in academic environments, private practice, or business settings; educators; clinical psychologists; and school psychologists. Psychiatrists and other physicians are also represented, thus giving the handbook a truly multidisciplinary approach. While the majority of contributors are from the United States, a number of chapters are by experts from Canada, Italy, Australia, New Zealand, and South Africa. The international authorship provides a broader perspective on recommended and adopted guidelines in the use of pharmacotherapy for certain disorders.

ORGANIZATION OF THIS VOLUME

The handbook is organized into three main parts. Part I, Fundamental Principles of Pharmacology and Psychopharmacology, presents an overview of key concepts in both pharmacology and psychopharmacology to provide readers with essential knowledge about the concepts and terminology utilized throughout the handbook. This part begins with a brief history of psychopharmacology and how it relates to psychology and psychiatry. Because psychopharmacology concerns the effects of drugs on the mind and behavior, the next chapter focuses on the key neurotransmitters and receptors involved in the actions of psychoactive drugs to provide a fundamental knowledge of brain structure and chemical neurotransmission. To illustrate these concepts, this chapter also includes links to some entertaining and instructive neuroscience video clips. The basic tenets of pharmacology are covered as well in the next chapter, including drug dosing, distribution, routes of administration, and drug interactions. The next two chapters focus on the role that animal and human laboratory research plays in understanding the functions of psychotropic medications within organisms. For instance, procedures have been developed to model various aspects of human pathologies in laboratory animals. These types of studies are important for assessing safety and mechanisms of action, and they can provide initial information on potential clinical efficacy. Human laboratory studies also have been useful in advancing psychiatric medication development and they fill an important translational gap between studies using laboratory models or animals and large-scale clinical trials testing the efficacy of medications in the patient population of interest. The last chapter in this part describes evidence-based pharmacotherapy, including the fundamentals of randomized clinical trials and the regulatory issues involved in bringing a drug to market, as well as the importance and utilization of additional efficacy and safety data collected during the postmarket phase.

Part II, Implementing Psychopharmacology for the Treatment of Psychological Disorders, Substance Use Disorders, and Addiction, is divided based on disorder to facilitate the use of this handbook as a desk reference tool. While there are several different approaches to classifying mental health disorders, we elected for a variety of reasons to align this handbook with the classification used in the *Diagnostic and Statistical Manual of Mental Disorders* (5th ed.; *DSM–5*; American Psychiatric Association, 2013). The *DSM–5* is organized by disorder, and each disorder has well-defined diagnostic criteria. This common language and these relatively specific criteria facilitate accurate and consistent diagnoses, which are crucial for the appropriate treatment of mental health disorders. Other advantages of using *DSM–5* criteria are that codes from the *International Classification of Diseases, 10th Revision, Clinical Modification* (ICD–10–CM; National Center for Health Statistics, 2018) are included, which providers can use in clinical practice for communication with other health care professionals and to convey reasons for treatment when communicating with third-party payment systems. For settings that use alternative classification frameworks, such as schools, chapter authors highlight diagnostic and assessment issues from a *DSM–5* as well as a behavioral (e.g., response to intervention) framework.

It was beyond the scope of this handbook to cover the entire *DSM–5*. Our intention was to focus on the disorders most likely to be encountered by clinicians and researchers for which pharmacological treatments with some evidence of effectiveness have been employed. Therefore, conditions such as dissociative disorders, somatic symptom disorders, gender dysphoria, elimination disorders, and paraphilic disorders are not covered in this handbook.

For neurodevelopmental disorders, we elected to focus on two conditions, each with a dedicated chapter: autism spectrum disorder and attention-deficit/hyperactivity disorder. For personality disorders, we focused solely on borderline personality disorder. With respect to sleep–wake disorders, there are approximately 10 disorders; however, most sleep–wake disorders rely on nonpharmacological treatments. Therefore, that chapter focuses on the pharmacological treatment of insomnia. The chapter on neurocognitive disorders focuses on Alzheimer's disease, frontotemporal dementia, Parkinson's disease, and Huntington's disease. Additional chapters in Part II include those on the pharmacological treatment of depressive disorders, bipolar disorder, anxiety disorders, schizophrenia and other psychotic disorders, obsessive-compulsive disorder and related disorders, impulse control disorders, trauma and stress-related disorders, and eating disorders. And, while pain isn't a distinct mental health disorder covered in the *DSM–5*, we felt that a chapter dedicated to the pharmacological treatment of pain and pain-related disorders is warranted and timely. A chapter on the pharmacological treatment of sexual disorders was also originally planned for the handbook but could not be included due to unforeseen complications that prevented its timely delivery.

Substance use and related disorders covers a range of substances, and many of these have different mechanisms of action and pharmacological treatments. Further, the use of pharmacological strategies (i.e., medication-assisted treatment) for the treatment of substance use disorders continues to be novel in the field and remains controversial in certain treatment circles. Therefore, this broad section begins with a general overview that touches on the historical context and rationale for medication-assisted treatment in this area, as well as the common processes targeted. This introduction is then followed by individual chapters dedicated to each major substance use disorder: alcohol, cannabis, psychostimulants, opioids, sedatives and anxiolytics, and tobacco. Within the section on substance use and related disorders, we also include a chapter dedicated to the pharmacological treatment of behavioral addictions.

As noted previously, the chapters in Part II follow a structured format to maintain cohesiveness across disorders. Each chapter begins with a short introduction, which is followed by information on the epidemiology and prevalence of the disorders. Each chapter then addresses the current best approaches for diagnosis, pharmacological treatment, assessing treatment response, management of side effects, and medication management issues. For every disorder, attempts are made to integrate the current understanding of the neurobiology and neurochemical mechanisms involved with the suggested pharmacological treatments. Each chapter also addresses other relevant issues that may need to be considered when using pharmacological treatments either across the lifespan (e.g., with children, elderly people) or with men and women.

Unfortunately, at this time, most of the evidence for pharmacological treatments for mental health disorders relies on adults, and primarily on men. Thus, an important outcome of this collaborative effort is the realization that there are important research gaps to fill across the disorders covered in this book. Given that psychotherapy and other nonpharmacological approaches are utilized to treat many mental health disorders and that they have a strong research foundation in the field of psychology, a section of each chapter in Part II is devoted to the integration of pharmacotherapy and nonpharmacological approaches, addressing the benefits and challenges of utilizing a combined approach. Each chapter also addresses common comorbidities and issues surrounding the pharmacological treatment of individuals with multiple mental health (or medical) disorders. We believe this is an important issue, given the prevalence of comorbidity and the clinical complexities often encountered by treatment providers in community settings. Also, given the rapidly changing landscape of drug development, each chapter in Part II concludes with a section on the most promising pharmacological—and sometimes nonpharmacological—treatments that are emerging.

Lastly, a unique aspect of Part II is that a Tool Kit of Resources is provided at the end of each chapter, consisting of recommended references and links to online sources that clinicians can use in practice. This information serves as an important educational and teaching tool so interested readers can stay abreast of the latest developments in the pharmacological treatments for each disorder. The Tool Kit also includes informational handouts for patients and their families. A number of chapters in Part I and Part III of this handbook also provide a Tool Kit of Resources.

Part III addresses several other topical issues that cut across all mental health disorders. Given the prevalence of psychiatric disorders that are treated with pharmacotherapy, psychologists frequently interact with patients and clients who are taking medications. Chapter 29 reviews the issues pertaining to the practice of psychology in the context of pharmacotherapy, such as guidelines related to providing information, collaborating with other professionals, and authority to actually prescribe pharmacotherapies. While prescriptive authority remains a controversial topic, this chapter presents a balanced perspective and emphasizes ethical issues as well as appropriate training and education. This chapter sets the stage for the subsequent chapter, which advocates for integrated behavioral health care within the primary care setting and the important role that psychologists with training in psychopharmacology can have within this framework. Part III of this handbook also addresses the complex role that pharmaceutical industries play in the treatment of mental health disorders, given that their focus is commercial rather than serving the public good, and it provides readers with an understanding of the steps involved in the drug approval process of the U.S. Food and Drug Administration.

Additionally, while this handbook is intended to provide a guide on the pharmacological treatment of mental health disorders, we felt that it would be shortsighted to not include a chapter in Part III on new nonpharmacological therapies directed at altering brain function. As brain stimulation therapy techniques are increasingly used to treat mental health disorders, it is important that psychologists be familiar with issues surrounding their development, testing, and clinical use. Lastly, we were fortunate to have former APA presidents Patrick H. DeLeon and Antonio E. Puente and their colleague Fernanda P. De Oliveira contribute the concluding chapter on the transformation of health care in the United States and the expanding roles of health care professionals.

ACKNOWLEDGMENTS

First, we want to extend our immense gratitude to all of the individuals who contributed a chapter for this handbook. We were overwhelmed by the positive responses we received from fellow colleagues as well as the experts we contacted for the very first time. We also are extremely appreciative of the collaborative stance of this community of authors. Everyone was incredibly responsive to our (sometimes extensive) feedback and made their best efforts to revise their chapters on time. We realize contributors' work was conducted in the broader context of their professional and personal lives, which placed demands on the finite hours of their day. The cooperative efforts of the authors allowed us to achieve our vision of a cohesive handbook that is easy to follow both in terms of structure and technical language.

Second, we want to thank Kristen Knight at the American Psychological Association. She was amazing at supporting both of us and the contributors to this handbook. Her availability and diligence helped keep deadlines on everyone's radar. Further, her gracious assistance and guidance during our learning process and struggles with the online manuscript tracking system facilitated a fairly soft and timely landing for each of the chapters.

During this process, we learned a great deal about mental health disorders that we had limited knowledge about; we also enjoyed a refresher on basic pharmacology and gained a better understanding of the issues surrounding prescriptive authority and the future of psychologists within health care systems. This project reminded us of the significant generosity and dedication within this community of professionals who have made it their life's work to better understand the processes and procedures that can help mitigate the suffering experienced by many individuals and their loved ones. Most importantly, we are grateful to our families for the many weekends and nights that they gave up with us while we made this handbook a reality.

Suzette M. Evans
Editor-in-Chief

Kenneth M. Carpenter
Associate Editor

References

American Psychiatric Association. (2013). *Diagnostic and statistical manual of mental disorders* (5th ed.). Washington, DC: Author.

National Center for Health Statistics. (2018). *ICD–10–CM official guidelines for coding and reporting—FY 2018*. Washington, DC: Author. https://www.cdc.gov/nchs/icd/icd10cm.htm

PART I

FUNDAMENTAL PRINCIPLES OF PHARMACOLOGY AND PSYCHOPHARMACOLOGY

A BRIEF HISTORY OF PSYCHOPHARMACOLOGY IN THE CONTEXT OF PSYCHOLOGY AND PSYCHIATRY

Robert E. McGrath

The history of psychopharmacology consists of two parallel stories. One is the story of the medications themselves, the discovery of the compounds that have come to be used for the amelioration of the mental disorders. This is a story that has been told multiple times from very different perspectives (e.g., Andreasen, 1984; Healy, 2004), and I will begin by summarizing some of the major milestones in the development of psychopharmacological agents. However, I use that history primarily as a backdrop for a second story, the story of how those discoveries have shaped and are shaping the professions of psychology and psychiatry. I will address the reinvention of psychiatry as a pharmacologically oriented discipline, culminating in a discussion of controversies surrounding the Research Domain Criteria (RDoC), the research framework the National Institute of Mental Health (NIMH) has adopted for research investigating mental disorders. Then I will move on to the growth of interest in psychopharmacology as a component of psychological practice, concluding with some final thoughts on the potential for psychology to ultimately follow the same path as psychiatry.

THE BIRTH OF PSYCHOPHARMACOLOGY

Historically, the understanding of mental disorders has been dominated by three perspectives. Perhaps the earliest of these perspectives attributed behavioral and emotional disturbances to the action of super-natural forces, a belief that provided justification for practices as chronologically distant as trephination—cutting holes in the skull, often with the goal of releasing evil spirits—in the Neolithic period and the burning of witches in 17th century Europe. With the emergence of a more secular culture, by the 19th century two other perspectives came to dominate our understanding of the mental disorders: the psychogenic and somatogenic. They have existed in tension ever since, both complementing and competing with each other.

The roots of the somatogenic perspective in fact run quite deep. The belief that emotional instability in women was due to a wandering uterus was widespread in the ancient Middle East, as was the use of various treatments such as exposure to strong odors to guide the uterus back to its rightful place. The theory first established by Hippocrates around 400 B.C.E. that mental disorders reflected an imbalance in the humors experienced intermittent popularity even in the modern era. It is strikingly similar in its essence to the parallel attribution in Chinese medicine to an imbalance between yin and yang, positive and negative forces in the body. Is it unreasonable to think of even modern biogenic models of mental disorders as suggesting an imbalance in the neurotransmitters of the brain?

The psychogenic perspective, focusing on life events and stressors, emerged slightly later. The Roman physician Galen, who was active in the

http://dx.doi.org/10.1037/0000133-001
APA Handbook of Psychopharmacology, S. M. Evans (Editor-in-Chief)

second century C.E., discussed the potential role of stress in abnormal behavior. Psychogenic models did not emerge as a strong alternative to the somatogenic until modern times, however.

The modern era in the understanding and treatment of the mental disorders begins around the start of the 19th century. Table 1.1 summarizes key turning points in that process, culminating in the emergence of psychopharmacology and its growing importance as a treatment for mental disorders.

Interest in mental disorders as a topic of study probably could not have flourished without the asylum movement that spread across Europe in the 19th century. Prior to that time, institutional-ization usually was, at best, warehousing, and at worst, cruel and inhumane. Quakers sponsored the founding of an asylum in York, England, that focused on compassionate care for "lunatics" under the guidance of William Tuke. Tuke's grandson later wrote a book about the so-called York Retreat (Tuke, 1813/1996) that popularized the concept of "moral treatment" for mental disorders, a term he borrowed from the writings of Philippe Pinel. The modern asylum movement, and the growing belief that individuals with severe mental disorders deserved to be treated with dignity, enhanced both the opportunity for and interest in studying the nature of such disorders.

TABLE 1.1

Milestones in Psychopharmacology in the United States

Year	Event
1796	The moral treatment movement spurs the founding of York Retreat by William Tuke. Offering compassionate treatment for individuals with SMIs, it was widely emulated. The aggregation of individuals with SMIs in asylums that adopted a humane treatment philosophy spurred research into the disorders.
1899	Bayer introduces Aspirin, the first widely successful medication.
1946	Veterans of World War II create a large population of patients needing help with emotional difficulties. The National Mental Health Act establishes the National Institute of Mental Health.
1951	The Humphrey-Durham amendment to the 1938 Food, Drug, and Cosmetic Act defines whole categories of drugs available only by prescription. Previously, prescriptions were largely limited to psychoactive drugs (e.g., cocaine; Temin, 1980).
1954	Lehmann and Hanrahan (1954) report dramatic effects administering chlorpromazine (Thorazine®) to individuals with schizophrenia, resulting in swift adoption in North America. The term *antipsychotic* comes into use. The second antipsychotic, reserpine, is also described for the first time.
1954	Schou, Juel-Nielsen, Strömgren, and Voldby (1954) publish the first controlled trial of lithium for mania.
1955	Meprobamate (Miltown®) is identified as a less sedating anxiolytic than the major tranquilizers, founding outpatient psychopharmacological treatment. It is quickly followed by the more popular chlordiazepoxide (Librium®).
1955	The Mental Health Study Act creates funding for psychopharmacology research.
1957	The first monoamine oxidase inhibitor, iproniazid, is described by Nathan Kline as a treatment for depression. Approved for use in 1958, it was withdrawn in 1961 because of hepatic effects.
1958	Kuhn's (1958) article on imipramine introduces the tricyclics to a wide audience. Among other firsts, Kuhn coins the term *antidepressant*.
1961	Amitriptyline follows. In a marketing innovation, it was introduced with the first book about depression written for nonphysicians (Ayd, 1961).
1962	Amendments to the Food, Drug, and Cosmetic Act establish randomized, placebo-controlled, double-blind studies as the gold standard for evaluating medications.
1965	Schildkraut (1965) introduces the catecholamine hypothesis of depression. Based on drug evidence, depression was associated with insufficient levels of catecholamines, and treatment effects with the inhibition of catecholamine uptake. Coppen (1967) made the parallel argument for serotonin, and later dopamine was implicated in schizophrenia on similar grounds (Creese, Burt, & Snyder, 1976).
1983	Fluvoxamine, the first so-called selective serotonin reuptake inhibitor, is marketed. It is followed four years later by fluoxetine (Prozac®).
1993	*Listening to Prozac* is published (Kramer, 1993), in which the author suggests psychotropic medications can help you feel "better than well."

Note. SMI = severe mental illness.

The biochemical foundations for the discovery of psychopharmacological agents began to emerge a century later. By the end of the 19th century, the dye industry was hiring large numbers of chemists with the goal of identifying new compounds with potential value as dyes. The development of new dyes during this period quickly led to studies on whether they could be used to stain bacteria, then to the finding that the dyes also interacted with bacteria, to evaluating their use as a form of treatment under the emerging belief that disease resulted from microscopic pathogens. By 1899, the German dye firm Bayer was marketing acetylsalicylic acid under the trade name Aspirin. The success of that compound inspired interest in the development of pharmaceutical agents.

With more than 1 million service members receiving diagnoses such as battle fatigue and psychoneurosis during and after World War II (Scull, 2011), the National Mental Health Act of 1946 identified the development of mental health treatments as a priority for the U.S. government, and established the NIMH to support those efforts. Interest in the possibility of biological interventions for mental disorders grew. The emergence of psychopharmacological agents in American psychiatry can be said to have begun in 1954, when Heinz Lehmann and Gorman Hanrahan first described the effects of chlorpromazine on individuals diagnosed with schizophrenia. This was followed shortly by Nathan Kline's description of reserpine. Both were particularly effective at reducing agitation in patients, an attribute that ultimately resulted in their labeling as "major tranquilizers." That was also the same year in which Schou, Juel-Nielsen, Strömgren, and Voldby (1954) described the use of lithium salts to reduce mania. Remarkably, the U.S. Food and Drug Administration (FDA) did not approve the use of lithium for the treatment of mania until 1970 (Shorter, 2009). Though central to the acceptance of these treatments in the United States, these early studies were often built on years of clinical observations by psychiatrists and other medical providers in Europe and Asia.

The public perception of psychopharmacological agents also began to take its modern shape in 1954. The simple choice of terminology for these new classes of medications would prove to have profound effects on how we think of them even today. As noted above, chlorpromazine's primary effect among individuals with schizophrenia was decreased activity and emotionality. That is, behavioral evidence suggested nothing more than that the medication reduced key symptoms of the disorder. However, by the end of 1954 chlorpromazine was being referred to as an "antipsychotic" (Healy, 2004). It is a term that subtly promises a direct effect, and perhaps even a curative effect, on the causal agent for the disorder. This pattern repeated several years later when Kuhn (1958) coined the term *antidepressant* to refer to imipramine. The widespread adoption of these terms is likely to have contributed to public perceptions about the efficacy of the medications.

A separate thread in the cultural acceptance of psychopharmacology emerged in 1955, when meprobamate was introduced under the trade name Miltown®. This was the first of the minor tranquilizers, a class of medications that was to have a profound effect on the future of psychiatry. Their milder sedating effect when compared with the major tranquilizers created an impression that meprobamate and its successors, particularly chlordiazepoxide (Librium®) and diazepam (Valium®), were safe to use even for relatively mild forms of anxiety and stress. Outpatient psychiatry prior to this time was almost exclusively devoted to the provision of psychotherapy. Psychotherapy remained largely equivalent to psychoanalysis, a treatment that required extensive additional training. The emergence of the minor tranquilizers substantially enhanced the economic base for outpatient psychiatry, a base that expanded further with the subsequent advent of medications for the alleviation of depression. Even at this early stage, economic forces were involved in psychiatry's widespread adoption of psychopharmacology as a treatment modality.

Amendments to the federal Food, Drug, and Cosmetic Act in 1962 subtly reinforced the equation of medications with cure. For the first time, drug trials used in applications to the FDA were required to focus on a specific diagnosis, and subsequent marketing was targeted to that diagnosis. This model has provided further support for perceiving medications as treatments for specific disorders rather than as palliatives for certain symptoms. Given the close equation of medications with a disorder, rather than the specific symptoms they treat, it is not surprising that by the mid-1960s, psychiatrists were looking to the neurobiological action of these medications as a guide to the biological mediators of the disorders. The emergence of various monoamine models for depression and schizophrenia (Coppen, 1967; Creese, Burt, & Snyder, 1976; Schildkraut, 1965), discussed further in the next section of this chapter, represented a natural next step in this process.

The 1962 amendments to the Food, Drug, and Cosmetic Act also established randomized, placebo-controlled, double-blind studies as the gold standard for evaluating medications (see Chapter 6, this volume, for more information on this topic). This was an important step in enhancing the rigor of the research supporting the introduction of new medications, but it had an important unanticipated social consequence. These amendments created substantial financial incentive for pharmaceutical companies to develop new medications. In recognition of the costs associated with the development of new medications, costs that can run in the billions, the FDA currently can award 5 years of exclusive marketing to the corporation selling the new drug, with an additional 6 months available for pediatric formulations (Lal, 2015). Since compounds are often patented many years before the drug is brought to market, the exclusivity period is important for protecting the investment in development. Medications have proven to be extremely lucrative during the period of exclusivity when compared with generic alternatives that subsequently become available (Haas, Phillips, Gerstenberger, & Seger, 2005). However, efficacy is defined as superiority to placebo, so there is no incentive to compare new compounds to existing medications. The result is that new medications are heavily marketed in comparison to existing medications during the exclusivity period, and are as a result widely adopted, even though many ultimately show no superiority over established medications. The adverse effects of many medications also do not fully come to light until they have been on the market for a few years (Lasser et al., 2002). A medication no better than existing medications with an uncertain side effect profile creates an unnecessary risk for the consumer. To offer a particularly

timely and relevant example, a recent study found no advantage to opioids over ibuprofen and acetaminophen for the alleviation of acute pain over a 2-hour period in an emergency department (Chang, Bijur, Esses, Barnaby, & Baer, 2017). One can only wonder how much of the opioid use epidemic in the United States could have been avoided had such research been required prior to their introduction to the market.

PSYCHOPHARMACOLOGY AND PSYCHIATRY

The various events outlined to this point provided the backdrop for an important process that began to build steam in the 1960s, which was the conversion of psychiatry from a profession that emphasized both medication and psychotherapy to one that focused largely on psychopharmacological interventions. The response rates reported in the literature even for individuals with severe and persistent mental illnesses were impressive, and clinical observation quickly convinced practitioners of their superiority to the existing alternatives. As noted previously, the introduction of the minor tranquilizers and the antidepressants created new opportunities for outpatient psychiatry. A number of other factors ultimately came to play a role in that transition, however.

One of the most important was the emergence of the monoamine hypotheses, beginning with Schildkraut's (1965) catecholamine hypothesis of depression. The monoamine hypotheses suggested that depression can be attributed to one of several neurotransmitters that involve a single amine group. Taking evidence that the antidepressants of the time were associated with the reuptake inhibition of certain neurotransmitters, the hypothesis equated a deficiency in the availability of catecholamines, a class of monoamine neurotransmitters that includes epinephrine, norepinephrine, and dopamine, with the etiology of depression. Coppen (1967) expanded this work to include serotonin, hence creating a general monoamine hypothesis.

This equation proved attractive for several reasons. It provided a simple model for depression and the effectiveness of the new medications that could be easily understood. It also completed the process of associating the medications with the root biological cause of the disorder that began with labeling these medications antidepressants. Subsequent research on new medications for depression has been largely driven by the search for compounds that elevate norepinephrine, dopamine, and/or serotonin. However, the monoamine model suffers from various difficulties. It is unclear why some chemicals that are known to elevate levels of various monoamines have been found to have an effect on depression while others have not. Also, the therapeutic effect of the medications takes several weeks to emerge even though the monoamine effects occur almost immediately (Hirschfeld, 2000; see Healy, 1997, for a fuller review). Finally, many depressed patients remain treatment refractory even after multiple monoamine trials (Gaynes et al., 2009). Even Coppen (1967) questioned whether the monoamine hypothesis could provide a sufficient theory of depression, and biomedical researchers have begun to consider other causes for at least some cases of depression, such as inflammation (Rosenblat, McIntyre, Alves, Fountoulakis, & Carvalho, 2015).

A second factor was the growth in marketing by pharmaceutical firms directly to physicians, a practice well-documented by Carlat (2010), and to consumers (see Chapter 31, this volume, for a more detailed discussion of this topic). This direct-to-consumer advertising (DTCA) of psychopharmacological agents took a major step forward in 1961. In introducing amitriptyline to the market as Elavil, Merck also sponsored publication of the first book appropriate for the general public on depression (Ayd, 1961). DTCA addressing both medications and the diagnoses targeted by those medications has been outlawed in all but a few countries. In contrast, the United States has few regulations concerning DTCA. DTCA remains a controversial topic, with research suggesting both primarily positive (Mukherji, Janakiraman, Dutta, & Rajiv, 2017) and negative (Mintzes, 2012) effects.

Third, the introduction of the psychotropic medications was followed by exaggerated claims to the general public about their power (e.g., Andreasen, 1984). Perhaps the most notorious example was Kramer's (1993) *Listening to Prozac*, which suggested that psychotropic medications can have profound effects on personality and general functioning. Though Kramer raised concerns about the use of medication for such purposes, it was his claim about the medications' effects that entered the public consciousness. In subsequent years, the popular literature has become more critical about psychotropic medication in particular (e.g., Kirsch, 2010; Whitaker, 2011) and the pharmaceutical industry in general (Carlat, 2010).

A fourth factor was the changing character of leadership in academic psychiatry (Sabshin, 2008). Where the majority of psychiatry departments were chaired by psychoanalysts in the 1960s, by the 2000s those positions were largely occupied by proponents of biological psychiatry, a transition that may in part be attributable to the concomitant growth in funding for pharmaceutical research (Moses, Dorsey, Matheson, & Thier, 2005).

A fifth factor was dissatisfaction with psychotherapy in comparison with medication. The literature available on psychotherapy in the 1960s was not kind to the practice, with Eysenck's (1952, 1966) negative summaries of the research on psychotherapy, and psychoanalysis in particular, playing a particularly important role in raising doubts about its efficacy (Wampold, 2013). It was only much later, with the emergence of meta-analysis (Smith, Glass, & Miller, 1980), that more positive conclusions about psychotherapy efficacy became widely disseminated. Psychoanalysis, which was the most popular therapy among psychiatrists, required years to master, and most popular therapies at the time required frequent contact with the primary provider. In terms of time commitment to an individual patient, it was reasonable for psychiatrists to consider medication a more efficient treatment modality, allowing them to serve a larger population of patients.

Finally, an anthropological study of the current state of psychiatry (Luhrmann, 2000) found that the emergence of managed care and related cost containment efforts has been particularly central to the relative decline of psychotherapy in psychiatry. With growing pressure to cut costs and maximize return, the result has been a shortening of the length of sessions, a decline in the use of psychotherapy, and the shift of psychotherapy to master's level providers. For example, Olfson and Marcus (2009) found that while the number of patients treated with anti-depressants doubled between 1996 and 2005, the percentage of those who were also receiving psychotherapy declined from 31.5% of surveyed respondents to 19.9%. Between 1985 and 1995, the mean length of office-based psychiatric visits declined from 42.8 minutes to 38.1 minutes, and the percent of sessions that were 10 minutes or less increased fourfold, from 2.9% to 12.1% (Olfson, Marcus, & Pincus, 1999). In contrast, the length of primary care visits demonstrated little change. Psychiatrists also reported that patients receiving psychotherapy as part of their services declined from 88.7% to 78.7%, while the percent receiving psychotropic medication increased from 43.6% to 69.4%.

The emphasis on biological conceptions of mental disorders exemplified by the monoamine hypothesis is unlikely to abate. In fact, recent efforts by the NIMH suggest that the emphasis on biological models for mental disorders in federal funding may even continue to grow. Since 2009, NIMH has committed a substantial portion of its resources to RDoC (Cuthbert & Insel, 2013; https://www.nimh.nih.gov/research-priorities/rdoc/constructs/rdoc-matrix.shtml). The RDoC is an attempt to characterize individuals with mental disorders in terms of five domains: negative valence systems, positive valence systems, cognitive systems, social processes, and arousal/regulatory systems. More relevant to the current discussion is the list of key units of analysis for studying the five domains: genes, molecules, cells, neural circuits, physiology, behaviors, self-reports, and paradigms (specific neurocognitive tasks). While this list includes the two primary sources of data used in *Diagnostic and Statistical Manual of Mental Disorders* (5th ed.; *DSM–5*; American Psychiatric Association, 2013) diagnosis—behaviors and self-report—the six additional units are largely biomedical, suggesting an increase in emphasis on the biological underpinnings of problematic behaviors. The initial goal of the RDoC initiative is to provide an integrated framework for research on mental disorders, but there is an implication that this approach will ultimately allow the development of a biologically informed diagnostic system that offers an advantage over the symptom-based diagnostic model embodied in the *DSM*.

Since the introduction of the RDoC, 15% of NIMH's translational research has been dedicated to RDoC projects (Cuthbert, 2015). Not surprisingly, such a radical revisioning of funding priorities has not been without its critics. Frances (2014) has pointed out its lack of relevance to the needs of patients today, when the biological substrates of mental disorders remain largely opaque. Goldfried (2016) has particularly warned about the dampening effect this adoption of biology as the core of mental disorders could have on funding for psychotherapy research and training. His comments raise significant concerns about the possibility that psychotherapy will continue to lose credibility in the face of efforts well-funded by both the federal government and the pharmaceutical industry to treat the biological elements of psychopathology as the most salient.

PSYCHOPHARMACOLOGY AND PSYCHOLOGY

Given the developments of the last 50 years in psychiatry, it should come as no surprise that health service psychologists have regularly grappled with the possibility of adding psychotropic medications to the psychological armamentarium. A later chapter (Chapter 29, this volume) will address the issue of psychologists and prescriptive authority. The remainder of this chapter will focus on the history of the movement for prescriptive authority within psychology.[1] A summary of some key developments in that movement can be found in Table 1.2. As early as 1981, a task force of the American Psychological Association (APA) Board of Professional Affairs concluded "physical" interventions are within the scope of practice of psychology so long as they are competently and appropriately administered. A second task force adopted similar conclusions 5 years later (APA, 1986).

---

[1] A terminological note is appropriate here. Much of what has been written about psychologists prescribing, particularly in the early days of the movement, referred to *prescription privileges*. When used to refer to state legislation permitting psychologists to prescribe, this term is a misnomer. States *authorize* psychologists to prescribe; hospitals and other health care organizations *privilege* health care providers. The correct term is prescriptive authority when talking about legislation, and prescription privileges only when talking about prescribing in some health care setting.

	TABLE 1.2	

A Chronology of Milestones in Prescriptive Authority for Psychologists

Year	Event
1981	The APA Board of Professional Affairs defines the conditions under which the use of "physical interventions" is within the scope of practice of psychology.
1984	Senator Daniel Inouye suggests at a meeting of the Hawaii Psychological Association that psychologists should adopt prescriptive authority as a legislative agenda.
1989	Congress funds a pilot training program for the DoD. The Psychopharmacology Demonstration Project begins two years later.
1992	An APA task force report identifies three levels of preparation for involvement in pharmacotherapy.
1993	The Prescribing Psychologists Register begins offering courses for civilian psychologists.
1993	Indiana permits prescriptive authority for psychologists in relevant federal programs.
1994	The Psychopharmacology Demonstration Project graduates its first two participants.
1995	The APA Council of Representatives votes to make obtaining prescriptive authority APA policy.
1997	The Psychopharmacology Demonstration Project is discontinued.
1999	Guam approves prescriptive authority for appropriately trained psychologists.
2002	New Mexico authorizes prescriptive authority for appropriately trained psychologists.
2004	Louisiana authorizes prescriptive authority for appropriately trained psychologists.
2005	The first prescription is signed by a civilian psychologist in Louisiana.
2014	Illinois authorizes prescriptive authority for appropriately trained psychologists.
2016	Iowa authorizes prescriptive authority for appropriately trained psychologists.
2017	Idaho authorizes prescriptive authority for appropriately trained psychologists.

Note. APA = American Psychological Association; DoD = Department of Defense. From "Prescriptive Authority for Psychologists," by R. E. McGrath, 2010, *Annual Review of Clinical Psychology*, 6, p. 23. Copyright 2010 by Annual Reviews. Adapted with permission.

Explicit discussion within the organization about the possibility of pursuing prescriptive authority for psychologists, commonly abbreviated as RxP, was first spurred by a speech Senator Daniel Inouye (D-HI) made to the Hawaii Psychological Association in 1984, in which he proposed RxP as a means of addressing the shortage of appropriately trained prescribers of psychotropic medications. That discussion ultimately resulted in the formation of an APA task force on psychopharmacology in 1990 (Smyer et al., 1993), and the adoption of RxP as APA policy in 1995 (Fox, 2003). Since that time, APA has sponsored a number of the key developments in RxP, as the following sections will describe.

The Psychopharmacology Demonstration Project

With support from Senator Inouye, Congress funded a pilot program called the Psychopharmacology Demonstration Project (PDP) in 1989 to train psychologists in the U.S. Department of Defense to prescribe. Opposition from physicians delayed the start, so the first cohort did not begin their training until 1991. Sammons and Brown (1997) outlined the evolution of the program. The first cohort began training equivalent to that of a physician's assistant. However, it was subsequently recognized that this approach was inconsistent with congressional intent, which was to prepare independent prescribers. The participants were then enrolled in a curriculum that overlapped heavily with one completed by medical students. This curriculum was also inconsistent with the mandated parameters of the program, as it required 3 years to complete both the didactic and practicum requirements, while the legislation called for a 2-year program. For subsequent cohorts the number of academic contact hours was slashed drastically, from 1,365 to 660 in the last two iterations. A second year was devoted to practicum, during which participants were expected to see at least 100 patients, though in practice they saw more.

Opposition to the program from physicians continued, and it was terminated in 1997. Even in that brief period, with only 10 graduates, it was the subject of four separate evaluations (Newman, Phelps, Sammons, Dunivin, & Cullen, 2000). In general, these evaluations were positive. An initial feasibility study found support among all categories of stakeholders, including primary care physicians and patients, with the exception of psychiatrists. It also concluded that training psychologists to prescribe would cost the military less than using physicians for the same purpose, even when including the one-time startup costs of the program. In contrast, a second study concluded that costs were excessive relative to need. A reanalysis of the findings (sponsored by APA) criticized this report for treating startup and evaluation costs as if they would remain constant, assuming the cost of training a psychologist to prescribe would be the same as that for a medical student even though the curriculum was abbreviated after the first cohort, and misestimating the need for psychiatrists once the United States had invaded Afghanistan and Iraq. Two more reports were completed after termination of the program, focusing on the performance of the PDP graduates. Overall the conclusions were positive. For example, it was noted that eight of the 10 had assumed positions as chiefs of mental health clinics, and their performance was rated positively even by psychiatrists. However, some statements identifying specific reservations about the graduates have been widely cited by psychologists who oppose prescriptive authority. For example, Robiner et al. (2002) focused on statements suggesting the PDP graduates demonstrated somewhat less medical and psychiatric knowledge than practicing psychiatrists.

Actions of the American Psychological Association

APA took a number of actions beginning in the 1990s to advance RxP. Based on the task force report by Smyer et al. (1993), three levels of education and training in psychopharmacology appropriate for psychologists were identified. Level 1 represented basic psychopharmacology education appropriate for all psychologists, for which a single course of 3 to 5 credits added to doctoral-level training in health service psychology was recommended. Level 2 referred to postdoctoral training for individuals who planned to collaborate actively with licensed prescribers in medication decision making. Level 3 referred to postdoctoral training in preparation for independent prescriptive authority. Model curricula were developed for all three levels, but only the Level 3 curriculum has continued to evolve (see APA Council of Representatives, 2009b, for the most recent version), and only programs for Level 3 training have emerged. Some psychologists are interested in psychopharmacology training in preparation for collaboration (i.e., Level 2), but in practice this is accomplished by completing the didactic portion of the Level 3 training.

The Level 3 model curriculum limits participation to currently licensed psychologists with a doctoral degree, and calls for at least 400 didactic contact hours in core content areas, a supervised clinical experience addressing eight clinical competencies, and a capstone competency evaluation. APA also developed model legislation for prescriptive authority (APA Council of Representatives, 2009a), established a committee to designate programs that are in compliance with the APA model curriculum as a quality assurance mechanism in training, and founded the Psychopharmacology Examination for Psychologists, or PEP, as a potential licensing examination for prescriptive authority. This examination is now overseen by the Association of State and Provincial Psychology Boards.

Programs specifically intended to train psychologists to prescribe outside the military have existed since 1993, with the founding of an organization called the Prescribing Psychologists Register. Currently, four programs are designated by APA as meeting the requirements of the model curriculum, at Alliant International University, the Southwestern Institute for the Advancement of Psychotherapy and New Mexico State University, Fairleigh Dickinson University, and the University of Hawai'i at Hilo Daniel K. Inouye College of Pharmacy. Though it is not a requirement of the APA model curriculum, all four programs culminate in awarding the degree Master of Science in Clinical Psychopharmacology. It was estimated at one point that more than 1,500 psychologists had completed didactic training in preparation for RxP (Ax, Fagan, & Resnick, 2009), a number that by now has probably risen above 2,000 given current enrollments in the existing programs.

Since 2001, APA has recognized psychopharmacology as a proficiency within psychology, a term that indicates a circumscribed activity within professional practice represented by a specific set of procedures or skills. The proficiency encompasses all three levels of applied training as well as training in psychopharmacology as a research endeavor. Finally, APA (2011) has promulgated guidelines for practitioners relevant to psychologists' involvement in pharmacotherapy either as information sources to patients, collaborators with prescribers, or independent prescribers. These are considered recommendations for best practices in an area of professional work, though they do not rise to the level of ethical standards. These guidelines are discussed in a later chapter (see Chapter 29, this volume).

Legislative and Regulatory Developments

The RxP movement's first legislative victory is rarely mentioned, because it was of greater symbolic than practical value. In 1993, the licensing law for psychologists in Indiana was amended to allow prescriptive authority for psychologists participating in a "federal government sponsored training or treatment program" (see Indiana Code § 25-33-1-2(c)). The revision was intended to extend prescriptive authority to graduates of the PDP. It represented the first recognition by a state legislature that psychologists need not pursue training in a second profession to become competent to prescribe. However, no psychologist has ever prescribed in Indiana, and that situation is unlikely to change unless federal agencies dramatically increase their training and/or hiring of psychologists to prescribe.

In 1999, the U.S. Territory of Guam was the first jurisdiction to award prescriptive authority to appropriately trained psychologists. Subsequent political struggles over the regulations governing professions in the territory delayed the implementation of the statute for many years, but a few psychologists are now eligible to prescribe there. Guam was followed in 2002 by New Mexico and in 2004 by Louisiana. Two aspects of prescriptive authority in Louisiana have been particularly controversial. One is the use of the term "medical psychologist" to refer to psychologists with prescriptive authority, a term some psychologists have considered confusing because it has historically been used within the discipline to refer to what is more commonly called health psy-

chology. Second, oversight of prescribing psychologists was transferred to the state Board of Medical Examiners.

After many years with no further legislative developments, three states have recently approved prescriptive authority for psychologists. In 2014, Illinois approved prescriptive authority. Iowa became the fourth state in 2016, Idaho the fifth in 2017.

The didactic requirements across the five states are similar, and allow for programs that follow the APA model curriculum (though Illinois has additional didactic requirements). All require a competency examination beyond the standard licensing examination for psychologists, a requirement that is met by the PEP. There are important differences in the required clinical experience across the states, however. At one extreme, Louisiana has no practicum requirement whatsoever. In contrast, New Mexico has a 480-hour clinical requirement, and Illinois requires a full-time practicum of 14 months. It is noteworthy that a review of license verification databases in summer 2017 revealed that about 100 out of 1,200 psychologists in Louisiana were medical psychologists (8%), while only 60 of 1,600 New Mexico licensed psychologists have achieved some level of prescriptive authority (4%) even though New Mexico approved prescriptive authority 2 years earlier than Louisiana. Since the primary difference between the two laws is in the practicum requirement, it is reasonable to hypothesize that the rigor of the practicum will be the strongest predictor of the extent to which psychologists obtain prescriptive authority in other states.

There are also differences in restrictions on practice. All states except Illinois have developed a two-stage model of practice, in which a period of restricted prescribing without incident allows the provider to advance to the full prescriptive authority allowed to psychologists. In most states, these are referred to as conditional prescribing psychologists versus prescribing psychologists. In Louisiana, the term medical psychologist applies to both stages, while the advanced stage is associated with a certificate of advanced practice. Idaho and Iowa both require direct supervision by a physician, while Illinois requires a collaborative agreement with a physician. Louisiana medical psychologists without a certificate of advanced standing and New Mexico prescribing psychologists can prescribe only in consultation and collaboration with the patient's primary or attending physician, so no formal arrangement with a physician is required.

Finally, states differ in the degree to which they have placed restrictions on the formulary and treatment populations for prescribing psychologists. The most common restriction on the former is a prohibition on the prescribing of narcotics. New Mexico and Illinois are more restrictive than other states in terms of who can be served by a prescribing psychologist, excluding individuals with certain medical conditions and pregnant women. Illinois also excluded youth and geriatric patients from the practice of the prescribing psychologist. The restrictions are significant enough to strongly recommend that psychologists familiarize themselves with the requirements concerning training and practice for a state before pursuing prescriptive authority. In the future, it is inevitable that these discrepancies will hinder the portability of prescriptive authority from one state to another.

Fourteen jurisdictions have also explicitly identified consultation on medications (Level 2) as within the scope of practice of psychology, either through the licensing law, regulation, or a clarifying statement from the board of psychology: California, District of Columbia, Florida, Louisiana (for psychologists without prescriptive authority), Maine, Massachusetts, Missouri, New Hampshire, New Jersey, New York, Ohio, Oklahoma, Tennessee, and Texas. On the other hand, several states—including Connecticut, Maryland, Illinois, Colorado, Minnesota, and Virginia—have passed legislation prohibiting school personnel from recommending the use of psychotropic medications, and this would include any psychologist employed by a school (Bentley & Collins, 2006). Psychologists who discuss medication decision making with their patients in other settings where the authority for such discussions has not been officially approved or denied should be aware that the legal or liability implications for doing so are ambiguous.

Changes have occurred in other settings besides the states. All three branches of the military that provide health care services (the Army, Navy, and Air Force) have officially recognized prescribing psychologists as independent prescribers whether trained through the PDP or a civilian program, so long as they meet certain standards set independently by each branch. These requirements are generally consistent with those found in bills that have been submitted at the state level. Though the commanding officer for a military medical treatment facility can still refuse to award prescribing privileges to a psychologist, the inclusion in regulation makes such an outcome less likely. As a result, the number of active-duty psychologists prescribing in the military seems to have been slowly increasing since the termination of the PDP, though the count is difficult to tally.

Success in the military has spurred efforts in other federal agencies, particularly the Commissioned Corps of the U.S. Public Health Service and the Indian Health Service. It was the Indian Health Service that first approved a psychologist to prescribe medications in 1988 in response to a shortage in the availability of appropriate psychiatric care in the Santa Fe, NM, region. The Indian Health Service actively recruits prescribing psychologists to address chronic gaps in the availability of appropriate care for individuals with mental disorders. These efforts have been less successful than desired because scope of practice in the Public Health Service and Indian Health Service is determined by the state of the psychologist's licensure. This restricts the pool of potential applicants to psychologists authorized to prescribe by their state of licensure. Some federally qualified health centers (community-based organizations that provide comprehensive primary care regardless of ability to pay or health insurance status), particularly in Hawaii, are also attempting to hire psychologists with postdoctoral training in psychopharmacotherapy even without prescriptive authority.

The Current Status of Prescriptive Practice

The very small population of psychologists actively prescribing places limitations on the generalizability to the future of any research on the current status of prescribing psychologists. That said, several articles have been published on this topic. Two studies have addressed attitudes towards prescribing psychologists among collaborating medical providers. The first asked 47 medical providers in a military hospital about their perceptions of a single prescribing psychologist (Shearer, Harmon, Seavey, & Tiu, 2012). The second surveyed a sample of 24 medical providers who had experience with at least one of 11 different prescribing psychologists (Linda & McGrath, 2017). In both studies, more than 90% of medical providers who worked with prescribing psychologists found them competent, safe prescribers who enhanced quality of care.

Three studies have been conducted evaluating various aspects of prescribing psychologists' professional practices (LeVine, Wiggins, & Masse, 2011; Linda & McGrath, 2017; Vento, 2014). Consistent findings included an increase in income, but also increased severity of diagnoses among patients being seen. Contrary to concerns raised by some critics of prescriptive authority for psychologists, prescribing psychologists seem to be increasing access to traditionally underserved populations. The surveys provided evidence of service to Medicaid and low-income patients, patients living in rural communities, and individuals of minority background. Unfortunately, consistent with the concern raised earlier, the largest of these studies included only 24 prescribing psychologists, which is inadequate and only represented 15% of the entire population of prescribers at that time. Clearly, the field will have to expand drastically before it is possible to get an accurate picture of the practices of prescribing psychologists.

CONCLUSION

The growing number of states awarding psychologists prescriptive authority suggests that a tipping point may well be emerging for this new professional identity. Prescriptive authority for psychologists creates a tremendous opportunity for the discipline while enhancing access to appropriately trained mental health prescribers. For those who pursue prescriptive authority, it will allow their patients to receive comprehensive behavioral health care from a single provider. For all psychologists, it will increase the population of prescribers with specialty training in the diagnosis of mental disorders and alternatives to medication. However, it also creates an important challenge for the profession of psychology.

Somatogenic explanations for mental disorders have historically predominated in the vernacular understanding of mental disorders. This preference may reflect the dramatic quality of some cases of severe mental illness, but another potential rationale is the understandable human desire to find a simple explanation for and efficient method of resolving distress. Psychiatrists incorporated psychotropic medications into their practices based on science. However, it can be argued that the degree to which these medications have become the predominant treatment in psychiatry may reflect social, economic, and political considerations as much as empirical ones. Psychologists as prescribers will face those same considerations. The question is whether psychologists can remain scientists, and recognize the value of both perspectives for the good of our patients. McGrath (2004) outlined various factors that can contribute to psychologists' being better prepared to resist those forces. These include the following:

- Psychologists' doctoral-level training traditionally focuses far more on psychosocial aspects of mental disorders than on the biological aspects.
- Psychologists are obtaining prescriptive authority in a period of increased skepticism over the effectiveness of psychotropic medications. The growing literature comparing psychosocial and biological interventions (e.g., Spielmans, Berman, & Usitalo, 2011), a literature that did not exist when psychiatry began its shift toward a heavily medication-oriented profession, can do a good deal to help psychologists remain balanced.
- There will always be a community dedicated to the science of psychology, and members of this community will inevitably turn their attention to the critical analysis of prescriptive practice within the field. The results of this work can play an important part in maintaining commitment to empirically based practice.

Despite these countervailing forces, social, political, and economic pressures are powerful shapers of human behavior. The challenge in RxP to this point has been obtaining authority to engage in biological interventions. Once that challenge has been addressed, the next challenge will be to ensure that psychologists maintain their investment in offering the full spectrum of services, championing the value of both psychogenic and somatogenic perspectives, and providing services based on the best interests of the patient.

References

American Psychiatric Association. (2013). *Diagnostic and statistical manual of mental disorders* (5th ed.). Arlington, VA: Author.

American Psychological Association. (1986). *Psychologists' Use of Physical Procedures Task Force report*. Washington, DC: Author.

American Psychological Association Board of Professional Affairs. (1981). *Task force report: Psychologists' use of physical interventions*. Washington, DC: American Psychological Association. Available at https://www.apa.org/about/policy/rxp-model-act.pdf

American Psychological Association Council of Representatives. (2009a). *American Psychological Association model legislation for prescriptive authority*. Washington, DC: American Psychological Association. Available at https://www.apa.org/about/policy/rxp-model-act.pdf

American Psychological Association Council of Representatives. (2009b). *American Psychological Association recommended postdoctoral education and training program in psychopharmacology for prescriptive authority*. Washington, DC: American Psychological Association. Available at https://www.apa.org/about/policy/rxp-model-curriculum.pdf

American Psychological Association Division 55 (American Society for the Advancement of Pharmacotherapy) Task Force on Practice Guidelines. (2011). Practice guidelines regarding psychologists' involvement in pharmacological issues. *American Psychologist, 66*, 835–849. http://dx.doi.org/10.1037/a0025890

Andreasen, N. (1984). *The broken brain: The biological revolution in psychiatry*. New York, NY: HarperCollins.

Ax, R. K., Fagan, T. J., & Resnick, R. J. (2009). Predoctoral prescriptive authority training: The rationale and a combined model. *Psychological Services, 6*, 85–95. http://dx.doi.org/10.1037/a0013824

Ayd, F. (1961). *Recognizing the depressed patient*. New York, NY: Grune & Stratton.

Bentley, K. J., & Collins, K. S. (2006). Psychopharmacological treatment for child and adolescent mental disorders. In C. Franklin, M. B. Harris, & P. Allen-Meares (Eds.), *The school services sourcebook: A guide for school-based professionals* (pp. 15–30). New York, NY: Oxford University Press.

Carlat, D. J. (2010). *Unhinged: The trouble with psychiatry—a doctor's revelations about a profession in crisis*. New York, NY: Free Press.

Chang, A. K., Bijur, P. E., Esses, D., Barnaby, D. P., & Baer, J. (2017). Effect of a single dose of oral opioid and nonopioid analgesics on acute extremity pain in the emergency department: A randomized clinical trial. *JAMA, 318*, 1661–1667. http://dx.doi.org/10.1001/jama.2017.16190

Coppen, A. (1967). The biochemistry of affective disorders. *The British Journal of Psychiatry, 113*, 1237–1264. http://dx.doi.org/10.1192/bjp.113.504.1237

Creese, I., Burt, D. R., & Snyder, S. H. (1976). Dopamine receptor binding predicts clinical and pharmacological potencies of antischizophrenic drugs. *Science, 192*, 481–483. http://dx.doi.org/10.1126/science.3854

Cuthbert, B. N. (2015). Research Domain Criteria: Toward future psychiatric nosologies. *Dialogues in Clinical Neuroscience, 17*, 89–97.

Cuthbert, B. N., & Insel, T. R. (2013). Toward the future of psychiatric diagnosis: The seven pillars of RDoC. *BMC Medicine, 11*, 126. http://dx.doi.org/10.1186/1741-7015-11-126

Eysenck, H. J. (1952). The effects of psychotherapy: An evaluation. *Journal of Consulting Psychology, 16*, 319–324. http://dx.doi.org/10.1037/h0063633

Eysenck, H. J. (1966). *The effects of psychotherapy*. New York, NY: International Science.

Fox, R. E. (2003). Early efforts by psychologists to obtain prescriptive authority. In M. T. Sammons, R. U. Paige, & R. F. Levant (Eds.), *Prescriptive authority for psychologists: A history and guide* (pp. 33–45). Washington, DC: American Psychological Association. http://dx.doi.org/10.1037/10484-002

Frances, A. (2014). RDoC is necessary, but very oversold. *World Psychiatry, 13*, 47–49. http://dx.doi.org/10.1002/wps.20102

Gaynes, B. N., Warden, D., Trivedi, M. H., Wisniewski, S. R., Fava, M., & Rush, A. J. (2009). What did STAR*D teach us? Results from a large-scale, practical, clinical trial for patients with depression. *Psychiatric Services, 60*, 1439–1445. http://dx.doi.org/10.1176/ps.2009.60.11.1439

Goldfried, M. R. (2016). On possible consequences of National Institute of Mental Health funding for psychotherapy research and training. *Professional Psychology: Research and Practice, 47*, 77–83. http://dx.doi.org/10.1037/pro0000034

Haas, J. S., Phillips, K. A., Gerstenberger, E. P., & Seger, A. C. (2005). Potential savings from substituting generic drugs for brand-name drugs: Medical expenditure panel survey, 1997–2000. *Annals of Internal Medicine, 142*, 891–897. http://dx.doi.org/10.7326/0003-4819-142-11-200506070-00006

Healy, D. (1997). *The antidepressant era*. Cambridge, MA: Harvard University Press.

Healy, D. (2004). *The creation of psychopharmacology* (rev. ed.). Cambridge, MA: Harvard University Press.

Hirschfeld, R. M. (2000). History and evolution of the monoamine hypothesis of depression. *The Journal of Clinical Psychiatry, 61*(Suppl. 6), 4–6.

Kramer, P. D. (1993). *Listening to Prozac: A psychiatrist explores antidepressant drugs and the remaking of the self.* New York, NY: Viking Press.

Kirsch, I. (2010). *The emperor's new drugs: Exploding the antidepressant myth.* New York, NY: Random House.

Kuhn, R. (1958). The treatment of depressive states with G 22355 (imipramine hydrochloride). *The American Journal of Psychiatry, 115,* 459–464. http://dx.doi.org/10.1176/ajp.115.5.459

Lal, R. (2015, May 19). Patents and exclusivity. *FDA/CDER SBIA Chronicles.* Available at https://www.fda.gov/downloads/drugs/developmentapprovalprocess/smallbusinessassistance/ucm447307.pdf

Lasser, K. E., Allen, P. D., Woolhandler, S. J., Himmelstein, D. U., Wolfe, S. M., & Bor, D. H. (2002). Timing of new black box warnings and withdrawals for prescription medications. *JAMA, 287,* 2215–2220. http://dx.doi.org/10.1001/jama.287.17.2215

Lehmann, H. E., & Hanrahan, G. E. (1954). Chlorpromazine; new inhibiting agent for psychomotor excitement and manic states. *Archives of Neurology and Psychiatry, 71,* 227–237. http://dx.doi.org/10.1001/archneurpsyc.1954.02320380093011

LeVine, E., Wiggins, J., & Masse, E. (2011). Prescribing psychologists in private practice: The dream and the reality of the experiences of prescribing psychologists. *Archives of Medical Psychology, 2,* 1–14.

Linda, W. P., & McGrath, R. E. (2017). The current status of prescribing psychologists: Practice patterns and medical professional evaluations. *Professional Psychology: Research and Practice, 48,* 38–45. http://dx.doi.org/10.1037/pro0000118

Luhrmann, T. M. (2000). *Of two minds: The growing disorder in American psychiatry.* New York, NY: Knopf.

McGrath, R. E. (2004). Saving our psychosocial souls. *American Psychologist, 59,* 644–645. http://dx.doi.org/10.1037/0003-066X.59.7.644

McGrath, R. E. (2010). Prescriptive authority for psychologists. *Annual Review of Clinical Psychology, 6,* 21–47. http://dx.doi.org/10.1146/annurev-clinpsy-090209-151448

Mintzes, B. (2012). Advertising of prescription-only medicines to the public: Does evidence of benefit counterbalance harm? *Annual Review of Public Health, 33,* 259–277. http://dx.doi.org/10.1146/annurev-publhealth-031811-124540

Moses, H., III, Dorsey, E. R., Matheson, D. H. M., & Thier, S. O. (2005). Financial anatomy of biomedical research. *JAMA, 294,* 1333–1342. http://dx.doi.org/10.1001/jama.294.11.1333

Mukherji, P., Janakiraman, R., Dutta, S., & Rajiv, S. (2017). How direct-to-consumer advertising for prescription drugs affects consumers' welfare: A natural experiment tests the impact of FDA legislation. *Journal of Advertising Research, 57,* 94–108. http://dx.doi.org/10.2501/JAR-2016-050

Newman, R., Phelps, R., Sammons, M. T., Dunivin, D. L., & Cullen, E. A. (2000). Evaluation of the Psychopharmacology Demonstration Project: A retrospective analysis. *Professional Psychology: Research and Practice, 31,* 598–603. http://dx.doi.org/10.1037/0735-7028.31.6.598

Olfson, M., & Marcus, S. C. (2009). National patterns in antidepressant medication treatment. *Archives of General Psychiatry, 66,* 848–856. http://dx.doi.org/10.1001/archgenpsychiatry.2009.81

Olfson, M., Marcus, S. C., & Pincus, H. A. (1999). Trends in office-based psychiatric practice. *The American Journal of Psychiatry, 156,* 451–457.

Robiner, W. N., Bearman, D. L., Berman, M., Grove, W. M., Colón, E., Mareck, S., & Armstrong, J. (2002). Prescriptive authority for psychologists: A looming health hazard? *Clinical Psychology: Science and Practice, 9,* 231–248. http://dx.doi.org/10.1093/clipsy.9.3.231

Rosenblat, J. D., McIntyre, R. S., Alves, G. S., Fountoulakis, K. N., & Carvalho, A. F. (2015). Beyond monoamines—Novel targets for treatment-resistant depression: A comprehensive review. *Current Neuropharmacology, 13,* 636–655. http://dx.doi.org/10.2174/1570159X13666150630175044

Sabshin, M. (2008). *Changing American psychiatry: A personal perspective.* Washington, DC: American Psychiatric Publishing.

Sammons, M. T., & Brown, A. B. (1997). The Department of Defense Psychopharmacology Demonstration Project: An evolving program for postdoctoral education in psychology. *Professional Psychology: Research and Practice, 28,* 107–112. http://dx.doi.org/10.1037/0735-7028.28.2.107

Schildkraut, J. J. (1965). The catecholamine hypothesis of affective disorders: A review of supporting evidence. *The American Journal of Psychiatry, 122,* 509–522. http://dx.doi.org/10.1176/ajp.122.5.509

Schou, M., Juel-Nielsen, N., Strömgren, E., & Voldby, H. (1954). The treatment of manic psychoses by the administration of lithium salts. *Journal of Neurology, Neurosurgery & Psychiatry, 17,* 250–260. http://dx.doi.org/10.1136/jnnp.17.4.250

Scull, A. (2011). The mental health sector and the social sciences in post-World War II USA. Part I: Total war and its aftermath. *History of Psychiatry, 22,* 3–19. http://dx.doi.org/10.1177/0957154X10388366

Shearer, D. S., Harmon, S. C., Seavey, B. M., & Tiu, A. Y. (2012). The primary care prescribing psychologist model: Medical provider ratings of the safety, impact and utility of prescribing psychology in a primary care setting. *Journal of Clinical Psychology in Medical Settings, 19,* 420–429. http://dx.doi.org/10.1007/s10880-012-9338-8

Shorter, E. (2009). The history of lithium therapy. *Bipolar Disorders, 11*(Suppl. 2), 4–9. http://dx.doi.org/10.1111/j.1399-5618.2009.00706.x

Smith, M. L., Glass, G. V., & Miller, T. I. (1980). *The benefits of psychotherapy.* Baltimore, MD: Johns Hopkins University Press.

Smyer, M. A., Balster, R. L., Egli, D., Johnson, D. L., Kilbey, M. M., Leith, N. J., & Puente, A. E. (1993). Summary of the report of the Ad Hoc Task Force on Psychopharmacology of the American Psychological Association. *Professional Psychology: Research and Practice, 24,* 394–403. http://dx.doi.org/10.1037/0735-7028.24.4.394

Spielmans, G. I., Berman, M. I., & Usitalo, A. N. (2011). Psychotherapy versus second-generation antidepressants in the treatment of depression: A meta-analysis. *Journal of Nervous and Mental Disease, 199,* 142–149. http://dx.doi.org/10.1097/NMD.0b013e31820caefb

Temin, P. (1980). *Taking your medicine: Drug regulation in the United States.* Cambridge, MA: Harvard University Press. http://dx.doi.org/10.4159/harvard.9780674592780

Tuke, S. (1996). *Description of the Retreat.* London, England: Process Press. (Original work published 1813)

Vento, C. (2014). Report from the trenches: Survey of New Mexico prescribing psychologists' outpatient practice characteristics and impact on mental health care disparities in calendar 2013. *Archives of Medical Psychology, 5,* 30–34.

Wampold, B. E. (2013). The good, the bad, and the ugly: A 50-year perspective on the outcome problem. *Psychotherapy, 50,* 16–24. http://dx.doi.org/10.1037/a0030570

Whitaker, R. (2011). *Anatomy of an epidemic: Magic bullets, psychiatric drugs, and the astonishing rise of mental illness in America.* New York, NY: Crown.

CHAPTER 2

BASIC INFORMATION ON PSYCHOTROPIC DRUGS, RECEPTOR SYSTEMS, AND THE BRAIN

Keith A. Trujillo

The brain is a remarkable multidimensional organ, with a rich complexity at multiple levels of analysis. One can examine its gross structure, microstructure, circuitry, neurochemistry, electrophysiology, molecular biology, genetics, genomics, behavior, or any combination of these. It is the organ that generates thoughts, feelings and behavior and gives us a sense of who we are. The brain is electrochemical in nature—electrical signals within brain cells (in the form of ion fluxes and action potentials) are converted to chemical signals between cells (synaptic neurotransmission). It is the chemical nature of the brain that allows it to be the target of drugs (chemicals) that can affect brain function, leading to changes in thoughts, feelings, and behavior, and serve as therapeutic interventions for psychiatric and neurological disorders. This chapter will offer a short summary of the structure of the brain and of chemical neurotransmission, with a particular focus on the key neurotransmitters and receptors involved in the actions of psychoactive drugs. The intent is not to be comprehensive, but instead to provide key examples that illustrate broader principles and give the reader an introduction that can be used as a foundation for further exploration. For deeper understanding, the following are excellent resources: Bohlen und Halbach and Dermietzel, 2006; Charney, Sklar, Buxbaum, and Nestler, 2013; Meyer and Quenzer, 2013; Schatzberg, Nemeroff, and American Psychiatric Association Publishing, 2017; and Stahl, 2013. In addition, the American College of Neuropsychopharmacology has made numerous chapters and articles available online, including the excellent books, *Psychopharmacology: The Fourth Generation of Progress* (https://acnp.org/digital-library/psychopharmacology-4th-generation-progress/) and *Neuropsychopharmacology: The Fifth Generation of Progress* (https://acnp.org/digital-library/neuropsychopharmacology-5th-generation-progress/), with chapters by leaders in the field, and several volumes of *Neuropsychopharmacology Reviews* (https://acnp.org/digital-library/neuropsychopharmacology-reviews/), which offers updates on specific topics in psychopharmacology (see the Tool Kit of Resources at end of chapter).

ORGANIZATION OF THE BRAIN

Upon gross dissection, it is immediately evident that the human brain is composed of multiple layers and structures. Historical work using simple visual observation identified individual nuclei (areas rich in cell bodies) that connected with other areas via fiber tracts (myelinated projections of neurons). Recent research using modern tools and techniques has identified complex circuitries, in which chemically distinct neurons from one region connect to neurons of another region to contribute to a particular behavior or function. A notable example is the mesocorticolimbic circuit, which consists of dopamine cells in the midbrain ventral tegmental area

http://dx.doi.org/10.1037/0000133-002
APA Handbook of Psychopharmacology, S. M. Evans (Editor-in-Chief)

that connect to the basal forebrain and frontal cortex and is involved in motivated behavior. Neurons in the terminal regions of the dopamine cells send connections to other areas of the brain, resulting in widespread impact of activation or inhibition of the circuit. Dysregulation of this circuit is thought to contribute to drug abuse, addiction, schizophrenia, and depression.

Chemical neuroanatomy, functional neuroanatomy, behavioral neuroscience and psychopharmacology are complementary areas of research that work to identify the neurochemistry of brain circuits and the contributions of these circuits to behavior and function. Although it is tempting to try to associate a particular brain region, circuit, or neurotransmitter with a specific behavior (in the past it was common to speak of "*the* brain center" or "*the* neurotransmitter" for a particular function), the brain is much more complex than that, with multiple areas and multiple neurotransmitters contributing to each function. It is best to think of the brain as a complicated mix of overlapping and intersecting circuits. Another layer of complexity is that neurons are modified by experience, so that the brain changes from moment to moment. A basic

principle of brain function is that of neuroplasticity—the brain is changed by experience and thus functioning is dynamic and constantly in flux (Citri & Malenka, 2008). Neuroplasticity is essential to brain function, most notably to learning and memory, but also in allowing the brain to respond and adapt to input from the environment.

The outermost convoluted layer of the brain is the cerebral cortex, which is dense with cell bodies and is gray in appearance (thus, called gray matter). Under the cortex are layers of white matter, which comprise myelinated tracts (neuronal axons) connecting regions of the cortex with one another and with subcortical areas. The four lobes of the cortex are associated with particular functions: frontal (planning and execution of movement), parietal (somatosensation), occipital (vision), and temporal (audition; see Figure 2.1). The frontal cortex is also important to psychopathology—specific areas of this cortical region have been found to contribute to major depression, bipolar disorder, obsessive-compulsive disorder, impulsivity, anxiety, and schizophrenia. As a result, numerous studies have been aimed at better understanding the neurobiology of the frontal cortex and the impact of psychotherapeutic drugs on this region.

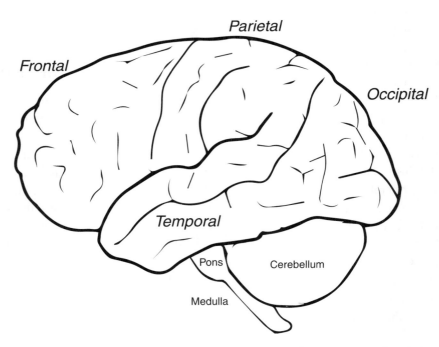

FIGURE 2.1.   Lateral view of a human brain. Lobes of the brain are identified, including frontal, parietal, occipital, and temporal. Also shown are cerebellum, pons, and medulla.

Below the cortex is the diencephalon, which is comprised of the thalamus and hypothalamus. The hypothalamus is especially important in behavior in that it is involved in a variety of functions, including temperature regulation, circadian rhythms, food and water intake, reproduction, stress, and emotional responses. It contains small molecule neurotransmitters, including dopamine, norepinephrine, serotonin, glutamate, gamma-aminobutyric acid (GABA), and acetylcholine, as well as several neuropeptides that regulate the pituitary gland. Below the diencephalon is the brainstem, which includes the midbrain, pons, and medulla, each with nuclei and fiber tracts that connect with other brain structures and containing a rich array of neurotransmitters. In particular, some of the key nuclei containing small molecule neurotransmitters, including dopamine, norepinephrine, serotonin, GABA, glutamate, and acetylcholine, are located in the brainstem and project throughout the central nervous system.

CELLS OF THE NERVOUS SYSTEM: NEURONS AND GLIA

Neurons are the brain cells most associated with information processing. Although they appear in many shapes and sizes, neurons typically have dendrites at their receiving end with neurotransmitter receptors for receiving chemical communication; these are connected to a cell body that contains much of the biosynthetic machinery for the cell. Extending from the cell body is an axon through which electrical signals are transmitted. At the end of the axon (the axon terminal) there is a gap, known as the synapse, across which chemical communication take place.

Glia have traditionally been viewed as "support cells" for neurons—offering structural and nutritional support, removing debris when damage occurs, and serving other housekeeping functions to help create an environment that assures optimal functioning of neurons. They are also responsible for synthesizing the myelin that surrounds and insulates neuronal fibers (axons) and facilitates electrical signaling in neurons. However, more recent work suggests that glia can have a much more central role in synaptic activity, including responding to neurotransmitters

and modulating neurotransmission. In recognition of the active role that glia can have in synaptic function, some have made reference to the *tripartite synapse*, which includes the presynaptic neuron, the postsynaptic neuron, and synapse-associated glia (Halassa, Fellin, & Haydon, 2007; Machado-Vieira, Manji, & Zarate, 2009; Quesseveur, Gardier, & Guiard, 2013; Schafer, Lehrman, & Stevens, 2013). The importance of glia to psychopharmacology is reflected in recent work that targets glia for potential therapeutic drugs (Machado-Vieira et al., 2009; Morris, Clark, Zinn, & Vissel, 2013; Salter & Stevens, 2017).

CHEMICAL COMMUNICATION AND DRUG TARGETS

One of the key tenets of psychopharmacology is that cells of the brain communicate via chemical signals. Neurotransmitters are synthesized and packaged in neurons and, upon an electrical signal, are released from the neuron and have the opportunity to affect adjacent neurons. The gap across which neurotransmitters flow is called the synapse, or synaptic cleft. When a neurotransmitter is released from a neuron (the presynaptic neuron), it can interact with receptors (large functional protein complexes) in the cell membrane on adjacent neurons (postsynaptic neurons). When a receptor on a postsynaptic neuron is activated by a neurotransmitter, chemical and/or electrical signals are generated, which thereby change the functional status of the neuron. The postsynaptic neuron will consequently be more likely or less likely to fire an action potential. If the postsynaptic neuron fires, it will then serve as the presynaptic neuron for the next neuron in the circuit, and so on.

Most neurotransmitters (some key exceptions are noted below) are packaged into small vesicles in neurons, which sit adjacent to the synapse in preparation for release. When an action potential fires, voltage-gated ion channels in the presynaptic membrane open, allowing for the influx of calcium ions. Calcium can then bind to specific proteins in the presynaptic terminal to mobilize the synaptic vesicles. The vesicles then fuse with the cell membrane and spill their contents into the synapse. The neurotransmitter can freely diffuse across the synapse and interact with receptor sites on the post-synaptic neuron.

Stages in the Life of a Neurotransmitter

Understanding the life of a neurotransmitter allows us to identify the various means by which psycho-active drugs can influence neurotransmission (Feldman, Meyer, & Quenzer, 1997). The key stages include (a) biosynthesis, (b) storage, (c) release, (d) receptor activation, and (e) inactivation/metabolism (see Figure 2.2). Cellular proteins that are key to each of these stages (such as enzymes and neurotransmitter receptors) can be targets for psychoactive drugs. By activating or inhibiting these proteins, a drug can activate or inhibit the actions of the neurotransmitter. Examples that follow help to

illustrate each of these stages and specific examples of drugs that can affect each step.

Biosynthesis.   Production of small molecule neuro-transmitters occurs through an enzyme-facilitated process. For example, in the biosynthesis of dopa-mine, tyrosine is converted to levodopa (L-dopa) by the enzyme tyrosine hydroxylase, and the L-dopa is converted to dopamine by the enzyme dopa decar-boxylase (also known as aromatic amino acid decar-boxylase). The drug alpha-methyl-para-tyrosine (AMPT) is an inhibitor of tyrosine hydroxylase. Blocking this enzyme decreases the production of dopamine and thereby acts to inhibit dopamine function. Therefore, in this case, tyrosine hydroxy-lase is the drug target. Conversely, L-dopa is an intermediate in the production of dopamine. By administering L-dopa, more of this intermediate

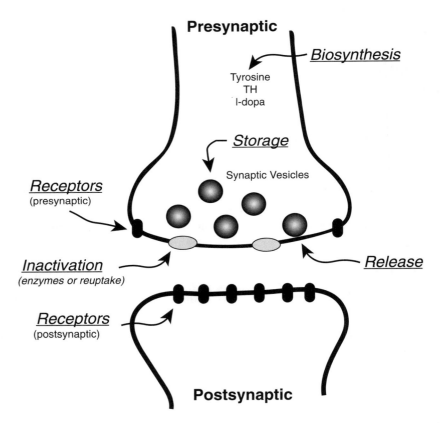

FIGURE 2.2.   Diagram of a synapse with potential targets for psychoactive drug action identified. A drug can enhance or inhibit neurotransmitter function by affecting any one of the following processes: (a) biosynthesis, (b) storage into synaptic vesicles, (c) release from the neuron, (d) receptor activation (either postsynaptic receptors or presynaptic receptors), or (e) neurotransmitter inactivation/metabolism. In this example, tyrosine is converted to levodopa (l-dopa) by the enzyme tyrosine hydroxylase (TH).

is available to be converted to dopamine, and an increase in dopamine function results. Increased dopamine activity by L-dopa is a treatment for Parkinson's disease, which results from a loss of dopamine neurons in a midbrain nucleus, the substantia nigra. In a similar manner, increasing or decreasing biosynthesis can facilitate or diminish the function of other neurotransmitters.

Storage. Storage of neurotransmitters into vesicles prepares them for release into the synapse. Reserpine is a drug that blocks the vesicular monoamine transporter (VMAT), which is responsible for transporting dopamine and related neurotransmitters into synaptic vesicles. Blockade of this transporter prevents the uptake of monoamines into the vesicles and leaves the vesicles without these neurotransmitters. When the neuron fires, the vesicles spill their contents, absent the monoamines, into the synapse. Since the vesicles are empty of neurotransmitter, no response occurs at the postsynaptic neuron. In this manner, reserpine inhibits the function of monoamine neurotransmitters, including dopamine, epinephrine, norepinephrine and serotonin.

Release. For a neurotransmitter to have an effect on the postsynaptic neuron it must be released from the presynaptic neuron. Increasing release facilitates action of the neurotransmitter, while preventing release blocks the action of the neurotransmitter. For example, black widow spider venom (latrotoxin) stimulates the release of the neurotransmitter acetylcholine, which causes excessive stimulation of muscle fibers. In contrast, botulinum toxin (Botox) irreversibly blocks the release of acetylcholine, which prevents nerves from activating muscle fibers, effectively paralyzing the muscles.

Receptor activation. Neurotransmitters impact on a postsynaptic neuron by binding to neurotransmitter receptors, large protein complexes that are embedded into the neuronal membrane. An analogy that is often used to explain receptor interactions is that of a lock and a key. The key is the neurotransmitter and the lock is a receptor activated by the neurotransmitter. There are specific receptors for each major neurotransmitter—for example, dopamine has receptors that it activates, which are different

from those activated by serotonin. According to the lock and key analogy, only specific keys can fit into the lock to activate the biochemical and electrical processes to impact on the cell. However, in addition to neurotransmitters, exogenous chemicals (drugs) can fit into specific locks, mimicking the actions of the neurotransmitter. Drugs that activate neurotransmitter receptors are known as agonists. A good example is morphine, which binds to opioid receptors, mimicking the actions of endogenous opioids. Alternatively, a drug can interact with a receptor and not activate the biochemical processes. By binding the receptor and preventing the action of the endogenous neurotransmitters, such a drug prevents neurotransmitter function. Drugs that block neurotransmitter receptors are referred to as antagonists. An example of this is naloxone (Narcan®), which is an opioid receptor antagonist. Because of its ability to potently block opioid receptors, naloxone is used for opioid overdoses since it rapidly reverses the effects of drugs that activate these receptors.

Autoreceptors are another type of neurotransmitter receptor that are critical to neurotransmitter function. These receptors are located on the presynaptic neuron and, when activated or blocked, regulate the biosynthesis and release of the neurotransmitter. In this respect they serve as a type of "thermostat," sensing the amount of neurotransmitter in the synapse. If these receptors are strongly stimulated, the receptor induces a biochemical response that reduces biosynthesis and/or release of the neurotransmitter. It is as if the presynaptic neuron senses that the circuit has been overactivated and compensates by reducing neurotransmitter activity. Conversely, if these receptors are not activated or are blocked, the biochemical cascade increases biosynthesis and/or release, compensating for underactivity.

Inactivation/metabolism. The final step in the life of a neurotransmitter is inactivation. If neuronal signaling is to be time-limited and discrete, there needs to be a process by which signaling is terminated. There are two general processes by which neurotransmitters are inactivated—reuptake and enzymatic inactivation. Some neurotransmitters utilize one of these processes, while others utilize both. Reuptake occurs via large protein complexes, known as transporters (sometimes referred to as reuptake sites), which are located on presynaptic terminals. These transporters actively remove the neurotransmitter from the synapse and thereby terminate its action, preventing it from further activating receptors. A good example of a drug class that acts via this mechanism is selective serotonin reuptake inhibitors. These drugs selectively block serotonin transporters, allowing serotonin to remain in the synapse longer so it can continue to activate the postsynaptic neuron.

The other process by which neurotransmitters are inactivated, enzymatic inactivation, transforms the neurotransmitter into a compound that can no longer interact with the receptors. A good example of a drug class that acts via enzymatic inactivation is monoamine oxidase inhibitors. These compounds block the enzyme that inactivates monoamines. When the enzyme is blocked, the monoamines (dopamine, norepinephrine, epinephrine and serotonin) have the ability to continue to be active in the synapse.

The actions of psychoactive drugs on biosynthesis, storage, release, receptors and inactivation will become evident in subsequent chapters as more examples are presented. The most important principle to remember is that psychoactive drugs act by stimulating, mimicking, blocking or otherwise modifying the actions of neurotransmitters.

Receptors

For a neurotransmitter to produce an electrical or chemical change in a cell, it must interact with a receptor. Neurotransmitter receptors are large protein complexes embedded in cell membranes. Referring back to the lock and key analogy, the neurotransmitter is the key and the receptor is the lock. The appropriate key will turn the tumblers of the lock, producing an electrical or chemical change in the cell. The electrical or chemical change produced by activation of a receptor is a process referred to as signal transduction. There are two main broad types of neurotransmitter receptors—ionotropic and metabotropic—each with a distinct signal transduction mechanism (see Figure 2.3).

Ionotropic receptors. The simplest signal transduction mechanism is mediated by ionotropic receptors.

These receptors, also known as ligand-gated ion channels or neurotransmitter-gated ion channels, are large protein complexes with a central ion channel (similar to a donut that can open and close the center hole). When a neurotransmitter activates the receptor, the ion channel opens, allowing for specific ions to flow through the channel (Figure 2.3). Because ions are unequally distributed between the inside and the outside of a neuron, electrical charges flow across the membrane, and these charges directly excite or inhibit the neuron. Since the opening of the ion channel is a direct response to binding of the neurotransmitter, the response is very rapid. As a result, these are sometimes called "fast receptors." The ion channel in an ionotropic receptor may be selective for sodium, potassium, chloride, or calcium. An ion channel that is selective for sodium will produce an excitatory effect on a neuron, whereas an ion channel that is selective for potassium or chloride will produce an inhibitory effect on a neuron. Calcium is unique in that it not only produces an electrical change (an excitatory effect), but can also activate specific enzymes in the neuron, initiating biochemical cascades that can modify the neuron in multiple ways.

Ionotropic receptors are made up of multiple protein subunits, and often different variants of the subunits can be synthesized and different combinations of subunits can make up a receptor. The pharmacology and the function of the receptors can vary, depending on the specific subunits that make up the receptor. As a result, there can be multiple subtypes of a particular ionotropic receptor produced by neurons in the brain.

Metabotropic receptors. The signal transduction mechanism for metabotropic receptors is more complex, involving biochemical cascades that can affect the cell electrically and chemically. Metabotropic receptors are also called G-protein-coupled receptors (GPCRs; due to their association with specific proteins in the cell) or 7-transmembrane receptors (due to their molecular shape in association with the neuronal membrane). They are large proteins that fold within and across the neuronal membrane, containing an external binding site for the neurotransmitter, and an internal tail that interacts with

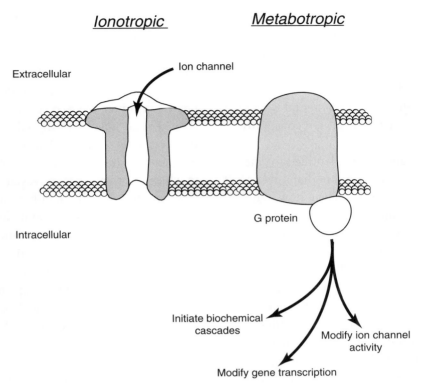

FIGURE 2.3.   Illustration of an ionotropic receptor and a metabotropic receptor. Ionotropic receptors are large protein complexes composed of multiple protein subunits that arrange to allow for a central ion channel. When a neurotransmitter activates the receptor, the ion channel opens, allowing for specific ions to flow through the channel. Metabotropic receptors (also known as G-protein-coupled receptors, or GPCRs) are large proteins that fold within and across the neuronal membrane. These receptors have an external binding site for the neurotransmitter, and an internal tail that interacts with intracellular signaling molecules that initiate biochemical cascades in the cell.

intracellular signaling molecules. Rather than multiple subunits (as in ionotropic receptors), a single protein makes up a metabotropic receptor. However, there may be different variants of the protein, resulting in receptors that differ in pharmacology and function.

When a neurotransmitter activates a metabotropic receptor, a conformational change in the receptor modifies an associated protein complex, known as a G-protein. This causes dissociation of the G-protein complex, allowing G-protein subunits to then trigger other events in the neuron (Figure 2.3). For example, a subunit of a G-protein may trigger the opening of an ion channel, allowing the flow of specific ions into or out of the neuron. As described previously for ionotropic receptors, excitation or inhibition

of the cell is dependent on the type of ion channel that is activated by the G-protein subunit. Given that there are biochemical steps between the binding of the neurotransmitter and the opening of the ion channel, these receptors can be a little slower than ionotropic receptors (although still very fast). In addition to activating an ion channel, a subunit of a G-protein can activate an enzymatic cascade that modifies the neuron in a longer-term manner—for example, by inserting receptors into the neuronal membrane or by activating the biosynthesis of new molecules that will modify the function of the neuron. The biochemical cascade initiated by activation of a metabotropic receptor is known as a second messenger system. However, this is often only the beginning of a potential cascade, as second messengers can activate third messengers, which can alter gene transcription in the cell. This can lead to increased or decreased production of key proteins, such as an enzyme or neurotransmitter receptor. Because of the ability of metabotropic receptor activation to change the biochemistry of a neuron in fundamental ways, it is a basic principle that neurons are constantly changing.

Nearly all neurotransmitters identified to date have multiple receptor types and perhaps even more subtypes. The receptors differ in how tightly the neurotransmitter binds and in the effects on the postsynaptic neuron. Activation of some may stimulate a neuron, while activation of others may inhibit a neuron. And, via activation of different metabotropic receptors, a neurotransmitter can have a variety of biochemical effects on a postsynaptic neuron. As an extreme example, at least 14 receptors for serotonin have been characterized, including a mix of metabotropic and ionotropic receptors (Aghajanian & Sanders-Bush, 2002; Baumgarten & Göthert, 2000). The use of multiple receptors allows for a myriad of effects of a particular neurotransmitter, depending on which specific receptor types and subtypes are available at a synapse.

OVERVIEW OF NEUROTRANSMITTERS AND OTHER SIGNALING MOLECULES

An analogy that is often used to describe neuronal functioning is that of a computer. According to this analogy, the brain is simply a digital device with 100 billion (or so) neurons that allow it to make complex computations. However, it is clear that this analogy falls short when you begin to consider the complexity of neuronal functioning. In a computer, a processor has two potential states, 0 or 1. At a very superficial glance, a neuron may be seen as similar, in that it fires an action potential or does not. But if neurons were simple digital devices, there would be a need for only a single neurotransmitter—or at most two neurotransmitters (one excitatory and the other inhibitory). The fact that there are more than a hundred neurotransmitters (and even more neurotransmitter receptors) tells us that much more information is encoded in neuronal communication

than simply firing or not (see Table 2.1 and Table 2.2). As noted previously, the activation of a receptor by a neurotransmitter can initiate biochemical cascades that modify a neuron from moment to moment. And the nature of that cascade depends on the neurotransmitter, the receptor, and the internal state (biochemical and electrical) of the neuron at the time the receptor is activated. The natural conclusion is that neurons are very complex biological "machines" in which information is conveyed in a constantly changing analog fashion, rather than digitally. The implications of this complexity are still not fully understood, but point to a rich future for research on neuronal functioning. This section summarizes the different types of neurotransmitters that are relevant to the actions of psychoactive drugs and their receptors.

Before discussing individual neurotransmitters, it is helpful to review the criteria that are necessary to identify a substance as a neurotransmitter. This gives an appreciation of the challenges that scientists face in identifying a new neurotransmitter and a better understanding of the physiological constraints of neurotransmission. The number of potential chemical compounds found in a cell are too numerous to count and many have multiple functional roles. Only a relatively small portion of these serve to provide chemical communication between neurons. To convince other scientists that a substance is a neurotransmitter, a research team must (a) demonstrate the biosynthesis of the substance in neurons; (b) show that the substance is released from these neurons when stimulated; (c) demonstrate that the substance mimics the actions of neuronal stimulation when applied exogenously at physiological concentrations; (d) identify specific receptors activated by the substance and show that the actions are blocked by receptor antagonists; and (e) identify the mechanisms for inactivation of the substance that results in termination of its signaling. These criteria are nearly identical to the stages in the life of a neurotransmitter described previously (Figure 2.2).

The discovery of neurotransmitters began in the early 20th century and continues today. Small molecule neurotransmitters, including monoamines and acetylcholine, were the first to be identified. This was followed by amino acid neurotransmitters and much later by peptide

TABLE 2.1

Classes of Neurotransmitters

Small molecules	Neuropeptides*	Others
Acetylcholine	**Opioid Family**	**Lipids**
	endorphins	endocannabinoids
Monoamines	enkephalins	
Catecholamines	dynorphins	**Gases**
dopamine	nociceptin (orphanin FQ)	nitric oxide
norepinephrine		carbon monoxide
epinephrine	**Vasopressin/Oxytocin Family**	hydrogen sulfide
	vasopressin	
Indoleamines	oxytocin	**Neurotrophins**
serotonin		Brain-derived neurotrophic factor (BDNF)
melatonin	**CCK/Gastrin Family**	Nerve growth factor (NGF)
	cholecystokinin (CCK)	Neurotrophin-3
Other monoamines	gastrin	Neurotrophin-4
histamine		
phenethylamine	**Somatostatin Family**	
tyramine	somatostatin	
octopamine	cortistatin	
Amino Acids	**Kinin/Tensin Family**	
Excitatory amino acids	substance P	
glutamate	neurokinin	
aspartate		
	CRH Family	
Inhibitory amino acids	corticotropin-releasing hormone	
GABA	urocortins	
glycine	urotensins	
	F- and Y-amide Family	
	gonadotropin inhibitory hormone	
	neuropeptide FF	
	neuropeptide Y	
	pancreatic polypeptide	
	peptide YY	
	prolactin-releasing peptide	
	Others	
	hypocretin/orexin	
	thyrotropin-releasing hormone	
	melanin-concentrating hormone	
	CART	
	AGRP	
	prolactin	

Note. *This list is not comprehensive. In particular, neuropeptides are too numerous to include all known substances, so key examples of families and members of these families are shown. GABA = gamma-aminobutyric acid.

neurotransmitters. More recently, gases and lipids have been found to serve as neurotransmitters (Table 2.1). The discovery of each new class of signaling molecules has been a revelation, humbling scientists and reminding us how much there is still to learn about neuronal function. Many neurotransmitters and signaling molecules have significant functions outside of the brain, in the gut, in the cardiovascular system, and in hormonal systems. However, full discussion of all of these roles is beyond the scope of the present chapter. Therefore, this work will focus primarily on neurotransmission in the brain, with occasional references to peripheral systems as warranted.

TABLE 2.2

Key Neurotransmitters That Are Targets for Psychoactive Drugs, Their Major Receptor Types, and Examples of Drugs

Neurotransmitter	Receptors	Selected psychoactive drugs*
Dopamine	D1, D2, D3, D4, D5	Amphetamines (+) Cocaine (+) Monoamine oxidase inhibitors (+) Traditional antipsychotics (−) Atypical antipsychotics (−)
Norepinephrine and epinephrine	α_1, α_2, β_1, β_2, β_3	Amphetamines (+) Tricyclic antidepressants (+) Serotonin and norepinephrine reuptake inhibitors (+) Monoamine oxidase inhibitors (+)
Serotonin	$5HT_{1A}$, $5HT_{1B}$, $5HT_{1D}$, $5HT_{1E}$, $5HT_{1F}$, $5HT_{2A}$, $5HT_{2B}$, $5HT_{2C}$, $5HT_3$, $5HT_4$, $5HT_{5A}$, $5HT_{5B}$, $5HT_6$, $5HT_7$	Amphetamines (+) Tricyclic antidepressants (+) Selective serotonin reuptake inhibitors (+) Monoamine oxidase inhibitors (+) Psychedelics (+/−) Atypical antipsychotics (−)
Acetylcholine	Nicotinic Muscarinic (M1, M2, M3, M4, M5)	Nicotine (+) Tacrine (+) Scopolamine (−)
Glutamate	NMDA, AMPA, kainate, mGluR (1–8)	Ketamine (−) Phencyclidine (−) Ethanol (−)
Gamma-aminobutyric acid (GABA)	GABA-A, GABA-B	Benzodiazepines (+) Z-drugs (+) Barbiturates (+) Ethanol (+)
Endocannabinoids	CB1, CB2	Delta-9-tetrahydrocannabinol (+) Rimonabant (−)
Endogenous opioid peptides	μ, δ, κ	Opioids (+) Naloxone (−)
Orexin/hypocretin	OX_1R, OX_2R	Suvorexant (−)

Note. *For drugs, (+) refers to a receptor agonist or a drug that activates the neurotransmitter; (−) refers to a receptor antagonist or a drug that inhibits the neurotransmitter. 5HT = 5-hydroxytryptamine (the chemical name for serotonin); NMDA = N-methyl-D-aspartate; AMPA = α-amino-3-hydroxy-5-methyl-4-isoxazolepropionic acid; CB = cannabinoid; OX = orexin.

Catecholamines

Catecholamines are a group of neurotransmitters—including dopamine, norepinephrine, and epinephrine—that share both chemical structure and a biosynthetic pathway (Aston-Jones, 2002; Bohlen und Halbach & Dermietzel, 2006; Di Chiara, 2002; Grace, 2002; Trendelenburg & Weiner, 1988).

These neurotransmitters are involved in a variety of behaviors and functions, ranging from movement, to wakefulness and attention, to feeding and reward. And, they are the targets of many psychoactive drugs (Table 2.2). These neurotransmitters belong to a broader class known as monoamines, which includes serotonin and melatonin, among others.

Biosynthesis and storage. Production of the catecholamines begins with the dietary amino acid tyrosine, which is transported into neurons and modified by a series of enzymes. The final product synthesized and released by a neuron is dependent on the specific enzymes that are active in the neurons. In dopamine neurons, tyrosine is converted to L-dopa by the enzyme tyrosine hydroxylase, and then L-dopa is converted to dopamine by the enzyme aromatic amino acid decarboxylase. If these are the only catecholamine biosynthetic enzymes active in the neuron, then the final neurotransmitter produced is dopamine. In a norepinephrine neuron there is an additional step—the enzyme dopamine-β-hydroxylase is active and converts dopamine to norepinephrine (this enzyme is not active in dopamine neurons). In an epinephrine neuron, norepinephrine is modified by the enzyme phenylethanolamine N-methyltransferase (PNMT) to produce epinephrine (this enzyme is not active in dopamine or norepinephrine neurons).

Catecholamines are stored in synaptic vesicles in axon terminals in preparation for release into the synapse. The storage in vesicles protects the catecholamines from degradation by enzymes and other molecules in the intracellular environment and allows for release of the neurotransmitters upon stimulation of the neuron. Synaptic vesicles in catecholamine neurons contain VMATs, which actively transport catecholamines from the cytoplasm of the cell and assure that the neurotransmitters are sequestered into the vesicles.

Receptors. There are specific receptors for each of the catecholamines, all metabotropic (Table 2.2). Five receptor types have been identified for dopamine: D1, D2, D3, D4 and D5. The receptors have been classified into two families based on the ways in which they affect biochemical cascades in neurons: D1-like receptors (which includes D1 and D5) and D2-like receptors (which includes D2, D3, and D4). The confusing numbering system is a historical accident reflecting the way the receptors were originally identified. Most of these receptors are traditional postsynaptic receptors; however, D2 receptors may be postsynaptic or presynaptic. When these receptors are located presynaptically they serve as autoreceptors, and upon activation inhibit the biosynthesis and release of dopamine.

Norepinephrine and epinephrine act on the same receptor types: alpha (α) and beta (β). There are two types of α receptors (α$_1$ and α$_2$) and three types of β receptors (β$_1$, β$_2$ and β$_3$); all are metabotropic. Each of these receptor types is postsynaptic, while α$_2$ receptors are both presynaptic (autoreceptors) and postsynaptic. These receptors are found throughout the brain and peripheral nervous system, with the exception of β$_3$ receptors, which are located principally in adipose tissue and are involved in thermogenesis and lipolysis.

Inactivation. Termination of the action of catecholamines occurs through a two-step process. The first step is reuptake—transporters located on presynaptic terminals actively transport catecholamines from the synaptic space and into the presynaptic neuron. Molecular biological research has revealed that there are two transporters for catecholamines, a dopamine transporter (DAT) that is expressed in dopamine-releasing neurons and a norepinephrine transporter (NET) that is expressed in norepinephrine-releasing neurons (an epinephrine transporter has not been found in the mammalian brain). Although the transporters are distinct, the selectivity for the catecholamines is low and each transporter can affect both dopamine and norepinephrine. The specificity appears to arise from localization of DAT into dopamine neurons and NET into norepinephrine neurons. When taken up back into neurons, the neurotransmitters can be recycled back into vesicles or inactivated by enzymes. Thus, the second step in the inactivation of catecholamines is enzymatic—specific enzymes in the presynaptic terminal metabolize the neurotransmitters, rendering them unable to interact with catecholamine receptors. The most important enzymes responsible for inactivation of the catecholamines in the brain are the monoamine oxidases (MAOs). However, catechol-O-methyltransferase (COMT) can also metabolize these neurotransmitters.

Brain localization. There are three major dopamine pathways in the brain. The nigrostriatal pathway has cell bodies located in the substantia nigra (a nucleus in the midbrain) and sends projections to the striatum (caudate nucleus and putamen). This pathway is involved in movement and habitual behavior, and loss of dopamine neurons in this pathway is causal in Parkinson's disease. The mesocorticolimbic pathway has cell bodies located in the ventral tegmental area (adjacent to the substantia nigra) and sends projections to the nucleus accumbens, olfactory tubercle, and prefrontal cortex. A major function of this pathway is reward, and the pathway is dysregulated in schizophrenia and addiction. The tuberoinfundibular pathway is located in the hypothalamus and regulates the release of the hormone prolactin by the pituitary gland. Blockade of dopamine receptors in this system by antipsychotic drugs can lead to mammary growth and lactation, even in males, and is one of the problematic side effects of these compounds.

Nuclei containing norepinephrine are located in the pons and medulla. The most prominent norepinephrine nucleus is the locus coeruleus, located in the dorsal pons (just below the cerebellum), which send projections throughout the cortex, forebrain, thalamus, hypothalamus, brainstem, and spinal cord. Due to its innervation of so many brain structures, it has the ability to widely influence brain function. The locus coeruleus is involved in arousal and attention, feeding, and other functions.

Epinephrine (sometimes referred to as adrenaline) is one of the key substances released by the adrenal glands in times of stress to prepare the body for "fight or flight." However, epinephrine is also found in the brain. Two epinephrine-containing nuclei have been identified in the medulla, but relatively little is known about their function.

Serotonin

Serotonin is a monoamine neurotransmitter (Aghajanian & Sanders-Bush, 2002; Baumgarten & Göthert, 2000; Bohlen und Halbach & Dermietzel, 2006). It is best known as the target of a popular class of antidepressant drugs known as selective serotonin reuptake inhibitors (SSRIs). Not surprisingly, it is involved in mood regulation, but also in a variety of other functions, including feeding, reward, anxiety, aggression, and sexual behavior. Additionally, serotonin is a target of atypical antipsychotics, which block serotonin $5HT_2$ receptors, and is prominent in the effects of psychedelic drugs, such as psilocybin and LSD (Table 2.2).

Biosynthesis and storage. The biosynthetic pathway for serotonin is similar to that of dopamine.

The dietary amino acid tryptophan is converted to 5-hydroxytryptophan by the enzyme tryptophan hydroxylase, and then 5-hydroxytryptophan is converted to serotonin (5-hydroxytryptamine) by the enzyme aromatic amino acid decarboxylase.

Like the catecholamines, serotonin is stored in synaptic vesicles in axon terminals. The storage in vesicles protects serotonin from degradation by enzymes and other molecules in the intracellular environment and allows for release upon stimulation of the neuron. Synaptic vesicles in serotonin neurons contain VMATs, which actively transport the neurotransmitter from the cytoplasm of the cell and assures that it is sequestered into the vesicles.

Receptors. There is a striking abundance of serotonin receptors—at least 14 have been identified thus far (Table 2.2). All serotonin receptors are metabotropic except $5HT_3$ receptors, which are ionotropic. It is currently unclear why there are so many serotonin receptors, but it suggests that serotonin can affect neurons biochemically and electrically in many ways. Moreover, it creates the opportunity for many different drugs to uniquely impact serotonin function.

Inactivation. Termination of serotonin parallels that of the catecholamines. The first step is reuptake—transporters located on presynaptic terminals actively transport serotonin from the synapse and into the presynaptic neuron. The serotonin transporter (SERT) is similar to, but distinct from, those that transport catecholamines. When taken up back into neurons, the serotonin can be recycled into vesicles or inactivated by enzymes. Specific enzymes in the presynaptic terminal metabolize serotonin so that it is unable to interact with its receptors. The most important enzymes in the brain for serotonin metabolism are the MAOs.

Brain localization. Serotonin is found in several nuclei, known as the raphe nuclei, in the medulla, pons, and upper brainstem. Raphe nuclei that are more caudal project to the brainstem and spinal cord, and among other functions, control pain responses. Raphe nuclei that are more rostral project to the forebrain and cerebral cortex and are involved in numerous functions, including mood, feeding, reward, anxiety, aggression, and sexual behavior.

Acetylcholine

Acetylcholine is most well-known for its role in mediating transmission at the neuromuscular junction. Release of acetylcholine from motor neurons, which innervate muscle fibers, acts on cholinergic receptors to evoke contraction. However, acetylcholine is also very important in brain function, where it is involved in learning and memory, wakefulness and attention, and other behaviors (Bohlen und Halbach & Dermietzel, 2006; Picciotto, Alreja, & Jentsch, 2002). Some drugs used in the treatment of Alzheimer's disease, such as donepezil and tacrine, facilitate acetylcholine neurotransmission. In addition, specific cholinergic receptors, known as nicotinic receptors, are the targets of nicotine, the primary psychoactive ingredient in tobacco (Table 2.2).

Biosynthesis and storage. Choline, which is normally consumed in the diet, is the starting material for acetylcholine. Choline is taken up into neurons via specific transporters. Within these neurons, the enzyme choline acetyltransferase transfers an acetate ion from acetyl coenzyme A to choline to produce acetylcholine.

Acetylcholine is stored in synaptic vesicles in axon terminals. Synaptic vesicles in acetylcholine neurons contain vesicular acetylcholine transporters (VAChTs), which actively transport the neurotransmitter from the cytoplasm of the cell and assures that it is sequestered into the vesicles for release into the synapse.

Receptors. The two major types of cholinergic receptors are nicotinic and muscarinic (Table 2.2). Nicotinic receptors are ionotropic and are made up of five protein subunits that come together to form the receptor complex. Since multiple proteins make up the subunits, there are multiple nicotinic receptor subtypes each comprised of a specific configuration of subunits. Activation of nicotinic receptors opens a sodium ion channel in the center of the receptor complex, resulting in activation of neurons. There are five different types of muscarinic receptors and all are metabotropic (M_1, M_2, M_3, M_4, and M_5). Most cholinergic receptors in the brain are muscarinic.

Inactivation. Acetylcholine is metabolized by the enzyme acetylcholinesterase. The enzyme is anchored to postsynaptic membranes in cholinergic synapses. The choline that results from the breakdown of acetylcholine can be recycled via reuptake into the presynaptic neuron from which acetylcholine was originally released.

Brain localization. Nuclei containing acetylcholine are found in the basal forebrain, septum, and brainstem. In the basal forebrain, cells in the nucleus basalis project throughout the cortex and therefore widely affect cortical function, whereas neurons in the septum innervate the hippocampus and other limbic structures. Loss of cholinergic neurons in the basal forebrain and septum is seen in Alzheimer's disease, which has led to the therapeutic use of drugs that activate acetylcholine for those with the disorder. In addition, acetylcholine is prominent in interneurons (cells that connect locally with neurons in a region) in the striatum. The balance between acetylcholine and dopamine is essential to proper function in this brain region, which is why some antimuscarinic drugs are used to treat Parkinson's disease and to combat tardive dyskinesia, both of which result from loss of dopamine in this region.

Amino Acid Neurotransmitters

Amino acids are ubiquitous in cells. They are the building blocks of proteins and are therefore found in abundance in every cell in the body. Because they are so widespread, it was a significant challenge for scientists to demonstrate their role as neurotransmitters. Nonetheless, research that focused on the biosynthesis, release, and other physiological properties of amino acids (see criteria necessary to identify a neurotransmitter listed previously) led to the identification of amino acid neurotransmitters. We now know that amino acid neurotransmitters function at a majority of synapses in the brain and serve as critical signaling molecules in numerous circuits. They have become the targets of significant research over the years, with much work aimed at understanding their functions and identifying therapeutic drugs for a variety of disorders.

Glutamate

Glutamate (glutamic acid) is the primary excitatory amino acid neurotransmitter in the brain (Bohlen und Halbach & Dermietzel, 2006; Coyle, Leski, & Morrison, 2002; Jonas & Monyer, 1999; Skolnick, 2010). It has been suggested that it is active at more than 90% of brain synapses. There is considerable interest in glutamate because of its pivotal role in neurotransmission. Functionally it is involved in behavioral and neural plasticity (changes in the brain induced by experience), including learning and memory, neural development, and drug tolerance and dependence. However, overactivity of glutamate can result in seizures and neuronal death. For example, brain ischemia leads to excessive release of glutamate, causing a type of neurotoxicity known as excitotoxicity. In addition, the seafood toxin domoic acid acts via activation of glutamate receptors. The club drugs ketamine and phencyclidine (PCP) act by blocking a type of glutamate receptors, known as N-methyl-D-aspartate (NMDA) receptors (Table 2.2).

Aspartate (aspartic acid) may also be an excitatory amino acid neurotransmitter; however, there is controversy over whether or not it meets all necessary criteria. It can activate the same receptors as glutamate, but further research is necessary to conclusively determine whether or not it normally functions as a neurotransmitter.

Biosynthesis and storage. The precursor for glutamate is glutamine, a dietary amino acid. Glutamine is converted to glutamate by the enzyme glutaminase located in mitochondria in presynaptic terminals. Glial cells work closely with neurons in the regulation of glutamate synthesis. Glutamate transporters (GLTs) located on glia remove the neurotransmitter from the extracellular space and supply the glutamine to neurons necessary for the production of glutamate.

Like other small molecule neurotransmitters, glutamate is sequestered into synaptic vesicles in the presynaptic terminal. Vesicular glutamate transporters (VGLUTs) located on vesicles in glutamatergic neurons transport glutamate into the vesicles so that it is protected from the intracellular environment and available for release.

Receptors. There are at least three major types of ionotropic receptors (AMPA, kainate, and NMDA) and eight metabotropic receptors (mGluRs; Table 2.1) for glutamate. AMPA (α-amino-3-hydroxy-5-methyl-4-isoxazolepropionic acid) receptors mediate much of the fast excitatory neurotransmission in the brain. Activation of AMPA receptors by glutamate allows

for the influx of sodium ions, resulting in an excitatory effect on postsynaptic neurons. As with AMPA receptors, activation of kainate receptors opens a sodium ion channel, producing an excitatory effect. Rather than a sodium ion channel, NMDA receptors have a central calcium ion channel. In addition, NMDA receptors have multiple sites that regulate the influx of calcium through the ion channel. A competitive site activated by glutamate is required for calcium channel opening; however, the ion channel will not open without glycine concurrently activating a coagonist site. Additionally, other sites for polyamines and zinc can also regulate the ability of glutamate to stimulate ion channel opening (see Figure 2.4). Calcium influx through

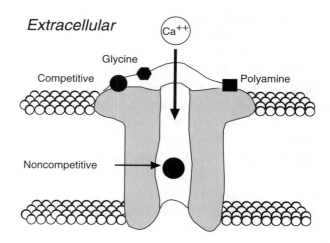

FIGURE 2.4. Diagram of an N-methyl-D-aspartate (NMDA) receptor. NMDA receptors are ionotropic receptors composed of multiple subunits, with an ion channel selective for calcium (Ca). There are multiple sites on the receptor that are targets for drugs: (a) the competitive site, at which the neurotransmitter glutamate binds; (b) the glycine site, which must be activated at the same time as the competitive site to open the ion channel, so is referred to as a coagonist; (c) a polyamine site, which, when activated, can modify receptor function; and (d) a noncompetitive site within the channel, at which the dissociatives ketamine and phencyclidine (and related drugs) act. GABA$_A$ receptors are similar in that they are composed of multiple subunits and have several binding sites at which drugs including barbiturates, benzodiazepines, alcohol, and others can influence receptor function. However, instead of a calcium ion channel, GABA$_A$ receptors contain a chloride channel. GABA = gamma-aminobutyric acid.

the NMDA receptor ion channel produces an excitatory effect on the postsynaptic neuron, and can also activate a variety of calcium-dependent enzymes that modify the biochemistry of the neuron. Through these calcium-dependent processes, activation of NMDA receptors contributes to behavioral and neural plasticity.

Metabotropic glutamate receptors make up three classes based on molecular structure and physiological effects: Group I, Group II, and Group III. Group I includes $mGluR_1$ and $mGluR_5$; Group II includes $mGluR_2$ and $mGluR_3$; and Group III includes $mGluR_4$, $mGluR_6$, $mGluR_7$, and $mGluR_8$.

Inactivation. The primary mechanism for inactivation of glutamate is via transporters that remove the neurotransmitter from the synapse. Transporters can be located on the presynaptic terminal or on glia adjacent to the synapse. The active role of glia in the regulation of glutamate contributed to the concept of the tripartite synapse, which includes the presynaptic neuron, the postsynaptic neuron, and the adjacent glia, each of which is critical to normal glutamate function. Once transported into the cell and removed from the synapse, glutamate can be converted back to glutamine by the enzyme glutamine synthetase, and then the glutamine can be recycled to once again be synthesized into glutamate. The central role of glia in glutamate regulation allows for pharmacotherapeutic targets not only on presynaptic and postsynaptic neurons but also on glial cells.

Brain localization. Glutamatergic cells and their receptors are widespread throughout the brain and are particularly evident in the cortex. They provide for communication across different regions of the cortex, and are prominent in key output pathways, such as from cortex to striatum.

GABA

Whereas glutamate is the primary excitatory neurotransmitter in the brain, GABA is the primary inhibitory neurotransmitter (Bohlen und Halbach & Dermietzel, 2006; Bowery & Smart, 2006; Möhler, 2001; Olsen, 2002; Uusi-Oukari & Korpi, 2010). Activation of GABA receptors reduces neuronal activity, and like glutamate, it is active at a large percentage of synapses in the brain. Underactivity of GABA can lead to seizures through a process known as disinhibition (low inhibitory activity allows for excessive excitation). Many sedative drugs, including alcohol, benzodiazepines, barbiturates, and the Z-drugs (drugs, such as zolpidem, that are used for sleep) act via activation of GABA receptors (Table 2.2).

Biosynthesis and storage. In a fascinating quirk of nature, glutamate is the starting material for synthesis of GABA. The enzyme glutamic acid decarboxylase (GAD) converts glutamate to GABA. Thus, the primary excitatory neurotransmitter in the brain is the precursor for the primary inhibitory neurotransmitter.

Like other small molecule neurotransmitters, GABA is taken up into synaptic vesicles via specific transporters, vesicular GABA transporters (VGATs), to protect it from the intracellular environment and prepare it for release.

Receptors. There are two major GABA receptors, $GABA_A$, which are ionotropic, and $GABA_B$, which are metabotropic (Table 2.2). $GABA_A$ receptors are the receptors most associated with the inhibitory effects of GABA. They are large protein complexes with a central chloride channel. Activation of the receptor opens the channel, allowing the influx of chloride ions into the cell and producing an inhibitory effect. In addition to the competitive site at which GABA binds, there are other sites that can modify receptor function, including a benzodiazepine site, a barbiturate site, and others. It is known that alcohol enhances function of $GABA_A$ receptors and work is ongoing to determine exactly how.

Inactivation. GABA transporters (GATs) on neurons and glia remove GABA from the synapse. Thus, similar to glutamate, regulation of extracellular GABA levels involves glia, in addition to presynaptic neurons. Intracellularly, GABA is broken down by the enzyme GABA-transaminase (GABA-T).

Brain localization. GABA is widespread throughout the brain. It is utilized as a neurotransmitter by many interneurons, but is also evident in some circuits with longer projections, such as from the striatum to the midbrain.

Glycine

Another inhibitory amino acid neurotransmitter is glycine (Bowery & Smart, 2006; Hernandes & Troncone, 2009). As with GABA, activation of glycine receptors reduces neuronal activity. Among the drugs that activate glycine receptors are alcohol and some general anesthetics. The toxin strychnine produces its effects by blocking glycine receptors. In another interesting quirk of nature, as noted above, glycine is a coagonist at NMDA receptors. As a result, this inhibitory neurotransmitter is required for activation of a major type of excitatory amino acid receptor.

Biosynthesis and storage. Glycine is a very simple molecule, among the simplest of amino acids. The dietary amino acid serine, in the presence of either glycine decarboxylase (GDC) or serine hydroxymethyltransferase (SHMT), is converted to glycine. Like other amino acid neurotransmitters, glycine is taken up into synaptic vesicles via vesicular transporters to protect it from the intracellular environment and prepare it for release. Glycine is transported into vesicles by the same vesicular transporters as for GABA (VGATs).

Receptors. Glycine receptors (GlyR) are ionotropic. Like GABA$_A$ receptors, they are large protein complexes with a central chloride channel. Activation of the receptor opens the channel, allowing the influx of chloride ions into the cell and an inhibitory effect.

Inactivation. Glycine transporters (GlyTs) on neurons and glia remove the neurotransmitter from the synapse. Thus, similar to other amino acid neurotransmitters, regulation of extracellular glycine levels involves glia, in addition to presynaptic neurons. GlyT1 is primarily located in glia, while GlyT2 is located in neurons. Intracellularly, glycine can be affected by different pathways.

Brain localization. Much of the research on glycine has traditionally focused on the retina and the spinal cord. However, more recently, the neurotransmitter has been found in other brain regions, including the basal ganglia, substantia nigra, pons, medulla, and cerebellum. Work continues on the role of glycine in these areas.

Neuropeptides

Peptides are small proteins. It was a revelation in the 1970s when it was determined that peptides could serve as neuronal signaling molecules. Up until that time, all of the known neurotransmitters (those described previously), as well as psychoactive drugs, were small molecules. It took extensive research to convince skeptics that much larger molecules

(up to 50 times larger than small molecule neurotransmitters) could be used by neurons for communication (Bohlen und Halbach & Dermietzel, 2006; Hökfelt, Bartfai, & Bloom, 2003; Holmes, Heilig, Rupniak, Steckler, & Griebel, 2003; Strand, 2003). As small proteins, neuropeptides are strings of amino acids ranging from three to 100 amino acids in length. There is evidence that the complexity in the structure of neuropeptides allows for more specificity than seen with small molecule neurotransmitters. It is also evident that there are more than 100 (and perhaps many more) individual neuropeptides in the brain (see Table 2.1 for a partial list). The variety of neuropeptides and their respective receptors allows for a myriad of unique and nuanced signals to be transmitted between neurons.

Some particularly noteworthy neuropeptides are the endogenous opioid peptides, which produce pleasurable effects and pain relief similar to morphine and other opioids. Another noteworthy neuropeptide is corticotrophin releasing hormone (CRH), which in the brain is involved in stress and anxiety. It is impossible to go through a comprehensive list, but it is clear that neuropeptides offer rich potential for therapeutic interventions in psychopharmacology (Griebel & Holsboer, 2012; Hökfelt et al., 2003; Holmes et al., 2003).

Biosynthesis and storage. The synthesis of neuropeptides differs significantly from that of small molecule neurotransmitters. As protein products, peptides go through the normal biosynthetic process for proteins: DNA is transcribed into RNA in the cell nucleus, RNA is translated into a protein precursor (a large protein from which the peptide product is cleaved) on ribosomes in the endoplasmic reticulum, and the protein undergoes posttranslational processing in the Golgi apparatus before being packaged into vesicles (posttranslational processing is the enzymatic modification of the protein precursor to create the final peptide products). The vesicles are then transported from the cell body (along with processing enzymes) to the synapse, where the peptide can be released. As a result, any new synthesis of neuropeptides must begin in the nucleus. If depletion of the peptide at the synapse occurs due to excessive release from the neuron, it takes time to replenish it due to the need to transport new peptide from the nucleus. This is in contrast to small molecule neurotransmitters, for which new synthesis can occur at the synapse (for small molecules, the biosynthetic enzymes and starting material are available in the presynaptic terminal, allowing for rapid replenishment).

A protein precursor can be the starting material for several different peptides. A good example of this is the precursor for the endogenous opioid peptide β-endorphin. This large protein, known as proopiomelanocortin (POMC), which is 241 amino acids in length, is the precursor not only for β-endorphin, but also for α-endorphin, γ-endorphin, β-lipoprotein, corticotropin-like intermediate peptide (CLIP), α-melanocyte-stimulating hormone, β-melanocyte-stimulating hormone, and adrenocorticotropic hormone (ACTH). Each of these peptides acts on different receptors and produces different functional effects. Since a single precursor can produce multiple peptide products, a diversity of effects can arise from a single starting protein.

Neuropeptides can be separated into families based on structural similarities in their protein precursors and physiological actions (Table 2.1). For example, there are four families of opioid peptides, each derived from an individual precursor: the POMC family, the prodynorphin family, the proenkephalin family, and the nociceptin (orphanin FQ) family. There is overlap in the functions of these peptides, but some also diverge in function and physiological action. The consequence is that a multifaceted, complex array of effects arises from peptide neurobiology. Interestingly, neuropeptides are often produced and released by the same neurons that produce and release small molecule neurotransmitters. The mechanisms and physiological consequences of cotransmission are not entirely understood, but they point toward a myriad of effects that can come from neuronal stimulation (Nusbaum, Blitz, & Marder, 2017).

Receptors. More than 100 neuropeptides have been identified, and most of these peptides can act at multiple receptors. Nearly all of the receptors for neuropeptides are metabotropic. Given the diversity of peptides and receptor types for each, it is impossible to summarize all of them. Some notable examples appear in Table 2.1 and Table 2.2.

Inactivation. Peptide neurotransmitters are inactivated via enzymatic degradation. Peptidases located in the extracellular space cleave the peptides, rendering the fragments unable to activate the peptide's receptors. Interestingly, however, in some cases peptidase actions can create a product that acts at the same receptor or at a different receptor than the original peptide. For example, one of the major products of the prodynorphin family is dynorphin A, which activates opioid receptors. In the synapse, removal of an amino acid from the end of the peptide results in a product known as des-tyrosine dynorphin, which produces potent functional effects, but does not activate opioid receptors. Instead, the actions of des-tyrosine dynorphin appear to be mediated by NMDA receptors. As a result, the final actions of a neuropeptide on a postsynaptic neuron can depend not only on the peptide released, but also on how it is enzymatically cleaved in the extracellular space. Peptides are large molecules that do not readily cross the blood–brain barrier so they are not good candidates for pharmacotherapy. However, targeting the peptidases responsible for the breakdown of specific peptides is a potential therapeutic strategy.

Brain localization. Neuropeptides and their receptors are located throughout the brain, with different peptides appearing in different nuclei and different circuits. Peptides also are important signaling molecules outside the brain, in the hypothalamic–pituitary–adrenal axis and the hypothalamic–pituitary–gonadal axis as well as in the gut. In fact, many peptides were first identified in these systems prior to being found in brain.

Gases
A striking discovery in the late 20th century was that gases can serve as neuronal signaling molecules (Boehning & Snyder, 2003; Bohlen und Halbach & Dermietzel, 2006; Mayer, 2000; Wu & Wang, 2005). These gases include nitric oxide, carbon monoxide, and hydrogen sulfide (Table 2.1). The most widely studied in the brain is nitric oxide, so it will serve here as an example for understanding gas neurotransmission more broadly. It is important to note that gases in the body are very labile, with a lifespan of only a few seconds. There are no means for storage, so upon biosynthesis they immediately

diffuse throughout the local region and activate their target molecules on adjacent neurons before they are inactivated. Because of their unique properties, gases do not fulfill the traditional criteria for identification of neurotransmitters. Nonetheless, they are now recognized as important neuronal signaling molecules. Given their unusual features, it has been suggested that gases should fall into a broad class termed *unconventional transmitters*.

It should also be noted that in the periphery, nitric oxide is involved in relaxing blood vessels. Erectile dysfunction drugs such as sildenafil act by activating nitric oxide in the vasculature, as do some drugs used in the treatment of cardiovascular disease.

Biosynthesis and storage. The amino acid arginine is converted to nitric oxide by the enzyme nitric oxide synthase. Nitric oxide synthase is activated by calcium influx through NMDA receptors. In this manner, nitric oxide is a downstream signaling molecule for the excitatory amino acid neurotransmitter glutamate. Thus, when glutamate is released and activates NMDA receptors, calcium enters the neuron and activates nitric oxide synthase, which results in the production of nitric oxide. As noted above, nitric oxide cannot be stored. However, it readily diffuses across cell membranes to reach its target. Following release of glutamate onto a postsynaptic neuron, the nearest target is the presynaptic neuron. As a result, nitric oxide serves as a *retrograde messenger* communicating a signal back to the presynaptic neuron. This retrograde signaling is important in different types of behavioral and neural plasticity, including learning and memory and drug tolerance and dependence, since nitric oxide synthase inhibitors can inhibit these phenomena. The concept of a retrograde messenger turned around conventional thinking that neurotransmission occurred unidirectionally, from a presynaptic neuron to a postsynaptic neuron.

Receptors. Nitric oxide does not act at traditional neurotransmitter receptors. Upon production it diffuses across cell membranes and activates the enzyme guanylyl cyclase. Activation of guanylyl cyclase generates cyclic guanosine monophosphate (cGMP), which can affect enzymes and other proteins in the presynaptic terminal, producing a functional change in the neuron.

Inactivation. There is no active process for inactivation of nitric oxide. However, it is very reactive with other molecules, which results in termination of its biological activity.

Brain localization. Given the short lifespan of nitric oxide, it cannot be visualized by traditional experimental techniques. Therefore, to determine where it might be active, researchers use approaches to visualize its biosynthetic enzyme, nitric oxide synthase. Nitric oxide synthase is scattered throughout the brain in both expected places based on glutamatergic function, and in unexpected places. Research is ongoing to determine the functional significance of its localization.

Lipids

Yet another striking discovery in the late 20th century was that lipids could serve as neurotransmitters. Scientists had long been searching for the receptors and endogenous substances that mediated the effects of cannabinoids (the active ingredients in cannabis). Once the receptors were identified in the late 1980s, this discovery accelerated the search for the endogenous ligands that activated the receptors. The search culminated in the discovery of a lipid, which the researchers called anandamide (ananda is the Sanscrit word for bliss). Chemically, anandamide is N-arachidonoylethanolamine (AEA). A second substance, 2-arachidonoylglycerol (2-AG) was soon found, and these substances were labeled endocannabinoids (endogenous cannabinoids; see Table 2.1; Hassan et al., 2017; Mechoulam & Parker, 2013; Pertwee, 2015). Like gases, lipids do not neatly fulfill the traditional criteria for identification of neurotransmitters; therefore, these too would fall into the broad class of unconventional transmitters.

Biosynthesis and storage. The endocannabinoids are synthesized from lipids found in the cell membrane. The processes are not completely understood, but it appears that production begins with increases in intracellular calcium in a postsynaptic cell, which activate enzymes responsible for endocannabinoid synthesis. For anandamide, phosphatidylethanolamine is converted to N-acylphosphatidylethanolamine (NAPE), and then this is converted to anandamide. There may be other pathways for anandamide synthesis, providing alternative routes to its production. For 2-AG, diacylglycerol (DAG) is converted by specific lipases into 2-AG.

Like gas neurotransmitters, lipid neurotransmitters are not stored in the cell. Because they are lipids, and lipids make up cell membranes, they readily diffuse from the site of production to their targets on adjacent neurons. And like gas neurotransmitters, they appear to have an important role as retrograde messengers, carrying a signal from the postsynaptic neuron to the presynaptic neuron. Evidence suggests that endocannabinoids are involved in cellular responses responsible for learning and memory. This may help to explain why flooding the brain with supraphysiological concentrations of exogenous cannabinoids from smoked or ingested cannabis interferes with memory formation.

Receptors. Two types of metabotropic receptors have been identified for endocannabinoids, CB_1 and CB_2 (Table 2.2). CB_1 receptors are most associated with brain function and are located in regions involved in reward and cognition, among others. Activation of CB_1 receptors on presynaptic terminals inhibits release of neurotransmitters, including glutamate, GABA, and acetylcholine. In contrast, CB_2 receptors are found primarily in the periphery in immune cells.

Inactivation. Endocannabinoids are inactivated via enzymatic processes. Anandamide is inactivated by the enzyme fatty acid amide hydrolase 1 (FAAH1), while 2-AG is inactivated by monoacylglycerol lipase (MAGL). Drug companies have been working to develop enzyme inhibitors to enhance endocannabinoid function for therapeutic potential.

Brain localization. Endocannabinoids and cannabinoid receptors are widespread throughout the brain (Pertwee, 2005, 2015). Interestingly, they are lacking in brainstem nuclei, especially areas involved in respiratory and cardiovascular function. This may help to explain why fatal overdose of cannabinoids is not seen—there is no direct targeting of processes fundamental for life, including breathing and heartbeat.

Neurotrophic Factors

A third class of signaling molecule has a role in retrograde messaging in the brain. Neurotrophic factors, sometimes referred to as growth factors, are proteins involved in the development, differentiation, growth, and survival of neurons, and they have a major role in neuroplasticity, including in learning and memory. There are multiple families of neurotrophic factors, and each of those contains multiple members; a family of particular importance to brain function is the neurotrophins (Lewin & Carter, 2014; Segal, 2003; Zweifel, Kuruvilla, & Ginty, 2005). There is growing interest in these molecules in psychopharmacology since there is evidence that they are involved in different psychiatric disorders. A case in point is brain-derived neurotrophic factor (BDNF). Among other actions, BDNF is thought to be involved in the therapeutic actions of antidepressants. In addition, BDNF has been linked to depression, schizophrenia, addiction, and several other disorders (Autry & Monteggia, 2012).

Biosynthesis and storage. Neurotrophins are proteins. Like the neuropeptides, they are synthesized through the normal biosynthetic process for proteins: DNA is transcribed into RNA, RNA is translated into a protein precursor, and the protein precursor is processed to produce the final product. They are then packaged into two types of vesicles. The first type, known as constitutive, is released independently of neuronal firing. The second type, known as regulated, is released upon neuronal stimulation. When released in the regulated manner, the neurotrophins, originating in the postsynaptic neuron cross the synapse and activate receptors on the presynaptic neuron.

Receptors. The major type of receptors responsible for the specific actions of neurotrophins are Trk (tropomyosin-receptor kinase) receptors. These receptors are large proteins embedded in the cell membrane. On the extracellular side of the membrane is a recognition site for the neurotrophin and on the intracellular side of the membrane is an enzymatic site. When a neurotrophin binds to the receptor, it activates the enzyme, which can then induce a variety of biochemical cascades that modify the cell. There are at least three Trk receptors, TrkA, TrkB and TrkC; TrkB is the one most prominent in the brain. A second type of receptor, known as p75, has been identified, but functions of this receptor are still unclear.

Inactivation. Upon binding, the neurotrophin and its receptor are internalized into the cell in vesicles. The neurotrophin-receptor complex can be degraded, or transported to the cell body where it has the ability to regulate gene transcription before it is degraded.

Brain localization.   Neurotrophins and their receptors are widely distributed in the brain, especially during development, reflecting their role in the development, differentiation, growth, and survival of neurons. In adults, specific factors remain concentrated in certain brain areas. For example, BDNF is found in the hippocampus, hypothalamus, amygdala, midbrain, pons, medulla, and cerebellum, among other brain regions.

MULTIPLE ACTIONS OF DRUGS

Almost everyone who has taken a drug for therapeutic or recreational purposes is familiar with both the target effects and side effects. It needs to be remembered that the distinction between target effects and side effects depends on the desire of the user. For example, one might use the antihistamine diphenhydramine for its ability to suppress allergy symptoms. In this case, sedation produced by the drug is a problematic side effect. However, some people use the same drug to promote sleep. In this case, sedation is the desired effect. Drugs can have multiple actions on neurotransmitter systems to produce target effects and side effects. A conceptual understanding of these multiple actions is summarized below.

Actions on Multiple Targets

No drug is specific in its actions, activating or inhibiting a single molecular target. Instead, a drug has differing abilities to affect multiple targets, such as different neurotransmitter receptors or enzymes. Ethanol is a great example of a promiscuous drug (one that interacts with multiple targets)—among several identified targets, it activates GABA and glycine receptors and inhibits glutamate receptors. By activating key inhibitory neurotransmitter receptors and inhibiting a key excitatory neurotransmitter receptor, ethanol's actions are multiplied, making it a potent sedative. Another example is the antipsychotic drug clozapine. This drug (and similar atypical antipsychotics) blocks both dopamine D_2 receptors and serotonin $5HT_{2A}$ receptors. Both

actions are thought to be involved in the therapeutic effects of clozapine, but through different means. Returning to the example of diphenhydramine, its ability to block histamine receptors is responsible for its antiallergy effects, whereas its blockade of muscarinic acetylcholine receptors produces sedation and dry mouth, and at high doses, confusion, agitation, and memory problems.

Actions on Multiple Circuits

A drug may not be particularly promiscuous, but can have diverse effects because of a neurotransmitter being active in multiple circuits. One example of this is the traditional antipsychotic drug haloperidol. Its therapeutic actions are mediated by blockade of dopamine receptors in the mesocorticolimbic circuit, a circuit involved in (among other things) positive symptoms of schizophrenia. However, haloperidol also blocks dopamine receptors in the nigrostriatal circuit, which is involved in movement, and the tuberoinfundibular circuit, which is involved in hormonal regulation. The actions of haloperidol in the nigrostriatal circuit produce the Parkinsonian side effects of the drug and its actions in the tuberoinfundibular circuit are responsible for hyperprolactinemia and breast enlargement. Another example is the opioid morphine, which produces many of its effects by activating μ-opioid receptors. Activation of these receptors in the spinal cord produces analgesia, activation in the mesolimbic system produces reward and euphoria, activation in the gut produces constipation, and activation in the medulla suppresses breathing. Thus, the same drug acting on the same receptor type in multiple circuits can produce a myriad of effects, both therapeutic and nontherapeutic.

NEUROTRANSMITTERS: PAST, PRESENT, AND FUTURE

Remarkable progress in the understanding of the brain, neurotransmitters, and psychopharmacology was made in the 20th century, and especially during the second half of the century. Each time scientists believed they had a good understanding of neurotransmission and cell signaling, a new discovery dramatically shifted thinking on the topic, as reflected in the identification of peptide neurotransmitters, gas neurotransmitters, lipid neurotransmitters, and neurotrophic factors. There are undoubtedly many more discoveries yet to be made. New tools, techniques, and approaches for studying the brain are being developed at a remarkable rate, leading to greater understanding of and better approaches to treating psychiatric disorders. This chapter provides a basic foundation for understanding neurotransmission, and the following chapters provide up-to-date knowledge of current thoughts about and approaches to pharmacotherapy. However, it must be remembered that this is a rapidly progressing field, and as a result, knowledge will change quickly. Thus, it is important to stay abreast of the latest findings to remain well-informed during this exciting era of scientific progress (see the Tool Kit of Resources).

TOOL KIT OF RESOURCES

Brain Structure Videos

2-Minute Neuroscience: Divisions of the Nervous System: https://www.neuroscientificallychallenged.com/blog/2-minute-neuroscience-divisions-of-the-nervous-system

2-Minute Neuroscience: Lobes and Landmarks of the Brain Surface: https://www.neuroscientifically challenged.com/blog/2-minute-neuroscience-lobes-landmarks-of-the-brain-surface-lateral-view

2-Minute Neuroscience: Medulla Oblongata: https://www.neuroscientificallychallenged.com/blog/2-minute-neuroscience-medulla-oblongata

Neurons and Glia Videos

2-Minute Neuroscience: The Neuron: https://www.neuroscientificallychallenged.com/blog/2-minute-neuroscience-neuron

2-Minute Neuroscience: Glial Cells: https://www.neuroscientificallychallenged.com/blog/2-minute-neuroscience-glial-cells

2-Minute Neuroscience: Action Potential: https://www.neuroscientificallychallenged.com/blog/2-minute-neuroscience-action-potential

2-Minute Neuroscience: Neurotransmitter Release: https://www.neuroscientificallychallenged.com/blog/2-minute-neuroscience-neurotransmitter-release

2-Minute Neuroscience: Synaptic Transmission: https://www.neuroscientificallychallenged.com/blog/2-minute-neuroscience-synaptic-transmission

Neurotransmitters and Drugs Videos

2-Minute Neuroscience: Receptors and Ligands: https://www.neuroscientificallychallenged.com/blog/2-minute-neuroscience-receptors-and-ligands

2-Minute Neuroscience: Dopamine: https://www.neuroscientificallychallenged.com/blog/2-minute-neuroscience-dopamine

2-Minute Neuroscience: Serotonin: https://www.neuroscientificallychallenged.com/blog/2-minute-neuroscience-serotonin

2-Minute Neuroscience: Selective Serotonin Reuptake Inhibitors: https://www.neuroscientifically challenged.com/blog/2-minute-neuroscience-selective-serotonin-reuptake-inhibitors-ssris

2-Minute Neuroscience: GABA: https://www.neuroscientificallychallenged.com/blog/2-minute-neuroscience-gaba

2-Minute Neuroscience: Benzodiazepines: https://www.neuroscientificallychallenged.com/blog/2-minute-neuroscience-benzodiazepines

Neurotransmitters and Drugs Online Resources

Psychopharmacology: The Fourth Generation of Progress: https://acnp.org/digital-library/psychopharmacology-4th-generation-progress/

Neuropsychopharmacology: The Fifth Generation of Progress: https://acnp.org/digital-library/neuropsychopharmacology-5th-generation-progress/

Neuropsychopharmacology Reviews: https://acnp.org/digital-library/neuropsychopharmacology-reviews/

References

Aghajanian, G. K., & Sanders-Bush, E. (2002). Serotonin. In K. L. Davis, D. Charney, J. T. Coyle, & C. Nemeroff (Eds.), *Neuropsychopharmacology: The fifth generation of progress* (pp. 15–34). Philadelphia, PA: Lippincott, Williams, & Wilkins.

*Asterisks indicate assessments or resources.

Aston-Jones, G. (2002). Norepinephrine. In K. L. Davis, D. Charney, J. T. Coyle, & C. Nemeroff (Eds.), *Neuropsychopharmacology: The fifth generation of progress* (pp. 47–58). Philadelphia, PA: Lippincott, Williams, & Wilkins.

Autry, A. E., & Monteggia, L. M. (2012). Brain-derived neurotrophic factor and neuropsychiatric disorders. *Pharmacological Reviews, 64,* 238–258. http://dx.doi.org/10.1124/pr.111.005108

Baumgarten, H. G., & Göthert, M. (Eds.). (2000). *Handbook of experimental pharmacology: Serotoninergic neurons and 5-HT receptors in the CNS* (Vol. 129). Berlin, Germany: Springer. http://dx.doi.org/10.1007/978-3-642-60921-3

Boehning, D., & Snyder, S. H. (2003). Novel neural modulators. *Annual Review of Neuroscience, 26,* 105–131. http://dx.doi.org/10.1146/annurev.neuro.26.041002.131047

*Bohlen und Halbach, O. V., & Dermietzel, R. (2006). *Neurotransmitters and neuromodulators: Handbook of receptors and biological effects* (2nd ed.). Weinheim, Germany: Wiley-VCH.

Bowery, N. G., & Smart, T. G. (2006). GABA and glycine as neurotransmitters: A brief history. *British Journal of Pharmacology, 147*(Suppl. 1), S109–S119. http://dx.doi.org/10.1038/sj.bjp.0706443

*Charney, D. S., Sklar, P. B., Buxbaum, J. D., & Nestler, E. J. (2013). *Neurobiology of Mental Illness* (4th ed.). New York, NY: Oxford University Press. http://dx.doi.org/10.1093/med/9780199934959.001.0001

Citri, A., & Malenka, R. C. (2008). Synaptic plasticity: Multiple forms, functions, and mechanisms. *Neuropsychopharmacology, 33,* 18–41. http://dx.doi.org/10.1038/sj.npp.1301559

Coyle, J. T., Leski, M. L., & Morrison, J. H. (2002). The diverse roles of l-glutamic acid in brain signal transduction. In K. L. Davis, D. Charney, J. T. Coyle, & C. Nemeroff (Eds.), *Neuropsychopharmacology: The fifth generation of progress* (pp. 71–90). Philadelphia, PA: Lippincott, Williams, & Wilkins.

Di Chiara, G. (Ed.). (2002). *Handbook of experimental pharmacology: Dopamine in the CNS* (Vol. 154). Berlin, Germany: Springer.

Feldman, R. S., Meyer, J. S., & Quenzer, L. F. (1997). *Principles of neuropsychopharmacology.* Sunderland, Mass: Sinauer Associates.

Grace, A. A. (2002). Dopamine. In K. L. Davis, D. Charney, J. T. Coyle, & C. Nemeroff (Eds.), *Neuropsychopharmacology: The fifth generation of progress* (pp. 119–132). Philadelphia, PA: Lippincott, Williams, & Wilkins.

Griebel, G., & Holsboer, F. (2012). Neuropeptide receptor ligands as drugs for psychiatric diseases: The end of the beginning? *Nature Reviews. Drug Discovery, 11,* 462–478. http://dx.doi.org/10.1038/nrd3702

Halassa, M. M., Fellin, T., & Haydon, P. G. (2007). The tripartite synapse: Roles for gliotransmission in health and disease. *Trends in Molecular Medicine, 13,* 54–63. http://dx.doi.org/10.1016/j.molmed.2006.12.005

Hassan, Z., Bosch, O. G., Singh, D., Narayanan, S., Kasinather, B. V., Seifritz, E., . . . Müller, C. P. (2017). Novel psychoactive substances—Recent progress on neuropharmacological mechanisms of action for selected drugs. *Frontiers in Psychiatry, 8,* 152. http://dx.doi.org/10.3389/fpsyt.2017.00152

Hernandes, M. S., & Troncone, L. R. (2009). Glycine as a neurotransmitter in the forebrain: A short review. *Journal of Neural Transmission, 116,* 1551–1560. http://dx.doi.org/10.1007/s00702-009-0326-6

Hökfelt, T., Bartfai, T., & Bloom, F. (2003). Neuropeptides: Opportunities for drug discovery. *Lancet Neurology, 2,* 463–472. http://dx.doi.org/10.1016/S1474-4422(03)00482-4

Holmes, A., Heilig, M., Rupniak, N. M., Steckler, T., & Griebel, G. (2003). Neuropeptide systems as novel therapeutic targets for depression and anxiety disorders. *Trends in Pharmacological Sciences, 24,* 580–588. http://dx.doi.org/10.1016/j.tips.2003.09.011

Jonas, P., & Monyer, H. (Eds.). (1999). *Handbook of experimental pharmacology: Ionotropic glutamate receptors in the CNS* (Vol. 141). Berlin, Germany: Springer. http://dx.doi.org/10.1007/978-3-662-08022-1

Lewin, G. R., & Carter, B. D. (Eds.). (2014). *Handbook of experimental pharmacology: Neurotrophic factors* (Vol. 220). Berlin, Germany: Springer. http://dx.doi.org/10.1007/978-3-642-45106-5

Machado-Vieira, R., Manji, H. K., & Zarate, C. A. (2009). The role of the tripartite glutamatergic synapse in the pathophysiology and therapeutics of mood disorders. *The Neuroscientist, 15,* 525–539. http://dx.doi.org/10.1177/1073858409336093

Mayer, B. (Ed.). (2000). *Handbook of experimental pharmacology: Nitric oxide* (Vol. 143). Berlin, Germany: Springer. http://dx.doi.org/10.1007/978-3-642-57077-3

Mechoulam, R., & Parker, L. A. (2013). The endocannabinoid system and the brain. *Annual Review of Psychology, 64,* 21–47. http://dx.doi.org/10.1146/annurev-psych-113011-143739

*Meyer, J. S., & Quenzer, L. F. (2013). *Psychopharmacology: Drugs, the brain, and behavior* (2nd ed.). Sunderland, MA: Sinauer Associates.

Möhler, H. (Ed.). (2001). *Handbook of experimental pharmacology: Pharmacology of GABA and glycine neurotransmission* (Vol. 150). Berlin, Germany: Springer. http://dx.doi.org/10.1007/978-3-642-56833-6

Morris, G. P., Clark, I. A., Zinn, R., & Vissel, B. (2013). Microglia: A new frontier for synaptic plasticity, learning and memory, and neurodegenerative disease research. *Neurobiology of Learning and Memory, 105,* 40–53. http://dx.doi.org/10.1016/j.nlm.2013.07.002

Nusbaum, M. P., Blitz, D. M., & Marder, E. (2017). Functional consequences of neuropeptide and small-molecule co-transmission. *Nature Reviews Neuroscience, 18,* 389–403. http://dx.doi.org/10.1038/nrn.2017.56

Olsen, R. W. (2002). GABA. In K. L. Davis, D. Charney, J. T. Coyle, & C. Nemeroff (Eds.), *Neuro-psychopharmacology: The fifth generation of progress* (pp. 159–168). Philadelphia, PA: Lippincott, Williams, & Wilkins.

Pertwee, R. G. (Ed.). (2005). *Handbook of experimental pharmacology: Cannabinoids* (Vol. 168). Berlin, Germany: Springer. http://dx.doi.org/10.1007/b137831

Pertwee, R. G. (Ed.). (2015). *Handbook of experimental pharmacology: Endocannabinoids* (Vol. 231). Cham, Switzerland: Springer. http://dx.doi.org/10.1007/978-3-319-20825-1

Picciotto, M. R., Alreja, M., & Jentsch, J. D. (2002). Acetylcholine. In K. L. Davis, D. Charney, J. T. Coyle, & C. Nemeroff (Eds.), *Neuropsychopharmacology: The fifth generation of progress* (pp. 3–14). Philadelphia, PA: Lippincott, Williams, & Wilkins.

Quesseveur, G., Gardier, A. M., & Guiard, B. P. (2013). The monoaminergic tripartite synapse: A putative target for currently available antidepressant drugs. *Current Drug Targets, 14,* 1277–1294. http://dx.doi.org/10.2174/13894501113149990209

Salter, M. W., & Stevens, B. (2017). Microglia emerge as central players in brain disease. *Nature Medicine, 23,* 1018–1027. http://dx.doi.org/10.1038/nm.4397

Schafer, D. P., Lehrman, E. K., & Stevens, B. (2013). The "quad-partite" synapse: Microglia-synapse interactions in the developing and mature CNS. *Glia, 61,* 24–36. http://dx.doi.org/10.1002/glia.22389

*Schatzberg, A. F., Nemeroff, C. B., & American Psychiatric Association Publishing. (2017). *The American Psychiatric Association Publishing textbook of psycho-pharmacology* (5th ed.). Arlington, VA: American Psychiatric Association Publishing.

Segal, R. A. (2003). Selectivity in neurotrophin signaling: Theme and variations. *Annual Review of Neuro-science, 26,* 299–330. http://dx.doi.org/10.1146/annurev.neuro.26.041002.131421

Skolnick, P. (Ed.). (2010). *Glutamate-based therapies for psychiatric disorders.* Basel, Switzerland: Springer. http://dx.doi.org/10.1007/978-3-0346-0241-9

*Stahl, S. M. (2013). *Stahl's essential psychopharmacology: Neuroscientific basis and practical application* (4th ed.). Cambridge, United Kingdom: Cambridge University Press.

Strand, F. L. (2003). Neuropeptides: General characteristics and neuropharmaceutical potential in treating CNS disorders. *Progress in Drug Research, 61,* 1–37.

Trendelenburg, U., & Weiner, N. (Eds.). (1988). *Handbook of experimental pharmacology: Catecholamines I* (Vol. 90). Berlin, Germany: Springer-Verlag. http://dx.doi.org/10.1007/978-3-642-46625-0

Uusi-Oukari, M., & Korpi, E. R. (2010). Regulation of $GABA_A$ receptor subunit expression by pharmacological agents. *Pharmacological Reviews, 62,* 97–135. http://dx.doi.org/10.1124/pr.109.002063

Wu, L., & Wang, R. (2005). Carbon monoxide: Endogenous production, physiological functions, and pharmacological applications. *Pharmacological Reviews, 57,* 585–630. http://dx.doi.org/10.1124/pr.57.4.3

Zweifel, L. S., Kuruvilla, R., & Ginty, D. D. (2005). Functions and mechanisms of retrograde neuro-trophin signalling. *Nature Reviews Neuroscience, 6,* 615–625. http://dx.doi.org/10.1038/nrn1727

CHAPTER 3

BASIC PSYCHOPHARMACOLOGY

Lorenz S. Neuwirth

The regularly occurring use of psychoactive substances by individuals has become deeply entrenched in today's society. Whether it is ingesting an Advil® to treat a headache, consuming an alcoholic beverage to toast at a family get-together, or smoking a cigar to celebrate the birth of a child, the increased socialization of psychoactive substances has evolved considerably over the last 50 years. Additionally, millions of Americans are prescribed a variety of drugs by mental and allied health care professionals for treating a range of mental health issues, such as depression (Kirsch et al., 2008), anxiety, and other psychiatric disorders (Olfson, Blanco, Liu, Moreno, & Laje, 2006; Whitaker, 2005), as a means to improve their quality of life. Notably, these interventions have in some cases resulted in the overprescribing of certain drugs (e.g., anti-depressive medications) that has disproportionately affected racial and ethnic minority populations within the United States (Alegría et al., 2008). Longitudinal studies further reveal that adolescent junior high (Chassin, Hussong, & Beltran, 2009), high school, and college student illicit drug use continues to upsurge (Johnston, O'Malley, Bachman, & Schulenberg, 2012, 2008). Further, illicit drug use among college students has substantially grown and evolved since the 1990s (Gledhill-Hoyt, Lee, Strote, & Wechsler, 2000). Most concerning has been prolific nonmedical prescription drug use by college students (McCabe, West, & Wechsler, 2007). A prime example would be a college student with attention-deficit/hyperactivity disorder (ADHD) selling his or her prescribed Adderall® (i.e., an amphetamine or psychostimulant) to another student without a mental health issue for the purpose of staying up later to cram for exams. Consequently, between the increased socialization of drugs and the acculturation of prescription and illicit drug use in society, mental and allied health care professionals face complex challenges in understanding, interpreting, and addressing the range of psychoactive substances used by their patients and their rationale for their drug use. Mental and allied health care professionals therefore need to be more educated about psychopharmacology than prior generations.

Historically, many mental and allied health care fields were less interdisciplinary than they are currently. Such independent health care provider specialties (e.g., social work, mental health counseling, neurology, psychiatry, psychology)—whereby general consultation occurred and subsequent referrals suggested patients seek treatment from other specialists—often left the coordination of the patient's medical information as the responsibility of the patient. This resulted at times in minimal or nonexistent person-centered-planning (e.g., the patient may restrict dialogue with the referred professionals and not address his or her presenting symptoms). Wang, Lane, and

Olfson (2005) conducted a 12-month survey of mental health service delivery in the United States, investigating patterns of patient needs in order to estimate needs left unmet or unserved. In their study, 41% of the patients received mental health service comprised of 22.8% treated by a primary/general care physician/doctor, 16% treated by a nonpsychiatrist mental health professional, 12.3% treated by a psychiatrist, 8.1% treated by a human services provider/social worker, and 6.8% treated by an alternative/complementary medical provider (Wang et al., 2005). Over time, these situations resulted in overburdening patients with excessive appointments, copays, consultations (which at times may have contradicted care), medications, and expected therapeutic outcomes. Notably, in some cases these experiences made patients question their trust of mental and allied health care professionals, resulting in suboptimal treatment outcomes and the subsequent choice by these individuals to abandon professional treatment and resort to self-medication or remain untreated (Wang et al., 2005), both of which contributed to mental health treatment dropout (Olfson et al., 2009; Wang, 2007).

As the health care system evolves in an attempt to incorporate better person-centered planning and more interdisciplinary discussion of patient needs between providers, patients may still drop out of treatment and opt to self-medicate despite these improvements (Bolton, Robinson, & Sareen, 2009). It is here where the problem lies for mental and allied health care professionals, such that a critical understanding of the basic principles of psychopharmacology regarding psychoactive substances is an inevitable requirement. Regardless of one's mental or allied health care specialty, communicating the basic principles of psychopharmacology to the layperson and the professional is arguably a key determining factor in identifying whether the patient is educated to seek professional help or may face the risks of choosing self-medication strategies to address their underlying biopsychological and mental health needs. It is important to note that the biopsychological mechanisms of any mental health issue, once activated, turned on, or triggered, cause the social expression of the disorder at the behavioral and psychological levels, which is

what we observe and experience with one another in society. This expression of the disorder is often what brings patients to a mental or allied health care professional for treatment. Moreover, when people self-medicate, they run the risk that they may either exacerbate current mental health symptoms—thereby increasing the severity of their disorder(s)—or bring on mental health symptoms despite having no prior history of mental illness. For these important reasons, a clear distinction is required between what is considered a drug versus a medication, so that mental and allied health care professionals can improve their understanding of the basic psychopharmacology of any substance deemed a drug. Through this understanding, mental and allied health care professionals can provide informed educational outcomes on such drug use through their service delivery.

MISCONCEPTIONS REGARDING DRUGS VERSUS MEDICATIONS

The major distinctions surrounding how and why individuals in society use drugs help professionals classify patient intent or rationale for using drugs. An individual's drug intent or motivation can be classified into either instrumental or recreational drug use. *Instrumental* drug use is defined as an individual's motivation to use a drug to address or treat a specific problem (e.g., using DayQuil™ to treat coughing, Xanax® to treat anxiety or panic disorder, or Adderall to treat ADHD). *Recreational* drug use is defined as an individual's use of a drug to experience specific effects (e.g., mixing DayQuil with alcohol to create "purple drank," taking nonprescription Xanax or Adderall to get high; Prus, 2018, pp. 5–6). Social misconceptions of drug use arise through these two motivational factors, as people erroneously use the word "drug" in conversation without distinguishing it from a purposeful medication and may be more inclined to classify most drugs as substances of abuse or eventual abuse. This can be problematic for mental and allied health care professionals in the field, as the goal is to educate patients and offer them a range of therapeutic options to address presenting symptoms. Such conversations, however, also require that mental and allied health care professionals are aware of personal biases regarding prescription medications. One way to avoid confounding mental and allied health care professional bias is to clearly educate the patient on the differences between instrumental and recreational medication use.

For example, instrumental use of Xanax to treat anxiety or a panic attack would be considered taking a medication to serve a medical purpose, whereas taking two or three times the prescribed amount of Xanax or taking Xanax without an underlying medical reason for doing so (i.e., nonprescribed purpose) would be considered recreational drug use and abuse. This latter situation is critical, as a medication can rapidly lose its instrumental definition and perhaps therapeutic value in society while its drug abuse potential increases. It is in this way that people often confuse how drugs enter society. They may accept the view that pharmaceutical companies and large corporations truly want to help address society's mental health issues and develop appropriate drugs with the goal of ameliorating those issues, or they may develop the alternative view that pharmaceutical companies and large corporations intentionally develop drugs for people to become addicted and dependent on their product at the expense of their mental health issues. Such skepticism of the rationale and purposefulness of drug development in addressing patient mental health outcomes requires careful, transparent discussion and an unbiased, informed education on the basics of psychopharmacology. Individuals and mental and allied health care professionals are equally important participants in this educational process if the population served is to be made aware of the reasons for using, as well as the risks associated with, any medication or drug that they consume.

At the other end of the spectrum, emergency medicine also informs us of specific examples that may alarm the public regarding growing drug problems that are less well-known in society. This is important to note, as most teenage and young adults engage intentionally or unintentionally with drugs in society during stressful transitionary times in their lifespan. At these critical time periods, social and peer pressures as well as real world demands can become difficult to manage, which may either evoke or exacerbate mental health issues in the population. As such, historical trends show that this particular age group is at high risk for recreational drug use and may opt to engage in such behaviors as an attempt to treat an underlying mental health issue or escape life's challenges. If the issues faced by teenagers and young adults remain unaddressed, they may result in early drug sensitization, dependence, and addiction, which may in turn increase future risks of drug overdose.

For example, Caldicott's and Kuhn's (2001) emergency medical report stated that gamma-hydroxybutyrate (GHB), otherwise known as the "date rape drug" and which in the 1960s was believed unlikely to cause an overdose in its victims, had substantially evolved through societal drug culture in very different ways from what was previously predicted. In their report, they detailed a few emergency cases in which they had to revive individuals from GHB overdoses with physostigmine (a drug used as an antidote against cholinergic poisoning; Caldicott & Kuhn, 2001). This suggested that drugs may be changing over time, either being manufactured as more potent (stronger) or being mixed with other drugs or agents (i.e., polydrug use), thus requiring emergency experts to anticipate reviving patients in the emergency room (Boyer, Quang, Woolf, & Shannon, 2001). Similarly, researchers are investigating and identifying the effects of naloxone in reviving patients who overdose on opioid-derived drugs (Dettmer, Saunders, & Strang, 2001; Kaplan et al., 1999; Sumner et al., 2016). Through early emergency medicine work on GHB overdoses, the medical field had to address these growing issues by developing reactive therapeutic treatment approaches to save lives, which could have been avoided if those individuals had been provided with proactive therapeutic psychotropic medications to address their mental health needs.

DRUG TERMINOLOGY FOR WORKING PROFESSIONALS

Some of the confusion surrounding what constitutes a drug versus a medication may result from the use of different names for a given substance—generic name, trade name, chemical name, and street name (see Table 3.1). People mostly know

TABLE 3.1

Clarifying What It Means When Using the Word Drug in Different Contexts

Drug name	OTC definition	Prescription definition
Trade name or brand name	A company has a proprietary trademarked name on a drug, but is used as an over-the-counter (OTC) medication (e.g., DayQuil™)	A company has a proprietary trademark and brand name for prescription medications that treat, for example, anxiety (Xanax®) or ADD/ADHD (Adderall®).
Generic name	A nonproprietary name that indicates the classification for an OTC medication to be used and distinguishes it from similar products in the same class (e.g., acetaminophen, dextromethorphan, pseudoephedrine)	A nonproprietary name that indicates the classification for the prescribed medication to be used and distinguishes it from other prescribed medications in the same class (e.g., alprazolam for Xanax, amphetamine and dextroamphetamine for Adderall).
Chemical name	A name that details a drug's or a medicine's chemical structure (i.e., how is it chemically derived or its molecular formula; e.g., acetaminophen [$C_8H_9NO_2$], dextromethorphan [$C_{18}H_{25}NO$], pseudoephedrine [$C_{10}H_{15}NO$])	A name that details a prescription medicine's chemical structure (e.g., alprazolam [$C_{17}H_{13}ClN_4$], amphetamine and dextroamphetamine [$C_9H_{13}N$])
Street name	A purposefully altered name for a medication created to disguise its name so that it can be used as a recreational drug for substance abuse (e.g., dextromethorphan's street name is Robo or Triple C)	For example, Xanax is known as benzos, blue v., candy, downers, sleeping pills, tranks; Rohypnol is known as roofies, roofinol, rope, and rophies; Adderall is known as addys, uppers, beans, black beauties, pep, pills, speed, dexies, zing, study buddies, smarties, and smart pills

Note. ADD = attention deficit disorder; ADHD = attention-deficit/hyperactivity disorder.

a drug by its street name and a medication by its trade name; fewer people know a medication by its generic name, and far less people know a drug by its chemical name. Thus, as individuals experience these terms for and definitions of a given drug, their perceptions of drug definitions can be rather limited or easily interchangeable. When people speak about drugs, they often refer to these substances by their street names (e.g., coke, meth, ecstasy, acid, weed) rather than calling them by their drug name (e.g., cocaine, methamphetamine, MDMA, LSD, marijuana). In addition, as younger generations use drugs and create more polydrug use, new street names are created, such as "sizzurp," "lean," or "purple drank." The latter polydrug mixture has emerged as an area of particular concern, as adolescents and young adults combine prescription cold medication (e.g., codeine, promethazine), alcohol, sugary soda (e.g., Sprite®, Mountain Dew®), and flavored candies (e.g., Jolly Rancher™) to achieve recreational highs at lower cost than other illicit drugs (as popularized in Houston's hip-hop music culture in the 1990s; Peters et al., 2003). This self-administered polydrug use creates the potential for very serious societal medical and mental health issues and new cultures evolving from such polydrug trends.

More troubling has been the rise in nonprescribed Adderall use and abuse by college students (Varga, 2012); as diagnoses of ADHD have become more common, students are more frequently prescribed Adderall or Vyvanse® to address their mental health issues. They may engage in illicit use, sales, and distribution of their medications, or they may illegally obtain, distribute, and sell these psychostimulant drugs on college campuses (Low & Gendaszek, 2002; Prudhomme White, Becker-Blease, & Grace-Bishop, 2010). The illicit use of these medications is most associated with cramming for tests, midterms, and finals, and writing papers (i.e., from 47.5% to 65.2%), as well as obtaining a recreational high (31%) and drug experimentation (29.9%; Teter, McCabe, LaGrange, Cranford, & Boyd, 2006). These trends have been promoted, reinforced, and popularized through social media such as Twitter (Hanson et al., 2013).

What many individuals fail to realize is that referring to a drug by its street name suggests that their experience and knowledge of the drug is limited to is recreational use or substance abuse, and not its potential medical purpose or its potential for harm. One can make the argument that there is no purpose in creating a polydrug such as purple drank except to get high. One can also argue that it is possible to have an educational conversation regarding the potential medical purposes of low-dose marijuana and MDMA for terminally ill people and those with posttraumatic stress disorder, but not about the potential medical purposes of weed or low-dose ecstasy. This latter point is rather critical, as younger generations continue to blur the lines in communicating about and advocating for drugs to be legalized when some prescription medications may already be available to address their psychological symptoms. In the case of students who have ADD/ADHD, prescribed medication helps them manage their focus while in school. However, other college students willingly engage in nonprescription use of Adderall and try to justify it as instrumental use as a means to focus in class and study for exams, while still others simply use it to get high. Despite current nonprescription drug use trends, it remains to be documented what proportion of these nonprescription psychostimulant college users are at risk for drug addiction (McCabe, West, Teter, & Boyd, 2014); misperceptions among college students of such addictions have been reported (McCabe, 2008). This may be further obfuscated by the "fear of being addicted to prescription drugs" created by the opioid epidemic, which is specific to opioid-derived medications and may not directly generalize to all prescription medications.

Notably, in the context of considerations around legalizing drugs (e.g., marijuana), one may ignore the possibility that just because a drug is legalized, its addictive potential and adverse risks or drug interactions are not reduced. Nor in the case of Adderall or opioid prescription medications does U.S. Food and Drug Administration (FDA) approval prevent individuals from misusing drugs. Therefore, it is prudent for mental and allied health care professionals to consider discussing recreational and instrumental drug use history or current behaviors with their patients to better understand the nature of their mental health issues as well as proper prescription drug management behaviors. Transparent dialogue between the patient and the professional may serve to foster a better understanding of the patient's pattern of behaviors, risks, and probabilities of abstaining from illicit drugs. Such invaluable information can be an effective counseling tool to follow the patient's commitment to their prescription drug therapy to address their underlying mental health issues. Alternatively, it can be used to predict how the patient may deviate from their prescription drug therapy or result in therapeutic dropout. A certain level of empathy is encouraged among mental and allied health care professionals, as an individual may not have a full perspective on drugs or medications described in this context, or might not have the education, tools, and effective means to manage his or her mental health issues. In addition, when professionals observe patient misconceptions or misperceptions, this presents a key opportunity for an important teaching moment within any intervention to supplement the services being provided. Although few mental and allied health care professionals will be tasked with prescribing psychotropic medications, as the health care system changes—with the hope of becoming more integrated—the more informed mental and allied health care professionals are regarding the role of psychopharmacology for treating mental health disorders, the more helpful they can be to their patients and society.

PSYCHOTROPIC DRUG DOSAGE

In this section and in those that follow, the term *drug* refers to a medication for psychotropic or mental health therapeutic purposes, as it enters the body and central nervous system (CNS) to cause a change in the physiological, psychological, and behavioral functions of an individual. The instrumental psychotropic effect of a drug (i.e., experiencing medical relief for a symptom) depends on the dose of the drug taken. This is important, as taking too much of any psychotropic drug—regardless of the intent—can result in a drug overdose, and too little of a psychotropic drug dose produces no beneficial medical effect or treatment gains. The regulation of the appropriate amount of a psychotropic drug that an individual should consume directly relates to an individual's body weight, and defines a drug dose. In other words, a drug dose is the ratio of the amount of drug an individual takes or is prescribed based on their body weight (i.e., typically measured as mg/kg [1 kg = 2.2 lb.]). Notably, most psychotropic medications are not prescribed on a mg/kg basis, nor are psychotropic drug doses individualized to any great extent. Patients are prescribed psychotropic drug doses using Latin-derived medical terms, such as q.d., qd, or QD, which stands for *quaque die* in Latin and translates to "once a day"; b.i.d. or BID, which stands for *bis in die* in Latin and translates to "two times a day"; t.i.d. or TID, which stands for *ter in die* in Latin and translates into "three times a day"; and q_h., where the "q" stands for "*quaque*," or "once," and the "h" stands for "hours" (e.g., "2 caps q6h" means "take two capsules once every 6 hours").

It is important to note that individuals are left to self-administer their psychotropic drugs following their prescriptions, but often do not consider dose or are unaware of related factors, and as a result may inadvertently place themselves at risk of over-consumption or over administration of a drug that could increase their chances of drug abuse and/or overdose (e.g., with benzodiazepines, opioids, psychostimulants). Often, individuals think of their psychotropic drug usage as a scale of quantity (e.g., as a pill a day or a pill every 6 hours) rather than by dosage, which presents another misconception or misperception that small quantities of psychotropic drugs might be socially acceptable to recreationally use and abuse since they are already medically beneficial. Yet, this by no means indicates that they cannot cause harm, and it further perpetuates the illicit use of nonprescribed medications. The lack of psychotropic drug education in society must be remedied to shift individual attitudes and perceptions regarding both drug acceptance and abstinence, and to improve mental health outcomes. Simons and Carey (2000) found that younger individuals, who had a more positive attitude about marijuana use and less so regarding drug-free experiences, were at the highest risk of using larger amounts of marijuana. Additionally, younger adolescent attitudes

towards psychotropic interventions may also contribute to maintaining their course of therapy or opting to move away from therapy. There is a debate as to whether the Drug Attitudinal Inventory assessment is a valid tool for elucidating such subjective experiences and their predictability of future drug use (Townsend, Floersch, & Findling, 2009). This latter point illustrates researchers' attempts to address and hone in on factors that could predict such perceptual drug addiction risks, but it is a very complex issue that has remained out of reach of most subjective screening tools. Further, individuals may also engage in prescription medication diversion, defined as "the unlawful channeling of regulated pharmaceuticals from legal sources to the illicit market place" (Inciardi, Surratt, Kurtz, & Burke, 2009, p. 2). Additionally, once prescribed a psychotropic medication, individuals may opt to sell it rather than use it, which contributes to two major societal issues: (a) mental health issues remain unaddressed, and (b) the illicit distribution and sale of these psychotropic medications may cause significant problems when used recreationally or with other drugs (Garnier et al., 2010).

To place the concept of psychotropic drug dosage into perspective, Figure 3.1 illustrates two hypothetical drugs that are compared as a function of dose (mg/kg) on the X-axis in relation to the individually experienced drug effect on the Y-axis. As in the case of chance when flipping a coin, with a 50% probability that there will be an outcome of heads or tails, there is also a drug dosage level at which there is a 50% chance that a drug will have an effect that can be observed in an individual (based on results from the population data) or that the individual will experience no effect. This phenomenon is called the *effective dose value*, or an ED_{50} value (or simply an ED_{50}), which represents the specific dose of a given drug that is effective in 50 percent of the population. As illustrated in Figure 3.1, the ED_{50} can be used to compare psychotropic drugs intended to treat the same mental health issue to determine which drug is more potent than another, or which drug may present with a wider therapeutic range to increase the treatment regimen drug dose to best meet an individual's mental health needs. The potency of a psychotropic drug

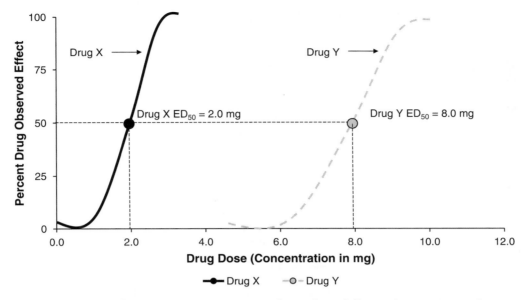

FIGURE 3.1.   An illustration comparing ED_{50} values of two different drugs to assess drug potency. Drug X (left) reaches its ED_{50} at 2.0 mg, in contrast to Drug Y (right), which reaches its ED_{50} at 8.0 mg. This suggests that Drug X is more potent than Drug Y, and that more caution should be used when prescribing and administering Drug X. Notably, both drugs have a restricted window for increasing medication dosage, as Drug X has a 1.0 mg range before reaching maximal drug effectiveness, and Drug Y has a 2 mg range before reaching its maximal effectiveness. Therefore, Drug Y may be potentially safer to use than Drug X.

is defined as the amount of a drug that produces a certain level or magnitude of the therapeutic effect observed (Prus, 2018). Thus, as Drug X shifts more towards the left it indicates that at lower doses this drug reaches its ED_{50} at 2.0 mg, when compared with Drug Y, which reaches its ED_{50} at 8.0 mg. This suggests that Drug X is perhaps stronger or more potent than Drug Y, since the individual can achieve the ED_{50} at 2.0 mg of Drug X versus 8.0 mg of Drug Y. It also suggests that taking more than approximately 3.0 mg of Drug X or 10.0 mg of Drug Y will not increase the drug's effectiveness, as these or higher doses may place the individual at risk for experiencing adverse side effects, toxic doses, or even overdose. To simplify this concept, the psychotropic drug potency (i.e., the binding affinity of the drug at the receptor level) refers to the amount of the drug required to produce a therapeutic effect (i.e., ED_{50}), whereas psychotropic drug efficacy (i.e., the activity that occurs between the drug and receptor interaction) refers to the maximal effect a drug can produce regardless of the dosage prescribed (see Figure 3.2). Thus, the ED_{50}

has been effective as a means to determine relative potency comparisons between different drugs.

It is equally important to note that drugs that are more potent can be dangerous at times, since higher potency levels or magnitudes can result in quicker drug sensitization and tolerance and be lethal when triggering an overdose. Drug sensitization refers to when, with each subsequent dose of psychotropic medication taken, an individual experiences an increasingly effective treatment outcome without increasing medication dosage. This suggests that the patient is rather sensitive to the medication and as such, is experiencing an increased psychotropic drug reaction; hence, drug sensitization (see Figure 3.3). Conversely, drug tolerance refers to when, following each subsequent dose of psychotropic medication, an individual experiences a reduction in his or her expected treatment outcomes without reducing medication dosage. This suggests that the patient is rather tolerant to the medication and as such, is experiencing a decreased psychotropic drug reaction; hence, drug tolerance (Figure 3.3). This concept is important, as drugs prescribed from

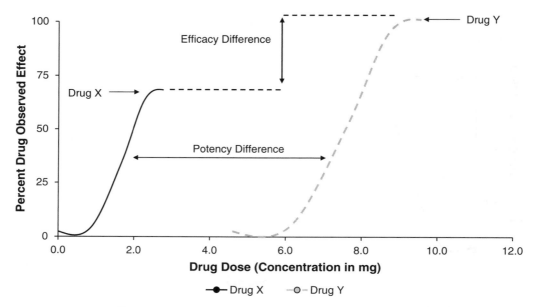

FIGURE 3.2.   An illustration comparing efficacy and potency values of two different psychotropic drugs. Drug potency refers to the amount of the drug required to produce a therapeutic effect (i.e., ED_{50}), whereas psychotropic drug efficacy refers to the maximal effect that a drug can produce regardless of the dosage prescribed. Drug X (left) reaches its ED_{50} at 2.0 mg, in contrast to Drug Y (right), which reaches its ED_{50} at 7.0 mg. This suggests that Drug X is more potent than Drug Y, and there is a difference of 4 mg in potency between the two drugs. Drug X reaches its efficacy between 2 to 3 mg, whereas Drug Y reaches its efficacy between 9 to 10 mg. This suggests that although Drug X is more potent, it has limited efficacy, and that Drug Y is less potent and has a greater degree of efficacy.

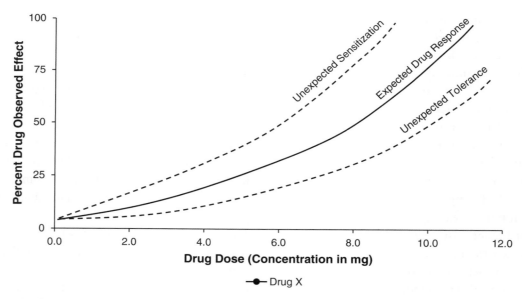

FIGURE 3.3.   An illustration comparing the expected drug response in contrast to unexpected drug sensitization and tolerance values for one psychotropic drug. Based on population data, an expected drug dose–response curve is used to guide prescription therapy to treat mental health issues. However, at times, some individuals' responses to such psychotropic medications may deviate leftward from the expected values and experience an increased drug potency effect called sensitization. In contrast, some individuals' responses may deviate rightward from expected values and experience a decreased drug potency effect called tolerance. Thus, mental and allied health care professionals should be mindful that, depending on the psychotropic medication and given patients' individual differences, patients' responsivity to such treatments should be carefully monitored over time.

the same class may not be sufficiently efficacious relative to others even at much higher doses. This can be due to a number of factors, such as competitive drug interactions or even receptor downregulation at the site of action in the synapses within the CNS. Both psychotropic drug sensitization and tolerance are important factors for mental and allied health care professionals to understand when working with patients. The way in which a drug enters the body and brain also can significantly influence the CNS through onset and duration of a drug's specific action, altering physiological, psychological, and behavioral functions.

DRUG ROUTES OF ADMINISTRATION

Although drug dosage is important in understanding how a drug will likely influence an individual's physiology, psychology, and behavior, it is also important to understand the speed at which drugs can influence the CNS. The potency of a drug can influence the immediacy of the impact on the CNS, which could be beneficial in the case of a therapeutic medication (e.g., epinephrine, amphetamines) or a drug revival agent (e.g., physostigmine, naloxone, Vivitrol®); in contrast, it can also be more harmful in illicit street drugs such as cocaine, opioids, LSD, or ecstasy. A drug must enter the body and be absorbed and distributed to reach the CNS in order to obtain the desired psychological changes.

The way in which a drug enters the body is defined as a route of drug exposure. Drugs can enter the body and affect brain functioning through the following routes: oral ingestion (i.e., swallowing a substance), sublingual (i.e., dissolving a substance under the tongue), nasal and mucosal membrane (i.e., absorbing the substance through the membranes of the nasal and oral cavities), inhalation (i.e., breathing the substance into the lungs), transdermal (i.e., absorbing the substance through the skin), subcutaneous (i.e., injecting the substance under the skin), intra-rectal (i.e., inserting a substance directly into the rectum or inserting the substance into another product and then inserting it directly into the rectum), intramuscular (i.e., injecting the substance directly into skeletal muscle), and intravenous (i.e., injecting the substance directly into a major vein of the body).

The routes of drug exposures are not limited to those described herein, any orifice of the body can be a potential route of drug exposure (e.g., eye drops within the mucous membranes of the eyelid). A clear understanding of drug dose and route of exposure is required to comprehend how they relate to drug safety and lethality.

DRUG SAFETY AND LETHALITY

Consistent with the concept of an ED_{50} described above, when drug and medication developers propose a new drug they are tasked to limit the potential for any inadvertent or adverse side effects. The goal of the researchers, medical experts, clinicians, and pharmaceutical scientists is to increase the benefits gained through a newly proposed drug therapy while concurrently reducing any foreseeable risks associated with such drug development. The key word here is "foreseeable," as not all side effects can be predicted nor can all polydrug or drug cross-talk interactions be determined, since human behavior is difficult to predict in these contexts and individual variability can involve ranges of neurobiological sensitivity or tolerance to certain drugs. Logically, a couple of questions arise: What is the probability that an individual would respond appropriately to these drugs during the course of therapy? What is the probability that an individual may stop taking a prescribed drug instrumentally and encounter the risk of abusing the drug recreationally? These issues, which have grown more concerning in society, further complicate matters for drug developers in treating mental health issues, and as such, remain highly controversial. The overarching goal in drug development is to provide people with a particular medication that instrumentally addresses their specific issues while helping to reduce their presenting psychological symptoms so that they can have a better quality of life. However, embedded in this drug development goal is the responsibility to create drugs that are only potent enough to achieve optimal treatment effectiveness in addressing a given mental health diagnosis, and to be mindful to reduce the potential for toxic drug doses.

Similar to a drug's ED_{50}, which suggests when a certain amount of a drug will have an observed therapeutic beneficial outcome in 50% of the population examined, a drug also has a toxic dose, or TD_{50}. The TD_{50} is very different from an ED_{50}, whereby a certain amount of a drug will no longer cause a therapeutic effect, but rather a toxic or adverse effect in 50% of the population tested. Notably, TD_{50} screenings are conducted in animal models (i.e., subjects rather than participants) prior to human clinical drug trials due to the severe risks associated with testing in humans, and for obvious reasons it could be considered unethical to test humans as a means to acquire such information. Therefore, animal studies are necessary to prevent inadvertent increases in health or disease issues. For example, in the 1960s thalidomide was prescribed to pregnant women to treat morning sickness, but it resulted in teratogenic effects (i.e., showed evidence of harming the developing fetus). To prevent the reoccurrence of such medical issues as presented in these most unfortunate historical examples, animal models are used (e.g., mice, rats, rabbits) often by pharmaceutical drug developers to screen and mini-

mize the TD_{50} risks associated with any drugs they create. Moreover, in order for drug developers to legally apply to the FDA to develop and undertake a human clinical trial, they are required to provide evidence based on objective data collected from animal models that the drug is sufficiently safe to responsibly conduct a clinical trial study in humans.

From these animal models, invaluable information can be obtained regarding the assessment of a therapeutic range in which drugs can be prescribed. Figure 3.4 illustrates another hypothetical comparison between a single drug's effective and lethal dose. In Figure 3.4, the ED_{50} and TD_{50} of Drug Y are shown. In this example, there is a narrow range from the 2.0 mg at which the drug shows effectiveness to increase the medication to maintain or improve its effectiveness, up to approximately 9.0 mg. Once Drug Y increases from 9.0 mg to 10.0 mg, it is reaching the TD_{50}, which will cause either toxicity or adverse effects in 50% of cases. In this situation, there is a far more restricted range from the 8.0 mg at which the drug shows

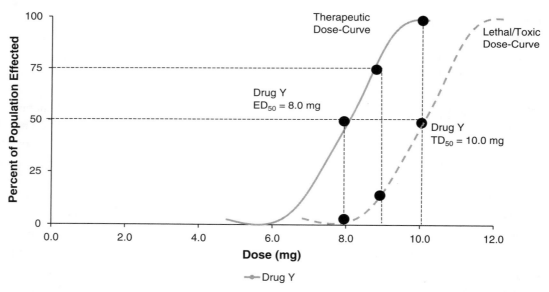

FIGURE 3.4. A hypothetical drug potency illustration comparing drug Y's effective dose (solid line) and lethal dose (dashed line) curves to assess the potential therapeutic versus toxic or adverse effects in a population. At an ED_{50}, the population experiences little to no toxic dose (i.e., TD_0). However, as the therapeutic dose increases to an ED_{75}, a population risk of a $TD_{12.5}$ is observed. As the therapeutic dose is increased to an ED_{100}, the population risk of a TD_{50} is observed. Thus, Drug Y is not an optimal drug therapy, as only 50% of the population may benefit from its therapy, and if a population requires an increase in the dose of this drug there is a risk of toxic or adverse side effects. Therefore, another drug alternative should be considered given the risks involved.

effectiveness to increase up to approximately 9.0 mg. Thus, Drug Y may be risky to administer, since it has less room for therapeutic improvement and may have more of a chance to produce a toxic or adverse drug effect with increases in dosage. Considering these two critical factors (i.e., the ED_{50} and the TD_{50}) and their respective dose–response curves (i.e., effectiveness and toxicity), it may be very challenging to decide which drug to administer to an individual in need. To appropriately determine a safe drug dose, a ratio between the ED_{50} and TD_{50} can be derived to assess the range that should be considered for administering a drug for therapeutic purposes, referred to as a therapeutic index.

The therapeutic index is calculated as shown in Figure 3.5. Using this calculation, the following question is approached responsibly: "How much of a given drug is safe to administer?" However, arguably this calculation is a tool to quantify a therapeutic index, but is still too liberal as it may inadvertently suggest that a drug with a smaller therapeutic index may be potentially safe. It is also limiting as it does not clarify whether a dose that is toxic below 50% is actually safe or potentially life threatening. For example, if we take the same hypothetical example from Figure 3.4 and relabel the Y-axis as the percent of drug effect observed we can generate Figure 3.6. In this example, Drug Y has an ED_{50} at 8.0 mg and at this dose there is a TD_0. However, once the dose is increased to an ED_{75} at 9.0 mg, the risk increases to a $TD_{12.5}$.

$$\frac{Toxic\ Dose\ or\ TD_{50}}{Effective\ Dose\ or\ ED_{50}} = Therapeutic\ Index\ \text{Ratio}$$

FIGURE 3.5. The formula used to calculate the therapeutic index of a given drug. To calculate a therapeutic index of any drug, divide the toxic dose (TD_{50}) by the effective dose (ED_{50}) to obtain the therapeutic index ratio. However, arguably this calculation is a tool to quantify a therapeutic index, but is still too liberal as it may inadvertently suggest that a drug with a smaller therapeutic index may be potentially safe. It is also limiting as it does not clarify whether a dose that is toxic below 50% is actually safe or potentially life threatening. Thus, extreme care and caution are advised.

Likewise, when the dose is increased to an ED_{100} at 10 mg, the risk proportionally increases to a TD_{50}. Thus, the intent to increase Drug Y's dose above the ED_{50} to improve therapeutic gains also increases the risk for an individual to experience a toxic or adverse effect. Although at first glance it may appear attractive that an ED_{100} can be used for Drug Y, it must be cautioned as this drug may cause adverse effects in 50% (i.e., TD_{50}) of individuals at that dose. Thus, extreme care and caution are advised when evaluating potent drugs. A more conservative formula, a certain safety index calculation, is employed to ensure that these critical factors are considered carefully (see Figure 3.7).

Thus, in adapting the concepts of the therapeutic index ratio (see Figure 3.5) to be more cautious and considerate of the potential toxic and adverse effects a given drug may produce, a safer calculation of the drug's maximal therapeutic benefit is weighed against the minimal dose at which the beginnings of a toxic or adverse effect can be carefully examined. This informs all parties of a given drug's benefits outweighing any potential risks to achieve the therapeutic outcomes desired and without inadvertently producing additional medical or mental health symptoms in an individual or patient. In addition to managing the certain safety index of a given drug, it is also necessary to understand how a drug is distributed in the body and CNS and how long it will remain before being eliminated.

DISTRIBUTION AND PHARMACOKINETICS

Pharmacokinetics refers to how a substance travels through the body and brain by absorption, distribution, metabolism, and elimination—often generally known through a mnemonic, ADME. Once drugs enter the body and are absorbed into the lungs and/or bloodstream, they are eventually distributed to other organs. In order for the drug to enter an organ and have an effect on any organ system, it requires a drug-specific penetration, passage, or transportation across biological membranes. In particular, the active metabolites of most drugs are broken down by specific enzymes within the liver or the CNS that cause the drug to act. For example,

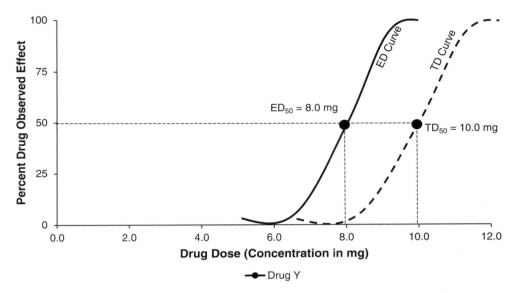

FIGURE 3.6.   A hypothetical illustration comparing one psychotropic drug's effective dose (solid line) and lethal dose (dashed line) curves to assess the potential therapeutic risks versus toxic or adverse effects in a population. At the ED_{50} for Drug Y, the population experiences little to no toxic dose (i.e., TD_0). However, as the therapeutic dose increases to 9.0 mg with an ED_{75}, now a population risk of a $TD_{12.5}$ is observed. Additionally, as the therapeutic dose is increased to 10 mg with an ED_{100}, the population risk of a TD_{50} is observed. Thus, caution must be used when evaluating the therapeutic gains that are desired, while maintaining careful attention to the potential increases in the TD values when drugs presenting with both issues are prescribed. This information can help both mental and allied health care professionals understand and perhaps detect abnormal client responses to therapeutic medication and their risks.

Zoloft® (i.e., sertraline, a selective serotonin reuptake inhibitor [SSRI]) is metabolized in the liver by P-450 enzymes, CYP 2D6 and 2B6, which can cause drug–drug interactions and produces the active metabolite desmethylsertraline and deposits it into the bloodstream. Desmethylsertraline will then be attracted to its target site through the bloodstream and inhibit reuptake of serotonin, thereby increasing the serotonin signal across the synapse and addressing anxiety and/or depression clinically. Once drug actions such as these occur, it is at this point that individuals either experience the desired effects of a given drug immediately or over time. The human body has drug absorption restrictions in that

$$\frac{\textit{Toxic Dose}\ (\text{TD})\ \text{in 1\% of Subjects or TD}_1}{\textit{Effective Dose}\ (\text{ED})\ \text{in 99\% of Subjects or ED}_{99}} = \textit{Certain Safety Index}\ \text{Ratio}$$

FIGURE 3.7.   The formula used to calculate a more conservative estimate, the certain safety index of a drug. To calculate a drug's certain safety index, divide the toxic dose observed in 1% of the subjects tested (i.e., TD_1) by the effective dose observed in 99% of the subjects tested (i.e., ED_{99}). This calculation is arguably a more appropriate tool to assess a drug's certain safety/therapeutic index, as it considers adding no more toxicity risk than is observed in 1% of the subjects in relation to the same drug's effectiveness in treating 99% of symptoms in the subjects. This proves most meaningful in maximizing the safety and minimizing the toxicity for subjects/participants tested, when used as a means to widen the therapeutic index range for treatment delivery.

only a certain amount can be absorbed at a given time. This helps to prevent a consequential drug "overloading" of any substance, minimizing toxicity via elimination. As such, if the body has reached its maximum capacity for any drug or its metabolites, the remaining circulating levels of the drug will be eliminated from the body. However, if the body has absorbed a small or moderate amount of a drug, then the drug will be eliminated based on its half-life (i.e., the amount of time it takes the body to eliminate half the amount of the drug circulating through the bloodstream; thus, drug concentration is measured as the amount of drug present in an individual's blood sample).

For example, if an adult takes two extra-strength capsules or 500 mg of Tylenol® instrumentally to address a headache and Tylenol has a half-life of 6 hours, the circulating drug concentration will be reduced to 250 mg at 6 hours, then to 125 mg at 12 hours, and so forth. Therefore, the half-life of a drug can be very informative as it can help guide mental and allied health care professionals in determining when it would be optimal to prescribe the next dose of a medication. This is important because if an individual takes another dose of a medication or drug too soon, he or she would inadvertently increase circulating drug concentration levels, risking toxic or adverse health effects. Cumulative drug effects refer to a continued building up of a drug concentration due to a combination of drug administration that is too frequent and not enough elimination to keep the drug at a steady state. A *therapeutic steady state* is defined as sustaining or maintaining a constant level of a drug or medication circulating through the bloodstream. Over time a drug can gradually build to levels that exceed a therapeutic steady state and approach a medically concerning state. Going back to the Tylenol example, according to the product's dosage information panel, taking 500 mg every 6 hours limits an individual to a maximum of six pills within a 24-hour period. However, if someone were to take more than this suggested safety limit, the individual may be at risk for acetaminophen toxicity or adverse effects associated with excessive amounts of circulating acetaminophen blood levels. The information provided by doctors and on prescription bottles or package inserts is meant to educate individuals regarding how to appropriately take medication to ensure an adequate level for ongoing therapy. This example can be generalized to psychiatric medications used in the same methodological way to treat individuals' underlying psychological symptoms so that they can experience similar relief. In the case of Zoloft for treatment of depression, the effective starting dose is 50 mg/day. If a patient is not showing any beneficial effects from this dosage in approximately 24 weeks, then the professional overseeing his or her care can safely increase the drug regimen monthly by 50 mg/day up to a maximum of 200 mg/day to effectively monitor for any adverse side effects while giving the drug enough time to produce therapeutic gains. Thus, once an optimal dose is reached (e.g., Zoloft 100 mg/day) whereby the patient subjectively reports less presenting symptoms and objectively shows fewer signs of mental health concerns, there is no need to further increase his or her medication. This would be an example of a single patient reaching his or her unique steady state of Zoloft for addressing depression (Prekorn & Lane, 1995).

PHARMACODYNAMICS

On a biological level, the actions of specific drugs and their targets (i.e., receptors between the neuronal synapses in the CNS) whereby they cause changes at the physiological, psychological, and behavioral levels are termed pharmacodynamics. As social biological beings, humans have a unique ability to adapt to their environments. Our brains also adapt to such changes in our external environment, and further adapt to changes that are caused by drug action within our internal CNS environment. Thus, medication or drug use can produce changes in the brain. These changes to a brain system can be minor or significant and either short- or long-lasting depending on the drug, the dose, and the duration of exposure (i.e., whether acute or chronic). In regard to pharmacodynamics, when a drug acts on its receptors it can change the ways in which neurons (i.e., individual nerve cells) within a given brain region communicate with other brain cells in the same region or different brain regions. Certain drugs can speed up or slow down both electrical potentials (i.e., local/graded potentials, action potential, excitatory postsynaptic potentials, or inhibitory postsynaptic potentials) and the rate of neurotransmission (i.e., the amount and duration in which neurochemical signals influence other neurons), depending on the dose and route of exposure (see Chapter 2, this volume, for more details on these topics). Therefore, these neurotransmitter events and the changes that occur in response to a drug or a medication provide meaningful information as to where the drug or medication is actually working within the CNS. This can help elucidate the biological mechanisms that underlie psychological and other mental health issues.

INDIVIDUAL FACTORS

As mentioned above, a number of factors have to be carefully considered when trying to determine the "optimal dose" of a drug. Individuals present with inherent variability regarding sensitivity or tolerance to certain drugs. Wilkinson (2005) suggested that one of the most difficult problems faced by mental and allied health care professionals is trying to determine how to optimize a person's dosage regimen, given that only 25% to 60% are effective in managing patient symptoms while a proportion of the remaining majority are either ineffective/benign or cause adverse effects. This is important, as not every person responds as predicted or intended, nor may he or she experience the desired positive effects of a given drug therapy. In some ways, this might account for why a certain percentage of the population may distrust synthetic drugs, and consider more natural or herbal drug therapies or perhaps even resort to illicit drugs. Wilkinson (2005) also indicated that the major enzymes within the liver that metabolize drugs—the cytochrome P-450 enzymes specifically—have become a very attractive area of investigation, as these enzymes may be able to best predict (i.e., as diagnostic/prognostic biomarkers) who would or would not respond particularly well to a given drug therapy, and they further suggest that populations can be examined for genetically linked drug response variability (Wilson et al., 2001). Moreover, such genetic patterning of a

population could prove useful in increasing the understanding of inheritance patterns for inter-individual differences (Evans & Johnson, 2001) and the role of pharmacogenetics as they relate to toxic and adverse drug reaction susceptibilities (Myer, 2000).

Consistent with these data, age can also impact pharmacogenetic factors, with increasing or decreasing drug absorption into the bloodstream and distribution within and across the body and brain, and can enhance or diminish the potential pharmacotherapy of a given prescription drug (Myer, 2000). Further, an individual's drug responsivity due to such pharmacogenetic factors can influence drug efficacy and the risk of an adverse drug reaction (Weinshilboum, 2003). This is important, as genetic inheritance patterns may predispose certain populations as drug resistant or exhibit a deficiency in metabolizing certain drug compounds, thereby limiting the range of psychotropic medications that can be prescribed. For example, Weinshilboum (2003) noted that, in Caucasian participants, 5% to 10% exhibited a deficiency in metabolizing the antihypertensive medication debrisoquin, which targets the CYP2D6 enzymes from the P-450 family. Additionally, P-450 enzymes are critical in identifying and breaking down endogenous chemical proteins that influence neurotransmission, which translates into an individual's clinical responsiveness to drug therapy (Cholerton, Daly, & Idle, 1992). Thus, if a person has genetic differences in his or her levels and/or activity of P-450 enzymes, he or she could perhaps have a very different profile in responding to drug therapy (i.e., a hypometabolizer or a hypermetabolizer). This could also result in a paradoxical profile in which the patient exhibits a response opposite of what is expected from the psychotropic therapy.

It is important to anticipate that drugs may not work the same for an individual across his or her lifespan. Since children are still undergoing brain development, neural network connectivity, and maturation as a function of age, mental and allied health care professionals must be cautious when working with and treating children with psychopharmacological interventions. Children weigh less than adults and are rapid metabolizers of substances, requiring that they take smaller drug doses to avoid adverse drug effects. However, at times there may be clear clinical need to prescribe children drugs; for example, to manage epilepsy. Despite children's inherent sensitivity to drugs, they can also be resistant to psychotropic therapies, prompting clinical and applied researchers to try to elucidate such phenomena (Kwan et al., 2010). Gender can also play a significant role in the metabolism of drugs, affecting both males and females differently as they develop, experience puberty, age—and in particular when women approach childbearing age and experience pregnancy. Thus, it is important to monitor the latter situation in women, as it remains controversial whether certain psychotropic treatments for pregnant women may have unexpected teratogenic or adverse side effects in babies during critical periods of gestational (in utero) and postnatal (via breast milk) development. For example, women are twice as likely to be diagnosed with depression, prescribed antidepressant psychotropic medications, and report more atypical variations in anxiety than are men, but due to interindividual variability and genetic differences, the explanation for this gender enigma has been elusive to scientists (Keers & Aitchison, 2010).

On the other side of the spectrum, as individuals age into the geriatric portion of the lifespan, they are faced with often inevitable medical complications that limit or reduce not only psychological function but functions of bodily organs such as the liver, kidney, and heart. The liver may fail to metabolize a drug, the kidney may fail to clear or eliminate a drug, and the heart may be too weak to circulate a drug to reach its targets. Thus, in the elderly, reduced drug delivery to intended targets and inability to efficiently remove a drug from the body require as much attention as is given to children, but for very different age-based reasons (Turnheim, 2003). Through the advancements of molecular biological techniques and data mining, a field of study has been established that precisely investigates patient responsivity and genetic information within pharmacogenetics and pharmacotherapeutics to provide the most individualized drug therapy possible. These medical advancements were not possible half a century ago, nor was it thought they could

revolutionize the way psychopharmacological therapies have been prescribed to patients ("trial-by-error" learning from patient feedback).

DRUG INTERACTIONS

It is noteworthy to mention the importance of drug-with-drug interactions, otherwise referred to as drug cross-talk. Certain drugs may have very peculiar outcomes when taken in combination. This is important as polydrug use occurs frequently in society. Certain medications or drugs when mixed together can have canceling effects, synergistic effects, or paradoxical effects. Often people may take more than one psychotropic medication to address their underlying mental health issues. The interactions resulting from such prescription polydrug use at the clinical level are termed drug–drug interactions. In frontline primary medicine, the prescribing of psychotropic prescription medications has increased by 48% over the last two decades; primary care physicians (PCPs) write 65% and 80% of all anxiolytic and antidepressant prescriptions, respectively (Lieberman, 2003). When patients take many prescription drugs, their liver is tasked with breaking down these chemicals into active metabolites that they can benefit from. However, when certain drugs require the same liver enzymes to break them down, a division of labor at the level of the liver enzymes may offset the intended psychotropic therapeutic outcomes. For example, mood stabilizing medication and antianxiety medication may require the same P-450 enzymes to create active metabolites to alleviate mental health issues, but may not produce desired outcomes if both active metabolites are not adequately generated to reach therapeutic levels within the patient (English, Dortch, Ereshefsky, & Jhee, 2012).

Thus, mental and allied health care professionals must be cautious not to overprescribe medications or prescribe medications without checking whether such known liver enzyme competition exists. Often a quick scan of a medication and its drug–drug interactions can be done using the http://www.drugs.com interaction checker function, which is a helpful tool for mental and allied health care professionals as well as the layperson. This topic requires considerable attention in the future of psychopharmacology, as PCPs may be more inclined to treat patient symptoms with less attention directed toward how these drugs actually work within the liver. The field finds these factors are increasingly an issue with drug–drug interactions within geriatric populations, which has prompted serious reconsideration of how and why medications should be prescribed in the elderly and an emerging need for a "drug appropriateness index" (Mallet, Spinewine, & Huang, 2007). Other drug interactions can occur with drug and nondrug mixtures, such as a prescription medication and grapefruit juice, which may counteract the prescription drug's intended effects (Bressler, 2006). Grapefruit juice interactions have been documented to have the most pronounced effects during first pass metabolism of heart medications (e.g., amiodarone and felodipine), which are often prescribed to the elderly in conjunction with psychotropic medications (Bressler, 2006). Alternative medicine approaches may combine natural herbs with drugs, creating an herb–drug interaction that causes undesirable side effects (e.g., taking St. John's wort with SSRIs may cause mild serotonin syndrome in patients [e.g., agitation, restlessness, confusion, rapid heart rate, high blood pressure]; Fugh-Berman, 2000). Moreover, studies have revealed that across the lifespan, approximately 19% of the population that takes prescription drugs that interact with alcohol take these medications while also engaging in alcohol consumption, causing alcohol–drug interactions that can have important clinical implications and complications as these individuals approach senescence (Pringle, Ahern, Heller, Gold, & Brown, 2005). Thus, caution should be taken when considering a situation in which drug interaction may be inevitable or suspected.

Further, individuals may be allergic to certain types of chemicals or may present with an allergic reaction to specific substances that make up the drug, or worse, the excipients (i.e., the other stabilizing, bulking, or filling agents within a drug; Narang et al., 2015). For example, some excipients are milk-based products that may inadvertently affect individuals who are lactose intolerant (Heyman & the Committee on Nutrition, 2006; Lomer, Parkes, & Sanderson, 2007), rather than an alternative chemi-

cally based agent to tolerate the stomach's acidic environment. This can be very problematic for patient and mental or allied health care professional treatment follow-up, as patients may unknowingly misinterpret excipient adverse side effects as side effects of the prescribed medication. This can result in patients and mental or allied health care professionals abandoning potentially therapeutic medications or drugs due to the issue of excipients. Thus, moving forward, the field should become more knowledgeable of excipient properties, and increase the transparency of filler ingredients and medication/drug interactions as a part of future therapies around mental health management.

CONCLUSION

Today, there is a growing need for mental and allied health care professionals to have a basic understanding of psychopharmacology, as many individuals receiving therapy or care from these service delivery professionals may require medication, are currently prescribed medication, or intentionally self-medicate to address their psychological needs. Thus, as mental and allied health care professionals frequently encounter individuals within society that present with such needs, it is important to provide them with an additional teaching moment addressing the fundamental differences between medications versus drugs and better informing the individual. Often, the basic concepts of a medication/drug dose, dose–response curve, toxic-dose–response curve, therapeutic index, safety index, pharmacokinetics, and pharmacodynamics are not apparent or formally taught. Additionally, many individuals do not understand the potential risks of self-medicating with drugs or nonprescription medications, as they can potentially exacerbate current underlying psychological disorders or even bring about a psychological disorder rather than treating one. Moreover, the definition of a drug has evolved to be rather ambiguous, with a wide array of potential social meanings causing increased confusion for the population, especially among those young in age and adolescents. Therefore, it is critical for mental and allied health care professionals to supplement their specialties with a basic working knowledge of psychopharmacology to further educate their clients and/or patients to make optimal and informed decisions with their medication and self-medication choices to improve their quality of life.

Although few psychologists are tasked with prescribing pharmacological medications to their patients, most will need to work with patients either currently taking psychotropic medications or who may benefit from such treatment. Further, as the health care system changes and hopefully becomes more integrated, the more informed psychologists are on the role of psychopharmacology in mental health disorders, the more helpful they can be to their patients and society. As advancements in molecular biology continue to occur and unravel the issues regarding genetic and individual variability, perhaps in the future researchers will begin to identify genetic tests relevant to psychological disorders, drug sensitivity, drug resistance, and drug-deficient biomarkers. Such an interdisciplinary approach will aid in the evolution from trial by error patient feedback pharmacological therapy to more of an individualized patient-matched therapy. However, as genes, biology, psychology, and behavior adapt to their environments, this pharmacogenetic approach has remained intriguing yet elusive. Further, one questions whether the development of such advanced pharmacogenetic technological tools and approaches will be swift enough to keep pace with ever-changing psychopharmacological needs.

In summary, navigating how individuals with mental health issues in society perceive drugs and psychopharmacological treatment from mental and allied health care professionals is a complex issue. Informing individuals about the most basic information regarding psychopharmacology can be just as challenging. Often, opportunities to introduce such dialogue may occur within service delivery interactions between individuals and their mental and allied health care professionals. Thus, there is a unique opportunity for a teaching moment to occur within such service delivery sessions to further supplement the primary service delivery objectives. The recommendation to provide a basic educational framework of psychopharmacology to individuals may function to ease patient/client concerns as they relate to medications and drug use, while also fostering the potential for transparent communication in the mental and allied health care professional and patient/client relationship regarding the individual's psychological symptoms and needs.

References

Alegría, M., Chatterji, P., Wells, K., Cao, Z., Chen, C. N., Takeuchi, D., . . . Meng, X. L. (2008). Disparity in depression treatment among racial and ethnic minority populations in the United States. *Psychiatric Services, 59*, 1264–1272. http://dx.doi.org/10.1176/ps.2008.59.11.1264

Bolton, J. M., Robinson, J., & Sareen, J. (2009). Self-medication of mood disorders with alcohol and drugs in the national epidemiologic survey on alcohol and related conditions. *Journal of Affective Disorders, 115*, 367–375. http://dx.doi.org/10.1016/j.jad.2008.10.003

Boyer, E. W., Quang, L., Woolf, A., & Shannon, M. (2001). Use of physostigmine in the management of gamma-hydroxybutyrate overdose. *Annals of Emergency Medicine, 38*, 346. http://dx.doi.org/10.1067/mem.2001.117502

Bressler, R. (2006). Grapefruit juice and prescription drug interactions. Exploring mechanisms of this interaction and potential toxicity for certain drugs. *Geriatrics, 61*, 12–18.

Caldicott, D. G. E., & Kuhn, M. (2001). Gamma-hydroxybutyrate overdose and physostigmine: Teaching new tricks to an old drug? *Annals of Emergency Medicine, 37*, 99–102. http://dx.doi.org/10.1067/mem.2001.111642

Chassin, L., Hussong, A., & Beltran, I. (2009). Adolescent substance use. In R. M. Lerner & L. Steinberg (Eds.), *Handbook of adolescent psychology* (pp. 723–764). Hoboken, NJ: Wiley.

Cholerton, S., Daly, A. K., & Idle, J. R. (1992). The role of individual human cytochromes P450 in drug metabolism and clinical response. *Trends in Pharmacological Sciences, 13*, 434–439. http://dx.doi.org/10.1016/0165-6147(92)90140-2

Dettmer, K., Saunders, B., & Strang, J. (2001). Take home naloxone and the prevention of deaths from opiate overdose: Two pilot schemes. *BMJ: British Medical Journal, 322*, 895–896. http://dx.doi.org/10.1136/bmj.322.7291.895

English, B. A., Dortch, M., Ereshefsky, L., & Jhee, S. (2012). Clinically significant psychotropic drug-drug interactions in the primary care setting. *Current Psychiatry Reports, 14*, 376–390. http://dx.doi.org/10.1007/s11920-012-0284-9

Evans, W. E., & Johnson, J. A. (2001). Pharmacogenomics: The inherited basis for interindividual differences in drug response. *Annual Review of Genomics and*

Human Genetics, 2, 9–39. http://dx.doi.org/10.1146/annurev.genom.2.1.9

Fugh-Berman, A. (2000). Herb-drug interactions. *Lancet, 355,* 134–138. http://dx.doi.org/10.1016/S0140-6736(99)06457-0

Garnier, L. M., Arria, A. M., Caldeira, K. M., Vincent, K. B., O'Grady, K. E., & Wish, E. D. (2010). Sharing and selling of prescription medications in a college student sample. *The Journal of Clinical Psychiatry, 71,* 262–269. http://dx.doi.org/10.4088/JCP.09m05189ecr

Gledhill-Hoyt, J., Lee, H., Strote, J., & Wechsler, H. (2000). Increased use of marijuana and other illicit drugs at US colleges in the 1990s: Results of three national surveys. *Addiction, 95,* 1655–1667. http://dx.doi.org/10.1046/j.1360-0443.2000.951116556.x

Hanson, C. L., Burton, S. H., Giraud-Carrier, C., West, J. H., Barnes, M. D., & Hansen, B. (2013). Tweaking and tweeting: Exploring Twitter for nonmedical use of a psychostimulant drug (Adderall) among college students. *Journal of Medical Internet Research, 15,* e62. http://dx.doi.org/10.2196/jmir.2503

Heyman, M. B., & the Committee on Nutrition. (2006). Lactose intolerance in infants, children, and adolescents. *Pediatrics, 118,* 1279–1286. http://dx.doi.org/10.1542/peds.2006-1721

Inciardi, J. A., Surratt, H. L., Kurtz, S. P., & Burke, J. J. (2009). The diversion of prescription drugs by health care workers in Cincinnati, Ohio. *Substance Use & Misuse, 41,* 255–264. http://dx.doi.org/10.1080/10826080500391829

Johnston, L. D., O'Malley, P. M., Bachman, J. G., & Schulenberg, J. E. (2008). Monitoring the future: National results on adolescent drug use: Overview of key findings, 2008 (NIH Publication No. 09-7401). Bethesda, MD: National Institute on Drug Abuse.

Johnston, L. D., O'Malley, P. M., Bachman, J. G., & Schulenberg, J. E. (2012). Monitoring the future national survey results on drug use 1975–2012: Overview 2012, Key findings on adolescent drug use. Ann Arbor, MI: Institute for Social Research, The University of Michigan.

Kaplan, J. L., Marx, J. A., Calabro, J. J., Gin-Shaw, S. L., Spiller, J. D., Spivey, W. L., . . . Harchelroad, F. P., Jr. (1999). Double-blind, randomized study of nalmefene and naloxone in emergency department patients with suspected narcotic overdose. *Annals of Emergency Medicine, 34,* 42–50. http://dx.doi.org/10.1016/S0196-0644(99)70270-2

Keers, R., & Aitchison, K. J. (2010). Gender differences in antidepressant drug response. *International Review of Psychiatry, 22,* 485–500. http://dx.doi.org/10.3109/09540261.2010.496448

Kirsch, I., Deacon, B. J., Huedo-Medina, T. B., Scoboria, A., Moore, T. J., & Johnson, B. T. (2008). Initial severity and antidepressant benefits: A meta-analysis of data submitted to the Food and Drug Administration. *PLoS Medicine, 5,* e45. http://dx.doi.org/10.1371/journal.pmed.0050045

Kwan, P., Arzimanoglou, A., Berg, A. T., Brodie, M. J., Allen Hauser, W., Mathern, G., . . . French, J. (2010). Definition of drug resistant epilepsy: Consensus proposal by the ad hoc Task Force of the ILAE Commission on Therapeutic Strategies. *Epilepsia, 51,* 1069–1077. http://dx.doi.org/10.1111/j.1528-1167.2009.02397.x

Lieberman, J. A. (2003). The use of antipsychotics in primary care. *Journal of Clinical Psychiatry, 5*(Suppl. 3), 3–8.

Lomer, M. C. E., Parkes, G. E., & Sanderson, J. D. (2007). Lactose intolerance in clinical practice: Myths and realities. *Alimentary Pharmacology & Therapeutics, 27,* 93–103. http://dx.doi.org/10.1111/j.1365-2036.2007.03557.x

Low, G. K., & Gendaszek, A. E. (2002). Illicit use of psychostimulants among college students: A preliminary study. *Journal of Psychology, Health & Medicine, 7,* 283–287. http://dx.doi.org/10.1080/13548500220139386

Mallet, L., Spinewine, A., & Huang, A. (2007). The challenge of managing drug interactions in elderly people. *The Lancet, 370,* 14–20. http://dx.doi.org/10.1016/S0140-6736(07)61092-7

McCabe, S. E. (2008). Misperceptions of non-medical prescription drug use: A web survey of college students. *Addictive Behaviors, 33,* 713–724. http://dx.doi.org/10.1016/j.addbeh.2007.12.008

McCabe, S. E., West, B. T., Teter, C. J., & Boyd, C. J. (2014). Trends in medical use, diversion, and nonmedical use of prescription medication among college students from 2003 to 2013: Connecting the dots. *Addictive Behaviors, 39,* 1176–1182. http://dx.doi.org/10.1016/j.addbeh.2014.03.008

McCabe, S. E., West, B. T., & Wechsler, H. (2007). Trends and college-level characteristics associated with the non-medical use of prescription drugs among US college students 1993 to 2001. *Addiction, 102,* 455–465. http://dx.doi.org/10.1111/j.1360-0443.2006.01733.x

Myer, U. A. (2000). Pharmacogenetics and adverse drug reactions. *The Lancet, 356,* 1667–1671. http://dx.doi.org/10.1016/S0140-6736(00)03167-6

Narang, A. S., Yamniuk, A., Zhang, L., Comezoglu, S. N., Bindra, D. S., Varia, S. A., Doyle, M., & Badawy, S. (2015). Drug excipient interactions. In A. Narang & S. Boddu (Eds.), *Excipient Applications in Formulation Design & Drug Delivery* (pp. 13–35). Cham, Switzerland: Springer.

Olfson, M., Blanco, C., Liu, L., Moreno, C., & Laje, G. (2006). National trends in the outpatient treatment of children and adolescents with antipsychotic drugs. *Archives of General Psychiatry, 63,* 679–685. http://dx.doi.org/10.1001/archpsyc.63.6.679

Olfson, M., Mojtabai, R., Sampson, N. A., Hwang, I., Druss, B., Wang, P. S., Wells, K. B., Pincus, H. A., & Kessler, R. C. (2009). Dropout from outpatient mental health care in the United States. *Psychiatric Services, 60,* 898–907. http://dx.doi.org/10.1176/ps.2009.60.7.898

Peters Jr., R. J., Keidler, S. H., Markham, C. M., Yacoubain, Jr., G. S., Peters, L. A., & Ellis, A. (2003). Beliefs and social norms about codeine and promethazine hydrochloride cough syrup (CPHCS) onset and perceived addiction among urban Houstonian adolescents: An addiction trend in the city of lean. *Journal of Drug Education, 33,* 415–425. http://dx.doi.org/10.2190/NXJ6-U60J-XTY0-09MP

Prekorn, S. H., & Lane, R. M. (1995). Sertraline 50 mg daily: The optimal dose in the treatment of depression. *International Clinical Pharmacology, 10*(3), 129–141.

Pringle, K. E., Ahern, F. M., Heller, D. A., Gold, C. H., & Brown, T. V. (2005). Potential for alcohol and prescription drug interactions in older people. *Journal of the American Geriatrics Society, 55,* 1930–1936. http://dx.doi.org/10.1111/j.1532-5415.2005.00474.x

Prudhomme White, B., Becker-Blease, K. A., & Grace-Bishop, K. (2010). Stimulant medication use, misuse, and abuse in an undergraduate and graduate student sample. *Journal of American College Health, 54,* 261–268. http://dx.doi.org/10.3200/JACH.54.5.261-268

Prus, A. (2018). *Drugs and the neuroscience of behavior* (2nd ed.). Los Angeles, CA: SAGE.

Simons, J., & Carey, K. B. (2000). Attitudes towards marijuana use and drug-free experience: Relationships and behavior. *Addictive Behaviors, 25*(3), 323–331.

Sumner, S. A., Mercado-Crespo, M. C., Spelke, B., Paulozzi, L., Sugarman, D. E., & Hills, S. D. (2016). Use of naloxone by emergency medical services during opioid drug overdose resuscitation efforts. *The Journal of Prehospital Emergency Care, 20,* 220–225. http://dx.doi.org/10.3109/10903127.2015.1076096

Teter, C. J., McCabe, S. E., LaGrange, K., Cranford, J. A., & Boyd, C. J. (2006). Illicit use of specific prescription stimulants among college students: Prevalence, motives, and routes of administration. *Pharmacotherapy, 26,* 1501–1510. http://dx.doi.org/10.1592/phco.26.10.1501

Townsend, L., Floersch, J., & Findling, R. L. (2009). The conceptual adequacy of the Drug Attitude Inventory for measuring youth attitudes toward psychotropic medications: A mixed methods evaluation. *Journal of Mixed Methods Research, 4,* 32–55. http://dx.doi.org/10.1177/1558689809352469

Turnheim, K. (2003). When drug therapy gets old: Pharmacokinetics and pharmacodynamics in the elderly. *Experimental Gerontology, 38*(8), 843–853.

Varga, M. (2012). Adderall abuse on college campuses: A comprehensive literature review. *Journal of Evidence-Based Social Work, 9,* 293–313. http://dx.doi.org/10.1080/15433714.2010.525402

Wang, J. (2007). Mental health treatment dropout and its correlates in a general population sample. *Medical Care, 45,* 224–229. http://dx.doi.org/10.1097/01.mlr.0000244506.86885.a5

Wang, P. S., Lane, M., & Olfson, M. (2005). Twelve-month use of mental health services in the United States: Results from the national comorbidity survey replication. *Archives of General Psychiatry, 65,* 629–640. http://dx.doi.org/10.1001/archpsyc.62.6.629

Weinshilboum, R. (2003). Inheritance and drug response. *The New England Journal of Medicine, 348,* 529–537. http://dx.doi.org/10.1056/NEJMra020021

Whitaker, R. (2005). Anatomy of an epidemic: Psychiatric drugs and the astonishing rise of mental illness in America. *Ethical Human Psychology and Psychiatry, 7*(1), 23–35.

Wilkinson, G. R. (2005). Drug metabolism and variability among patients in drug response. *The New England Journal of Medicine, 352,* 2211–2221. http://dx.doi.org/10.1056/NEJMra032424

Wilson, J. F., Weale, M. E., Smith, A. C., Gratix, F., Fletcher, B., Thomas, M. G., Bradman, N., & Goldstein, D. B. (2001). Population genetic structure of variable drug response. *Nature Genetics, 29,* 265–269.

Chapter 4

THE ROLE OF ANIMAL LABORATORY RESEARCH IN PSYCHOPHARMACOLOGY

Susan Schenk, Maree Hunt, Anne Macaskill, and Michaela Pettie

There is tremendous between subject variability in the response to drugs. Even for drugs with a very selective pharmacological target—and even in the absence of pharmacokinetic variation—variability in potency or efficacy in terms of producing a given behavioral response is often quite large. This variability indicates that the magnitude of the pharmacodynamic response must be impacted by other variables. Indeed, there is a wealth of information showing that genetic and environmental factors are important determinants of drug effects. This chapter will present some of these factors with a particular emphasis on how animal studies have helped in understanding the impact of these variables on drug responses. Additionally, we will present some specific advantages of using animals to study drug effects. Finally, we have selected some examples of animal behaviors that have been examined and procedures that have been developed to model various aspects of human pathologies. In the final section, we present some limitations of animal research and opportunities for improvements.

VALUE OF ANIMAL RESEARCH IN PSYCHOPHARMACOLOGY

The most commonly used laboratory animals are rodents (primarily rats and mice) and nonhuman primates. Rodents are small, and inexpensive to purchase or breed. Rodent-based studies do not require extensive space for housing. Thus, there are economic advantages to using rodents for research purposes. They have many similarities to humans in terms of neuroanatomy and physiology. Importantly, the rat and mouse genome have been sequenced and the ability to manipulate genes provides a means of examining the role of genetic factors in behavior. Rodents have short lifespans (about 2 years), which precludes them as being good species for studying diseases associated with aging. Further, rodents have limited cognitive abilities, which limits their value in terms of translation to human cognitive disorders. Finally, rodents are usually inbred, which makes the genetic contribution to disease difficult to study unless genetic manipulations (described later in this chapter) are conducted.

Nonhuman primates, on the other hand, are large and require significantly greater space. Further, nonhuman primates are expensive to procure. Often, this leads to studies with small sample sizes that might not provide sufficient power. Nonetheless, nonhuman primates are biologically more similar to humans, so that studies in these species produce results that are sometimes more valid, particularly when determining effects of manipulations on reproduction, social behavior, and cognition. Nonhuman primates have a longer lifespan than rodents but shorter than humans, which makes studies across the lifespan more feasible than studies in humans.

http://dx.doi.org/10.1037/0000133-004
APA Handbook of Psychopharmacology, S. M. Evans (Editor-in-Chief)

It has been well established that both nature (genetics) and nurture (environment) interact to impact behavior. Thus, even within genetically identical twins, there is substantial variability in concordance rates for various psychiatric illnesses (Huang et al., 2000). Animal subjects provide an ability to manipulate a number of environmental and genetic factors individually and to determine the effect of each single manipulation as well as potential interactions between nature and nurture on behavior.

Ability to Determine Factors That Impact the Response to Drugs

A number of different environmental or genetic variables can influence the behavioral and neurochemical response to drugs. In the following section, we describe some of those variables

Diet.   Diet can be manipulated to alter the synthesis of neurotransmitters and behavior (Wurtman, 1987). For example, tryptophan is an essential amino acid and is a precursor in the synthesis of serotonin (5-HT). Humans receive all of their tryptophan from dietary sources (Moore et al., 2000), so tryptophan in the diet can be manipulated and changes in behavior measured. In humans, tryptophan loading or depletion appears to modify social behavior (Steenbergen, Jongkees, Sellaro, & Colzato, 2016), impulsive behavior (Worbe, Savulich, Voon, Fernandez-Egea, & Robbins, 2014) and mood (S. N. Young, 2013), to name a few factors. Supplemental nutrients, including omega-3 and vitamin D, have been suggested to augment the effects of antidepressant drugs (Sarris et al., 2016). In laboratory animals, the diet can be manipulated to alter neurotransmitter synthesis over long periods of time, correlations with behavior can be produced, and the relationship can be determined. For example, tryptophan rich or tryptophan depleted diets modulated aggressive behavior in mice (Kantak, Hegstrand, & Eichelman, 1980) and rats (Kantak, Hegstrand, Whitman, & Eichelman, 1980).

Genetics.   Pharmacogenetics/pharmacogenomics refers to inherited genetic differences in drug metabolic pathways. Physiological responses to drugs occur as the drug is absorbed and distributed to target areas where it interacts with receptors and enzymes, and ultimately the drug is metabolized and excreted. At any point in the process genetic variation can alter the physiological and behavioral response.

Multiple forms of different genes can be produced amongst members of the same species, an effect called polymorphism. These differences in some genes predict responses to various medications. Animal studies have successfully modeled conditions with recognizable causes, but neurocognitive disorders are difficult because they have multiple causes. Researchers can take the information derived from humans with certain disease states and try to reproduce the genetic variant in a mouse model, for example, by knocking out or knocking down the gene of interest, and use sophisticated behavioral tests to determine effects on behaviors of interest. Examples of such an approach are described below for Alzheimer's disease (AD), substance use disorders, post-traumatic stress disorder (PTSD), and autism spectrum disorders (ASDs).

Epigenetic factors.   Epigenetics is the study of gene expression alterations that are heritable but do not involve alterations in the DNA sequence. Mechanisms include DNA methylation and post-translational histone modifications. Epigenetic mechanisms regulate gene promotion as well as silencing. The balance is important for normal functioning. The epigenome is dynamic and is influenced by many factors, and several genes and drug targets are under epigenetic control (Fisel, Schaeffeler, & Schwab, 2016). These epigenetic factors contribute to interindividual variability in response to drugs and are subject to environmental modification (Sng & Meaney, 2009). For example, glucocorticoid receptor methylation in the hippocampus in rat pups has been demonstrated in response to maternal grooming (Weaver et al., 2004). This epigenetic modification is retained through to adulthood. Excessive alcohol drinking was also associated with epigenetic modifications of genes (Nieratschker et al., 2014) and epigenetic mechanisms have been shown to play a role in synaptic plasticity and in memory formation (Levenson & Sweatt, 2005).

Other environmental variables. Social isolation and other forms of stress are risk factors for the development of various disorders. Early rearing environments exert neurobiological changes that persist into adulthood. Deprivation produces cognitive deficits and anxiety, among other behavioral deficits including increased stress responses and decreased social behavior (Dinkler et al., 2017). These deficits might be tied to epigenetic factors in combination with experiences of maltreatment (Weder et al., 2014). These are difficult to study in humans given the limited number of case studies and their diversity. Animal studies on rearing conditions and other stressors can, and have, revealed a number of consequences of impoverished social housing and other stressors on drug responses (Drury, Sánchez, & Gonzalez, 2016; Schenk, Lacelle, Gorman, & Amit, 1987; Stairs & Bardo, 2009). For example, the response to diazepam, desipramine, and amphetamine was, in part, determined by whether male rats were housed in isolated or enriched conditions (Simpson, Bree, & Kelly, 2012).

Ability to Administer Drugs Acutely as Well as Chronically

The doses and number of exposures to drugs that can be administered to humans are often limited by concern raised by potential safety factors. These factors are not as relevant in studies of laboratory animals, and a wider range of both acute and chronic doses of drugs can be administered to determine behavioral and other effects. Preclinical studies have shown that many drug effects change as a function of repeated exposure. Depending on the treatment regimen and the behavior that is measured, drug effects can undergo either tolerance—a decreased behavioral response—or sensitization—an increased behavioral response (Harper, Kay, & Hunt, 2013; Maier, Abdalla, Ahrens, Schallert, & Duvauchelle, 2012). These effects of repeated exposure reflect changes in pharmacodynamic responses to the drugs or in pharmacokinetics.

Repeated agonist administration produces receptor downregulation, a decrease in the number of receptors that are able to respond to a neurotransmitter, as a compensatory mechanism to maintain homeostasis. This is most often produced through phosphorylation of the receptor, internalization, or degradation of cell surface receptors. Similarly, repeated antagonist administration produces receptor upregulation, an increase in the number of receptors that are able to respond to a neurotransmitter. The density of receptors is determined by rates of gene expression, protein synthesis, and receptor trafficking to and from the membrane. However, upregulation or downregulation is also dependent on the regimen of drug exposure.

Repeated drug effects can also be observed in terms of pharmacokinetics. Changes in drug absorption, distribution, and metabolism can be altered by repeated drug exposure. Repeated drug exposures can induce synthesis of P450s, which results in lower plasma drug concentrations for a given dose of drug and an increase in the dose of drug that is required to produce the behavioral or neurochemical effect.

Ability to Test Experimental Drugs With High Selectivity

During the process of drug development, a number of tests are conducted to determine potential toxic effects, pharmacokinetics, pharmacodynamics, and metabolism. At any point in the process, the drug may be abandoned for further testing. Thus, although the drug might not be appropriate for use in humans, it still might provide a valuable tool for basic research. As an example, the selective dopamine D_1-like antagonist, SCH 23390, was initially developed as an antipsychotic drug, but because of its very short duration of action in nonhuman primates it never progressed to clinical trials (Chipkin, 1990). Nonetheless SCH 23390 has been an extraordinarily useful drug for examining the role of dopamine D_1-like receptors in a variety of behaviors, as indicated by almost 5,000 hits in a PubMed search (conducted on July 6, 2017).

Ability to Determine Potential Side Effects and Toxicity of Drugs

Unwanted or adverse effects can also be produced by drugs that have therapeutic effects. It is important to determine what the adverse drug reaction is, whether it occurs following administration of therapeutic doses, and whether the adverse reaction is of significant concern to preclude introduction of the drug for human consumption. For example, selective serotonin reuptake inhibitors (SSRIs) are effective for treating depression, but they also can produce unwanted effects called serotonin syndrome, with symptoms including agitation, confusion, increased heart rate and blood pressure, loss of muscle control, and heavy sweating.

Before a drug can be introduced for use in humans, there is an extensive screening which includes, among other things, determination of the lethal dose following acute or multiple exposures. Preclinical tests include those aimed at identifying potential toxic effects, carcinogenic effects, mutagenic effects and adverse reactions.

Ability to Measure Drug Effects Throughout the Lifespan

Lifespan studies can be quite advantageous since some effects are only observed when manipulations are conducted later in life, and others when manipulations are conducted early in life. Rats and mice have a lifespan of about 2 years, and nonhuman primates have lifespans of 20 to 30 years. Rodents, therefore, provide only a limited window of opportunity in terms of investigating effects of drugs on behavior at different phases of life. Nonhuman primates provide a larger window.

The first phase of life, weaning, is about 6 months in humans and nonhuman primates and 3 weeks for rodents. Sexual maturity occurs in humans at about 11.5 years, nonhuman primates at about 5 years of age, and rats at about 50 days. Humans are considered adults at about 20 years of age, nonhuman primates at about 15 years of age, and rodents at about 7 to 8 months of age. Aged rodents are older than 24 months, aged nonhuman primates are older than 20 years, and aged humans are 60 years or older (Dutta & Sengupta, 2016; Sengupta, 2013). It is therefore relatively time efficient to investigate the effects of early and later manipulations on behavior throughout the lifespan by conducting within-subject longitudinal studies in laboratory rodents, but less so in no-human primates. Lifespan studies can generally only be conducted using

between-group designs in humans, since longitudinal studies are typically of lengthy duration, time consuming, and very expensive.

Example of Drug Development That Has Benefitted From Animal Research

Animal models of disease must capture the etiology and neurobiological mechanisms of the disorder and be able to predict treatment efficacy. Accordingly, an appropriate model has to have construct, face, and predictive validity (Willner, 1986). Construct validity refers to whether the model disease state has similar neurobiological mechanisms to the human disease state. Face validity refers to how well the model produces symptoms of the human disease. Predictive validity refers to how well treatments that are effective in the human disease are also effective in the animal model. Construct validity is often difficult to ascertain, because the neurobiological bases of a psychological disease is often not known. Therefore, models frequently rely on face and predictive validity and try to translate to determine construct validity.

AD is one disorder that has been successfully modeled in animal studies, and these models satisfy criteria for construct and face validity. It has a well-understood neurobiological mechanism and a well-defined cluster of symptoms. The field of psychopharmacology has been instrumental in uncovering treatments for AD.

AD is characterized by memory deficits and eventual deterioration of cognitive functioning. The earliest studies suggested that the memory deficits were due to presynaptic cholinergic deficits (Coyle, Price, & DeLong, 1983). In contrast to other disease states that are also characterized by memory and other cognitive deficits, AD is additionally diagnosed by the extensive loss of localized brain cells and synaptic connections as well as the development of β-amyloid plaques and neurofibrillary lesions (Katzman & Saitoh, 1991).

Animal studies contributed a great deal to understanding the basis for the development of amyloid plaques and the mechanisms of neurotoxicity (Yamada & Nabeshima, 2000). Studies in humans suffering from the disease have suggested various genetic polymorphisms that might interact with environmental circumstances to produce AD (Tanzi et al., 1996). This provided a framework for developing animals with the same genetic polymorphisms (Yamada & Nabeshima, 2000). It became clear, however, that only a small proportion of AD cases could be attributed to genetic mutations. At the same time, some of the brain and behavior changes associated with AD could be produced pharmacologically (Murray & Fibiger, 1986), and pharmacological manipulations were proposed to reverse the specific degeneration of cholinergic neurons in AD (Scott & Crutcher, 1994).

In particular, the role of the animal laboratory in developing treatments for AD has involved various models (both genetic and pharmacological), large numbers of behavioral tests to assess the effect of the manipulations on cognitive functioning, and, on the basis of those results, tests of the impact of drugs aimed at either slowing the progression of the disease or decreasing the cognitive deficits (Bachurin, Bovina, & Ustyugov, 2017). These drugs have focused primarily on boosting endogenous acetylcholine function by preventing degradation by acetylcholinesterase. These acetylcholinesterase inhibitors seemed to provide transient prevention of cognitive decline in AD patients, but alone did not provide long-term beneficial results (Galimberti & Scarpini, 2016). This disappointing outcome probably reflects the fact that the neurodegenerative disease encompasses more than simply a loss of cholinergic neurotransmission. Other attempts to develop effective pharmacotherapies have been equally unimpressive despite enormous preclinical effort (Bachurin et al., 2017).

How can animal research provide better candidates for treatments for this disease? One thing that must be considered is the ability to produce a model that reflects the progressive neurodegeneration that occurs with this disease. However, this process is not understood. Additionally, some of the cognitive deficits that are apparent in the early stages of the disease might be due to different mechanisms than deficits that are produced in the later stages. This could indicate that different treatment options might be desirable depending on the stage of the disease.

EXAMPLES OF ANIMAL BEHAVIORS USED TO DEVELOP DRUGS TO TREAT HUMAN DISORDERS

Animal behaviors have been validated in terms of capturing aspects of human behavior related to mental health as per the *Diagnostic and Statistical Manual of Mental Disorders* (5th ed.; *DSM–5*) and Research Domain Criteria (RDoC). They are often validated on the basis of their sensitivity to drugs with known clinical efficacy and insensitivity to drugs that lack clinical efficacy. The idea is to use these behavioral assays to understand the basis of the symptom and to develop novel pharmacotherapeutics.

Currently, there is an important distinction between *DSM* criteria and the RDoC. The *DSM* represents a spectrum of behavioral abnormalities to provide a most likely diagnosis. It provides a descriptive classification of psychological disorders, but there is no clear etiology based on *DSM* criteria. There is tremendous comorbidity, and so pharmacological treatments might not be specific to a disorder. This makes it difficult, if not impossible, to model various diseases in animals according to *DSM* symptomology.

The RDoC was initiated to concentrate on maladaptive behaviors and on their underlying causal mechanisms, rather than the syndrome that might include those behaviors (Clark, Cuthbert, Lewis-Fernández, Narrow, & Reed, 2017; Lilienfeld & Treadway, 2016; J. W. Young, Winstanley, Brady, & Hall, 2017). This is of great importance, since individuals often meet *DSM* criteria for more than one disorder because of the overlap in symptoms. This might explain why antidepressant drugs such as SSRIs are effective not only in treating affective disorders but also eating and anxiety disorders, as well as others including autism (see the discussion later in this chapter).

It is apparent that many psychological disorders are not discrete entities, but have overlapping etiologies. Because we lack sufficient understanding of the biological bases for various *DSM*-classified disorders, and because one behavioral anomaly can often lead to or result from other behavioral anomalies that comprise the *DSM* classification, as noted previously, it becomes difficult, if not impossible, to develop valid animal models of the disorders (Nestler & Hyman, 2010). Behavioral processes that contribute to a disorder can, however, be produced reliably in animal models (Kaffman & Krystal, 2012; Sarnyai et al., 2011).

One disease that has proven impossible to model in animals is schizophrenia, a uniquely human disorder that comprises deficits in cognitive processing as well as a range of other symptoms, and for which a large number of putative genetic and environmental processes have been implicated (Birnbaum & Weinberger, 2017; Farrell et al., 2015; Sawa & Snyder, 2002). Although schizophrenia as a syndrome cannot be modeled in animals, many of the behavioral symptoms of the disorder have been successfully produced following administration of drugs, brain lesions, or genetic manipulations, and these can provide testable hypotheses concerning the biological and environmental determinants of the disease (Mitchell, Huang, Moghaddam, & Sawa, 2011).

Animal models of human disorders use assays to mimic and mirror the symptoms that define the *DSM* and RDoC criteria of disorders, particularly those of disorders such as anxiety (Ennaceur & Chazot, 2016; Harro, 2018; Hart et al., 2016), affective disorders (Beyer & Freund, 2017; Logan & McClung, 2016; Willner & Belzung, 2015), attention-deficit/hyperactivity disorder (ADHD; Hayward, Tomlinson, & Neill, 2016), and schizophrenia (Ayhan, McFarland, & Pletnikov, 2016). Here we provide descriptions of some measures of disorders that have been less well documented.

Measures of Social Behavior

Social behavior refers to behavior that occurs in the presence of and in relation to conspecifics (animals of the same species). This includes sociability, play behavior, aggression, and interaction. In order to investigate social behavior, a variety of behavioral measures have been developed. These measures take advantage of the complex social structure and natural behaviors exhibited by a variety of animal species.

Interaction. The social interaction assay involves the observation of behavior during the interaction of conspecifics. The behaviors observed and investigated depend on the species in question. In nonhuman primates, measures focus on behaviors such as vocalizations that communicate identity, sex, and status (Watson & Platt, 2012); complex social behavior; rule learning; deception; alliances; and pair-bonding (Digby & Barreto, 1993; Sutcliffe & Poole, 1984). These social behaviors are also observed in humans (Miller et al., 2016).

In contrast, social play with litter mates is the first non–mother-directed behavior to emerge in rats (Vanderschuren, Niesink, & Van Ree, 1997). The exaggerated behaviors are referred to as "rough and tumble" play behavior (Pellis & Pellis, 2007), and they diminish after sexual maturity. The frequency, duration, and onset latency of "pouncing" and "pinning" behaviors make up the standard methods with which to measure play behavior.

Pinning refers to instances in which one animal in a pair stands over the exposed ventral surface of playmate lying prostrate with their back against the floor of the enclosure (Meaney & Stewart, 1981; Melotti, Bailoo, Murphy, Burman, & Wurbel, 2014). Pouncing refers to instances in which one animal in a pair pounces atop the dorsal surface of a playmate whose anterior surface faces the floor of the enclosure (Meaney & Stewart, 1981). These measures are contrasted to subjects' time spent alone or in contact with conspecifics without engaging in pinning or pouncing behaviors (passive behaviors).

Resident intruder. The resident–intruder assay measures the social aggression exhibited by a male "resident" animal when encountering a novel "intruder" conspecific. Males are typically subjects in this assay as they consistently display aggressive and territorial behaviors compared with females, who generally display these behaviors only when pregnant or lactating (Albert, Jonik, & Walsh, 1992). A resident male rat or mouse is housed within a test enclosure for a predetermined duration. A novel intruder male conspecific is then introduced to the same enclosure, and the frequency and duration of threatening behaviors are measured (such as upright postures, appearing larger, and biting the defender; Blanchard, Blanchard, Takahashi, & Kelley, 1977). The behaviors observed can be grouped into three categories. The first category is nonsocial activity, in which animals maintain a distance from each other and may engage in self-grooming, environmental exploration, or resting. The second category is social activity, in which animals exhibit behaviors such as following, walking away, and body and genital sniffing (Fernández-Espejo & Mir, 1990). The third is aggressive behavior, in which animals exhibit lateral threat (piloerection, standing side on to the defender with a hunched back), biting, and "clinching" or aggressive fighting (see Koolhaas et al., 2013, for a detailed description).

Social approach avoidance. Proximity tests such as the social approach avoidance assay measure the time spent with a social stimulus (the familiar conspecific), when compared with time spent with a novel social stimulus (the novel conspecific; Brodkin, Hagemann, Nemetski, & Silver, 2004). These tests typically comprise a two-phase approach.

In the first phase, following habituation to the testing apparatus, the primary social stimulus is introduced. Social stimuli are often conspecific juvenile animals (around weaning age) of the same sex. They are contained or restricted to an area within the testing chamber, often by being placed in an enclosure from which they cannot escape. The test animal can smell and see the social stimulus and this phase provides an opportunity for the conspecific to become familiar.

During the second phase, a novel conspecific is introduced in a different place in the test chamber. The test animal is provided with the opportunity to interact with either the familiar or the novel conspecific. The test animal is observed for time spent with the known primary social stimulus (social familiarity), and time spent with the novel conspecific represents social novelty. Animals with social deficits spend more time with the known conspecific or alone when compared with animals without deficits, who spend more time exploring or interacting with the novel stimulus (Hrabovska & Salyha, 2016).

Communication
Laboratory animals typically use ultrasonic vocalizations (USVs; N. Takahashi, Kashino, & Hironaka, 2010) and odorants (Arakawa, Blanchard, Arakawa, Dunlap, & Blanchard, 2008) to communicate environmental and emotional information. Odorants, or scent marks, communicate health, fertility, and territory through small deposits of urine in the surroundings. Deposit of odorants is an adaptive behavior for the establishment and continuance of social relationships with conspecifics.

Vocalizations. Rats and mice vocalize at frequencies beyond the human hearing range. These USVs can be grouped by average frequency and duration (Portfors, 2007). The frequency range of 30 to 90 kilohertz (kHz) during 10 to 200 milliseconds (ms) reflects the neural and social development of preweaned rodent pups (Scattoni, Crawley, & Ricceri, 2009). These vocalizations play an important role in mother–pup communication. For example, rat pups emit a significant number of vocalizations with an average frequency of 40 kHz when isolated from their litter and mother (Hofer, 1996).

USVs within 18 to 32 kHz range that occur for 300 to 4000 ms (commonly known as 22 kHz calls) reflect negative affective states in adult rodents (Knutson, Burgdorf, & Panksepp, 1999). These low frequency USVs are emitted under a number of conditions: in fear- and anxiety-related contexts (Jelen, Soltysik, & Zagrodzka, 2003), following some drug administration (Knutson et al., 1999), during drug withdrawal (Miczek & Barros, 1996; Sales, 1972; Vivian & Miczek, 1991), during aggressive interactions (Miczek, Weerts, Vivian, & Barros, 1995; L. K. Takahashi, Thomas, & Barfield, 1983), and during exposure to predator odor (Blanchard, Blanchard, Agullana, & Weiss, 1991).

USVs in the frequency range of 48 to 70 kHz and with a duration of 60 ms reflect positive affective states in adult rodents. These vocalizations occur during mating (Sales, 1972), play behavior (Knutson, Burgdorf, & Panksepp, 1998), and following the administration of drugs of abuse (Simola, Frau, Plumitallo, & Morelli, 2014).

Odorant communication. Odorants are a deliberate signaling, whereby animals deposit urinary droplets and anogenital scent from glands (Roberts, 2007) that guide the behaviors of the receiver to approach or avoid the marker. Scent marking is most frequent for dominant adult males, but also occurs with the odors of "in-heat" females. Increased frequency in scent marking in males is attributed to territorial and sexual behaviors (Arakawa et al., 2008). Dominant male mice mark more than subordinates (Lumley, Sipos, Charles, Charles, & Meyerhoff, 1999), and marks from dominate males are preferred by females (Rich & Hurst, 1998).

Reward

Deficits in processing of rewarding information are common across many *DSM* disorders, including depressive disorders, bipolar and related disorders, feeding and eating disorders, substance-related and addictive disorders, gender dysphoria, and a range of neurodegenerative disorders.

Self-stimulation. The seminal paper by Olds and Milner (Olds & Milner, 1954) showed that electrical stimulation of certain brain regions was positively reinforcing and that animals would learn a number of different tasks to obtain the stimulation. This discovery opened the door to the possibility of measuring reward systems in the brain. That behavior has been termed intracranial brain stimulation or self-stimulation. Researchers found that brain stimulation is also rewarding in humans (Bishop, Elder, & Heath, 1963). It has been suggested that the activity in brain systems that reinforces behavior is also produced when other, natural rewards are encountered and is also the basis for pathological responses to "normally" rewarding situations.

Accordingly, researchers are asking: Can an understanding of the brain circuitry underlying self-stimulation help us to understand pathological responses to rewarding stimuli? Deficits in learning and memory? Cognition? Can we develop drugs to improve behavior based on effects on self-simulation behavior?

Sucrose preference test. Most animal species have an innate preference for sweet flavors, and laboratory animals rapidly learn to perform tasks that will result in delivery of those solutions. The sucrose preference test measures the relative consumption of a sweetened solution compared with water. The preference is easy to measure objectively by presenting water and sweetened solution and comparing consumption. Anhedonia is reflected in a lack of preference for the sweetened solution.

Conditioned place preference. The conditioned place preference paradigm assesses whether animals acquire a preference for an environment that has repeatedly been paired with a positive reinforcer. Typically, on one day animals will receive an injection of a drug and then be confined to one distinctive environment, and on alternate days they will receive a placebo injection and be confined to a different environment. After a number of such pairings the animal is allowed to choose the environment it prefers by having access to both. If the animal spends more time in the drug-paired environment, it indicates that the environment has acquired positive effects through the pairing with a rewarding event. Alternatively, the animal might spend less time in the drug-paired environment, which may indicate an aversive, or anhedonic, effect of the drug.

Self-administration. The reinforcing effects of drugs can be demonstrated by providing laboratory animals with the opportunity to self-inject drugs contingent on the performance of an operant response, like pressing a lever, nose-poking into an opening, or running a runway. With few exceptions, drugs that are misused or abused by humans support the acquisition of this self-administration behavior by laboratory animals. The various behavioral paradigms used to measure acquisition and maintenance of self-administration have been reviewed in detail elsewhere (see Belin, Belin-Rauscent, Everitt, & Dalley, 2016). Several manipulations have been shown facilitate the acquisition of self-administration, suggesting that they increase the potency and/or efficacy of drug reinforcement, providing potential predisposing factors in drug abuse. The important question becomes "Why?," and this question is easily addressed in animal studies since variables can be manipulated in a controlled manner in laboratory animals.

Cognition

Many disorders are characterized by deficits in cognition and animal models have been developed in order to measure cognitive ability. Some of these are described below.

Delayed matching to sample task. One commonly used animal model of cognition is the delayed matching to sample (DMTS) task (Blough, 1959). The rat version of this task uses an operant chamber with two levers and a food dispenser. Subjects complete repeated trials consisting of the following sequence: (a) one lever (left or right) is inserted into the chamber—this is the *sample* stimulus, and the rat must remember whether the left or right lever was inserted to receive food later; (b) the rat presses the lever, causing the chamber to retract the lever so that it disappears from view; (c) both levers are absent from the chamber for a delay—the retention interval; (d) both levers are inserted into the chamber; (e) if the rat presses the sample lever presented earlier, making an accurate response, it receives food. As the retention interval is increased in length, accuracy degrades, indicating a forgetting function. Some pharmacological manipulations degrade performance on the DMTS task while others improve performance. This demonstrates the sensitivity of the DMTS task to differential drug effects.

Two dimensions of memory are initial encoding and rate of forgetting over time. The DMTS task allows the effect of pharmacological manipulations on these two dimensions of memory to be separated. Some manipulations alter rate of forgetting, indexed by the slope of the forgetting function, and others alter encoding, indexed by the height of the forgetting function (level of accuracy at very short delays). The DMTS task can also be used to characterize the particular type of error increased by drug administration. For example, errors may be caused by increased proactive interference from previous trials. This manifests as increased disruption to trials in which the correct response in the current trial differs from the response made on the previous trial. In other words, proactive interference occurs when the rat becomes confused about whether it saw a given sample during this trial or during the previous trial.

A shopper might experience a similar proactive interference error when they return to the location in which they parked their car on a previous visit to the supermarket.

Eight-arm radial arm maze. The eight-arm radial arm maze (RAM; Olton, Collison, & Werz, 1977) provides another example of an animal behavioral model that can be used to investigate the effects of pharmacological manipulations on different types of memory. The radial arm maze consists of a central area with eight arms radiating from the center. Researchers can place food at the end of any or all of the arms, and the rat is placed in the central area at the start of each trial. In the standard version of this task, typically used with rats, all eight arms are baited with food on each session. If the rat travels to the end of an arm for the first time, it receives food (a correct response). If the rat reenters an arm it has already visited on that session, it does not receive food and this is counted as an error. Rats are only able to enter eight arms on each session, meaning that reentering arms reduces the amount of food they receive. Thus, the RAM assesses memory because rats must remember which arms they have already entered to perform the task correctly.

A variant in which only four of eight arms are baited at random can be used to determine whether a manipulation of interest increases reference memory errors, working memory errors, or both (Kay, Harper, & Hunt, 2010). The rat is able to enter four arms each day before they are removed from the maze. The same four arms contain food each day, thus the rat must use reference memory to recall which four arms have previously been baited and working memory to track which arms they have visited on the current session. Therefore, pharmacological manipulations that increase entries to arms that have never been baited likely disrupt reference memory, while those that increase entries to arms already visited on the current session disrupt working memory. The DMTS task and the RAM are two of a range of possible animal models of different memory processes (see Dudchenko, 2004, for discussion of the advantages and disadvantages of other animal memory models).

Behavioral flexibility. Behavioral inflexibility can be defined as continuing with a course of action when it is no longer rewarding, productive, or successful; conversely, flexibility allows individuals to modify their behavior in approach to feedback about changing environmental conditions. In humans this type of inflexibility has been assessed using set-shifting tasks such as the Wisconsin Card Sorting Test (Berg, 1948), and deficits are associated with a range of disorders including problematic cocaine use (Madoz-Gúrpide, Blasco-Fontecilla, Baca-García, & Ochoa-Mangado, 2011) and ADHD (Seidman, Biederman, Faraone, Weber, & Ouellette, 1997).

Behavioral flexibility can be captured by various animal models (Izquierdo & Jentsch, 2012). One example is a set-shifting task for rats developed by Floresco, Block, and Tse (2008). This set-shifting task uses an operant chamber with two levers, a light over each lever, and a food dispenser. On each trial, the light above one lever is illuminated at random, and the rat chooses one lever to respond on. Animals must first respond based on one rule; for example, a visual-cue discrimination rule in which they must respond to the lever under the illuminated light in order to receive food. After a few sessions, the rule switches; for example, it may switch to a response-discrimination rule, and now the rat must respond to one of the levers (e.g., left) and disregard the location of the light in order to receive food. Rapid changes from one rule to the other indicate high levels of flexibility.

Flexibility tasks can separate impairments in initial rule acquisition, reversal learning, and set shifting (Floresco et al., 2008). Reversal learning requires an intradimensional shift—for example, from the rule "respond on the lever on the left" to the rule "respond on the lever on the right." Set shifting requires an extradimensional shift—for example, from the rule "respond on the lever on the left" to the rule "respond on the lever under the light." People demonstrate different patterns of impairment across these types of learning tasks depending on their condition or diagnosis (Pantelis et al., 1999). Animal models have also indicated pharmacological approaches to increasing flexibility (Nikiforuk & Popik, 2011).

Impulsivity. Impulsivity has multiple dimensions, and different animal models capture different facets. Some researchers have used set-shifting tasks to investigate impulsivity, as flexibly responding to new rules requires impulse control to inhibit responses based on previous rules (Izquierdo & Jentsch, 2012). Similarly, other animal models assess impulsivity as an inability to override a high probability response when environmental conditions signal it is not appropriate. For example, in the go/no-go task, rats must make a response when they see one more frequent cue, and withhold a response when they see another less frequent cue.

Five-choice serial reaction time task. Another animal model of impulsivity, the five-choice serial reaction time task (5-CSRTT; Robbins, 2002), uses a chamber with multiple response alternatives, such as nose-poke apertures for rats. On each trial, a light within one randomly selected aperture flashes (typically for 0.5 seconds). If the rat responds in that particular aperture within a brief interval, it receives food. Responses in the wrong location or at the wrong time produce a brief time out during which subjects cannot receive food. Responses before the light flashes are considered impulsive because the rat failed to inhibit a highly probable response (nose poking) when the stimulus context (absence of a light) indicated that it would not be rewarded. Impulsivity on this measure is correlated with other behaviors indicating impulsivity, such as cocaine self-administration (Dalley et al., 2007). Other types of errors indicate deficits in other processes, such as attention.

Delay discounting. Impulsivity can also be measured as the selection of smaller immediate rewards over larger but delayed rewards. The impact of delay on reward value is referred to as "delay discounting" (or "temporal discounting"); choices of smaller, sooner rewards over larger, later rewards reflect the fact that the value of the rewards decreases (i.e., is discounted) as a function of the delay to their receipt. In studies with people, participants make (typically hypothetical) choices between smaller, sooner rewards and larger, later rewards; for example choosing between receiving $100 immediately and $200 in 6 months

(Du, Green, & Myerson, 2002). In a parallel animal task, a rat might choose between pressing one lever that produces two pellets immediately and another lever that produces five pellets after a delay of 10 seconds (Mazur, 1987). Using these tasks, the *indifference point* for a particular reinforcer at a given delay is determined. For example, an individual rat might be indifferent between receiving one pellet immediately and receiving two pellets in 5 seconds. This indicates that, for that subject, delaying the receipt of two pellets by 5 seconds causes it to lose half its value. By determining indifference points at a range of delays, a *delay discounting function* can be identified for each subject. Steeper delay discounting functions indicate that delay has a larger impact on choice and reinforcer value, and therefore that individual is relatively impulsive, while shallower discounting functions indicate relative self-control. People who use drugs of abuse, smoke, and drink excessively show steeper delay discounting on this type of task in cross-sectional studies (MacKillop et al., 2011). Measures of delay discounting can also predict treatment outcome (Sheffer et al., 2012). Bickel, Jarmolowicz, Mueller, Koffarnus, and Gatchalian (2012) argued that steep discounting of delayed reinforcers is a "transdisease process" that contributes to a wide range of diseases and disorders with behavioral components.

EXAMPLES OF ANIMAL MODELS THAT HAVE BEEN DEVELOPED TO MODEL *DSM–5* DISORDERS

A large number of animal models of *DSM–5* disorders have been developed. Below we outline some of the more recent advances in models of substance use, autism spectrum, and posttraumatic stress disorders. We describe the models and then provide pharmacological and genetic contributions to the disorders that have been uncovered as a result of research conducted using the animal model.

Substance Use Disorders

A major advantage of animal studies of substance misuse is the ability to examine factors that might impact drug-taking during all phases from initiation,

to maintenance, to extensive use. Animal models also provide the opportunity to assess the impact of drug-taking when initiated at different times during the lifespan. Additionally, animal studies provide the opportunity to perform pharmacological and genetic manipulations in order to understand factors that might predispose individuals to and maintain drug-taking. Animal studies, therefore, provide information concerning risk factors that might predispose individuals to initiation into drug-taking and those that might predispose individuals to misuse.

The *DSM–5* provides criteria for substance misuse (Hasin et al., 2013). Some of these have been demonstrated using drug self-administration procedures (Deroche-Gamonet & Piazza, 2014; Piazza & Deroche-Gamonet, 2013; Vanderschuren & Ahmed, 2013). For example, a progressive increase in the amount of self-administered drug can be demonstrated under some conditions for some rats, and this has been suggested to reflect the criterion of using larger amounts of a drug for longer periods of time (Edwards & Koob, 2013; Vendruscolo et al., 2011). Other studies have shown that drug self-administration by some laboratory animals is not impacted by association with negative stimuli such as the presentation of a shock (Deroche-Gamonet, Belin, & Piazza, 2004; Torres et al., 2017; Pelloux, Everitt, & Dickinson, 2007) or adulteration of drug solutions with bitter tasting quinine (Galli & Wolffgramm, 2004).

Substance misuse is a chronic–relapsing disorder and relapse is often precipitated by craving. An understanding of the factors that lead to craving and the development of treatments to mitigate craving has therefore been a focus of intense investigation.

Craving. Craving is a subjective response and so it cannot be measured in animal subjects. As a correlate of relapse, drug seeking is often measured (Venniro, Caprioli, & Shaham, 2016). Drug seeking is inferred when performance of the task that has previously led to drug infusions persists even when the drug is no longer available. Thus, following self-administration during which lever presses have led to the delivery of a drug infusion, an extinction phase ensues during which lever pressing no longer results in drug delivery. Reinstatement of this extinguished behavior indicates a drug-seeking response.

Some studies investigate context-induced drug seeking as a model of craving that occurs when individuals are confronted with contexts in which they used to take drugs (Khoo, Gibson, Prasad, & McNally, 2017). Others provide more specific cues that had been associated with self-administered drugs, such as a visual, olfactory, or auditory stimulus, to determine whether exposure can precipitate a drug-seeking response. Finally, other studies measure drug seeking following administration of a single injection of the drug in order to mimic craving that can be produced by drug exposure (Jaffe, Cascella, Kumor, & Sherer, 1989).

The drug-seeking response is often persistent and resistant to extinction. Resistance to extinction of the drug-seeking response has also been used to identify factors that might impact relapse. These studies have shown that only some animals develop compulsive drug seeking that is resistant to extinction and is resistant to decreases in drug taking produced by punishment.

Pharmacological manipulations.   Pharmacological manipulations have been conducted in order to determine factors that might predispose an individual to the initial positive effects of drugs and to determine neurochemical mechanisms underlying the maintenance of drug taking and drug seeking. Controlled studies in laboratory animals support the idea that exposure to some drugs might predispose to repeated drug use (Horger, Giles, & Schenk, 1992; Horger, Wellman, Morien, Davies, & Schenk, 1991; Schenk & Izenwasser, 2002). Various neuroplastic changes in reward-relevant brain regions produced by preexposure have been proposed to underlie this predisposition and have suggested various environmental factors that might enhance susceptibility to repeated drug taking.

Other studies have examined the pharmacological basis of self-administration by determining the effects of selective agonists and antagonists on drug taking and drug seeking. The use of optogenetic procedures that use light to activate or inhibit selective neurochemical systems is now providing additional data concerning changes in the brain that underlie the transition from drug use to misuse.

Genetic manipulations.   A genetic predisposition for drug self-administration has been demonstrated by developing rat lines with a preference for alcohol (Li, Lumeng, McBride, & Murphy, 1987) and nicotine (Nesil, Kanit, Li, & Pogun, 2013), and with low or high novelty responses (García-Fuster, Perez, Clinton, Watson, & Akil, 2010) or different preferences for saccharin (Carroll, Morgan, Anker, Perry, & Dess, 2008). Different rat and mouse strains also appear differentially sensitive to the reinforcing effects of some drugs (Giorgi, Piras, & Corda, 2007; Phillips, 1993; Shuster, 1990), supporting a genetic basis. More recent advances in gene technology have examined the development and maintenance of self-administration following knockout, knock-down, or conditional knockout of various genes (Mayfield, Arends, Harris, & Blednov, 2016; Phillips, Mootz, & Reed, 2016).

Autism Spectrum Disorders

ASDs are characterized and defined by deficits in social interaction and communication, and repetitive, restricted behavior, interests, or activities. Individuals with ASD have difficulty with social interaction and verbal and nonverbal cues (including eye contact, facial expressions, and gestures). Furthermore, there are restricted interests, movement, behavior, and speech patterns. These deficits frequently prevent engagement in socially typical interactions. Animal models have been developed to provide the behavioral symptomology of ASD by way of genetic or pharmacological manipulations.

Social interaction deficits.   Various animal models have been developed and the subsequent defects in social interaction demonstrated using the aforementioned social interaction and social approach assays (see the Measures of Social Behavior section earlier in this chapter). Mice demonstrating ASD-like behaviors show reduced social grooming and contact, including nose-to-nose sniffing or crawling over or under a social mate (McFarlane et al., 2008). Rats modeling ASD-like behaviors show decreased investigation of other rats when compared with controls (Dufour-Rainfray et al., 2010).

Communication deficits. Ultrasonic vocalizations have been extensively studied in relation to ASD-like behaviors in animals. Animals modeling ASD communication deficits show reductions in the overall number of vocalizations, as seen in mice with mutations to the SHANK genes (SHANK are involved in the scaffolding proteins in the postsynaptic cells; Ey et al., 2013) or serotonin genes (Mosienko, Beis, Alenina, & Wöhr, 2015). In addition, some animal models show increased latencies to vocalize when compared with control animals (Radyushkin et al., 2009).

Repetitive behaviors. There are multiple measures to examine ASD-like stereotyped behavior in animals. Rats displaying ASD-like behavior demonstrated increased repetitive beam breaks (interruption of invisible infrared beams to measure the body movements) in an open field test chamber (T. Schneider & Przewłocki, 2005), and increased self-grooming, cage climbing, and rearing onto their hind legs (Won et al., 2012).

Early life manipulations. Pharmacological manipulations, lesioning techniques, or prenatal treatments are utilized to examine ASD-like behaviors in animals. Decreases in social interaction (pinning, exploration, and approach behaviors) have been observed in rats following lesions to the amygdala or hippocampus during the early postnatal period (Postnatal Day [PND] 7) or later on (PND 21; Wolterink et al., 2001). Furthermore, lesions of the medial prefrontal cortex led to a reduction in play behavior and social exploration in rats (M. Schneider & Koch, 2005).

A pharmacological manipulation to model ASD is to treat rodents prenatally with valproate (VPA). VPA is an antiepileptic and anticonvulsant medication. The children of women exposed to this drug during pregnancy were more prone to develop ASD and other congenital deficits. Rats or mice prenatally treated with VPA produced offspring with ASD-like reductions in social interaction and communication, along with increased repetitive movements (Raza et al., 2015; T. Schneider & Przewłocki, 2005; T. Schneider, Turczak, & Przewłocki, 2006). Decreases in the frequency of pinning, increases in the latency to interact, and decreases in the overall number of

interactions were produced when this model was employed (T. Schneider & Przewłocki, 2005). Rats prenatally exposed to VPA at gestational day 12 demonstrated small repetitive movements, stereotyped behavior, and repeated exploration of previously explored arms of the testing enclosure (Mabunga, Gonzales, Kim, Kim, & Shin, 2015).

Genetic manipulations. Genetic manipulations are a different approach to examining ASD-like behaviors in laboratory animals. Extensive focus has been placed on the BTBR T+tf/J (BTBR) mouse model (a genetically altered strain with complete lack of the corpus callosum) for examining ASD-like behaviors, as these animals consistently exhibit decreased sociability and unusual vocalizations (McFarlane et al., 2008; Moy et al., 2007). These behavioral deficits have been suggested to result from reductions in size of the hippocampus and an absent corpus callosum (Wahlsten, Metten, & Crabbe, 2003).

BTBR mice show deficits in behavioral flexibility as identified with an olfactory hole board assay. The apparatus uses 16 depressions or "holes" in the floor to measure the effect of odor on behavior. The deficit identified in the BTBR mice is comparable to the restrictive interests that is one of the core symptoms of ASD (Moy et al., 2008). Defensor et al. (2011) utilized the BTBR mouse model compared with standard laboratory mice (B6 strain) in the social interaction assay, and found reduced sociability as reflected in avoidance of direct nose-to-nose behaviors from other mice (McFarlane et al., 2008; Scattoni, Martire, Cartocci, Ferrante, & Ricceri, 2013). Furthermore, administration of fluoxetine (an SSRI, typically used to treat depression and anxiety) to BTBR mice increased their sociability to match that of controls (Chadman, 2011; Gould et al., 2011).

In addition to the BTBR mice, male mice with a genetic mutation in the neuroligin gene (neuroligin is involved in presynaptic cell adhesion) demonstrate increased latencies to vocalize and decreased vocalizations when interacting with a sexually receptive (in heat) female (El-Kordi et al., 2013; Radyushkin et al., 2009). Mice with abnormal SHANK genes were also dysfunctional in these assays (Ey et al., 2013; Wöhr, 2014). Mice with

SHANK mutations also demonstrated increased self-grooming, behavioral inflexibility, and locomotor activity, which is comparable to a core symptom of ASD (restrictive behaviors and interests; Jiang & Ehlers, 2013; Wang et al., 2011).

Posttraumatic Stress Disorders

PTSD is included in the *DSM–5* as a trauma- and stressor-related disorder. The *DSM–5* criteria require as part of the diagnosis that the disorder arises from experiencing a severe traumatic event. Other criteria for the diagnosis include the presence of symptoms related to the event that intrude on the individual's ongoing life. These symptoms may include reexperiencing the traumatic event and intense psychological and/or physiological responses to cues related to the event.

PTSD diagnosis further requires evidence of persistent avoidance of trauma-related stimuli and other examples of decreased psychological functioning, such as diminished interest or participation, irritable behavior or aggression, hypervigilance, and exaggerated startle responses. These symptoms must last for at least 1 month and create functional impairments. Animal models have been useful in determining mechanisms that contribute to this type of persistent response to a stressful event.

Animal models of posttraumatic stress disorder development. All animal models capture the essential feature of the disorder in that it develops as a direct result of experiencing an extremely traumatic event. The traumatic event usually involves a stressor of some sort. Stressors include electric shock (e.g., Olson et al., 2011), exposure to predators or predator cues, forced water immersion, single prolonged exposure to a succession of stressors, or acute exposure to a strong stressor after a period of chronic exposure to weaker stressors. Typically, the stressful event occurs in a distinct context. This maps the dominant idea that abnormalities in associative learning processes, such as Pavlovian conditioning, underlie this disorder. In conditioned place preference, described previously, cues are usually associated with a positive reinforcer, while in PTSD, environmental cues become strongly

associated with the stressor. Models that include predators or predator cues have added ethological validity, as they resemble trauma that might be encountered in the wild and for which there may be evolutionary vulnerability.

To capture the long-term rather than acute fear response, behavioral and pathophysiological responses are assessed some days or weeks after exposure to the stressor. This also models the idea that PTSD can, in part, be conceptualized as both a failure of fear extinction and an enhancement of fear learning. Many of the models successfully produce pathophysiological abnormalities comparable to those observed in patients with PTSD. As an example, stress activates the hypothalamic–pituitary–adrenal axis (HPA axis), causing the release of corticotropin-releasing factor (CRF) from the hypothalamus, which triggers adrenocorticotropic hormone (ACTH) from the anterior pituitary. ACTH triggers the release of glucocorticoids from the adrenal gland. PTSD may in part result from a deficit in this stress response. Liberzon, Abelson, Flagel, Raz, and Young (1999), using a single prolonged stress model, and Roth et al. (2012), using a chronic and acute stress paradigm, showed that these animal models of PTSD produce a deficit in this axis.

Selectivity of posttraumatic stress disorder development. One noted feature of PTSD development is that not all individuals exposed to the same environmental stressor develop the disorder. When people are exposed to highly aversive events that produce acute fear, some will go on to develop PTSD while others will not. Animal models, particularly those that use predator stress, have successfully modeled this variability in response across individuals. Potential genetic and epigenetic factors can be manipulated with animal subjects in ways not feasible with human participants, and thus can identify potential genetic and epigenetic factors that underlie susceptibility to the disorder.

Abnormal fear responses. In addition to showing fear in the presence of the context experienced during exposure to the stressor, animals exposed to a PTSD model show enhanced fear learning in new contexts. As an example, rats were exposed to repeated shock in one context to model a traumatic event, but then were exposed to a mild stressor in a completely new context (Rau, DeCola, & Fanselow, 2005). Subsequently, rats showed excessive fear in the new context even in the absence of the stressor. This fear response persisted up to 3 months following the initial stressor.

Other persistent generalized fear or anxiety responses are commonly reported. These generalized impairments to function have been assessed across a range of apparatuses, including measuring time spent on open arms of an elevated maze and in central areas of an open field using the social interaction test described earlier as well as the acoustic startle test, which assesses animal responses to an unexpected noise. Abnormal reactivity in these tests resemble the avoidance behavior and social isolation common in patients with PTSD.

Other intrusions into ongoing life. Animal models have also been used to model other behavioral problems involved with PTSD. These showed deficits in spatial memory and recognition memory (Kohda et al., 2007), deficits in acquisition or memory of cues that represent safe environments (Cohen, Liberzon, & Richter-Levin, 2009), increased acquisition of voluntary alcohol consumption (Meyer, Long, Fanselow, & Spigelman, 2013), and increased aggression in a resident–intruder paradigm for mice following exposure to a shock-based PTSD model (Olson et al., 2011).

Pharmacological manipulations. A large number of brain regions involved in fear acquisition and extinction and other memory processes have been implicated in PTSD. These include the hippocampus, prefrontal cortex, and amygdala (Dahlgren et al., 2018; Kitayama, Vaccarino, Kutner, Weiss, & Bremner, 2005). Animal studies show that several neurochemical systems mediate PTSD symptomology, including abnormal glutamatergic, serotonergic, and brain-derived neurotrophic factor levels (Pitman et al., 2012). Abnormalities in immune mechanisms have also been implicated in PTSD development (Deslauriers, Powell, & Risbrough, 2017).

Given the extensive pathophysiological abnormalities identified so far, it is not surprising that a number of pharmacological interventions have been examined in preclinical trials, with some progressing to clinical trials. As an example, methylphenidate (Ritalin®, a dopamine reuptake inhibitor), particularly when given in combination with a noradrenergic reuptake inhibitor, mitigated impairments in fear extinction, avoidance, and hyperarousal in a rat model (Aga-Mizrachi et al., 2014).

Currently SSRIs are approved for treatment of PTSD, but their success in practice is equivocal. Acute administration of SSRIs may in fact enhance associative fear learning while also facilitating fear extinction (Bowers & Ressler, 2015). In contrast, chronic administration may impair fear learning, but unfortunately also fear extinction (Burghardt, Sigurdsson, Gorman, McEwen, & LeDoux, 2013). These findings are consistent with the equivocal success of SSRI treatment.

Other promising pharmacological therapies examined in preclinical trials and introduced into clinical trials include D-cycloserine (an antibiotic used to treat tuberculosis), aimed at facilitating long-term fear extinction and corticosterone which might, if given in a timely manner, reduce the risk of developing PTSD in the face of trauma (Bowers & Ressler, 2015).

Genetic manipulations. Although there are rat and mice genetic models of high trait anxiety and other abnormal fear responses, there is not an accepted genetic model of PTSD as a disorder that arises out of trauma. However, across-strain variation in rats' susceptibility to PTSD symptoms suggests that genetic factors may have a role in this disorder. When the inbred Lewis rat strain is exposed to a predator stress model, about half the rats show excess fear. This strain, therefore, has potential as a genetic model to investigate gene–environment interactions (Goswami, Rodríguez-Sierra, Cascardi, & Paré, 2013). More recently it has been suggested that a binding protein, FKBP5, may mediate responses to stress (Schöner, Heinz, Endres, Gertz, & Kronenberg, 2017). FKBP5 knock out mice showed less fear type responses after, but not before, exposure to stressors. Therefore, this may be a promising model capturing the role of experiencing trauma in the disorder.

LIMITATIONS OF ANIMAL STUDIES

While there are successes, there are also limitations with animal research used to model human pathologies. Some of these limitations arise out of the sound scientific decision to control variables that contribute to variability and thus ensure replicability of results. Males and females respond differently to drugs, and differences in both pharmacokinetic (bioavailability, distribution, metabolism, and excretion) and pharmacodynamic responses have been observed (Soldin, Chung, & Mattison, 2011; Soldin & Mattison, 2009; Tanaka, 1999; Waxman & Holloway, 2009). Aging results in a large number of changes in cardiac, renal, gastrointestinal, and neuroendocrine systems (Fernandez et al., 2011). These changes also can impact drug pharmacokinetics. Some studies have suggested that drug absorption, distribution, metabolism, and clearance are reduced as a function of age, but others have suggested an increase (Mangoni & Jackson, 2004), and the effect of age might be dependent on the particular drug characteristics. Drug absorption, distribution, and metabolism can also vary considerably between species.

These realities and the desire to control variation has led to the majority of animal models using rodent species and adult males as test subjects. The reduction in variability afforded by this choice has satisfied ethical concerns to minimize subject numbers, while also providing sufficient statistical power to answer the first important questions around the potential of animal models. However, this choice also presents challenges to the face, construct, and predictive validity of the research that the field now needs to address. Indeed, the 1994 mandate of the National Institutes of Health to ensure inclusion of women in clinical research was expanded in 2014 to require testing of more female animal subjects.

Reliance on Males in Models

The reliance on males in animal models is particularly problematic, as there are sex differences in the prevalence of almost all mental health disorders whether represented by the *DSM–5* or by RDoC. With reference to the disorders described previously, there are sex differences in prevalence and form of substance use disorders (Kuhn, 2015; Riley, Hempel, & Clasen, 2018), autism (Lai et al., 2011; May, Cornish, & Rinehart, 2016), and PTSD (Ibáñez, Blanco, Moreryra, & Sáiz-Ruiz, 2003; Wong, Zane, Saw, & Chan, 2013). While some disorders are male dominated, such as autism, and thus warrant the use of male subjects, women are more susceptible to other *DSM–5* disorders, such as PTSD or substance use disorders.

Additionally, studies suggest that at least in some cases, both the disorder itself, response to treatment, and/or the validity of the animal models commonly used may be moderated by sex. As an example, a single prolonged stress model of PTSD in female rats, as opposed to male rats, did not show a deficit in cued fear extinction, but did show an upregulation of hippocampal glucocorticoid receptors (Keller, Schreiber, Staib, & Knox, 2015). Animal models that have examined sex differences have also shown marked sex differences in quantitative measures of drug misuse and in the mechanisms that might underpin these differences (Becker & Koob, 2016).

In more recent years, studies have included females and examined sex as an independent variable, but there remains a discrepancy between studies that include females and those that only use males (Becker & Koob, 2016; Glover, Jovanovic, & Norrholm, 2015; Kokras et al., 2015; Lind et al., 2017).

Most Studies Done in Adults

As noted previously, most animal models have used adult subjects; however, brain systems develop from childhood through to adulthood (Giedd, 2004; Lewis, Cruz, Eggan, & Erickson, 2004; van den Bos, Rodriguez, Schweitzer, & McClure, 2015). For example, there is considerable plasticity in brain dopamine and serotonin systems throughout development (Benes, Taylor, & Cunningham, 2000), and these differences are reflected in different drug responses (Dwyer & Leslie, 2016). The prevalence of mental disorders also varies across the lifespan, with some disorders more common in adults, but others appearing in childhood, adolescence, or in later life.

Animal models of developmental disorders such as autism and Alzheimer's disease discussed previously have used appropriately aged animal models that target the development of the disorder. However, there is evidence that there can be a developmental trajectory of many adult mental health disorders (Kaffman & Krystal, 2012). As an example, PTSD studies suggests that childhood trauma may contribute to the selective vulnerability to this disorder (Yehuda, Halligan, & Grossman, 2001). Similarly, the age at which alcohol consumption begins has been associated with vulnerability to addiction, with children exposed to alcohol at younger ages being more likely to have a substance use disorder as adolescents and in later life (e.g., Blomeyer et al., 2013). The contribution of animal models to our understanding of such disorders may be improved by including a wider age range in animal models.

Species Differences

More than 90% of biomedical research uses rodent models because of the relatively short lifespan and the resulting potential for a large number of tests to be conducted. As a result, allometric approaches have been developed to allow translation of drug doses between species (Nair & Jacob, 2016; Sharma & McNeill, 2009). While this type of scaling might allay the concern of obtaining appropriate translational doses, it fails to account for basic differences between mice and rats and between these animals and humans in the behavioral responses to various drugs (Ellenbroek & Youn, 2016).

The use of nonhuman primates to model certain disease states is also advantageous because of the close phylogenetic relationship with humans. Thus, especially for disorders that have a strong cognitive component or involve verbal behavior, nonhuman primates provide advantages in terms of modeling the human condition. This close relationship has also raised ethical concerns specific to these species, and therefore research with these species is now highly regulated.

Recently, the use of invertebrates has also provided models that might be useful for understanding the potential mechanisms of some disorders. Drosophila have been used to study the genetic basis of certain phenotypes (Narayanan & Rothenfluh, 2016), and C. elegans has been used to study molecular mechanisms underlying various neurological disorders (Bessa, Maciel, & Rodrigues, 2013).

Zebrafish have also emerged as a promising vertebrate species. While less complex, this fish has comparable neuroanatomy and neurotransmitter systems to other vertebrates. They have advantages over rodents and mice in terms of the number that can be bred in a short period of time; females can produce hundreds of eggs multiple times per week, and the developmental time from fertilization to adulthood is around 3 months.

Zebrafish have complex social interactions that show disruption as a result of environmental or genetic manipulations. These fish therefore have the potential as models for disorders that affect social behavior. As an example, shoaling (the behavior of remaining with other fish for social reasons) in adulthood can be disrupted by providing short-term exposure of an egg to a small dosage of alcohol. This has been put forward as a model of milder forms of fetal alcohol syndrome (Shams, Rihel, Ortiz, & Gerlai, 2018). Assays developed to assess fear and anxiety in these fish that are analogous to the open field and light–dark emergence paradigms used with rodents might serve in a model of PTSD (Caramillo et al., 2015). The fish also show conditioned place preference effects that could be used in models of substance use disorders (Caramillo, Khan, Collier, & Echevarria, 2015).

References

Aga-Mizrachi, S., Cymerblit-Sabba, A., Gurman, O., Balan, A., Shwam, G., Deshe, R., . . . Avital, A. (2014). Methylphenidate and desipramine combined treatment improves PTSD symptomatology in a rat model. *Translational Psychiatry, 4*, e447. http://dx.doi.org/10.1038/tp.2014.82

Albert, D. J., Jonik, R. H., & Walsh, M. L. (1992). Hormone-dependent aggression in male and female rats: Experiential, hormonal, and neural foundations. *Neuroscience and Biobehavioral Reviews, 16*, 177–192. http://dx.doi.org/10.1016/S0149-7634(05)80179-4

Arakawa, H., Blanchard, D. C., Arakawa, K., Dunlap, C., & Blanchard, R. J. (2008). Scent marking behavior as an odorant communication in mice. *Neuroscience and Biobehavioral Reviews, 32*, 1236–1248. http://dx.doi.org/10.1016/j.neubiorev.2008.05.012

Ayhan, Y., McFarland, R., & Pletnikov, M. V. (2016). Animal models of gene–environment interaction in schizophrenia: A dimensional perspective. *Progress in Neurobiology, 136*, 1–27. http://dx.doi.org/10.1016/j.pneurobio.2015.10.002

Bachurin, S. O., Bovina, E. V., & Ustyugov, A. A. (2017). Drugs in clinical trials for Alzheimer's disease: The major trends. *Medicinal Research Reviews*, 1186–1225. http://dx.doi.org/10.1002/med.21434

Becker, J. B., & Koob, G. F. (2016). Sex differences in animal models: Focus on addiction. *Pharmacological Reviews, 68*, 242–263. http://dx.doi.org/10.1124/pr.115.011163

Belin, D., Belin-Rauscent, A., Everitt, B. J., & Dalley, J. W. (2016). In search of predictive endophenotypes in addiction: Insights from preclinical research. *Genes, Brain & Behavior, 15*, 74–88. http://dx.doi.org/10.1111/gbb.12265

Benes, F. M., Taylor, J. B., & Cunningham, M. C. (2000). Convergence and plasticity of monoaminergic systems in the medial prefrontal cortex during the postnatal period: Implications for the development of psychopathology. *Cerebral Cortex, 10*, 1014–1027. http://dx.doi.org/10.1093/cercor/10.10.1014

Berg, E. A. (1948). A simple objective technique for measuring flexibility in thinking. *Journal of General Psychology, 39*, 15–22. http://dx.doi.org/10.1080/00221309.1948.9918159

Bessa, C., Maciel, P., & Rodrigues, A. J. (2013). Using *C. elegans* to decipher the cellular and molecular mechanisms underlying neurodevelopmental disorders. *Molecular Neurobiology, 48*, 465–489. http://dx.doi.org/10.1007/s12035-013-8434-6

Beyer, D. K. E., & Freund, N. (2017). Animal models for bipolar disorder: From bedside to the cage. *International Journal of Bipolar Disorders, 5*, 35. http://dx.doi.org/10.1186/s40345-017-0104-6

Bickel, W. K., Jarmolowicz, D. P., Mueller, E. T., Koffarnus, M. N., & Gatchalian, K. M. (2012). Excessive discounting of delayed reinforcers as a trans-disease process contributing to addiction and other disease-related vulnerabilities: Emerging evidence. *Pharmacology & Therapeutics, 134*, 287–297. http://dx.doi.org/10.1016/j.pharmthera.2012.02.004

Birnbaum, R., & Weinberger, D. R. (2017). Genetic insights into the neurodevelopmental origins of schizophrenia. *Nature Reviews Neuroscience, 18*, 727–740. http://dx.doi.org/10.1038/nrn.2017.125

Bishop, M. P., Elder, S. T., & Heath, R. G. (1963). Intracranial self-stimulation in man. *Science, 140*, 394–396. http://dx.doi.org/10.1126/science.140.3565.394

Blanchard, R. J., Blanchard, D. C., Agullana, R., & Weiss, S. M. (1991). Twenty-two kHz alarm cries to presentation of a predator, by laboratory rats living in visible burrow systems. *Physiology & Behavior, 50*, 967–972. http://dx.doi.org/10.1016/0031-9384(91)90423-L

Blanchard, R. J., Blanchard, D. C., Takahashi, T., & Kelley, M. J. (1977). Attack and defensive behaviour in the albino rat. *Animal Behaviour, 25*, 622–634. http://dx.doi.org/10.1016/0003-3472(77)90113-0

Blomeyer, D., Friemel, C. M., Buchmann, A. F., Banaschewski, T., Laucht, M., & Schneider, M. (2013). Impact of pubertal stage at first drink on adult drinking behavior. *Alcoholism: Clinical and Experimental Research, 37*, 1804–1811.

Blough, D. S. (1959). Delayed matching in the pigeon. *Journal of the Experimental Analysis of Behavior, 2*, 151–160.

Bowers, M. E., & Ressler, K. J. (2015). An overview of translationally informed treatments for post-traumatic stress disorder: Animal models of Pavlovian fear conditioning to human clinical trials. *Biological Psychiatry, 78*, E15–E27. http://dx.doi.org/10.1016/j.biopsych.2015.06.008

Brodkin, E. S., Hagemann, A., Nemetski, S. M., & Silver, L. M. (2004). Social approach–avoidance behavior of inbred mouse strains towards DBA/2 mice. *Brain Research, 1002*, 151–157. http://dx.doi.org/10.1016/j.brainres.2003.12.013

Burghardt, N. S., Sigurdsson, T., Gorman, J. M., McEwen, B. S., & LeDoux, J. E. (2013). Chronic antidepressant treatment impairs the acquisition of fear extinction. *Biological Psychiatry, 73*, 1078–1086. http://dx.doi.org/10.1016/j.biopsych.2012.10.012

Caramillo, E. M., Khan, K. M., Collier, A. D., & Echevarria, D. J. (2015). Modeling PTSD in the zebrafish: Are we there yet? *Behavioural Brain Research, 276*, 151–160. http://dx.doi.org/10.1016/j.bbr.2014.05.005

Carroll, M. E., Morgan, A. D., Anker, J. J., Perry, J. L., & Dess, N. K. (2008). Selective breeding for differential saccharin intake as an animal model of drug abuse. *Behavioural Pharmacology, 19*, 435–460. http://dx.doi.org/10.1097/FBP.0b013e32830c3632

Chadman, K. K. (2011). Fluoxetine but not risperidone increases sociability in the BTBR mouse model of autism. *Pharmacology, Biochemistry, and Behavior, 97*, 586–594. http://dx.doi.org/10.1016/j.pbb.2010.09.012

Chipkin, R. E. (1990). D$_1$ antagonist in clinical trial. *Trends in Pharmacological Sciences, 11*, 185. http://dx.doi.org/10.1016/0165-6147(90)90111-K

Clark, L. A., Cuthbert, B., Lewis-Fernández, R., Narrow, W. E., & Reed, G. M. (2017). Three approaches to understanding and classifying mental disorder: ICD–11, *DSM–5*, and the National Institute of Mental Health's Research Domain Criteria (RDoC).

Psychological Science in the Public Interest, 18, 72–145. http://dx.doi.org/10.1177/1529100617727266

Cohen, H., Liberzon, I., & Richter-Levin, G. (2009). Exposure to extreme stress impairs contextual odour discrimination in an animal model of PTSD. *International Journal of Neuropsychopharmacology, 12*, 291–303. http://dx.doi.org/10.1017/S146114570800919X

Coyle, J. T., Price, D. L., & DeLong, M. R. (1983). Alzheimer's disease: A disorder of cortical cholinergic innervation. *Science, 219*, 1184–1190. http://dx.doi.org/10.1126/science.6338589

Dahlgren, M. K., Laifer, L. M., VanElzakker, M. B., Offringa, R., Hughes, K. C., Staples-Bradley, L. K., . . . Shin, L. M. (2018). Diminished medial prefrontal cortex activation during the recollection of stressful events is an acquired characteristic of PTSD. *Psychological Medicine, 48*, 1128–1138.

Dalley, J. W., Fryer, T. D., Brichard, L., Robinson, E. S., Theobald, D. E., Lääne, K., . . . Robbins, T. W. (2007). Nucleus accumbens D2/3 receptors predict trait impulsivity and cocaine reinforcement. *Science, 315*, 1267–1270. http://dx.doi.org/10.1126/science.1137073

Defensor, E. B., Pearson, B. L., Pobbe, R. L., Bolivar, V. J., Blanchard, D. C., & Blanchard, R. J. (2011). A novel social proximity test suggests patterns of social avoidance and gaze aversion-like behavior in BTBR T+ tf/J mice. *Behavioural Brain Research, 217*, 302–308. http://dx.doi.org/10.1016/j.bbr.2010.10.033

Deroche-Gamonet, V., Belin, D., & Piazza, P. V. (2004). Evidence for addiction-like behavior in the rat. *Science, 305*(5686), 1014–1017. http://dx.doi.org/10.1126/science.1099020

Deroche-Gamonet, V., & Piazza, P. V. (2014). Psychobiology of cocaine addiction: Contribution of a multi-symptomatic animal model of loss of control. *Neuropharmacology, 76*(Pt B), 437–449. http://dx.doi.org/10.1016/j.neuropharm.2013.07.014

Deslauriers, J., Powell, S., & Risbrough, V. B. (2017). Immune signaling mechanisms of PTSD risk and symptom development: Insights from animal models. *Current Opinion in Behavioral Sciences, 14*, 123–132. http://dx.doi.org/10.1016/j.cobeha.2017.01.005

Digby, L. J., & Barreto, C. E. (1993). Social organization in a wild population of *Callithrix jacchus*: I. Group composition and dynamics. *Folia Primatologica, 61*, 123–134. http://dx.doi.org/10.1159/000156739

Dinkler, L., Lundström, S., Gajwani, R., Lichtenstein, P., Gillberg, C., & Minnis, H. (2017). Maltreatment-associated neurodevelopmental disorders: A co-twin control analysis. *Journal of Child Psychology and Psychiatry, 58*, 691–701. http://dx.doi.org/10.1111/jcpp.12682

Drury, S. S., Sánchez, M. M., & Gonzalez, A. (2016). When mothering goes awry: Challenges and opportunities for utilizing evidence across rodent, nonhuman primate and human studies to better define the biological consequences of negative early caregiving. *Hormones and Behavior, 77*, 182–192. http://dx.doi.org/10.1016/j.yhbeh.2015.10.007

Du, W. J., Green, L., & Myerson, J. (2002). Cross-cultural comparisons of discounting delayed and probabilistic rewards. *The Psychological Record, 52*, 479–492. http://dx.doi.org/10.1007/BF03395199

Dudchenko, P. A. (2004). An overview of the tasks used to test working memory in rodents. *Neuroscience and Biobehavioral Reviews, 28*, 699–709. http://dx.doi.org/10.1016/j.neubiorev.2004.09.002

Dufour-Rainfray, D., Vourc'h, P., Le Guisquet, A. M., Garreau, L., Ternant, D., Bodard, S., . . . Guilloteau, D. (2010). Behavior and serotonergic disorders in rats exposed prenatally to valproate: A model for autism. *Neuroscience Letters, 470*, 55–59. http://dx.doi.org/10.1016/j.neulet.2009.12.054

Dutta, S., & Sengupta, P. (2016). Men and mice: Relating their ages. *Life Sciences, 152*, 244–248. http://dx.doi.org/10.1016/j.lfs.2015.10.025

Dwyer, J. B., & Leslie, F. M. (2016). Adolescent maturation of dopamine D1 and D2 receptor function and interactions in rodents. *PLoS One, 11*, e0146966. http://dx.doi.org/10.1371/journal.pone.0146966

Edwards, S., & Koob, G. F. (2013). Escalation of drug self-administration as a hallmark of persistent addiction liability. *Behavioural Pharmacology, 24*, 356–362. http://dx.doi.org/10.1097/FBP.0b013e3283644d15

El-Kordi, A., Winkler, D., Hammerschmidt, K., Kästner, A., Krueger, D., Ronnenberg, A., . . . Ehrenreich, H. (2013). Development of an autism severity score for mice using *Nlgn4* null mutants as a construct-valid model of heritable monogenic autism. *Behavioural Brain Research, 251*, 41–49. http://dx.doi.org/10.1016/j.bbr.2012.11.016

Ellenbroek, B., & Youn, J. (2016). Rodent models in neuroscience research: Is it a rat race? *Disease Models & Mechanisms, 9*, 1079–1087. http://dx.doi.org/10.1242/dmm.026120

Ennaceur, A., & Chazot, P. L. (2016). Preclinical animal anxiety research—Flaws and prejudices. *Pharmacology Research & Perspectives, 4*, e00223. http://dx.doi.org/10.1002/prp2.223

Ey, E., Torquet, N., Le Sourd, A. M., Leblond, C. S., Boeckers, T. M., Faure, P., & Bourgeron, T. (2013). The autism *ProSAP1/Shank2* mouse model displays quantitative and structural abnormalities in ultra-sonic vocalisations. *Behavioural Brain Research, 256*, 677–689. http://dx.doi.org/10.1016/j.bbr.2013.08.031

Farrell, M. S., Werge, T., Sklar, P., Owen, M. J., Ophoff, R. A., O'Donovan, M. C., . . . Sullivan, P. F. (2015).

Evaluating historical candidate genes for schizophrenia. *Molecular Psychiatry, 20,* 555–562. http://dx.doi.org/10.1038/mp.2015.16

Fernandez, E., Perez, R., Hernandez, A., Tejada, P., Arteta, M., & Ramos, J. T. (2011). Factors and mechanisms for pharmacokinetic differences between pediatric population and adults. *Pharmaceutics, 3,* 53–72. http://dx.doi.org/10.3390/pharmaceutics3010053

Fernández-Espejo, E., & Mir, D. (1990). Ethological analysis of the male rat's socioagonistic behavior in a resident-intruder paradigm. *Aggressive Behavior, 16,* 41–55. http://dx.doi.org/10.1002/1098-2337 (1990)16:1<41::AID-AB2480160106>3.0.CO;2-V

Fisel, P., Schaeffeler, E., & Schwab, M. (2016). DNA methylation of ADME genes. *Clinical Pharmacology and Therapeutics, 99,* 512–527. http://dx.doi.org/10.1002/cpt.343

Floresco, S. B., Block, A. E., & Tse, M. T. (2008). Inactivation of the medial prefrontal cortex of the rat impairs strategy set-shifting, but not reversal learning, using a novel, automated procedure. *Behavioural Brain Research, 190,* 85–96. http://dx.doi.org/10.1016/j.bbr.2008.02.008

Galimberti, D., & Scarpini, E. (2016). Old and new acetylcholinesterase inhibitors for Alzheimer's disease. *Expert Opinion on Investigational Drugs, 25,* 1181–1187. http://dx.doi.org/10.1080/13543784.2016.1216972

Galli, G., & Wolffgramm, J. (2004). Long-term voluntary D-amphetamine consumption and behavioral predictors for subsequent D-amphetamine addiction in rats. *Drug and Alcohol Dependence, 73,* 51–60. http://dx.doi.org/10.1016/j.drugalcdep.2003.09.003

García-Fuster, M. J., Perez, J. A., Clinton, S. M., Watson, S. J., & Akil, H. (2010). Impact of cocaine on adult hippocampal neurogenesis in an animal model of differential propensity to drug abuse. *European Journal of Neuroscience, 31,* 79–89. http://dx.doi.org/10.1111/j.1460-9568.2009.07045.x

Giedd, J. N. (2004). Structural magnetic resonance imaging of the adolescent brain. *Annals of the New York Academy of Sciences, 1021,* 77–85. http://dx.doi.org/10.1196/annals.1308.009

Giorgi, O., Piras, G., & Corda, M. G. (2007). The psychogenetically selected Roman high- and low-avoidance rat lines: A model to study the individual vulnerability to drug addiction. *Neuroscience and Biobehavioral Reviews, 31,* 148–163. http://dx.doi.org/10.1016/j.neubiorev.2006.07.008

Glover, E. M., Jovanovic, T., & Norrholm, S. D. (2015). Estrogen and extinction of fear memories: Implications for posttraumatic stress disorder treatment. *Biological Psychiatry, 78,* 178–185. http://dx.doi.org/10.1016/j.biopsych.2015.02.007

Goswami, S., Rodríguez-Sierra, O., Cascardi, M., & Paré, D. (2013). Animal models of post-traumatic stress disorder: Face validity. *Frontiers in Neuroscience, 7,* 89. http://dx.doi.org/10.3389/fnins.2013.00089

Gould, G. G., Hensler, J. G., Burke, T. F., Benno, R. H., Onaivi, E. S., & Daws, L. C. (2011). Density and function of central serotonin (5-HT) transporters, 5-HT$_{1A}$ and 5-HT$_{2A}$ receptors, and effects of their targeting on BTBR T+tf/J mouse social behavior. *Journal of Neurochemistry, 116,* 291–303. http://dx.doi.org/10.1111/j.1471-4159.2010.07104.x

Harper, D. N., Kay, C., & Hunt, M. (2013). Prior MDMA exposure inhibits learning and produces both tolerance and sensitization in the radial-arm maze. *Pharmacology, Biochemistry, and Behavior, 105,* 34–40. http://dx.doi.org/10.1016/j.pbb.2013.01.018

Harro, J. (2018). Animals, anxiety, and anxiety disorders: How to measure anxiety in rodents and why. *Behavioural Brain Research, 352,* 81–93. http://dx.doi.org/10.1016/j.bbr.2017.10.016

Hart, P. C., Bergner, C. L., Smolinsky, A. N., Dufour, B. D., Egan, R. J., LaPorte, J. L., & Kalueff, A. V. (2016). Experimental models of anxiety for drug discovery and brain research. In G. Proetzel & M. Wiles (Eds.), *Mouse models for drug discovery: Methods in molecular biology* (Vol. 1438; pp. 271–291). New York, NY: Humana Press. http://dx.doi.org/10.1007/978-1-4939-3661-8_16

Hasin, D. S., O'Brien, C. P., Auriacombe, M., Borges, G., Bucholz, K., Budney, A., . . . Grant, B. F. (2013). *DSM–5* criteria for substance use disorders: Recommendations and rationale. *The American Journal of Psychiatry, 170,* 834–851. http://dx.doi.org/10.1176/appi.ajp.2013.12060782

Hayward, A., Tomlinson, A., & Neill, J. C. (2016). Low attentive and high impulsive rats: A translational animal model of ADHD and disorders of attention and impulse control. *Pharmacology & Therapeutics, 158,* 41–51. http://dx.doi.org/10.1016/j.pharmthera.2015.11.010

Hofer, M. A. (1996). Multiple regulators of ultrasonic vocalization in the infant rat. *Psychoneuroendocrinology, 21,* 203–217. http://dx.doi.org/10.1016/0306-4530(95)00042-9

Horger, B. A., Giles, M. K., & Schenk, S. (1992). Preexposure to amphetamine and nicotine predisposes rats to self-administer a low dose of cocaine. *Psychopharmacology, 107,* 271–276. http://dx.doi.org/10.1007/BF02245147

Horger, B. A., Wellman, P. J., Morien, A., Davies, B. T., & Schenk, S. (1991). Caffeine exposure sensitizes rats to the reinforcing effects of cocaine. *Neuroreport: An International Journal for the Rapid Communication of Research in Neuroscience, 2,* 53–56. http://dx.doi.org/10.1097/00001756-199101000-00013

Hrabovska, S., & Salyha, Y. T. (2016). Animal models of autism spectrum disorders and behavioral techniques of their examination. *Neurophysiology, 48*, 380–388. http://dx.doi.org/10.1007/s11062-017-9613-2

Huang, W. Y., Maier, W., Murelle, L., Cory, L. A., Eaves, L. J., & Shepherd, N. S. (2000). Concordance among monozygotic and dizygotic twins from a population-based sample for self-reported atopic triad, syndrome x, and psychiatric conditions. *Genetics in Medicine, 2*, 79. http://dx.doi.org/10.1097/00125817-200001000-00098

Ibáñez, A., Blanco, C., Moreryra, P., & Sáiz-Ruiz, J. (2003). Gender differences in pathological gambling. *The Journal of Clinical Psychiatry, 64*, 295–301. http://dx.doi.org/10.4088/JCP.v64n0311

Izquierdo, A., & Jentsch, J. D. (2012). Reversal learning as a measure of impulsive and compulsive behavior in addictions. *Psychopharmacology, 219*, 607–620. http://dx.doi.org/10.1007/s00213-011-2579-7

Jaffe, J. H., Cascella, N. G., Kumor, K. M., & Sherer, M. A. (1989). Cocaine-induced cocaine craving. *Psychopharmacology, 97*, 59–64. http://dx.doi.org/10.1007/BF00443414

Jelen, P., Soltysik, S., & Zagrodzka, J. (2003). 22-kHz ultrasonic vocalization in rats as an index of anxiety but not fear: Behavioral and pharmacological modulation of affective state. *Behavioural Brain Research, 141*, 63–72. http://dx.doi.org/10.1016/S0166-4328(02)00321-2

Jiang, Y. H., & Ehlers, M. D. (2013). Modeling autism by *SHANK* gene mutations in mice. *Neuron, 78*, 8–27. http://dx.doi.org/10.1016/j.neuron.2013.03.016

Kaffman, A., & Krystal, J. H. (2012). New frontiers in animal research of psychiatric illness. In F. Kobeissy (Ed.), *Methods in molecular biology: Psychiatric disorders* (Vol. 829, pp. 3–30). New York, NY: Humana Press. http://dx.doi.org/10.1007/978-1-61779-458-2_1

Kantak, K. M., Hegstrand, L. R., & Eichelman, B. (1980). Dietary tryptophan modulation and aggressive behavior in mice. *Pharmacology, Biochemistry, and Behavior, 12*, 675–679. http://dx.doi.org/10.1016/0091-3057(80)90147-1

Kantak, K. M., Hegstrand, L. R., Whitman, J., & Eichelman, B. (1980). Effects of dietary supplements and a tryptophan-free diet on aggressive behavior in rats. *Pharmacology, Biochemistry, and Behavior, 12*, 173–179. http://dx.doi.org/10.1016/0091-3057(80)90351-2

Katzman, R., & Saitoh, T. (1991). Advances in Alzheimer's disease. *The FASEB Journal, 5*, 278–286. http://dx.doi.org/10.1096/fasebj.5.3.2001787

Kay, C., Harper, D. N., & Hunt, M. (2010). Differential effects of MDMA and scopolamine on working versus reference memory in the radial arm maze task. *Neurobiology of Learning and Memory, 93*, 151–156. http://dx.doi.org/10.1016/j.nlm.2009.09.005

Keller, S. M., Schreiber, W. B., Staib, J. M., & Knox, D. (2015). Sex differences in the single prolonged stress model. *Behavioural Brain Research, 286*, 29–32.

Khoo, S. Y., Gibson, G. D., Prasad, A. A., & McNally, G. P. (2017). How contexts promote and prevent relapse to drug seeking. *Genes, Brain & Behavior, 16*, 185–204. http://dx.doi.org/10.1111/gbb.12328

Kitayama, N., Vaccarino, V., Kutner, M., Weiss, P., & Bremner, J. D. (2005). Magnetic resonance imaging (MRI) measurement of hippocampal volume in post-traumatic stress disorder: A meta-analysis. *Journal of Affective Disorders, 88*, 79–86. http://dx.doi.org/10.1016/j.jad.2005.05.014

Knutson, B., Burgdorf, J., & Panksepp, J. (1998). Anticipation of play elicits high-frequency ultrasonic vocalizations in young rats. *Journal of Comparative Psychology, 112*, 65–73. http://dx.doi.org/10.1037/0735-7036.112.1.65

Knutson, B., Burgdorf, J., & Panksepp, J. (1999). High-frequency ultrasonic vocalizations index conditioned pharmacological reward in rats. *Physiology & Behavior, 66*, 639–643. http://dx.doi.org/10.1016/S0031-9384(98)00337-0

Kohda, K., Harada, K., Kato, K., Hoshino, A., Motohashi, J., Yamaji, T., . . . Kato, N. (2007). Glucocorticoid receptor activation is involved in producing abnormal phenotypes of single-prolonged stress rats: A putative post-traumatic stress disorder model. *Neuroscience, 148*, 22–33. http://dx.doi.org/10.1016/j.neuroscience.2007.05.041

Kokras, N., Antoniou, K., Mikail, H. G., Kafetzopoulos, V., Papadopoulou-Daifoti, Z., & Dalla, C. (2015). Forced swim test: What about females? *Neuropharmacology, 99*, 408–421. http://dx.doi.org/10.1016/j.neuropharm.2015.03.016

Koolhaas, J. M., Coppens, C. M., de Boer, S. F., Buwalda, B., Meerlo, P., & Timmermans, P. J. (2013). The resident-intruder paradigm: A standardized test for aggression, violence and social stress. *Journal of Visualized Experiments, 77*, e4367. http://dx.doi.org/10.3791/4367

Kuhn, C. (2015). Emergence of sex differences in the development of substance use and abuse during adolescence. *Pharmacology & Therapeutics, 153*, 55–78. http://dx.doi.org/10.1016/j.pharmthera.2015.06.003

Lai, M. C., Lombardo, M. V., Pasco, G., Ruigrok, A. N., Wheelwright, S. J., Sadek, S. A., . . . Baron-Cohen, S., & the MRC AIMS Consortium. (2011). A behavioral comparison of male and female adults with high functioning autism spectrum conditions. *PLoS One, 6*, e20835. http://dx.doi.org/10.1371/journal.pone.0020835

Levenson, J. M., & Sweatt, J. D. (2005). Epigenetic mechanisms in memory formation. *Nature Reviews Neuroscience, 6*, 108–118. http://dx.doi.org/10.1038/nrn1604

Lewis, D. A., Cruz, D., Eggan, S., & Erickson, S. (2004). Postnatal development of prefrontal inhibitory circuits and the pathophysiology of cognitive dysfunction in schizophrenia. *Annals of the New York Academy of Sciences, 1021*, 64–76. http://dx.doi.org/10.1196/annals.1308.008

Li, T. K., Lumeng, L., McBride, W. J., & Murphy, J. M. (1987). Rodent lines selected for factors affecting alcohol consumption. *Alcohol and Alcoholism (Oxford, Oxfordshire), Supplement, 1*, 91–96.

Liberzon, I., Abelson, J. L., Flagel, S. B., Raz, J., & Young, E. A. (1999). Neuroendocrine and psychophysiologic responses in PTSD: A symptom provocation study. *Neuropsychopharmacology, 21*, 40–50. http://dx.doi.org/10.1016/S0893-133X(98)00128-6

Lilienfeld, S. O., & Treadway, M. T. (2016). Clashing diagnostic approaches: *DSM-ICD* versus RDoC. *Annual Review of Clinical Psychology, 12*, 435–463. http://dx.doi.org/10.1146/annurev-clinpsy-021815-093122

Lind, K. E., Gutierrez, E. J., Yamamoto, D. J., Regner, M. F., McKee, S. A., & Tanabe, J. (2017). Sex disparities in substance abuse research: Evaluating 23 years of structural neuroimaging studies. *Drug and Alcohol Dependence, 173*, 92–98. http://dx.doi.org/10.1016/j.drugalcdep.2016.12.019

Logan, R. W., & McClung, C. A. (2016). Animal models of bipolar mania: The past, present and future. *Neuroscience, 321*, 163–188. http://dx.doi.org/10.1016/j.neuroscience.2015.08.041

Lumley, L. A., Sipos, M. L., Charles, R. C., Charles, R. F., & Meyerhoff, J. L. (1999). Social stress effects on territorial marking and ultrasonic vocalizations in mice. *Physiology & Behavior, 67*, 769–775. http://dx.doi.org/10.1016/S0031-9384(99)00131-6

Mabunga, D. F., Gonzales, E. L., Kim, J. W., Kim, K. C., & Shin, C. Y. (2015). Exploring the validity of valproic acid animal model of autism. *Experimental Neurobiology, 24*, 285–300. http://dx.doi.org/10.5607/en.2015.24.4.285

MacKillop, J., Amlung, M. T., Few, L. R., Ray, L. A., Sweet, L. H., & Munafò, M. R. (2011). Delayed reward discounting and addictive behavior: A meta-analysis. *Psychopharmacology, 216*, 305–321. http://dx.doi.org/10.1007/s00213-011-2229-0

Madoz-Gúrpide, A., Blasco-Fontecilla, H., Baca-García, E., & Ochoa-Mangado, E. (2011). Executive dysfunction in chronic cocaine users: An exploratory study. *Drug and Alcohol Dependence, 117*, 55–58. http://dx.doi.org/10.1016/j.drugalcdep.2010.11.030

Maier, E. Y., Abdalla, M., Ahrens, A. M., Schallert, T., & Duvauchelle, C. L. (2012). The missing variable: Ultrasonic vocalizations reveal hidden sensitization and tolerance-like effects during long-term cocaine administration. *Psychopharmacology, 219*, 1141–1152. http://dx.doi.org/10.1007/s00213-011-2445-7

Mangoni, A. A., & Jackson, S. H. D. (2004). Age-related changes in pharmacokinetics and pharmacodynamics: Basic principles and practical applications. *British Journal of Clinical Pharmacology, 57*, 6–14. http://dx.doi.org/10.1046/j.1365-2125.2003.02007.x

May, T., Cornish, K., & Rinehart, N. J. (2016). Gender profiles of behavioral attention in children with autism spectrum disorder. *Journal of Attention Disorders, 20*, 627–635. http://dx.doi.org/10.1177/1087054712455502

Mayfield, J., Arends, M. A., Harris, R. A., & Blednov, Y. A. (2016). Genes and alcohol consumption: Studies with mutant mice. *International Review of Neurobiology, 126*, 293–355. http://dx.doi.org/10.1016/bs.irn.2016.02.014

Mazur, J. E. (1987). An adjusting procedure for studying delayed reinforcement. In J. E. M. M. L. Commons, J. A. Nevin, & H. Rachlin (Eds.), *Quantitative analysis of behavior: Vol. 5. The effect of delay and of intervening events on reinforcement value*. Hillsdale, NJ: Erlbaum.

McFarlane, H. G., Kusek, G. K., Yang, M., Phoenix, J. L., Bolivar, V. J., & Crawley, J. N. (2008). Autism-like behavioral phenotypes in BTBR T+tf/J mice. *Genes, Brain & Behavior, 7*, 152–163. http://dx.doi.org/10.1111/j.1601-183X.2007.00330.x

Meaney, M. J., & Stewart, J. (1981). A descriptive study of social development in the rat (*Rattus norvegicus*). *Animal Behaviour, 29*, 34–45. http://dx.doi.org/10.1016/S0003-3472(81)80149-2

Melotti, L., Bailoo, J. D., Murphy, E., Burman, O., & Wurbel, H. (2014). Play in rats: Association across contexts and types, and analysis of structure. *Animal Behavior and Cognition, 1*, 489–501. http://dx.doi.org/10.12966/abc.11.06.2014

Meyer, E. M., Long, V., Fanselow, M. S., & Spigelman, I. (2013). Stress increases voluntary alcohol intake, but does not alter established drinking habits in a rat model of posttraumatic stress disorder. *Alcoholism: Clinical and Experimental Research, 37*, 566–574. http://dx.doi.org/10.1111/acer.12012

Miczek, K. A., & Barros, H. M. T. (1996). Withdrawal from oral cocaine in rats: Ultrasonic vocalizations and tactile startle. *Psychopharmacology, 125*, 379–384. http://dx.doi.org/10.1007/BF02246021

Miczek, K. A., Weerts, E. M., Vivian, J. A., & Barros, H. M. (1995). Aggression, anxiety and vocalizations in animals: GABA$_A$ and 5-HT anxiolytics. *Psychopharmacology, 121*, 38–56. http://dx.doi.org/10.1007/BF02245590

Miller, C. T., Freiwald, W. A., Leopold, D. A., Mitchell, J. F., Silva, A. C., & Wang, X. (2016). Marmosets: A neuroscientific model of human social behavior. *Neuron, 90*, 219–233. http://dx.doi.org/10.1016/j.neuron.2016.03.018

Mitchell, K. J., Huang, Z. J., Moghaddam, B., & Sawa, A. (2011). Following the genes: A framework for animal modeling of psychiatric disorders. *BMC Biology, 9*, 76. http://dx.doi.org/10.1186/1741-7007-9-76

Moore, P., Landolt, H. P., Seifritz, E., Clark, C., Bhatti, T., Kelsoe, J., . . . Gillin, J. C. (2000). Clinical and physiological consequences of rapid tryptophan depletion. *Neuropsychopharmacology, 23*, 601–622. http://dx.doi.org/10.1016/S0893-133X(00)00161-5

Mosienko, V., Beis, D., Alenina, N., & Wöhr, M. (2015). Reduced isolation-induced pup ultrasonic communication in mouse pups lacking brain serotonin. *Molecular Autism, 6*, 13. http://dx.doi.org/10.1186/s13229-015-0003-6

Moy, S. S., Nadler, J. J., Young, N. B., Nonneman, R. J., Segall, S. K., Andrade, G. M., . . . Magnuson, T. R. (2008). Social approach and repetitive behavior in eleven inbred mouse strains. *Behavioural Brain Research, 191*, 118–129. http://dx.doi.org/10.1016/j.bbr.2008.03.015

Moy, S. S., Nadler, J. J., Young, N. B., Perez, A., Holloway, L. P., Barbaro, R. P., . . . Crawley, J. N. (2007). Mouse behavioral tasks relevant to autism: Phenotypes of 10 inbred strains. *Behavioural Brain Research, 176*, 4–20. http://dx.doi.org/10.1016/j.bbr.2006.07.030

Murray, C. L., & Fibiger, H. C. (1986). Pilocarpine and physostigmine attenuate spatial memory impairments produced by lesions of the nucleus basalis magnocellularis. *Behavioral Neuroscience, 100*, 23–32. http://dx.doi.org/10.1037/0735-7044.100.1.23

Nair, A. B., & Jacob, S. (2016). A simple practice guide for dose conversion between animals and human. *Journal of Basic and Clinical Pharmacy, 7*, 27–31. http://dx.doi.org/10.4103/0976-0105.177703

Narayanan, A. S., & Rothenfluh, A. (2016). I believe I can fly!: Use of *drosophila* as a model organism in neuropsychopharmacology research. *Neuropsychopharmacology, 41*, 1439–1446. http://dx.doi.org/10.1038/npp.2015.322

Nesil, T., Kanit, L., Li, M. D., & Pogun, S. (2013). Nine generations of selection for high and low nicotine intake in outbred Sprague–Dawley rats. *Behavior Genetics, 43*, 436–444. http://dx.doi.org/10.1007/s10519-013-9605-y

Nestler, E. J., & Hyman, S. E. (2010). Animal models of neuropsychiatric disorders. *Nature Neuroscience, 13*, 1161–1169. http://dx.doi.org/10.1038/nn.2647

Nieratschker, V., Grosshans, M., Frank, J., Strohmaier, J., von der Goltz, C., El-Maarri, O., . . . Rietschel, M. (2014). Epigenetic alteration of the dopamine transporter gene in alcohol-dependent patients is associated with age. *Addiction Biology, 19*, 305–311. http://dx.doi.org/10.1111/j.1369-1600.2012.00459.x

Nikiforuk, A., & Popik, P. (2011). Long-lasting cognitive deficit induced by stress is alleviated by acute administration of antidepressants. *Psychoneuroendocrinology, 36*, 28–39. http://dx.doi.org/10.1016/j.psyneuen.2010.06.001

Olds, J., & Milner, P. (1954). Positive reinforcement produced by electrical stimulation of septal area and other regions of rat brain. *Journal of Comparative and Physiological Psychology, 47*, 419–427. http://dx.doi.org/10.1037/h0058775

Olson, V. G., Rockett, H. R., Reh, R. K., Redila, V. A., Tran, P. M., Venkov, H. A., . . . Raskind, M. A. (2011). The role of norepinephrine in differential response to stress in an animal model of posttraumatic stress disorder. *Biological Psychiatry, 70*, 441–448. http://dx.doi.org/10.1016/j.biopsych.2010.11.029

Olton, D. S., Collison, C., & Werz, M. A. (1977). Spatial memory and radial arm maze performance of rats. *Learning and Motivation, 8*, 289–314. http://dx.doi.org/10.1016/0023-9690(77)90054-6

Pantelis, C., Barber, F. Z., Barnes, T. R. E., Nelson, H. E., Owen, A. M., & Robbins, T. W. (1999). Comparison of set-shifting ability in patients with chronic schizophrenia and frontal lobe damage. *Schizophrenia Research, 37*, 251–270. http://dx.doi.org/10.1016/S0920-9964(98)00156-X

Pellis, S. M., & Pellis, V. C. (2007). Rough-and-tumble play and the development of the social brain. *Current Directions in Psychological Science, 16*, 95–98. http://dx.doi.org/10.1111/j.1467-8721.2007.00483.x

Pelloux, Y., Everitt, B. J., & Dickinson, A. (2007). Compulsive drug seeking by rats under punishment: Effects of drug taking history. *Psychopharmacology, 194*, 127–137. http://dx.doi.org/10.1007/s00213-007-0805-0

Phillips, T. J. (1993). Use of genetically distinct mouse populations to explore ethanol reinforcement. *Alcohol and Alcoholism (Oxford, Oxfordshire). Supplement, 2*, 451–455.

Phillips, T. J., Mootz, J. R., & Reed, C. (2016). Identification of treatment targets in a genetic mouse model of voluntary methamphetamine drinking. *International Review of Neurobiology, 126*, 39–85. http://dx.doi.org/10.1016/bs.irn.2016.02.001

Piazza, P. V., & Deroche-Gamonet, V. (2013). A multistep general theory of transition to addiction. *Psychopharmacology, 229*, 387–413. http://dx.doi.org/10.1007/s00213-013-3224-4

Pitman, R. K., Rasmusson, A. M., Koenen, K. C., Shin, L. M., Orr, S. P., Gilbertson, M. W., . . . Liberzon, I. (2012). Biological studies of post-traumatic stress disorder. *Nature Reviews Neuroscience, 13*, 769–787. http://dx.doi.org/10.1038/nrn3339

Portfors, C. V. (2007). Types and functions of ultrasonic vocalizations in laboratory rats and mice. *Journal of the American Association for Laboratory Animal Science; JAALAS, 46*(1), 28–34.

Radyushkin, K., Hammerschmidt, K., Boretius, S., Varoqueaux, F., El-Kordi, A., Ronnenberg, A., . . . Ehrenreich, H. (2009). Neuroligin-3-deficient mice: Model of a monogenic heritable form of autism with an olfactory deficit. *Genes, Brain & Behavior, 8,* 416–425. http://dx.doi.org/10.1111/j.1601-183X.2009.00487.x

Rau, V., DeCola, J. P., & Fanselow, M. S. (2005). Stress-induced enhancement of fear learning: An animal model of posttraumatic stress disorder. *Neuroscience and Biobehavioral Reviews, 29,* 1207–1223. http://dx.doi.org/10.1016/j.neubiorev.2005.04.010

Raza, S., Himmler, B. T., Himmler, S. M., Harker, A., Kolb, B., Pellis, S. M., & Gibb, R. (2015). Effects of prenatal exposure to valproic acid on the development of juvenile-typical social play in rats. *Behavioural Pharmacology, 26,* 707–719. http://dx.doi.org/10.1097/fbp.0000000000000169

Rich, T. J., & Hurst, J. L. (1998). Scent marks as reliable signals of the competitive ability of mates. *Animal Behaviour, 56,* 727–735. http://dx.doi.org/10.1006/anbe.1998.0803

Riley, A. L., Hempel, B. J., & Clasen, M. M. (2018). Sex as a biological variable: Drug use and abuse. *Physiology & Behavior, 187,* 79–96. http://dx.doi.org/10.1016/j.physbeh.2017.10.005

Robbins, T. W. (2002). The 5-choice serial reaction time task: Behavioural pharmacology and functional neurochemistry. *Psychopharmacology, 163,* 362–380. http://dx.doi.org/10.1007/s00213-002-1154-7

Roberts, S. C. (2007). Scent marking. *Rodent societies: An ecological and evolutionary perspective,* 255–266.

Roth, M. K., Bingham, B., Shah, A., Joshi, A., Frazer, A., Strong, R., & Morilak, D. A. (2012). Effects of chronic plus acute prolonged stress on measures of coping style, anxiety, and evoked HPA-axis reactivity. *Neuropharmacology, 63,* 1118–1126. http://dx.doi.org/10.1016/j.neuropharm.2012.07.034

Sales, G. (1972). Ultrasound and mating behaviour in rodents with some observations on other behavioural situations. *Journal of Zoology, 168,* 149–164.

Sarnyai, Z., Alsaif, M., Bahn, S., Ernst, A., Guest, P. C., Hradetzky, E., . . . Wesseling, H. (2011). Behavioral and molecular biomarkers in translational animal models for neuropsychiatric disorders. *International Review of Neurobiology, 101,* 203–238. http://dx.doi.org/10.1016/B978-0-12-387718-5.00008-0

Sarris, J., Murphy, J., Mischoulon, D., Papakostas, G. I., Fava, M., Berk, M., & Ng, C. H. (2016). Adjunctive nutraceuticals for depression: A systematic review and meta-analyses. *The American Journal of Psychiatry, 173,* 575–587. http://dx.doi.org/10.1176/appi.ajp.2016.15091228

Sawa, A., & Snyder, S. H. (2002). Schizophrenia: Diverse approaches to a complex disease. *Science,* 296(5568), 692–695. http://dx.doi.org/10.1126/science.1070532

Scattoni, M. L., Crawley, J., & Ricceri, L. (2009). Ultrasonic vocalizations: A tool for behavioural phenotyping of mouse models of neurodevelopmental disorders. *Neuroscience and Biobehavioral Reviews, 33,* 508–515. http://dx.doi.org/10.1016/j.neubiorev.2008.08.003

Scattoni, M. L., Martire, A., Cartocci, G., Ferrante, A., & Ricceri, L. (2013). Reduced social interaction, behavioural flexibility and BDNF signalling in the BTBR T+ tf/J strain, a mouse model of autism. *Behavioural Brain Research, 251,* 35–40. http://dx.doi.org/10.1016/j.bbr.2012.12.028

Schenk, S., & Izenwasser, S. (2002). Pretreatment with methylphenidate sensitizes rats to the reinforcing effects of cocaine. *Pharmacology, Biochemistry, and Behavior, 72,* 651–657. http://dx.doi.org/10.1016/S0091-3057(02)00735-9

Schenk, S., Lacelle, G., Gorman, K., & Amit, Z. (1987). Cocaine self-administration in rats influenced by environmental conditions: Implications for the etiology of drug abuse. *Neuroscience Letters, 81,* 227–231. http://dx.doi.org/10.1016/0304-3940(87)91003-2

Schneider, M., & Koch, M. (2005). Deficient social and play behavior in juvenile and adult rats after neonatal cortical lesion: Effects of chronic pubertal cannabinoid treatment. *Neuropsychopharmacology, 30,* 944–957. http://dx.doi.org/10.1038/sj.npp.1300634

Schneider, T., & Przewłocki, R. (2005). Behavioral alterations in rats prenatally exposed to valproic acid: Animal model of autism. *Neuropsychopharmacology, 30,* 80–89. http://dx.doi.org/10.1038/sj.npp.1300518

Schneider, T., Turczak, J., & Przewłocki, R. (2006). Environmental enrichment reverses behavioral alterations in rats prenatally exposed to valproic acid: Issues for a therapeutic approach in autism. *Neuropsychopharmacology, 31,* 36–46. http://dx.doi.org/10.1038/sj.npp.1300767

Schöner, J., Heinz, A., Endres, M., Gertz, K., & Kronenberg, G. (2017). Post-traumatic stress disorder and beyond: An overview of rodent stress models. *Journal of Cellular and Molecular Medicine, 21,* 2248–2256. http://dx.doi.org/10.1111/jcmm.13161

Scott, S. A., & Crutcher, K. A. (1994). Nerve growth factor and Alzheimer's disease. *Reviews in the Neurosciences, 5,* 179–211. http://dx.doi.org/10.1515/REVNEURO.1994.5.3.179

Seidman, L. J., Biederman, J., Faraone, S. V., Weber, W., & Ouellette, C. (1997). Toward defining a neuropsychology of attention deficit-hyperactivity disorder: Performance of children and adolescents from a large clinically referred sample. *Journal of Consulting and Clinical Psychology, 65,* 150–160. http://dx.doi.org/10.1037/0022-006X.65.1.150

Sengupta, P. (2013). The laboratory rat: Relating its age with human's. *International Journal of Preventive Medicine, 4*(6), 624–630.

Shams, S., Rihel, J., Ortiz, J. G., & Gerlai, R. (2018). The zebrafish as a promising tool for modeling human brain disorders: A review based upon an IBNS symposium. *Neuroscience & Biobehavioral Reviews, 85,* 176–190

Sharma, V., & McNeill, J. H. (2009). To scale or not to scale: The principles of dose extrapolation. *British Journal of Pharmacology, 157,* 907–921. http://dx.doi.org/10.1111/j.1476-5381.2009.00267.x

Sheffer, C., Mackillop, J., McGeary, J., Landes, R., Carter, L., Yi, R., . . . Bickel, W. (2012). Delay discounting, locus of control, and cognitive impulsiveness independently predict tobacco dependence treatment outcomes in a highly dependent, lower socioeconomic group of smokers. *The American Journal on Addictions, 21,* 221–232. http://dx.doi.org/10.1111/j.1521-0391.2012.00224.x

Shuster, L. (1990). Genetics of responses to drugs of abuse. *The International Journal of Addictions, 25,* 57–79. http://dx.doi.org/10.3109/10826089009067005

Simola, N., Frau, L., Plumitallo, A., & Morelli, M. (2014). Direct and long-lasting effects elicited by repeated drug administration on 50-kHz ultrasonic vocalizations are regulated differently: Implications for the study of the affective properties of drugs of abuse. *International Journal of Neuropsychopharmacology, 17,* 429–441. http://dx.doi.org/10.1017/S1461145713001235

Simpson, J., Bree, D., & Kelly, J. P. (2012). Effect of early life housing manipulation on baseline and drug-induced behavioural responses on neurochemistry in the male rat. *Progress in Neuro-Psychopharmacology & Biological Psychiatry, 37,* 252–263. http://dx.doi.org/10.1016/j.pnpbp.2012.02.008

Sng, J., & Meaney, M. J. (2009). Environmental regulation of the neural epigenome. *Epigenomics, 1,* 131–151. http://dx.doi.org/10.2217/epi.09.21

Soldin, O. P., Chung, S. H., & Mattison, D. R. (2011). Sex differences in drug disposition. *Journal of Biomedicine & Biotechnology, 2011,* 1. http://dx.doi.org/10.1155/2011/187103

Soldin, O. P., & Mattison, D. R. (2009). Sex differences in pharmacokinetics and pharmacodynamics. *Clinical Pharmacokinetics, 48,* 143–157. http://dx.doi.org/10.2165/00003088-200948030-00001

Stairs, D. J., & Bardo, M. T. (2009). Neurobehavioral effects of environmental enrichment and drug abuse vulnerability. *Pharmacology, Biochemistry, and Behavior, 92,* 377–382. http://dx.doi.org/10.1016/j.pbb.2009.01.016

Steenbergen, L., Jongkees, B. J., Sellaro, R., & Colzato, L. S. (2016). Tryptophan supplementation modulates social behavior: A review. *Neuroscience and Biobehavioral Reviews, 64,* 346–358. http://dx.doi.org/10.1016/j.neubiorev.2016.02.022

Sutcliffe, A., & Poole, T. (1984). Intragroup agonistic behavior in captive groups of the common marmoset *Callithrix jacchus jacchus. International Journal of Primatology, 5,* 473–489. http://dx.doi.org/10.1007/BF02692270

Takahashi, L. K., Thomas, D. A., & Barfield, R. J. (1983). Analysis of ultrasonic vocalizations emitted by residents during aggressive encounters among rats (*Rattus norvegicus*). *Journal of Comparative Psychology, 97,* 207–212. http://dx.doi.org/10.1037/0735-7036.97.3.207

Takahashi, N., Kashino, M., & Hironaka, N. (2010). Structure of rat ultrasonic vocalizations and its relevance to behavior. *PLoS One, 5*(11), e14115. http://dx.doi.org/10.1371/journal.pone.0014115

Tanaka, E. (1999). Gender-related differences in pharmacokinetics and their clinical significance. *Journal of Clinical Pharmacy and Therapeutics, 24,* 339–346. http://dx.doi.org/10.1046/j.1365-2710.1999.00246.x

Tanzi, R. E., Kovacs, D. M., Kim, T. W., Moir, R. D., Guenette, S. Y., & Wasco, W. (1996). The gene defects responsible for familial Alzheimer's disease. *Neurobiology of Disease, 3,* 159–168. http://dx.doi.org/10.1006/nbdi.1996.0016

Torres, O. V., Jayanthi, S., Ladenheim, B., McCoy, M. T., Krasnova, I. N., & Cadet, J. L. (2017). Compulsive methamphetamine taking under punishment is associated with greater cue-induced drug seeking in rats. *Behavioural Brain Research, 326,* 265–271. http://dx.doi.org/10.1016/j.bbr.2017.03.009

van den Bos, W., Rodriguez, C. A., Schweitzer, J. B., & McClure, S. M. (2015). Adolescent impatience decreases with increased frontostriatal connectivity. *PNAS: Proceedings of the National Academy of Sciences of the United States of America, 112,* E3765–E3774. http://dx.doi.org/10.1073/pnas.1423095112

Vanderschuren, L. J., & Ahmed, S. H. (2013). Animal studies of addictive behavior. *Cold Spring Harbor Perspectives in Medicine, 3,* a011932. http://dx.doi.org/10.1101/cshperspect.a011932

Vanderschuren, L. J., Niesink, R. J., & Van Ree, J. M. (1997). The neurobiology of social play behavior in rats. *Neuroscience and Biobehavioral Reviews, 21,* 309–326. http://dx.doi.org/10.1016/S0149-7634(96)00020-6

Vendruscolo, L. F., Schlosburg, J. E., Misra, K. K., Chen, S. A., Greenwell, T. N., & Koob, G. F. (2011). Escalation patterns of varying periods of heroin access. *Pharmacology, Biochemistry, and Behavior, 98,* 570–574. http://dx.doi.org/10.1016/j.pbb.2011.03.004

Venniro, M., Caprioli, D., & Shaham, Y. (2016). Animal models of drug relapse and craving: From drug priming-induced reinstatement to incubation of craving after voluntary abstinence. *Progress in Brain Research, 224*, 25–52. http://dx.doi.org/10.1016/bs.pbr.2015.08.004

Vivian, J. A., & Miczek, K. A. (1991). Ultrasounds during morphine withdrawal in rats. *Psychopharmacology, 104*, 187–193. http://dx.doi.org/10.1007/BF02244177

Wahlsten, D., Metten, P., & Crabbe, J. C. (2003). Survey of 21 inbred mouse strains in two laboratories reveals that BTBR T/+ tf/tf has severely reduced hippocampal commissure and absent corpus callosum. *Brain Research, 971*, 47–54. http://dx.doi.org/10.1016/S0006-8993(03)02354-0

Wang, X., McCoy, P. A., Rodriguiz, R. M., Pan, Y., Je, H. S., Roberts, A. C., . . . Jiang, Y. H. (2011). Synaptic dysfunction and abnormal behaviors in mice lacking major isoforms of *Shank3*. *Human Molecular Genetics, 20*, 3093–3108. http://dx.doi.org/10.1093/hmg/ddr212

Watson, K. K., & Platt, M. L. (2012). Of mice and monkeys: Using non-human primate models to bridge mouse- and human-based investigations of autism spectrum disorders. *Journal of Neurodevelopmental Disorders, 4*, 01. http://dx.doi.org/10.1186/1866-1955-4-21

Waxman, D. J., & Holloway, M. G. (2009). Sex differences in the expression of hepatic drug metabolizing enzymes. *Molecular Pharmacology, 76*, 215–228. http://dx.doi.org/10.1124/mol.109.056705

Weaver, I. C., Cervoni, N., Champagne, F. A., D'Alessio, A. C., Sharma, S., Seckl, J. R., . . . Meaney, M. J. (2004). Epigenetic programming by maternal behavior. *Nature Neuroscience, 7*, 847–854. http://dx.doi.org/10.1038/nn1276

Weder, N., Zhang, H., Jensen, K., Yang, B. Z., Simen, A., Jackowski, A., . . . Kaufman, J. (2014). Child abuse, depression, and methylation in genes involved with stress, neural plasticity, and brain circuitry. *Journal of the American Academy of Child & Adolescent Psychiatry, 53*, 417–24.e5. http://dx.doi.org/10.1016/j.jaac.2013.12.025

Willner, P. (1986). Validation criteria for animal models of human mental disorders: Learned helplessness as a paradigm case. *Progress in Neuro-Psychopharmacology & Biological Psychiatry, 10*, 677–690. http://dx.doi.org/10.1016/0278-5846(86)90051-5

Willner, P., & Belzung, C. (2015). Treatment-resistant depression: Are animal models of depression fit for purpose? *Psychopharmacology, 232*, 3473–3495. http://dx.doi.org/10.1007/s00213-015-4034-7

Wöhr, M. (2014). Ultrasonic vocalizations in *Shank* mouse models for autism spectrum disorders: Detailed spectrographic analyses and developmental profiles. *Neuroscience and Biobehavioral Reviews, 43*, 199–212. http://dx.doi.org/10.1016/j.neubiorev.2014.03.021

Wolterink, G., Daenen, L. E., Dubbeldam, S., Gerrits, M. A., van Rijn, R., Kruse, C. G., . . . Van Ree, J. M. (2001). Early amygdala damage in the rat as a model for neurodevelopmental psychopathological disorders. *European Neuropsychopharmacology, 11*, 51–59. http://dx.doi.org/10.1016/S0924-977X(00)00138-3

Won, H., Lee, H.-R., Gee, H. Y., Mah, W., Kim, J.-I., Lee, J., . . . Kim, E. (2012). Autistic-like social behaviour in *Shank2*-mutant mice improved by restoring NMDA receptor function. *Nature, 486*, 261–265. http://dx.doi.org/10.1038/nature11208

Wong, G., Zane, N., Saw, A., & Chan, A. K. K. (2013). Examining gender differences for gambling engagement and gambling problems among emerging adults. *Journal of gambling studies / co-sponsored by the National Council on Problem Gambling and Institute for the Study of Gambling and Commercial Gaming, 29*, 171–189. http://dx.doi.org/10.1007/s10899-012-9305-1

Worbe, Y., Savulich, G., Voon, V., Fernandez-Egea, E., & Robbins, T. W. (2014). Serotonin depletion induces "waiting impulsivity" on the human four-choice serial reaction time task: Cross-species translational significance. *Neuropsychopharmacology, 39*, 1519–1526. http://dx.doi.org/10.1038/npp.2013.351

Wurtman, R. J. (1987). Nutrients affecting brain composition and behavior. *Integrative Psychiatry, 5*(4), 226–238.

Yamada, K., & Nabeshima, T. (2000). Animal models of Alzheimer's disease and evaluation of anti-dementia drugs. *Pharmacology & Therapeutics, 88*, 93–113. http://dx.doi.org/10.1016/S0163-7258(00)00081-4

Yehuda, R., Halligan, S. L., & Grossman, R. (2001). Childhood trauma and risk for PTSD: Relationship to intergenerational effects of trauma, parental PTSD, and cortisol excretion. *Development and Psychopathology, 13*, 733–753.

Young, J. W., Winstanley, C. A., Brady, A. M., & Hall, F. S. (2017). Research Domain Criteria versus *DSM V*: How does this debate affect attempts to model corticostriatal dysfunction in animals? *Neuroscience & Biobehavioral Reviews, 76*(Pt B), 301–316. http://dx.doi.org/10.1016/j.neubiorev.2016.10.029

Young, S. N. (2013). The effect of raising and lowering tryptophan levels on human mood and social behaviour. *Philosophical Transactions of the Royal Society of London. Series B, Biological Sciences, 368*, 20110375. http://dx.doi.org/10.1098/rstb.2011.0375

CHAPTER 5

THE ROLE OF CLINICAL (HUMAN) LABORATORY RESEARCH IN PSYCHOPHARMACOLOGY

Robert Miranda, Jr., Lara A. Ray, and Stephanie S. O'Malley

Pharmacotherapy is a key component of evidence-based treatments for many mental health and substance use disorders. One in six adults in the United States takes a psychiatric drug, with higher rates among women (Moore & Mattison, 2017), and one in 13 children and adolescents is prescribed medication for emotional or behavioral difficulties (Howie, Pastor, & Lukacs, 2014). Yet, despite widespread use of psychotropic drugs to abate psychiatric symptoms, the efficacy of most medications is modest and there is considerable person-to-person variability in treatment responsiveness. Moreover, advances in pharmacotherapy for psychiatric disorders have progressed more slowly than those for other health conditions. One reason for this lag is that innovations in medication development rely almost exclusively on traditional clinical trial methods that are costly, take years to inform the potential efficacy of candidate medications, and often yield null findings. Developing new ways to accelerate the drug discovery process is key to advancing clinical care.

Human laboratory paradigms encompass an array of methods for collecting data on central features of psychiatric disorders in experimentally controlled conditions. These methods are increasingly leveraged to advance psychiatric medication development and fill an important translational gap between preclinical analogues and large-scale clinical trials. This chapter starts with a discussion of the value of human laboratory paradigms in the medications development pipeline and in psychopharmacological research more broadly. Next, some of the unique advantages of medication development research in the human laboratory are presented through an illustrative case focused on alcohol use disorder. This example is followed by a review of validated paradigms for capturing clinically relevant intermediate phenotypes that cut across many forms of psychopathology, including reward sensitivity, impulsivity, anxiety, and craving. These transdiagnostic constructs apply to several psychiatric conditions and are considered prime treatment targets for pharmacotherapy for myriad disorders. Next, specific examples of human laboratory paradigms developed to model illnesses in the *Diagnostic and Statistical Manual of Mental Disorders* (5th ed.; *DSM–5*; American Psychiatric Association, 2013)—namely substance use disorders, depression, eating disorders, and posttraumatic stress disorder (PTSD)—are described. Finally, challenges and shortcomings of existing methods are reviewed and recommendations for future directions are provided.

It is important to consider that human laboratory paradigms are rapidly advancing and broadening to address a host of clinical applications. A comprehensive and detailed review of the numerous methodological issues involved in human laboratory paradigms across myriad disorders and

The National Institute of Alcohol Abuse and Alcoholism supported this work (AA007850).

http://dx.doi.org/10.1037/0000133-005
APA Handbook of Psychopharmacology, S. M. Evans (Editor-in-Chief)

facets of psychiatry is beyond the scope of any one chapter. The goal of this chapter is to provide an overview of the application of human laboratory paradigms to advance medication development for psychiatric disorders, including addiction.

RELEVANCE OF LABORATORY PARADIGMS TO PSYCHOPHARMACOLOGICAL RESEARCH

Traditional approaches to discovering new drugs are predicated on culling knowledge gained from preclinical animal models to select novel compounds for investigation in large-scale clinical trials with humans. Although the randomized controlled trial (RTC) remains the gold standard for evaluating the efficacy of new interventions, RTC methods are costly and time-consuming (Perkins & Lerman, 2011). Each new medication costs an estimated two billion dollars and takes an average of 14 years to move from initial drug discovery through human testing to U.S. Food and Drug Administration (FDA) approval (Paul et al., 2010). Furthermore, at least one third of investigational drugs tested in clinical trials fail to show benefit beyond control conditions and do not proceed in the development process (Kola, 2008). The slow-moving pace of advancing available treatment options presents an urgent public health challenge, as prevalence rates of psychiatric disorders continues to rise while treatment effects remain modest.

Human laboratory paradigms are one way to accelerate medication development for psychiatric disorders. By bridging preclinical analogue models and large-scale clinical trials, laboratory paradigms provide a mechanistic evaluation of how novel compounds affect clinically relevant constructs or intermediate phenotypes—that is, reliably measured dynamic neurobehavioral processes underlying psychopathology—and fill a critical gap in the medication development pipeline (McKee, Weinberger, Shi, Tetrault, & Coppola, 2012). Identifying medication effects on intermediate phenotypes associated with clinical efficacy affords a practical approach to screening novel medications to determine whether additional testing in a large-scale clinical trial is warranted.

Modeling medication effects in the human laboratory has several fundamental advantages. Perhaps the most distinct advantage is the high level of experimental control, which maximizes scientific rigor and affords greater confidence that changes observed in the target variables were caused by the experimental medication. Another advantage is that laboratory tests of medication effects on key intermediate phenotypes afford fine-grained and multidimensional assessment of core features of psychiatric disorders. These methods, which span objective behavioral and neurocognitive assessments, psychophysiological recordings, and neuroimaging techniques, provide important information about medication effects that is not otherwise available. Laboratory paradigms can also elucidate how efficacious interventions exert their beneficial effects on key outcomes, thus informing the most promising molecular targets. Human laboratory approaches are less costly than clinical trials and more efficient for screening pharmacotherapies (i.e., can be conducted in a shorter amount of time with fewer participants). Furthermore, laboratory methods capture important person-to-person variability in medication responsiveness and identify the types of patients mostly likely to respond to a given treatment. These methods afford substantial reproducibility, and the careful consideration of procedures and measurements allows for replication of findings across studies and laboratories.

AN ILLUSTRATIVE CASE: THE ALCOHOL CUE REACTIVITY PARADIGM

Human laboratory paradigms are arguably most advanced and widely used in the addiction field, especially in terms of psychopharmacological research (Bujarski & Ray, 2016). Here we demonstrate the application of human laboratory methods to advance medication development for alcohol use disorder. Our goal is to illustrate how laboratory paradigms can elucidate mechanisms of medication effects and capture information about how individuals will respond to interventions. We focus on four key merits of the paradigm, including the ability to detect individual variability, reproducibility, sensitivity to detect differences between experimental medications and placebo, and predictability of clinical trial success. In doing so, it is important to recognize central psychometric constructs such as face validity, predictive validity, and construct validity. Specifically, face validity refers to degree to which the paradigm appears effective at its stated goal. In this case, cue reactivity (e.g., in vivo exposure to alcohol beverage cues) benefits from strong face validity as it captures craving using real-world cues and standardized procedures. Construct validity, in turn, refers to the degree to which a test measures what it claims to measure. As described in this chapter, alcohol cue reactivity represents a gold-standard for capturing alcohol craving in the laboratory and has been subjected to construct validation through comparisons with multiple methodologies. Lastly, predictive validity refers to the extent to which cue reactivity scores predict outcomes on a given criterion measure. As reviewed next, there is strong evidence of predictive validity for cue reactivity, including in the domain of treatment response.

We chose the cue reactivity paradigm because its phenomenology is well characterized across both substance use and eating disorders and among adolescents and adults, it is amenable to a variety of experimental manipulations (e.g., mood/stress induction) and assessment measures (e.g., subjective, physiological, and neuroimaging), and emerging data show it predicts treatment effects in clinical trials. The alcohol cue reactivity paradigm involves systematic exposure to cues (i.e., visual, tactile, olfactory, proprioceptive, etc.) that elicit responses presumed to relate to the motivational processes that underlie drinking. Similar methods are used to study eating disorders. Reactivity can be assessed across multiple domains, including subjective (e.g., craving, mood) and physiological (e.g., heart rate, skin conductance, facial electromyograms, hormones) responses, and neuroimaging studies show that exposure to alcohol and other drug cues reliably produces activation in neural circuits involved in learning and memory (Courtney, Schacht, Hutchison, Roche, & Ray, 2016). In addition, this paradigm can be combined with an emotional overlay via mood induction procedures to broaden the scope of possible mechanisms evaluated (Koob &

Mason, 2016). By doing so, this cue reactivity paradigm can simulate common interoceptive and exteroceptive triggers for relapse, and thus presumably maximize the predictability of outcomes in clinical trials.

During a standard in vivo cue reactivity paradigm, participants complete baseline subjective and physiological measures to capture their current state prior to experimental procedures. Following baseline assessments, participants are presented with a glass half full of water accompanied by a commercially labeled bottle of water. Audio recordings instruct participants to sniff the glass when high tones signaled and stop sniffing when low tones signaled; olfactory exposures occur in variable intervals during each trial. In this way, exposures span visual, tactile, olfactory, and proprioceptive stimuli. Following the water trial, participants undergo a brief relaxation period followed by two alcohol cue exposure trials, which are identical to the water trial except the glass contains their most commonly consumed alcoholic beverage and is accompanied by its commercially labeled bottle. Two alcohol trials ensure a stable estimate of participants' reactions to alcohol cues. At the end of each trial, participants rate their subjective craving. Trials are presented in the same order for all participants because of known carryover effects (Monti et al., 1987).

Reactivity to alcohol and other drug cues varies from person to person, with some individuals showing little or no increase in target variables (e.g., craving) from the baseline or neutral cue trials to alcohol/drug cue trials. Some researchers have operationalized "responders" to cues as individuals who show any change (Monti et al., 1999; Monti et al., 1993), whereas others have specified an exact minimum change (e.g., > 1-point increase in average craving; Shiffman et al., 2003; Tidey, Rohsenow, Kaplan, Swift, & Adolfo, 2008). Potential sources of variability include sex (Rubonis et al., 1994), genetic factors (Bach, Kirsch, et al., 2015; Bach, Vollstädt-Klein, et al., 2015), personality (Bradizza et al., 1999; Litvin & Brandon, 2010), and substance use factors, such as lifetime alcohol use and parental drinking problems (Curtin, Barnett, Colby, Rohsenow, & Monti, 2005), and these individual differences may moderate medication effects

(Hutchison et al., 2006; McGeary et al., 2006; Ooteman et al., 2009).

This paradigm demonstrates a high level of reproducibility. A widely cited meta-analysis of cue reactivity studies reported robust effects for self-reported craving in response to cues and a somewhat smaller, albeit still meaningful, effect size for physiological responses to cues (Carter & Tiffany, 1999). The autonomic profile of cue reactivity is fairly similar across drugs of abuse and is often characterized by increases in heart rate and sweat gland activity and decreases in peripheral temperature. These physiological reactions are sensitive to medication effects (Monti et al., 1999; Ooteman, Koeter, Verheul, Schippers, & van den Brink, 2007).

The cue reactivity paradigm reliably detects significant medication–placebo differences for most medications studied. Cue-induced craving is blunted by a variety of medications, such as naltrexone (Miranda et al., 2014; Monti et al., 1999; O'Malley, Krishnan-Sarin, Farren, Sinha, & Kreek, 2002), gabapentin (Mason, Light, Williams, & Drobes, 2009), mifepristone (Vendruscolo et al., 2015), prazosin (Fox et al., 2012), D-cycloserine (MacKillop et al., 2015), quetiapine (Ray, Chin, Heydari, & Miotto, 2011), and olanzapine (Hutchison et al., 2001), as well as combinations of these medications (Myrick et al., 2008; Ray et al., 2014). Moreover, cue reactivity effects are generally consistent with decreases in craving observed in clinical trials of these medications (Mason et al., 2014; O'Malley et al., 1992; Vendruscolo et al., 2015).

Although few studies have directly examined whether cue reactivity measured in the laboratory prospectively predicts clinical trial success, mounting evidence suggests it may be a powerful tool for understanding how interventions work and for identifying promising new treatment options for addiction (Abrams, Monti, Carey, Pinto, & Jacobus, 1988; Koob & Mason, 2016). Craving in response to alcohol or affective cues is predictive of subsequent drinking outcomes, including relapse (Drummond & Glautier, 1994; Sinha et al., 2011; Spagnolo et al., 2014). Researchers have also examined the association between physiological cue reactivity and relapse, and many studies show physiological reactivity (e.g., salivation, heart rate) predicts relapse

(Drummond & Glautier, 1994; Grüsser et al., 2004; Rohsenow et al., 1994).

This illustration demonstrates the applicability of the cue reactivity paradigm to advancing our understanding of alcohol use disorder on both theoretical and practical levels. Much of this work helped solidify the role of craving in models of addiction and underscored its relevance as an important treatment target. These studies also highlight its utility for comparing a variety of medications using the same methods.

VALIDATED PARADIGMS FOR CAPTURING CLINICALLY RELEVANT ASPECTS OF PSYCHOPATHOLOGY

Neuropsychiatric disorders are pleomorphic with considerable heterogeneity among individuals with the same diagnosis in terms of pathogenesis, symptom presentation, and clinical course. Consequently, there is growing recognition of the importance of identifying dimensional pathophysiological mechanisms, or intermediate phenotypes, that are common across myriad psychiatric disorders (Insel et al., 2010). Aligned with this transdiagnostic approach, several human laboratory models are designed to capture key constructs shared by multiple forms of psychopathology.

Reward Sensitivity

The concept of reward sensitivity is steeped in animal learning research and refers to individual variability in initial responses to reward as well as approach behaviors involved in reward seeking (e.g., incentive salience; Fowles, 1980; Gray, 1970). This propensity is linked to frontostriatal neural circuitry that responds to interoceptive and exteroceptive goal- or reward-relevant cues and governs goal-directed behavior and approach motivation. Several experimental paradigms are available to capture reward sensitivity in the human laboratory. Measures of responsiveness to rewards include performance on gambling, decision making, operant tasks, and neuroimaging paradigms. Common to these tasks is the focus on respondents' subjective, behavioral, or physiological responsiveness to stimuli that experimentally vary in reward salience.

Examples include self-report measures of enjoyment or positive affect in response to presented stimuli; behavioral measures of how hard participants will work during laboratory tasks to obtain rewarding stimuli (e.g., money or preferred music) or how frequently participants respond to higher magnitude or more probable rewards; and physiological measures of reactivity, such as startle or cortisol reactivity, or brain imaging to visual, olfactory, auditory, imaginal stimuli (e.g., guided imagery).

Individual differences in reward sensitivity are associated with specific types of psychopathology. Hypersensitivity to reward, which promotes increased incentive motivation and goal-directed behavior, is associated with mania, hypomania, and the early stages of addiction, while blunted sensitivity, marked by decreased motivation and withdrawal, is characteristic of unipolar depression and more progressed substance use disorders (Alloy, Olino, Freed, & Nusslock, 2016; Volkow, Koob, & McLellan, 2016; Yip & Potenza, 2018). Moreover, abnormalities in reward sensitivity appear to mark vulnerability to certain psychiatric disorders, such as depression (Nelson et al., 2013). For example, youth ages 16 to 20 years at risk for depression based on their family history of major depressive disorder, as compared with low-risk controls, showed reduced sensitivity to reward on a decision-making gambling paradigm administered in the human laboratory (Mannie, Williams, Browning, & Cowen, 2015). Specifically, youth at risk for depression took fewer risks in their wagers on the task as compared with their low-risk counterparts, regardless of the probability of a favorable outcome. This conservative behavioral response style, which is consistent with response patterns observed among individuals with major depression (Forbes & Dahl, 2012), implicates reward sensitivity as a clinically relevant marker for psychiatric liability.

Researchers have examined the effects of a variety of psychotropic agents on these tasks, including drugs of abuse and pharmacotherapies (Adida et al., 2015; Perkins & Karelitz, 2013; White, Lejuez, & de Wit, 2007). For example, recent studies highlight a link between impaired decision making, reflective of heightened reward sensitivity, and bipolar disorder (Adida et al., 2011; Yechiam, Hayden, Bodkins,

O'Donnell, & Hetrick, 2008). Results of a recent open-label study found that lithium treatment was dose-dependently associated with improved performance on a laboratory gambling task (Adida et al., 2015). In addition, emerging evidence suggests that neural activation to reward cues predicts responsiveness to medications in clinical trials. For example, efficacy analyses from a clinical trial that compared varenicline and bupropion for smoking cessation showed that smokers with greater neural activation to naturally rewarding stimuli than to cigarette-related stimuli had a similar benefit from either medication. By contrast, smokers with larger neural responses to cigarette-related stimuli as compared with naturally rewarding cues had greater benefit from varenicline at all time points through the trial (Cinciripini et al., 2017).

Impulsivity

From a behavioral and cognitive neuroscience perspective, impulsivity or low behavioral inhibition refers to two interrelated processes (Peters & Büchel, 2011; Robbins, Gillan, Smith, de Wit, & Ersche, 2012; Winstanley, Olausson, Taylor, & Jentsch, 2010). The first is impulsive action or behavioral/motor impulsivity, which is characterized by difficulty preventing the initiation of a behavior or stopping a behavior already in action (Hamilton, Littlefield, et al., 2015; Hamilton, Mitchell, et al., 2015). The second is impulsive choice or cognitive impulsivity, which is characterized by the tendency to prefer small immediate rewards rather than larger delayed ones. These two constructs are weakly correlated, supporting their unique contributions to understanding impulsivity (Hamilton, Littlefield, et al., 2015; Reynolds, Penfold, & Patak, 2008).

Aspects of impulsive behavior are central to many forms of psychopathology, such as neuro-developmental disorders, disruptive disorders, impulse-control disorders, conduct disorders, and addiction. Examples of paradigms used to measure behavioral inhibition in the human laboratory, along with the effects of medications on these phenotypes, include continuous performance tasks, go/no-go tasks, and stop-signal tasks. Continuous performance tasks involve continuous monitoring of target stimuli and provide a measure of inhibition and inattention. Acute doses of stimulant medications generally improve performance on these tasks (Hall et al., 2016). Go/no-go tasks provide a behavioral measure of impulse control by capturing the ability to inhibit prepotent responses to a specified stimulus, and there are a number of variations of the basic paradigm (Fillmore, 2003; Newman, Widom, & Nathan, 1985). Studies with individuals with attention-deficit/hyperactivity disorder (ADHD) show that performance on a variety of go/no-go tasks is sensitive to psychostimulants (Chamberlain et al., 2011). In addition, studies have paired this behavioral paradigm with the assessment of event-related potentials (ERPs) to capture brain activity during the task (Luijten et al., 2014). Stimulant medications typically increase amplitudes of certain ERP components (i.e., P3), and emerging data suggest that brain activity recorded during the task predicts stimulant treatment response among children and adolescents with ADHD (Ogrim et al., 2014). Stop-signal tasks are reaction time assessments that measure the speed of inhibitory processing during a discrimination test (Alderson, Rapport, & Kofler, 2007). Stimulant medications generally improve performance on these tasks in a dose-dependent manner (Coghill et al., 2014; Rosch et al., 2016).

Anxiety

Fear conditioning has long been applied as an etiological model for anxiety disorders (Craske et al., 2009). Specifically, enhanced acquisition of conditioned fear and deficits in extinction are believed to contribute to long-lasting anxiety (Mineka & Zinbarg, 2006). In support, a meta-analysis (Lissek et al., 2005) and most subsequent studies (Craske et al., 2008; Liberman, Lipp, Spence, & March, 2006; Otto et al., 2007; Waters, Henry, & Neumann, 2009) suggested that, compared with healthy controls, those with anxiety disorders exhibit stronger responding to the conditioned stimulus (CS+) in simple fear conditioning (reflecting enhanced conditioning) and during extinction (reflecting impaired extinction). In general, the differences from controls are stronger during extinction than during acquisition, and the extinction effects appear to be not solely due to elevated acquisition responding (Liberman et al., 2006; Otto et al., 2007).

Elevations in responding to the CS+ persist at extinction recall (Milad et al., 2008). Although the various forms of fear learning represent complex processes involving multiple brain regions, evidence in rodents, nonhuman primates, and humans most consistently implicates the amygdala in the instantiation of stimulus–reinforcement associations and the ventral medial prefrontal cortex in fear extinction and recall of extinction learning (Shin & Liberzon, 2010; Sotres-Bayon, Cain, & LeDoux, 2006). In the laboratory, participants are trained to acquire a fear response to a given stimuli, and psychophysiological measures (i.e., galvanic skin response) and subjective ratings are often used as dependent measures of fear acquisition, fear extinction, and extinction recall, with each level of analysis having distinct clinical significance (Vervliet, Craske, & Hermans, 2013). Importantly, fear-conditioning models can be applied across species, thus facilitating translational research in anxiety and related disorders. Further, these models have been used in the context of treatment development, particularly extinction-derived strategies for optimizing exposure therapy for anxiety disorders and augmentation of consolidation through NMDA receptor antagonists (Rodrigues et al., 2014).

Craving

Craving, or the urge/desire to use a drug or consume certain foods, is central to contemporary models of addiction, binge eating, and obesity (Drummond, 2000; Sinha, 2018). Alcohol and other drugs of abuse as well as highly palatable foods (e.g., processed foods high in saturated fats or carbohydrates) produce a host of pleasurable effects by stimulating brain reward circuitry (Sinha, 2018; Volkow et al., 2016). This activation of reward pathways promotes associative learning that over time triggers activation of the brain's reward and appetitive motivational systems in response to environmental stimuli paired with substance use and food consumption. This anticipatory response (i.e., cue reactivity) to conditioned stimuli elicits craving and heightens the probability and intensity of subsequent substance use and food intake (Ramirez & Miranda, 2014). Indeed, subjective and physiological reactivity to drug and food cues are thought to reflect motivational processes that maintain maladaptive drug and food consumption.

Exposure to alcohol and food cues can simulate a high-risk situation for relapse or excessive food consumption, especially when performed with recently abstinent individuals or those with a higher body mass index (Sinha, 2018). Craving and other indices of cue reactivity are strong predictors of substance use and greater food intake in the human laboratory (Hilbert et al., 2018; Leeman, Corbin, & Fromme, 2009; O'Malley et al., 2002) and the natural environment (Chao, Jastreboff, White, Grilo, & Sinha, 2017; Miranda et al., 2016; Ramirez & Miranda, 2014). As such, they are considered clinically relevant intermediate phenotypes predictive of clinical outcomes.

Numerous studies have examined the ability of medications to dampen this craving response. Medications (e.g., gabapentin, naltrexone) that decrease alcohol cue-elicited craving in the laboratory typically also reduce craving and drinking in clinical trials (Mason et al., 2014; Miranda et al., 2014). Findings from persons with eating disorders show a similar pattern (Davis et al., 2012; Davis, Levitan, Kaplan, Carter-Major, & Kennedy, 2016). On the whole, human studies and animal models suggest that individuals for whom drug or food cues attain incentive motivational value or incentive salience are most likely to exhibit relapse to excessive drug or food consumption.

EXAMPLES OF PARADIGMS DEVELOPED TO MODEL *DSM–5* DISORDERS

For the past two decades, researchers have increasingly leveraged human laboratory paradigms to advance pharmacotherapy for a variety of psychiatric disorders. As we have emphasized, on the whole this work has transformed how we screen novel medications for potential efficacy and improved our understanding of the mechanisms by which efficacious medications exert their beneficial effects. The next section describes examples of paradigms used to study substance use disorders, major depressive disorder, eating disorders, and PTSD. In addition, we review evidence that supports their utility.

Substance Use Disorders

Addiction is chronic brain disease characterized by a compulsive cycle of intoxication, craving, bingeing, and withdrawal that persists despite negative consequences (Litten et al., 2015; Volkow et al., 2016). Contemporary models stress the importance of the transition from controlled to excessive maladaptive alcohol and other substance use, and researchers have theorized two key pathogenic mechanisms that may explain why individuals, especially adolescents and young adults, are especially susceptible to this shift (Koob, 2009; Volkow & Li, 2005; Volkow et al., 2016). Alcohol and other drugs disrupt "bottom-up" motivational processes that evaluate the reward/incentive salience of environmental stimuli and sensitize the brain to the acute effects of substance use and drug-related cues. At the same time, impaired "top-down" executive control over prepotent responses compromises inhibitory control and reward processing. Together, these two important facets of neurocognitive dysfunction appear to both heighten sensitivity to substance use and drug cues and compromise impulse control, thereby promoting excessive and maladaptive use.

There are multiple paradigms for studying addiction pathology in the human laboratory, and researchers have leveraged nearly all of these tasks to study medication effects on key intermediate phenotypes (Ray, Bujarski, & Roche, 2016; Yardley & Ray, 2017). Beyond the cue reactivity paradigm reviewed earlier in this chapter, these paradigms often include alcohol (and drug) administration paradigms, also known as alcohol (or drug) challenges. They consist of controlled administration of alcohol or drugs under laboratory conditions and typically involve psychophysiological and subjective ratings of intoxication as primary endpoints. In addition to the forced administration (or challenge) paradigm, self-administration and progression ratio administration models have also been used. Self-administration consists of allowing individuals to decide whether or not to self-administer alcohol (or drugs), typically choosing between the alcohol/drug and a monetary reward. The endpoint for the self-administration model consists of total number of self-administrations or time to first self-administration.

In turn, progressive ratio self-administration consists of asking individuals to "work" for a given reinforcer in ways such that the required workload increases systematically. Breakpoint, defined as the point at which individuals stop working for the reinforcer, is the typical outcome measure for progressive ratio models. In addition to the experimental manipulations capturing the binge-intoxication stage (administration, self-administration, and progressive ratio administration), a host of behavioral tasks have been recently employed to capture dimensions of binge-intoxication and loss of control. These are measures such as delay discounting (in which individuals choose between smaller immediate reinforcers and later larger reinforcers) and the stop-signal task (in which individuals are asked to inhibit a prepotent response in the presence of an inhibitory cue such as a loud sound).

Rather than focusing on a single paradigm, more recent studies have combined a host of paradigms to more effectively screen pharmacotherapies (e.g., alcohol administration combined with alcohol self-administration; Ray, Green, et al., 2018). This may be particularly useful in screening novel compounds whereby the mechanisms of action may be less clear, thus requiring a more comprehensive assessment of multiple putative mechanisms in the laboratory. For example, a recent human laboratory study of a novel neuro-immune modulator (ibudilast) for the treatment of alcoholism combined alcohol cue reactivity, stress reactivity, and alcohol administration methodologies to assess the initial efficacy of the drug (Ray, Bujarski, Shoptaw, et al., 2017). While taking ibudilast, compared with placebo, participants reported mood improvements during stress exposure and alcohol cue exposure, as well as reductions in tonic levels of alcohol craving. As the field of medication development for alcoholism progresses towards elucidating novel targets and compounds (Litten et al., 2012; Litten, Falk, Ryan, & Fertig, 2016), a flexible application of a wide range of human laboratory models to screen pharmacotherapies for early efficacy will become more prevalent.

Major Depressive Disorder

Major depressive disorder (MDD) is a complex psychiatric condition that develops from the dynamic interplay between myriad neurobiological, genetic, and psychosocial factors. Researchers have applied several behavioral paradigms to study core features of MDD, including reward sensitivity and processing. Studies of reward sensitivity show that adolescents and adults with depression consistently fail to approach rewards in behavioral tasks. These effects are observed in tasks that involve explicit approach (Cella, Dymond, & Cooper, 2010; Han et al., 2012), such as the Iowa Gambling Task (Bechara, Damasio, Damasio, & Anderson, 1994) and the Effort Expenditure for Rewards Task (Treadway, Buckholtz, Schwartzman, Lambert, & Zald, 2009), and where rewards are implicitly learned, such as signal detection tasks (Morris, Bylsma, Yaroslavsky, Kovacs, & Rottenberg, 2015; Pizzagalli, Iosifescu, Hallett, Ratner, & Fava, 2008; Pizzagalli, Jahn, & O'Shea, 2005).

Clinical neuroscience investigations of reward processing in depression have included resting state frontal electroencephalography (EEG), ERPs, and functional magnetic resonance imaging (fMRI). For example, a meta-analytic review concluded that depression is characterized by patterns of frontal asymmetry, with heightened right activation, which is indicative of heightened withdrawal-related affect (Thibodeau, Jorgensen, & Kim, 2006). Studies also show that only early-onset depression is associated with reduced left frontal asymmetry during a laboratory-based gambling task (Shankman, Klein, Tenke, & Bruder, 2007), which suggests that frontal asymmetry may represent a subtype of MDD. Others have found blunted feedback negativity in ERPs—electrical potentials elicited by specific stimuli that measures reward sensitivity—among individuals with more severe depression (Foti & Hajcak, 2009; Liu et al., 2014). These findings afford an objective index of reward hyposensitivity in MDD. Finally, researchers have paired reward sensitivity tasks with fMRI to assess brain reactivity to a variety of rewards. Numerous studies have demonstrated that individuals with depression, as compared with nondepressed controls, exhibit reduced neural activity to rewarding stimuli

(Chantiluke et al., 2012; Forbes et al., 2009; Smoski, Rittenberg, & Dichter, 2011).

Few studies have applied laboratory paradigms to investigate medication effects in persons with MDD, but research in this area is growing and early findings are compelling. Several EEG studies found that SSRI treatment is associated with changes in prefrontal oscillatory activity (Bares et al., 2010; Leuchter, Cook, Gilmer, et al., 2009; Leuchter, Cook, Marangell, et al., 2009), and changes in oscillatory activity observed early in medication treatment predicted remission of depressive symptoms 7 weeks later (Leuchter et al., 2017).

Eating Disorders

Binge-eating disorder (BED) is characterized by recurrent episodes of excessive food intake and occurs in 2% to 5% of the adult population, making it the most common eating disorder (Dingemans, Bruna, & van Furth, 2002; Kessler et al., 2013). Research implicates several interconnected intermediate phenotypes at the core of BED, including attentional bias towards food cues, cognitive flexibility, and perseverative or compulsive behavior. Researchers have studied binge eating in the human laboratory, where individuals with BED engage in binge eating in a standardized setting, and findings showed that participants with BED consumed significantly more food and ate at a faster rate than control participants (Sysko, Devlin, Walsh, Zimmerli, & Kissileff, 2007; Walsh, 2011; Walsh & Boudreau, 2003; Yanovski et al., 1992).

Theoretical models posit that negative affect plays a central role in the pathogenesis of BED, and mounting evidence from the human laboratory supports this link. For example, negative affect elicited in the human laboratory was associated with increased urge to binge eat (Zeeck, Stelzer, Linster, Joos, & Hartmann, 2011). In addition, adults with BED consume larger amounts of food, exhibit greater loss of control, and consume food more quickly following the negative mood induction relative to a relaxed condition and compared with individuals without BED. Examples of experimental procedures used to elicit negative affect include viewing sad video clips (Svaldi, Tuschen-Caffier, Trentowska, Caffier, & Naumann, 2014)

and performing a stress-inducing behavioral task, namely the Trier Social Stress Test (Kirschbaum, Pirke, & Hellhammer, 1993; Laessle & Schulz, 2009). During this well-established stress induction task, research participants prepare a speaking monologue and complete a verbal math test in front of an audience that provides no positive feedback while subjective, cardiovascular, and hormone responses are typically recorded.

Although laboratory studies have advanced our understanding of the link between negative affect and binge eating, application of these methods to pharmacotherapy research is at a nascent stage. The FDA recently approved lisdexamfetamine dimesylate (Vyvanse), a d-amphetamine prodrug indicated for the treatment of ADHD, for the treatment of adults with moderate to severe BED (McElroy, Hudson, et al., 2016; McElroy, Mitchell, et al., 2016), and other medications are commonly prescribed off-label (Grilo, Reas, & Mitchell, 2016). Studies have shown the psychostimulant methylphenidate, as compared with placebo, reduces subjective appetite, cravings, and food consumption in the human laboratory, especially among women (Davis et al., 2012; Davis et al., 2016). In addition, pharmacotherapies for obesity have been evaluated for effects on brain reactivity to food cues (Wang et al., 2014) and eating behavior (Spiegel et al., 1987) in the laboratory.

Posttraumatic Stress Disorder

Substantial knowledge exists about the pathophysiology of PTSD. But advances in our understanding of PTSD have not yet translated into new pharmacotherapies, and currently approved treatments for PTSD, namely paroxetine and sertraline, are suboptimal (Kelmendi et al., 2016). PTSD occurs following exposure to traumatic events and is defined in the *DSM–5* by symptoms of reexperiencing the event (e.g., distressing thoughts, dreams, flashbacks), persistent avoidance of stimuli associated with the event, negative cognitions and mood (e.g., feelings of detachment, inability to experience positive feelings, distorted cognitions about the event), and hyperarousal and reactivity associated with the event (e.g., exaggerated startle reactions, poor concentration, irritability and jumpiness, insomnia, and hypervigilance; Shalev, Liberzon, & Marmar, 2017). Functional neuroimaging studies in animals and human subjects have implicated neural systems in the pathophysiology of PTSD, including fear learning, threat detection, executive function, and emotion regulation and contextual processing (Shalev et al., 2017).

Laboratory paradigms—both preclinical and human studies—have been used to understand PTSD. In human subjects, the most common laboratory paradigm exposes participants to trauma-related stimuli (e.g., sounds, pictures, mental imagery) and compares their responses to those elicited by neutral control stimuli (Keane et al., 1998; Pitman, Orr, Forgue, de Jong, & Claiborn, 1987). Measured outcomes include psychophysiological responses (heart rate, heart rate variability, blood pressure, skin conductance, cortisol, startle response), self-reports of distress, and ratings of emotions. Using this approach, research suggests that heart rate increases to trauma-related cues is a distinguishing feature of PTSD (Keane et al., 1998), and a recent meta-analysis concluded that skin conductance is the most sensitive measure of hyperarousal (Pineles et al., 2013). An innovation in the presentation of trauma-related stimuli is the use of virtual reality, which researches have applied to study medication effects. For example, researchers have studied the effects of D-cycloserine or alprazolam in combination with exposure therapy using virtual reality to present trauma-related cues, and measured startle and cortisol responses to combat stimuli pretherapy and post-therapy as outcomes (Rothbaum et al., 2014).

Individuals with PTSD show exaggerated psycho-physiological responses not only to aversive stimuli but also to safety cues not previously paired with the aversive outcome, and they show heightened fear responses during extinction when the aversive stimulus is no longer paired with the aversive outcome. This pattern of findings suggests an inability to regulate fear and relates to reexperiencing symptoms of PTSD (Jovanovic, Rauch, Rothbaum, & Rothbaum, 2017). This paradigm shows promise for screening pharmacotherapies; in one study, dexamethasone was demonstrated to reverse deficits in fear extinction and to improve discrimination of safety cues (Michopoulos et al., 2017).

Although several paradigms are available to screen medications for PTSD, it is unlikely that any one paradigm will be sufficient to predict a drug's potential efficacy for treating PTSD in clinical trials. Drug approval by the FDA is based on significant differences on the Clinician-Administered PTSD Scale for DSM–5 (CAPS5) Total, an interviewer-based assessment of the frequency and severity of PTSD symptoms (Weathers et al., 2013), with good response often defined by a specific threshold (e.g., 30% improvement) for improvement (Davidson, Rothbaum, van der Kolk, Sikes, & Farfel, 2001). As a result, a medication development program for PTSD should consider incorporating several paradigms to screen for effects on the varied symptoms associated with PTSD.

LIMITATIONS AND RECOMMENDATIONS FOR FUTURE RESEARCH

Human laboratory paradigms have proven useful for screening novel medications and elucidating the mechanisms by which efficacious medications produce beneficial effects. As with all research methods, however, these paradigms must be considered in the context of their shortcomings. There are several important considerations, including ecological validity, delineation of temporal associations between putative mechanisms of pharmacotherapy action and actual changes in target behaviors, sensitivity to between-person variability, including the ability to capture age and sex differences, detection of differences between experimental medications and placebo, and predictability of clinical trial success.

Lack of Ecological Validity

What laboratory research gains in terms of experimental control it loses in terms of ecological validity. Rapid advances in knowledge about promising medications require not only data from controlled laboratory settings but also essential information about how laboratory findings generalize to behavior in the natural environment. At present, our understanding of how observations from the human laboratory relate to real-world behaviors is at an early stage (Ramirez & Miranda, 2014), and few studies have directly tested whether medication effects on intermediate phenotypes captured via laboratory paradigms predict treatment responsiveness (Leuchter et al., 2017). In addition, not all medications with demonstrated efficacy to treat psychopathology produce observable effects on human laboratory paradigms. For example, certain medications that reduce alcohol consumption in clinical trials do not reliably affect cue reactivity in the human laboratory (Hammarberg, Jayaram-Lindström, Beck, Franck, & Reid, 2009; Miranda et al., 2008; Miranda et al., 2016; Ooteman et al., 2007). These findings highlight that not all candidate paradigms are suited to detect relevant intermediate phenotypes for a given medication. Careful consideration is necessary when selecting paradigms to study specific experimental medications, and assessing multiple possible mechanisms is often advantageous.

In this regard, greater attention may need to be paid to prioritizing intermediate outcomes that are most highly predictive of the outcomes on which pharmacotherapies are approved. At present, the only efficacy outcomes accepted by the FDA for substance use disorders are abstinence and no heavy drinking for alcohol use disorder and abstinence for smoking cessation; most recently, the approval of lisdexamfetamine dimesylate for BED was based on reductions in the frequency of binge eating. Thus, it is important to consider face, predictive, and construct validity of human laboratory models to clinical relevance and application. Inasmuch as laboratory paradigms are leveraged to screen novel medications and expedite the drug discovery process, it is critical that any signal on intermediate phenotypes measured in the laboratory predict clinical outcomes in real-world settings. Thus, for addictive and eating behaviors, the predictive utility of laboratory paradigms might benefit from inclusion of behavioral outcomes, such as number of drinks or number of calories consumed, or the ability to delay use (Leeman et al., 2010; O'Malley et al., 2002; Udo, Harrison, Shi, Tetrault, & McKee, 2013). Similarly, for mood and anxiety disorders, laboratory paradigms might benefit from the inclusion of measures that best align with the types of outcomes used to evaluate the efficacy of medication

in clinical trials and by regulatory agencies such as the FDA.

Inadequate Attention to Individual Differences

Despite disparities across many neuropsychiatric disorders, much of the laboratory research to date has included only limited numbers of women and persons from diverse backgrounds. Even studies that include balanced numbers of women and minorities often either do not provide analyses specific to these subgroups or do not have sufficient statistical power to provide meaningful information about whether the effects of the experimental medication differ by gender or minority status.

This shortcoming arises, in part, from the considerable statistical power afforded by the experimental control in laboratory paradigms, which allows for smaller sample sizes. Although this quality is a notable advantage, researchers should consider whether studies are adequately powered to assess whether findings generalize across genders and minority groups. This limitation is particularly concerning in light of mounting evidence for important sex differences in treatment responsiveness (O'Malley et al., 2018). For example, research shows that methylphenidate suppresses appetite ratings, food cravings, and food consumption in the human laboratory among women who are overweight/obese, but not among men (Davis et al., 2016). Others have shown that guanfacine, an alpha-2 agonist, enhanced cognitive inhibitory function following a cue reactivity paradigm among treatment-seeking women with cocaine dependence (Milivojevic, Fox, Jayaram-Lindstrom, Hermes, & Sinha, 2017). But, this effect was not observed in their male counterparts. The issue of sex-differences in human laboratory models warrants attention in future research, particularly because human laboratory models have typically enrolled small samples that are not adequately powered to detect sex differences. As the National Institutes of Health has increased its focus on sex-differences research and provided more clear guidelines for the expected consideration of sex as a biological variable in research (https://grants.nih.gov/grants/guide/notice-files/NOT-OD-15-102.html), we expect that human laboratory models will become increasingly relevant to elucidating sex differences across a host of pertinent clinical phenotypes.

Similarly, most laboratory studies are restricted to adults despite clear evidence that the onset of nearly all psychiatric disorders occurs during adolescence and young adulthood. The relevance of pharmaco-therapies to the development of more effective, comprehensive care for adolescents with certain disorders is unclear, in part, because the quality of evidence on which to make recommendations is limited. Indeed, compelling evidence from several branches of medicine demonstrate that the safety and efficacy of medication use with adolescents cannot be inferred from adult data (Bridge et al., 2007; Mayes et al., 2007; Safer, 2004). Consequently, recent legislative changes require that medications indicated for adults also be tested with pediatric populations. Lastly, differences between treatment-seeking individuals and nontreatment seekers have been recently highlighted as a potential source of variability that hinders the integration of human laboratory data and clinical trials outcomes (Ray, Bujarski, Yardley, Roche, & Hartwell, 2017; Rohn et al., 2017).

Unknown Predictability of Treatment Responsiveness

Laboratory paradigms are also limited in their ability to elucidate mechanisms of beneficial treatment effects, even though they are commonly used for this purpose. Data collected in the laboratory, which often comprises a static measure assessed at a single time point, typically cannot inform the temporal sequence of putative mechanisms on behavioral changes in the real world. Even when laboratory studies show medication effects on a putative mechanism of action (e.g., reward sensitivity, alcohol or other drug craving), such findings only test the first link of the proposed causal chain from medication to putative mechanism of action, and leave the second link from the mechanism to the clinical outcome (e.g., depressive symptoms, alcohol and other drug use) to be assumed from other research. In addition, clinical scientists have argued that the most useful intermediate phenotypes are likely to be state-dependent and dynamic (Leuchter, Hunter, Krantz, & Cook, 2014), and this may be especially

salient when intermediate phenotypes fluctuate rapidly over time and vary greatly (e.g., duration, intensity) within the same individual, such as with mood states (e.g., stress or anxiety and depressive symptoms); impulsivity; reward sensitivity; craving for highly palatable food, alcohol, or other drugs of abuse; and subjective responses of substance and food consumption. Thus, the reproducibility and generalizability of measures captured in the laboratory may be limited.

One way to maximize clinical utility is to pair human laboratory research with ecological momentary assessment (EMA) methods. Using EMA methods, also referred to as experience sampling, data on momentary events are collected in real time in participants' natural environments, affording a truly prospective analysis of the relationship between specific events and target behaviors, such as stressful events, food consumption, and alcohol and other drug use (Connolly & Alloy, 2018; Haynos et al., 2017; Miranda et al., 2016; Wonderlich et al., 2017). Capturing momentary events in natural settings allows for the gathering of real-time data on dynamic constructs (e.g., affective states, craving, eating behaviors, substance use) and of temporal and contextual data, which are difficult and at times impossible to simulate in the human laboratory. Unlike other methods, EMA is an inherently idiographic approach uniquely suited for examining individual variability in dynamic constructs that evolve over time, testing the strength of associations with contextual factors, and parsing within- and between-subjects variance (Shiffman, 2014). Thus, although human laboratory studies are the standard for understanding medication mechanisms, pairing EMA methods with laboratory paradigms can provide important information not obtainable from laboratory paradigms alone.

CONCLUSION

Laboratory paradigms can screen medications for treating psychopathology across the lifespan in rapid fashion and can also help elucidate how efficacious medications exert their beneficial effects, thus informing the types of medications that are most promising as well as the types of individuals most likely to benefit from a given treatment. Medication development research in the human laboratory is most comprehensively studied using multiple paradigms that target an array of behavioral, physiological, and neurocognitive phenotypes. Further, efforts to refine human laboratory methods to harness their full translational potential are underway and focus on obtaining a highly representative clinical sample and a well characterized set of behavioral and biological markers that are most relevant to mechanisms of psychopathology maintenance and recovery.

References

Abrams, D. B., Monti, P. M., Carey, K. B., Pinto, R. P., & Jacobus, S. I. (1988). Reactivity to smoking cues and relapse: Two studies of discriminant validity. *Behaviour Research and Therapy, 26,* 225–233. http://dx.doi.org/10.1016/0005-7967(88)90003-4

Adida, M., Jollant, F., Clark, L., Besnier, N., Guillaume, S., Kaladjian, A., . . . Courtet, P. (2011). Trait-related decision-making impairment in the three phases of bipolar disorder. *Biological Psychiatry, 70,* 357–365. http://dx.doi.org/10.1016/j.biopsych.2011.01.018

Adida, M., Jollant, F., Clark, L., Guillaume, S., Goodwin, G. M., Azorin, J. M., & Courtet, P. (2015). Lithium might be associated with better decision-making performance in euthymic bipolar patients. *European Neuropsychopharmacology, 25,* 788–797. http://dx.doi.org/10.1016/j.euroneuro.2015.03.003

Alderson, R. M., Rapport, M. D., & Kofler, M. J. (2007). Attention-deficit/hyperactivity disorder and behavioral inhibition: A meta-analytic review of the stop-signal paradigm. *Journal of Abnormal Child Psychology, 35,* 745–758. http://dx.doi.org/10.1007/s10802-007-9131-6

Alloy, L. B., Olino, T., Freed, R. D., & Nusslock, R. (2016). Role of reward sensitivity and processing in major depressive and bipolar spectrum disorders. *Behavior Therapy, 47,* 600–621. http://dx.doi.org/10.1016/j.beth.2016.02.014

American Psychiatric Association. (2013). *Diagnostic and statistical manual of mental disorders* (5th ed.). Washington, DC: American Psychiatric Association.

Bach, P., Kirsch, M., Hoffmann, S., Jorde, A., Mann, K., Frank, J., . . . Vollstädt-Klein, S. (2015). The effects of single nucleotide polymorphisms in glutamatergic neurotransmission genes on neural response to alcohol cues and craving. *Addiction Biology, 20,* 1022–1032. http://dx.doi.org/10.1111/adb.12291

Bach, P., Vollstädt-Klein, S., Kirsch, M., Hoffmann, S., Jorde, A., Frank, J., . . . Kiefer, F. (2015). Increased

mesolimbic cue-reactivity in carriers of the mu-opioid-receptor gene *OPRM1* A118G polymorphism predicts drinking outcome: A functional imaging study in alcohol dependent subjects. *European Neuropsychopharmacology, 25,* 1128–1135. http://dx.doi.org/10.1016/j.euroneuro.2015.04.013

Bares, M., Brunovsky, M., Novak, T., Kopecek, M., Stopkova, P., Sos, P., . . . Höschl, C. (2010). The change of prefrontal QEEG theta cordance as a predictor of response to bupropion treatment in patients who had failed to respond to previous antidepressant treatments. *European Neuropsychopharmacology, 20,* 459–466. http://dx.doi.org/10.1016/j.euroneuro.2010.03.007

Bechara, A., Damasio, A. R., Damasio, H., & Anderson, S. W. (1994). Insensitivity to future consequences following damage to human prefrontal cortex. *Cognition, 50,* 7–15. http://dx.doi.org/10.1016/0010-0277(94)90018-3

Bradizza, C. M., Gulliver, S. B., Stasiewicz, P. R., Torrisi, R., Rohsenow, D. J., & Monti, P. M. (1999). Alcohol cue reactivity and private self-consciousness among male alcoholics. *Addictive Behaviors, 24,* 543–549. http://dx.doi.org/10.1016/S0306-4603(98)00093-8

Bridge, J. A., Iyengar, S., Salary, C. B., Barbe, R. P., Birmaher, B., Pincus, H. A., . . . Brent, D. A. (2007). Clinical response and risk for reported suicidal ideation and suicide attempts in pediatric antidepressant treatment: A meta-analysis of randomized controlled trials. *JAMA, 297,* 1683–1696. http://dx.doi.org/10.1001/jama.297.15.1683

Bujarski, S., & Ray, L. A. (2016). Experimental psychopathology paradigms for alcohol use disorders: Applications for translational research. *Behaviour Research and Therapy, 86,* 11–22. http://dx.doi.org/10.1016/j.brat.2016.05.008

Carter, B. L., & Tiffany, S. T. (1999). Meta-analysis of cue-reactivity in addiction research. *Addiction, 94,* 327–340. http://dx.doi.org/10.1046/j.1360-0443.1999.9433273.x

Cella, M., Dymond, S., & Cooper, A. (2010). Impaired flexible decision-making in major depressive disorder. *Journal of Affective Disorders, 124,* 207–210. http://dx.doi.org/10.1016/j.jad.2009.11.013

Chamberlain, S. R., Robbins, T. W., Winder-Rhodes, S., Müller, U., Sahakian, B. J., Blackwell, A. D., & Barnett, J. H. (2011). Translational approaches to frontostriatal dysfunction in attention-deficit/hyperactivity disorder using a computerized neuropsychological battery. *Biological Psychiatry, 69,* 1192–1203. http://dx.doi.org/10.1016/j.biopsych.2010.08.019

Chantiluke, K., Halari, R., Simic, M., Pariante, C. M., Papadopoulos, A., Giampietro, V., & Rubia, K. (2012). Fronto-striato-cerebellar dysregulation in adolescents with depression during motivated attention. *Biological Psychiatry, 71,* 59–67. http://dx.doi.org/10.1016/j.biopsych.2011.09.005

Chao, A. M., Jastreboff, A. M., White, M. A., Grilo, C. M., & Sinha, R. (2017). Stress, cortisol, and other appetite-related hormones: Prospective prediction of 6-month changes in food cravings and weight. *Obesity, 25,* 713–720. http://dx.doi.org/10.1002/oby.21790

Cinciripini, P. M., Green, C. E., Robinson, J. D., Karam-Hage, M., Engelmann, J. M., Minnix, J. A., . . . Versace, F. (2017). Benefits of varenicline vs. bupropion for smoking cessation: A Bayesian analysis of the interaction of reward sensitivity and treatment. *Psychopharmacology, 234,* 1769–1779. http://dx.doi.org/10.1007/s00213-017-4580-2

Coghill, D. R., Seth, S., Pedroso, S., Usala, T., Currie, J., & Gagliano, A. (2014). Effects of methylphenidate on cognitive functions in children and adolescents with attention-deficit/hyperactivity disorder: Evidence from a systematic review and a meta-analysis. *Biological Psychiatry, 76,* 603–615. http://dx.doi.org/10.1016/j.biopsych.2013.10.005

Connolly, S. L., & Alloy, L. B. (2018). Negative event recall as a vulnerability for depression: Relationship between momentary stress-reactive rumination and memory for daily life stress. *Clinical Psychological Science, 6,* 32–47. http://dx.doi.org/10.1177/2167702617729487

Courtney, K. E., Schacht, J. P., Hutchison, K., Roche, D. J., & Ray, L. A. (2016). Neural substrates of cue reactivity: Association with treatment outcomes and relapse. *Addiction Biology, 21* 3–22.

Craske, M. G., Rauch, S. L., Ursano, R., Prenoveau, J., Pine, D. S., & Zinbarg, R. E. (2009). What is an anxiety disorder? *Depression and Anxiety, 26,* 1066–1085. http://dx.doi.org/10.1002/da.20633

Craske, M. G., Waters, A. M., Lindsey Bergman, R., Naliboff, B., Lipp, O. V., Negoro, H., & Ornitz, E. M. (2008). Is aversive learning a marker of risk for anxiety disorders in children? *Behaviour Research and Therapy, 46,* 954–967. http://dx.doi.org/10.1016/j.brat.2008.04.011

Curtin, J. J., Barnett, N. P., Colby, S. M., Rohsenow, D. J., & Monti, P. M. (2005). Cue reactivity in adolescents: Measurement of separate approach and avoidance reactions. *Journal of Studies on Alcohol, 66,* 332–343. http://dx.doi.org/10.15288/jsa.2005.66.332

Davidson, J. R., Rothbaum, B. O., van der Kolk, B. A., Sikes, C. R., & Farfel, G. M. (2001). Multicenter, double-blind comparison of sertraline and placebo in the treatment of posttraumatic stress disorder. *Archives of General Psychiatry, 58,* 485–492. http://dx.doi.org/10.1001/archpsyc.58.5.485

Davis, C., Fattore, L., Kaplan, A. S., Carter, J. C., Levitan, R. D., & Kennedy, J. L. (2012). The suppression of

appetite and food consumption by methylphenidate: The moderating effects of gender and weight status in healthy adults. *International Journal of Neuropsychopharmacology, 15,* 181–187. http://dx.doi.org/10.1017/S1461145711001039

Davis, C., Levitan, R. D., Kaplan, A. S., Carter-Major, J. C., & Kennedy, J. L. (2016). Sex differences in subjective and objective responses to a stimulant medication (methylphenidate): Comparisons between overweight/obese adults with and without binge-eating disorder. *International Journal of Eating Disorders, 49,* 473–481. http://dx.doi.org/10.1002/eat.22493

Dingemans, A. E., Bruna, M. J., & van Furth, E. F. (2002). Binge eating disorder: A review. *International Journal of Obesity, 26,* 299–307. http://dx.doi.org/10.1038/sj.ijo.0801949

Drummond, D. C. (2000). What does cue-reactivity have to offer clinical research? *Addiction, 95*(Suppl. 2), S129–S144. http://dx.doi.org/10.1046/j.1360-0443.95.8s2.2.x

Drummond, D. C., & Glautier, S. (1994). A controlled trial of cue exposure treatment in alcohol dependence. *Journal of Consulting and Clinical Psychology, 62,* 809–817. http://dx.doi.org/10.1037/0022-006X.62.4.809

Fillmore, M. T. (2003). Drug abuse as a problem of impaired control: Current approaches and findings. *Behavioral and Cognitive Neuroscience Reviews, 2,* 179–197. http://dx.doi.org/10.1177/1534582303257007

Forbes, E. E., & Dahl, R. E. (2012). Research Review: Altered reward function in adolescent depression: What, when and how? *Journal of Child Psychology and Psychiatry, 53,* 3–15. http://dx.doi.org/10.1111/j.1469-7610.2011.02477.x

Forbes, E. E., Hariri, A. R., Martin, S. L., Silk, J. S., Moyles, D. L., Fisher, P. M., . . . Dahl, R. E. (2009). Altered striatal activation predicting real-world positive affect in adolescent major depressive disorder. *The American Journal of Psychiatry, 166,* 64–73. http://dx.doi.org/10.1176/appi.ajp.2008.07081336

Foti, D., & Hajcak, G. (2009). Depression and reduced sensitivity to non-rewards versus rewards: Evidence from event-related potentials. *Biological Psychology, 81,* 1–8. http://dx.doi.org/10.1016/j.biopsycho.2008.12.004

Fowles, D. C. (1980). The three arousal model: Implications of gray's two-factor learning theory for heart rate, electrodermal activity, and psychopathy. *Psychophysiology, 17,* 87–104. http://dx.doi.org/10.1111/j.1469-8986.1980.tb00117.x

Fox, H. C., Anderson, G. M., Tuit, K., Hansen, J., Kimmerling, A., Siedlarz, K. M., . . . Sinha, R. (2012). Prazosin effects on stress- and cue-induced craving and stress response in alcohol-dependent individuals:

Preliminary findings. *Alcoholism: Clinical and Experimental Research, 36,* 351–360. http://dx.doi.org/10.1111/j.1530-0277.2011.01628.x

Gray, J. A. (1970). The psychophysiological basis of introversion-extraversion. *Behaviour Research and Therapy, 8,* 249–266. http://dx.doi.org/10.1016/0005-7967(70)90069-0

Grilo, C. M., Reas, D. L., & Mitchell, J. E. (2016). Combining pharmacological and psychological treatments for binge eating disorder: Current status, limitations, and future directions. *Current Psychiatry Reports, 18,* 55. http://dx.doi.org/10.1007/s11920-016-0696-z

Grüsser, S. M., Wrase, J., Klein, S., Hermann, D., Smolka, M. N., Ruf, M., . . . Heinz, A. (2004). Cue-induced activation of the striatum and medial prefrontal cortex is associated with subsequent relapse in abstinent alcoholics. *Psychopharmacology, 175,* 296–302. http://dx.doi.org/10.1007/s00213-004-1828-4

Hall, C. L., Valentine, A. Z., Groom, M. J., Walker, G. M., Sayal, K., Daley, D., & Hollis, C. (2016). The clinical utility of the continuous performance test and objective measures of activity for diagnosing and monitoring ADHD in children: A systematic review. *European Child & Adolescent Psychiatry, 25,* 677–699. http://dx.doi.org/10.1007/s00787-015-0798-x

Hamilton, K. R., Littlefield, A. K., Anastasio, N. C., Cunningham, K. A., Fink, L. H., Wing, V. C., . . . Potenza, M. N. (2015). Rapid-response impulsivity: Definitions, measurement issues, and clinical implications. *Personality Disorders: Theory, Research, and Treatment, 6,* 168–181. http://dx.doi.org/10.1037/per0000100

Hamilton, K. R., Mitchell, M. R., Wing, V. C., Balodis, I. M., Bickel, W. K., Fillmore, M., . . . Moeller, F. G. (2015). Choice impulsivity: Definitions, measurement issues, and clinical implications. *Personality Disorders: Theory, Research, and Treatment, 6,* 182–198. http://dx.doi.org/10.1037/per0000099

Hammarberg, A., Jayaram-Lindström, N., Beck, O., Franck, J., & Reid, M. S. (2009). The effects of acamprosate on alcohol-cue reactivity and alcohol priming in dependent patients: A randomized controlled trial. *Psychopharmacology, 205,* 53–62. http://dx.doi.org/10.1007/s00213-009-1515-6

Han, G., Klimes-Dougan, B., Jepsen, S., Ballard, K., Nelson, M., Houri, A., . . . Cullen, K. (2012). Selective neurocognitive impairments in adolescents with major depressive disorder. *Journal of Adolescence, 35,* 11–20. http://dx.doi.org/10.1016/j.adolescence.2011.06.009

Haynos, A. F., Berg, K. C., Cao, L., Crosby, R. D., Lavender, J. M., Utzinger, L. M., . . . Crow, S. J. (2017). Trajectories of higher- and lower-order dimensions of negative and positive affect relative to restrictive

eating in anorexia nervosa. *Journal of Abnormal Psychology, 126,* 495–505. http://dx.doi.org/10.1037/abn0000202

Hilbert, A., Kurz, S., Dremmel, D., Weihrauch Blüher, S., Munsch, S., & Schmidt, R. (2018). Cue reactivity, habituation, and eating in the absence of hunger in children with loss of control eating and attention-deficit/hyperactivity disorder. *International Journal of Eating Disorders, 51,* 223–232. http://dx.doi.org/10.1002/eat.22821

Howie, L. D., Pastor, P. N., & Lukacs, S. L. (2014). *Use of medication prescribed for emotional and behavioral difficulties among children aged 6–17 years in the United States, 2011–2012.* Hyattsville, MD: National Center for Health Statistics.

Hutchison, K. E., Ray, L., Sandman, E., Rutter, M. C., Peters, A., Davidson, D., & Swift, R. (2006). The effect of olanzapine on craving and alcohol consumption. *Neuropsychopharmacology, 31,* 1310–1317. http://dx.doi.org/10.1038/sj.npp.1300917

Hutchison, K. E., Swift, R., Rohsenow, D. J., Monti, P. M., Davidson, D., & Almeida, A. (2001). Olanzapine reduces urge to drink after drinking cues and a priming dose of alcohol. *Psychopharmacology, 155,* 27–34. http://dx.doi.org/10.1007/s002130000629

Insel, T., Cuthbert, B., Garvey, M., Heinssen, R., Pine, D. S., Quinn, K., . . . Wang, P. (2010). Research domain criteria (RDoC): Toward a new classification framework for research on mental disorders. *The American Journal of Psychiatry, 167,* 748–751. http://dx.doi.org/10.1176/appi.ajp.2010.09091379

Jovanovic, T., Rauch, S. A., Rothbaum, A. O., & Rothbaum, B. O. (2017). Using experimental methodologies to assess posttraumatic stress. *Current Opinion in Psychology, 14,* 23–28. http://dx.doi.org/10.1016/j.copsyc.2016.10.001

Keane, T. M., Kolb, L. C., Kaloupek, D. G., Orr, S. P., Blanchard, E. B., Thomas, R. G., . . . Lavori, P. W. (1998). Utility of psychophysiological measurement in the diagnosis of posttraumatic stress disorder: Results from a Department of Veterans Affairs Cooperative Study. *Journal of Consulting and Clinical Psychology, 66,* 914–923. http://dx.doi.org/10.1037/0022-006X.66.6.914

Kelmendi, B., Adams, T. G., Yarnell, S., Southwick, S., Abdallah, C. G., & Krystal, J. H. (2016). PTSD: From neurobiology to pharmacological treatments. *European Journal of Psychotraumatology, 7,* 31858. http://dx.doi.org/10.3402/ejpt.v7.31858

Kessler, R. C., Berglund, P. A., Chiu, W. T., Deitz, A. C., Hudson, J. I., Shahly, V., . . . Xavier, M. (2013). The prevalence and correlates of binge eating disorder in the World Health Organization World Mental Health Surveys. *Biological Psychiatry, 73,* 904–914. http://dx.doi.org/10.1016/j.biopsych.2012.11.020

Kirschbaum, C., Pirke, K. M., & Hellhammer, D. H. (1993). The "Trier Social Stress Test"—A tool for investigating psychobiological stress responses in a laboratory setting. *Neuropsychobiology, 28,* 76–81. http://dx.doi.org/10.1159/000119004

Kola, I. (2008). The state of innovation in drug development. *Clinical Pharmacology and Therapeutics, 83*(2), 227–230. http://dx.doi.org/10.1038/sj.clpt.6100479

Koob, G. F. (2009). Neurobiological substrates for the dark side of compulsivity in addiction. *Neuropharmacology, 56*(Suppl. 1), 18–31. http://dx.doi.org/10.1016/j.neuropharm.2008.07.043

Koob, G. F., & Mason, B. J. (2016). Existing and future drugs for the treatment of the dark side of addiction. *Annual Review of Pharmacology and Toxicology, 56,* 299–322. http://dx.doi.org/10.1146/annurev-pharmtox-010715-103143

Laessle, R. G., & Schulz, S. (2009). Stress-induced laboratory eating behavior in obese women with binge eating disorder. *International Journal of Eating Disorders, 42,* 505–510. http://dx.doi.org/10.1002/eat.20648

Leeman, R. F., Corbin, W. R., & Fromme, K. (2009). Craving predicts within session drinking behavior following placebo. *Personality and Individual Differences, 46,* 693–698. http://dx.doi.org/10.1016/j.paid.2009.01.024

Leeman, R. F., Heilig, M., Cunningham, C. L., Stephens, D. N., Duka, T., & O'Malley, S. S. (2010). Ethanol consumption: How should we measure it? Achieving consilience between human and animal phenotypes. *Addiction Biology, 15,* 109–124. http://dx.doi.org/10.1111/j.1369-1600.2009.00192.x

Leuchter, A. F., Cook, I. A., Gilmer, W. S., Marangell, L. B., Burgoyne, K. S., Howland, R. H., . . . Greenwald, S. (2009). Effectiveness of a quantitative electroencephalographic biomarker for predicting differential response or remission with escitalopram and bupropion in major depressive disorder. *Psychiatry Research, 169,* 132–138. http://dx.doi.org/10.1016/j.psychres.2009.04.004

Leuchter, A. F., Cook, I. A., Marangell, L. B., Gilmer, W. S., Burgoyne, K. S., Howland, R. H., . . . Greenwald, S. (2009). Comparative effectiveness of biomarkers and clinical indicators for predicting outcomes of SSRI treatment in major depressive disorder: Results of the BRITE-MD study. *Psychiatry Research, 169,* 124–131. http://dx.doi.org/10.1016/j.psychres.2009.06.004

Leuchter, A. F., Hunter, A. M., Jain, F. A., Tartter, M., Crump, C., & Cook, I. A. (2017). Escitalopram but not placebo modulates brain rhythmic oscillatory activity in the first week of treatment of major depressive disorder. *Journal of Psychiatric Research, 84,* 174–183. http://dx.doi.org/10.1016/j.jpsychires.2016.10.002

Leuchter, A. F., Hunter, A. M., Krantz, D. E., & Cook, I. A. (2014). Intermediate phenotypes and biomarkers of treatment outcome in major depressive disorder. *Dialogues in Clinical Neuroscience, 16,* 525–537.

Liberman, L. C., Lipp, O. V., Spence, S. H., & March, S. (2006). Evidence for retarded extinction of aversive learning in anxious children. *Behaviour Research and Therapy, 44,* 1491–1502. http://dx.doi.org/10.1016/j.brat.2005.11.004

Lissek, S., Powers, A. S., McClure, E. B., Phelps, E. A., Woldehawariat, G., Grillon, C., & Pine, D. S. (2005). Classical fear conditioning in the anxiety disorders: A meta-analysis. *Behaviour Research and Therapy, 43,* 1391–1424. http://dx.doi.org/10.1016/j.brat.2004.10.007

Litten, R. Z., Egli, M., Heilig, M., Cui, C., Fertig, J. B., Ryan, M. L., . . . Noronha, A. (2012). Medications development to treat alcohol dependence: A vision for the next decade. *Addiction Biology, 17,* 513–527. http://dx.doi.org/10.1111/j.1369-1600.2012.00454.x

Litten, R. Z., Falk, D. E., Ryan, M. L., & Fertig, J. B. (2016). Discovery, development, and adoption of medications to treat alcohol use disorder: Goals for the phases of medications development. *Alcoholism: Clinical and Experimental Research, 40,* 1368–1379. http://dx.doi.org/10.1111/acer.13093

Litten, R. Z., Ryan, M. L., Falk, D. E., Reilly, M., Fertig, J. B., & Koob, G. F. (2015). Heterogeneity of alcohol use disorder: Understanding mechanisms to advance personalized treatment. *Alcoholism: Clinical and Experimental Research, 39,* 579–584. http://dx.doi.org/10.1111/acer.12669

Litvin, E. B., & Brandon, T. H. (2010). Testing the influence of external and internal cues on smoking motivation using a community sample. *Experimental and Clinical Psychopharmacology, 18,* 61–70. http://dx.doi.org/10.1037/a0017414

Liu, W. H., Wang, L. Z., Shang, H. R., Shen, Y., Li, Z., Cheung, E. F., & Chan, R. C. (2014). The influence of anhedonia on feedback negativity in major depressive disorder. *Neuropsychologia, 53,* 213–220. http://dx.doi.org/10.1016/j.neuropsychologia.2013.11.023

Luijten, M., Machielsen, M. W., Veltman, D. J., Hester, R., de Haan, L., & Franken, I. H. (2014). Systematic review of ERP and fMRI studies investigating inhibitory control and error processing in people with substance dependence and behavioural addictions. *Journal of Psychiatry & Neuroscience, 39,* 149–169. http://dx.doi.org/10.1503/jpn.130052

MacKillop, J., Few, L. R., Stojek, M. K., Murphy, C. M., Malutinok, S. F., Johnson, F. T., . . . Monti, P. M. (2015). D-cycloserine to enhance extinction of cue-elicited craving for alcohol: A translational approach. *Translational Psychiatry, 5,* e544. http://dx.doi.org/10.1038/tp.2015.41

Mannie, Z. N., Williams, C., Browning, M., & Cowen, P. J. (2015). Decision making in young people at familial risk of depression. *Psychological Medicine, 45*, 375–380. http://dx.doi.org/10.1017/S0033291714001482

Mason, B. J., Light, J. M., Williams, L. D., & Drobes, D. J. (2009). Proof-of-concept human laboratory study for protracted abstinence in alcohol dependence: Effects of gabapentin. *Addiction Biology, 14*, 73–83. http://dx.doi.org/10.1111/j.1369-1600.2008.00133.x

Mason, B. J., Quello, S., Goodell, V., Shadan, F., Kyle, M., & Begovic, A. (2014). Gabapentin treatment for alcohol dependence: A randomized clinical trial. *JAMA Internal Medicine, 174*, 70–77. http://dx.doi.org/10.1001/jamainternmed.2013.11950

Mayes, T. L., Tao, R., Rintelmann, J. W., Carmody, T., Hughes, C. W., Kennard, B. D., . . . Emslie, G. J. (2007). Do children and adolescents have differential response rates in placebo-controlled trials of fluoxetine? *CNS Spectrums, 12*, 147–154. http://dx.doi.org/10.1017/S1092852900020666

McElroy, S. L., Hudson, J., Ferreira-Cornwell, M. C., Radewonuk, J., Whitaker, T., & Gasior, M. (2016). Lisdexamfetamine dimesylate for adults with moderate to severe binge eating disorder: Results of two pivotal phase 3 randomized controlled trials. *Neuropsychopharmacology, 41*, 1251–1260. http://dx.doi.org/10.1038/npp.2015.275

McElroy, S. L., Mitchell, J. E., Wilfley, D., Gasior, M., Ferreira-Cornwell, M. C., McKay, M., . . . Hudson, J. I. (2016). Lisdexamfetamine dimesylate effects on binge eating behaviour and obsessive-compulsive and impulsive features in adults with binge eating disorder. *European Eating Disorders Review, 24*, 223–231. http://dx.doi.org/10.1002/erv.2418

McGeary, J. E., Monti, P. M., Rohsenow, D. J., Tidey, J., Swift, R., & Miranda, R., Jr. (2006). Genetic moderators of naltrexone's effects on alcohol cue reactivity. *Alcoholism: Clinical and Experimental Research, 30*, 1288–1296. http://dx.doi.org/10.1111/j.1530-0277.2006.00156.x

McKee, S. A., Weinberger, A. H., Shi, J., Tetrault, J., & Coppola, S. (2012). Developing and validating a human laboratory model to screen medications for smoking cessation. *Nicotine & Tobacco Research, 14*, 1362–1371. http://dx.doi.org/10.1093/ntr/nts090

Michopoulos, V., Norrholm, S. D., Stevens, J. S., Glover, E. M., Rothbaum, B. O., Gillespie, C. F., . . . Jovanovic, T. (2017). Dexamethasone facilitates fear extinction and safety discrimination in PTSD: A placebo-controlled, double-blind study. *Psychoneuroendocrinology, 83*, 65–71. http://dx.doi.org/10.1016/j.psyneuen.2017.05.023

Milad, M. R., Orr, S. P., Lasko, N. B., Chang, Y., Rauch, S. L., & Pitman, R. K. (2008). Presence and acquired origin of reduced recall for fear extinction in PTSD: Results of a twin study. *Journal of Psychiatric Research, 42*, 515–520. http://dx.doi.org/10.1016/j.jpsychires.2008.01.017

Milivojevic, V., Fox, H. C., Jayaram-Lindstrom, N., Hermes, G., & Sinha, R. (2017). Sex differences in guanfacine effects on stress-induced stroop performance in cocaine dependence. *Drug and Alcohol Dependence, 179*, 275–279. http://dx.doi.org/10.1016/j.drugalcdep.2017.07.017

Mineka, S., & Zinbarg, R. (2006). A contemporary learning theory perspective on the etiology of anxiety disorders: It's not what you thought it was. *American Psychologist, 61*, 10–26. http://dx.doi.org/10.1037/0003-066X.61.1.10

Miranda, R., Jr., MacKillop, J., Monti, P. M., Rohsenow, D. J., Tidey, J., Gwaltney, C., . . . McGeary, J. (2008). Effects of topiramate on urge to drink and the subjective effects of alcohol: A preliminary laboratory study. *Alcoholism: Clinical and Experimental Research, 32*, 489–497. http://dx.doi.org/10.1111/j.1530-0277.2007.00592.x

Miranda, R., Jr., MacKillop, J., Treloar, H., Blanchard, A., Tidey, J. W., Swift, R. M., . . . Monti, P. M. (2016). Biobehavioral mechanisms of topiramate's effects on alcohol use: An investigation pairing laboratory and ecological momentary assessments. *Addiction Biology, 21*, 171–182. http://dx.doi.org/10.1111/adb.12192

Miranda, R., Jr., Ray, L., Blanchard, A., Reynolds, E. K., Monti, P. M., Chun, T., . . . Ramirez, J. (2014). Effects of naltrexone on adolescent alcohol cue reactivity and sensitivity: An initial randomized trial. *Addiction Biology, 19*, 941–954. http://dx.doi.org/10.1111/adb.12050

Monti, P. M., Binkoff, J. A., Abrams, D. B., Zwick, W. R., Nirenberg, T. D., & Liepman, M. R. (1987). Reactivity of alcoholics and nonalcoholics to drinking cues. *Journal of Abnormal Psychology, 96*, 122–126. http://dx.doi.org/10.1037/0021-843X.96.2.122

Monti, P. M., Rohsenow, D. J., Hutchison, K. E., Swift, R. M., Mueller, T. I., Colby, S. M., . . . Abrams, D. B. (1999). Naltrexone's effect on cue-elicited craving among alcoholics in treatment. *Alcoholism: Clinical and Experimental Research, 23*(8), 1386–1394.

Monti, P. M., Rohsenow, D. J., Rubonis, A. V., Niaura, R. S., Sirota, A. D., Colby, S. M., & Abrams, D. B. (1993). Alcohol cue reactivity: Effects of detoxification and extended exposure. *Journal of Studies on Alcohol, 54*, 235–245. http://dx.doi.org/10.15288/jsa.1993.54.235

Moore, T. J., & Mattison, D. R. (2017). Adult utilization of psychiatric drugs and differences by sex, age, and race. *JAMA Internal Medicine, 177*, 274–275. http://dx.doi.org/10.1001/jamainternmed.2016.7507

Morris, B. H., Bylsma, L. M., Yaroslavsky, I., Kovacs, M., & Rottenberg, J. (2015). Reward learning in pediatric depression and anxiety: Preliminary findings in a high-risk sample. *Depression and Anxiety, 32*, 373–381. http://dx.doi.org/10.1002/da.22358

Myrick, H., Anton, R. F., Li, X., Henderson, S., Randall, P. K., & Voronin, K. (2008). Effect of naltrexone and ondansetron on alcohol cue-induced activation of the ventral striatum in alcohol-dependent people. *Archives of General Psychiatry, 65*, 466–475. http://dx.doi.org/10.1001/archpsyc.65.4.466

Nelson, B. D., McGowan, S. K., Sarapas, C., Robison-Andrew, E. J., Altman, S. E., Campbell, M. L., . . . Shankman, S. A. (2013). Biomarkers of threat and reward sensitivity demonstrate unique associations with risk for psychopathology. *Journal of Abnormal Psychology, 122*, 662–671. http://dx.doi.org/10.1037/a0033982

Newman, J. P., Widom, C. S., & Nathan, S. (1985). Passive avoidance in syndromes of disinhibition: Psychopathy and extraversion. *Journal of Personality and Social Psychology, 48*, 1316–1327. http://dx.doi.org/10.1037/0022-3514.48.5.1316

Ogrim, G., Kropotov, J., Brunner, J. F., Candrian, G., Sandvik, L., & Hestad, K. A. (2014). Predicting the clinical outcome of stimulant medication in pediatric attention-deficit/hyperactivity disorder: Data from quantitative electroencephalography, event-related potentials, and a go/no-go test. *Neuropsychiatric Disease and Treatment, 10*, 231–242. http://dx.doi.org/10.2147/NDT.S56600

O'Malley, S. S., Jaffe, A. J., Chang, G., Schottenfeld, R. S., Meyer, R. E., & Rounsaville, B. (1992). Naltrexone and coping skills therapy for alcohol dependence. A controlled study. *Archives of General Psychiatry, 49*, 881–887. http://dx.doi.org/10.1001/archpsyc.1992.01820110045007

O'Malley, S. S., Krishnan-Sarin, S., Farren, C., Sinha, R., & Kreek, M. J. (2002). Naltrexone decreases craving and alcohol self-administration in alcohol-dependent subjects and activates the hypothalamo-pituitary-adrenocortical axis. *Psychopharmacology, 160*, 19–29. http://dx.doi.org/10.1007/s002130100919

O'Malley, S. S., Zweben, A., Fucito, L. M., Wu, R., Piepmeier, M. E., Ockert, D. M., . . . Gueorguieva, R. (2018). Effect of varenicline combined with medical management on alcohol use disorder with comorbid cigarette smoking: A randomized clinical trial. *JAMA Psychiatry, 75*, 129–138.

Ooteman, W., Koeter, M. W., Verheul, R., Schippers, G. M., & van den Brink, W. (2007). The effect of naltrexone and acamprosate on cue-induced craving, autonomic nervous system and neuroendocrine reactions to alcohol-related cues in alcoholics. *European Neuropsychopharmacology, 17*, 558–566. http://dx.doi.org/10.1016/j.euroneuro.2007.02.012

Ooteman, W., Naassila, M., Koeter, M. W., Verheul, R., Schippers, G. M., Houchi, H., . . . van den Brink, W. (2009). Predicting the effect of naltrexone and acamprosate in alcohol-dependent patients using genetic indicators. *Addiction Biology, 14*, 328–337. http://dx.doi.org/10.1111/j.1369-1600.2009.00159.x

Otto, M. W., Leyro, T. M., Christian, K., Deveney, C. M., Reese, H., Pollack, M. H., & Orr, S. P. (2007). Prediction of "fear" acquisition in healthy control participants in a de novo fear-conditioning paradigm. *Behavior Modification, 31*, 32–51. http://dx.doi.org/10.1177/0145445506295054

Paul, S. M., Mytelka, D. S., Dunwiddie, C. T., Persinger, C. C., Munos, B. H., Lindborg, S. R., & Schacht, A. L. (2010). How to improve R&D productivity: The pharmaceutical industry's grand challenge. *Nature Reviews. Drug Discovery, 9*, 203–214. http://dx.doi.org/10.1038/nrd3078

Perkins, K. A., & Karelitz, J. L. (2013). Influence of reinforcer magnitude and nicotine amount on smoking's acute reinforcement enhancing effects. *Drug and Alcohol Dependence, 133*, 167–171. http://dx.doi.org/10.1016/j.drugalcdep.2013.05.016

Perkins, K. A., & Lerman, C. (2011). Early human screening of medications to treat drug addiction: Novel paradigms and the relevance of pharmacogenetics. *Clinical Pharmacology and Therapeutics, 89*, 460–463. http://dx.doi.org/10.1038/clpt.2010.254

Peters, J., & Büchel, C. (2011). The neural mechanisms of inter-temporal decision-making: Understanding variability. *Trends in Cognitive Sciences, 15*, 227–239. http://dx.doi.org/10.1016/j.tics.2011.03.002

Pineles, S. L., Suvak, M. K., Liverant, G. I., Gregor, K., Wisco, B. E., Pitman, R. K., & Orr, S. P. (2013). Psychophysiologic reactivity, subjective distress, and their associations with PTSD diagnosis. *Journal of Abnormal Psychology, 122*, 635–644. http://dx.doi.org/10.1037/a0033942

Pitman, R. K., Orr, S. P., Forgue, D. F., de Jong, J. B., & Claiborn, J. M. (1987). Psychophysiologic assessment of posttraumatic stress disorder imagery in Vietnam combat veterans. *Archives of General Psychiatry, 44*, 970–975. http://dx.doi.org/10.1001/archpsyc.1987.01800230050009

Pizzagalli, D. A., Iosifescu, D., Hallett, L. A., Ratner, K. G., & Fava, M. (2008). Reduced hedonic capacity in major depressive disorder: Evidence from a probabilistic reward task. *Journal of Psychiatric Research, 43*, 76–87. http://dx.doi.org/10.1016/j.jpsychires.2008.03.001

Pizzagalli, D. A., Jahn, A. L., & O'Shea, J. P. (2005). Toward an objective characterization of an anhedonic phenotype: A signal-detection approach. *Biological Psychiatry, 57*, 319–327. http://dx.doi.org/10.1016/j.biopsych.2004.11.026

Ramirez, J., & Miranda, R., Jr. (2014). Alcohol craving in adolescents: Bridging the laboratory and natural environment. *Psychopharmacology*, *231*, 1841–1851. http://dx.doi.org/10.1007/s00213-013-3372-6

Ray, L. A., Bujarski, S., & Roche, D. J. (2016). Subjective response to alcohol as a research domain criterion. *Alcoholism: Clinical and Experimental Research*, *40*, 6–17. http://dx.doi.org/10.1111/acer.12927

Ray, L. A., Bujarski, S., Shoptaw, S., Roche, D. J., Heinzerling, K., & Miotto, K. (2017). Development of the neuroimmune modulator ibudilast for the treatment of alcoholism: A randomized, placebo-controlled, human laboratory trial. *Neuropsychopharmacology*, *42*, 1776–1788. http://dx.doi.org/10.1038/npp.2017.10

Ray, L. A., Bujarski, S., Yardley, M. M., Roche, D. J. O., & Hartwell, E. E. (2017). Differences between treatment-seeking and non-treatment-seeking participants in medication studies for alcoholism: Do they matter? *The American Journal of Drug and Alcohol Abuse*, *43*, 703–710. http://dx.doi.org/10.1080/00952990.2017.1312423

Ray, L. A., Chin, P. F., Heydari, A., & Miotto, K. (2011). A human laboratory study of the effects of quetiapine on subjective intoxication and alcohol craving. *Psychopharmacology*, *217*, 341–351. http://dx.doi.org/10.1007/s00213-011-2287-3

Ray, L. A., Courtney, K. E., Ghahremani, D. G., Miotto, K., Brody, A., & London, E. D. (2014). Varenicline, low dose naltrexone, and their combination for heavy-drinking smokers: Human laboratory findings. *Psychopharmacology*, *231*, 3843–3853. http://dx.doi.org/10.1007/s00213-014-3519-0

Ray, L. A., Green, R., Roche, D. J. O., Bujarski, S., Hartwell, E. E., Lim, A. C., . . . Miotto, K. (2018). Pharmacogenetic effects of naltrexone in individuals of East Asian descent: Human laboratory findings from a randomized trial. *Alcoholism: Clinical and Experimental Research*, *42*, 613–623.

Reynolds, B., Penfold, R. B., & Patak, M. (2008). Dimensions of impulsive behavior in adolescents: Laboratory behavioral assessments. *Experimental and Clinical Psychopharmacology*, *16*, 124–131. http://dx.doi.org/10.1037/1064-1297.16.2.124

Robbins, T. W., Gillan, C. M., Smith, D. G., de Wit, S., & Ersche, K. D. (2012). Neurocognitive endophenotypes of impulsivity and compulsivity: Towards dimensional psychiatry. *Trends in Cognitive Sciences*, *16*, 81–91. http://dx.doi.org/10.1016/j.tics.2011.11.009

Rodrigues, H., Figueira, I., Lopes, A., Gonçalves, R., Mendlowicz, M. V., Coutinho, E. S., & Ventura, P. (2014). Does D-cycloserine enhance exposure therapy for anxiety disorders in humans? A meta-analysis. *PLoS ONE*, *9*(7), e93519. http://dx.doi.org/10.1371/journal.pone.0093519

Rohn, M. C., Lee, M. R., Kleuter, S. B., Schwandt, M. L., Falk, D. E., & Leggio, L. (2017). Differences between treatment-seeking and nontreatment-seeking alcohol-dependent research participants: An exploratory analysis. *Alcoholism: Clinical and Experimental Research*, *41*, 414–420. http://dx.doi.org/10.1111/acer.13304

Rohsenow, D. J., Monti, P. M., Rubonis, A. V., Sirota, A. D., Niaura, R. S., Colby, S. M., . . . Abrams, D. B. (1994). Cue reactivity as a predictor of drinking among male alcoholics. *Journal of Consulting and Clinical Psychology*, *62*, 620–626. http://dx.doi.org/10.1037/0022-006X.62.3.620

Rosch, K. S., Fosco, W. D., Pelham, W. E., Jr., Waxmonsky, J. G., Bubnik, M. G., & Hawk, L. W., Jr. (2016). Reinforcement and stimulant medication ameliorate deficient response inhibition in children with attention-deficit/hyperactivity disorder. *Journal of Abnormal Child Psychology*, *44*, 309–321. http://dx.doi.org/10.1007/s10802-015-0031-x

Rothbaum, B. O., Price, M., Jovanovic, T., Norrholm, S. D., Gerardi, M., Dunlop, B., . . . Ressler, K. J. (2014). A randomized, double-blind evaluation of D-cycloserine or alprazolam combined with virtual reality exposure therapy for posttraumatic stress disorder in Iraq and Afghanistan War veterans. *The American Journal of Psychiatry*, *171*, 640–648. http://dx.doi.org/10.1176/appi.ajp.2014.13121625

Rubonis, A. V., Colby, S. M., Monti, P. M., Rohsenow, D. J., Gulliver, S. B., & Sirota, A. D. (1994). Alcohol cue reactivity and mood induction in male and female alcoholics. *Journal of Studies on Alcohol*, *55*, 487–494. http://dx.doi.org/10.15288/jsa.1994.55.487

Safer, D. J. (2004). A comparison of risperidone-induced weight gain across the age span. *Journal of Clinical Psychopharmacology*, *24*, 429–436. http://dx.doi.org/10.1097/01.jcp.0000130558.86125.5b

Shalev, A., Liberzon, I., & Marmar, C. (2017). Post-traumatic stress disorder. *The New England Journal of Medicine*, *376*, 2459–2469. http://dx.doi.org/10.1056/NEJMra1612499

Shankman, S. A., Klein, D. N., Tenke, C. E., & Bruder, G. E. (2007). Reward sensitivity in depression: A biobehavioral study. *Journal of Abnormal Psychology*, *116*, 95–104. http://dx.doi.org/10.1037/0021-843X.116.1.95

Shiffman, S. (2014). Conceptualizing analyses of ecological momentary assessment data. *Nicotine & Tobacco Research*, *16*(Suppl. 2), S76–S87. http://dx.doi.org/10.1093/ntr/ntt195

Shiffman, S., Shadel, W. G., Niaura, R., Khayrallah, M. A., Jorenby, D. E., Ryan, C. F., & Ferguson, C. L. (2003). Efficacy of acute administration of nicotine gum in relief of cue-provoked cigarette craving. *Psychopharmacology*, *166*, 343–350. http://dx.doi.org/10.1007/s00213-002-1338-1

Shin, L. M., & Liberzon, I. (2010). The neurocircuitry of fear, stress, and anxiety disorders. *Neuropsychopharmacology, 35*, 169–191. http://dx.doi.org/10.1038/npp.2009.83

Sinha, R. (2018). Role of addiction and stress neurobiology on food intake and obesity. *Biological Psychology, 131*, 5–13. http://dx.doi.org/10.1016/j.biopsycho.2017.05.001

Sinha, R., Fox, H. C., Hong, K. I., Hansen, J., Tuit, K., & Kreek, M. J. (2011). Effects of adrenal sensitivity, stress- and cue-induced craving, and anxiety on subsequent alcohol relapse and treatment outcomes. *Archives of General Psychiatry, 68*, 942–952. http://dx.doi.org/10.1001/archgenpsychiatry.2011.49

Smoski, M. J., Rittenberg, A., & Dichter, G. S. (2011). Major depressive disorder is characterized by greater reward network activation to monetary than pleasant image rewards. *Psychiatry Research: Neuroimaging, 194*, 263–270. http://dx.doi.org/10.1016/j.pscychresns.2011.06.012

Sotres-Bayon, F., Cain, C. K., & LeDoux, J. E. (2006). Brain mechanisms of fear extinction: Historical perspectives on the contribution of prefrontal cortex. *Biological Psychiatry, 60*, 329–336. http://dx.doi.org/10.1016/j.biopsych.2005.10.012

Spagnolo, P. A., Ramchandani, V. A., Schwandt, M. L., Zhang, L., Blaine, S. K., Usala, J. M., . . . Heilig, M. (2014). Effects of naltrexone on neural and subjective response to alcohol in treatment-seeking alcohol-dependent patients. *Alcoholism: Clinical and Experimental Research, 38*, 3024–3032. http://dx.doi.org/10.1111/acer.12581

Spiegel, T. A., Stunkard, A. J., Shrager, E. E., O'Brien, C. P., Morrison, M. F., & Stellar, E. (1987). Effect of naltrexone on food intake, hunger, and satiety in obese men. *Physiology & Behavior, 40*, 135–141. http://dx.doi.org/10.1016/0031-9384(87)90198-3

Svaldi, J., Tuschen-Caffier, B., Trentowska, M., Caffier, D., & Naumann, E. (2014). Differential caloric intake in overweight females with and without binge eating: Effects of a laboratory-based emotion-regulation training. *Behaviour Research and Therapy, 56*, 39–46. http://dx.doi.org/10.1016/j.brat.2014.02.008

Sysko, R., Devlin, M. J., Walsh, B. T., Zimmerli, E., & Kissileff, H. R. (2007). Satiety and test meal intake among women with binge eating disorder. *International Journal of Eating Disorders, 40*, 554–561. http://dx.doi.org/10.1002/eat.20384

Thibodeau, R., Jorgensen, R. S., & Kim, S. (2006). Depression, anxiety, and resting frontal EEG asymmetry: A meta-analytic review. *Journal of Abnormal Psychology, 115*, 715–729. http://dx.doi.org/10.1037/0021-843X.115.4.715

Tidey, J. W., Rohsenow, D. J., Kaplan, G. B., Swift, R. M., & Adolfo, A. B. (2008). Effects of smoking abstinence, smoking cues and nicotine replacement in smokers with schizophrenia and controls. *Nicotine & Tobacco Research, 10*, 1047–1056. http://dx.doi.org/10.1080/14622200802097373

Treadway, M. T., Buckholtz, J. W., Schwartzman, A. N., Lambert, W. E., & Zald, D. H. (2009). Worth the "EEfRT"? The effort expenditure for rewards task as an objective measure of motivation and anhedonia. *PLoS ONE, 4*, e6598. http://dx.doi.org/10.1371/journal.pone.0006598

Udo, T., Harrison, E. L., Shi, J., Tetrault, J., & McKee, S. A. (2013). A preliminary study on the effect of combined nicotine replacement therapy on alcohol responses and alcohol self-administration. *The American Journal on Addictions, 22*, 590–597. http://dx.doi.org/10.1111/j.1521-0391.2013.12014.x

Vendruscolo, L. F., Estey, D., Goodell, V., Macshane, L. G., Logrip, M. L., Schlosburg, J. E., . . . Mason, B. J. (2015). Glucocorticoid receptor antagonism decreases alcohol seeking in alcohol-dependent individuals. *The Journal of Clinical Investigation, 125*, 3193–3197. http://dx.doi.org/10.1172/JCI79828

Vervliet, B., Craske, M. G., & Hermans, D. (2013). Fear extinction and relapse: State of the art. *Annual Review of Clinical Psychology, 9*, 215–248. http://dx.doi.org/10.1146/annurev-clinpsy-050212-185542

Volkow, N., & Li, T. K. (2005). The neuroscience of addiction. *Nature Neuroscience, 8*, 1429–1430. http://dx.doi.org/10.1038/nn1105-1429

Volkow, N. D., Koob, G. F., & McLellan, A. T. (2016). Neurobiologic advances from the brain disease model of addiction. *The New England Journal of Medicine, 374*, 363–371. http://dx.doi.org/10.1056/NEJMra1511480

Walsh, B. T. (2011). The importance of eating behavior in eating disorders. *Physiology & Behavior, 104*, 525–529. http://dx.doi.org/10.1016/j.physbeh.2011.05.007

Walsh, B. T., & Boudreau, G. (2003). Laboratory studies of binge eating disorder. *International Journal of Eating Disorders, 34*(Suppl.), S30–S38. http://dx.doi.org/10.1002/eat.10203

Wang, G. J., Tomasi, D., Volkow, N. D., Wang, R., Telang, F., Caparelli, E. C., & Dunayevich, E. (2014). Effect of combined naltrexone and bupropion therapy on the brain's reactivity to food cues. *International Journal of Obesity, 38*, 682–688. http://dx.doi.org/10.1038/ijo.2013.145

Waters, A. M., Henry, J., & Neumann, D. L. (2009). Aversive Pavlovian conditioning in childhood anxiety disorders: Impaired response inhibition and resistance to extinction. *Journal of Abnormal Psychology, 118*, 311–321. http://dx.doi.org/10.1037/a0015635

Weathers, F. W., Blake, D. D., Schnurr, P. P., Kaloupek, D. G., Marx, B. P., & Keane, T. M. (2013).

The Clinician-Administered PTSD Scale for DSM–5 (CAPS-5). Retrieved from https://www.ptsd.va.gov

White, T. L., Lejuez, C. W., & de Wit, H. (2007). Personality and gender differences in effects of d-amphetamine on risk taking. *Experimental and Clinical Psychopharmacology, 15,* 599–609.

Winstanley, C. A., Olausson, P., Taylor, J. R., & Jentsch, J. D. (2010). Insight into the relationship between impulsivity and substance abuse from studies using animal models. *Alcoholism: Clinical and Experimental Research, 34,* 1306–1318.

Wonderlich, J. A., Breithaupt, L. E., Crosby, R. D., Thompson, J. C., Engel, S. G., & Fischer, S. (2017). The relation between craving and binge eating: Integrating neuroimaging and ecological momentary assessment. *Appetite, 117,* 294–302. http://dx.doi.org/10.1016/j.appet.2017.07.005

Yanovski, S. Z., Leet, M., Yanovski, J. A., Flood, M., Gold, P. W., Kissileff, H. R., & Walsh, B. T. (1992). Food selection and intake of obese women with binge-eating disorder. *The American Journal of Clinical Nutrition, 56,* 975–980. http://dx.doi.org/10.1093/ajcn/56.6.975

Yardley, M. M., & Ray, L. A. (2017). Medications development for the treatment of alcohol use disorder: Insights into the predictive value of animal and human laboratory models. *Addiction Biology, 22,* 581–615. http://dx.doi.org/10.1111/adb.12349

Yechiam, E., Hayden, E. P., Bodkins, M., O'Donnell, B. F., & Hetrick, W. P. (2008). Decision making in bipolar disorder: A cognitive modeling approach. *Psychiatry Research, 161,* 142–152. http://dx.doi.org/10.1016/j.psychres.2007.07.001

Yip, S. W., & Potenza, M. N. (2018). Application of Research Domain Criteria to childhood and adolescent impulsive and addictive disorders: Implications for treatment. *Clinical Psychology Review, 64,* 41–56. http://dx.doi.org/10.1016/j.cpr.2016.11.003

Zeeck, A., Stelzer, N., Linster, H. W., Joos, A., & Hartmann, A. (2011). Emotion and eating in binge eating disorder and obesity. *European Eating Disorders Review, 19,* 426–437.

CHAPTER 6

EVIDENCE-BASED PHARMACOTHERAPY

F. Scott Kraly

Evidence based medicine is the conscientious, explicit, and judicious use of current best evidence in making decisions about the care of individual patients. The practice of evidence based medicine means integrating individual clinical expertise with the best available external clinical evidence from systematic research.

—*Sackett et al.*, 1996, p. 71

Evidence-based medicine may be defined as the systematic, quantitative, preferentially experimental approach to obtaining and using medical information.

—*Haidich*, 2010, p. 29

Convincing evidence to support a claim results from sustained systematic scientific inquiry. Comprehensive research typically includes findings from observational, correlational, and, most importantly, experimental studies that provide converging evidence to support or to reject a hypothesis. To what extent does this type of comprehensive study form the evidence base supporting the use of pharmacotherapy for treatment of specific psychiatric diagnoses?

The evidence base supporting the eventual use of a psychiatric medication builds upon the results of preclinical studies in animals and early clinical

trials in humans. The evidence base is subsequently strengthened by findings from large-scale placebo-controlled randomized clinical trials (RCTs). Those methodologically rigorous experiments play a decisive role, standing at the intersection of early trials that provide data to support the request for regulatory approval and the subsequent entry of that newly approved medication to the market. Regulatory approval immediately permits widespread clinical use of the new medication for its approved indication as well as for off-label usage for unapproved indications. Postmarketing research continues to produce important findings relevant to whether the various uses of that new drug constitute judicious usage. Just how good is the evidence base constructed prior to regulatory approval, and subsequently expanded during the postmarketing period?

To address that question, consider as a frame of reference the scientific study of the relation between brain processes and behavior. That is a suitable context for comparison, because pharmacotherapy for psychiatric problems is certainly a brain and behavior enterprise. For example, a search for the mechanism of action for a drug that improves symptoms of a psychiatric disorder is one kind of research project undertaken by some behavioral neuroscientists.

What kind of evidence is required to convincingly support an idea such as, "A neurotransmitter in a

http://dx.doi.org/10.1037/0000133-006
APA Handbook of Psychopharmacology, S. M. Evans (Editor-in-Chief)

specific site in brain contributes to the control of a specific behavior"?

A program of research that takes on that hypothesis would employ multiple research strategies and a wide variety of techniques, many of which would be used in experiments in animals. This broad approach would evaluate whether the phenomenon under study was robust, whether it was present under many or under limited circumstances, and whether it was functional in other species, including humans. Extended study likely would produce apparently conflicting findings. But when the preponderance of results and their interpretations are largely consistent, they would represent converging evidence to accept or reject the original hypothesis. Taken together, converging evidence from extended study using multiple research strategies in a variety of experimental conditions could establish the core of an evidence base to support (or refute) a hypothesis regarding a brain process and behavior.

That kind of broad evidence base stands in contrast to the amount of evidence signifying efficacy, clinical effectiveness, safety, and tolerability at the time a drug is being scrutinized for approval by the U.S. Food and Drug Administration (FDA). The early foundation of an evidence base to support regulatory approval of a new drug is normally the result of relatively limited findings from preclinical (i.e., animal) studies, small-scale experiments in patients, and the results from typically one or two larger-scale rigorously conducted experiments (the RCTs).

Of those various sources of evidence, the results of experiments conducted in humans provide the most valuable findings for establishing the core of an evidence base for pharmacotherapy. The artful clinical use of those findings toward a favorable balance of benefits and risks requires wisdom acquired from clinical experience and knowledge gained from a critical appreciation of the relevant research. Pharmacotherapy may further improve a benefits/risks balance when the best of evidence-based psychotherapy is combined with judicious use of evidence-based pharmacotherapy (Baldessarini, 2013). A judicious use of pharmacotherapy begins with a critical

understanding of the relative value of clinical drug trials.

RANDOMIZED CLINICAL DRUG TRIALS: PURPOSES AND STRENGTHS

The clinical drug trial has provided the primary data for initial evaluations of the efficacy and safety of new psychiatric medications for more than 50 years. Standards and expectations for rigorous experimental design attempt to ensure that clinical drug trials at least meet minimum requirements (see Tool Kit of Resources). The FDA website (http://www.FDA.gov) provides guidelines intended to facilitate the use of rigorous experimental design, and the full and effective presentation of the results of those experiments. A clinical drug trial is expected to bear the hallmarks of good science; it should posit a testable hypothesis, be placebo-controlled with random assignment of participants into treatment conditions or groups, use manipulations of carefully selected independent variables (e.g., dosage), have measurable and reliable dependent variables (e.g., primary and secondary outcome measures), and objectively scrutinize the data using appropriate statistical analysis (Kraemer & Schatzberg, 2009).

When well-planned and well-executed, an excellent clinical trial can offer evidence that supports a claim that a drug has efficacy and is relatively safe. For that single trial, however, efficacy and relative safety are demonstrated for the limited circumstances of that particular experiment. In other words, a reasonable conclusion from a methodologically rigorous clinical drug trial generally takes the following form: This has been demonstrated to be the case under the limited conditions in which the phenomenon has been studied.

The minimum requirements for a well-constructed drug trial have been established and are periodically modified by a group of scientists and editors to ensure that RCT data are collected in a manner that permits interpretable findings. These Consolidated Standards of Reporting Trials (CONSORT; Altman et al., 2001; Zwarenstein et al., 2008) attempt to ensure that rigorous scientific methodology is used to collect and report data. The objective of RCTs is clear and narrow: The principal goal is to support the request to begin sale and use of a new medication.

Generally, a minimum of two RCTs, but sometimes only one RCT, is sufficient to support FDA approval for entry into the market for treatment of a specific psychiatric condition or behavioral disorder. Two carefully conducted RCTs represent two pieces of good scientific work, but they are merely two pieces of converging evidence demonstrating efficacy and relative safety. In contrast, if only two carefully conducted experiments supported a hypothesis regarding brain and behavior, that situation would never be taken as convincing evidence to support an idea. The results of those two experiments would be taken as preliminary evidence—merely a start toward years of further investigation.

Why would limited clinical trial evidence be considered sufficient to support regulatory approval for a new medication? It represents a compromise among parties having differing interests in successful development and use of pharmacotherapy. The compromise appears rather big, favoring some interests over others. But it may be a reasonable compromise. After all, currently available pharmacotherapy offers rather nonspecific, unpredictable, and only partial improvement for any specific category of psychiatric disorder (Baldessarini, 2013). In fact, some patients prescribed a medication fail to improve. Therefore, there is pressing need for new, better medications. Patients and their families, physicians, psychiatrists, psychologists, other prescribing professionals, and the pharmaceutical industry and their stockholders surely want new, more effective psychiatric medications sooner rather than later. The demand to fulfill those needs outweighs the demand for more extensive scientific investigation that would certainly delay availability of those medications. Moreover, conducting more extensive and expensive investigations may or may not produce products that are appreciably more effective and more safe than the medications currently available. Perhaps some of those more extensive investigations can wait until after the drug has been approved and is made available, and those two RCTs are just enough to presume that it is reasonable that further studies can take place while the new medication is being used as a treatment option.

Those few preapproval clinical drug trials provide essential evidence representing a pivotal point in the development of a new pharmacotherapy: The moment of regulatory approval not only brings prescribers and patients a new therapeutic option, but also brings the drug to a context in which the medication's effectiveness and safety can begin to be evaluated in a clinically more meaningful set of circumstances. The postmarketing study of a drug's effectiveness is expected to ask more clinically meaningful questions than those addressed during the typical preapproval RCT—questions such as whether the medication is effective in patients showing comorbidity, or whether the drug combined with psychotherapy or behavioral therapy is more effective than the pharmacotherapy alone.

By the time the results of RCTs support successful consideration of a drug by the FDA, the evidence base includes preclinical (animal) and clinical research evaluating toxicity (the FDA Phase I), small sample studies identifying effective dosages in humans with a specific disorder (Phase II), and the RCT experiments in humans (Phase III). This collection of evidence will be supplemented after regulatory approval by academic and industry-supported research efforts, including practical clinical trials (Phase IV), clinical anecdotal evidence regarding effectiveness and safety, and postmarketing information regarding adverse events. Among these various components of the evidence base, the Phase III RCTs create the foundation of the evidence base and introduce the drug into the market. Those few RCTs certainly are useful, but are they good enough? This question requires considering in some detail the limitations of clinical drug trials and assessing their effects on the use of an approved medication in a clinical setting.

RANDOMIZED CLINICAL DRUG TRIALS: LIMITATIONS

A methodologically rigorous experiment requires control of independent variables that are manipulated, as well as careful selection, measurement, and analysis of sensitive and reliable dependent variables. Potential sources of confounding must be eliminated or controlled. These expectations regarding experimental design determine the extent to which the results of an RCT are valuable for evidence-based pharmacotherapy. Will a demonstration of efficacy in an RCT predict effectiveness in a clinical setting?

A demonstration of efficacy in an RCT is typically satisfied by showing that the effects of a drug treatment upon primary or secondary outcome measures are statistically significant compared with a control treatment condition (placebo). A statistically significant difference between drug and placebo can sometimes be achieved with merely a marginal difference between those two treatment groups— a difference so small as to be relatively unimportant in a clinical setting. A modest yet statistically significant improvement indicates that patients have improved to some degree, but it does not necessarily mean that the improvement is clinically meaningful or that patients feel completely well again.

Regardless of the magnitude of a drug's effect size (i.e., measured effect of drug minus effect of placebo), the majority of RCTs assess efficacy for a group of patients in a study, and do not evaluate effectiveness measured as remission or a return to wellness. There are examples for how to structure a study that measures whether a medication restores wellness (e.g., Goldbloom & Olmsted, 1993), but such demonstrations are not required of RCTs to support requests for regulatory approval. Obviously, a demonstration of a medication-induced return to wellness must clear a higher bar than a demonstration of a drug-induced effect that is merely statistically greater than placebo treatment. When the magnitude-of-effect bar is set lower for an RCT, it may well increase the likelihood the results can support a request for regulatory approval. But, that lower standard threatens the clinical utility of the findings from the RCT.

Characteristics of the typical RCT that impose limits on a study's utility are not necessarily weaknesses of experimental design. An RCT can have a tight, efficient experimental design that provides a rigorous test of a clearly specified hypothesis regarding drug efficacy, but have limited ability to predict that drug's clinical effectiveness. These limitations are often attributable to one or more of the following issues:

- Exclusion factors often create an atypical sample of patients. The most common example of this is to exclude individuals who satisfy diagnostic criteria for any disorder other than the one under investigation in the study. In fact, most RCTs do not study the effects of a drug in patients who demonstrate a comorbid psychiatric condition. This maneuver eliminates potential sources of confounding attributable to comorbidity, thereby decreasing variability in measures of outcome and increasing the power of statistical analysis. This can increase the likelihood of a statistically significant demonstration of drug efficacy, but will limit the generalizability of the findings to those patients who do not present comorbidity in a clinical setting.

- Exclusion factors often deny access to individuals currently or recently being treated with a psychotropic drug. This removes potential sources of confounding due to drug interactions or to previous medication-induced neuroadaptations in brain neurochemistry. This can decrease variability in measures of outcome, thereby increasing the likelihood of a statistically significant demonstration of drug efficacy. But it also means that the results of the RCT may not be sufficiently predictive of the effect of the drug being studied on patients who are using (or have previously used) other psychiatric medications.

- Exclusion factors can deny access to individuals who have been previously treated for the psychiatric disorder being studied. This maneuver excludes from the trial individuals who previously had been refractory to treatment for the psychiatric condition being studied. Excluding patients who may be among the most difficult to treat successfully may increase the potential for demonstrating efficacy for the drug being investigated, and may overestimate the drug's potential clinical effectiveness.

- Use of a single dose of drug. The choice of single dose can favor the selection of dose that is likely to have a measurable desired effect, while at the same time have relatively lesser potential for producing adverse events. An RCT that employs only a single dose provides little or no information regarding an effective dosage for an individual patient. Such single-dose RCTs reveal the average response to a dose of medication that might be too small or too large to be the ideal dose for an individual patient.

- Short duration of study. Practical considerations certainly make long-term studies extremely difficult. But short-term studies cannot reveal whether efficacy increases or decreases over a longer duration of treatment that may be more probable in a clinical setting. Shorter-duration studies typically are not designed to measure consequences of discontinuation of pharmacotherapy or intervals of recovery between relapses. Moreover, shorter-duration RCTs are likely to underestimate the incidence and the impact of adverse events when that medication ultimately is used more chronically.

There are other characteristics related to the methodology or execution of an RCT that can limit the utility of the results for predicting clinical effectiveness of a drug. These include the following:

- Participant drop-outs. Any RCT can have the power of its statistical analysis compromised by premature dropouts of individuals in the study. Although there are strategies and statistical techniques for dealing with the dropout problem, important information will be lost and that missing information can result in decreased assessment of adverse events and/or exaggerated measure of effect size. In addition, disproportionate dropout rates can result from randomized assignment of participants to treatment groups (Corrigan & Salzer, 2003), because randomization typically fails to take into account the preferences for treatments of patients entering the study. This problem can decrease the internal validity of the clinical trial and make difficult the interpretation of a measure of drug efficacy.
- Selection of outcome measures. Some RCTs use measures of clinical outcome rarely or never used in clinical practice. The typical RCT is more likely to use clinical scales and surrogate outcome (i.e., presumed predictors of eventual clinical

improvement) measures than it is to measure clinical outcome or quality of life.

- Lack of drug versus drug comparisons in Phase III RCTs. Although it has become conventional that an RCT intended to support a request for FDA approval employ a placebo control (Kraemer & Schatzberg, 2009), it is not generally expected that an RCT compare the efficacy of the drug being investigated with an active control drug previously approved for clinical use. This means that the typical RCT provides little or no information about whether a new medication will be more or less effective than an older medication (Streiner, 2007).
- Ethical concerns presented by placebo control treatment. Ethical concerns arise when placebo is considered to be a treatment expected to have no effect. Although there is evidence that placebo can be active treatment causing measurable changes in brain (Benedetti et al., 2011; Pollo & Benedetti, 2009), ethical concerns remain regarding whether patients experience coercion when granting informed consent (Weimer et al., 2015), or when treatment with placebo might result in deterioration of a patient's condition.
- Alternatives to placebo control treatment. Although it has been asserted that the use of placebo control treatment in clinical drug trials is necessary and irreplaceable (Leber, 2000), various alternatives to placebo control have been used in clinical trials (Kraemer & Schatzberg, 2009). These alternative control treatments can be considered as two categories—reasonable alternatives and unacceptable alternatives that damage the methodological rigor of a clinical test of drug efficacy. Several reasonable alternatives address the ethical concern that placebo may do nothing, but they do not establish a methodology that enables a true drug versus placebo comparison. These alternatives include (a) combining some form of supportive counseling together with medication and together with placebo, respectively, in the treated groups of participants in a clinical trial; (b) using treatment-as-usual control instead of placebo control, that is, patients in the control condition receive whichever clinical treatment they would normally have received had they not

entered the clinical trial; and (c) using standard-of-treatment control instead of placebo control, that is, patients in the control condition receive what is considered to be the most effective treatment currently in use. Other alternatives to placebo control are considered to be generally unacceptable because they diminish the methodological rigor (e.g., diminished blinding regarding treatment, increased heterogeneity, decreased statistical power) of a clinical trial (Kraemer & Schatzberg, 2009). These include (a) a pre-post treatment comparison in which each participant provides data before medication and subsequently after medication; (b) a historical control group—data from a placebo-control group not being treated concurrently with the drug-treated group; and (c) a waiting list control group—participants in a clinical trial who are offered medication only after the trial has ended.

- Complications of placebo efficacy in the assessment of drug efficacy. The results of RCTs and practical clinical trials might be more useful if the interpretation of drug versus placebo comparisons were not confronted by high rates of response to placebo treatment. The efficacy of placebo in a double-blind RCT can be appreciable—for example, as high as 10% to 50% improvement in symptoms of depression (Walsh et al., 2002).
- Less rigorous methodology that may increase apparent placebo efficacy. Factors other than drug or placebo are kept equivalent and constant in each of two treatment groups in a well-constructed and carefully executed RCT. This should remove or control for potentially confounding variables to ensure that the comparison between the drug-treated group and the placebo-treated group is interpretable. But it is difficult to control all potential confounding variables within the environmental context of the drug or placebo treatments in a clinical trial, and it may not be possible to fully control factors that contribute to a placebo effect (and to a drug effect), such as the interaction between the patient and clinician or experimenter and other aspects of the treatment environment (Ernst, 2007; Finniss, Kaptchuk, Miller, & Benedetti, 2010). Accordingly, large measured placebo effects are more likely in some

experiments than in others, particularly in multi-center studies (Undurraga & Baldessarini, 2012), when it is difficult to implement uniform protocol across multiple research sites. Apparently RCTs conducted by the National Institute of Mental Health have better success at diminishing variability in outcome measures, therefore increasing statistical power, compared with trials conducted by industry; more rigorous methodology and more careful execution can result in smaller measured effects of placebo treatment, enhancing the assessment of a drug's efficacy for improving symptoms of depression (Li et al., 2017; Walkup, 2017).

- Numerous challenges with multicenter studies. A successful multicenter or multinational RCT requires successful implementation of protocol concerning inclusion and exclusion criteria and the measurement of outcomes that are common to each site providing data for the RCT. Differences in language, resources, and expertise of staff conducting the study, however, can introduce inconsistencies in the implementation of diagnostic criteria used to select participants, resulting in increased heterogeneity of the patient sample. Despite various sites in different countries agreeing to implementation of a common protocol, multicenter studies are also more likely to present inconsistencies in the measurement of ordinarily sensitive and reliable outcome measures and differences in participant dropout rates across sites owing to methodological inconsistencies or cultural attitudes regarding treatments (Baldessarini, 2013). These problems can diminish the methodological rigor and the power of statistical analysis of data, despite the advantage of larger numbers of participants available in multicenter studies.
- Manipulation of placebo effect size to create bias. Employing a placebo-washout criterion that excludes patients who demonstrate some measure of improvement to placebo can reduce the magnitude of a placebo effect in a clinical drug trial. Such an exclusion criterion then leaves a sample of patients who are less likely to demonstrate placebo efficacy and perhaps more likely to demonstrate apparently greater efficacy

of drug. Alternatively, those patients who do not wash out (i.e., those who are less responsive to placebo) may be less responsive to any treatment, and therefore less likely to show appreciable drug efficacy.

In short, a placebo control treatment functions best when the drug trial's methodology is rigorous and procedures in the clinical trial are carefully implemented (Walkup, 2017). Those circumstances should reduce variability in measures of outcome, increase the power of statistical analysis of data, and facilitate interpretation of findings. So long as there is the expectation for a placebo control in a clinical drug trial, however, it will be difficult to measure a so-called *pure* drug effect, because a drug is administered within a social therapeutic context that interacts with the drug's pharmacological attributes as well as with those of the pharmacologically inert placebo (Ernst, 2007; Finniss et al., 2010). This means that the measured efficacies of drug and of placebo are affected by factors such as experimenter–participant interaction and other aspects of a clinical drug trial's procedures (e.g., requiring that a participant keep a diary self-reporting medication/placebo compliance or outcome measures). Moreover, the social environment of a drug trial experiment is not likely to resemble the social environment for clinical use of that drug. Those differences in social context challenge the external validity of a clinical drug trial, limiting the usefulness of efficacy in a clinical trial for predicting effectiveness in a clinical setting.

In summary, even when the experimental design of an RCT meets minimum standards required by a regulatory agency, there can be considerable variability in the quality and utility of the data that an RCT collects. Moreover, there is little incentive for an RCT to do more than meet minimum standards, when the express goal of Phase III RCTs is to provide enough "pivotal" evidence to achieve regulatory approval. After all, it is the regulatory agency that sets the expectations and the standards for RCTs. So long as the regulatory agency enables RCTs to remain relatively minimal, their ability to predict clinical effectiveness will be limited. It then becomes the post–regulatory approval, postmarketing Phase IV

experiments that provide the more important findings for effective clinical use of a new medication.

PRACTICAL CLINICAL TRIALS IN PSYCHOPHARMACOLOGY

Practical clinical trials—also called pragmatic, effectiveness, or management trials—randomly assign real-world patients into experiments designed to evaluate the effectiveness of an approved medication under conditions in which patients are likely to be treated. These Phase IV experiments are less likely to be funded by pharmaceutical industry resources and are likely to have greater value than Phase III RCTs for identifying the circumstances under which a specific medication can be expected to be clinically useful.

As with RCTs, practical clinical trials are bolstered by guidelines for experimental design (e.g., Treweek et al., 2006). Examples of large-scale practical clinical trials include the Clinical Antipsychotic Trials of Intervention Effectiveness (CATIE; e.g., Lieberman et al., 2005), the Cost Utility of the Latest Antipsychotic Drugs in Schizophrenia Study (CUtLASS; e.g., Jones et al., 2006), and the Sequenced Treatment Alternatives to Relieve Depression (STAR*D; e.g., Sinyor et al., 2010) trials. The STAR*D trials were sponsored by the National Institute of Mental Health at a cost of $65 million over a period of 6 years. It included comparisons of effectiveness of monotherapy, combined treatments, and augmentation strategies for a variety of medications. Assessment of effectiveness included measures of the primary outcome of remission (using the Hamilton Depression Rating Scale) and secondary outcomes including physician and patient self-reports and measures of patients' levels of function and quality of life.

Given the magnitude of resources required to administer practical clinical trials, it is not surprising that there are comparatively fewer such trials than there are RCTs. The case for providing resources to support more practical clinical trials in psychiatry is compelling (March et al., 2005; Vitiello, 2015), as is the need for high standards (Barbui & Cipriani, 2007; Tansella et al., 2006). Specific ways in which practical clinical drug trials compensate for the limitations of RCTs include the following:

- Fewer exclusion factors. Excluding fewer individuals increases the likelihood that the sample is representative of patients who seek treatment, including patients showing comorbidity.
- Larger sample size. A larger, more heterogeneous sample size may require a multicenter clinical trial. This can provide sufficiently large subgroups of treatment conditions that may give the study enough statistical power to permit comparisons of effectiveness of several different drugs, different modes of behavioral or psychotherapy, and combinations of treatments.
- Setting. Practical clinical trials are more likely to be conducted in the setting of clinical practice, increasing the generalizability of the findings.
- Outcome measures. Measures of clinical effectiveness are more likely to include the kind of assessment tools commonly used in clinical practice.
- Goals. Because gaining regulatory approval of a product is not the principal goal of a practical clinical trial, there is less likelihood of bias that might influence experimental design, exclusion criteria, analysis of data, selection of data reported, and interpretation of results.
- Dosage of drug. Selection of dosages of drug are determined by clinical judgment, and not unduly influenced by a desire to minimize the likelihood of drug-induced adverse events.
- Duration of study. A practical clinical trial is likely to run longer than an RCT, because the participants are patients in treatment. This increases the likelihood of measuring effectiveness of treatment in the short term as well as during discontinuation of medication, and of measuring duration of remission prior to relapse.

Does a comparison between the results of an RCT and the results of a randomized practical clinical trial demonstrate that drug efficacy demonstrated in an RCT might not adequately predict clinical effectiveness? It can, as illustrated from data obtained in STAR*D research studying depressed patients in a practical clinical trial (Wisniewski et al., 2009). The analysis compared results from the subgroup

of depressed patients who would have successfully met inclusion/exclusion criteria for a typical RCT with those individuals in the practical clinical trial who would have been excluded from a typical RCT. Comparing the "efficacy sample" of participants to the larger, more heterogeneous "nonefficacy sample" revealed notable differences suggesting inflated assessment of drug efficacy in the RCT/efficacy sample of participants: Only 22.2% of individuals in the total sample ($n = 2,855$) met typical criteria for inclusion in an efficacy (RCT) sample. Individuals in this efficacy sample were more likely to be younger, White, employed, married, more educated, privately insured, and have higher income. They also were generally more healthy at onset of the study, revealing shorter average duration of illness, lower rates of family history of substance abuse, and fewer prior suicide attempts. The efficacy sample generally better tolerated the drug treatment, reporting fewer severe or intolerable side effects and fewer serious psychiatric adverse events. The efficacy sample had a higher average rate of favorable response to the drug (51.6%) than did the nonefficacy sample (39.1%). The efficacy sample also had a higher average rate of remission (34.4%) than did the nonefficacy sample (24.7%). Taken together, these findings generally suggest that drug trials that have more expansive inclusion criteria are more likely to measure efficacy in a sample of individuals that are more representative of real-life patients, and therefore the results of those drug trials are more likely to predict the magnitude of clinical effectiveness for that medication.

In summary, practical clinical trials enrich the evidence base for pharmacotherapy. That is their principal goal. Because practical clinical trials measure drug efficacy in a sample of individuals that is more representative of real-life patients and also are more likely to compare the effectiveness of a medication to other treatments in clinical use, the results of practical trials are more likely to facilitate the application of personalized medicine (Goldberger & Buxton, 2013)—that is, tailoring the use of medication to patients showing particular characteristics of diagnosis, comorbidity, polypharmacy, and history of previous treatment. Whereas Phase III RCTs are pivotal for bringing a drug to market, Phase IV practical clinical trials may provide evidence that is more useful for predicting the effectiveness of a drug under the various circumstances experienced by individual patients.

BASIC RESEARCH COMPLEMENTING THE EVIDENCE BASE

A mix of clinical anecdotal evidence, case studies, clinical drug trials, and practical clinical trials contribute in different measure to an evidence base for pharmacotherapy. That evidence base can be extended by results from a variety of basic research strategies. The variety of strategies is too broad to review here, but examples of some of those research approaches show how their findings can enhance the evidence base.

Neuroimaging

One approach employs neuroimaging techniques to identify pathophysiology contributing to symptoms of a psychiatric disorder. An example of this strategy used positron emission tomography (PET) to indirectly measure availability of endogenous dopamine in synapses in dorsal striatum of the human brain during craving for cocaine. This work (Volkow et al., 2006) demonstrated that increased availability of synaptic dopamine in a specific region of the brain correlates with intensity of craving for cocaine. These findings identify a potential specific neurochemical target for medications that might diminish craving.

A second example (Volkow et al., 2012) used PET neuroimaging to reveal a correlation between long-term (12 months) oral methylphenidate-induced improvement in symptoms of attention-deficit/hyperactivity disorder (ADHD) and decreased availability of D2/D3 dopamine receptors in ventral striatum of adults. These findings provide evidence for a presumed brain site-specific mechanism of action of methylphenidate for treatment of ADHD.

Neuroimaging using PET technology can also measure changes in glucose utilization in the brain that accompany improvement in symptoms induced by pharmacotherapy or nondrug therapies. For example, brain region-specific changes in glucose metabolism correlate with improvement in symptoms of major depression during cognitive behavioral therapy (CBT) or pharmacotherapy (paroxetine) for major depression (Goldapple et al., 2004), demonstrating (a) similar changes in glucose metabolism in the same select regions of brain following either pharmacotherapy or CBT, (b) directionally different changes in glucose metabolism in the same select regions of brain for pharmacotherapy or CBT, and (c) changes in glucose metabolism in select regions of brain that are unique to either pharmacotherapy or CBT. Such findings contribute to the evidence base by supporting the general idea that pharmacotherapy can, under some conditions, be expected to affect brain in some of the same ways as can CBT, and that some of the ways in which pharmacotherapy affects brain differ from changes produced by CBT.

Between-Sex Measure of Drug Efficacy

Another example is research designed to compare effectiveness of two different drugs used in men and women meeting *Diagnostic and Statistical Manual of Mental Disorders* (DSM) diagnosis of major depression. That work (Kornstein et al., 2000) revealed that the tricyclic imipramine can be more effective for treatment of major depression in men than in women, as evidenced in shorter latency to show improvement, greater improvement in primary outcome measures, and fewer reports of adverse events. In addition, the selective serotonin reuptake inhibitor (SSRI) sertraline was measured to be more effective in women than in men in the 12-week study. In contrast, postmenopausal women showed better responsiveness to imipramine than to sertraline. Although this experiment did not meet the expectations for experimental design for practical clinical trials (e.g., Treweek et al., 2006), the findings extend the evidence base in ways that would benefit decisions for pharmacotherapy based upon gender and age of patients.

Combined Medication and Psychotherapy

Other work that can expand the evidence base includes experiments that compare effectiveness of combined medication and nondrug approaches. One example is a study using a two-stage medication treatment (desipramine first, followed by fluoxetine if necessary) combined with CBT or supportive psychotherapy for bulimia nervosa (Walsh et al., 1997). The results demonstrated CBT to be superior to supportive psychotherapy, and that CBT combined with medication was superior to medication (or placebo) alone whereas supportive psychotherapy combined with medication was not superior to medication alone. In addition, combining CBT with medication appeared to decrease the average dosage of desipramine that was required to be effective. Another example is a study in which naltrexone was combined with either CBT or motivational enhancement therapy for treatment of alcohol dependence (Anton et al., 2005). It demonstrated superior effectiveness of naltrexone combined with CBT compared to monotherapy, or to drug combined with motivational enhancement therapy. Although these two experiments did not meet the expectations for experimental design of practical clinical trials, this type of research expands the evidence base for pharmacotherapy by identifying specific circumstances in which combined drug and nondrug therapies may be more beneficial than drug or behavioral monotherapy.

In summary, there are numerous experiments in humans that study various aspects of pharmacotherapy for psychiatric indications. Much of that research is conducted after regulatory approval for a new medication. That basic research, together with published RCTs and practical clinical trials, provides an enormous collection of research findings that can be very difficult to integrate and prioritize regarding their relative utility for the treatment of an individual patient. Moreover, many prescribing professionals lack the expertise to critically read original research reports that span diverse areas of neuroscience, psychiatry, psychopharmacology, and clinical psychology. Meta-analysis of published research offers some relief, but not without controversy.

META-ANALYSIS OF RESEARCH MEASURING DRUG EFFICACY OR EFFECTIVENESS

Meta-analysis provides a type of systematic review intended to address a specific research question. The publication of meta-analyses has demonstrated

exponential growth over the past 40 years (Haidich, 2010), and the findings of meta-analyses now play an important role in evidence-based medicine. The citation impact of published meta-analysis research has been impressive (Patsopoulos et al., 2005), supporting the perceived importance and clinical utility of the findings of meta-analysis research.

The major goal of meta-analysis is to quantify a synthesis of effect sizes reported from individual experiments (see Figure 6.1). The results of meta-analysis ostensibly could offer a prescribing clinician a summary objective assessment of research in order to facilitate decisions regarding the appropriate treatment for an individual patient. Meta-analysis of the relevant published work can be seen as an alternative to information that could be acquired by reading a published traditional narrative summary of that work—a review paper. In contrast to a review paper, quantitative meta-analysis can have the advantage of being able to objectively detect patterns of effects of psychiatric medications; for example, the specific conditions in which a drug induces larger effect sizes.

Meta-analysis is not exempt from problems in methodological design and implementation. Standards for meta-analysis of high quality are made explicit in various guidelines (Liberati et al., 2009; Moher et al., 2010). Given the increasing reliance on meta-analysis in psychopharmacology—and more broadly in the health sciences—it is important to consider some of the issues and problems that confront meta-analysis (Haidich, 2010; Tharyan, 1998), including the following:

■ Careful and complete selection of data is essential. The utility of meta-analysis for clinical pharmacotherapy is limited by the researcher's ability to thoroughly and judiciously search the relevant published literature and access unpublished relevant data (Hart et al., 2012). One obstacle to this is that Phase III RCTs are more likely to report positive findings of efficacy for drugs being investigated, whereas negative findings or findings of smaller effect sizes are more likely to remain unpublished (Page et al., 2014) or unreported (Anderson et al., 2015). Moreover, prospective registration of clinical trials in

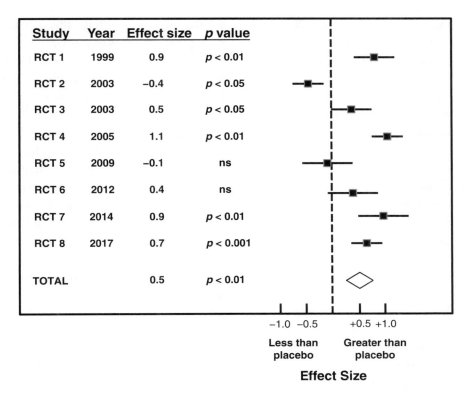

Study	Year	Effect size	*p* value
RCT 1	1999	0.9	*p* < 0.01
RCT 2	2003	–0.4	*p* < 0.05
RCT 3	2003	0.5	*p* < 0.05
RCT 4	2005	1.1	*p* < 0.01
RCT 5	2009	–0.1	ns
RCT 6	2012	0.4	ns
RCT 7	2014	0.9	*p* < 0.01
RCT 8	2017	0.7	*p* < 0.001
TOTAL		0.5	*p* < 0.01

–1.0 –0.5   +0.5 +1.0

Less than placebo   Greater than placebo

Effect Size

FIGURE 6.1.   A schematic representation of a forest plot for results from a fictional meta-analysis applied to eight randomized clinical drug trials (RCTs 1–8) published during the year indicated. A black square represents the effect size (d = [drug efficacy – placebo efficacy]/combined variance for drug and placebo) for each one of the eight RCTs. A positive effect size indicates drug had a greater effect than placebo upon outcome measures. A negative effect size indicates placebo had a greater effect than drug. Horizontal lines represent 95% confidence intervals. The *p* values report level of statistical significance for effect size. The open diamond represents the mean effect size and confidence interval for all eight RCTs; the mean effect size essentially represents the average of the mean effect sizes (black squares). The summary results of meta-analysis for drug versus placebo comparisons often report alternative computations of effect size, such as relative risk ratio (RR) or odds ratio (OR). ns = not significant.

psychiatry has had mixed success (Miller et al., 2015; Mulder et al., 2018; Scott et al., 2015), thereby diminishing awareness of unpublished, potentially negative findings.

■ Inclusion and exclusion criteria are pivotal. The careful selection and implementation of inclusion and exclusion criteria regarding the methodology of selected studies is decisive in determining the quality and utility of meta-analysis. Careful implementation of criteria decreases bias and heterogeneity, improves the power of statistical analysis of effect sizes, and facilitates interpretation and generalizability of the overall findings.

■ Quality of selected studies must be considered. Inclusion criteria should incorporate assessment of the quality of the individual studies considered for the meta-analysis, the meta-analysis should compare effect sizes for subgroups of studies that differ in methodological rigor, or higher quality studies should have greater weight for determining overall effect size.

Given the difficulty of designing, implementing, and ultimately evaluating a meta-analysis, there are methods (e.g., A MeaSurement Tool to Assess systematic Reviews [AMSTAR]) for assessing the quality of systematic reviews (Shea et al., 2009). Assessment of quality of a meta-analysis is important because some consider meta-analyses to be at the top of the hierarchy of a clinical evidence base (Haidich, 2010; Leucht et al., 2016), presumably unburdened by biases associated with other research (e.g., translational animal research, clinical case studies, RCTs, narrative systematic reviews).

Multiple treatments or network meta-analysis searches published (and unpublished) data to make indirect comparisons between different drugs used as pharmacotherapy (Leucht et al., 2016). Network meta-analysis can compare mean effect sizes for two medications by comparing the efficacies of each of those drugs to the efficacy of a third (reference) drug. This approach is used to rank drugs based on direct and indirect comparisons of mean effect sizes. For example, network meta-analysis of 15 antipsychotic medications studied in 212 published and unpublished RCTs revealed substantial differences among drugs for side effects, but relatively smaller differences for efficacy (Leucht et al., 2013). In addition, rank ordering of effect sizes differed for various domains (e.g., weight gain vs. extrapyramidal side-effects, etc.). Demonstrating that there can be different hierarchies for drug efficacy depending on the desired outcome can be useful for prescribing guidelines. Network meta-analysis can also compare multiple drug and nondrug treatments. For example, a network meta-analysis was used to perform a large-scale comparison of medication efficacy, tolerability, and safety, along with CBT and placebo treatments for major depression in children and adolescents in RCTs or in unpublished sets of data (Ma et al., 2014).

Some meta-analysis studies expand the evidence base despite having goals that are somewhat more academic than clinical. One example is a meta-analysis of neuroimaging studies that examined the characteristics of the dopamine dysfunction in schizophrenia. This work (Howes et al., 2012), considering results of 44 neuroimaging studies, revealed a significant increase in presynaptic dopamine function that could contribute to excessive synaptic dopamine neurotransmission. This finding suggests a novel pharmacotherapeutic approach

for treating schizophrenia that inhibits presynaptic dopamine synthesis or release.

Meta-analysis also has provided a unique approach for identifying effective dosages in men and women being treated for schizophrenia (Eugene & Masiak, 2017) by analyzing data reported for 70 patients in four published studies using PET neuroimaging measures of dopamine D2 receptor occupancy by olanzapine. The meta-analysis identified the lowest dosage of olanzapine necessary to produce at least 70% occupancy of D2 receptors—the minimum D2 receptor antagonism necessary for clinical effectiveness that avoids specific serious adverse events. This pharmacodynamics modeling study predicted that women would require a 10 mg/day dosage of olanzapine, while men would require a 20 mg/day dosage both for initiation and for maintenance treatment. This expands the evidence base for pharmacotherapy by identifying sex-specific, minimum average clinical dosages based on the effectiveness of the drug for targeting a characteristic of brain pathophysiology for schizophrenia.

Meta-analysis can provide information useful for establishing guidelines for decisions regarding pharmacotherapy. The results of meta-analyses can be misinterpreted, however, resulting in inappropriate generalizations applied to decisions regarding clinical treatment. This kind of mistake can be avoided with careful assessment of the quality of methodology of a meta-analysis (Shea et al., 2009), the judicious interpretation of results (Chaimani et al., 2017), and prudent application of findings to develop guidelines for treatment (Guyatt et al., 2008).

Meta-analysis and network meta-analysis are vulnerable to the criticism that those quantitative reviews of experiments bring, at best, indirect evidence to the evidence base, because they are comparing data for effect sizes across multiple experiments. The RCT or a practical clinical trial measures a mean effect size for a drug under specific experimental conditions. In contrast, meta-analysis computes an average value of mean effect sizes for a group of clinical trials that are likely to have some differences in experimental conditions. Although the meta-analysis assessment of effect size has the advantage of working with a larger set of data, its measure of the average of mean effect sizes may be no more valuable for predicting effectiveness in an individual patient than is mean effect size measured in an individual RCT.

Finally, the most rigorous, methodologically sound meta-analysis can only be as good as the quality of the research it is reviewing. The methodological or technological shortcomings of RCTs, practical clinical trials, and unpublished data delimit the usefulness of subsequent meta-analyses for helping to assemble clinical guidelines and inform clinical decisions (Chaimani et al., 2017).

REGULATORY AGENCY POLICIES SHAPE THE EVIDENCE BASE

As touched on previously, a drug in development moves toward approval at the FDA in this manner (Ciociola et al., 2014; Murphy & Roberts, 2006): Following collection of data ranging from pharmacokinetics to safety, an application for an Investigational New Drug (IND) is filed. The FDA evaluates the application, assessing the drug's potential to ultimately be approved for marketing and clinical use. From this point on, the FDA has oversight of continuing development through Phases I, II, and III studies prior to regulatory approval, and during Phase IV postmarketing studies. Prior to approval, smaller-scale RCTs are conducted in Phase II, and RCTs with greater numbers of participants are conducted in Phase III.

Approval by the FDA is generally understood to signal effectiveness and safety for new medications, because regulatory approval requires that substantial evidence has been obtained from adequate and well-controlled investigations of that drug (Laughren, 2010). This evidence is gathered from various types of investigations, but it is principally the randomized clinical trials that provide the substantial or pivotal evidence for supporting a decision to approve.

With data from at least two (and sometimes only one) Phase III randomized, placebo-controlled clinical drug trials, the manufacturer submits a new drug application (NDA) to the FDA. Approval of the NDA permits the drug's entry into the market with the expectation that postmarketing studies will further evaluate efficacy and safety in a larger, more heterogeneous sample of patients being treated, or

patients being studied in practical clinical trials. Postmarketing reports of serious side effects can result in the FDA requiring that "black box" labeling warn about potential for serious adverse events (Lasser et al., 2002). Black box warnings negatively affect prescribing (O'Brien et al., 2017). Once a drug has reached the marketplace for its approved use for treating a specific condition, the drug becomes available for off-label clinical use.

For psychiatric medications approved through this process between 2005 and 2012, 100% of the 43 new drugs approved had been studied in double-blind RCTs, 56% were compared with a placebo control, 44% were compared with an active drug control, 88% had efficacy measured either by a clinical rating scale (72%) or by clinical outcome (16%), and 12% had efficacy assessed using a surrogate outcome measure (Downing et al., 2014). It is fairly common for clinical drug trials to use an outcome measure assumed to be a valid indicator of eventual clinical improvement, thereby shortening the duration of the trial (Fleming & DeMets, 1996). An example of a surrogate outcome measure in a clinical trial of a psychiatric medication would be the use of standardized rating scales of symptoms as a surrogate for clinical assessment of full remission.

The approval process can be abbreviated when drugs are evaluated under expedited review, but concerns regarding assessments of efficacy and safety often arise (Chary & Pandian, 2017; Moore & Furberg, 2014). Drugs considered under expedited approval are more likely to use surrogate outcome measures in trials of short duration, some shorter than 6 weeks (Downing et al., 2014), thereby risking underestimating the incidence of adverse events that may require longer latency to appear.

Requiring only a single pivotal RCT also can shorten the time for drug development leading to approval. This arrangement typically anticipates that postapproval research will further evaluate efficacy and safety. This strategy can be disappointing. For example, for 20 FDA-approved medications in 2008, only 31% of the promised postapproval studies were conducted within the 5 years following approval (Moore & Furberg, 2014). Of those 20 approved medications (only one was a psychiatric medication), five received new or enhanced black box warnings, and eight drugs subsequently were required to have risk-management plans. In a study of 117 drugs that had been approved based on the results of a single pivotal RCT, 35% failed to receive the expected postapproval clinical trials (Pease et al., 2017). Perhaps more concerning, less than 10% of those 117 drugs subsequently had at least one published postapproval RCT that demonstrated efficacy based upon measures of clinical outcome.

Because Phase III RCTs are pivotal for decisions regarding approval, it is important to consider the limitations that the requirement of only one or two early RCTs might impose: At minimum, a drug studied in an RCT is expected to be statistically significantly better than placebo treatment under the limited experimental conditions of those one or two RCTs. This rather modest supporting clinical evidence allows a newly approved medication to be used with patients whose situations may or may not resemble those of the individuals studied in the early RCTs. This means that at the initial entry of that new medication into the clinical arena, its effectiveness and tolerability in an individual patient can represent essentially an educated guess. In addition, at initial entry into the market there typically is little or no evidence to predict the new medication's effectiveness or tolerability for those patients who present comorbidity, or for those being treated with multiple medications (O'Hara et al., 2017). In addition, because many early RCTs may study participants for short durations, may use surrogate outcome measures, and are less likely to use clinical outcome as the primary outcome measure, there is little known about effectiveness or tolerability for those patients using the medication for the long term, including using it for maintenance treatment. Nor is there likely to be much if any useful information regarding discontinuation of treatment.

Can the shortcomings regarding the usefulness of the early evidence base be rectified by changes to the regulatory approval process? What regulatory practices hinder or help the evidence base at the time of entry into the market?

The practice of accelerating the approval process by employing a minimum standard of only one pivotal RCT, supplemented by supporting evidence

from less valuable sources of data, can speed entry into the market. But this expedited review ultimately slows development of the evidence base: One full-scale RCT of high quality provides less data and pertinent information than two high quality full-scale RCTs, provides less supporting evidence to the base, and limits ideas for hypotheses that can be subsequently tested in important early postmarketing Phase IV practical clinical trials. Accelerating the approval process by permitting the use of surrogate endpoints or the use of clinical scales instead of measures of clinical outcome or quality of life certainly shortens the duration of studies and reduces costs. But this practice also constrains the utility of the evidence base at the time the new medication enters the marketplace (Fleming & DeMets, 1996). Moreover, drugs approved through an accelerated process appear more likely to earn a black box warning or to be withdrawn from the market for safety reasons (Frank et al., 2014).

Finally, permitting the use of direct-to-consumer advertising—typically beginning within 1 year of regulatory approval (Donohue et al., 2007)—facilitates early usage of new medications (Gaudiano & Miller, 2013; Gilbody et al., 2005) at a rate that can outpace important growth of the evidence base generated by Phase IV clinical trials. This increased prescribing and usage that transcends advances in the evidence base magnifies shortcomings of the early evidence base and of the educated guesswork inherent to off-label prescribing.

In summary, the standards for approval of a new medication by the FDA represent a compromise among the competing interests of the pharmaceutical industry, prescribing professionals, patients, consumers, and advocacy groups. This compromise is evidently intended to facilitate both making a new medication available as soon as reasonably possible, and basing the use of that medication on scientific evidence. The prevailing balance between early availability versus strength of the evidence base decidedly favors early availability. Most of the more clinically useful information about effectiveness of a new medication is learned after it begins to be sold and widely prescribed, magnifying the importance of postmarketing research. Important information for judicious prescribing is discovered through postapproval Phase IV practical clinical trials, anecdotal clinical evidence, and trial-and-error indicated use or off-label use of the medication in individual patients. Thus, current FDA regulatory practices result in approved-indicated use and off-label use of newer medications supported by a relatively weak evidence base that has the potential to be strengthened with continuing use and investigation. In short, important research on effectiveness, tolerability, and safety trails the drug's entry into the market, and the preapproval evidence from measures of drug efficacy in RCTs is not a robust or reliable predictor of clinical effectiveness or tolerability.

OFF-LABEL PRESCRIBING

Regulatory approval of a medication permits off-label use for purposes other than the approved indication. This off-label avenue of consent piggybacks on the limited evidence base that supported the request for regulatory approval for a specific indication. This permits the clinical judgment of the prescriber to supersede evidence that might later be obtained from systematic scientific inquiry in Phase IV RCTs and practical clinical trials. Ensuring the autonomy to treat according to the best judgment of the clinician to serve the best interests of the patient, regardless of the quality of the evidence base, nonetheless raises concern about the wisdom of increasingly widespread use of off-label prescribing.

This concern is heightened by the fact that psychiatric medications are increasingly being prescribed by professionals lacking training in psychiatry or clinical psychology, or without sufficient knowledge of psychopharmacology (Mark et al., 2009; Olfson, Blanco, Wang, Laje, & Correll, 2014; Olfson, Kroenke, Wang, & Blanco, 2014). In addition, some physicians appear to not be adequately informed about approved versus off-label status of some psychiatric medications, or about the extent of evidence demonstrating efficacy of psychiatric medications that they are prescribing (Chen et al., 2009).

Of further concern is the fact that regulatory approval of a medication for a specific indication in adults allows off-label prescribing of that drug to treat children and adolescents. Such off-label usage begins to create an evidence base for pharmacotherapy in children and adolescents for both the originally approved indication and for any other disorder. This off-label-generated expansion of the evidence base for a drug, founded mostly upon clinical anecdotes and small-scale trials, is even less substantive than the evidence base created by the original few Phase II and Phase III RCTs in adults that were scrutinized during the regulatory approval process (American Academy of Pediatrics Committee on Drugs, 2014).

The incidence of off-label prescribing of psychiatric medications is striking and it is growing: Representative national data for 2001 (Radley et al., 2006) estimate that approximately 31% of 18 million psychiatric drug prescriptions were for off-label purposes. This appears to be higher than the rate of off-label prescribing for prescription drugs overall (Field, 2008). In addition (Radley et al., 2006), off-label use of psychiatric medications showed the greatest disparity (compared with nonpsychiatric medications) between the incidence of off-label usage supported by scientific evidence (4%) compared with off-label usage not supported by scientific evidence (96%). This is consistent with findings from 2005 through 2007 in which antidepressants, antipsychotics, and anxiolytics/sedatives predominated among the top 25 drugs ranked by incidence of off-label usage (Walton et al., 2008).

These statistics for off-label use of psychotropic drugs are not so surprising when considering that for each class of medications approved to treat *DSM–IV* categories of psychiatric conditions, the number of different off-label uses exceeds the FDA-approved indications (Devulapalli & Nasrallah, 2009). Factors that contribute to high incidences of off-label usage include polypharmacy to treat comorbidities and pharmacotherapy that targets symptoms, many of which appear in diagnostic criteria for multiple psychiatric indications (Walton et al., 2008). This latter fact encourages use of drugs to treat symptoms of the approved indications and also to treat off-label the analogous symptoms of other (unapproved) indications.

Despite these concerns, off-label prescribing of psychiatric medications serves a variety of useful purposes (Stahl, 2013), including treating an unapproved indication, using an unapproved or unlabeled dosage, treating for an unapproved or unlabeled duration, treating an unapproved or unlabeled age group, and treating in combination with a second drug not approved in the label. Each of those purposes represents the use of an approved medication, but without supporting scientific evidence. This gives physicians the latitude to act in what they believe to be the best interests of the patient. A patient certainly would want a prescribing physician to have this autonomy for delivering personalized medical treatment (Gupta & Nayak, 2014). But what does it say about evidence-based pharmacotherapy when more than 90% of the psychiatric drugs that are prescribed off-label have relatively little or no scientific evidence to support that unapproved use (Radley et al., 2006)?

Off-label prescribing can benefit all stakeholders—clinicians, clients, and industry. All win if and when the off-label usage improves quality of treatment. But, it is reasonable to contend that off-label prescribing of psychiatric medications is more akin to educated guesswork, or experimentation without informed consent, than it is convincingly evidence-based treatment.

DISPARITY IN THE EVIDENCE BASE FOR AGE, SEX, AND ETHNICITY

Those most vulnerable to the shortcomings of off-label use of psychiatric medications are child, adolescent, and elderly patients (Vitiello, 2007). Off-label pharmacotherapy with these patient groups raises ethical concerns (Spetie & Arnold, 2007; Welisch & Altamirano-Diaz, 2015) as well as misgivings regarding the use of treatments lacking a solid evidence base. The evidence base for pharmacotherapy in these groups is relatively weak principally because the majority of RCTs in Phases II and III use adults as participants. Recent (mid-1990s) changes in FDA policies (and also in those of European regulatory agencies), as well as incentives, have increased the use of patients in these vulnerable age groups as participants in studies evaluating efficacy and safety of psychiatric medications (Spetie & Arnold, 2007; Welisch & Altamirano-Diaz, 2015).

The ensuing strengthening of the evidence base obviates some of the concerns of off-label treatment of these age groups, but it remains the case that the use of psychiatric medications in young patients is outpacing the research that might validate such practice (Vitiello, 2007).

Children and Adolescents
In the United Kingdom, where psychotherapy has been the first-line treatment for ADHD in children and adolescents, prescriptions for medications for ADHD increased by 800% from 2000 to 2015 (Renoux et al., 2016). During the same period in the United States, the use of medications for major depression in adolescents and young adults increased by 21% despite no significant increase in the use of counseling or psychotherapy (Mojtabai, Olfson, & Han, 2016).

Specifically regarding off-label prescribing, data (from 2001–2004) for outpatient pediatric (less than 18 years of age) visits that included prescription of psychotropic medication revealed that more than 50% of those prescriptions were off-label for indication or for dosage (Bazzano et al., 2009). Off-label use in patients younger than 20 years increased at a pace greater than increases in prescribing for adults, nearly doubling between 1999 and 2010 (Olfson, Blanco, et al., 2014); this increase in prescribing was coincident with a decline in the use of psychotherapy, and an increasing proportion of those prescriptions were written by nonpsychiatrist practitioners. Moreover, across a 12-year period (from 1996–2007) the frequency of psychiatric drug polypharmacy in children and adolescents nearly doubled (Comer, Olfson, & Mojtabai, 2010).

Carrying out clinical drug trials using children and adolescents as participants has been slowed by a need for solving methodological issues (Vitiello, 2007) related to using young patients in experiments (e.g., informed consent, difficulty diagnosing, placebo control) and also because of ethical concerns (Spetie & Arnold, 2007; Welisch & Altamirano-Diaz, 2015). Success in addressing some of those issues has increased the incidence of RCTs in children and adolescents, but the developing evidence base for pharmacotherapy in young people is unlikely to have kept pace with increasing off-label prescribing in those groups (Vitiello, 2007).

Addressing methodological and ethical concerns has done little to remove worry regarding another important issue: Exposing a still developing brain and nervous system to potent psychotropic drugs can alter the course of development (Andersen, 2003). Whether psychotropic medications have negative or positive consequences on the development of the human brain remains an open question (Singh & Chang, 2012). This fact presents legitimate concern to researchers wanting to perform RCTs and practical clinical trials intended to expand the evidence base, and to clinicians prescribing psychotropic medications for young patients.

With these issues taken together, it is not surprising that the evidence base from the results of RCTs or practical clinical trials performed in children and adolescents is inferior to the evidence base for pharmacotherapy in adults. Consequently, the numbers of drugs that are FDA-approved for treating children or adolescents are fewer, practically compelling off-label use of medications for treatment—assuming that a drug is more likely to be effective as treatment than would psycho- therapy or behavioral therapy. That assumption is consistent with recent trends for use of different treatment modalities for psychiatric diagnoses (Olfson, Kroenke, et al., 2014).

As pharmacotherapy becomes increasingly commonplace, the operational evidence base for off-label pharmacotherapy in children and adolescents is to a great extent the evidence base established for FDA-approved use and off-label use in adults. The justification for this is the false assumption that what is learned about efficacy and safety in adults predicts what could be learned about efficacy and safety in children and adolescents. This means off-label use of psychiatric medications in children and adolescents generally poses uncertain benefits and risks.

Elderly Patients

Risks also attend the use of psychiatric medications to treat elderly patients, including adverse events due to drug interactions made more likely by polypharmacy (Maust et al., 2017). An elderly patient requiring treatment also presents difficulty for predicting the effectiveness and safety of a medication, owing to age-related differences in pharmacokinetics and pharmacodynamics (Howland, 2009; Trifirò & Spina, 2011), age-related changes in brain neurochemistry (Anyanwu, 2007; Meltzer et al., 2003), difficulty following instructions for use of medication due to drug-induced or age- related impairment in cognition, and unpredictable drug interactions (Hilmer et al., 2007). A reduction in the potential for harm from drug interactions may require deprescribing—"systematically identifying and tapering, reducing or stopping medications that are not indicated (either because of previous misdiagnosis or evidence of no benefit or harm for a true diagnosis), or are causing, or have consider- able potential to cause, adverse effects" (Scott & Le Couteur, 2015).

Although elderly patients are represented in RCTs, statistical analyses of data to determine the efficacy of a drug in that specific subgroup of patients are infrequently reported. Moreover, the incidence of polypharmacy diminishes the ability to produce guidelines for prescribing that are useful, given the heterogeneity of the physiological status of elderly patients. Thus, the evidence base from most clinical drug trials is of relatively little use for predicting clinical effectiveness specifically for the elderly (Pollock et al., 2009).

Women

Women are also underserved by the evidence base. Very little research prior to the middle 1990s measured and compared efficacy for psychiatric medications in women versus men in clinical drug trials (Yonkers & Brawman-Mintzer, 2002; Yonkers, Kando, Cole, & Blumenthal, 1992). To address this neglect, the FDA loosened restrictions on the use of women of childbearing potential in research, and the FDA and the National Institutes of Health issued requirements for including women in clinical trials and for performing statistical analyses to assess for differences between sexes (Merkatz et al., 1993). The representation of women in clinical drug trials subsequently has shown only modest improvement (Eshera et al., 2015; Liu & DiPietro Mager, 2016; Poon et al., 2013). There now is evidence for sex differences in the brain (Cosgrove et al., 2007) and in pharmacokinetics and pharmacodynamics for psychiatric medications (Marazziti et al., 2013). There are RCTs and practical clinical trials that compare efficacy of medications in women versus men (Franconi & Campesi, 2014), in particular for antidepressant and antipsychotic medications. The evidence base remains inadequate, however, to provide guidelines that facilitate tailoring pharmacotherapy to women and men, except perhaps for isolated instances (e.g., Kornstein et al., 2000).

A consideration of reasons why women (and ethnic minority persons) are not yet being adequately represented in clinical trials suggests potential remedies, including (Coakley et al., 2012) (a) engaging local community organizations and their trusted leaders to facilitate recruitment of participants by emphasizing the importance of clinical trials for underrepresented groups; (b) having administrators of clinical trials communicate with increased transparency and without being condescending, which may diminish distrust and concern regarding stigma for potential participants; (c) encouraging patients to demand quality health care while educating physicians, health care providers, and patients regarding the ways in which clinical research of high quality ultimately benefits all; (d) understanding geographic differences regarding the incidence of disorders that disproportionally affect women or minority persons, which can facilitate recruitment of participants; (e) employing more stringent regulatory requirements for design of clinical trials that include sufficient representation of sex and ethnicity; (f) employing technological tools that improve the ability to collect, store, and analyze data to reveal sex or ethnic differences; and (g) increasing the use of web-based direct-to-participant venues for clinical trials, allowing participants to contribute from their homes at their convenience, which could diminish problems related to transportation and distance from trial sites that make participation difficult.

Minority Ethnic Groups

The evidence base for differences in efficacy of psychiatric medications for different ethnicities also is deficient (Malik et al., 2010; Moore &

Mattison, 2017). Published research describes differences in pharmacokinetics and pharmacodynamics for several classes of medications, but the findings support little more than broad generalizations, such as Whites typically require larger dosages of psychiatric medications than do people of color.

The ethnic diversity within sample sizes in most clinical drug trials is not representative of the proportions of minority racial or ethnic groups in the population of the United States (Coakley et al., 2012; Eshera et al., 2015). In societies experiencing a shift in the majority ethnicity, it will become important to construct RCTs and practical drug trials that measure efficacy for various racial groups and ethnicities. Research should also assess the impact of social and cultural factors that can contribute to differences in effectiveness of medications, such as religious beliefs or attitudes toward using psychotropic drugs or herbal remedies (Rey, 2006).

In summary, when an evidence base is relatively weak, increased off-label prescribing and educated guesswork play greater roles in prescribing medications for children, adolescent, elderly, and non-White patients.

THE EVIDENCE BASE AS GUIDE FOR PRESCRIBING

Do all prescribing professionals expertly use the evidence base for judicious prescribing of psychiatric mediations? Probably not (Chen et al., 2009). The capacity—the experience and the available time—for critically reading the primary literature in professional journals in psychiatry, clinical psychology, psychopharmacology, behavioral medicine, and neuroscience is relatively uncommon. But the ability to appreciate the strengths and the weaknesses of the evidence base for pharmacotherapy can be acquired with an investment of time. Several excellent sources provide advice useful for beginning to tackle the primary literature in clinical psychopharmacology (Dubovsky & Dubovsky, 2007; McGrath, 2010, 2012).

The most effective way to acquire critical reading skills is to participate in a seminar, reading published articles along with a person who has sufficient expertise to create a reading list that includes a broad range of research papers, review articles, pertinent essays, case studies, meta-analyses, and editorials. Reading two papers every other week for a year should be sufficient. The ability to read critically becomes evident when a person needs to read only methods and results sections of research papers to understand the strengths and limitations of a study and to appreciate alternative interpretations of the results. The problem then becomes finding the time for reading the primary literatures on a regular basis for an extended period of time—the length of one's career, as the evidence base for pharmacotherapy continues to evolve.

Critical reading of research papers affords a working knowledge of what the results of RCTs and practical clinical trials can actually deliver. The critical reader should have a full appreciation for whether a demonstration of efficacy might or might not predict clinical effectiveness. That appreciation should help in crafting an individualized treatment program.

It is unrealistic to expect that every professional with the responsibility of prescribing psychotropic drugs will be able to hold to a commitment to develop and continue to use critical reading skills. An alternative is to rely on guidance from resources that summarize findings from clinical trials, academic research, and meta-analyses with the goal of recommending treatment options based on the authors' critical reading of the published findings. The best of these resources present not only a summary of findings, but also an assessment of the quality of types of research that provide evidence relevant for a variety of treatment options, including pharmacotherapy (e.g., Nathan & Gorman, 2015; Stein et al., 2012). An online resource of significant value is the Cochrane Library (www.cochranelibrary.com).

Treatment guidelines are not an equivalent substitute for having a working knowledge about principles of psychopharmacology, drug development, regulatory agency standards and practices, experimental design, statistical analysis of data, and the ways in which legislation and industry influence access and pricing for medications

(Goldberger & Buxton, 2013). In fact, the principal goal of prescribing guidelines and the principal goal of individualized treatment are at odds: Guidelines recommend what might be best for the average patient, whereas most patients are not average. In addition, the quality of a prescribing guideline is limited by the quality of the research used to construct the guideline (Guyatt et al., 2008), and it is vulnerable to influence from industry, which raises concern about the fidelity of some guidelines (Healy, 2009).

IMPROVING THE EVIDENCE BASE FOR PHARMACOTHERAPY

The evidence base for pharmacotherapy begins as preclinical studies using animal models facilitate development of new drugs to be tested in Phases II, III, and IV in humans. The operational clinical utility of the evidence base subsequently evolves from pre–regulatory approval continuing through postapproval clinical use and research. Across that period of time, the research supporting regulatory approval for a new medication is the pivotal, fateful element. The preapproval RCTs are important for more than merely authorizing a new drug to reach the market. They also determine the relative importance and necessity of subsequent post-marketing research, and the extent to which clinical practices can claim to be principally evidence based. How might the evidence base be improved to make pharmacotherapy more effective?

The preclinical translational research is most useful when not hindered by lack of knowledge regarding pathophysiology that underlies symptoms for psychiatric disorders (Berk & Nierenberg, 2015). An ideal animal model would have good construct validity and predictive validity, making it useful for forecasting the potential for a new drug's clinical effectiveness (Hyman, 2016; Kraly, 2014; Sarter & Tricklebank, 2012). When validity of an animal model is hindered by ignorance regarding patho-physiology, it frustrates development of novel pharmacotherapeutics. That problem has contributed to the recent reduction of pharmaceutical industry resources spent on research using animal models, consequently curtailing development of psychiatric medications having novel mechanisms of action (Cowen, 2011; Hyman, 2016). Thus, it is important that animal models incorporate discoveries regarding pathophysiology to facilitate development of drugs that are ultimately tested in Phases II, III, and IV in humans. (See Chapter 4, this volume.)

Academic research in humans can drive formulation of hypotheses tested and methodologies used in clinical drug trials. The quality and utility of Phases II, III, and IV clinical trials depend to some extent on the quality of diagnostic criteria used to select participants for trials. Nosology for psychiatric disorders in *DSM–5* continues to depend almost entirely on criteria based on behavior, and not upon pathophysiology related to symptoms. Moreover, current diagnostic categories are characterized by heterogeneity that might be diminished if criteria included measurable pathophysiology (Gorman & Nathan, 2015) such as neuroimaging measures or biomarkers (Laughren, 2010). Dividing current categories into subcategories that incorporate identified pathophysiology should reduce heterogeneity. Using these revised diagnostic criteria for subcategories of disorders for selection of participants should also reduce variability for measures of clinical outcome, and those participants should be more representative of subgroups of patients who seek treatment. This should improve the predictive validity of the results from RCTs (Norquist & Hyman, 1999).

The value of RCTs can be improved in ways that expand or strengthen the evidence base, such as raising the standards and expectations for regulatory approval (which certainly will be easier said than done), increasing the regulatory requirement for proportionate representation in clinical trials of currently underrepresented groups (e.g., children, adolescents, women, racial and ethnic groups), providing greater incentives for industry-sponsored practical clinical drug trials to offset the incentive that off-label prescribing practices afford for not conducting postmarketing research, and increasing the working knowledge that prescribing professionals have for judicious implementation of the scientific evidence that supports (or does not support) the use of medication as monotherapy or as adjunct to psychotherapy.

CONCLUSION: WHAT THE EVIDENCE BASE CURRENTLY PROVIDES

The current evidence base for pharmacotherapy provides the opportunity to leap from experiments that demonstrate efficacy in a group of patients to attempts to provide effective individualized treatment for patients. The length of that leap shortens as postmarketing practical clinical trials enrich the evidence base with information that is more pertinent for tailoring the use of a drug to a patient's unique set of circumstances. New knowledge about efficacy of newer and older medications is important, but it does not purge contemporary pharmacotherapy of its trial-and-error nature, because the evidence base is not yet good enough to enable a clinician to reliably predict effectiveness and tolerability for a specific medication prescribed for an individual patient. But the evidence base can support a well-informed judicious speculation, following up, and making the necessary adjustments to treatment.

The current status of the evidence base represents a compromise among the competing interests of those who prescribe, those who approve, those who sell, and those who use psychiatric medications. Of those participating groups, the pharmaceutical industry has the superior resources to influence that compromise. This has produced a compromise that prioritizes making new medications available as soon as reasonably possible, following regulatory approval based upon the results of experiments principally designed to demonstrate drug efficacy for a limited, specific set of circumstances (Singal et al., 2014). Regulatory approval sanctions usage for a specific indication and allows off-label prescribing for unapproved indications, with the understanding that research will expand the evidence base as patients are being treated with a drug that continues to be investigated. These circumstances can only ensure that a patient may or may not improve. On the reasonable probability that the patient might benefit, the patient effectively becomes the single subject in a unique clinical experiment.

Prescribing that "experiment" may be the best treatment for a patient who is suffering and wanting and expecting to get better. Given the current unpredictability of pharmacotherapy for effectiveness and tolerability, however, it may be best to consider medication as well as evidence-based psychotherapy (Huhn et al., 2014; Nathan & Gorman, 2015).

The evidence base for pharmacotherapy and the no-less-important evidence base for psychotherapy (Cook et al., 2017) are limited, but useful. The evidence base for pharmacotherapy will be improved if the concerned parties can agree to alter priorities in such a way as to better profit the prescriber and the patient. Without an adjustment of priorities, the experimental science that constructs the evidence base will continue to run behind the clinical use of psychotropic drugs. When more of the scientific evidence precedes and guides the use of those drugs, prescribers and patients will be better served.

TOOL KIT OF RESOURCES

Clinical Trials Guidelines and Reporting Standards

Sponsor and Researcher Resources

U.S. Food and Drug Administration
https://www.fda.gov/ScienceResearch/
SpecialTopics/RunningClinicalTrials/
GuidancesInformationSheetsandNotices/
ucm219433.htm

World Health Organization
http://apps.who.int/iris/bitstream/10665/76705/1/
9789241504294_eng.pdf

Consolidated Standards of Reporting Trials (CONSORT)
http://www.consort-statement.org

American Psychological Association
http://www.apastyle.org/manual/related/
JARS-MARS.pdf

Standard Protocol Items: Recommendations for Interventional Trials (SPIRIT)
http://www.bmj.com/content/bmj/346/
bmj.e7586.full.pdf

Clinical Trials Registries

Researcher Resources

U.S. National Institutes of Health
https://clinicaltrials.gov

Health Canada
https://www.canada.ca/en/health-canada/services/
drugs-health-products/drug-products/
health-canada-clinical-trials-database.html

European Medicines Agency
https://www.clinicaltrialsregister.eu

World Health Organization
http://www.who.int/ictrp/en/

Clinical Trials Participation

Sponsor and Patient Resources

U.S. National Institute of Mental Health
https://www.nimh.nih.gov/health/trials/
index.shtml

Citizens for Responsible Care and Research (CIRCARE)
http://www.circare.org/registries.htm

Reviews of the Evidence Base

Prescriber and Patient Resources

Cochrane Library
http://www.cochranelibrary.com/about/
about-cochrane-systematic-reviews.html

Nathan, P. E., & Gorman, J. M. (Eds.). (2015). A guide to treatments that work (4th ed.). New York, NY: Oxford University Press.

Stein, D. J., Lerer, B., & Stahl, S. M. (Eds.). (2012). Essential evidence-based psychopharmacology (2nd ed.). New York, NY: Cambridge University Press.

Meta-Analysis

Researcher and Prescriber Resources

Preferred Reporting Items for Systematic Reviews and Meta-Analyses (PRISMA)
http://prisma-statement.org

A MeaSurement Tool to Assess systematic Reviews (AMSTAR)
https://amstar.ca/index.php

Continuing Education in Clinical Psychopharmacology

Prescriber Resources

American Society of Clinical Psychopharmacology
https://www.ascpp.org

American Psychiatric Nurses Association
https://e-learning.apna.org

References

Altman, D. G., Schulz, K. F., Moher, D., Egger, M., Davidoff, F., Elbourne, D., . . . Lang, T., & the CONSORT GROUP (Consolidated Standards of Reporting Trials). (2001). The revised CONSORT statement for reporting randomized trials: Explanation and elaboration. *Annals of Internal Medicine, 134,* 663–694. http://dx.doi.org/10.7326/0003-4819-134-8-200104170-00012

American Academy of Pediatrics Committee on Drugs. (2014). Policy Statement: Off-label use of drugs in children. *Pediatrics, 133,* 563–567.

Andersen, S. L. (2003). Trajectories of brain development: Point of vulnerability or window of opportunity? *Neuroscience and Biobehavioral Reviews, 27,* 3–18. http://dx.doi.org/10.1016/S0149-7634(03)00005-8

Anderson, M. L., Chiswell, K., Peterson, E. D., Tasneem, A., Topping, J., & Califf, R. M. (2015). Compliance with results reporting at ClinicalTrials.gov. *The New England Journal of Medicine, 372,* 1031–1039. http://dx.doi.org/10.1056/NEJMsa1409364

Anton, R. F., Moak, D. H., Latham, P., Waid, L. R., Myrick, H., Voronin, K., . . . Woolson, R. (2005). Naltrexone combined with either cognitive behavioral or motivational enhancement therapy for alcohol dependence. *Journal of Clinical Psychopharmacology, 25,* 349–357. http://dx.doi.org/10.1097/01.jcp.0000172071.81258.04

Anyanwu, E. C. (2007). Neurochemical changes in the aging process: Implications in medication in the elderly. *The Scientific World Journal, 7,* 1603–1610. http://dx.doi.org/10.1100/tsw.2007.112

Baldessarini, R. J. (2013). *Chemotherapy in psychiatry: Pharmacologic basis of treatments for major mental illness* (3rd ed.). New York, NY: Springer. http://dx.doi.org/10.1007/978-1-4614-3710-9

Barbui, C., & Cipriani, A. (2007). Evidence-based psychopharmacology: An agenda for the future. *Evidence-Based Mental Health, 10,* 4–6. http://dx.doi.org/10.1136/ebmh.10.1.4-a

Bazzano, A. T. F., Mangione-Smith, R., Schonlau, M., Suttorp, M. J., & Brook, R. H. (2009). Off-label prescribing to children in the United States outpatient setting. *Academic Pediatrics, 9,* 81–88. http://dx.doi.org/10.1016/j.acap.2008.11.010

Benedetti, F., Carlino, E., & Pollo, A. (2011). How placebos change the patient's brain. *Neuropsychopharmacology, 36,* 339–354. http://dx.doi.org/10.1038/npp.2010.81

Berk, M., & Nierenberg, A. A. (2015). Three paths to drug discovery in psychiatry. *The American Journal of Psychiatry, 172,* 412–414. http://dx.doi.org/10.1176/appi.ajp.2014.14070858

Chaimani, A., Salanti, G., Leucht, S., Geddes, J. R., & Cipriani, A. (2017). Common pitfalls and mistakes in the set-up, analysis and interpretation of results in network meta-analysis: What clinicians should look for in a published article. *Evidence-Based Mental Health, 20,* 88–94. http://dx.doi.org/10.1136/eb-2017-102753

Chary, K. V., & Pandian, K. (2017). Accelerated approval of drugs: Ethics versus efficacy. *Indian Journal of Medical Ethics, 2,* 244–247. http://dx.doi.org/10.20529/IJME.2017.062

Chen, D. T., Wynia, M. K., Moloney, R. M., & Alexander, G. C. (2009). U.S. physician knowledge of the FDA-approved indications and evidence base for commonly prescribed drugs: Results of a national survey. *Pharmacoepidemiology and Drug Safety, 18,* 1094–1100. http://dx.doi.org/10.1002/pds.1825

Ciociola, A. A., Cohen, L. B., Kulkarni, P., & the FDA-Related Matters Committee of the American College of Gastroenterology. (2014). How drugs are developed and approved by the FDA: Current process and future directions. *The American Journal of Gastroenterology, 109,* 620–623. http://dx.doi.org/10.1038/ajg.2013.407

Coakley, M., Fadiran, E. O., Parrish, L. J., Griffith, R. A., Weiss, E., & Carter, C. (2012). Dialogues on diversifying clinical trials: Successful strategies for engaging women and minorities in clinical trials. *Journal of Women's Health, 21,* 713–716. http://dx.doi.org/10.1089/jwh.2012.3733

Cook, S. C., Schwartz, A. C., & Kaslow, N. J. (2017). Evidence-based psychotherapy: Advantages and challenges. *Neurotherapeutics: The Journal of the American Society for Experimental Neuro-Therapeutics, 14,* 537–545. http://dx.doi.org/10.1007/s13311-017-0549-4

Comer, J. S., Olfson, M., & Mojtabai, R. (2010). National trends in child and adolescent psychotropic polypharmacy in office-based practice, 1996–2007. *Journal of the American Academy of Child & Adolescent Psychiatry, 49,* 1001–1010. http://dx.doi.org/10.1016/j.jaac.2010.07.007

*Asterisks indicate assessments or resources.

Corrigan, P. W., & Salzer, M. S. (2003). The conflict between random assignment and treatment preference: Implications for internal validity. *Evaluation and Program Planning, 26,* 109–121. http://dx.doi.org/10.1016/S0149-7189(03)00014-4

Cosgrove, K. P., Mazure, C. M., & Staley, J. K. (2007). Evolving knowledge of sex differences in brain structure, function, and chemistry. *Biological Psychiatry, 62,* 847–855. http://dx.doi.org/10.1016/j.biopsych.2007.03.001

Cowen, P. J. (2011). Has psychopharmacology got a future? *The British Journal of Psychiatry, 198,* 333–335. http://dx.doi.org/10.1192/bjp.bp.110.086207

Devulapalli, K. K., & Nasrallah, H. A. (2009). An analysis of the high psychotropic off-label use in psychiatric disorders: The majority of psychiatric diagnoses have no approved drug. *Asian Journal of Psychiatry, 2,* 29–36. http://dx.doi.org/10.1016/j.ajp.2009.01.005

Donohue, J. M., Cevasco, M., & Rosenthal, M. B. (2007). A decade of direct-to-consumer advertising of prescription drugs. *The New England Journal of Medicine, 357,* 673–681. http://dx.doi.org/10.1056/NEJMsa070502

Downing, N. S., Aminawung, J. A., Shah, N. D., Krumholz, H. M., & Ross, J. S. (2014). Clinical trial evidence supporting FDA approval of novel therapeutic agents, 2005–2012. *JAMA, 311,* 368–377. http://dx.doi.org/10.1001/jama.2013.282034

Dubovsky, S. L., & Dubovsky, A. N. (2007). *Psychotropic drug prescriber's guide: Ethical mental health treatment in the age of big pharma.* New York, NY: W. W. Norton.

Ernst, E. (2007). Placebo: New insights into an old enigma. *Drug Discovery Today, 12*(9–10), 413–418. http://dx.doi.org/10.1016/j.drudis.2007.03.007

Eshera, N., Itana, H., Zhang, L., Soon, G., & Fadiran, E. O. (2015). Demographics of clinical trials participants in pivotal clinical trials for new molecular entity drugs and biologics approved by FDA from 2010 to 2012. *American Journal of Therapeutics, 22,* 435–455. http://dx.doi.org/10.1097/MJT.0000000000000177

Eugene, A. R., & Masiak, J. (2017). A pharmacodynamic modelling and simulation study identifying gender differences of daily olanzapine dose and dopamine D2-receptor occupancy. *Nordic Journal of Psychiatry, 71,* 417–424. http://dx.doi.org/10.1080/08039488.2017.1314011

Field, R. I. (2008). The FDA's new guidance for off-label promotion is only a start. *Pharmacology and Therapeutics, 33*(4), 220, 249.

Finniss, D. G., Kaptchuk, T. J., Miller, F., & Benedetti, F. (2010). Biological, clinical, and ethical advances of placebo effects. *Lancet, 375,* 686–695. http://dx.doi.org/10.1016/S0140-6736(09)61706-2

Fleming, T. R., & DeMets, D. L. (1996). Surrogate end points in clinical trials: Are we being misled? *Annals of Internal Medicine, 125,* 605–613. http://dx.doi.org/10.7326/0003-4819-125-7-199610010-00011

Franconi, F., & Campesi, I. (2014). Sex and gender influences on pharmacological response: An overview. *Expert Review of Clinical Pharmacology, 7,* 469–485. http://dx.doi.org/10.1586/17512433.2014.922866

Frank, C., Himmelstein, D. U., Woolhandler, S., Bor, D. H., Wolfe, S. M., Heymann, O., . . . Lasser, K. E. (2014). Era of faster FDA drug approval has also seen increased black-box warnings and market withdrawals. *Health Affairs, 33,* 1453–1459. http://dx.doi.org/10.1377/hlthaff.2014.0122

Gaudiano, B. A., & Miller, I. W. (2013). The evidence-based practice of psychotherapy: Facing the challenges that lie ahead. *Clinical Psychology Review, 33,* 813–824. http://dx.doi.org/10.1016/j.cpr.2013.04.004

Gilbody, S., Wilson, P., & Watt, I. (2005). Benefits and harms of direct to consumer advertising: A systematic review. *Quality & Safety in Health Care, 14,* 246–250. http://dx.doi.org/10.1136/qshc.2004.012781

Goldapple, K., Segal, Z., Garson, C., Lau, M., Bieling, P., Kennedy, S., & Mayberg, H. (2004). Modulation of cortical-limbic pathways in major depression: Treatment-specific effects of cognitive behavior therapy. *Archives of General Psychiatry, 61,* 34–41. http://dx.doi.org/10.1001/archpsyc.61.1.34

Goldberger, J. J., & Buxton, A. E. (2013). Personalized medicine vs guideline-based medicine. *JAMA, 309*(24), 2559–2560. http://dx.doi.org/10.1001/jama.2013.6629

Goldbloom, D. S., & Olmsted, M. P. (1993). Pharmacotherapy of bulimia nervosa with fluoxetine: Assessment of clinically significant attitudinal change. *The American Journal of Psychiatry, 150,* 770–774. http://dx.doi.org/10.1176/ajp.150.5.770

Gorman, J. M., & Nathan, P. E. (2015). Challenges to implementing evidence-based treatments. In P. E. Nathan & J. M. Gorman (Eds.), *A guide to treatments that work* (4th ed., pp. 1–21). New York, NY: Oxford University Press.

Gupta, S. K., & Nayak, R. P. (2014). Off-label use of medicine: Perspective of physicians, patients, pharmaceutical companies and regulatory authorities. *Journal of Pharmacology & Pharmacotherapeutics, 5,* 88–92. http://dx.doi.org/10.4103/0976-500X.130046

Guyatt, G. H., Oxman, A. D., Vist, G. E., Kunz, R., Falck-Ytter, Y., Alonso-Coello, P., Schünemann, H. J., & the GRADE Working Group. (2008). GRADE: An emerging consensus on rating quality of evidence and strength of recommendations. *British Medical Journal, 336,* 924–926. http://dx.doi.org/10.1136/bmj.39489.470347.AD

Haidich, A. B. (2010). Meta-analysis in medical research. *Hippokratia, 14*(Suppl. 1), 29–37.

Hart, B., Lundh, A., & Bero, L. (2012). Effect of reporting bias on meta-analyses of drug trials: Reanalysis of meta-analyses. *BMJ, 344*, d7202. http://dx.doi.org/10.1136/bmj.d7202

Healy, D. (2009). Trussed in evidence? Ambiguities at the interface between clinical evidence and clinical practice. *Transcultural Psychiatry, 46*, 16–37. http://dx.doi.org/10.1177/1363461509102285

Hilmer, S. N., McLachlan, A. J., & Le Couteur, D. G. (2007). Clinical pharmacology in the geriatric patient. *Fundamental & Clinical Pharmacology, 21*, 217–230. http://dx.doi.org/10.1111/j.1472-8206.2007.00473.x

Howes, O. D., Kambeitz, J., Kim, E., Stahl, D., Slifstein, M., Abi-Dargham, A., & Kapur, S. (2012). The nature of dopamine dysfunction in schizophrenia and what this means for treatment. *Archives of General Psychiatry, 69*, 776–786. http://dx.doi.org/10.1001/archgenpsychiatry.2012.169

Howland, R. H. (2009). Effects of aging on pharmacokinetic and pharmacodynamics drug processes. *Journal of Psychosocial Nursing and Mental Health Services, 47*(10), 15–18.

Huhn, M., Tardy, M., Spineli, L. M., Kissling, W., Förstl, H., Pitschel-Walz, G., . . . Leucht, S. (2014). Efficacy of pharmacotherapy and psychotherapy for adult psychiatric disorders: A systematic overview of meta-analyses. *JAMA Psychiatry, 71*, 706–715. http://dx.doi.org/10.1001/jamapsychiatry.2014.112

Hyman, S. E. (2016). Back to basics: Luring industry back into neuroscience. *Nature Neuroscience, 19*(11), 1383–1384. http://dx.doi.org/10.1038/nn.4429

Jones, P. B., Barnes, T. R. E., Davies, L., Dunn, G., Lloyd, H., Hayhurst, K. P., . . . Lewis, S. W. (2006). Randomized controlled trial of the effect on quality of life of second- vs first-generation antipsychotic drugs in schizophrenia: Cost Utility of the Latest Antipsychotic Drugs in Schizophrenia Study (CUtLASS 1). *Archives of General Psychiatry, 63*, 1079–1087. http://dx.doi.org/10.1001/archpsyc.63.10.1079

Kornstein, S. G., Schatzberg, A. F., Thase, M. E., Yonkers, K. A., McCullough, J. P., Keitner, G. I., . . . Keller, M. B. (2000). Gender differences in treatment response to sertraline versus imipramine in chronic depression. *The American Journal of Psychiatry, 157*, 1445–1452. http://dx.doi.org/10.1176/appi.ajp.157.9.1445

Kraemer, H. C., & Schatzberg, A. F. (2009). Statistics, placebo response, and clinical trial design in psychopharmacology. In A. F. Schatzberg & C. B. Nemeroff (Eds.), *Textbook of Psychopharmacology* (4th ed., pp. 243–258). Washington, DC: American Psychiatric Publishing. http://dx.doi.org/10.1176/appi.books.9781585623860.as11

Kraly, F. S. (2014). *Psychopharmacology problem solving: Principles and practices to get it right.* New York, NY: W. W. Norton.

Lasser, K. E., Allen, P. D., Woolhandler, S. J., Himmelstein, D. U., Wolfe, S. M., & Bor, D. H. (2002). Timing of new black box warnings and withdrawals for prescription medications. *JAMA, 287*, 2215–2220. http://dx.doi.org/10.1001/jama.287.17.2215

Laughren, T. P. (2010). What's next after 50 years of psychiatric drug development: An FDA perspective. *The Journal of Clinical Psychiatry, 71*(9), 1196–1204. http://dx.doi.org/10.4088/JCP.10m06262gry

Leber, P. (2000). The use of placebo control groups in the assessment of psychiatric drugs: An historical context. *Biological Psychiatry, 47*, 699–706. http://dx.doi.org/10.1016/S0006-3223(99)00321-2

Leucht, S., Chaimani, A., Cipriani, A. S., Davis, J. M., Furukawa, T. A., & Salanti, G. (2016). Network meta-analyses should be the highest level of evidence in treatment guidelines. *European Archives of Psychiatry and Clinical Neuroscience, 266*, 477–480. http://dx.doi.org/10.1007/s00406-016-0715-4

Leucht, S., Cipriani, A., Spineli, L., Mavridis, D., Orey, D., Richter, F., . . . Davis, J. M. (2013). Comparative efficacy and tolerability of 15 antipsychotic drugs in schizophrenia: A multiple-treatments meta-analysis. *Lancet, 382*, 951–962. http://dx.doi.org/10.1016/S0140-6736(13)60733-3

Li, L., Li, Y., & Zheng, Q. (2017). High placebo response rates hamper the discovery of antidepressants for depression in children and adolescents. *The American Journal of Psychiatry, 174*, 696–697. http://dx.doi.org/10.1176/appi.ajp.2017.17030347

Liberati, A., Altman, D. G., Tetzlaff, J., Mulrow, C., Gøtzsche, P. C., Ioannidis, J. P. A., . . . Moher, D. (2009). The PRISMA statement for reporting systematic reviews and meta-analyses of studies that evaluate healthcare interventions: Explanation and elaboration. *BMJ, 339*, b2700. http://dx.doi.org/10.1136/bmj.b2700

Lieberman, J. A., Stroup, T. S., McEvoy, J. P., Swartz, M. S., Rosenheck, R. A., Perkins, D. O., . . . Hsiao, J. K., & the Clinical Antipsychotic Trials of Intervention Effectiveness (CATIE) Investigators. (2005). Effectiveness of antipsychotic drugs in patients with chronic schizophrenia. *The New England Journal of Medicine, 353*, 1209–1223. http://dx.doi.org/10.1056/NEJMoa051688

Liu, K. A., & DiPietro Mager, N. A. (2016). Women's involvement in clinical trials: Historical perspective and future implications. *Pharmacy Practice, 14*, 708. http://dx.doi.org/10.18549/PharmPract.2016.01.708

Ma, D., Zhang, Z., Zhang, X., & Li, L. (2014). Comparative efficacy, acceptability, and safety of medicinal, cognitive-behavioral therapy, and placebo treatments for acute major depressive disorder in children and adolescents: A multiple-treatments meta-analysis. *Current Medical Research and Opinion, 30*, 971–995. http://dx.doi.org/10.1185/03007995.2013.860020

Malik, M., Lake, J., Lawson, W. B., & Joshi, S. V. (2010). Culturally adapted pharmacotherapy and the integrative formulation. *Child and Adolescent Psychiatric Clinics of North America, 19,* 791–814. http://dx.doi.org/10.1016/j.chc.2010.08.003

Marazziti, D., Baroni, S., Picchetti, M., Piccinni, A., Carlini, M., Vatteroni, E., . . . Dell'Osso, L. (2013). Pharmacokinetics and pharmacodynamics of psychotropic drugs: Effect of sex. *CNS Spectrums, 18,* 118–127. http://dx.doi.org/10.1017/S1092852912001010

March, J. S., Silva, S. G., Compton, S., Shapiro, M., Califf, R., & Krishnan, R. (2005). The case for practical clinical trials in psychiatry. *The American Journal of Psychiatry, 162,* 836–846. http://dx.doi.org/10.1176/appi.ajp.162.5.836

Mark, T. L., Levit, K. R., & Buck, J. A. (2009). Datapoints: Psychotropic drug prescriptions by medical specialty. *Psychiatric Services, 60,* 1167. http://dx.doi.org/10.1176/ps.2009.60.9.1167

Maust, D. T., Gerlach, L. B., Gibson, A., Kales, H. C., Blow, F. C., & Olfson, M. (2017). Trends in central nervous system-active polypharmacy among older adults seen in outpatient care in the United States. *JAMA Internal Medicine, 177,* 583–585. http://dx.doi.org/10.1001/jamainternmed.2016.9225

McGrath, R. E. (2010). Evaluating drug research. In R. E. McGrath & B. A. Moore (Eds.), *Pharmacotherapy for psychologists: Prescribing and collaborative roles* (pp. 133–150). Washington, DC: American Psychological Association. http://dx.doi.org/10.1037/12167-007

McGrath, R. E. (2012). Research in clinical psychopharmacology. In M. Muse & B. A. Moore (Eds.), *Handbook of clinical psychopharmacology for psychologists* (pp. 431–456). Hoboken, NJ: John Wiley & Sons, Inc.

Meltzer, C. C., Becker, J. T., Price, J. C., & Moses-Kolko, E. (2003). Positron emission tomography imaging of the aging brain. *Neuroimaging Clinics of North America, 13,* 759–767. http://dx.doi.org/10.1016/S1052-5149(03)00108-4

Merkatz, R. B., Temple, R., Sobel, S., Feiden, K., Kessler, D. A., & the Working Group on Women in Clinical Trials. (1993). Women in clinical trials of new drugs. A change in Food and Drug Administration policy. *The New England Journal of Medicine, 329,* 292–296. http://dx.doi.org/10.1056/NEJM199307223290429

Miller, J. E., Korn, D., & Ross, J. S. (2015). Clinical trial registration, reporting, publication and FDAAA compliance: A cross-sectional analysis and ranking of new drugs approved by the FDA in 2012. *BMJ Open, 5,* e009758. http://dx.doi.org/10.1136/bmjopen-2015-009758

Moher, D., Liberati, A., Tetzlaff, J., Altman, D. G., & the PRISMA Group. (2010). Preferred reporting items for systematic reviews and meta-analyses: The PRISMA statement. *International Journal of Surgery, 8,* 336–341. http://dx.doi.org/10.1016/j.ijsu.2010.02.007

Mojtabai, R., Olfson, M., & Han, B. (2016). National trends in the prevalence and treatment of depression in adolescents and young adults. *Pediatrics, 138,* e2016-1878. http://dx.doi.org/10.1542/peds.2016-1878

Moore, T. J., & Furberg, C. D. (2014). Development times, clinical testing, postmarket follow-up, and safety risks for the new drugs approved by the US food and drug administration: The class of 2008. *JAMA: Internal Medicine, 174,* 90–95. http://dx.doi.org/10.1001/jamainternmed.2013.11813

Moore, T. J., & Mattison, D. R. (2017). Adult utilization of psychiatric drugs and differences by sex, age, and race. *JAMA: Internal Medicine, 177,* 274–275. http://dx.doi.org/10.1001/jamainternmed.2016.7507

Mulder, R., Singh, A. B., Hamilton, A., Das, P., Outhred, T., Morris, G., . . . Malhi, G. S. (2018). The limitations of using randomized controlled trials as a basis for developing treatment guidelines. *Evidence-Based Mental Health, 21,* 4–6.

Murphy, S., & Roberts, R. (2006). "Black box" 101: How the Food and Drug Administration evaluates, communicates, and manages drug benefit/risk. *The Journal of Allergy and Clinical Immunology, 117,* 34–39. http://dx.doi.org/10.1016/j.jaci.2005.10.031

*Nathan, P. E., & Gorman, J. M. (Eds.). (2015). *A guide to treatments that work* (4th ed.). New York, NY: Oxford University Press. http://dx.doi.org/10.1093/med:psych/9780195304145.001.0001

Norquist, G., & Hyman, S. E. (1999). Advances in understanding and treating mental illness: Implications for policy. *Health Affairs, 18,* 32–47. http://dx.doi.org/10.1377/hlthaff.18.5.32

O'Brien, P. L., Cummings, N., & Mark, T. L. (2017). Off-label prescribing of psychotropic medication, 2005–2013: An examination of potential influences. *Psychiatric Services, 68,* 549–558. http://dx.doi.org/10.1176/appi.ps.201500482

O'Hara, R., Beaudreau, S. A., Gould, C. E., Froehlich, W., & Kraemer, H. C. (2017). Handling clinical comorbidity in randomized clinical trials in psychiatry. *Journal of Psychiatric Research, 86,* 26–33. http://dx.doi.org/10.1016/j.jpsychires.2016.11.006

Olfson, M., Blanco, C., Wang, S., Laje, G., & Correll, C. U. (2014). National trends in the mental health care of children, adolescents, and adults by office-based physicians. *JAMA: Psychiatry, 71,* 81–90. http://dx.doi.org/10.1001/jamapsychiatry.2013.3074

Olfson, M., Kroenke, K., Wang, S., & Blanco, C. (2014). Trends in office-based mental health care provided by psychiatrists and primary care physicians. *The Journal of Clinical Psychiatry, 75,* 247–253. http://dx.doi.org/10.4088/JCP.13m08834

Page, M. J., McKenzie, J. E., Kirkham, J., Dwan, K., Kramer, S., Green, S., & Forbes, A. (2014). Bias due to selective inclusion and reporting of outcomes and analyses in systematic reviews of randomised trials of healthcare interventions. *Cochrane Database of Systematic Reviews, 10*, MR000035.

Patsopoulos, N. A., Analatos, A. A., & Ioannidis, J. P. A. (2005). Relative citation impact of various study designs in the health sciences. *JAMA, 293*, 2362–2366. http://dx.doi.org/10.1001/jama.293.19.2362

Pease, A. M., Krumholz, H. M., Downing, N. S., Aminawung, J. A., Shah, N. D., & Ross, J. S. (2017). Postapproval studies of drugs initially approved by the FDA on the basis of limited evidence: Systematic review. *British Medical Journal, 357*, j1680. http://dx.doi.org/10.1136/bmj.j1680

Pollo, A., & Benedetti, F. (2009). The placebo response: Neurobiological and clinical issues of neurological relevance. *Progress in Brain Research, 175*, 283–294. http://dx.doi.org/10.1016/S0079-6123(09)17520-9

Pollock, B., Forsyth, C., & Bies, R. (2009). The critical role of clinical pharmacology in geriatric psychopharmacology. *Clinical Pharmacology and Therapeutics, 85*, 89–93. http://dx.doi.org/10.1038/clpt.2008.229

Poon, R., Khanijow, K., Umarjee, S., Fadiran, E., Yu, M., Zhang, L., & Parekh, A. (2013). Participation of women and sex analyses in late-phase clinical trials of new molecular entity drugs and biologics approved by the FDA in 2007–2009. *Journal of Women's Health, 22*, 604–616. http://dx.doi.org/10.1089/jwh.2012.3753

Radley, D. C., Finkelstein, S. N., & Stafford, R. S. (2006). Off-label prescribing among office-based physicians. *Archives of Internal Medicine, 166*, 1021–1026. http://dx.doi.org/10.1001/archinte.166.9.1021

Renoux, C., Shin, J.-Y., Dell'Aniello, S., Fergusson, E., & Suissa, S. (2016). Prescribing trends of attention-deficit hyperactivity disorder (ADHD) medications in UK primary care, 1995–2015. *British Journal of Clinical Pharmacology, 82*, 858–868. http://dx.doi.org/10.1111/bcp.13000

Rey, J. A. (2006). The interface of multiculturalism and psychopharmacology. *Journal of Pharmacy Practice, 19*, 379–385. http://dx.doi.org/10.1177/0897190007300734

Sackett, D. L., Rosenberg, W. M., Gray, J. A., Haynes, R. B., & Richardson, W. S. (1996). Evidence based medicine: What it is and what it isn't. *British Medical Journal, 312*, 71–72. http://dx.doi.org/10.1136/bmj.312.7023.71

Sarter, M., & Tricklebank, M. (2012). Revitalizing psychiatric drug discovery. *Nature Reviews. Drug Discovery, 11*, 423–424. http://dx.doi.org/10.1038/nrd3755

Scott, A., Rucklidge, J. J., & Mulder, R. T. (2015). Is mandatory prospective trial registration working to prevent publication of unregistered trials and selective outcome reporting? An observational study of five psychiatry journals that mandate prospective clinical trial registration. *PLoS One, 10*, e0133718. http://dx.doi.org/10.1371/journal.pone.0133718

Scott, I. A., & Le Couteur, D. G. (2015). Physicians need to take the lead in deprescribing. *Internal Medicine Journal, 45*, 352–356. http://dx.doi.org/10.1111/imj.12693

Shea, B. J., Hamel, C., Wells, G. A., Bouter, L. M., Kristjansson, E., Grimshaw, J., . . . Boers, M. (2009). AMSTAR is a reliable and valid measurement tool to assess the methodological quality of systematic reviews. *Journal of Clinical Epidemiology, 62*, 1013–1020. http://dx.doi.org/10.1016/j.jclinepi.2008.10.009

Singal, A. G., Higgins, P. D. R., & Waljee, A. K. (2014). A primer on effectiveness and efficacy trials. *Clinical and Translational Gastroenterology, 5*, e45. http://dx.doi.org/10.1038/ctg.2013.13

Singh, M. K., & Chang, K. D. (2012). The neural effects of psychotropic medications in children and adolescents. *Child and Adolescent Psychiatric Clinics of North America, 21*, 753–771. http://dx.doi.org/10.1016/j.chc.2012.07.010

Sinyor, M., Schaffer, A., & Levitt, A. (2010). The sequenced treatment alternatives to relieve depression (STAR*D) trial: A review. *Canadian Journal of Psychiatry, 55*, 126–135. http://dx.doi.org/10.1177/070674371005500303

Spetie, L., & Arnold, L. E. (2007). Ethical issues in child psychopharmacology research and practice: Emphasis on preschoolers. *Psychopharmacology, 191*, 15–26. http://dx.doi.org/10.1007/s00213-006-0685-8

Stahl, S. M. (2013). Off-label prescribing: Best practice or malpractice? *CNS Spectrums, 18*, 1–4. http://dx.doi.org/10.1017/S1092852913000011

*Stein, D. J., Lerer, B., & Stahl, S. M. (Eds.). (2012). *Essential evidence-based psychopharmacology* (2nd ed.). New York, NY: Cambridge University Press. http://dx.doi.org/10.1017/CBO9780511910395

Streiner, D. L. (2007). Alternatives to placebo-controlled trials. *The Canadian Journal of Neurological Sciences, 34*(Suppl. 1), S37–S41. http://dx.doi.org/10.1017/S0317167100005540

Tansella, M., Thornicroft, G., Barbui, C., Cipriani, A., & Saraceno, B. (2006). Seven criteria for improving effectiveness trials in psychiatry. *Psychological Medicine, 36*, 711–720. http://dx.doi.org/10.1017/S003329170600715X

Tharyan, P. (1998). The relevance to meta-analysis, systematic reviews and the Cochrane collaboration to clinical psychiatry. *Indian Journal of Psychiatry*, *40*(2), 135–148.

Treweek, S., McCormack, K., Abalos, E., Campbell, M., Ramsay, C., Zwarenstein, M., & the PRACTIHC Collaboration. (2006). The Trial Protocol Tool: The PRACTIHC software tool that supported the writing of protocols for pragmatic randomized controlled trials. *Journal of Clinical Epidemiology, 59*, 1127–1133. http://dx.doi.org/10.1016/j.jclinepi.2005.12.019

Trifirò, G., & Spina, E. (2011). Age-related changes in pharmacodynamics: Focus on drugs acting on central nervous and cardiovascular systems. *Current Drug Metabolism, 12*, 611–620. http://dx.doi.org/10.2174/138920011796504473

Undurraga, J., & Baldessarini, R. J. (2012). Randomized, placebo-controlled trials of antidepressants for acute major depression: Thirty-year meta-analytic review. *Neuropsychopharmacology, 37*, 851–864. http://dx.doi.org/10.1038/npp.2011.306

Vitiello, B. (2007). Research in child and adolescent psychopharmacology: Recent accomplishments and new challenges. *Psychopharmacology, 191*, 5–13. http://dx.doi.org/10.1007/s00213-006-0414-3

Vitiello, B. (2015). Practical clinical trials in psychopharmacology: A systematic review. *Journal of Clinical Psychopharmacology, 35*, 178–183. http://dx.doi.org/10.1097/JCP.0000000000000295

Volkow, N. D., Wang, G.-J., Telang, F., Fowler, J. S., Logan, J., Childress, A.-R., . . . Wong, C. (2006). Cocaine cues and dopamine in dorsal striatum: Mechanism of craving in cocaine addiction. *The Journal of Neuroscience, 26*, 6583–6588. http://dx.doi.org/10.1523/JNEUROSCI.1544-06.2006

Volkow, N. D., Wang, G.-J., Tomasi, D., Kollins, S. H., Wigal, T. L., Newcorn, J. H., . . . Swanson, J. M. (2012). Methylphenidate-elicited dopamine increases in ventral striatum are associated with long-term symptom improvement in adults with attention deficit hyperactivity disorder. *The Journal of Neuroscience, 32*, 841–849. http://dx.doi.org/10.1523/JNEUROSCI.4461-11.2012

Walkup, J. T. (2017). Antidepressant efficacy for depression in children and adolescents: Industry- and NIMH-funded studies. *The American Journal of Psychiatry, 174*, 430–437. http://dx.doi.org/10.1176/appi.ajp.2017.16091059

Walsh, B. T., Seidman, S. N., Sysko, R., & Gould, M. (2002). Placebo response in studies of major depression: Variable, substantial, and growing. *JAMA, 287*, 1840–1847. http://dx.doi.org/10.1001/jama.287.14.1840

Walsh, B. T., Wilson, G. T., Loeb, K. L., Devlin, M. J., Pike, K. M., Roose, S. P., . . . Waternaux, C. (1997). Medication and psychotherapy in the treatment of bulimia nervosa. *The American Journal of Psychiatry, 154*, 523–531. http://dx.doi.org/10.1176/ajp.154.4.523

Walton, S. M., Schumock, G. T., Lee, K.-V., Alexander, G. C., Meltzer, D., & Stafford, R. S. (2008). Prioritizing future research on off-label prescribing: Results of a quantitative evaluation. *Pharmacotherapy, 28*, 1443–1452. http://dx.doi.org/10.1592/phco.28.12.1443

Weimer, K., Colloca, L., & Enck, P. (2015). Placebo effects in psychiatry: Mediators and moderators. *The Lancet Psychiatry, 2*, 246–257. http://dx.doi.org/10.1016/S2215-0366(14)00092-3

Welisch, E., & Altamirano-Diaz, L. A. (2015). Ethics of pharmacological research involving adolescents. *Paediatric Drugs, 17*, 55–59. http://dx.doi.org/10.1007/s40272-014-0114-0

Wisniewski, S. R., Rush, A. J., Nierenberg, A. A., Gaynes, B. N., Warden, D., Luther, J. F., . . . Trivedi, M. H. (2009). Can phase III trial results of antidepressant medications be generalized to clinical practice? A STAR*D report. *The American Journal of Psychiatry, 166*, 599–607. http://dx.doi.org/10.1176/appi.ajp.2008.08071027

Yonkers, K. A., & Brawman-Mintzer, O. (2002). The pharmacologic treatment of depression: Is gender a critical factor? *The Journal of Clinical Psychiatry, 63*, 610–615. http://dx.doi.org/10.4088/JCP.v63n0714

Yonkers, K. A., Kando, J. C., Cole, J. O., & Blumenthal, S. (1992). Gender differences in pharmacokinetics and pharmacodynamics of psychotropic medication. *The American Journal of Psychiatry, 149*, 587–595. http://dx.doi.org/10.1176/ajp.149.5.587

Zwarenstein, M., Treweek, S., Gagnier, J. J., Altman, D. G., Tunis, S., Haynes, B., . . . Moher, D., the CONSORT group, & the Pragmatic Trials in Healthcare (Practihc) group. (2008). Improving the reporting of pragmatic trials: An extension of the CONSORT statement. *British Medical Journal, 337*, a2390. http://dx.doi.org/10.1136/bmj.a2390

IMPLEMENTING PSYCHOPHARMACOLOGY FOR THE TREATMENT OF PSYCHOLOGICAL DISORDERS, SUBSTANCE USE DISORDERS, AND ADDICTION

PHARMACOLOGICAL TREATMENT OF PSYCHOLOGICAL DISORDERS

CHAPTER 7

PHARMACOLOGICAL TREATMENT OF DEPRESSIVE DISORDERS

Liisa Hantsoo and Sarah Mathews

The depressive disorders are among the most commonly diagnosed psychiatric disorders in the United States (Kessler, Chiu, Demler, & Walters, 2005), and antidepressants are among the most prescribed drugs in U.S. outpatient medical practices (Olfson & Marcus, 2009). The *Diagnostic and Statistical Manual of Mental Disorders* (5th ed.; *DSM–5*; American Psychiatric Association, 2013) includes eight depressive disorders: major depressive disorder (MDD), persistent depressive disorder (PDD; dysthymia), premenstrual dysphoric disorder (PMDD), disruptive mood dysregulation disorder (a pediatric diagnosis), substance- or medication-induced depressive disorder, depressive disorder due to another medical condition, other specified depressive disorder, and unspecified depressive disorder. The *DSM–5* also includes specifiers, such as "with peripartum onset," "with seasonal pattern," and "with anxious distress." In this chapter, the focus will be on MDD, PDD, PMDD, and peripartum depression (PD), as these are the more prevalent types of depression. As pharmacologic treatment of depression becomes more widely available, allied providers should be well-versed in psychopharmacologic management of depressive symptoms. This chapter focuses on pharmacologic treatment of the depressive disorders, and is geared toward nonpsychiatrists.

EPIDEMIOLOGY AND PREVALENCE

MDD's hallmark is the major depressive episode, a period of at least 2 weeks of low mood or anhedonia, accompanied by neurovegetative symptoms (e.g., changes in appetite, sleep patterns, energy level) that causes impairment in functioning. MDD is relatively common, with a lifetime prevalence in the United States of 16% (Kessler et al., 2003). Onset is often between late adolescence and the early 40s, with a median age of onset of 25 years (Bromet et al., 2011). The disorder is chronic in many people; 50% who remitted after one episode experienced at least one recurrence (Burcusa & Iacono, 2007). Each additional episode has a compounding effect, increasing the likelihood of experiencing another episode (Solomon et al., 2000).

Less common than MDD, PDD is a *DSM–5* diagnosis that consolidates *DSM–IV* chronic major depressive disorder and dysthymic disorder. PDD is defined in *DSM–5* as a depressed mood lasting most of the day, more days than not, for at least 2 years, accompanied by at least two additional symptoms: low self-esteem, difficulty concentrating or decision making, hopelessness, or the neurovegetative symptoms of depression. The lifetime prevalence rate is around 2.5% (Kessler et al., 2005), and many people with PDD also will experience a

We thank Samantha Linhares for assistance in preparing the resources toolkit, and Heather M. Pederson, PhD for constructive feedback on drafts. We would also like to acknowledge our funding sources, including the National Institutes of Health Mentored Patient-Oriented Research Career Development Award (K23MH107831; Hantsoo) and Brain and Behavior Research Foundation NARSAD Young Investigator Award (Hantsoo).

http://dx.doi.org/10.1037/0000133-007
APA Handbook of Psychopharmacology, S. M. Evans (Editor-in-Chief)

major depressive episode or other psychiatric diagnosis (Blanco et al., 2010; Klein, Schwartz, Rose, & Leader, 2000). Risk factors for PDD are similar to those for MDD (Blanco et al., 2010).

Premenstrual dysphoric disorder (PMDD) is a cyclic mood disorder, characterized by cognitive–affective symptoms in the week before menses (American Psychiatric Association, 2013). PMDD affects about 3% to 8% of women (Halbreich, 2008). Diagnosis is based on a perimenstrual pattern of at least five physical, affective, and/or behavioral symptoms, with at least one key affective symptom (marked depressed mood, hopelessness, or self-deprecating thoughts; affective lability, tearfulness, sensitivity to rejection; irritability or anger; or anxiety or tension; American Psychiatric Association, 2013). Many women experience milder premenstrual symptoms, often referred to as premenstrual syndrome (PMS). Organizations including the American College of Obstetricians and Gynecologists (ACOG) and the World Health Organization (WHO) have published criteria for these milder premenstrual mood changes (American College of Obstetricians and Gynecologists, 2001; WHO, 2004). ACOG's PMS criteria include one physical or psychological symptom in the 5 days prior to menses, which must occur in three consecutive menstrual cycles and must subside within four days of menses onset. As with PMDD, the symptoms must cause impairment, and must be verified by prospective rating. Of note for the clinician, PMDD and PMS are the only depressive disorders that require prospective symptom tracking for diagnosis. Recommendations for prospective symptom tracking will be presented in the Assessment section of this chapter (see also the Tool Kit of Resources at the end of the chapter).

PD includes antenatal depression (depression during pregnancy) and postpartum depression. The *DSM–5* includes PD not as its own diagnosis, but as a diagnostic specifier ("with peripartum onset"), indicating a depressive episode occurring during pregnancy or in the 4 weeks following delivery. Antenatal depression affects about 7% of pregnant women and postpartum depression occurs in roughly 10% of postpartum women (Gavin et al., 2005), although estimates are imprecise since many studies

use a 3-, 6-, or 12-month postdelivery timeframe (Kim, Epperson, Weiss, & Wisner, 2014) as opposed to the 4 weeks predicated by the *DSM–5*.

HISTORIC BACKGROUND OF PSYCHOPHARMACOLOGIC TREATMENT

Descriptions of depression date back to ancient texts, but it was not until the 1950s that the first medications for depression were developed (Hillhouse & Porter, 2015; also see Chapter 1, this volume, for more details). This first generation of medications included tricyclic antidepressants (TCAs, such as clomipramine [e.g., Anafranil®], imipramine [e.g., Tofranil®], nortriptyline [e.g., Pamelor®], doxepin [e.g., Sinequan®], amitriptyline [e.g., Elavil®]) and monoamine oxidase inhibitors (MAOIs, such as phenelzine [e.g., Nardil®], tranyl-cypromine [e.g., Parnate®], and selegiline [e.g., Emsam®]). These medications were developed in the era of the monoamine hypothesis of depression, which held that deficiencies in serotonin, epineph-rine, norepinephrine, and dopamine underpinned depression. MAOIs inhibit monoamine oxidase, the enzyme that catabolizes monoamine neuro-transmitters in the synapse. By preventing the breakdown of monoamines, their availability in the synaptic cleft is increased. The tricyclics, so named for their three-ring chemical structure, acted as serotonin and norepinephrine reuptake inhibitors (SNRIs), similarly increasing the length of activity of these monoamines, with antimuscarinic, anti-histamine, and anticholinergic effects as well. The MAOIs and tricyclics had a number of undesirable side effects. For instance, MAOI users had to avoid consuming the amine tyramine, found in common foods, to avoid a potentially lethal hypertensive crisis. Tricyclics could produce dry mouth, blurry vision, altered gastrointestinal motility, urinary retention, or cognitive side effects, as well as cardiovascular side effects or seizures.

As the serotonin hypothesis of depression took hold in the 1970s, the second generation of anti-depressants, selective serotonin reuptake inhibitors (SSRIs), were introduced. These medications bound postsynaptic serotonin receptors, allowing more serotonin to accumulate in the synaptic cleft. Fluoxetine (e.g., Prozac®, Sarafem®) was the first

SSRI approved by the U.S. Food and Drug Administration (FDA), and went on the U.S. market in 1988 (Hillhouse & Porter, 2015). This was followed by other SSRIs including paroxetine (e.g., Paxil®), sertraline (e.g., Zoloft®), citalopram (e.g., Celexa®), and escitalopram (e.g., Lexapro®). In 1989, bupropion (e.g., Wellbutrin®), a dopamine-norepinephrine reuptake inhibitor, was approved by the FDA. The first of the SNRIs, venlafaxine (e.g., Effexor®), was introduced in 1993, followed by duloxetine (e.g., Cymbalta®) and milnacipran (e.g., Savella®). With more specific mechanisms of action, the SSRIs and SNRIs had more acceptable side effect profiles than the MAOIs and tricyclics. SSRIs are still the most commonly prescribed antidepressants, given their good safety and tolerability profiles (Dupuy, Ostacher, Huffman, Perlis, & Nierenberg, 2011). For more detail on the history of antidepressant medications, Hillhouse and Porter (2015) provide a thorough review.

DIAGNOSING DEPRESSIVE DISORDERS

When diagnosing a depressive disorder, a thorough clinical assessment by a mental health provider should evaluate symptoms, past depressive episodes, comorbid disorders, and medication trials and responses. Assessment should rule out medical conditions that mimic depressive symptoms, such as hypothyroidism, a sleep disorder, or treatment side effects from a medication. Brief screenings, including self-report or those administered by a provider, may serve as a starting point for more detailed assessment. Here, we describe well-validated tools that can be used to assess depressive symptoms, aiding in diagnosis of MDD, PDD, PMDD, or PD.

Assessment of Major Depression and Persistent Depressive Disorder

Clinician administered scales. The Hamilton Depression Rating Scale (HAM-D) is a 21- or 17-item measure administered by a health care professional (Hamilton, 1960). A structured interview guide is available to foster reliable administration (Williams, 1988). The scoring range suggests absence of depression (score 0–6), mild depression

(score 7–17), moderate depression (score 18–24), or severe depression (score >24). The Inventory of Depressive Symptomatology (IDS) was developed as an alternative to the HAM-D, with a 16-item Quick IDS (QIDS; Rush et al., 2003) available. The Montgomery-Åsberg Depression Rating Scale (MADRS) is a 10-item clinician-administered scale that is more focused on the psychological symptoms of depression than the neurovegetative symptoms (Montgomery & Åsberg, 1979).

Self-report scales. The Beck Depression Inventory (BDI) is a well-established 21-item self-report measure assessing depressive symptoms in the past 2 weeks (Beck, Steer, Ball, & Ranieri, 1996). The freely available Patient Health Questionnaire–9 (PHQ-9; Kroenke, Spitzer, & Williams, 2001) similarly assesses depressive symptoms over the past 2 weeks and provides cutoffs for likely mild, moderate, or severe depression.

Assessment of Premenstrual Dysphoric Disorder

To be diagnosed with PMDD, symptoms must be confirmed with at least two menstrual cycles of prospective daily ratings. The Daily Record of Severity of Problems (DRSP) is the gold standard tool for prospectively assessing PMDD symptoms (Endicott, Nee, & Harrison, 2006). A scoring rubric guides the clinician in diagnosing PMDD via comparison of number and severity of symptoms in the follicular (asymptomatic) versus luteal (premenstrual) phase of the menstrual cycle. An alternative, the Carolina Premenstrual Assessment Scoring System (C-PASS), was published in 2016 (Eisenlohr-Moul et al., 2016) and assesses whether the individual meets full PMDD criteria versus another menstrually-related mood disorder, providing a more dimensional approach than the Endicott scoring rubric for the DRSP (Epperson & Hantsoo, 2017).

Assessment of Peripartum Depression

Rating scales used to assess depression in the general population may not be appropriate for assessing PD. Pregnancy and postpartum include physical symptoms that are considered normal perinatally, yet overlap with depressive symptoms, such as changes in energy, weight, appetite, and sleep. The clinician-rated Pregnancy Depression Scale (PDS) is a 7-item scale derived from the HAM-D (Altshuler et al., 2008). The Edinburgh Postnatal Depression Scale (EPDS; Cox, Holden, & Sagovsky, 1987) is a well-established 10-item self-report scale that assesses symptoms of postpartum depression occurring in the past week. While initially developed for use in the postpartum period, studies have established its validity during pregnancy as well (Flynn, Sexton, Ratliff, Porter, & Zivin, 2011). The Perinatal Depression Inventory (PDI) is a 14-item scale that, unlike the EPDS, assesses depressive symptoms in the antenatal *or* postpartum period (Brodey et al., 2016). When assessing PD, the clinician should ask the patient about depressive symptoms during or following other pregnancies, as this is a risk factor for subsequent episodes. The provider may also ask about whether the pregnancy was planned, whether it was desired, how the patient feels about motherhood, support from her partner, and whether she has any concerns about the transition to motherhood, as these factors may influence depressive symptoms or risk.

EVIDENCE-BASED PHARMACOLOGICAL TREATMENTS OF DEPRESSIVE DISORDERS

Pharmacologic treatment is recommended for moderate to severe MDD (Fournier et al., 2010), and is also an option for PMDD or PD that has not responded to nonpharmacologic treatments. When deciding whether psychopharmacologic treatment is appropriate, severity of symptoms should be considered, along with the potential for side effects, treatment history, patient preference, and medical comorbidities.

Major Depression and Persistent Depressive Disorder

As mentioned, SSRIs are the most commonly prescribed medications for depression. At a general level, SSRIs exert their therapeutic effect by inhibiting reuptake of synaptic serotonin (5-HT) by the presynaptic neuron. With serotonin remaining in the synapse for a longer period of

time, the neurotransmitter is able to repeatedly stimulate its postsynaptic receptors. There are more than 15 different serotonin receptor subtypes (e.g., 5-HT$_{1A}$) found throughout the brain and an SSRI may have more or less affinity for a particular receptor subtype. In addition, SSRIs impact muscarinic, adrenergic, serotonergic, and cholinergic receptors to various degrees (Owens, Morgan, Plott, & Nemeroff, 1997). This can influence a patient's response to or side effects experienced with a particular SSRI. Pharmacokinetics, such as half-life and metabolites produced, are also an important consideration when selecting an antidepressant due to potential for discontinuation symptoms if doses are missed. There is typically a lag between SSRI initiation and improvement in symptoms, which can be 1 to 6 weeks (van Calker et al., 2009). This is generally understood to be due to effects on postsynaptic function, consistent with a reformulation of the monoamine hypothesis that proposed depression was not due to a serotonin deficit, but to dysregulated serotonergic postsynaptic receptor function (Hindmarch, 2002).

The newer generation antidepressants include SNRIs (e.g., venlafaxine, desvenlafaxine [e.g., Pristiq®], duloxetine), norepinephrine-dopamine reuptake inhibitors (NDRIs, e.g., bupropion), α2-adrenergic receptor antagonists (e.g., mirtazapine [e.g., Remeron®]), and serotonin antagonist and reuptake inhibitors (e.g., trazodone [e.g., Desyrel®]). While serotonin has been linked to depressive symptoms including anxiety, dopamine has been linked with symptoms related to motivation, pleasure, and reward, and norepinephrine has been linked with alertness and energy (Nutt, 2008). Thus, these medications that impact dopamine and norepinephrine may address a wider range of symptoms than those impacting serotonin alone.

Meta-analyses have found that SSRIs have similar efficacy to tricyclics (Anderson, 2000; Geddes, Freemantle, Mason, Eccles, & Boynton, 2000), but that SSRIs have superior acceptability and tolerability (Guaiana, Barbui, & Hotopf, 2007). There are fewer studies comparing SSRIs with newer generation antidepressants. One meta-analysis concluded that while there were no significant differences among newer generation antidepressants in terms of efficacy or effectiveness, there were differences in side effect profiles that should be considered in treatment planning (Gartlehner et al., 2008). For instance, paroxetine had greater mean weight gain and sexual dysfunction than some other drugs, and venlafaxine had a higher mean incidence of nausea and vomiting than SSRIs. A meta-analysis in *The Lancet* compared 12 newer generation antidepressants (bupropion, citalopram, duloxetine, escitalopram, fluoxetine, fluvoxamine [e.g., Luvox®], milnacipran, mirtazapine, paroxetine, reboxetine [e.g., Edronax®], sertraline, and venlafaxine) and included six SSRIs (citalopram, escitalopram, fluoxetine, fluvoxamine, paroxetine, sertraline; Cipriani et al., 2009). It found that mirtazapine, escitalopram, venlafaxine, and sertraline were significantly more efficacious than duloxetine, fluoxetine, fluvoxamine, paroxetine, and reboxetine. The meta-analysis concluded that sertraline may be the best first-line treatment for moderate to severe major depression, considering its efficacy, acceptability, and cost. However, this recommendation was not without controversy, with some researchers pointing out that there may have been methodologic issues (e.g., failure to account for potential confounders such as psychiatric comorbidity, starting dose, titration schedule, or concomitant benzodiazepine use) or publication bias (Seyringer & Kasper, 2009). There is no one-size-fits-all treatment for MDD, making broad recommendations such as these challenging. However, insights from large-scale treatment studies such as the Sequenced Treatment Alternatives to Relieve Depression (STAR*D) trials, discussed in a following section of this chapter, can provide useful information on treatment approaches. While there is less literature on the pharmacologic treatment of PDD, it is treated similarly to MDD, with SSRIs being a common treatment choice (Meister et al., 2016).

Premenstrual Dysphoric Disorder

ACOG (American College of Obstetricians and Gynecologists, 2001) and the International Society for Premenstrual Disorders (Ismaili et al., 2016) recommend pharmacotherapy as a first-line treatment for PMDD and severe mood-related PMS. A meta-analysis of randomized placebo-controlled trials found that daily SSRI is an effective treatment for PMDD (Marjoribanks, Brown, O'Brien, & Wyatt, 2013). In addition to such "continuous" pharmacotherapy, PMDD may be treated with dosing schemes restricted to the luteal phase (Marjoribanks et al., 2013). Intermittent dosing refers to administering the medication only during the luteal phase (ovulation to menstruation onset; Freeman, 2004), while symptom-onset treatment initiates medication each cycle when the patient notices symptoms (usually a week or so before menses onset) and continues daily until menstruation (Steinberg, Cardoso, Martinez, Rubinow, & Schmidt, 2012). Interestingly, PMDD symptoms respond to SSRIs within days, as opposed to the weeks required for symptom reduction in MDD, and at lower doses (Landén & Thase, 2006; Steinberg et al., 2012), allowing luteal phase dosing regimens. The rapid onset of action is likely due to the SSRIs' interaction with enzymes involved in neurosteroid synthesis, as opposed to purely serotonergic mechanisms (Griffin & Mellon, 1999). Meta-analyses indicate a moderate to large effect size for both continuous and luteal phase SSRI treatment (Marjoribanks et al., 2013; Shah et al., 2008), and no clear difference in symptom response between the two dosing regimens (Marjoribanks et al., 2013). Luteal phase dosing with a shorter half-life SSRI, such as sertraline, paroxetine controlled release (CR), or citalopram, may most benefit women who experience SSRI side effects such as nausea, decreased libido, or drowsiness.

However, more than one third of women with PMDD do not respond to an SSRI (Halbreich, 2008). For these women, hormonal treatment (e.g., an oral contraceptive) for PMDD may be an option, but findings are mixed (Cunningham, Yonkers, O'Brien, & Eriksson, 2009). Combined oral contraceptives (COCs) are a daily pill used for pregnancy prevention that include a combination of estrogen and progestogen (a synthetic equivalent to progesterone). There are numerous generic and brand-name formulations of COCs containing different amounts of these hormones. COCs have been shown to somewhat reduce PMDD symptoms, but often with a large placebo effect (Eisenlohr-Moul, Girdler, Johnson, Schmidt, & Rubinow, 2017; Freeman et al., 2012; Lopez, Kaptein, & Helmerhorst,

2012). Progesterone monotherapy for PMS was not supported by strong evidence in a Cochrane review (Ford, Lethaby, Roberts, & Mol, 2012). Gonadotropin-releasing hormone (GnRH) agonists or inhibitors induce postmenopausal levels of ovarian hormones (Pincus, Alam, Rubinow, Bhuvaneswar, & Schmidt, 2011). GnRH drugs are typically used only when women with PMDD have failed multiple trials of SSRIs, as extended hypoestrogenism in premenopausal women may have negative health effects. A last-resort option for severe treatment-resistant PMDD is oophorectomy, or surgical meno-pause (Wyatt, Dimmock, Ismail, Jones, & O'Brien, 2004). As this treatment induces sudden menopause and prohibits further childbearing, it is only used in the most severe cases.

Peripartum Depression

Pharmacologic treatment of PD including during pregnancy, postpartum, or while breastfeeding requires special considerations. During pregnancy, many women are reluctant to take medication due to fear of causing harm to the fetus. However, the potential risks to the fetus from medication must be considered with the potential risks to the fetus of untreated depression (Nulman et al., 2012). There are few randomized controlled trials (RCTs) of antidepressants during pregnancy, given potential ethical issues. In a report on psychopharmaco-therapy during pregnancy, the American Psychiatric Association and ACOG published practice guide-lines regarding medication use during pregnancy (Yonkers et al., 2009). These guidelines review potential risks of antidepressant use during preg-nancy and weigh these against the risks of untreated depression.

Among women with a previous episode of post-partum depression, antidepressants are sometimes started prophylactically to prevent recurrence (Wisner et al., 2004). SSRIs are generally considered safe during breastfeeding (Davanzo, Copertino, De Cunto, Minen, & Amaddeo, 2011). Citalopram, venlafaxine, and fluoxetine may not be the first choice for breastfeeding mothers due to their maternal milk to plasma ratio and relative infant dose (Berle & Spigset, 2011; Davanzo et al., 2011). However, the patient's history of medication response should

be considered when selecting pharmacotherapy. If a patient who is breastfeeding has had a favorable response to these agents in the past, they may be a treatment option. Due to altered drug metabolism postpartum (Sit, Perel, Helsel, & Wisner, 2008), antidepressant dosages should start low and be titrated slowly in the postpartum period (Kim, Epperson et al., 2014).

There are few placebo-controlled antidepressant treatment studies in postpartum women specifically. An open-label prospective study of escitalopram in nonbreastfeeding depressed postpartum women found a 93% response rate (Misri, Abizadeh, Albert, Carter, & Ryan, 2012). A small pilot study of bupropion sustained release (SR) in women with MDD onset within 3 months of childbirth found a 75% response rate (Nonacs et al., 2005). One placebo-controlled RCT of paroxetine found a significantly greater proportion of remissions in the active medication group, but no significant difference between paroxetine and placebo in responder rate (Yonkers, Lin, Howell, Heath, & Cohen, 2008). Sertraline produced similar improvement in symp-toms compared with nortriptyline (Wisner et al., 2006). An RCT of sertraline in women with post-partum depression found better response and remission rates than placebo, particularly in women who had developed postpartum depression within 4 weeks of childbirth (Hantsoo et al., 2014).

PD may result from atypical response of the central nervous system to hormonal fluctuations during or following pregnancy. However, there are few studies assessing hormonal treatment of PD symptoms. Women who received a medroxy-progesterone acetate injection following delivery did not have significantly lower EPDS scores at 6 weeks postpartum compared with women who did not receive the hormonal injection (Tsai & Schaffir, 2010). Women who received an intra-muscular injection of norethisterone enanthate, a progestogen-only contraceptive, within 2 days post-delivery actually had worse depressive symptoms than a placebo group at 6 weeks postpartum, and no difference at 3 months postpartum (Lawrie et al., 1998). A recent double-blind RCT suggested that an intravenous formulation of allopregnanolone, a progesterone metabolite, may be an emerging option for treating severe postpartum depression (Kanes et al., 2017). Women with severe postpartum depression who received intravenous allopregnanolone treatment over the course of 60 hours had a significant reduction in depression scores (based on the HAM-D) compared with placebo. Further work is needed to determine whether other formulations (e.g., oral) are as effective.

BEST APPROACHES FOR ASSESSING TREATMENT RESPONSE AND MANAGING SIDE EFFECTS

Major Depression and Persistent Depressive Disorder

Symptoms should be monitored regularly to assess treatment response during the initial weeks of treatment. It is recommended that providers administer a standardized depression rating tool to augment their clinical judgment when assessing treatment response. Otherwise, they may fail to detect patients' lack of improvement or symptom worsening (Hatfield, McCullough, Frantz, & Krieger, 2010). The PHQ-9 is well-suited to assess depression treatment response, as it measures the cardinal symptoms of major depression, is sensitive to change over time, and provides easily interpretable score ranges (Fortney et al., 2017). A suggested guideline is to assess the patient 4 to 6 weeks after medication initiation. If the PHQ-9 score is five or more points lower than the pretreatment baseline, the individual is responding and current medication should be continued (Bentley, Pagalilauan, & Simpson, 2014). For a score reduction of two to four points, the provider may consider continuing this medication at a higher dosage. For score reductions of less than two points, the provider should consider initiating a trial of a second medication, alone or in combination with the initial medication prescribed. Cross-tapering may be used to simultaneously wean the patient off of one medication while titrating up the other, especially if the medications are of different neurochemical classes (Keks, Hope, & Keogh, 2016).

Thirty-eight percent of more than 700 patients taking citalopram, escitalopram, fluoxetine, paroxetine, or sertraline reported at least one side effect (Cascade, Kalali, & Kennedy, 2009). The most commonly reported side effects were sexual dysfunction, sleepiness, and weight gain (Cascade et al., 2009). Nausea, insomnia, and headache are other common short-lived side effects of SSRIs (Marjoribanks et al., 2013), while weight gain and sexual dysfunction are longer term side effects (Deshmukh & Franco, 2003; Montgomery, Baldwin, & Riley, 2002). Other common side effects of the SSRIs and newer generation antidepressants include headache, dry mouth, insomnia, and dizziness (Mackay et al., 1999). Some of these may be mitigated by reducing the dose (Sienaert, 2014). Hepatotoxicity and cardiovascular changes are rare but serious side effects of some antidepressants. A 2014 review includes useful tables of antidepressant side effects and the associated neurotransmitter systems (Bentley et al., 2014).

Premenstrual Dysphoric Disorder

Unlike MDD, treatment response to SSRIs often occurs rapidly in PMDD, within a few days (Steinberg et al., 2012). In order to monitor treatment response, patients should continue to rate their menstrual mood symptoms daily throughout their menstrual cycle using the DRSP or C-PASS. Response is often operationalized as a 50% reduction in symptoms from pretreatment luteal phase to treated luteal phase (Steinberg et al., 2012).

Peripartum Depression

Experts recommend administering the EPDS monthly to monitor treatment response (Kim, Epperson et al., 2014). As the items on the EPDS are geared toward the perinatal period, they are more sensitive to month-to-month changes in perinatal depressive symptoms than a more general measure, such as the PHQ-9.

MEDICATION MANAGEMENT ISSUES

There are a number of potential challenges in the pharmacologic treatment of depression, including medication adherence, partial symptom response, unsupervised medication discontinuation, and relapse. Medication adherence refers to taking the medication as prescribed by the provider—the appropriate dose at the appropriate time. Individuals who are adherent with their medication over the long term have better outcomes than nonadherent patients (Åkerblad, Bengtsson, von Knorring, & Ekselius, 2006). Numerous factors can influence medication adherence, including side effects, comorbidity, age, and availability of follow-up care, to name a few (Akincigil et al., 2007). Data from chart reviews and insurance claims have found antidepressant adherence ranging from 12% to 72%, suggesting that many individuals discontinue their antidepressant before the recommended 6 months following symptom remission (Keyloun et al., 2017; Mårdby et al., 2016).

The STAR*D study, which ran at multiple sites across the United States from 2001 to 2006, assessed pharmacologic treatment approaches for individuals whose symptoms had not responded to the initial medication trial. The study found that more than half of the participants achieved remission after multiple medication trials (Rush et al., 2006). Generally, if a patient fails two antidepressants from different neurochemical classes at therapeutic doses, she or he is considered to have treatment-resistant depression (M. Fava & Davidson, 1996). With severe depression, approaches may include augmentation of antidepressant with an atypical antipsychotic (Han et al., 2015) or high-dose antidepressant treatment (e.g., rapidly doubling or tripling the dose; Jakubovski, Varigonda, Freemantle, Taylor, & Bloch, 2016). For perinatal treatment-resistant depression, including partial response to SSRI, experts recommend three trials of different antidepressants or augmenting agents; for a thorough review see Robakis and Williams (2013).

Relapse is common, as MDD is considered a chronic condition. Individuals with a history of a major depressive episode have a significantly elevated risk of experiencing additional episodes (Burcusa & Iacono, 2007). Antidepressant maintenance therapy is often used to prevent relapse. However, some patients relapse despite remaining on an antidepressant (Gueorguieva, Chekroud, & Krystal, 2017). Reasons for this are unclear, but could include pharmacokinetic tolerance. If the clinician is able to rule out treatment nonadherence or inadequate dose as causative factors, she or he

could consider approaches including dosage change, switching to another antidepressant, or augmentation with another medication (Targum, 2014).

Once remission is achieved, tapering off of an antidepressant should occur under the guidance of a clinician, who can determine readiness to discontinue medication based on length of symptom remission, and monitor for emergent symptoms such as self-harm, suicidal ideation, or panic attacks. When creating a tapering schedule, the prescribing provider will consider the medication dose, half-life, and withdrawal potential. If a patient has been on the medication for more than 1 month, it is recommended that the taper occur over at least 4 weeks (Ogle & Akkerman, 2013), as more abrupt cessation of an SSRI or SNRI is associated with "withdrawal" or discontinuation symptoms including insomnia, headache, nausea, dizziness, or mood changes (Black, Shea, Dursun, & Kutcher, 2000). However, some contend that discontinuation symptoms may occur regardless of length of taper (G. A. Fava, Gatti, Belaise, Guidi, & Offidani, 2015). Providers should discuss potential withdrawal effects with the patient before tapering begins.

When treating perinatal depression, there are special considerations regarding medication management. A woman who is taking antidepressants and learns she is pregnant should discuss options with her clinician before self-tapering or abruptly stopping medication on her own. This will allow the provider and patient to weigh the risks of potential discontinuation symptoms or relapse, and the impact of untreated depression during pregnancy versus prenatal exposure of the fetus to an antidepressant. Some women who discontinue antidepressants around the time of conception opt to reinitiate the medication at some point during pregnancy (Cohen, Altshuler, Stowe, & Faraone, 2004).

EVALUATION OF PHARMACOLOGICAL APPROACHES ACROSS THE LIFESPAN

Childhood and Adolescence

The prevalence of depression is around 2% to 11% in children and in adolescents (Kashani et al., 1983; Merikangas et al., 2010). The American Academy of Child and Adolescent Psychiatry (AACAP) practice parameters for children and adolescents with depressive disorders recommend that treatment is initiated with psychoeducation on depression for the child and caregivers, supportive management or psychotherapy, and family and school involvement (Birmaher & Brent, 2007). In mild to moderate depression, these measures, cognitive behavioral therapy (CBT), or interpersonal psychotherapy (IPT) are often efficacious (Birmaher & Brent, 2007). However, if a patient does not respond to these measures or has significant impairment, suicidality, or agitation, then pharmacologic treatment should be considered. The AACAP practice parameters note that there may be limited availability of pediatric mental health providers, and that some families may have objections to medication use in children. Fluoxetine and escitalopram are FDA approved for treatment of pediatric depression (U.S. Food and Drug Administration, 2014). Other SSRIs are commonly used, but considered off-label for pediatric patients. The tricyclics are not recommended as a first-line pediatric treatment, as they have not been shown to be more efficacious than placebo and have a greater number of side effects and potential for fatality after overdose (Birmaher & Brent, 2007). Antidepressant dosing in children is similar to that in adults, although initial doses should be lower in children; see Birmaher and Brent (2007) for basic dosage guidelines. Because the half-life of some medications may be shorter in children than in adults, the AACAP recommends that pediatric patients are monitored for withdrawal symptoms if they are taking medication only once per day (Birmaher & Brent, 2007). They recommend that patients are seen weekly for the first month, and that symptoms are assessed at 4-week intervals to monitor treatment response. The Children's Depression Rating Scale (CDRS; Poznanski, Cook, & Carroll, 1979) or Children's Depression Inventory (CDI; Kovacs, 1992) are options for monitoring treatment response in children ages 6 to 12 years and 7 to 17 years, respectively. For adolescents, scales used with adults, such as the Center for Epidemiologic Studies Depression Scale (CES-D), may be used (Stockings et al., 2015). If response is not achieved by 8 to 12 weeks of treatment, the guidelines suggest that other treatment options be

considered. Once response is achieved, it is recommended that the patient remain on medication for 6 to 12 months to prevent relapse. When the patient does discontinue medication, tapering should occur very slowly. For those who develop depression in childhood, particularly in adolescence, there is an increased risk of having additional depressive episodes in adulthood (Birmaher, Arbelaez, & Brent, 2002).

Adulthood

As this chapter is already focused on treatment of depressive disorders in adulthood, we will highlight here only a few key points in the adult lifespan that are particularly relevant to consider in treatment. First, during childhood the prevalence of depressive disorders is similar in boys and girls; however, with puberty, the prevalence in adolescent and adult females is double that of males (Burt & Stein, 2002). It is also at this time that females may begin to experience PMS, PMDD, or premenstrual worsening of a depressive disorder; however, this often does not present until a woman's 20s or 30s. Women with a history of depressive episodes are at risk for perimenopausal depression, although even women with no history of depression are two to three times more likely to develop depression perimenopausally (Bromberger et al., 2011; Freeman, Sammel, Lin, & Nelson, 2006). Recent research suggests that women who experienced significant stress during adolescence are more likely to have incident depression in the menopausal transition (Epperson et al., 2017). SSRIs are the first-line treatment for perimenopausal depression, particularly in women with a past history of depression, and emerging evidence suggests adjunct estradiol treatment may also be an option (Soares, 2017).

Older Adulthood

Depressive disorders are more prevalent among those aged 85 and older or among those in nursing homes (Luppa et al., 2012; Seitz, Purandare, & Conn, 2010), but depression is often undertreated in older adults (Barry, Abou, Simen, & Gill, 2012). Older patients with depression may present with complaints including fatigue, weight loss, or unexplained physical symptoms; cognitive complaints; social withdrawal; refusal to eat or engage in self-care; or use of alcohol or sedatives (Kok & Reynolds, 2017). Diagnosis may be more challenging if there are cognitive or medical comorbidities. If a patient is experiencing cognitive difficulties, it is recommended that a caregiver report on the patient's symptoms, and a cognitive assessment such as the Mini-Mental State Examination should be performed (Kok & Reynolds, 2017). A 2017 *JAMA* review suggested the Geriatric Depression Scale Short Form, a 15-item measure that can be administered by a provider or completed as self-report (Kok & Reynolds, 2017). Meta-analyses indicate that SSRIs, SNRIs, and TCAs may be efficacious for depression in older adults (Calati et al., 2013; Kok, Nolen, & Heeren, 2012). Side effects and tolerability are a concern, particularly if the patient is taking other medications for physical illness, in which case it is also important to consider whether cognitive or functional capacity will influence ability to be adherent to medication (Kok & Reynolds, 2017).

CONSIDERATION OF POTENTIAL SEX DIFFERENCES

In adulthood, women are twice as likely as men to have MDD (Bromet et al., 2011). Reasons for this are complex, and likely include a combination of social and biological contributors (Derry, Padin, Kuo, Hughes, & Kiecolt-Glaser, 2015; Nolen-Hoeksema, Larson, & Grayson, 1999). Women may present with different symptomatology than men; for instance, increased tearfulness or appetite (Romans, Tyas, Cohen, & Silverstone, 2007). The STAR*D studies found that women had less suicidal ideation but more past suicide attempts than men; men were more likely to have substance or alcohol abuse comorbidity, while women had more comorbid anxiety and eating disorders (Marcus et al., 2008). In a study of 1,401 opposite-sex dizygotic twin pairs who met criteria for MDD, the females reported increased fatigue, hypersomnia, and psychomotor retardation, while the males reported more insomnia and agitation (A. A. Khan, Gardner, Prescott, & Kendler, 2002). In a sample of older adults, women more commonly had changes in appetite and expe-

rienced joylessness during depression, while men more often experienced agitation (Kockler & Heun, 2002). Another important sex difference in depressive disorders is postpartum depression, which has traditionally been understood to occur only in women. There is some evidence that men may also experience depression following the birth of a child, although this is distinct from the hormonally-mediated changes in mood that women may experience perinatally (Paulson & Bazemore, 2010). In men, these symptoms of depression are more likely to be associated with psychosocial factors.

Women and men may also differ in their response to treatments. This may be due in part to pharmacokinetics, which can be influenced by factors including gut transit time, stomach pH (a measure of acidity), body fat, fluid distribution, metabolism, and renal function, all of which vary between the sexes (Damoiseaux, Proost, Jiawan, & Melgert, 2014). Women may require a lower dose of some medications, such as sertraline (Thiels, Linden, Grieger, & Leonard, 2005), while other medications show no difference in therapeutic dose between men and women (A. Khan, Brodhead, Schwartz, Kolts, & Brown, 2005; Young et al., 2009). In the STAR*D studies, women had a better treatment response to open-label citalopram than men, with no significant differences in dose or side effects (Young et al., 2009). Response rates were similar between women and men for placebo and SNRIs, but there were significantly more female responders to SSRIs than males (A. Khan et al., 2005). However, other studies have failed to find sex differences in treatment response for fluoxetine (Quitkin et al., 2002), sertraline (Thiels et al., 2005), clomipramine, citalopram, paroxetine, and moclobemide (e.g., Amira; Hildebrandt et al., 2003). All studies mentioned in this section were designed to specifically assess sex differences. However, some of these studies were open label, providing weaker evidence than a placebo-controlled study would. While sex differences may be modified by age, there is little research on this. Women were more responsive to sertraline, but only among those age 40 years and older (Morishita & Kinoshita, 2008). Women aged 50 years or older taking an SSRI had a lower chance of remission compared with women under 50 and men (Thase, Entsuah, Cantillon, & Kornstein, 2005). It may not be age or sex per se that causes differences, but hormonal status, although more research is needed in this area.

INTEGRATION OF PHARMACOTHERAPY WITH NONPHARMACOLOGICAL APPROACHES: BENEFITS AND CHALLENGES

Major Depression and Persistent Depressive Disorder

Pharmacologic treatment of depressive disorders is often combined with nonpharmacologic treatments, such as psychotherapy. In depressive disorders, CBT targets dysfunctional cognitions and behaviors, while IPT targets an individual's interpersonal environment. CBT combined with antidepressant medication had better recovery rates for MDD than antidepressants alone, but only in individuals with severe or nonchronic MDD (Hollon et al., 2014). This result is similar to a meta-analysis that found that individuals with milder depression had similar response rates to combined medication and psychotherapy versus psychotherapy alone (CBT or IPT), but those with more severe, recurrent depression had significantly better outcomes when on the combined treatment (Thase et al., 1997). The Cognitive Behavioural Therapy as an Adjunct to Pharmacotherapy for Treatment Resistant Depression in Primary Care (CoBalT) trial assessed CBT as an adjunct to treatment as usual for individuals with treatment-resistant depression in a primary care setting. The study recruited more than 400 participants who continued to meet criteria for depression after being on an antidepressant for at least 6 weeks from 73 primary care practices in the United Kingdom. CoBalT found that CBT significantly improved treatment response among pharmacotherapy nonresponders (Wiles et al., 2013). Combined treatment may produce more durable response (Karyotaki et al., 2016) and be more effective in preventing relapse (Guidi, Tomba, & Fava, 2016) than pharmacotherapy alone.

Additional forms of adjunct psychotherapy include IPT and mindfulness-based techniques. However, these trials are fewer in number and are smaller than the CBT augmentation trials. IPT did not provide benefit above and beyond pharmacotherapy for patients with MDD (Souza et al., 2016), with similar findings in adults with dysthymic disorder (de Mello, Myczcowisk, & Menezes, 2001). There was no difference in time to relapse or remission in a pharmacotherapy group versus a pharmacotherapy plus mindfulness-based cognitive therapy group (Kuyken et al., 2016). However, individuals with inadequate response to antidepressants had an improvement in depressive symptoms with an 8-week breathing-based meditation intervention compared with a waitlist control group (Sharma, Barrett, Cucchiara, Gooneratne, & Thase, 2017).

Other additions to pharmacotherapy may include telephone-administered therapy, Internet-based therapies, exercise, and bright light therapy, although there are fewer studies on these practices, or electroconvulsive therapy (ECT) or transcranial magnetic stimulation (TMS) for severe, treatment-resistant depression. Six counseling and support sessions delivered weekly over the telephone, in addition to pharmacotherapy, significantly reduced depressive symptoms at 3- and 6-month follow-up compared with pharmacotherapy alone (Tutty, Simon, & Ludman, 2000). A larger study of individuals starting an antidepressant found that an eight-session telephone CBT program improved depression symptoms compared with antidepressant alone (Simon, Ludman, Tutty, Operskalski, & Von Korff, 2004). Interpersonal and social rhythm therapy (a form of behavioral therapy often used in bipolar disorder that focuses on interpersonal relationships and maintaining consistent patterns in daily activities such as sleeping, eating, and exercise) or intensive clinical management delivered once per week over the telephone for 30 to 45 minutes in combination with an antidepressant produced larger percentages of responders over an 8-week trial than an antidepressant alone (Corruble et al., 2016). A meta-analysis of 10 randomized trials of bright light therapy at 5000 lux or greater for at least 30 minutes combined with antidepressant suggested an added benefit of bright light therapy over medication alone (Penders et al., 2016). Exercise as an adjunct to pharmacotherapy may provide a small benefit, but studies have typically used small sample sizes (Danielsson, Noras, Waern, & Carlsson, 2013). Finally, ECT or TMS are options for severe, treatment-resistant depression. Both are brain stimulation therapies, meaning that currents are applied to stimulate the brain and are administered several times per week until response is achieved. ECT involves applying an electrical current to induce a brief seizure, and TMS uses magnetic fields to induce electrical currents in specific areas of the brain. A meta-analysis suggested that ECT alone or in conjunction with an antidepressant provided better symptom improvement than antidepressant alone among individuals with treatment-resistant depression (Song et al., 2015). ECT may impact some aspects of memory and executive function, particularly in the first few days following treatment (Semkovska & McLoughlin, 2010). Like ECT, TMS may be used alone or in conjunction with pharmacotherapy (Perera et al., 2016). However, a large randomized, double-blind, sham-controlled study found no additional benefit of TMS beyond that provided by antidepressant alone (Herwig et al., 2007).

Premenstrual Dysphoric Disorder

Nonpharmacologic treatments for PMDD include psychotherapy, changes in diet or exercise, and complementary treatments such as vitamin B6 or calcium supplements (Yonkers & Simoni, 2018). However, there is little evidence for efficacy of these measures in conjunction with pharmacologic treatment. The Royal College of Obstetricians and Gynaecologists treatment guidelines indicate that simple interventions should be tried prior to pharmacotherapy, including exercise, vitamin B6 (100 mg), diet (complex carbohydrates during the late luteal phase), or calcium (1,000 mg daily), but there are no trials assessing these used in conjunction with an antidepressant or hormonal treatment. CBT is also recommended as an intervention for milder cases of PMDD, but there are no existing studies comparing CBT with pharmacotherapy or in conjunction with pharmacotherapy in PMDD.

Peripartum Depression

Pregnancy and the postpartum period represent a unique psychosocial and biological milieu. Stressors such as parenting (Misri et al., 2010) and role changes (Logsdon, Wisner, Hanusa, & Phillips, 2003) may impact willingness to seek psychiatric care. If antidepressant treatment alone is not sufficient to treat PD, psychotherapy is a common adjunct. While meta-analysis suggests that CBT and IPT are both beneficial for PD (Sockol, Epperson, & Barber, 2011), findings on psychotherapy as an adjunct to medication in peripartum women are mixed. In a pragmatic, open-label RCT, women with postpartum depression were randomized to antidepressant pharmacotherapy (general practitioner's choice) or supportive therapy with the option of antidepressant (Sharp et al., 2010). After 4 weeks of treatment, the pharmacotherapy group had twice the improvement rate of the supportive therapy group, but at 18 weeks, there was no statistically significant difference between the two treatments. Postpartum women with MDD and comorbid anxiety randomized to paroxetine monotherapy or paroxetine with CBT showed significant improvement (Misri, Reebye, Corral, & Milis, 2004). Other studies have shown that combined treatment is equivalent to pharmacotherapy alone (Appleby, Warner, Whitton, & Faragher, 1997; Milgrom et al., 2015; Misri et al., 2004). Placebo-controlled studies that compare medication with psychotherapy in the PD population are lacking. As the peripartum phase may involve barriers to psychotherapy treatment, such as limited mobility, schedule, childcare, or transportation, another option may be computer-based therapies such as therapy sessions via video chat, computer-assisted therapy, or self-guided online therapy (Hantsoo, Podcasy, Sammel, Epperson, & Kim, 2017; Kim, Hantsoo, Thase, Sammel, & Epperson, 2014). However, there are no studies looking specifically at these treatments in combination with pharmacotherapy.

INTEGRATED APPROACHES FOR ADDRESSING COMMON COMORBID DISORDERS

The depressive disorders are often comorbid with other psychiatric disorders. In the U.S. National Comorbidity Survey Replication, 72% of those with a lifetime MDD diagnosis had a psychiatric comorbidity (Kessler et al., 2003). This included 59.2% with a comorbid anxiety disorder, 30% with comorbid impulse control disorder, and 24% with a comorbid substance use disorder. Patients with comorbid disorders may require higher doses of medication or require more time for treatment response (Silverstone & Salinas, 2001).

SSRIs and SNRIs are used not only to treat depressive disorders, but also anxiety disorders, making them an ideal choice for patients with these comorbidities. Beyond SSRIs or SNRIs, benzodiazepines with a long half-life, such as clonazepam, may be used for rapid control of anxiety symptoms (Coplan, Aaronson, Panthangi, & Kim, 2015). For patients with a history of substance abuse, atypical antipsychotics are an option instead of benzodiazepines to manage anxiety (Coplan et al., 2015). In terms of nonpharmacologic treatments, the Unified Protocol for Transdiagnostic Treatment of Emotional Disorders (UP) is a transdiagnostic CBT protocol, meaning that it can be used across several related diagnoses (Barlow, Allen, & Choate, 2016). Thus, for someone with a depressive disorder and a secondary anxiety disorder diagnosis, this may be a useful approach. UP includes standard CBT techniques, such as cognitive reappraisal and exposure with five core modules: emotion awareness, cognitive flexibility, emotion avoidance, emotion-related physical sensations, and emotion-focused exposures.

For those with depression and a comorbid substance use disorder diagnosis, psychosocial treatment is typically used to address the substance abuse concern (Pettinati, O'Brien, & Dundon, 2013). It may be useful to reduce the patient's substance use early in treatment to determine the severity of affective symptoms in the absence of the substance (Pettinati et al., 2013). However, if the depressive episode is exacerbating substance use, it may make sense to address the depressive symptoms first via pharmacotherapy (Pettinati, 2004). While antidepressant medications such as SSRIs will address the depressive symptoms, they do not necessarily improve the substance use symptoms (Kranzler et al., 2006; Pettinati, 2004). Further, chronic alcohol

use may affect the pharmacokinetics of prescribed psychiatric medications, especially in patients who have liver damage resulting from chronic alcohol use. To address both depressive symptoms and alcoholism, adding a medication such as naltrexone (which reduces alcohol use) to the antidepressant pharmacotherapy may be effective (Pettinati et al., 2010).

EMERGING TRENDS

While the monoamine hypothesis of depression drove drug development initially, recent efforts have concentrated on refining the specific receptors or transporters targeted within the monoamine system, shifting the focus to other neurotransmitter systems such as glutamate or gamma-aminobutyric acid (GABA), and even moving beyond neurotransmitters to study inflammation or neurogenesis. Multimodal antidepressants are designed to affect a wider range of monoamine receptors and transporters. For instance, vilazodone (e.g., Viibryd®) is a serotonin transporter (SERT) inhibitor and 5-HT_{1A} partial agonist approved by the FDA in 2011 (Laughren et al., 2011). Vortioxetine (e.g., Brintellix®) is a SERT inhibitor, 5-HT_{1A} agonist and 5-HT_3 receptor antagonist that was approved by the FDA in 2013 (Bang-Andersen et al., 2011). Both medications have shown efficacy similar to that of traditional antidepressants, but there is little data on long-term treatment outcomes (Citrome, 2016; Connolly & Thase, 2016). Triple reuptake inhibitors have been another recent area of research. These agents block 5-HT, norepinephrine, and dopamine reuptake, hence the acronym SNDRIs. However, there are few successful clinical trials of these agents, and more research is needed (Learned et al., 2012; Zhang et al., 2014).

Ketamine, which affects the glutamate system as an *N*-methyl-d-aspartate (NMDA) receptor antagonist, produces a rapid antidepressant effect in patients with treatment-resistant depression (Berman et al., 2000). Ketamine was initially developed as an anesthetic, but has been studied off-label at low doses to produce antidepressant effects within hours of intravenous administration. However, the antidepressant effects of ketamine for depression only last a few days (Kishimoto et al., 2016) so patients need to go to their treatment facility every few days for additional ketamine infusions. Ketamine also has abuse potential and can elicit psychotomimetic side effects such as delirium, disorientation, or hallucinations (Short, Fong, Galvez, Shelker, & Loo, 2018).

There is a large body of research demonstrating links between depression and inflammation (Kiecolt-Glaser, Derry, & Fagundes, 2015). Thus, efforts are emerging to develop medications that may treat depressive symptoms by targeting the immune system, particularly proinflammatory cytokines such as tumor necrosis factor-alpha (TNF-α). A trial of infliximab (an anti-TNF-α antibody) in individuals with depression showed that for those who started the study with higher levels of inflammation, infliximab improved depressive symptoms (Raison et al., 2013). However, those who did not have elevated inflammation before treatment did not show improvement with infliximab over placebo. Further work is needed in this area. Neurogenesis stimulators are another potential avenue for depression treatment. These agents, such as NSI-189 (a benzylpiperizine-aminopyridine compound), stimulate neurogenesis—the production of new neurons—in the hippocampus. A preliminary double-blind RCT in depressed outpatients showed significant improvement in depressive symptoms among those taking NSI-189 versus placebo (M. Fava et al., 2016); however, more studies are needed. Another developing treatment area is personalized medicine. Pharmacogenomics assesses how a person's genes might influence his or her response to pharmacotherapy. Among individuals whose medication for depression was based on pharmacogenomics testing, some had better remission rates, but results were mixed across studies (Rosenblat, Lee, & McIntyre, 2017). Thus, to date there is only limited evidence for pharmacogenomics-guided treatment. However, these are among many potential pathways for improvements in the pharmacologic treatment of depression that may provide new options in the coming decades.

TOOL KIT OF RESOURCES

Major Depression

Patient Resources

Anxiety and Depression Association of America (ADAA), Screening for Depression: https://adaa.org/iving-with-anxiety/ask-and-learn/screenings/screening-depression

Mayo Clinic Patient Care & Health Information, Diseases & Conditions: Depression (Major Depressive Disorder): http://www.mayoclinic.org/diseases-conditions/depression/home/ovc-20321449

National Institute of Mental Health (NIMH), Health and Education, Mental Health Information: Depression: https://www.nimh.nih.gov/health/topics/depression/index.shtml

National Institute of Mental Health. (2015). *Depression: What you need to know* (NIH Publication No. 15-3561). Bethesda, MD: U.S. Government Printing Office. Available at https://www.nimh.nih.gov/health/publications/depression-what-you-need-to-know/index.shtml

Provider Resources

American Psychiatric Association. (2010). Treating major depressive disorder: A quick reference guide. Washington, DC: Author. http://psychiatryonline.org/pb/assets/raw/sitewide/practice_guidelines/guidelines/mdd-guide.pdf

Anxiety and Depression Association of America (ADAA), Clinical Practice Review for Major Depressive Disorder: https://adaa.org/resources-professionals/practice-guidelines-mdd

Gartlehner, G., Gaynes, B. N., Amick, H. R., Asher, G. N., Morgan, L. C., Coker-Schwimmer, E., . . . Lohr, K. N. (2016). Comparative benefits and harms of antidepressant, psychological, complementary, and exercise treatments for major depression: An evidence report for a clinical practice guideline from the American College of Physicians. *Annals of Internal Medicine, 164,* 331–341. http://dx.doi.org/10.7326/M15-1813

Gelenberg, A. J., Freeman, M. P., Markowitz, J. C., Rosenbaum, J. F., Thase, M. E., Trivedi, M. H., & Van Rhoads, R. S. (2010). Practice guideline for the treatment of patients with major depressive disorder, third edition. *The American Journal of Psychiatry, 167*(10), 1. Retrieved from https://psychiatryonline.org/pb/assets/raw/sitewide/practice_guidelines/guidelines/mdd.pdf

Premenstrual Dysphoric Disorder

Patient Resources

American Academy of Family Physicians (2002). Information from your family doctor: Premenstrual dysphoric disorder (PMDD). *American Family Physician, 66*(7), 1253–1254. Retrieved from http://www.aafp.org/afp/2002/1001/p1253.html

American College of Obstetricians and Gynecologists, Frequently Asked Questions, Gynecologic Problems: Premenstrual Syndrome (PMS): https://www.acog.org/Patients/FAQs/Premenstrual-Syndrome-PMS

Cleveland Clinic, PMS and PMDD: https://my.cleveland clinic.org/health/articles/pms-and-pmdd

MedlinePlus Medical Encyclopedia, Premenstrual Dysphoric Disorder: https://medlineplus.gov/ency/article/007193.htm

Johns Hopkins Medicine Health Library, What Is Premenstrual Dysphoric Disorder (PMDD)? http://www.hopkinsmedicine.org/healthlibrary/conditions/gynecological_health/premenstrual_dysphoric_disorder_pmdd_85,P00580

U.S. Department of Health and Human Services, Office on Women's Health, Premenstrual Syndrome: https://www.womenshealth.gov/a-z-topics/premenstrual-syndrome

Provider Resources

Association of Reproductive Health Professionals, Managing Premenstrual Symptoms: Treatment: https://www.arhp.org/quick-reference-guide-or-clinicians/managing-premenstrual-symptoms/treatment

Braverman, P. K. (2007). Premenstrual syndrome and premenstrual dysphoric disorder. *Journal of Pediatric and Adolescent Gynecology, 20*, 3–12. http://dx.doi.org/10.1016/j.jpag.2006.10.007

Halbreich, U., Borenstein, J., Pearlstein, T., & Kahn, L. S. (2003). The prevalence, impairment, impact, and burden of premenstrual dysphoric disorder (PMS/PMDD). *Psychoneuroendocrinology, 28*(Suppl. 3), 1–23.

Hantsoo, L., & Epperson, C. N. (2015). Premenstrual dysphoric disorder: Epidemiology and treatment. *Current Psychiatry Reports, 17*, 87. http://dx.doi.org/10.1007/s11920-015-0628-3

Rapkin, A. (2003). A review of treatment of premenstrual syndrome and premenstrual dysphoric disorder. *Psychoneuroendocrinology, 28*(Suppl. 3), 39–53.

Peripartum Depression

Patient Resources

American College of Obstetricians and Gynecologists, Frequently Asked Questions, Gynecologic Problems: Postpartum Depression: https://www.acog.org/Patients/FAQs/Postpartum-Depression

Council on Patient Safety in Women's Healthcare, Maternal Mental Health: Depression and Anxiety: http://safehealthcareforeverywoman.org/patient-safety-bundles/maternal-mental-health-depression-and-anxiety/

March of Dimes, Postpartum Depression: http://www.marchofdimes.org/pregnancy/postpartum-depression.aspx

Postpartum Support International (PSI): http://www.postpartum.net/

U.S. Department of Health and Human Services, Office on Women's Health, Postpartum Depression: https://www.womenshealth.gov/a-z-topics/depression-during-and-after-pregnancy

Provider Resources

American College of Obstetricians and Gynecologists. (2018). *Screening for perinatal depression.* Albany, NY: Author. Available at https://www.acog.org/Clinical-Guidance-and-Publications/Committee-Opinions/Committee-on-Obstetric-Practice/Screening-for-Perinatal-Depression

Gaynes, B. N., Gavin, N., Meltzer-Brody, S., Lohr, K. N., Swinson, T., Gartlehner, G., . . . Miller, W. C. (2005). *Perinatal depression: Prevalence, screening accuracy, and screening outcomes* (Evidence Reports/Technology Assessments, No. 119). Rockville, MD: Agency for Healthcare Research and Quality. Available at https://www.ncbi.nlm.nih.gov/books/NBK37740/

Goodman, J. H., & Tyer-Viola, L. (2010). Detection, treatment, and referral of perinatal depression and anxiety by obstetrical providers. *Journal of Women's Health, 19*, 477–490. http://dx.doi.org/10.1089/jwh.2008.1352

New York State Department of Health, Screening for Maternal Depression: https://www.health.ny.gov/community/pregnancy/health_care/perinatal/maternal_depression/providers/screening.htm

Sockol, L. E., Epperson, C. N., & Barber, J. P. (2011). A meta-analysis of treatments for perinatal depression. *Clinical Psychology Review, 31*, 839–849. http://dx.doi.org/10.1016/j.cpr.2011.03.009

References

Åkerblad, A.-C., Bengtsson, F., von Knorring, L., & Ekselius, L. (2006). Response, remission and relapse in relation to adherence in primary care treatment of depression: A 2-year outcome study. *International Clinical Psychopharmacology, 21,* 117–124. http://dx.doi.org/10.1097/01.yic.0000199452.16682.b8

Akincigil, A., Bowblis, J. R., Levin, C., Walkup, J. T., Jan, S., & Crystal, S. (2007). Adherence to antidepressant treatment among privately insured patients diagnosed with depression. *Medical Care, 45,* 363–369. http://dx.doi.org/10.1097/01.mlr.0000254574.23418.f6

*Altshuler, L. L., Cohen, L. S., Vitonis, A. F., Faraone, S. V., Harlow, B. L., Suri, R., . . . Stowe, Z. N. (2008). The Pregnancy Depression Scale (PDS): A screening tool for depression in pregnancy. *Archives of Women's Mental Health, 11,* 277–285. http://dx.doi.org/10.1007/s00737-008-0020-y

American College of Obstetricians and Gynecologists. (2001). ACOG practice bulletin: Premenstrual syndrome. Clinical management guidelines for obstetrician-gynecologists. *International Journal of Obstetrics & Gynecology, 73,* 183–191. http://dx.doi.org/10.1016/S0020-7292(01)00400-3

American Psychiatric Association. (2013). *Diagnostic and statistical manual of mental disorders* (5th ed.). Arlington, VA: American Psychiatric Association Publishing.

Anderson, I. M. (2000). Selective serotonin reuptake inhibitors versus tricyclic antidepressants: A meta-analysis of efficacy and tolerability. *Journal of Affective Disorders, 58,* 19–36. http://dx.doi.org/10.1016/S0165-0327(99)00092-0

Appleby, L., Warner, R., Whitton, A., & Faragher, B. (1997). A controlled study of fluoxetine and cognitive-behavioural counselling in the treatment of postnatal depression. *BMJ, 314,* 932–936. http://dx.doi.org/10.1136/bmj.314.7085.932

Bang-Andersen, B., Ruhland, T., Jørgensen, M., Smith, G., Frederiksen, K., Jensen, K. G., . . . Stensbøl, T. B. (2011). Discovery of 1-[2-(2,4-dimethylphenyl-sulfanyl)phenyl]piperazine (Lu AA21004): A novel multimodal compound for the treatment of major depressive disorder. *Journal of Medicinal Chemistry, 54,* 3206–3221. http://dx.doi.org/10.1021/jm101459g

Barlow, D. H., Allen, L. B., & Choate, M. L. (2016). Toward a unified treatment for emotional disorders–Republished article. *Behavior Therapy, 47,* 838–853. http://dx.doi.org/10.1016/j.beth.2016.11.005

Barry, L. C., Abou, J. J., Simen, A. A., & Gill, T. M. (2012). Under-treatment of depression in older persons. *Journal of Affective Disorders, 136,* 789–796. http://dx.doi.org/10.1016/j.jad.2011.09.038

Beck, A. T., Steer, R. A., Ball, R., & Ranieri, W. (1996). Comparison of Beck Depression Inventories-IA and -II in psychiatric outpatients. *Journal of Personality Assessment, 67,* 588–597. http://dx.doi.org/10.1207/s15327752jpa6703_13

Bentley, S. M., Pagalilauan, G. L., & Simpson, S. A. (2014). Major depression. *The Medical Clinics of North America, 98*(5), 981–1005. http://dx.doi.org/10.1016/j.mcna.2014.06.013

Berle, J. Ø., & Spigset, O. (2011). Antidepressant use during breastfeeding. *Current Women's Health Reviews, 7,* 28–34. http://dx.doi.org/10.2174/157340411794474784

Berman, R. M., Cappiello, A., Anand, A., Oren, D. A., Heninger, G. R., Charney, D. S., & Krystal, J. H. (2000). Antidepressant effects of ketamine in depressed patients. *Biological Psychiatry, 47,* 351–354. http://dx.doi.org/10.1016/S0006-3223(99)00230-9

Birmaher, B., Arbelaez, C., & Brent, D. (2002). Course and outcome of child and adolescent major depressive disorder. *Child and Adolescent Psychiatric Clinics of North America, 11,* 619–637. http://dx.doi.org/10.1016/S1056-4993(02)00011-1

Birmaher, B., & Brent, D. (2007). Practice parameter for the assessment and treatment of children and adolescents with depressive disorders. *Journal of the American Academy of Child & Adolescent Psychiatry, 46,* 1503–1526. http://dx.doi.org/10.1097/chi.0b013e318145ae1c

Black, K., Shea, C., Dursun, S., & Kutcher, S. (2000). Selective serotonin reuptake inhibitor discontinuation syndrome: Proposed diagnostic criteria. *Journal of Psychiatry & Neuroscience, 25*(3), 255–261.

Blanco, C., Okuda, M., Markowitz, J. C., Liu, S.-M., Grant, B. F., & Hasin, D. S. (2010). The epidemiology of chronic major depressive disorder and dysthymic disorder: Results from the National Epidemiologic Survey on Alcohol and Related Conditions. *The Journal of Clinical Psychiatry, 71,* 1645–1656. http://dx.doi.org/10.4088/JCP.09m05663gry

Brodey, B. B., Goodman, S. H., Baldasaro, R. E., Brooks-DeWeese, A., Wilson, M. E., Brodey, I. S. B., & Doyle, N. M. (2016). Development of the Perinatal Depression Inventory (PDI)-14 using item response theory: A comparison of the BDI-II, EPDS, PDI, and PHQ-9. *Archives of Women's Mental Health, 19,* 307–316. http://dx.doi.org/10.1007/s00737-015-0553-9

Bromberger, J. T., Kravitz, H. M., Chang, Y.-F., Cyranowski, J. M., Brown, C., & Matthews, K. A. (2011). Major depression during and after the menopausal transition: Study of Women's Health Across the Nation (SWAN). *Psychological Medicine, 41,* 1879–1888. http://dx.doi.org/10.1017/S003329171100016X

*Asterisks indicate assessments or resources.

Bromet, E., Andrade, L. H., Hwang, I., Sampson, N. A., Alonso, J., de Girolamo, G., . . . Kessler, R. C. (2011). Cross-national epidemiology of *DSM–IV* major depressive episode. *BMC Medicine, 9*, 90. http://dx.doi.org/10.1186/1741-7015-9-90

Burcusa, S. L., & Iacono, W. G. (2007). Risk for recurrence in depression. *Clinical Psychology Review, 27*(8), 959–985. http://dx.doi.org/10.1016/j.cpr.2007.02.005

Burt, V. K., & Stein, K. (2002). Epidemiology of depression throughout the female life cycle. *The Journal of Clinical Psychiatry, 63*(Suppl. 7), 9–15.

Calati, R., Salvina Signorelli, M., Balestri, M., Marsano, A., De Ronchi, D., Aguglia, E., & Serretti, A. (2013). Antidepressants in elderly: Metaregression of double-blind, randomized clinical trials. *Journal of Affective Disorders, 147*, 1–8. http://dx.doi.org/10.1016/j.jad.2012.11.053

Cascade, E., Kalali, A. H., & Kennedy, S. H. (2009). Real-world data on SSRI antidepressant side effects. *Psychiatry, 6*(2), 16–18.

Cipriani, A., Furukawa, T. A., Salanti, G., Geddes, J. R., Higgins, J. P., Churchill, R., . . . Barbui, C. (2009). Comparative efficacy and acceptability of 12 new-generation antidepressants: A multiple-treatments meta-analysis. *The Lancet, 373*, 746–758. http://dx.doi.org/10.1016/S0140-6736(09)60046-5

Citrome, L. (2016). Vortioxetine for major depressive disorder: An indirect comparison with duloxetine, escitalopram, levomilnacipran, sertraline, venlafaxine, and vilazodone, using number needed to treat, number needed to harm, and likelihood to be helped or harmed. *Journal of Affective Disorders, 196*, 225–233. http://dx.doi.org/10.1016/j.jad.2016.02.042

Cohen, L. S., Altshuler, L. L., Stowe, Z. N., & Faraone, S. V. (2004). Reintroduction of antidepressant therapy across pregnancy in women who previously discontinued treatment. A preliminary retrospective study. *Psychotherapy and Psychosomatics, 73*, 255–258. http://dx.doi.org/10.1159/000077745

Connolly, K. R., & Thase, M. E. (2016). Vortioxetine: A new treatment for major depressive disorder. *Expert Opinion on Pharmacotherapy, 17*, 421–431. http://dx.doi.org/10.1517/14656566.2016.1133588

Coplan, J. D., Aaronson, C. J., Panthangi, V., & Kim, Y. (2015). Treating comorbid anxiety and depression: Psychosocial and pharmacological approaches. *World Journal of Psychiatry, 5*, 366–378. http://dx.doi.org/10.5498/wjp.v5.i4.366

Corruble, E., Swartz, H. A., Bottai, T., Vaiva, G., Bayle, F., Llorca, P.-M., . . . Gorwood, P. (2016). Telephone-administered psychotherapy in combination with antidepressant medication for the acute treatment of major depressive disorder. *Journal of Affective Disorders, 190*, 6–11. http://dx.doi.org/10.1016/j.jad.2015.07.052

Cox, J. L., Holden, J. M., & Sagovsky, R. (1987). Detection of postnatal depression. Development of the 10-item Edinburgh Postnatal Depression Scale. *The British Journal of Psychiatry, 150*, 782–786. http://dx.doi.org/10.1192/bjp.150.6.782

Cunningham, J., Yonkers, K. A., O'Brien, S., & Eriksson, E. (2009). Update on research and treatment of premenstrual dysphoric disorder. *Harvard Review of Psychiatry, 17*, 120–137. http://dx.doi.org/10.1080/10673220902891836

Damoiseaux, V. A., Proost, J. H., Jiawan, V. C. R., & Melgert, B. N. (2014). Sex differences in the pharmacokinetics of antidepressants: Influence of female sex hormones and oral contraceptives. *Clinical Pharmacokinetics, 53*, 509–519. http://dx.doi.org/10.1007/s40262-014-0145-2

Danielsson, L., Noras, A. M., Waern, M., & Carlsson, J. (2013). Exercise in the treatment of major depression: A systematic review grading the quality of evidence. *Physiotherapy Theory and Practice, 29*, 573–585. http://dx.doi.org/10.3109/09593985.2013.774452

Davanzo, R., Copertino, M., De Cunto, A., Minen, F., & Amaddeo, A. (2011). Antidepressant drugs and breastfeeding: A review of the literature. *Breastfeeding Medicine, 6*, 89–98. http://dx.doi.org/10.1089/bfm.2010.0019

de Mello, M. F., Myczcowisk, L. M., & Menezes, P. R. (2001). A randomized controlled trial comparing moclobemide and moclobemide plus interpersonal psychotherapy in the treatment of dysthymic disorder. *Journal of Psychotherapy Practice and Research, 10*, 117–123.

Derry, H. M., Padin, A. C., Kuo, J. L., Hughes, S., & Kiecolt-Glaser, J. K. (2015). Sex differences in depression: Does inflammation play a role? *Current Psychiatry Reports, 17*, 78. http://dx.doi.org/10.1007/s11920-015-0618-5

Deshmukh, R., & Franco, K. (2003). Managing weight gain as a side effect of antidepressant therapy. *Cleveland Clinic Journal of Medicine, 70*(7), 614–623.

*Dupuy, J. M., Ostacher, M. J., Huffman, J., Perlis, R. H., & Nierenberg, A. A. (2011). A critical review of pharmacotherapy for major depressive disorder. *International Journal of Neuropsychopharmacology, 14*, 1417–1431. http://dx.doi.org/10.1017/S1461145711000083

Eisenlohr-Moul, T. A., Girdler, S. S., Johnson, J. L., Schmidt, P. J., & Rubinow, D. R. (2017). Treatment of premenstrual dysphoria with continuous versus intermittent dosing of oral contraceptives: Results of a three-arm randomized controlled trial. *Depression and Anxiety, 34*, 908–917. http://dx.doi.org/10.1002/da.22673

*Eisenlohr-Moul, T. A., Girdler, S. S., Schmalenberger, K. M., Dawson, D. N., Surana, P., Johnson, J. L.,

& Rubinow, D. R. (2016). Toward the reliable diagnosis of *DSM–5* premenstrual dysphoric disorder: The Carolina Premenstrual Assessment Scoring System (C-PASS). *The American Journal of Psychiatry, 174*, 51–59. http://dx.doi.org/10.1176/appi.ajp.2016.15121510

*Endicott, J., Nee, J., & Harrison, W. (2006). Daily Record of Severity of Problems (DRSP): Reliability and validity. *Archives of Women's Mental Health, 9*, 41–49. http://dx.doi.org/10.1007/s00737-005-0103-y

Epperson, C. N., & Hantsoo, L. V. (2017). Making strides to simplify diagnosis of premenstrual dysphoric disorder. *The American Journal of Psychiatry, 174*, 6–7. http://dx.doi.org/10.1176/appi.ajp.2016.16101144

Epperson, C. N., Sammel, M. D., Bale, T. L., Kim, D. R., Conlin, S., Scalice, S., . . . Freeman, E. W. (2017). Adverse childhood experiences and risk for first-episode major depression during the menopause transition. *The Journal of Clinical Psychiatry, 78*, e298–e307. http://dx.doi.org/10.4088/JCP.16m10662

Fava, G. A., Gatti, A., Belaise, C., Guidi, J., & Offidani, E. (2015). Withdrawal symptoms after selective serotonin reuptake inhibitor discontinuation: A systematic review. *Psychotherapy and Psychosomatics, 84*, 72–81. http://dx.doi.org/10.1159/000370338

Fava, M., & Davidson, K. G. (1996). Definition and epidemiology of treatment-resistant depression. *Psychiatric Clinics of North America, 19*, 179–200. http://dx.doi.org/10.1016/S0193-953X(05)70283-5

Fava, M., Johe, K., Ereshefsky, L., Gertsik, L. G., English, B. A., Bilello, J. A., . . . Freeman, M. P. (2016). A Phase 1B, randomized, double blind, placebo controlled, multiple-dose escalation study of NSI-189 phosphate, a neurogenic compound, in depressed patients. *Molecular Psychiatry, 21*, 1372–1380. http://dx.doi.org/10.1038/mp.2015.178

Flynn, H. A., Sexton, M., Ratliff, S., Porter, K., & Zivin, K. (2011). Comparative performance of the Edinburgh Postnatal Depression Scale and the Patient Health Questionnaire-9 in pregnant and postpartum women seeking psychiatric services. *Psychiatry Research, 187*, 130–134. http://dx.doi.org/10.1016/j.psychres.2010.10.022

Ford, O., Lethaby, A., Roberts, H., & Mol, B. W. J. (2012). Progesterone for premenstrual syndrome. *The Cochrane Database of Systematic Reviews, 3*, CD003415.

Fortney, J. C., Unützer, J., Wrenn, G., Pyne, J. M., Smith, G. R., Schoenbaum, M., & Harbin, H. T. (2017). A tipping point for measurement-based care. *Psychiatric Services, 68*, 179–188. http://dx.doi.org/10.1176/appi.ps.201500439

Fournier, J. C., DeRubeis, R. J., Hollon, S. D., Dimidjian, S., Amsterdam, J. D., Shelton, R. C., & Fawcett, J. (2010). Antidepressant drug effects and depression severity: A patient-level meta-analysis. *JAMA, 303*, 47–53. http://dx.doi.org/10.1001/jama.2009.1943

Freeman, E. W. (2004). Luteal phase administration of agents for the treatment of premenstrual dysphoric disorder. *CNS Drugs, 18*, 453–468. http://dx.doi.org/10.2165/00023210-200418070-00004

Freeman, E. W., Halbreich, U., Grubb, G. S., Rapkin, A. J., Skouby, S. O., Smith, L., . . . Constantine, G. D. (2012). An overview of four studies of a continuous oral contraceptive (levonorgestrel 90 mcg/ethinyl estradiol 20 mcg) on premenstrual dysphoric disorder and premenstrual syndrome. *Contraception, 85*, 437–445. http://dx.doi.org/10.1016/j.contraception.2011.09.010

Freeman, E. W., Sammel, M. D., Lin, H., & Nelson, D. B. (2006). Associations of hormones and menopausal status with depressed mood in women with no history of depression. *Archives of General Psychiatry, 63*, 375–382. http://dx.doi.org/10.1001/archpsyc.63.4.375

Gartlehner, G., Thieda, P., Hansen, R. A., Gaynes, B. N., Deveaugh-Geiss, A., Krebs, E. E., & Lohr, K. N. (2008). Comparative risk for harms of second-generation antidepressants: A systematic review and meta-analysis. *Drug Safety, 31*, 851–865. http://dx.doi.org/10.2165/00002018-200831100-00004

Gavin, N. I., Gaynes, B. N., Lohr, K. N., Meltzer-Brody, S., Gartlehner, G., & Swinson, T. (2005). Perinatal depression: A systematic review of prevalence and incidence. *Obstetrics and Gynecology, 106*(5, Pt. 1), 1071–1083. http://dx.doi.org/10.1097/01.AOG.0000183597.31630.db

Geddes, J. R., Freemantle, N., Mason, J., Eccles, M. P., & Boynton, J. (2000). SSRIs versus other anti-depressants for depressive disorder. *Cochrane Database of Systematic Reviews, 2*, CD001851.

Griffin, L. D., & Mellon, S. H. (1999). Selective serotonin reuptake inhibitors directly alter activity of neuro-steroidogenic enzymes. *Proceedings of the National Academy of Sciences of the United States of America, 96*, 13512–13517. http://dx.doi.org/10.1073/pnas.96.23.13512

Guaiana, G., Barbui, C., & Hotopf, M. (2007). Amitriptyline for depression. *Cochrane Database of Systematic Reviews, 3*, CD004186.

Gueorguieva, R., Chekroud, A. M., & Krystal, J. H. (2017). Trajectories of relapse in randomised, placebo-controlled trials of treatment discontinuation in major depressive disorder: An individual patient-level data meta-analysis. *The Lancet Psychiatry, 4*, 230–237. http://dx.doi.org/10.1016/S2215-0366(17)30038-X

Guidi, J., Tomba, E., & Fava, G. A. (2016). The sequential integration of pharmacotherapy and psychotherapy in the treatment of major depressive disorder: A meta-analysis of the sequential model and a critical review of the literature. *The American Journal of Psychiatry, 173*, 128–137. http://dx.doi.org/10.1176/appi.ajp.2015.15040476

Halbreich, U. (2008). Selective serotonin reuptake inhibitors and initial oral contraceptives for the treatment of PMDD: Effective but not enough. *CNS Spectrums, 13,* 566–572. http://dx.doi.org/10.1017/S1092852900016849

Hamilton, M. (1960). A rating scale for depression. *Journal of Neurology, Neurosurgery, & Psychiatry, 23,* 56–62. http://dx.doi.org/10.1136/jnnp.23.1.56

Han, C., Wang, S.-M., Kwak, K.-P., Won, W.-Y., Lee, H., Chang, C. M., . . . Pae, C.-U. (2015). Aripiprazole augmentation versus antidepressant switching for patients with major depressive disorder: A 6-week, randomized, rater-blinded, prospective study. *Journal of Psychiatric Research, 66–67,* 84–94. http://dx.doi.org/10.1016/j.jpsychires.2015.04.020

Hantsoo, L., Podcasy, J., Sammel, M., Epperson, C. N., & Kim, D. R. (2017). Pregnancy and the acceptability of computer-based versus traditional mental health treatments. *Journal of Women's Health, 26,* 1106–1113. http://dx.doi.org/10.1089/jwh.2016.6255

Hantsoo, L., Ward-O'Brien, D., Czarkowski, K. A., Gueorguieva, R., Price, L. H., & Epperson, C. N. (2014). A randomized, placebo-controlled, double-blind trial of sertraline for postpartum depression. *Psychopharmacology, 231,* 939–948. http://dx.doi.org/10.1007/s00213-013-3316-1

Hatfield, D., McCullough, L., Frantz, S. H. B., & Krieger, K. (2010). Do we know when our clients get worse? An investigation of therapists' ability to detect negative client change. *Clinical Psychology & Psychotherapy, 17,* 25–32.

Herwig, U., Fallgatter, A. J., Höppner, J., Eschweiler, G. W., Kron, M., Hajak, G., . . . Schönfeldt-Lecuona, C. (2007). Antidepressant effects of augmentative transcranial magnetic stimulation: Randomised multicentre trial. *The British Journal of Psychiatry, 191,* 441–448. http://dx.doi.org/10.1192/bjp.bp.106.034371

Hildebrandt, M. G., Steyerberg, E. W., Stage, K. B., Passchier, J., Kragh-Soerensen, P., & the Danish University Antidepressant Group. (2003). Are gender differences important for the clinical effects of antidepressants? *The American Journal of Psychiatry, 160,* 1643–1650. http://dx.doi.org/10.1176/appi.ajp.160.9.1643

Hillhouse, T. M., & Porter, J. H. (2015). A brief history of the development of antidepressant drugs: From monoamines to glutamate. *Experimental and Clinical Psychopharmacology, 23,* 1–21. http://dx.doi.org/10.1037/a0038550

Hindmarch, I. (2002). Beyond the monoamine hypothesis: Mechanisms, molecules and methods. *European Psychiatry, 17*(Suppl. 3), 294–299. http://dx.doi.org/10.1016/S0924-9338(02)00653-3

Hollon, S. D., DeRubeis, R. J., Fawcett, J., Amsterdam, J. D., Shelton, R. C., Zajecka, J., . . . Gallop, R. (2014). Effect of cognitive therapy with antidepressant medications vs antidepressants alone on the rate of recovery in major depressive disorder: A randomized clinical trial. *JAMA Psychiatry, 71,* 1157–1164. http://dx.doi.org/10.1001/jamapsychiatry.2014.1054

Ismaili, E., Walsh, S., O'Brien, P. M. S., Bäckström, T., Brown, C., Dennerstein, L., . . . Consensus Group of the International Society for Premenstrual Disorders. (2016). Fourth consensus of the International Society for Premenstrual Disorders (ISPMD): Auditable standards for diagnosis and management of premenstrual disorder. *Archives of Women's Mental Health, 19,* 953–958. http://dx.doi.org/10.1007/s00737-016-0631-7

Jakubovski, E., Varigonda, A. L., Freemantle, N., Taylor, M. J., & Bloch, M. H. (2016). Systematic review and meta-analysis: Dose-response relationship of selective serotonin reuptake inhibitors in major depressive disorder. *The American Journal of Psychiatry, 173,* 174–183. http://dx.doi.org/10.1176/appi.ajp.2015.15030331

Kanes, S., Colquhoun, H., Gunduz-Bruce, H., Raines, S., Arnold, R., Schacterle, A., . . . Meltzer-Brody, S. (2017). Brexanolone (SAGE-547 injection) in postpartum depression: A randomised controlled trial. *The Lancet, 390*(10093), 480–489. http://dx.doi.org/10.1016/S0140-6736(17)31264-3

Karyotaki, E., Smit, Y., Holdt Henningsen, K., Huibers, M. J. H., Robays, J., de Beurs, D., & Cuijpers, P. (2016). Combining pharmacotherapy and psychotherapy or monotherapy for major depression? A meta-analysis on the long-term effects. *Journal of Affective Disorders, 194,* 144–152. http://dx.doi.org/10.1016/j.jad.2016.01.036

Kashani, J. H., McGee, R. O., Clarkson, S. E., Anderson, J. C., Walton, L. A., Williams, S., . . . McKnew, D. H. (1983). Depression in a sample of 9-year-old children, Prevalence and associated characteristics. *Archives of General Psychiatry, 40,* 1217–1223. http://dx.doi.org/10.1001/archpsyc.1983.01790100063009

Keks, N., Hope, J., & Keogh, S. (2016). Switching and stopping antidepressants. *Australian Prescriber, 39*(3), 76–83.

Kessler, R. C., Berglund, P., Demler, O., Jin, R., Koretz, D., Merikangas, K. R., . . . Wang, P. S., & the National Comorbidity Survey Replication. (2003). The epidemiology of major depressive disorder: Results from the National Comorbidity Survey Replication (NCS-R). *JAMA, 289,* 3095–3105. http://dx.doi.org/10.1001/jama.289.23.3095

Kessler, R. C., Chiu, W. T., Demler, O., & Walters, E. E. (2005). Prevalence, severity, and comorbidity of 12-month *DSM–IV* disorders in the National Comorbidity Survey Replication. *Archives of General Psychiatry, 62,* 617–627. http://dx.doi.org/10.1001/archpsyc.62.6.617

Keyloun, K. R., Hansen, R. N., Hepp, Z., Gillard, P., Thase, M. E., & Devine, E. B. (2017). Adherence and persistence across antidepressant therapeutic classes: A retrospective claims analysis among insured US patients with major depressive disorder (MDD). *CNS Drugs, 31*, 421–432. http://dx.doi.org/10.1007/s40263-017-0417-0

Khan, A. A., Gardner, C. O., Prescott, C. A., & Kendler, K. S. (2002). Gender differences in the symptoms of major depression in opposite-sex dizygotic twin pairs. *The American Journal of Psychiatry, 159*, 1427–1429. http://dx.doi.org/10.1176/appi.ajp.159.8.1427

Khan, A., Brodhead, A. E., Schwartz, K. A., Kolts, R. L., & Brown, W. A. (2005). Sex differences in antidepressant response in recent antidepressant clinical trials. *Journal of Clinical Psychopharmacology, 25*, 318–324. http://dx.doi.org/10.1097/01.jcp.0000168879.03169.ce

Kiecolt-Glaser, J. K., Derry, H. M., & Fagundes, C. P. (2015). Inflammation: Depression fans the flames and feasts on the heat. *The American Journal of Psychiatry, 172*, 1075–1091. http://dx.doi.org/10.1176/appi.ajp.2015.15020152

Kim, D. R., Epperson, C. N., Weiss, A. R., & Wisner, K. L. (2014). Pharmacotherapy of postpartum depression: An update. *Expert Opinion on Pharmacotherapy, 15*, 1223–1234. http://dx.doi.org/10.1517/14656566.2014.911842

Kim, D. R., Hantsoo, L., Thase, M. E., Sammel, M., & Epperson, C. N. (2014). Computer-assisted cognitive behavioral therapy for pregnant women with major depressive disorder. *Journal of Women's Health (2002), 23*, 842–848. http://dx.doi.org/10.1089/jwh.2014.4867

Kishimoto, T., Chawla, J. M., Hagi, K., Zarate, C. A., Kane, J. M., Bauer, M., & Correll, C. U. (2016). Single-dose infusion ketamine and non-ketamine N-methyl-d-aspartate receptor antagonists for unipolar and bipolar depression: A meta-analysis of efficacy, safety and time trajectories. *Psychological Medicine, 46*, 1459–1472. http://dx.doi.org/10.1017/S0033291716000064

Klein, D. N., Schwartz, J. E., Rose, S., & Leader, J. B. (2000). Five-year course and outcome of dysthymic disorder: A prospective, naturalistic follow-up study. *The American Journal of Psychiatry, 157*, 931–939. http://dx.doi.org/10.1176/appi.ajp.157.6.931

Kockler, M., & Heun, R. (2002). Gender differences of depressive symptoms in depressed and nondepressed elderly persons. *International Journal of Geriatric Psychiatry, 17*, 65–72. http://dx.doi.org/10.1002/gps.521

Kok, R. M., Nolen, W. A., & Heeren, T. J. (2012). Efficacy of treatment in older depressed patients: A systematic review and meta-analysis of double-blind randomized controlled trials with antidepressants. *Journal of Affective Disorders, 141*, 103–115. http://dx.doi.org/10.1016/j.jad.2012.02.036

Kok, R. M., & Reynolds, C. F., III. (2017). Management of depression in older adults: A review. *JAMA, 317*, 2114–2122. http://dx.doi.org/10.1001/jama.2017.5706

Kovacs, M. (1992). *The Children's Depression Inventory*. Tonawanda, NY: Multi-Health Systems.

Kranzler, H. R., Mueller, T., Cornelius, J., Pettinati, H. M., Moak, D., Martin, P. R., . . . Keller, M. (2006). Sertraline treatment of co-occurring alcohol dependence and major depression. *Journal of Clinical Psychopharmacology, 26*, 13–20. http://dx.doi.org/10.1097/01.jcp.0000194620.61868.35

*Kroenke, K., Spitzer, R. L., & Williams, J. B. (2001). The PHQ-9: Validity of a brief depression severity measure. *Journal of General Internal Medicine, 16*, 606–613. http://dx.doi.org/10.1046/j.1525-1497.2001.016009606.x

Kuyken, W., Warren, F. C., Taylor, R. S., Whalley, B., Crane, C., Bondolfi, G., . . . Dalgleish, T. (2016). Efficacy of mindfulness-based cognitive therapy in prevention of depressive relapse: An individual patient data meta-analysis from randomized trials. *JAMA Psychiatry, 73*, 565–574. http://dx.doi.org/10.1001/jamapsychiatry.2016.0076

Landén, M., & Thase, M. E. (2006). A model to explain the therapeutic effects of serotonin reuptake inhibitors: The role of 5-HT$_2$ receptors. *Psychopharmacology Bulletin, 39*, 147–166.

Laughren, T. P., Gobburu, J., Temple, R. J., Unger, E. F., Bhattaram, A., Dinh, P. V., . . . Zineh, I. (2011). Vilazodone: Clinical basis for the US Food and Drug Administration's approval of a new antidepressant. *The Journal of Clinical Psychiatry, 72*, 1166–1173. http://dx.doi.org/10.4088/JCP.11r06984

Lawrie, T. A., Hofmeyr, G. J., De Jager, M., Berk, M., Paiker, J., & Viljoen, E. (1998). A double-blind randomised placebo controlled trial of postnatal norethisterone enanthate: The effect on postnatal depression and serum hormones. *British Journal of Obstetrics and Gynaecology, 105*, 1082–1090. http://dx.doi.org/10.1111/j.1471-0528.1998.tb09940.x

Learned, S., Graff, O., Roychowdhury, S., Moate, R., Krishnan, K. R., Archer, G., . . . Ratti, E. (2012). Efficacy, safety, and tolerability of a triple reuptake inhibitor GSK372475 in the treatment of patients with major depressive disorder: Two randomized, placebo- and active-controlled clinical trials. *Journal of Psychopharmacology, 26*, 653–662. http://dx.doi.org/10.1177/0269881111424931

Logsdon, M. C., Wisner, K., Hanusa, B. H., & Phillips, A. (2003). Role functioning and symptom remission in women with postpartum depression after antidepressant treatment. *Archives of Psychiatric Nursing, 17*, 276–283. http://dx.doi.org/10.1053/j.apnu.2003.10.004

Lopez, L. M., Kaptein, A. A., & Helmerhorst, F. M. (2012). Oral contraceptives containing drospirenone for premenstrual syndrome. *The Cochrane Database of Systematic Reviews, 2,* CD006586.

Luppa, M., Sikorski, C., Luck, T., Ehreke, L., Konnopka, A., Wiese, B., . . . Riedel-Heller, S. G. (2012). Age- and gender-specific prevalence of depression in latest-life—systematic review and meta-analysis. *Journal of Affective Disorders, 136,* 212–221. http://dx.doi.org/10.1016/j.jad.2010.11.033

Mackay, F. R., Dunn, N. R., Martin, R. M., Pearce, G. L., Freemantle, S. N., & Mann, R. D. (1999). Newer antidepressants: A comparison of tolerability in general practice. *The British Journal of General Practice: The Journal of the Royal College of General Practitioners, 49*(448), 892–896.

Marcus, S. M., Kerber, K. B., Rush, A. J., Wisniewski, S. R., Nierenberg, A., Balasubramani, G. K., . . . Trivedi, M. H. (2008). Sex differences in depression symptoms in treatment-seeking adults: Confirmatory analyses from the Sequenced Treatment Alternatives to Relieve Depression study. *Comprehensive Psychiatry, 49,* 238–246. http://dx.doi.org/10.1016/j.comppsych.2007.06.012

Mårdby, A.-C., Schiöler, L., Sundell, K. A., Bjerkeli, P., Lesén, E., & Jönsson, A. K. (2016). Adherence to antidepressants among women and men described with trajectory models: A Swedish longitudinal study. *European Journal of Clinical Pharmacology, 72,* 1381–1389. http://dx.doi.org/10.1007/s00228-016-2106-1

Marjoribanks, J., Brown, J., O'Brien, P. M. S., & Wyatt, K. (2013). Selective serotonin reuptake inhibitors for premenstrual syndrome. *Cochrane Database of Systematic Reviews, 2013*(6), CD001396. http://dx.doi.org/10.1002/14651858.CD001396.pub3

Meister, R., von Wolff, A., Mohr, H., Härter, M., Nestoriuc, Y., Hölzel, L., & Kriston, L. (2016). Comparative safety of pharmacologic treatments for persistent depressive disorder: A systematic review and network meta-analysis. *PLoS One, 11,* e0153380. http://dx.doi.org/10.1371/journal.pone.0153380

Merikangas, K. R., He, J.-P., Burstein, M., Swanson, S. A., Avenevoli, S., Cui, L., . . . Swendsen, J. (2010). Lifetime prevalence of mental disorders in U.S. adolescents: Results from the National Comorbidity Survey Replication—Adolescent Supplement (NCS-A). *Journal of the American Academy of Child & Adolescent Psychiatry, 49,* 980–989. http://dx.doi.org/10.1016/j.jaac.2010.05.017

Milgrom, J., Gemmill, A. W., Ericksen, J., Burrows, G., Buist, A., & Reece, J. (2015). Treatment of postnatal depression with cognitive behavioural therapy, sertraline and combination therapy: A randomised controlled trial. *Australian and New Zealand Journal of Psychiatry, 49,* 236–245. http://dx.doi.org/10.1177/0004867414565474

Misri, S., Abizadeh, J., Albert, G., Carter, D., & Ryan, D. (2012). Restoration of functionality in postpartum depressed mothers: An open-label study with escitalopram. *Journal of Clinical Psychopharmacology, 32,* 729–732. http://dx.doi.org/10.1097/JCP.0b013e31826867c9

Misri, S., Kendrick, K., Oberlander, T. F., Norris, S., Tomfohr, L., Zhang, H., & Grunau, R. E. (2010). Antenatal depression and anxiety affect postpartum parenting stress: A longitudinal, prospective study. *The Canadian Journal of Psychiatry, 55,* 222–228. http://dx.doi.org/10.1177/070674371005500405

Misri, S., Reebye, P., Corral, M., & Milis, L. (2004). The use of paroxetine and cognitive-behavioral therapy in postpartum depression and anxiety: A randomized controlled trial. *The Journal of Clinical Psychiatry, 65,* 1236–1241. http://dx.doi.org/10.4088/JCP.v65n0913

Montgomery, S. A., & Åsberg, M. (1979). A new depression scale designed to be sensitive to change. *The British Journal of Psychiatry, 134,* 382–389. http://dx.doi.org/10.1192/bjp.134.4.382

Montgomery, S. A., Baldwin, D. S., & Riley, A. (2002). Antidepressant medications: A review of the evidence for drug-induced sexual dysfunction. *Journal of Affective Disorders, 69,* 119–140. http://dx.doi.org/10.1016/S0165-0327(01)00313-5

Morishita, S., & Kinoshita, T. (2008). Predictors of response to sertraline in patients with major depression. *Human Psychopharmacology: Clinical and Experimental, 23,* 647–651. http://dx.doi.org/10.1002/hup.969

Nolen-Hoeksema, S., Larson, J., & Grayson, C. (1999). Explaining the gender difference in depressive symptoms. *Journal of Personality and Social Psychology, 77,* 1061–1072. http://dx.doi.org/10.1037/0022-3514.77.5.1061

Nonacs, R. M., Soares, C. N., Viguera, A. C., Pearson, K., Poitras, J. R., & Cohen, L. S. (2005). Bupropion SR for the treatment of postpartum depression: A pilot study. *International Journal of Neuropsychopharmacology, 8,* 445–449. http://dx.doi.org/10.1017/S1461145705005079

Nulman, I., Koren, G., Rovet, J., Barrera, M., Pulver, A., Streiner, D., & Feldman, B. (2012). Neurodevelopment of children following prenatal exposure to venlafaxine, selective serotonin reuptake inhibitors, or untreated maternal depression. *The American Journal of Psychiatry, 169,* 1165–1174. http://dx.doi.org/10.1176/appi.ajp.2012.11111721

Nutt, D. J. (2008). Relationship of neurotransmitters to the symptoms of major depressive disorder. *The Journal of Clinical Psychiatry, 69*(Suppl. E1), 4–7.

Ogle, N. R., & Akkerman, S. R. (2013). Guidance for the discontinuation or switching of antidepressant therapies in adults. *Journal of Pharmacy Practice,*

26, 389–396. http://dx.doi.org/10.1177/
0897190012467210

Olfson, M., & Marcus, S. C. (2009). National patterns in antidepressant medication treatment. *Archives of General Psychiatry*, 66, 848–856. http://dx.doi.org/10.1001/archgenpsychiatry.2009.81

Owens, M. J., Morgan, W. N., Plott, S. J., & Nemeroff, C. B. (1997). Neurotransmitter receptor and transporter binding profile of antidepressants and their metabolites. *The Journal of Pharmacology and Experimental Therapeutics*, 283, 1305–1322.

Paulson, J. F., & Bazemore, S. D. (2010). Prenatal and postpartum depression in fathers and its association with maternal depression: A meta-analysis. *JAMA*, 303, 1961–1969. http://dx.doi.org/10.1001/jama.2010.605

Penders, T. M., Stanciu, C. N., Schoemann, A. M., Ninan, P. T., Bloch, R., & Saeed, S. A. (2016). Bright light therapy as augmentation of pharmacotherapy for treatment of depression: A systematic review and meta-analysis. *The Primary Care Companion for CNS Disorders*, 18. http://dx.doi.org/10.4088/PCC.15r01906

Perera, T., George, M. S., Grammer, G., Janicak, P. G., Pascual-Leone, A., & Wirecki, T. S. (2016). The Clinical TMS Society consensus review and treatment recommendations for TMS therapy for major depressive disorder. *Brain Stimulation*, 9, 336–346. http://dx.doi.org/10.1016/j.brs.2016.03.010

Pettinati, H. M. (2004). Antidepressant treatment of co-occurring depression and alcohol dependence. *Biological Psychiatry*, 56, 785–792. http://dx.doi.org/10.1016/j.biopsych.2004.07.016

Pettinati, H. M., O'Brien, C. P., & Dundon, W. D. (2013). Current status of co-occurring mood and substance use disorders: A new therapeutic target. *The American Journal of Psychiatry*, 170, 23–30. http://dx.doi.org/10.1176/appi.ajp.2012.12010112

Pettinati, H. M., Oslin, D. W., Kampman, K. M., Dundon, W. D., Xie, H., Gallis, T. L., . . . O'Brien, C. P. (2010). A double-blind, placebo-controlled trial combining sertraline and naltrexone for treating co-occurring depression and alcohol dependence. *The American Journal of Psychiatry*, 167, 668–675. http://dx.doi.org/10.1176/appi.ajp.2009.08060852

Pincus, S. M., Alam, S., Rubinow, D. R., Bhuvaneswar, C. G., & Schmidt, P. J. (2011). Predicting response to leuprolide of women with premenstrual dysphoric disorder by daily mood rating dynamics. *Journal of Psychiatric Research*, 45, 386–394. http://dx.doi.org/10.1016/j.jpsychires.2010.07.006

Poznanski, E. O., Cook, S. C., & Carroll, B. J. (1979). A depression rating scale for children. *Pediatrics*, 64(4), 442–450.

Quitkin, F. M., Stewart, J. W., McGrath, P. J., Taylor, B. P., Tisminetzky, M. S., Petkova, E., . . . Klein, D. F. (2002). Are there differences between women's and men's antidepressant responses? *The American Journal of Psychiatry*, 159, 1848–1854. http://dx.doi.org/10.1176/appi.ajp.159.11.1848

Raison, C. L., Rutherford, R. E., Woolwine, B. J., Shuo, C., Schettler, P., Drake, D. F., . . . Miller, A. H. (2013). A randomized controlled trial of the tumor necrosis factor antagonist infliximab for treatment-resistant depression: The role of baseline inflammatory biomarkers. *JAMA Psychiatry*, 70, 31–41. http://dx.doi.org/10.1001/2013.jamapsychiatry.4

Robakis, T. K., & Williams, K. E. (2013). Biologically based treatment approaches to the patient with resistant perinatal depression. *Archives of Women's Mental Health*, 16, 343–351. http://dx.doi.org/10.1007/s00737-013-0366-7

Romans, S. E., Tyas, J., Cohen, M. M., & Silverstone, T. (2007). Gender differences in the symptoms of major depressive disorder. *Journal of Nervous and Mental Disease*, 195, 905–911. http://dx.doi.org/10.1097/NMD.0b013e3181594cb7

Rosenblat, J. D., Lee, Y., & McIntyre, R. S. (2017). Does pharmacogenomic testing improve clinical outcomes for major depressive disorder? A systematic review of clinical trials and cost-effectiveness studies. *The Journal of Clinical Psychiatry*, 78, 720–729. http://dx.doi.org/10.4088/JCP.15r10583

*Rush, A. J., Trivedi, M. H., Ibrahim, H. M., Carmody, T. J., Arnow, B., Klein, D. N., . . . Keller, M. B. (2003). The 16-Item Quick Inventory of Depressive Symptomatology (QIDS), clinician rating (QIDS-C), and self-report (QIDS-SR): A psychometric evaluation in patients with chronic major depression. *Biological Psychiatry*, 54, 573–583. http://dx.doi.org/10.1016/S0006-3223(02)01866-8

Rush, A. J., Trivedi, M. H., Wisniewski, S. R., Nierenberg, A. A., Stewart, J. W., Warden, D., . . . Fava, M. (2006). Acute and longer-term outcomes in depressed outpatients requiring one or several treatment steps: A STAR*D report. *The American Journal of Psychiatry*, 163, 1905–1917. http://dx.doi.org/10.1176/ajp.2006.163.11.1905

Seitz, D., Purandare, N., & Conn, D. (2010). Prevalence of psychiatric disorders among older adults in long-term care homes: A systematic review. *International Psychogeriatrics*, 22, 1025–1039. http://dx.doi.org/10.1017/S1041610210000608

Semkovska, M., & McLoughlin, D. M. (2010). Objective cognitive performance associated with electroconvulsive therapy for depression: A systematic review and meta-analysis. *Biological Psychiatry*, 68, 568–577. http://dx.doi.org/10.1016/j.biopsych.2010.06.009

Seyringer, M.-E., & Kasper, S. (2009). Ranking antidepressants. *The Lancet, 373,* 1760–1761. http://dx.doi.org/10.1016/S0140-6736(09)60976-4

Shah, N. R., Jones, J. B., Aperi, J., Shemtov, R., Karne, A., & Borenstein, J. (2008). Selective serotonin reuptake inhibitors for premenstrual syndrome and premenstrual dysphoric disorder: A meta-analysis. *Obstetrics and Gynecology, 111,* 1175–1182. http://dx.doi.org/10.1097/AOG.0b013e31816fd73b

Sharma, A., Barrett, M. S., Cucchiara, A. J., Gooneratne, N. S., & Thase, M. E. (2017). A Breathing-based meditation intervention for patients with major depressive disorder following inadequate response to antidepressants: A randomized pilot study. *The Journal of Clinical Psychiatry, 78,* e59–e63. http://dx.doi.org/10.4088/JCP.16m10819

Sharp, D. J., Chew-Graham, C., Tylee, A., Lewis, G., Howard, L., Anderson, I., . . . Peters, T. J. (2010). A pragmatic randomised controlled trial to compare antidepressants with a community-based psychosocial intervention for the treatment of women with postnatal depression: The RESPOND trial. *Health Technology Assessment, 14,* 1–153. http://dx.doi.org/10.3310/hta14430

Short, B., Fong, J., Galvez, V., Shelker, W., & Loo, C. K. (2018). Side-effects associated with ketamine use in depression: A systematic review. *The Lancet Psychiatry, 5,* 65–78. http://dx.doi.org/10.1016/S2215-0366(17)30272-9

Sienaert, P. (2014). Managing the adverse effects of antidepressants. *Psychiatric Times, 31*(7). Retrieved from http://www.psychiatrictimes.com/special-reports/managing-adverse-effects-antidepressants

Silverstone, P. H., & Salinas, E. (2001). Efficacy of venlafaxine extended release in patients with major depressive disorder and comorbid generalized anxiety disorder. *The Journal of Clinical Psychiatry, 62,* 523–529. http://dx.doi.org/10.4088/JCP.v62n07a04

Simon, G. E., Ludman, E. J., Tutty, S., Operskalski, B., & Von Korff, M. (2004). Telephone psychotherapy and telephone care management for primary care patients starting antidepressant treatment: A randomized controlled trial. *JAMA, 292,* 935–942. http://dx.doi.org/10.1001/jama.292.8.935

Sit, D. K., Perel, J. M., Helsel, J. C., & Wisner, K. L. (2008). Changes in antidepressant metabolism and dosing across pregnancy and early postpartum. *The Journal of Clinical Psychiatry, 69,* 652–658. http://dx.doi.org/10.4088/JCP.v69n0419

Soares, C. N. (2017). Depression and menopause: Current knowledge and clinical recommendations for a critical window. *Psychiatric Clinics of North America, 40,* 239–254. http://dx.doi.org/10.1016/j.psc.2017.01.007

Sockol, L. E., Epperson, C. N., & Barber, J. P. (2011). A meta-analysis of treatments for perinatal depression. *Clinical Psychology Review, 31,* 839–849. http://dx.doi.org/10.1016/j.cpr.2011.03.009

Solomon, D. A., Keller, M. B., Leon, A. C., Mueller, T. I., Lavori, P. W., Shea, M. T., . . . Endicott, J. (2000). Multiple recurrences of major depressive disorder. *The American Journal of Psychiatry, 157,* 229–233. http://dx.doi.org/10.1176/appi.ajp.157.2.229

Song, G.-M., Tian, X., Shuai, T., Yi, L.-J., Zeng, Z., Liu, S., . . . Wang, Y. (2015). Treatment of adults with treatment-resistant depression: Electroconvulsive therapy plus antidepressant or electroconvulsive therapy alone? Evidence from an indirect comparison meta-analysis. *Medicine, 94*(26), e1052. http://dx.doi.org/10.1097/MD.0000000000001052

Souza, L. H., Salum, G. A., Mosqueiro, B. P., Caldieraro, M. A., Guerra, T. A., & Fleck, M. P. (2016). Interpersonal psychotherapy as add-on for treatment-resistant depression: A pragmatic randomized controlled trial. *Journal of Affective Disorders, 193,* 373–380. http://dx.doi.org/10.1016/j.jad.2016.01.004

Steinberg, E. M., Cardoso, G. M. P., Martinez, P. E., Rubinow, D. R., & Schmidt, P. J. (2012). Rapid response to fluoxetine in women with premenstrual dysphoric disorder. *Depression and Anxiety, 29,* 531–540. http://dx.doi.org/10.1002/da.21959

Stockings, E., Degenhardt, L., Lee, Y. Y., Mihalopoulos, C., Liu, A., Hobbs, M., & Patton, G. (2015). Symptom screening scales for detecting major depressive disorder in children and adolescents: A systematic review and meta-analysis of reliability, validity and diagnostic utility. *Journal of Affective Disorders, 174,* 447–463. http://dx.doi.org/10.1016/j.jad.2014.11.061

Targum, S. D. (2014). Identification and treatment of antidepressant tachyphylaxis. *Innovations in Clinical Neuroscience, 11*(3–4), 24–28.

Thase, M. E., Entsuah, R., Cantillon, M., & Kornstein, S. G. (2005). Relative antidepressant efficacy of venlafaxine and SSRIs: Sex-age interactions. *Journal of Women's Health, 14,* 609–616. http://dx.doi.org/10.1089/jwh.2005.14.609

Thase, M. E., Greenhouse, J. B., Frank, E., Reynolds, C. F., III, Pilkonis, P. A., Hurley, K., . . . Kupfer, D. J. (1997). Treatment of major depression with psychotherapy or psychotherapy-pharmacotherapy combinations. *Archives of General Psychiatry, 54,* 1009–1015. http://dx.doi.org/10.1001/archpsyc.1997.01830230043006

Thiels, C., Linden, M., Grieger, F., & Leonard, J. (2005). Gender differences in routine treatment of depressed outpatients with the selective serotonin reuptake inhibitor sertraline. *International Clinical Psychopharmacology, 20,* 1–7. http://dx.doi.org/10.1097/00004850-200501000-00001

Tsai, R., & Schaffir, J. (2010). Effect of depot medroxy-progesterone acetate on postpartum depression. *Contraception, 82*, 174–177. http://dx.doi.org/10.1016/j.contraception.2010.03.004

Tutty, S., Simon, G., & Ludman, E. (2000). Telephone counseling as an adjunct to antidepressant treatment in the primary care system. A pilot study. *Effective Clinical Practice, 3*(4), 170–178.

U.S. Food and Drug Administration. (2014). Consumer updates - FDA: Don't leave childhood depression untreated [Web content]. Retrieved from https://www.fda.gov/forconsumers/consumerupdates/ucm413161.htm

van Calker, D., Zobel, I., Dykierek, P., Deimel, C. M., Kech, S., Lieb, K., . . . Schramm, E. (2009). Time course of response to antidepressants: Predictive value of early improvement and effect of additional psychotherapy. *Journal of Affective Disorders, 114*, 243–253. http://dx.doi.org/10.1016/j.jad.2008.07.023

Wiles, N., Thomas, L., Abel, A., Ridgway, N., Turner, N., Campbell, J., . . . Lewis, G. (2013). Cognitive behavioural therapy as an adjunct to pharmacotherapy for primary care based patients with treatment resistant depression: Results of the CoBalT randomised controlled trial. *The Lancet, 381*, 375–384. http://dx.doi.org/10.1016/S0140-6736(12)61552-9

Williams, J. B. (1988). A structured interview guide for the Hamilton Depression Rating Scale. *Archives of General Psychiatry, 45*, 742–747. http://dx.doi.org/10.1001/archpsyc.1988.01800320058007

Wisner, K. L., Hanusa, B. H., Perel, J. M., Peindl, K. S., Piontek, C. M., Sit, D. K. Y., . . . Moses-Kolko, E. L. (2006). Postpartum depression: A randomized trial of sertraline versus nortriptyline. *Journal of Clinical Psychopharmacology, 26*, 353–360. http://dx.doi.org/10.1097/01.jcp.0000227706.56870.dd

Wisner, K. L., Perel, J. M., Peindl, K. S., Hanusa, B. H., Piontek, C. M., & Findling, R. L. (2004). Prevention of postpartum depression: A pilot randomized clinical trial. *The American Journal of Psychiatry*, 161, 1290–1292. http://dx.doi.org/10.1176/appi.ajp.161.7.1290

World Health Organization. (2004). *ICD–10: International statistical classification of diseases and related health problems* (10th rev., 2nd ed.). Geneva, Switzerland: Author.

Wyatt, K. M., Dimmock, P. W., Ismail, K. M. K., Jones, P. W., & O'Brien, P. M. S. (2004). The effectiveness of GnRHa with and without "add-back" therapy in treating premenstrual syndrome: A meta analysis. *BJOG, 111*, 585–593. http://dx.doi.org/10.1111/j.1471-0528.2004.00135.x

Yonkers, K. A., Lin, H., Howell, H. B., Heath, A. C., & Cohen, L. S. (2008). Pharmacologic treatment of postpartum women with new-onset major depressive disorder: A randomized controlled trial with paroxetine. *The Journal of Clinical Psychiatry, 69*, 659–665. http://dx.doi.org/10.4088/JCP.v69n0420

Yonkers, K. A., & Simoni, M. K. (2018). Premenstrual disorders. *American Journal of Obstetrics and Gynecology, 218*, 68–74. http://dx.doi.org/10.1016/j.ajog.2017.05.045

Yonkers, K. A., Wisner, K. L., Stewart, D. E., Oberlander, T. F., Dell, D. L., Stotland, N., . . . Lockwood, C. (2009). The management of depression during pregnancy: A report from the American Psychiatric Association and the American College of Obstetricians and Gynecologists. *Obstetrics and Gynecology, 114*, 703–713. http://dx.doi.org/10.1097/AOG.0b013e3181ba0632

Young, E. A., Kornstein, S. G., Marcus, S. M., Harvey, A. T., Warden, D., Wisniewski, S. R., . . . John Rush, A. (2009). Sex differences in response to citalopram: A STAR*D report. *Journal of Psychiatric Research, 43*, 503–511. http://dx.doi.org/10.1016/j.jpsychires.2008.07.002

Zhang, R., Li, X., Shi, Y., Shao, Y., Sun, K., Wang, A., . . . Li, Y. (2014). The effects of LPM570065, a novel triple reuptake inhibitor, on extracellular serotonin, dopamine and norepinephrine levels in rats. *PLoS One, 9*, e91775. http://dx.doi.org/10.1371/journal.pone.0091775

CHAPTER 8

PHARMACOLOGICAL TREATMENT OF BIPOLAR DISORDER

Joshua D. Rosenblat and Roger S. McIntyre

Pharmacological interventions are the primary modality of treatment for bipolar disorder (BD). Numerous medications are currently approved in the treatment of BD; however, medication selection must be tailored to the specific patient and illness phase. Careful medication selection and monitoring is required to effectively treat BD, with numerous patient and medication factors to consider when selecting an optimal treatment plan. This chapter provides an overview of currently available pharmacological treatments for BD, along with a discussion of factors that should be considered when initiating and continuing treatment. Additionally, the limitations of current treatments are reviewed, with a brief discussion of future treatments currently under investigation.

EPIDEMIOLOGY AND PREVALENCE

BD is a severe and persistent mental illness associated with significant morbidity and mortality. In the United States, the estimated lifetime prevalence of BD is 4% (Blanco et al., 2017; Kessler et al., 2005). Onset of illness is typically early in life, with initial symptoms often experienced during adolescence (Chengappa et al., 2003). The median age of onset for BD is 25, which is substantially earlier compared with major depressive disorder (MDD; median age of onset is 32; Kessler et al., 2005). From the first onset of initial mood symptoms, BD is character-

ized by a relapsing and remitting course, typically requiring lifelong pharmacological treatment.

Over the past several decades, numerous pharmacological treatments for BD have been identified. As with many treatments in psychiatry, the historical identification and development of treatments for BD primarily emerged through serendipitous discoveries. For BD, essentially all treatments are medications that were initially developed to treat a different disorder that were subsequently repurposed to be used in the treatment of BD. The exclusive use of repurposed medications is somewhat unique to BD compared with other major mental illnesses, as numerous pharmacological treatments have been developed specifically for other psychiatric disorders, such as selective serotonin reuptake inhibitors (SSRIs) for MDD or antipsychotics for schizophrenia. In contrast, as noted, all BD treatments were initially used for other indications. Lithium, anticonvulsants (e.g., valproate, carbamazepine, lamotrigine), and second-generation antipsychotics (SGAs) are currently the primary treatments for BD; however, lithium was first used in the treatment of gout (Shorter, 2009), anticonvulsants for epilepsy, and SGAs for schizophrenia.

The lack of de novo BD treatments speaks to some of the complexity and difficulties of understanding and treating BD. While decades of research have revealed numerous potential contributing mechanisms to the onset and progression of BD, the field

http://dx.doi.org/10.1037/0000133-008
APA Handbook of Psychopharmacology, S. M. Evans (Editor-in-Chief)

still lacks a unifying hypothesis to adequately explain the pathoetiology of BD. The absence of clear hypotheses has limited drug discovery, since BD treatment advances have been forced to rely exclusively on serendipity and repurposing of treatments initially designed for other disorders rather than designing and testing hypothesis-driven interventions.

The current chapter highlights evidence-based pharmacological treatments of BD. The effective use of pharmacological treatments may allow many patients to achieve full remission of symptoms; however, currently available treatments are still associated with high rates of relapse, recurrence, treatment resistance, and poor tolerability. As such, new treatments with improved efficacy and tolerability are still desperately needed. Further, the goal of new treatments should move beyond remission of symptoms and strive for disease-modifying effects that may allow for full recovery and the experience of wellness, rather than only the absence of mood symptoms (Brown, McIntyre, Rosenblat, & Hardeland, 2018).

DIAGNOSING BIPOLAR DISORDER

Similar to other psychiatric disorders, BD is a clinical diagnosis based primarily on a thorough, complete psychiatric assessment. In the *Diagnostic and Statistical Manual of Mental Disorders* (5th edition; *DSM–5*), Bipolar and Related Disorders has now been given its own chapter between the Schizophrenia Spectrum and Other Psychotic Disorders chapter and the Depressive Disorders chapter in recognition that BD is a distinct illness existing on the spectrum between psychotic disorders and unipolar depressive disorders (American Psychiatric Association, 2013). As in the *DSM–IV–TR*, the diagnosis of BD is further subcategorized into bipolar I disorder (BD-I) and bipolar II disorder (BD-II). The diagnosis of BD-I requires the history of at least one manic episode with no requirement of previous major depressive episodes (MDEs). For BD-II, a history of at least one hypomanic episode and one MDE is required (American Psychiatric Association, 2013).

When a patient presents with a current manic or hypomanic episode, the diagnosis of BD is usually clear; however, more commonly, patients will present with a current MDE and an unclear history of potential previous manic or hypomanic episodes. The assessor then has the difficult task of differentiating bipolar from unipolar depression. The correct diagnosis of bipolar versus unipolar depression is of critical importance, as it directly impacts treatment selection along with predicted illness course (Forty et al., 2008). Retrospective studies have shown that patients with BD are frequently initially diagnosed with MDD (i.e., unipolar depression), leading to approximately 70% of BD patients being initially misdiagnosed (Angst et al., 2011; Hirschfeld, Lewis, & Vornik, 2003). Furthermore, one third of patients do not receive the correct diagnosis of BD for more than 10 years after initial symptom onset, leading to a significant delay in the initiation of appropriate evidence-based pharmacological treatments (Hirschfeld et al., 2003).

The misdiagnosis of BD as MDD frequently leads to treatment with a first-line antidepressant (as described in Chapter 7, this volume). Antidepressants pose the immediate risk of a manic switch (i.e., causing a "switch" from an MDE to a manic episode), which may have significant and potentially irreversible medical, financial, social, and occupational consequences (Wehr & Goodwin, 1987). Moreover, even in the absence of a manic switch, the greater concern in the long term is inadequate and inappropriate treatment, as initiation of evidence-based treatment (e.g., mood stabilizers) is delayed. With a missed diagnosis of BD, patients may be trialed on several treatments for MDD and be labelled as treatment refractory, when in reality the lack of symptomatic improvement is secondary to inappropriate treatment (e.g., receiving antidepressants instead of mood stabilizers; Ghaemi, Hsu, Soldani, & Goodwin, 2003).

A thorough evaluation of potential previous hypomanic/manic episodes is paramount for an accurate and timely diagnosis of BD. Delineating an accurate timeline and the quality and severity of manic symptoms through history obtained directly from the patient along with collateral history from people who might have witnessed previous episodes is often helpful for clarifying the diagnosis. Where the history of mania or hypomania is absent or unclear, several clinical characteristics may help predict an increased likelihood of a diagnosis of BD (Forty et al., 2008). Using these clinical characteristics, the International Society for Bipolar Disorders (ISBD) has created a probabilistic model to help predict the risk of BD based on several factors that increase the probability of a diagnosis of bipolar depression, including hypersomnia, hyperphagia, recurrence (i.e., greater than five MDEs), psychotic symptoms, and a family history of BD, as summarized in Table 8.1 (Mitchell, Goodwin, Johnson, & Hirschfeld, 2008).

In addition to a thorough psychiatric assessment, as previously described, the use of several screening and diagnostic tools may aid in the recognition of BD. Validated screening and assessment tools are summarized in Table 8.2. The Mood Disorder Questionnaire (MDQ) is often preferred for clinical use given its validity and brevity. The MDQ is a five minute clinically validated screening tool that is publicly available and has been shown to increase detection rates for both BD-I and BD-II (Hirschfeld et al., 2000). If an assessor lacks confidence or experience in diagnosing BD, a positive MDQ screen would indicate that a referral to a mood disorder specialist is recommended to increase the likelihood of an accurate diagnosis and initiation of appropriate treatment.

EVIDENCE-BASED PHARMACOLOGICAL TREATMENTS OF BIPOLAR DISORDER

Pharmacological therapies are the primary form of treatment in BD, with lifelong pharmacotherapy usually indicated due to the high risk of relapse and recurrence when treatment is discontinued (McIntyre, 2015; Yatham et al., 2013). Pharmacological treatment of BD is unique compared with most other psychiatric disorders, as efficacy and U.S. Food and Drug Administration (FDA) approval is specific to illness phase. As such, BD treatments are specifically approved for the acute treatment of bipolar depressive, manic, or mixed episodes, or for maintenance treatment, as shown in Table 8.3. Of note, many treatments are still commonly and appropriately used during other phases (i.e., prescribed "off-label") in the absence of FDA approval (e.g., lithium or lamotrigine for treatment of bipolar depression).

TABLE 8.1

Proposed Probabilistic Approach to the Diagnosis of Bipolar I Depression in a Person Experiencing a Major Depressive Episode With No Clear Prior Episodes of Mania

The greater likelihood of the diagnosis of bipolar I depression should be considered if >4 of the following features are present[a]	The greater likelihood of the diagnosis of unipolar depression should be considered if >3 of the following features are present[a]
Symptomatology and mental state signs	
▪ Hypersomnia and/or increased daytime napping	▪ Initial insomnia
▪ Hyperphagia and/or increased weight	▪ Appetite and/or weight loss
▪ Other "atypical" depressive symptoms such as "leaden paralysis"	▪ Normal or increased activity levels
▪ Psychomotor retardation	▪ Somatic complaints
▪ Psychotic features and/or pathological guilt	
▪ Lability of mood/manic symptoms	
Course of illness	
▪ Early onset of first depression (<25 years)[a]	▪ Later onset of first depression (>25 years)[a]
▪ Multiple prior episodes of depression (>4 episodes)[a]	▪ Long duration of current episode (>6 months)[a]
Family History	
▪ Positive family history of bipolar disorder	▪ Negative family history of bipolar disorder

Note. From "Diagnostic Guidelines for Bipolar Depression: A Probabilistic Approach," by P. B. Mitchell, G. M. Goodwin, G. F. Johnson, and R. M. Hirschfeld, 2008, *Bipolar Disorders*, *10*, p. 150. Copyright 2008 by Wiley. Reprinted with permission.
[a]Confirmation of the specific numbers to be used requires further study and consideration.

TABLE 8.2

Screening and Diagnostic Tools to Aid in the Recognition of Bipolar Disorder

Tool	Description
Mood Disorder Questionnaire (Hirschfeld et al., 2000)	Clinically validated self-report screening tool for bipolar I disorder and bipolar II disorder
Hypomania Checklist (HCL-32; Altinbas et al., 2014)	Patient self-report that screens for lifetime hypomanic symptoms
Bipolar Depression Rating Scale (Galvão et al., 2013)	Clinician-administered assessment of current symptoms
Mini International Neuropsychiatric Interview (Hergueta & Weiller, 2013)	Patient self-report assessing current manic symptoms
Clinically Useful Depression Outcome Scale with DSM–5 Mixed (Zimmerman, Chelminski, Young, Dalrymple, & Martinez, 2014)	Patient self-report assessing current manic symptoms as part of mixed features

FDA approval based on illness phase (e.g., rather than approving treatments for all phases of BD) occurs because of the substantial differences in efficacy depending on illness phase. For example, numerous agents have been shown to be efficacious in the acute treatment of manic episodes (Yildiz, Nikodem, Vieta, Correll, & Baldessarini, 2015); however, consider-ably fewer agents have demonstrated efficacy in the acute treatment of bipolar depression (Selle, Schalkwijk, Vázquez, & Baldessarini, 2014). With these differences in efficacy depending on illness phase, the treatment of BD is often considered the most complex, with numerous factors and caveats to consider when selecting and optimizing treatment.

TABLE 8.3

FDA-Approved Treatments for Bipolar Disorder

Drug (generic name)	Common trade names	Depression	Mania	Mixed	Maintenance
Lithium	Eskalith®, Lithobid®		X		X
Anticonvulsants					
Valproate	Depakote®, Epival®		X	X	
Carbamazepine	Tegretol®, Carbatrol®		X	X	
Lamotrigine	Lamictal®				X
Antipsychotics/neuroleptics					
Quetiapine[a]	Seroquel®	X	X		X
Lurasidone	Latuda®	X			
Aripiprazole[a]	Abilify®		X	X	X
Risperidone[a]	Risperdal®		X	X	
Ziprasidone	Geodon®, Zeldox®		X	X	
Cariprazine	Vraylar®		X	X	
Olanzapine[a]	Zyprexa®		X	X	X
Olanzapine/fluoxetine combination (OFC)	Symbyax®	X			
Asenapine[a]	Saphris®, Sycrest®		X	X	
Chlorpromazine[a]	Largactil®, Thorazine®		X		

Note. Listed approval is for adults (age 18–65), unless otherwise specified ([a]also approved for adolescents age 13–17). Approval information obtained from http://www.fda.gov, as of October 2017.

The complexity of treatment is further increased as medications that may help to alleviate one pole of symptoms may simultaneously exacerbate symptoms of the opposite mood pole, thus increasing the risk of relapse or recurrence of the opposite mood state. For example, SSRIs and stimulants may sometimes be beneficial in the acute treatment of bipolar depression, however, they carry significant risk of causing a manic switch. Similarly, many effective treatments of mania may lead to depressive symptoms, such as hypersomnia and low energy secondary to the sedating effects of many antimanic agents. Several other factors contribute to the complexity of treating BD, such as high rates of psychiatric and medical comorbidity and the poor tolerability of many BD treatments.

While the treatment of BD is often challenging, an organized and structured approach may allow for effective treatment to alleviate current symptoms and decrease the risk of relapse and recurrence. Towards this end, in this section we will summarize the following: (a) basic principles of BD treatment, (b) descriptions of commonly prescribed mood stabilizers, and (c) an approach to treatment of specific illness phases (i.e., acute treatment of mania and depression and maintenance treatment).

Principles of Pharmacological Treatment

Numerous factors must be considered when selecting pharmacological treatments for BD. The following section reviews these considerations, along with general principles required to effectively and safely treat patients with BD. Both phase-specific efficacy and tolerability must be considered in selecting a treatment. Understanding unique patient and medication factors is also important to find the best treatment for each individual patient.

Considerations for phase-specific efficacy. In medication selection, several factors must be considered, as summarized in Exhibit 8.1. Central to medication selection is consideration of expected efficacy and tolerability. Current symptomatology often largely dictates treatment selection. As shown in Tables 8.4 and 8.5, different mood stabilizers have variable efficacy in the treatment and prevention of major depressive and manic episodes. As such, in an acute mood episode, specifically selecting a mood stabilizer with demonstrated efficacy in that specific mood state is required.

The use of monotherapy (i.e., use of only one medication) should be prioritized when possible to minimize the risk of additional side effects, drug–drug interactions, and increasing costs. However, the use of combination therapies is often required due

---

EXHIBIT 8.1

Key Consideration and Principles in the selection of Pharmacological Treatment for Bipolar Disorder

- Prior to prescribing treatment, a thorough psychiatric assessment is required.
- A medical evaluation with relevant baseline bloodwork is usually indicated.
- Once a diagnosis of *bipolar disorder* has been confirmed, treatment with a mood stabilizer (e.g., lithium, anticonvulsants, or antipsychotics) is indicated, regardless of phase of illness.
- The informed consent discussion should include evaluation of phase-specific efficacy, along with short- and long-term side effect profiles.
- Considerations of medication costs and drug coverage should be part of the informed consent discussion.
- Selection of medications with both demonstrated efficacy in the current phase of illness and favorable tolerability/safety profiles should be prioritized.
- Monotherapy should be used if possible; however, combination therapy may be required when severe symptoms, psychotic features, or treatment resistance is evident.
- Use of metabolically neutral (e.g., no weight gain) treatments should be prioritized.
- Sedating treatments should be dosed once daily at night time, if possible.
- The potential for drug–drug interactions should be considered.
- Simplicity of use (e.g., once daily oral dosing) should be considered.
- Patient preference should be elicited in the medication selection process.
- Lifelong pharmacological treatment is usually required, with few exceptions.
- Use of adjunctive psychosocial interventions should be considered; however, they should only be used in combination with adequate pharmacological treatment.

TABLE 8.4

Overview of Efficacy and Tolerability of Lithium and Anticonvulsants (Based on Evidence and Expert Consensus)

Drug	Efficacy in mania		Efficacy in depression		Notable safety/tolerability concerns*
	Acute	Relapse prevention	Acute	Relapse prevention	
Lithium	+++	+++	++	++	Renal, thyroid, metabolic
Divalproex	+++	++	+	+/–	Bone marrow suppression, metabolic, PCOS, teratogenicity
Carbamazepine	++	++	+	+	Blood marrow suppression, sedation, teratogenicity
Oxcarbazepine	+	+	+/–	+/–	Sedation
Lamotrigine	+/–	+/–	++	++	Risk of severe rash
Topiramate	–	–	+	+	Cognitive dysfunction
Gabapentin	–	–	–	–	Sedation

Note. For efficacy during specified illness phase: +++ = highly efficacious, ++ = moderately efficacious, + = mildly efficacious, +/– = minimal or unclear efficacy, – = evidence for lack of efficacy. PCOS = polycystic ovarian syndrome. *Not a complete list of side effects, only highlighting key concerns. "Metabolic" refers generally to all metabolic effects (e.g., weight gain, dyslipidemia, insulin resistance).

TABLE 8.5

Overview of Efficacy and Tolerability of Antipsychotic Efficacy (Including Only Select Agents Commonly Used in North America)

Drug	Efficacy in mania		Efficacy in depression		Notable safety/tolerability concerns*
	Acute	Relapse prevention	Acute	Relapse prevention	
First-generation antipsychotics					
Haloperidol**	+++	++	+	+/–	Parkinsonism
Chlorpromazine	++	+	+/–	+/–	Parkinsonism, sedation
Second-generation antipsychotics					
Quetiapine	+++	+++	+++	+++	Sedation, metabolic
Olanzapine	+++	+++	+	+	Sedation, metabolic
Clozapine	++	++	+	+	Sedation, metabolic, myocarditis, agranulocytosis, seizures
Risperidone**	+++	+++	+	+	Parkinsonism
Paliperidone**a	+++	+++	+	+	Parkinsonism
Lurasidone	+	+	+++	++	Akathisia
Asenapine	++	++	+/–	+	Sedation
Ziprasidone	++	+	–	+/–	Akathisia, QTc prolongation
Partial dopamine agonists					
Aripiprazole**	++	+	+/–	+	Akathisia
Cariprazine	++	+	+	+/–	Akathisia
Brexipiprazole	+/–	+/–	+/–	+/–	Akathisia

Note. For efficacy during specified illness phase: +++ = highly efficacious, ++ = moderately efficacious, + = mildly efficacious, +/– = minimal or unclear efficacy, – = evidence for lack of efficacy. QTc = corrected QT interval. *Not a complete list of side effects, only highlighting key concerns. "Metabolic" refers generally to all metabolic effects (e.g., weight gain, dyslipidemia, insulin resistance). **Also available as long-acting depot injection. aSuggested efficacy for paliperidone largely extrapolated from risperidone data.

to the high rates of relapse and treatment resistance with monotherapies. Combination therapies should be considered within the context of severe symptoms, treatment resistance, and/or psychotic features. For example, with a severe manic episode with psychotic features, the use of dual therapy with an antipsychotic plus a conventional mood stabilizer (e.g., lithium or anticonvulsant) is usually indicated. Clinical trials have focused on combining SGAs with lithium or divalproex, and as such are the most evidence-based and commonly used combinations (Parker, Graham, & Tavella, 2017). Table 8.6 summarizes specific common and efficacious combinations used for the acute treatment of mania and depression along with combinations used for maintenance therapy.

Considerations for tolerability and safety. The importance of considering tolerability and safety has been increasingly emphasized by both patients

---

TABLE 8.6

Common Effective Combinations Used During Specific Illness Phases of Bipolar Disorder

Illness phase	Combinations
Mania	Lithium + antipsychotic (quetiapine, risperidone, olanzapine, aripiprazole, asenapine)
	Divalproex + antipsychotic (quetiapine, risperidone, olanzapine, aripiprazole, asenapine)
	Lithium + divalproex
Depression	Lurasidone + lithium
	Lurasidone + divalproex
	Olanzapine + fluoxetine* (available in combination pill)
	Quetiapine + SSRI* (except paroxetine)
	Lithium + lamotrigine
	Lithium + antidepressant* (bupropion or SSRIs, except paroxetine)
Euthymia (maintenance)	Lithium + antipsychotic (quetiapine, risperidone, olanzapine, aripiprazole, ziprasidone, lurasidone)
	Divalproex +antipsychotic (quetiapine, risperidone, olanzapine, aripiprazole, ziprasidone, lurasidone)
	Lithium + lamotrigine

Note. *Avoid use of antidepressant with mixed features or history of rapid cycling or propensity for manic/hypomanic episodes.

and clinicians (McIntyre, 2015). In the short term, poor tolerability may lead to early treatment discontinuation and a potential rupture in the therapeutic alliance with the treatment provider. Further, for patients who continue poorly tolerated treatment, given that treatment is usually lifelong, the significant side effects of many BD treatments may lead to significant long-term medical sequelae. Most notably, several treatments are associated with significant metabolic side effects, leading to features of metabolic syndrome, such as significant weight gain, dyslipidemia, insulin resistance, and resultant cardiovascular disease (Solmi et al., 2017). As such, treatment guidelines now emphasize the importance of prioritizing metabolically neutral agents (Parker et al., 2017). Figure 8.1 illustrates the relative metabolic effects of various mood stabilizers. If metabolic changes are observed, switching to a more metabolically neutral agent should be considered in conjunction with evaluating the risk of relapse with a switch in treatment (Kemp, 2014).

Common and problematic side effects also include excessive sedation and risk of extrapyramidal symptoms (EPS). Table 8.7 summarizes the variable effects of various mood stabilizing treatments on wakefulness. Notably, individual patients may have different reactions and report experiencing sedative effects with any mood stabilizing agent. As such, a thorough inquiry of potential side effects, especially the impact on sleep and wakefulness, should be assessed for every patient individually and treatment timing tailored accordingly (e.g., sedating medications taken at night). For antipsychotics, EPS is another common side effect with variable prevalence (e.g., common with risperidone, rare with quetiapine) and quality (e.g., parkinsonism with risperidone, akathisia with aripiprazole) depending on agent. Relative rates and characteristics of EPS are further reviewed in Chapter 10, this volume.

Taken together, as summarized in Exhibit 8.1, several factors should be considered when selecting a treatment for BD. Current symptom profile, severity of symptoms, history of response (including personal and family history of response), treatment resistance, and side effect profiles should be considered.

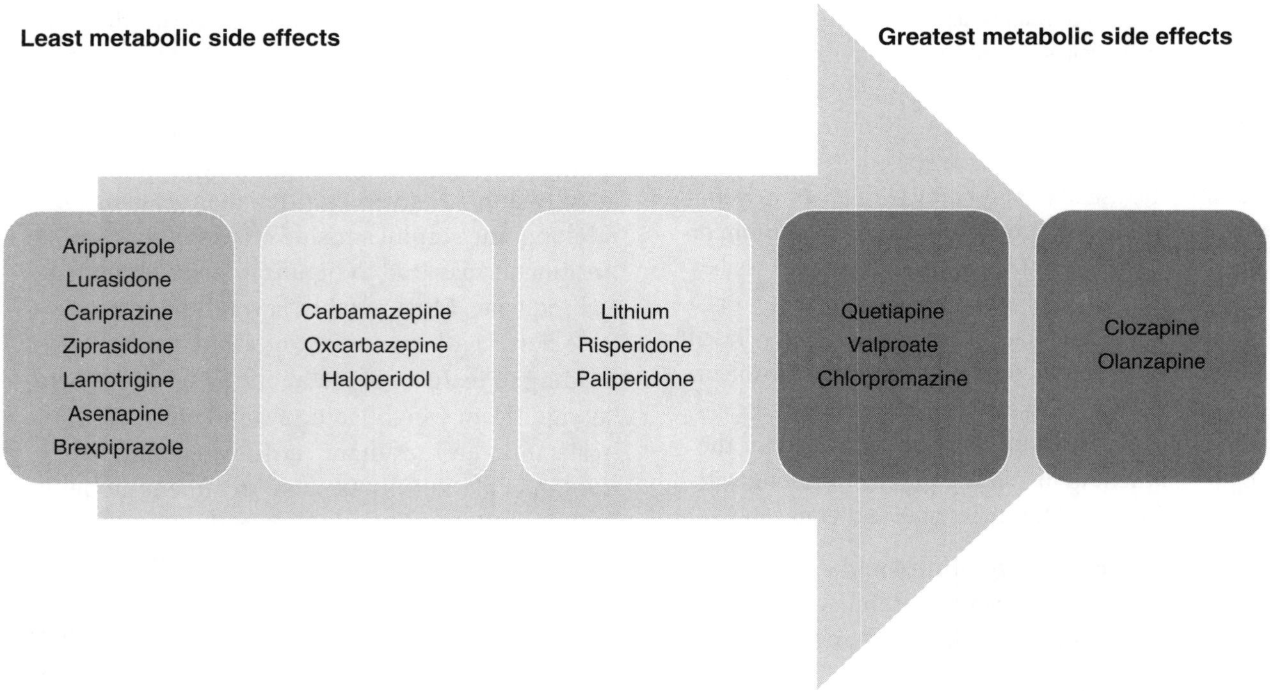

Least metabolic side effects

Greatest metabolic side effects

| Aripiprazole
Lurasidone
Cariprazine
Ziprasidone
Lamotrigine
Asenapine
Brexpiprazole | Carbamazepine
Oxcarbazepine
Haloperidol | Lithium
Risperidone
Paliperidone | Quetiapine
Valproate
Chlorpromazine | Clozapine
Olanzapine |

FIGURE 8.1. Relative metabolic effects of mood stabilizing treatments.

Summary of Select Mood Stabilizing Agents: Mechanisms of Action, Efficacy, and Tolerability

As previously described, there is no "anti-BD" medication, but rather, various classes of medications that have been repurposed to target BD symptoms, with variable efficacy depending on illness phase. The following section summarizes the mechanism of action, efficacy and tolerability of lithium, anticonvulsants, antipsychotics and

antidepressants. Notably, the mechanism of action leading to mood stabilizing effects remains largely unknown for several of these medications.

Lithium.   Lithium is known as the "classic mood stabilizer" and has been routinely used in the treatment of BD for more than 50 years (Shorter, 2009). As one of the oldest treatments for BD, lithium remains a key treatment option during all phases of illness. The definitive mechanism of action remains unclear; however, several plausible hypotheses have emerged. The most studied targets of lithium are signal transduction sites beyond neurotransmitter receptors. Lithium has been shown to inhibit messenger enzymes, such as inositol monophosphate, glycogen synthase kinase 3 (GSK-3), and protein kinase C (PKC), along with modulating G proteins (Jope, 1999). The net effect of these molecular changes is the alteration of neuronal signaling cascades to promote neuroprotection and neuroplasticity, which may facilitate the mood stabilizing effects of lithium (Malhi, Tanious, Das, Coulston, & Berk, 2013). An additional hypothesis that has emerged is that the immunomodulatory effects of lithium may play a significant role (Horrobin &

TABLE 8.7

Sedating Effects of Mood Stabilizing Agents

Sedating	Sleep-wake neutral	Wake-promoting
Clozapine	Lamotrigine	Aripiprazole
Olanzapine	Risperidone	Cariprazine
Quetiapine	Paliperidone	Brexpiprazole
Asenapine	Ziprasidone	
Chlorpromazine	Lurasidone	
Valproate	Haloperidol	
Lithium		
Carbamazepine		
Oxcarbazepine		

Lieb, 1981). Replicated evidence has demonstrated a clear role of immune dysfunction in the pathophysiology of BD (Rosenblat & McIntyre, 2017a). As such, the immunomodulatory effect of lithium has been suggested to be another potential mechanism of action facilitating lithium's mood stabilizing effects.

Regardless of the mechanism of action, replicated evidence has demonstrated a robust antimanic effect with lithium (Storosum et al., 2007). Lithium has also been shown to have antidepressant effects (in BD and MDD) and to be highly efficacious in the prevention of future manic episodes, and, to a lesser extent, depressive episodes (Young & Newham, 2006). Further, lithium has been shown to have a mood-independent (in BD and other disorders) antisuicide effect and continues to be one of the only medications proven to decrease suicide rates (Cipriani, Hawton, Stockton, & Geddes, 2013). Lithium may be effectively used as a monotherapy during any illness phase or in combination with most antipsychotics, valproate, or lamotrigine.

Despite the ample evidence of numerous benefits of prescribing lithium in BD, the use of lithium has significantly decreased in the United States as the use of SGAs has become more popular in the treatment of BD (Pillarella, Higashi, Alexander, & Conti, 2012). This change in prescribing patterns is likely partly related to the perceived simplicity in prescribing SGAs versus the anticipated complexity of prescribing lithium. Indeed, there is added complexity in prescribing lithium as serum levels of the drug, along with thyroid and renal function, must be monitored regularly (Ng et al., 2009). The rare but potentially lethal risk of lithium toxicity may also discourage prescribers from using lithium (McKnight et al., 2012). However, with adequate monitoring, side effects and toxicity (as summarized in Exhibit 8.2) may be detected early and treated appropriately, making lithium a safe and often well tolerated treatment option. Of note, SGAs also require regular monitoring and carry significant risk for metabolic effects (Ng et al., 2009). As such, lithium use should not be avoided simply based on perceived complexity of prescribing and monitoring compared with SGAs. Rather, lithium should be more frequently considered in the treatment of BD.

EXHIBIT 8.2

LITHIVM Mnemonic for Side Effects and Signs of Lithium Toxicity

---

Leukocytosis/**L**ethargy
Insipidus (nephrogenic diabetes insipidus)
Tremor/**T**eratogenicity (Ebstein's anomaly)
Hypothyroidism/**H**yperparathyroidism
Increased weight
Vomiting
Metallic taste/**M**yocardial (ECG changes)

Note. ECG = electrocardiogram.

Anticonvulsants. Along with lithium, anticonvulsants are also considered conventional mood stabilizers. Anticonvulsants were initially repurposed for the treatment of mania given the theoretical parallels between seizures and manic episodes. The phenomenon of *kindling* has been proposed in both epilepsy and BD, as seizures and mood episodes respectively have a kindling effect in that every episode or seizure leads to neurobiological changes that increase the risk of future occurrences (Berk et al., 2017). Additionally, both mania and seizures are associated with inappropriately overactive neural circuits (i.e., imbalance between activating glutamate signaling and inhibitory gamma-aminobutyric acid [GABA] signaling). Valproate and carbamazepine were among the first anticonvulsants assessed for the acute treatment of mania and both proved to be efficacious antimanic treatments (Yildiz et al., 2015). A potential class effect was initially assumed, leading to clinical trials assessing the antimanic effects of numerous other anticonvulsants (e.g., pregabalin, gabapentin, levetiracetam, topiramate, oxcarbazepine). These yielded mostly disappointing results, with valproate and carbamazepine being the only anticonvulsants to demonstrate a consistent antimanic effect (Grunze, 2010). Given this variability in efficacy, the anticonvulsant effect in itself is unlikely to be the only or primary mechanism of action for the antimanic effects of valproate and carbamazepine. Similar to lithium, the mechanism of action remains unclear, with several unproven hypotheses.

Divalproex (the long-acting formulation of valproate recommended for BD) is the most commonly used anticonvulsant in BD. Proposed mechanisms of action include inhibiting neuronal sodium channels, increasing the action of GABA, and modulating downstream signaling cascades (i.e., similar to lithium's effect on second messenger systems; Williams, Cheng, Mudge, & Harwood, 2002). Divalproex has robust evidence for use in the acute treatment of mania, in which it may be used as a monotherapy or in combination with an SGA or lithium (Yildiz et al., 2015). Divalproex also has evidence to support use during maintenance therapy; however, divalproex has a greater effect in preventing future manic episodes with less of an effect in preventing depressive episodes (Vieta et al., 2011). Notably, divalproex has minimal efficacy in the acute treatment of bipolar depression. Similar to lithium, the use of divalproex has decreased as the use of SGAs has become more popular. Divalproex also requires monitoring of serum levels, blood counts, and liver function, and for metabolic side effects (Figure 8.2; Ng et al., 2009). From a safety and tolerability perspective, the greatest concerns with divalproex are the risk for polycystic ovarian syndrome (PCOS), weight gain, and teratogenicity (i.e., risk of fetal neural tube defects if taken during pregnancy). The recommended and most well tolerated formulation of valproate is the long-acting formulation, divalproex, which should be used preferentially instead of other formulations (e.g., valproic acid) when possible (Yatham et al., 2013).

Carbamazepine was the first anticonvulsant shown to have an antimanic effect; however, it is currently used less frequently compared with divalproex, given differences in efficacy and tolerability. Similar to divalproex, efficacy has primarily been established for the acute treatment of mania along with prevention of future manic episodes, and to a lesser extent, prevention of depressive episodes (Vieta et al., 2011). Significant safety concerns for carbamazepine include risk of bone marrow suppression leading to hematological complications, hepatic dysfunction, and risk of severe rash (i.e., Stevens–Johnson syndrome). Of note, the dosing of carbamazepine may also be challenging as it autoinduces CYP450 3A4, the primary enzyme responsible for its own metabolism. As such, serum levels may decrease even if the dose is unchanged.

Regular monitoring of serum levels is thus required, as shown in Figure 8.5.

The mechanism of action of carbamazepine also remains unclear; the mechanism is likely related to modulating sodium channels, but in a different manner compared with divalproex (Williams et al., 2002). Oxcarbazepine and eslicarbazepine likely have similar mechanisms of action with less safety concerns; however, the efficacy of these alternative mood stabilizers has yet to be adequately demonstrated in BD (Popova, Leighton, Bernabarre, Bernardo, & Vieta, 2007).

Lamotrigine is another commonly prescribed anticonvulsant in BD; however, in contrast to other anticonvulsants, lamotrigine is primarily prescribed for the treatment and prevention of depressive episodes, with limited benefit in the treatment and prevention of manic episodes (Amann, Born, Crespo, Pomarol-Clotet, & McKenna, 2011). Lamotrigine is generally well tolerated with minimal propensity for metabolic effects. The main side effect of concern is the risk of a severe drug rash (e.g., Stevens–Johnson syndrome). To minimize the risk of developing this severe rash, a slow titration (e.g., 6 weeks to reach a therapeutic dose) with regular monitoring for rashes is required. With this necessary slow titration, lamotrigine requires weeks to months before showing antidepressant effects (Amann et al., 2011). The delayed effect is also one of the reasons lamotrigine is only FDA approved for maintenance treatment, although it is commonly and appropriately prescribed for bipolar depressive episodes with adequate patient counseling about the delayed antidepressant effects. For patients with a propensity to have recurrent manic or hypomanic episodes, mixed features, or rapid cycling, lamotrigine should be combined with a treatment with good efficacy in the prevention of manic episodes, such as lithium or an SGA. The combination of lamotrigine with divalproex should be avoided, as there is a significant drug–drug interaction that increases the risk of a severe rash as lamotrigine levels are increased. As such, lamotrigine dosages should be decreased by half during the titration (e.g., starting with 12.5 mg instead of 25 mg) if coprescribing divalproex.

Antipsychotics. Soon after the effects of antipsychotics were discovered for the treatment of schizophrenia, antipsychotics were utilized in the

Level 1A Established efficacy:

Mild to moderate severity and/or not requiring hospitalization
- ✦ Optimize mood stabilizer (lithium*, divalproex*, or carbamazepine*) if already prescribed. Check blood levels if appropriate.
- ✦ Lithium* monotherapy
- ✦ Monotherapy with aripiprazole, asenapine, divalproex*, quetiapine, risperidone, ziprasidone, or cariprazine.

Severe and/or requiring hospitalization
- ✦ Lithium* or divalproex* + aripiprazole, asenapine, quetiapine, or risperidone
- ✦ Electroconvulsive therapy (ECT) is recommended if medical emergency/patient welfare at risk and pharmacotherapy is insufficient.

Level 1B Established efficacy, but with safety concerns:**

Mild to moderate severity and/or not requiring hospitalization
- ✦ Monotherapy with either haloperidol or olanzapine

Severe and/or requiring hospitalization
- ✦ Lithium* or divalproex* + either haloperidol or olanzapine

 Level 2   If Levels 1A and 1B are ineffective and/or not well tolerated:
- ✦ Combination treatment with lithium* + divalproex*
- ✦ Combination with lithium* and/or divalproex* + second generation antipsychotic (SGA) other than clozapine
- ✦ Carbamazepine* monotherapy

 Level 3   If Levels 1 and 2 are ineffective and/or not well tolerated:
- ✦ Electroconvulsive therapy (ECT)
- ✦ Clozapine + lithium* or divalproex*
- ✦ Lithium* + carbamazepine*
- ✦ Divalproex* + carbamazepine*

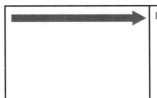 **Level 4   If Levels 1–3 are ineffective and/or not well tolerated:**
- ✦ A three-drug combination of Level 1, 2, and 3. Drugs may include first generation antipsychotic (FGA) or second generation antipsychotic (SGA) but **NOT TWO** antipsychotic medications.

  Example: lithium* + (divalproex* or carbamazepine*) + antipsychotic

Notes:

*Caution should be used when prescribing lithium, lamotrigine, divalproex or carbamazepine to women of reproductive age due to increased risks to the fetus with use during pregnancy, including neural tube and other major birth defects. Please see Florida Best Practice Recommendations for Women of Reproductive Age with Serious Mental Illness and Comorbid Substance Use Disorders and online guideline on the Pharmacological Treatment of Mood Disorders During Pregnancy.

**Side-effect concerns with these agents include weight gain, metabolic syndrome, and extrapyramidal symptoms (EPS). Side-effects warrant vigilance and close monitoring on the part of the clinicians.

Data for use of paliperidone to treat bipolar mania are mixed. Paliperidone >6 mg has some data supporting efficacy.

Benzodiazepines may be used as an adjunct treatment for acute treatment of bipolar mania.

FIGURE 8.2.   Algorithm for treatment of mania and hypomania based on Florida Medicaid guidelines. From "2017–2018 Florida Best Practice Psychotherapeutic Medication Guidelines for Adults," by R. S. McIntyre, 2018, pp. 16–17 (http://www. medicaidmentalhealth.org/_assets/file/Guidelines/2018-Psychotherapeutic%20 Medication%20Guidelines%20for%20Adults%20with%20References.pdf). Copyright 2018 by the USF Medicaid Drug Therapy Management Program for Behavioral Health. Reprinted with permission.

acute treatment of mania, particularly when psychotic features were present. Early on, antipsychotics were found to be helpful in the acute treatment of mania with quick effects, as monotherapy or in combination with a conventional mood stabilizer (e.g., lithium or anticonvulsant). As with schizophrenia, currently the use of SGAs is predominant, with first-generation antipsychotics infrequently prescribed given the risk of tardive dyskinesia with long-term use. Details about mechanism of action and side effect profiles are further discussed in Chapter 10, this volume.

For the acute treatment of mania, it is likely that all antipsychotics have an effect; as shown in Table 8.3, almost all are FDA indicated for the acute treatment of manic and mixed episodes. A comparative network meta-analysis comparing the antimanic effects of all treatments found the following order of efficacy of antimanic antipsychotics (from most efficacious to least, with all antipsychotics being more effective compared with placebo): haloperidol, risperidone, olanzapine, aripiprazole, quetiapine, asenapine, and ziprasidone (Yildiz et al., 2015). Given that all antipsychotics appear to be effective antimanic treatments, focusing on short- and long-term tolerability is a key factor in deciding treatment selection.

For the acute treatment of bipolar depression, only lurasidone, quetiapine, and olanzapine–fluoxetine combination pill (OFC) are FDA approved with evidence for efficacy. Of these three SGAs, lurasidone may be preferentially selected given that quetiapine and OFC have significant metabolic effects and sedation. Quetiapine is the only agent with evidence for efficacy in the acute treatment of BD-II depression. It is possible that other SGAs may be effective (for both BD-I or BD-II depression), but bipolar depression is very understudied, with evidence limited to these three agents.

For maintenance treatment, it is likely that all antipsychotics have an effect for relapse prevention of mania and, to a lesser extent, depression; however, only quetiapine, aripiprazole, and olanzapine are FDA-approved maintenance treatments. If an antipsychotic is being used as a monotherapy for maintenance, it will likely need to be continued; however, if it is being used adjunctively with a conventional mood stabilizer, a careful assessment of why the antipsychotic was initiated is required. When used adjunctively, given the potential long-term effects of antipsychotic use, discontinuation of the antipsychotic a year after the most recent mood episode should be considered. However, if the patient's condition is brittle, with a known history of treatment resistance and frequent relapses, continuing the combination therapy indefinitely may be indicated due to the elevated risk of destabilization when discontinuing the antipsychotic.

Antidepressants. The use of antidepressants in BD continues to be controversial. Antidepressants may trigger or worsen manic symptoms (Altshuler et al., 1995). As such, during an acute manic or hypomanic episode or when mixed features are present, all antidepressants should be discontinued (McIntyre, 2015). Further, in patients with a history of antidepressant treatment-emergent manic switches, antidepressants should be avoided. Similarly, if a patient has rapid cycling or a propensity for manic or hypomanic episodes, antidepressants should be avoided.

The use of antidepressants should be limited to the acute treatment of bipolar depression, with a greater role likely in BD-II compared with BD-I (Altshuler et al., 2017; Yatham et al., 2013). When using antidepressants in BD, two specific concerns arise: (a) the risk of a potential manic switch (Viktorin et al., 2014) and (b) the risk of inefficacy (Ostacher, Tandon, & Suppes, 2016). Most prescribers are more hypervigilant about the first risk (i.e., causing a manic episode, a manic switch), but the risk of inefficacy is of greater long-term concern, especially with antidepressant monotherapy. Mood stabilizers have greater effect for the acute treatment of bipolar depression as well as for relapse prevention. As such, if a patient is being treated instead with antidepressant monotherapy, they are not receiving the most evidence-based treatment, thus potentially delaying remission and recovery (Pacchiarotti et al., 2013). Taken together, antidepressants should not be used first line, but they may have a role for augmenting mood stabilizers when an inadequate response is found with evidence-based mood stabilizer treatments. Indeed, while their use remains controversial, replicated evidence has shown antidepressant effects of adjunctive antidepressants in the acute treatment of bipolar depression (Liu et al., 2017).

Patients with BD-II, low propensity for manic/hypomanic episodes, or previous history of response to antidepressants may be more likely to benefit from antidepressant treatment (Pacchiarotti et al., 2013). Antidepressant monotherapy should be discouraged. In general, tricyclics and tetracyclics, along with SSRIs and norepinephrine inhibitors (SNRIs), have elevated risk of manic switches and should be avoided (Salvi, Fagiolini, Swartz, Maina, & Frank, 2008). Bupropion and SSRIs (except for paroxetine) have evidence to support an antidepressant effect in BD and are likely have the best risk–benefit profile of the antidepressants (McInerney & Kennedy, 2014).

While not an approved treatment for MDD or BD, modafinil is indicated for improving wakefulness in patients with excessive sleepiness, a symptom that is common and functionally impairing in bipolar depression. Further, adjunctive modafinil treatment was demonstrated in one randomized controlled trial (RCT) to have an acute antidepressant effect in participants with bipolar depression that were resistant to mood stabilizers (Frye et al., 2007). Additionally, adjunctive modafinil was not associated with increased risk of mania compared with the adjunctive placebo group. As such, modafinil presents an additional option in the treatment of bipolar depression.

Algorithm for Treatment of Bipolar Disorder

In the following section, we describe current evidence-based recommendations for the treatment of BD during its various illness phases. Of note, the most recent American Psychiatric Association guidelines for the treatment of BD were published in 2002 (American Psychiatric Association, 2002). Since 2002, a large number of BD clinical trials have been conducted. Thus, the current recommendations are in accordance with the 2017–2018 Florida Best Practice Psychotherapeutic Medication Guidelines for Adults (Florida Medicaid guidelines; University of South Florida, Florida Medicaid Drug Therapy Management Program, 2018), which have integrated the results from more recent clinical trials.

These guidelines may differ from other treatment guidelines, as a greater emphasis has been placed on balancing efficacy with tolerability. As such, certain treatments that have robust evidence of efficacy may be lower in the treatment algorithm (as compared with previous treatment guidelines) because of concerns around tolerability and safety (Parker et al., 2017). Readers are encouraged to compare and contrast other recent international BD treatment guidelines (references provided in the Tool Kit of Resources at the end of this chapter). However, for clarity, only the Florida Medicaid guidelines for the pharmacological treatment of BD are summarized here. The following flow diagrams focus on pharmacological interventions. Prior to initiating any pharmacological interventions, all the factors involved in treatment selection summarized previously (Exhibit 8.1) should be considered. Additionally, the use of measurement-based care using validated scales, as summarized in Table 8.8, is merited to more accurately evaluate treatment response. The primary goals of BD treatment are remission, maintenance of remission, prevention of relapse/recurrence, and full functional recovery while experiencing good medication tolerability. Selection of acute treatment should take maintenance treatment goals into account.

During the acute treatment of mania or hypomania, the algorithm in Figure 8.2 may be followed. In addition to starting an evidence-based antimanic

---

TABLE 8.8

Validated Measures to Evaluate Treatment Response in Bipolar Disorder

Scales evaluating manic symptoms	Scales evaluating depressive symptoms
Young Mania Rating Scale	Beck Depression Inventory
Bech-Rafaelsen Mania Rating Scale	Hamilton Rating Scale for Depression
Altman Self-Rating Mania Scale	Montgomery-Åsberg Depression Rating Scale
Self-Report Manic Inventory	Patient Health Questionnaire (PHQ-9)
	Quick Inventory of Depression Symptomatology

agent as described in that algorithm, all anti-depressants and stimulants should be discontinued as these agents may worsen symptoms of mania or hypomania. Of note, there is no separate section included on the treatment of hypomania due to limited availability of data. As such, treatment of hypomania should be extrapolated from evidence and guidelines for treatment of mania. The algorithm for the acute treatment of bipolar depression and for maintenance treatment are summarized in Figure 8.3 and Figure 8.4, respectively.

In addition to diagnosing current illness phase, the *DSM–5* allows for the specification of the presence of specific features (American Psychiatric Association, 2013). In BD, the most important features that directly impact treatment selection are *mixed features*, *psychotic features* and, to a lesser extent, *anxious distress*. If psychotic features are present during any phase of illness, the addition of an SGA is indicated (i.e., during depression or mania with psychotic features). Compared with psychotic features, the treatment of mixed features remains less clear, as the *DSM–IV–TR* definition of mixed states was changed in 2013 with the publication of the *DSM–5*, thus limiting the number of studies conducted with *DSM–5*-defined mixed features (Rosenblat & McIntyre, 2017b). As such, treatment of mixed features in BD is based on (a) the relatively few completed studies using *DSM–5*-defined mixed features, (b) extrapolation of results from studies assessing treatments of *DSM–IV–TR*-defined mixed episodes, and (c) expert opinion (Grunze et al., 2018; Stahl et al., 2017).

Integrating these three sources of data, consensus guidelines on the treatment of mood episodes with mixed features were recently published (Stahl et al., 2017). When mixed features are identified, anti-depressants and stimulants should be discontinued as they may worsen symptoms of mania. Recommended treatments of mixed states include agents that may simultaneously improve symptoms of depression and mania. Mixed states comprised of syndromal mania and subsyndromal depression are best treated with SGAs (e.g., asenapine, cariprazine, quetiapine) and mixed states comprised of syndromal depression and subsyndromal hypomania are best treated specifically with lurasidone or quetiapine. Divalproex is an additional alternative if SGAs provide inadequate control of symptoms; however, divalproex's anti-depressant effects are less robust and therefore may be less helpful to simultaneously treat both mood poles. Short-term use of benzodiazepines or hypnotics may also be of benefit if decreased sleep, irritability, or agitation is present. Notably, when mixed features are identified, patients should be monitored closely, as mixed states are associated with increased risk of suicidality and other risky behaviors (Seo, Wang, Jun, Woo, & Bahk, 2016).

BEST APPROACHES FOR ASSESSING TREATMENT RESPONSE AND MANAGING SIDE EFFECTS

When initiating any of the previously described treatments, a systematic approach to assessing treatment response and side effects is imperative to providing optimal care. Measurement-based care using validated scales is required to accurately evaluate treatment response (Fortney et al., 2017). Validated scales are summarized in Table 8.8. Baseline symptoms severity of both manic and depressive symptoms should be evaluated along with reassessment of symptom severity at each visit. Given the high prevalence of mixed features, evaluating symptoms of both mania and depression at each visit is required, even when treatment is currently targeted at alleviating symptoms of one mood pole. As smart phone technology develops, it may allow for the potential use of daily symptom monitoring to aid in evaluation of treatment response and side effects (Grünerbl et al., 2015).

As with the evaluation of treatment response, a systematic approach to the evaluation of treatment emergent side effects is indicated, as summarized in Figure 8.5 (Ng et al., 2009). Mild, tolerable side effects emerging early in the course of treatment (e.g., mild gastrointestinal side effects, mild headache) may provide reassurance, and treatment should be continued as many of these side effects may spontaneously subside after the first few days to weeks of treatment. If significant or intolerable treatment emergent side effects are identified (e.g., severe rash, significant weight gain, dyslipidemia, insulin resistance), discontinuation of the likely offending agent may be required, balancing the need

Level 1 **Established efficacy:**

✦ Optimize index mood stabilizer if already prescribed a mood stabilizer. Check blood levels if appropriate.

✦ Quetiapine or lurasidone monotherapy*

Notes: Only quetiapine has established efficacy for bipolar II disorder. Lurasidone has a better metabolic profile than quetiapine.

✦ Lamotrigine monotherapy

✦ Lurasidone or lamotrigine** adjunctive to lithium or divalproex if index mood stabilizer has been optimized.

**Caution:* There is a drug-drug interaction with use of lamotrigine and divalproex together that requires reducing the lamotrigine dose by 50% of the typical lamotrigine dose.

✦ Do not utilize conventional antidepressants (e.g., SSRIs, SNRIs, TCAs, MAOIs) as a first-line therapy.

Level 2A **Established efficacy, but with safety concerns*:**

✦ Olanzapine + fluoxetine (bipolar I disorder)

Note: Tolerability limitations include weight gain and metabolic concerns.

Level 2B **Better tolerability, but limited efficacy*:**

✦ Lithium (bipolar 1 disorder)

✦ 2 drug combination of above medications. Drugs may include either a first generation antipsychotic (FGA) or second generation antipsychotic (SGA) but **NOT TWO** antipsychotic medications

Note: Efficacy limitations, relatively few positive randomized controlled trials.

Level 3 **If Levels 1 and 2 are ineffective and/or not well tolerated*:**

✦ Electroconvulsive therapy (ECT)

Note: Consideration is merited due to clinical need, despite even greater efficacy/tolerability limitations than Level 1 and 2 treatments.

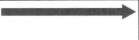

Level 4 **If Levels 1–3 are ineffective and/or not well tolerated:**

✦ Cariprazine

✦ FDA-approved agent for bipolar disorder + conventional antidepressant (e.g., SSRI)*

✦ Pramipexole

✦ Adjunctive: modafinil, thyroid hormone (T3), or stimulants

✦ 3 drug combination

✦ Transcranial magnetic stimulation (TMS)

Notes:

▪ There is inadequate information (including negative trials) to recommend adjunctive antidepressants, aripiprazole, ziprasidone, levetiracetam, armodafinil, or omega-3 fatty acids for bipolar depression.

▪ Preliminary evidence is available for cariprazine in the treatment for bipolar I depression.

▪ Antidepressant monotherapy is not recommended in bipolar I depression; recommendation is for adjunctive mood stabilizer with antidepressant.

▪ Superiority (in other words, efficacy and safety) of antidepressant monotherapy versus adjunctive mood stabilizer with antidepressant for treatment of bipolar II depression is uncertain.

FIGURE 8.3. Algorithm for the acute treatment of bipolar depression based on Florida Medicaid guidelines. From "2017–2018 Florida Best Practice Psychotherapeutic Medication Guidelines for Adults," by R. S. McIntyre, 2018, pp. 14–15 (http://www.medicaidmentalhealth.org/_assets/file/Guidelines/2018-Psychotherapeutic%20Medication%20Guidelines%20for%20Adults%20with%20References.pdf). Copyright 2018 by the USF Medicaid Drug Therapy Management Program for Behavioral Health. Reprinted with permission.

Level 1   Established efficacy:

- ✦ Periodic evaluation: frequency based on clinical needs
- ✦ Continue with effective and well-tolerated treatment
- ✦ Lithium* monotherapy
- ✦ Quetiapine monotherapy
- ✦ Lamotrigine* (evidence strongest for prevention of depression)
- ✦ If initially stabilized on divalproex*†, maintain.
- ✦ Aripiprazole or aripiprazole long-acting injectable, long-acting risperidone monotherapy
- ✦ Quetiapine (for recurrence prevention) or ziprasidone (for relapse prevention) adjunctive to (lithium* or divalproex*†)
- ✦ Asenapine monotherapy

†*Note: Be aware that there are limited data on long-term efficacy of divalproex.*

 Level 2A   Established efficacy, but with safety concerns:**

- ✦ Olanzapine monotherapy
- ✦ Olanzapine adjunctive to lithium* or divalproex*†

Level 2B   If Level 1 is ineffective and/or not well tolerated:

- ✦ Continue effective and well-tolerated acute treatment(s) if not listed in Level 1
- ✦ Lithium* and divalproex*† combination
- ✦ Follow acute mania/bipolar depression guidelines to achieve remission or partial remission

 Level 3   If Levels 1 and 2 are ineffective and/or not well tolerated:

- ✦ Adjunctive clozapine (avoid combining with another antipsychotic)
- ✦ Electroconvulsive therapy (ECT)†

Notes:

*Caution should be used when prescribing lithium, lamotrigine, divalproex or carbamazepine to women of reproductive age due to increased risks to the fetus with use during pregnancy, including neural tube and other major birth defects. Please see Florida Best Practice Recommendations for Women of Reproductive Age with Serious Mental Illness and Comorbid Substance Use Disorders and online guideline on the Pharmacological Treatment of Mood Disorders During Pregnancy.

**Side-effect concerns with these agents include weight gain, metabolic syndrome, and extrapyramidal symptoms (EPS). Side-effects warrant vigilance and close monitoring on the part of the clinician.

†Long-term efficacy data are limited for the following: divalproex monotherapy, carbamazepine (drug interaction risk), antidepressants, and electroconvulsive therapy (inconvenience/expense).

FIGURE 8.4.   Algorithm for the maintenance of bipolar disorder treatment based on Florida Medicaid guidelines. From "2017–2018 Florida Best Practice Psychotherapeutic Medication Guidelines for Adults," by R. S. McIntyre, 2018, p. 18 (http://www. medicaidmentalhealth.org/_assets/file/Guidelines/2018-Psychotherapeutic%20 Medication%20Guidelines%20for%20Adults%20with%20References.pdf). Copyright 2018 by the USF Medicaid Drug Therapy Management Program for Behavioral Health. Reprinted with permission.

for efficacy with tolerability. Switching to another evidence-based agent with a decreased risk of the same problematic side effect would be advised.

MEDICATION MANAGEMENT ISSUES

The majority of this chapter focuses on initial pharmacological management strategies in BD. However, BD has a relapsing and remitting course with high rates of treatment resistance. Determining the most

likely underlying causes of treatment resistance is paramount in deciding how to optimize treatment. The cause of apparent treatment resistance (i.e., not improving with initially prescribed treatments) can be secondary to (a) inadequate medication trials (i.e., the mood stabilizer has not been prescribed at an adequate dose or for an adequate duration), (b) nonadherence to the prescribed treatment (i.e., the patient is not taking the treatment as prescribed), (c) previously unidentified perpetuating factors

'Basic' parameters for all patients prior to treatment implementation

History: medical comorbidities (including CVD risk factors), smoking status, alcohol use, pregnancy status, family history of CVD risk factors

Investigations: waist circumference and/or BMI (weight & height), BP, FBC, EUC, LFTs, fasting glucose, fasting lipid profile

Manage any identified medical conditions as appropriate

Selection of medication, taking into consideration overall health risk profile

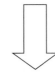

'Add-on' parameters according to treatment selected

Lithium

Baseline: TSH, Ca

Serum level: 2 levels to establish therapeutic dose, then every 3–6 months, after dose increases and as clinically indicated

Longitudinal monitoring
- EUC every 3–6 months
- Ca, TSH, and weight after 6 months, then annually

Valproate and carbamazepine

Baseline: Haematological and hepatic history

Serum level: 2 levels to establish therapeutic dose (4 weeks apart for carbamazepine), then as clinically indicated

Longitudinal monitoring
- ***Valproate:*** Weight, FBC LFT, menstrual history every 3 months for the first year, then annually; BP, fasting glucose, and lipid profile if risk factors; bone densitometry if risk factors
- ***Carbamazepine:*** FBC, LFT, EUC monthly for first 3 months, then annually; alert to rash especially in first few months of treatment; bone densitometry if risk factors; review contraceptive efficacy where applicable

Lamotrigine
- Alert to rash

Atypical antipsychotics[a]

Longitudinal monitoring
- Weight monthly for first 3 months, then every 3 months
- BP and fasting glucose every 3 months for first year, then annually
- Fasting lipid profile after 3 months, then annually
- ECG and prolactin level as clinically indicated

[a]Clozapine an exception

CVD = cardiovascular disease; BMI = body mass index; BP = blood pressure; FBC = full blood count; EUC = electrolytes, urea, and creatinine; LFTs = liver function tests; TSH = thyroid stimulating hormone; Ca = calcium; ECG = electrocardiogram.

FIGURE 8.5. The International Society for Bipolar Disorders consensus guidelines for the safety monitoring of bipolar disorder treatments. From "The International Society for Bipolar Disorders (ISBD) Consensus Guidelines for the Safety Monitoring of Bipolar Disorder Treatments," by F. Ng, O. K. Mammen, I. Wilting, G. S. Sachs, I. N. Ferrier, F. Cassidy, . . . International Society for Bipolar Disorders, 2009, *Bipolar Disorders*, *11*, p. 562. Copyright 2009 by Wiley. Reprinted with permission.

that are driving the illness course (e.g., substance misuse, other medications, worsening psychosocial environment, comorbid psychiatric or medical diagnoses), or (d) biological treatment resistance (i.e., the appropriate medication combination has yet to be identified; Gitlin, 2006; Nemeroff, 2007).

If nonadherence occurs, understanding the reasons behind nonadherence is essential for improving adherence. For example, often patients stop taking prescribed medications because of intolerable side effects (e.g., sexual side effects, weight gain, sedation) that they have not disclosed to their prescriber. In this scenario, providing appropriate psychoeducation and switching to a more well-tolerated medication may quickly correct the difficulties with adherence, and subsequently lead to treatment response when serum levels are consistently therapeutic (i.e., when the patient is taking the medication as prescribed). Other factors, such as cost or remembering to take the medication, should also be considered when nonadherence is suspected. If remembering to take the medications is identified as a barrier, simplifying the medication regimen and collaborating with the pharmacy (e.g., use of blister packs or other medication reminders) may be helpful. Alternatively, if nonadherence is secondary to lack of capacity to make the appropriate treatment decision, assertive treatment with a substitute decision maker may be required.

When nonadherence is identified, the use of depot antipsychotics (i.e., long acting injectable antipsychotics) may also be explored. Of the SGA depots, risperidone (given every 2 weeks) and aripiprazole (given every 4 weeks) have specifically been demonstrated to be efficacious in BD (Calabrese et al., 2017; Kishi, Oya, & Iwata, 2016). Additionally, many clinicians extrapolate the efficacy results of risperidone to assume that paliperidone is similarly efficacious, given that it is an active metabolite of risperidone. As such, the off-label use of long acting paliperidone (available in two formulations, given every 4 weeks or every 12 weeks) may also be appropriate; however, there is minimal direct evidence to support efficacy in BD (Nikolić, Page, Akram, & Khan, 2017).

The presence of previously unidentified perpetuating biological and psychosocial factors may contribute to the inhibition of remission and recovery. From a biological perspective, commonly unidentified perpetuating factors include the use and misuse of substances (e.g., cocaine, alcohol), coprescribed medications (e.g., antidepressants, stimulants, steroids, interferon), and unidentified contributing medical disorders (e.g., sleep apnea, anemia, hypothyroidism or hyperthyroidism) and psychiatric disorders (e.g., personality disorders, eating disorders, anxiety). Careful attention to each of these categories may reveal the underlying etiology of the apparent treatment resistance. Identifying and then correcting the underlying cause may lead to significant improvements in overall treatment outcomes (Gitlin, 2006; Nemeroff, 2007). Numerous psychosocial factors also may perpetuate the mood episode, especially with treatment-resistant bipolar depression. Evidence-based psychosocial interventions are further discussed in the Integration of Pharmacotherapy With Nonpharmacological Approaches section of this chapter.

Some patients may still experience persistent symptoms, even with perfect adherence and treatment of other perpetuating factors. The Florida Medicaid guidelines presented above show an algorithm to follow when adequate trials of first-line treatments fail. Unfortunately, the evidence base for treatment resistant and treatment refractory BD is limited, as most RCTs have either assessed monotherapies or dual therapy dual therapy with various combinations of divalproex, lithium, lamotrigine, SGAs, and antidepressants. As such, after a few failed medication trials, the prescriber is often left to try off-label combinations based on expert opinion, as there is minimal evidence to guide treatment at this stage.

EVALUATION OF PHARMACOLOGICAL APPROACHES ACROSS THE LIFESPAN

The current chapter has focused on the treatment of BD in the adult population (i.e., age 18–65), as the majority of available evidence is for this age group. However, there are notable differences in the treatment of geriatric (i.e., older than 65) and pediatric (i.e., younger than 18) populations. Over the past decade, there has been a substantial increase in the amount of research being conducted in the treatment of BD with both of these age categories. There has been increasing interest in and need for understanding the efficacy and tolerability of psychiatric treatments in older patients (Sajatovic et al., 2015), and interest has also grown in evaluating treatments for pediatric BD. Historically, there has been significant debate about the existence of pediatric BD. Critics of pediatric BD have suggested that symptoms of mania in this population are better explained by other childhood disorders, such as impulse control disorders (e.g., attention-deficit/hyperactivity disorder [ADHD]) and behavioral disorders (i.e., conduct disorder and oppositional defiant disorder). However, more recently the existence of pediatric BD has become widely accepted as replicated evidence has demonstrated the importance of recognizing, diagnosing, and treating BD in this age group (Goldstein et al., 2017).

Given the previous controversy and recent accumulation of evidence regarding diagnosis and treatment of pediatric BD, the ISBD formed a task force to summarize and contextualize findings in pediatric BD (Goldstein et al., 2017). From a treatment perspective, there is Level I evidence (i.e., positive effect demonstrated by at least one well-designed RCT) to support the use of SGAs in the treatment of manic and mixed episodes in pediatric BD. Risperidone, aripiprazole, quetiapine, olanzapine, and asenapine are FDA-approved for the acute treatment of mania in youth (age 10–17). Notably, however, children and adolescents appear to be more prone to metabolic side effects with SGAs and require close metabolic monitoring (Correll, Sheridan, & DelBello, 2010). Another important difference observed in pediatric BD is that conventional mood stabilizers (i.e., lithium and anticonvulsants) are less effective in the acute treatment of mania compared with adults (Correll et al., 2010).

Significantly less data is available for the treatment of bipolar depression and maintenance treatment in pediatric BD. Only OFC is FDA approved for the acute treatment of bipolar depression in youth. Additionally, in a published RCT of 347 youth (age 10–17), lurasidone was found to have a significant antidepressant effect at the end of a 6-week trial (DelBello et al., 2017). Quetiapine has also been evaluated for bipolar depression in youth in two large RCTs, but with negative results, showing no benefit above

the placebo response rate (DelBello et al., 2009; Findling, Pathak, Earley, Liu, & DelBello, 2014). As with adults, the use of antidepressant monotherapy is discouraged, especially in youth as there is an increased risk of treatment emergent suicidality (Goldstein et al., 2017).

In older patients, continuing treatment that was effective and well tolerated during earlier adulthood is usually indicated (Aziz, Lorberg, & Tampi, 2006). However, lower doses may be required, as there is increased risk of toxicity (Valiengo, Stella, & Forlenza, 2016). The risk of treatment-emergent cardiac arrhythmia and resultant sudden cardiac death is also increased, and therefore electrocardiograms are indicated with any changes in medications (Straus et al., 2006). Lower serum levels of lithium are also indicated. Older patients are at increased risk for falls and therefore medication associated with heavy sedation (summarized in Table 8.7) or orthostatic hypotension (e.g., quetiapine and olanzapine) should be avoided or used with caution (Woolcott et al., 2009).

CONSIDERATION OF POTENTIAL SEX DIFFERENCES

The relative prevalence of BD in men and women is similar, with a male-to-female prevalence ratio of 1.1:1 (Blanco et al., 2017). Studies investigating sex differences in BD are notably sparse compared with those for MDD (Kawa et al., 2005). Recommended treatments for BD are the same in men and women, with no consistently reported differences in efficacy; however, there are some differences in side effect profiles (Diflorio & Jones, 2010). For example, women are at risk of treatment-emergent PCOS with divalproex, with significant potential sequelae such as amenorrhea, hyperandrogenism, weight gain, and insulin resistance (Zhang, Li, Li, & Zou, 2016). Other mood stabilizers with significant metabolic effects (see Figure 8.1) may also increase the risk of developing PCOS.

Additionally, special considerations must be made for women of childbearing age within the context of pregnancy and breastfeeding (Payne, 2017). Preconception counseling is recommended to evaluate treatment options prior to becoming pregnant (Temming, Cahill, & Riley, 2016). Adequate discussion and planning may allow for folate supplementation and, if needed, medication changes prior to conception to minimize risk of teratogenicity. With BD, the postpartum period is high risk for relapse of severe mood episodes and psychosis (Wesseloo et al., 2016). As such, having adequate mood stabilizing treatment is usually advised.

Lithium and anticonvulsants have known risks for causing fetal abnormalities when taken during pregnancy. Early poorly designed studies showed a 400-fold increase in risk of cardiac malformation with fetal exposure to lithium; however, more recent studies with improved study design suggest that lithium poses a low absolute risk, with only 1% to 4% of lithium-exposed fetuses developing cardiac malformation (McKnight et al., 2012). As such, lithium may often be continued during pregnancy with an adequate informed consent discussion (Wald, Muzyk, & Clark, 2016). If lithium is continued during pregnancy, the serum lithium levels should be monitored closely and adjusted accordingly to maintain therapeutic levels, given the changes in blood volume during pregnancy. Additionally, lithium use is contraindicated while breastfeeding as high levels of lithium may be found in breast milk. As such, either bottle feeding or discontinuation of lithium would be advised.

Anticonvulsants pose a greater risk and are usually advised against in women planning to become pregnant, as valproate and carbamazepine are associated with significantly elevated risk of fetal neural tube defects (Tomson et al., 2011). Conversely, anticonvulsants are frequently used during lactation as a relatively safe option with added monitoring of the newborn, with monitoring of infant blood levels if concerns arise (Temming et al., 2016).

Among the BD treatment options, SGAs are likely the safest during both pregnancy and lactation; however, effects of SGAs on infants when used during pregnancy and lactation remain understudied (Smith & Dubovsky, 2017). One concern with some SGAs is increasing the risk of gestational diabetes, but this risk is usually less of a concern and is treatable compared with potential irreversible fetal malformations with anticonvulsants. Similar to anticonvulsants, SGAs may be used during lactation with added monitoring of the newborn.

There are also notable phenomenological differences, which will only be briefly summarized herein. Compared with men, women with BD are more prone to depressive episodes, suicide attempts, mixed features, and rapid cycling (Diflorio & Jones, 2010). Similar to MDD, women may also experience exacerbations of mood symptoms during the premenstrual period, which may be associated with a more severe illness course (Perich et al., 2017). The perimenopausal period is also associated with worsening depressive symptoms (Freeman et al., 2002). Women are more likely to have atypical depressive symptoms as well, with increased appetite and weight gain being common symptoms associated with depressive episodes (Miller et al., 2015). Rates of comorbidity also vary between men and women, as comorbid anxiety and eating disorders are more common in women and substance use disorders are more common in men (Baldassano, 2006).

INTEGRATION OF PHARMACOTHERAPY WITH NONPHARMACOLOGICAL APPROACHES: BENEFITS AND CHALLENGES

Pharmacotherapy remains the cornerstone of treatment for BD. Adjunctive nonpharmacological treatments should also be considered during all phases of illness. Nonpharmacological approaches can broadly be categorized into (a) brain stimulation and (b) psychosocial interventions. Both categories have evidence supporting efficacy in BD, with specific interventions demonstrating antidepressive and antimanic effects along with preventing relapse and recurrence.

Brain stimulation represents one of the oldest treatment modalities of BD. More specifically, electroconvulsive therapy (ECT) was the earliest treatment for acute mania that demonstrated a potent and rapid antimanic effect (Mukherjee, Sackeim, & Schnur, 1994). While ECT is still effective, pharmacotherapy has largely replaced ECT in the acute treatment of manic and mixed episodes given the invasiveness, cost, and cognitive dysfunction associated with ECT. However, ECT may still be indicated if manic or mixed symptoms are refractory to medications or if the use of medications is contraindicated, as there are no absolute contraindications to ECT. For treatment resistant/refractory bipolar depression, ECT has demonstrated antidepressant efficacy (Medda, Toni, & Perugi, 2014). ECT is also indicated for severe depression with acute suicidality when a rapid effect is needed and oral medications might not be feasible. Additionally, ECT is usually the treatment of choice for catatonia secondary to BD (Luchini et al., 2015).

More recently, the role of repetitive transcranial magnetic stimulation (rTMS) has been investigated with mixed results. While initial observational data and open label studies showed promising results (Pallanti et al., 2014; Rachid, Moeglin, & Sentissi, 2017; Rostami, Kazemi, Nitsche, Gholipour, & Salehinejad, 2017; Zendjidjian et al., 2014), RCTs have failed to demonstrate efficacy compared with placebo (Fitzgerald et al., 2016). There also have been concerns about potential rTMS treatment-emergent mania/hypomania in the absence of adequate mood stabilizer treatment, suggesting that rTMS monotherapy (or in combination with an antidepressant) should be avoided in BD (Rachid, 2017). Magnetic seizure therapy has also been of interest, but has only case report-level evidence (Noda et al., 2014).

Psychosocial interventions are important and efficacious adjunctive treatments of BD as well. Most current BD treatment guidelines suggest that all patients should receive, at a minimum, comprehensive psychoeducation (Parker et al., 2017). Psychoeducation should provide patients with information about the signs and symptoms of relapse along with strategies to decrease risk of relapse. Key counseling topics include, but are not limited to, the importance of sleep hygiene, exercise, maintaining a healthy diet, avoiding substance use, and encouraging social interaction. In addition to psychoeducation, the use of evidence-based psychotherapy may be of great benefit, especially for the treatment and prevention of bipolar depressive episodes (Miklowitz, 2008). In the treatment of bipolar depression specifically, cognitive behavioral therapy (CBT), mindfulness, interpersonal and social rhythm therapy, and family-focused therapy have demonstrated antidepressant efficacy along with anxiolytic effects (Salcedo et al.,

2016). Taken together, a comprehensive treatment plan for patients with bipolar depression includes these therapies in addition to appropriate pharmacotherapy.

INTEGRATED APPROACHES FOR ADDRESSING COMMON COMORBID DISORDERS

In BD, psychiatric and medical comorbidity is the rule rather than the exception. The effective treatment of comorbidities starts with adequate screening of common comorbidities. Replicated evidence has demonstrated high rates of comorbidity with anxiety disorders, ADHD, substance use disorders, eating disorders, and personality disorders (McIntyre et al., 2012; Rosenbluth et al., 2012). As per the Canadian Network for Mood and Anxiety Treatments (CANMAT) guidelines on management of comorbidity in mood disorders, several principles should be considered including, but are not limited to: establishing the diagnosis, risk assessment, establishing the appropriate setting for treatment, chronic disease management, concurrent treatment, and measurement-based care (McIntyre et al., 2012). Importantly, comorbid psychiatric disorders should be concurrently managed during the treatment of BD. For example, providers should not wait for comorbid substance use to be adequately treated prior to providing BD treatment, and vice versa. Toward this end, both psychosocial and psychopharmacological treatments should be utilized to treat comorbid conditions.

For comorbid anxiety disorders, CBT and mindfulness are effective options, if available. Pharmacologically, doses of SGAs and/or conventional mood stabilizers may be further optimized to control comorbid symptoms of anxiety. SGAs are particularly effective at mitigating anxiety during all illness phases, including during euthymic periods. Gabapentin and pregabalin represent alternative treatments for comorbid anxiety without the risk of manic switches associated with antidepressant treatment (Rakofsky & Dunlop, 2011). Intermediate or longer half-life benzodiazepines may be required for short-term utilization only for moderate to severe anxiety. If these approaches inadequately alleviate symptoms of anxiety, first-line antidepressants for anxiety (e.g., sertraline, escitalopram) may be required with the risk of a manic switch.

For ADHD, first-line stimulants (e.g., methylphenidate, lisdexamfetamine) may still be effectively and safely used with the added caution to monitor for potential manic/hypomanic switches (McIntyre et al., 2012). A key consideration is that stimulants should be used in combination with an adequate dose of a mood stabilizer. Stimulants should be avoided in patients with rapid cycling, mixed features, or active psychosis. Stimulants (e.g., lisdexamfetamine) may also be cautiously prescribed for comorbid binge eating disorder with a relatively low risk of treatment-emergent mania (McIntyre et al., 2013).

For comorbid personality disorders, dialectical behavioral therapy may be particularly effective, specifically for borderline personality disorder (BPD). In some cases, long-term psychodynamic psychotherapy may also be indicated (Rosenbluth et al., 2012). Of note, a careful assessment is required in patients with BD with comorbid BPD, as manic symptoms or mixed features may at times be confused with BPD-related affective dysregulation (Bayes, Parker, & McClure, 2016).

EMERGING TRENDS

Several novel treatments for BD are currently being investigated, providing hope for improved efficacy and tolerability. Novel emerging treatments for bipolar depression are of particular interest and importance, as they may satisfy an essential unmet need in the treatment of BD. Modulation of the glutamate system as well as the immune system are particularly promising treatment targets for bipolar depression.

Over the past decade, mounting evidence has strongly implicated immune dysfunction in the pathoetiology of numerous neuropsychiatric disorders, including BD (Rosenblat & McIntyre, 2017a). Targeting the immune system has been proposed as a potential way to modify the disease course of BD by targeting the underlying cause (i.e., inflammation) of BD rather than only the downstream effects (e.g., neurotransmitter levels; Rosenblat & McIntyre, 2016). Several proof-of-

concept clinical trials have demonstrated antidepressant effects of anti-inflammatory agents when used in BD (Rosenblat et al., 2016). Of the anti-inflammatories, N-acetylcysteine (NAC) has shown the most consistent results for demonstrating an antidepressant effect in BD and is already recommended as adjunctive treatment in some guidelines (Yatham et al., 2013). Minocycline, infliximab, celecoxib, pioglitazone, and liraglutide have shown promising antidepressant effects in preliminary studies as well.

There has also been significant interest in omega-3 fatty acids given their anti-inflammatory effects and excellent tolerability profile (Bloch & Hannestad, 2012). In BD, results have been mixed, with some trials showing an antidepressant effect (Frangou, Lewis, & McCrone, 2006; Stoll et al., 1999) and others reporting no effect compared with conventional therapy alone (Frangou, Lewis, Wollard, & Simmons, 2007; Hirashima et al., 2004; Keck et al., 2006). The mixed results of these studies may suggest that omega-3s (and likely all anti-inflammatory agents) are beneficial in only a subset of those with BD. In an RCT with unipolar depression, omega-3s were found to have a significant antidepressant effect in the subset of participants with elevated inflammatory markers (Rapaport et al., 2016). Intriguingly, in participants with normal inflammatory marker levels, placebo had a greater antidepressant effect compared with omega-3s, leading to an overall negative study outcome (i.e., no significant antidepressant effect was found when including the entire sample). While this study was on unipolar depression, it is likely that a similar effect may be observed in BD in that only patients with elevated inflammatory markers may benefit from anti-inflammatory treatments such as omega-3s, but further study is still required to confirm or refute this hypothesis in the BD population.

Targeting the glutamate system has also become of great interest in recent years with both bipolar and unipolar depression (Caddy et al., 2015). Interest in the glutamate system grew out of the identification of ketamine as a rapid acting antidepressant with potent antidepressant effects in both bipolar and unipolar depression (Kishimoto et al., 2016). Ketamine, a dissociative anesthetic, modulates the glutamate system as an N-methyl-D-aspartate (NMDA) antagonist. Modulation of the glutamate system is believed to be ketamine's primary mechanism of action mediating its antidepressant effects (Tokita, Yamaji, & Hashimoto, 2012). Replicated RCTs have provided Level I evidence (e.g., established efficacy) for the use of ketamine in the acute treatment of depression (Kishimoto et al., 2016), but several limitations prevent its use (Sanacora et al., 2017). Gold standard ketamine treatments for depression are via the intravenous (IV) route (ketamine 0.5 mg/kg IV infused over 40 minutes) and therefore are resource intensive and more invasive compared with other BD treatments (i.e., orally administered medications). Additionally, most RCTs assessed only a one-time dose of IV ketamine and therefore the long-term risks and benefits are yet to be adequately studied. As such, providing long-term ketamine treatments for depression is an inappropriate extrapolation of currently available evidence (Sanacora et al., 2017). The risk for misuse (given that ketamine also has abuse liability) and potential dissociative effects are also of concern.

Given these concerns, other agents targeting the glutamate system (e.g., D-cycloserine, riluzole, CP-101,606, CERC-301, basimglurant, JNJ-40411813, dextromethorphan, nitrous oxide, rapastinel, esketamine) are also currently under investigation (Lener, Kadriu, & Zarate, 2017). For example, dextromethorphan, an oral over-the-counter cough suppressant, is also an NMDA antagonist and has been evaluated in the acute treatment of bipolar depression with promising preliminary results (Kelly & Lieberman, 2014; Lee et al., 2017). However, compared with ketamine, no other glutamate modulating agent has demonstrated the same reproducible and robust rapid antidepressant effects (Lener et al., 2017).

Another emerging area in BD is evaluating treatments specifically for BD-II. As shown in Figure 8.3, only quetiapine has robust evidence for efficacy in the treatment of BD-II depression. Results from RCTs in BD-I are often extrapolated in the treatment of BD-II, but emerging evidence suggests that these distinct disorders may require different treatment approaches (Grande, Berk, Birmaher, & Vieta, 2016).

TOOL KIT OF RESOURCES

Bipolar Disorder

Patient Resources

Depression and Bipolar Support Alliance: http://www.dbsalliance.org/

MindShift phone app: https://www.anxietybc.com/resources/mindshift-app

Moodgym phone app: https://moodgym.com.au/

Mayo Clinic Patient Care & Health Information, Diseases & Conditions: Bipolar Disorder: https://www.mayoclinic.org/diseases-conditions/bipolar-disorder/symptoms-causes/syc-20355955

National Institute of Mental Health, Health and Education, Mental Health Information: Bipolar Disorder: https://www.nimh.nih.gov/health/topics/bipolar-disorder/index.shtml

Clinician Resources

2017–2018 Florida Best Practice Psychotherapeutic Medication Guidelines for Adults (Florida Medicaid guidelines): http://www.medicaidmentalhealth.org/_assets/file/Guidelines/2018-Psychotherapeutic%20Medication%20Guidelines%20for%20Adults%20with%20References.pdf

CANMAT Treatment Guidelines: http://dx.doi.org/10.1111/bdi.12025

World Federation of Societies of Biological Psychiatry Treatment Guidelines: http://dx.doi.org/10.1080/15622975.2017.1384850

Consensus guidelines for mixed depression: http://dx.doi.org/10.1017/S1092852917000165

Mood Disorder Questionnaire (MDQ): http://www.sadag.org/images/pdf/mdq.pdf

Hypomania Checklist (HCL-32): http://www.oacbdd.org/clientuploads/Docs/2010/Spring%20Handouts/Session%20220b.pdf

Young Mania Rating Scale (YMRS): https://www.outcometracker.org/library/YMRS.pdf

Altman Self-Rating Mania Scale (ASRM): http://www.cqaimh.org/pdf/tool_asrm.pdf

References

*Altinbas, K., Ozerdem, A., Prieto, M. L., Fuentes, M. E., Yalin, N., Ersoy, Z., . . . Frye, M. A. (2014). A multinational study to pilot the modified Hypomania Checklist (mHCL) in the assessment of mixed depression. *Journal of Affective Disorders, 152–154,* 478–482. http://dx.doi.org/10.1016/j.jad.2013.07.032

Altshuler, L. L., Post, R. M., Leverich, G. S., Mikalauskas, K., Rosoff, A., & Ackerman, L. (1995). Antidepressant-induced mania and cycle acceleration: A controversy revisited. *The American Journal of Psychiatry, 152,* 1130–1138. http://dx.doi.org/10.1176/ajp.152.8.1130

Altshuler, L. L., Sugar, C. A., McElroy, S. L., Calimlim, B., Gitlin, M., Keck, P. E., Jr., . . . Suppes, T. (2017). Switch rates during acute treatment for bipolar ii depression with lithium, sertraline, or the two combined: A randomized double-blind comparison. *The American Journal of Psychiatry, 174,* 266–276. http://dx.doi.org/10.1176/appi.ajp.2016.15040558

Amann, B., Born, C., Crespo, J. M., Pomarol-Clotet, E., & McKenna, P. (2011). Lamotrigine: When and where does it act in affective disorders? A systematic review. *Journal of Psychopharmacology, 25,* 1289–1294. http://dx.doi.org/10.1177/0269881110376695

American Psychiatric Association. (2002). Practice guideline for the treatment of patients with bipolar disorder (revision). *The American Journal of Psychiatry, 159*(4, Suppl.), 1–50.

American Psychiatric Association. (2013). *Diagnostic and statistical manual of mental disorders* (5th ed.). Washington, DC: Author.

Angst, J., Azorin, J. M., Bowden, C. L., Perugi, G., Vieta, E., Gamma, A., Young, A. H., & the BRIDGE Study Group. (2011). Prevalence and characteristics of undiagnosed bipolar disorders in patients with a major depressive episode: The BRIDGE study. *Archives of General Psychiatry, 68,* 791–798. http://dx.doi.org/10.1001/archgenpsychiatry.2011.87

Aziz, R., Lorberg, B., & Tampi, R. R. (2006). Treatments for late-life bipolar disorder. *American Journal of Geriatric Pharmacotherapy, 4,* 347–364. http://dx.doi.org/10.1016/j.amjopharm.2006.12.007

Baldassano, C. F. (2006). Illness course, comorbidity, gender, and suicidality in patients with bipolar disorder. *The Journal of Clinical Psychiatry, 67*(Suppl. 11), 8–11.

Bayes, A., Parker, G., & McClure, G. (2016). Emotional dysregulation in those with bipolar disorder, borderline personality disorder and their comorbid expression. *Journal of Affective Disorders, 204,* 103–111. http://dx.doi.org/10.1016/j.jad.2016.06.027

Berk, M., Post, R., Ratheesh, A., Gliddon, E., Singh, A., Vieta, E., . . . Dodd, S. (2017). Staging in bipolar disorder: From theoretical framework to clinical utility. *World Psychiatry, 16*(3), 236–244. http://dx.doi.org/10.1002/wps.20441

Blanco, C., Compton, W. M., Saha, T. D., Goldstein, B. I., Ruan, W. J., Huang, B., & Grant, B. F. (2017). Epidemiology of *DSM–5* bipolar I disorder: Results from the National Epidemiologic Survey on Alcohol and Related Conditions—III. *Journal of Psychiatric Research, 84,* 310–317. http://dx.doi.org/10.1016/j.jpsychires.2016.10.003

Bloch, M. H., & Hannestad, J. (2012). Omega-3 fatty acids for the treatment of depression: Systematic review and meta-analysis. *Molecular Psychiatry, 17,* 1272–1282. http://dx.doi.org/10.1038/mp.2011.100

Brown, G. M., McIntyre, R. S., Rosenblat, J., & Hardeland, R. (2018). Depressive disorders: Processes leading to neurogeneration and potential novel treatments. *Progress in Neuro-Psychopharmacology & Biological Psychiatry, 80*(Pt C), 189–204. http://dx.doi.org/10.1016/j.pnpbp.2017.04.023

Caddy, C., Amit, B. H., McCloud, T. L., Rendell, J. M., Furukawa, T. A., McShane, R., . . . Cipriani, A. (2015). Ketamine and other glutamate receptor modulators for depression in adults. *Cochrane Database of Systematic Reviews, 2015*(9), CD011612. http://dx.doi.org/10.1002/14651858.CD011612.pub2

Calabrese, J. R., Sanchez, R., Jin, N., Amatniek, J., Cox, K., Johnson, B., . . . Carson, W. H. (2017). Efficacy and safety of aripiprazole once-monthly in the maintenance treatment of bipolar I disorder: A double-blind, placebo-controlled, 52-week randomized withdrawal study. *The Journal of Clinical Psychiatry, 78,* 324–331. http://dx.doi.org/10.4088/JCP.16m11201

Chengappa, K. N., Kupfer, D. J., Frank, E., Houck, P. R., Grochocinski, V. J., Cluss, P. A., & Stapf, D. A. (2003). Relationship of birth cohort and early age at onset of illness in a bipolar disorder case registry. *The American Journal of Psychiatry, 160,* 1636–1642. http://dx.doi.org/10.1176/appi.ajp.160.9.1636

Cipriani, A., Hawton, K., Stockton, S., & Geddes, J. R. (2013). Lithium in the prevention of suicide in mood disorders: Updated systematic review and

*Asterisks indicate assessments or resources.

meta-analysis. *BMJ: British Medical Journal, 346,* f3646. http://dx.doi.org/10.1136/bmj.f3646

Correll, C. U., Sheridan, E. M., & DelBello, M. P. (2010). Antipsychotic and mood stabilizer efficacy and tolerability in pediatric and adult patients with bipolar I mania: A comparative analysis of acute, randomized, placebo-controlled trials. *Bipolar Disorders, 12,* 116–141. http://dx.doi.org/10.1111/j.1399-5618.2010.00798.x

DelBello, M. P., Chang, K., Welge, J. A., Adler, C. M., Rana, M., Howe, M., . . . Strakowski, S. M. (2009). A double-blind, placebo-controlled pilot study of quetiapine for depressed adolescents with bipolar disorder. *Bipolar Disorders, 11,* 483–493. http://dx.doi.org/10.1111/j.1399-5618.2009.00728.x

DelBello, M. P., Goldman, R., Phillips, D., Deng, L., Cucchiaro, J., & Loebel, A. (2017). Efficacy and safety of lurasidone in children and adolescents with bipolar I depression: A double-blind, placebo-controlled study. *Journal of the American Academy of Child & Adolescent Psychiatry, 56,* 1015–1025. http://dx.doi.org/10.1016/j.jaac.2017.10.006

Diflorio, A., & Jones, I. (2010). Is sex important? Gender differences in bipolar disorder. *International Review of Psychiatry, 22,* 437–452. http://dx.doi.org/10.3109/09540261.2010.514601

Findling, R. L., Pathak, S., Earley, W. R., Liu, S., & DelBello, M. P. (2014). Efficacy and safety of extended-release quetiapine fumarate in youth with bipolar depression: An 8 week, double-blind, placebo-controlled trial. *Journal of Child and Adolescent Psychopharmacology, 24,* 325–335. http://dx.doi.org/10.1089/cap.2013.0105

Fitzgerald, P. B., Hoy, K. E., Elliot, D., McQueen, S., Wambeek, L. E., & Daskalakis, Z. J. (2016). A negative double-blind controlled trial of sequential bilateral rTMS in the treatment of bipolar depression. *Journal of Affective Disorders, 198,* 158–162. http://dx.doi.org/10.1016/j.jad.2016.03.052

Fortney, J. C., Unützer, J., Wrenn, G., Pyne, J. M., Smith, G. R., Schoenbaum, M., & Harbin, H. T. (2017). A tipping point for measurement-based care. *Psychiatric Services, 68,* 179–188. http://dx.doi.org/10.1176/appi.ps.201500439

Forty, L., Smith, D., Jones, L., Jones, I., Caesar, S., Cooper, C., . . . Craddock, N. (2008). Clinical differences between bipolar and unipolar depression. *The British Journal of Psychiatry, 192,* 388–389. http://dx.doi.org/10.1192/bjp.bp.107.045294

Frangou, S., Lewis, M., & McCrone, P. (2006). Efficacy of ethyl-eicosapentaenoic acid in bipolar depression: Randomised double-blind placebo-controlled study. *The British Journal of Psychiatry, 188,* 46–50. http://dx.doi.org/10.1192/bjp.188.1.46

Frangou, S., Lewis, M., Wollard, J., & Simmons, A. (2007). Preliminary in vivo evidence of increased N-acetyl-aspartate following eicosapentanoic acid

treatment in patients with bipolar disorder. *Journal of Psychopharmacology, 21,* 435–439. http://dx.doi.org/10.1177/0269881106067787

Freeman, M. P., Smith, K. W., Freeman, S. A., McElroy, S. L., Kmetz, G. E., Wright, R., & Keck, P. E., Jr. (2002). The impact of reproductive events on the course of bipolar disorder in women. *The Journal of Clinical Psychiatry, 63,* 284–287. http://dx.doi.org/10.4088/JCP.v63n0403

Frye, M. A., Grunze, H., Suppes, T., McElroy, S. L., Keck, P. E., Jr., Walden, J., . . . Post, R. M. (2007). A placebo-controlled evaluation of adjunctive modafinil in the treatment of bipolar depression. *The American Journal of Psychiatry, 164,* 1242–1249. http://dx.doi.org/10.1176/appi.ajp.2007.06060981

*Galvão, F., Sportiche, S., Lambert, J., Amiez, M., Musa, C., Nieto, I., . . . Lepine, J. P. (2013). Clinical differences between unipolar and bipolar depression: Interest of BDRS (Bipolar Depression Rating Scale). *Comprehensive Psychiatry, 54,* 605–610. http://dx.doi.org/10.1016/j.comppsych.2012.12.023

Ghaemi, S. N., Hsu, D. J., Soldani, F., & Goodwin, F. K. (2003). Antidepressants in bipolar disorder: The case for caution. *Bipolar Disorders, 5,* 421–433. http://dx.doi.org/10.1046/j.1399-5618.2003.00074.x

Gitlin, M. (2006). Treatment-resistant bipolar disorder. *Molecular Psychiatry, 11,* 227–240. http://dx.doi.org/10.1038/sj.mp.4001793

Goldstein, B. I., Birmaher, B., Carlson, G. A., DelBello, M. P., Findling, R. L., Fristad, M., . . . Youngstrom, E. A. (2017). The International Society for Bipolar Disorders Task Force report on pediatric bipolar disorder: Knowledge to date and directions for future research. *Bipolar Disorders, 19,* 524–543. http://dx.doi.org/10.1111/bdi.12556

Grande, I., Berk, M., Birmaher, B., & Vieta, E. (2016). Bipolar disorder. *The Lancet, 387,* 1561–1572. http://dx.doi.org/10.1016/S0140-6736(15)00241-X

Grünerbl, A., Muaremi, A., Osmani, V., Bahle, G., Ohler, S., Tröster, G., . . . Lukowicz, P. (2015). Smartphone-based recognition of states and state changes in bipolar disorder patients. *IEEE Journal of Biomedical and Health Informatics, 19,* 140–148. http://dx.doi.org/10.1109/JBHI.2014.2343154

Grunze, H., Vieta, E., Goodwin, G. M., Bowden, C., Licht, R. W., Azorin, J. M., . . . Members of the WFSBP Task Force on Bipolar Affective Disorders working on this topic. (2018). The World Federation of Societies of Biological Psychiatry (WFSBP) Guidelines for the Biological Treatment of Bipolar Disorders: Acute and long-term treatment of mixed states in bipolar disorder. *The World Journal of Biological Psychiatry, 19,* 2–58.

Grunze, H. C. (2010). Anticonvulsants in bipolar disorder. *Journal of Mental Health (Abingdon, England), 19,* 127–141. http://dx.doi.org/10.3109/09638230903469186

*Hergueta, T., & Weiller, E. (2013). Evaluating depressive symptoms in hypomanic and manic episodes using a structured diagnostic tool: Validation of a new Mini International Neuropsychiatric Interview (M.I.N.I.) module for the *DSM–5* "With Mixed Features" specifier. *International Journal of Bipolar Disorders, 1,* 21. http://dx.doi.org/10.1186/2194-7511-1-21

Hirashima, F., Parow, A. M., Stoll, A. L., Demopulos, C. M., Damico, K. E., Rohan, M. L., . . . Renshaw, P. F. (2004). Omega-3 fatty acid treatment and T(2) whole brain relaxation times in bipolar disorder. *The American Journal of Psychiatry, 161,* 1922–1924. http://dx.doi.org/10.1176/ajp.161.10.1922

Hirschfeld, R. M., Lewis, L., & Vornik, L. A. (2003). Perceptions and impact of bipolar disorder: How far have we really come? Results of the national depressive and manic-depressive association 2000 survey of individuals with bipolar disorder. *The Journal of Clinical Psychiatry, 64,* 161–174. http://dx.doi.org/10.4088/JCP.v64n0209

*Hirschfeld, R. M., Williams, J. B., Spitzer, R. L., Calabrese, J. R., Flynn, L., Keck, P. E., Jr., . . . Zajecka, J. (2000). Development and validation of a screening instrument for bipolar spectrum disorder: The Mood Disorder Questionnaire. *The American Journal of Psychiatry, 157,* 1873–1875. http://dx.doi.org/10.1176/appi.ajp.157.11.1873

Horrobin, D. F., & Lieb, J. (1981). A biochemical basis for the actions of lithium on behaviour and on immunity: Relapsing and remitting disorders of inflammation and immunity such as multiple sclerosis or recurrent herpes as manic-depression of the immune system. *Medical Hypotheses, 7,* 891–905. http://dx.doi.org/10.1016/0306-9877(81)90044-X

Jope, R. S. (1999). Anti-bipolar therapy: Mechanism of action of lithium. *Molecular Psychiatry, 4*(2), 117–128. http://dx.doi.org/10.1038/sj.mp.4000494

Kawa, I., Carter, J. D., Joyce, P. R., Doughty, C. J., Frampton, C. M., Wells, J. E., . . . Olds, R. J. (2005). Gender differences in bipolar disorder: Age of onset, course, comorbidity, and symptom presentation. *Bipolar Disorders, 7,* 119–125. http://dx.doi.org/10.1111/j.1399-5618.2004.00180.x

Keck, P. E., Jr., Mintz, J., McElroy, S. L., Freeman, M. P., Suppes, T., Frye, M. A., . . . Post, R. M. (2006). Double-blind, randomized, placebo-controlled trials of ethyl-eicosapentanoate in the treatment of bipolar depression and rapid cycling bipolar disorder. *Biological Psychiatry, 60,* 1020–1022. http://dx.doi.org/10.1016/j.biopsych.2006.03.056

Kelly, T. F., & Lieberman, D. Z. (2014). The utility of the combination of dextromethorphan and quinidine in the treatment of bipolar II and bipolar NOS. *Journal of Affective Disorders, 167,* 333–335. http://dx.doi.org/10.1016/j.jad.2014.05.050

Kemp, D. E. (2014). Managing the side effects associated with commonly used treatments for bipolar depression. *Journal of Affective Disorders, 169*(Suppl. 1), S34–S44. http://dx.doi.org/10.1016/S0165-0327(14)70007-2

Kessler, R. C., Berglund, P., Demler, O., Jin, R., Merikangas, K. R., & Walters, E. E. (2005). Lifetime prevalence and age-of-onset distributions of *DSM–IV* disorders in the National Comorbidity Survey Replication. *Archives of General Psychiatry, 62,* 593–602. http://dx.doi.org/10.1001/archpsyc.62.6.593

Kishi, T., Oya, K., & Iwata, N. (2016). Long-acting injectable antipsychotics for prevention of relapse in bipolar disorder: A systematic review and meta-analyses of randomized controlled trials. *International Journal of Neuropsychopharmacology, 19,* pyw038. http://dx.doi.org/10.1093/ijnp/pyw038

Kishimoto, T., Chawla, J. M., Hagi, K., Zarate, C. A., Kane, J. M., Bauer, M., & Correll, C. U. (2016). Single-dose infusion ketamine and non-ketamine N-methyl-d-aspartate receptor antagonists for unipolar and bipolar depression: A meta-analysis of efficacy, safety and time trajectories. *Psychological Medicine, 46,* 1459–1472. http://dx.doi.org/10.1017/S0033291716000064

Lee, S. Y., Chen, S. L., Wang, T. Y., Chang, Y. H., Chen, P. S., Huang, S. Y., . . . Lu, R. B. (2017). The COMT Val158Met polymorphism is associated with response to add-on dextromethorphan treatment in bipolar disorder. *Journal of Clinical Psychopharmacology, 37,* 94–98. http://dx.doi.org/10.1097/JCP.0000000000000633

Lener, M. S., Kadriu, B., & Zarate, C. A., Jr. (2017). Ketamine and beyond: Investigations into the potential of glutamatergic agents to treat depression. *Drugs, 77,* 381–401. http://dx.doi.org/10.1007/s40265-017-0702-8

Liu, B., Zhang, Y., Fang, H., Liu, J., Liu, T., & Li, L. (2017). Efficacy and safety of long-term antidepressant treatment for bipolar disorders - A meta-analysis of randomized controlled trials. *Journal of Affective Disorders, 223,* 41–48. http://dx.doi.org/10.1016/j.jad.2017.07.023

Luchini, F., Medda, P., Mariani, M. G., Mauri, M., Toni, C., & Perugi, G. (2015). Electroconvulsive therapy in catatonic patients: Efficacy and predictors of response. *World Journal of Psychiatry, 5,* 182–192. http://dx.doi.org/10.5498/wjp.v5.i2.182

Malhi, G. S., Tanious, M., Das, P., Coulston, C. M., & Berk, M. (2013). Potential mechanisms of action of lithium in bipolar disorder. Current understanding. *CNS Drugs, 27,* 135–153. http://dx.doi.org/10.1007/s40263-013-0039-0

McInerney, S. J., & Kennedy, S. H. (2014). Review of evidence for use of antidepressants in bipolar depression. *The Primary Care Companion for CNS Disorders, 16.* http://dx.doi.org/10.4088/PCC.14r01653

McIntyre, R. S. (2015). 2015 Florida Best Practice Psycho-therapeutic Medication Guidelines for Adults. Retrieved from http://medicaidmentalhealth.org/ViewGuideline.cfm?GuidelineID=97

*McIntyre, R. S. (2018). 2017–2018 Florida Best Practice Psychotherapeutic Medication Guidelines for Adults. Retrieved from http://www.medicaidmentalhealth.org/_assets/file/Guidelines/2018-Psychotherapeutic%20Medication%20Guidelines%20for%20Adults%20with%20References.pdf

McIntyre, R. S., Alsuwaidan, M., Soczynska, J. K., Szpindel, I., Bilkey, T. S., Almagor, D., . . . Kennedy, S. H. (2013). The effect of lisdexamfetamine dimesylate on body weight, metabolic parameters, and attention deficit hyperactivity disorder symptomatology in adults with bipolar I/II disorder. *Human Psychopharmacology: Clinical and Experimental, 28,* 421–427. http://dx.doi.org/10.1002/hup.2325

McIntyre, R. S., Rosenbluth, M., Ramasubbu, R., Bond, D. J., Taylor, V. H., Beaulieu, S., & Schaffer, A., & the Canadian Network for Mood and Anxiety Treatments (CANMAT) Task Force. (2012). Managing medical and psychiatric comorbidity in individuals with major depressive disorder and bipolar disorder. *Annals of Clinical Psychiatry, 24,* 163–169.

McKnight, R. F., Adida, M., Budge, K., Stockton, S., Goodwin, G. M., & Geddes, J. R. (2012). Lithium toxicity profile: A systematic review and meta-analysis. *Lancet, 379,* 721–728. http://dx.doi.org/10.1016/S0140-6736(11)61516-X

Medda, P., Toni, C., & Perugi, G. (2014). The mood-stabilizing effects of electroconvulsive therapy. *The Journal of ECT, 30*(4), 275–282.

Miklowitz, D. J. (2008). Adjunctive psychotherapy for bipolar disorder: State of the evidence. *The American Journal of Psychiatry, 165,* 1408–1419. http://dx.doi.org/10.1176/appi.ajp.2008.08040488

Miller, L. J., Ghadiali, N. Y., Larusso, E. M., Wahlen, K. J., Avni-Barron, O., Mittal, L., & Greene, J. A. (2015). Bipolar disorder in women. *Health Care for Women International, 36,* 475–498. http://dx.doi.org/10.1080/07399332.2014.962138

Mitchell, P. B., Goodwin, G. M., Johnson, G. F., & Hirschfeld, R. M. (2008). Diagnostic guidelines for bipolar depression: A probabilistic approach. *Bipolar Disorders, 10*(1p2), 144–152. http://dx.doi.org/10.1111/j.1399-5618.2007.00559.x

Mukherjee, S., Sackeim, H. A., & Schnur, D. B. (1994). Electroconvulsive therapy of acute manic episodes: A review of 50 years' experience. *The American Journal of Psychiatry, 151,* 169–176. http://dx.doi.org/10.1176/ajp.151.2.169

Nemeroff, C. B. (2007). Prevalence and management of treatment-resistant depression. *The Journal of Clinical Psychiatry, 68*(Suppl. 8), 17–25.

Ng, F., Mammen, O. K., Wilting, I., Sachs, G. S., Ferrier, I. N., Cassidy, F., . . . International Society for Bipolar Disorders. (2009). The International Society for Bipolar Disorders (ISBD) consensus guidelines for the safety monitoring of bipolar disorder treatments. *Bipolar Disorders, 11,* 559–595. http://dx.doi.org/10.1111/j.1399-5618.2009.00737.x

Nikolić, N., Page, N., Akram, A., & Khan, M. (2017). The impact of paliperidone palmitate long-acting injection on hospital admissions in a mental health setting. *International Clinical Psychopharmacology, 32,* 95–102. http://dx.doi.org/10.1097/YIC.0000000000000155

Noda, Y., Daskalakis, Z. J., Downar, J., Croarkin, P. E., Fitzgerald, P. B., & Blumberger, D. M. (2014). Magnetic seizure therapy in an adolescent with refractory bipolar depression: A case report. *Neuropsychiatric Disease and Treatment, 10,* 2049–2055.

Ostacher, M. J., Tandon, R., & Suppes, T. (2016). Florida best practice psychotherapeutic medication guidelines for adults with bipolar disorder: A novel, practical, patient-centered guide for clinicians. *The Journal of Clinical Psychiatry, 77,* 920–926. http://dx.doi.org/10.4088/JCP.15cs09841

Pacchiarotti, I., Bond, D. J., Baldessarini, R. J., Nolen, W. A., Grunze, H., Licht, R. W., . . . Vieta, E. (2013). The International Society for Bipolar Disorders (ISBD) task force report on antidepressant use in bipolar disorders. *The American Journal of Psychiatry, 170,* 1249–1262. http://dx.doi.org/10.1176/appi.ajp.2013.13020185

Pallanti, S., Grassi, G., Antonini, S., Quercioli, L., Salvadori, E., & Hollander, E. (2014). rTMS in resistant mixed states: An exploratory study. *Journal of Affective Disorders, 157,* 66–71. http://dx.doi.org/10.1016/j.jad.2013.12.024

Parker, G. B., Graham, R. K., & Tavella, G. (2017). Is there consensus across international evidence-based guidelines for the management of bipolar disorder? *Acta Psychiatrica Scandinavica, 135,* 515–526. http://dx.doi.org/10.1111/acps.12717

Payne, J. L. (2017). Psychopharmacology in pregnancy and breastfeeding. *Psychiatric Clinics of North America, 40,* 217–238. http://dx.doi.org/10.1016/j.psc.2017.01.001

Perich, T. A., Roberts, G., Frankland, A., Sinbandhit, C., Meade, T., Austin, M. P., & Mitchell, P. B. (2017). Clinical characteristics of women with reproductive cycle-associated bipolar disorder symptoms. *Australian and New Zealand Journal of Psychiatry, 51,* 161–167. http://dx.doi.org/10.1177/0004867416670015

Pillarella, J., Higashi, A., Alexander, G. C., & Conti, R. (2012). Trends in use of second-generation antipsychotics for treatment of bipolar disorder in the United States, 1998–2009. *Psychiatric Services, 63,* 83–86. http://dx.doi.org/10.1176/appi.ps.201100092

Popova, E., Leighton, C., Bernabarre, A., Bernardo, M., & Vieta, E. (2007). Oxcarbazepine in the treatment of bipolar and schizoaffective disorders. *Expert Review of Neurotherapeutics*, 7, 617–626. http://dx.doi.org/10.1586/14737175.7.6.617

Rachid, F. (2017). Repetitive transcranial magnetic stimulation and treatment-emergent mania and hypomania: A review of the literature. *Journal of Psychiatric Practice*, 23(2), 150–159. http://dx.doi.org/10.1097/PRA.0000000000000219

Rachid, F., Moeglin, C., & Sentissi, O. (2017). Repetitive Transcranial Magnetic Stimulation (5 and 10?Hz) With Modified Parameters in the Treatment of Resistant Unipolar and Bipolar Depression in a Private Practice Setting. *Journal of Psychiatric Practice*, 23, 92–100. http://dx.doi.org/10.1097/PRA.0000000000000213

Rakofsky, J. J., & Dunlop, B. W. (2011). Treating nonspecific anxiety and anxiety disorders in patients with bipolar disorder: A review. *The Journal of Clinical Psychiatry*, 72, 81–90. http://dx.doi.org/10.4088/JCP.09r05815gre

Rapaport, M. H., Nierenberg, A. A., Schettler, P. J., Kinkead, B., Cardoos, A., Walker, R., & Mischoulon, D. (2016). Inflammation as a predictive biomarker for response to omega-3 fatty acids in major depressive disorder: A proof-of-concept study. *Molecular Psychiatry*, 21, 71–79. http://dx.doi.org/10.1038/mp.2015.22

Rosenblat, J. D., Kakar, R., Berk, M., Kessing, L. V., Vinberg, M., Baune, B. T., . . . McIntyre, R. S. (2016). Anti-inflammatory agents in the treatment of bipolar depression: A systematic review and meta-analysis. *Bipolar Disorders*, 18, 89–101. http://dx.doi.org/10.1111/bdi.12373

Rosenblat, J. D., & McIntyre, R. S. (2016). Bipolar Disorder and Inflammation. *Psychiatric Clinics of North America*, 39, 125–137. http://dx.doi.org/10.1016/j.psc.2015.09.006

Rosenblat, J. D., & McIntyre, R. S. (2017a). Bipolar disorder and immune dysfunction: Epidemiological findings, proposed pathophysiology and clinical implications. *Brain Sciences*, 7, E144. http://dx.doi.org/0.3390/brainsci7110144

Rosenblat, J. D., & McIntyre, R. S. (2017b). Treatment of mixed features in bipolar disorder. *CNS Spectrums*, 22, 141–146. http://dx.doi.org/10.1017/S1092852916000547

Rosenbluth, M., Macqueen, G., McIntyre, R. S., Beaulieu, S., Schaffer, A., & the Canadian Network for Mood and Anxiety Treatments (CANMAT) Task Force. (2012). The Canadian Network for Mood and Anxiety Treatments (CANMAT) task force recommendations for the management of patients with mood disorders and comorbid personality disorders. *Annals of Clinical Psychiatry*, 24(1), 56–68.

Rostami, R., Kazemi, R., Nitsche, M. A., Gholipour, F., & Salehinejad, M. A. (2017). Clinical and demographic predictors of response to rTMS treatment in unipolar and bipolar depressive disorders. *Clinical Neurophysiology*, 128, 1961–1970. http://dx.doi.org/10.1016/j.clinph.2017.07.395

Sajatovic, M., Strejilevich, S. A., Gildengers, A. G., Dols, A., Al Jurdi, R. K., Forester, B. P., . . . Shulman, K. I. (2015). A report on older-age bipolar disorder from the International Society for Bipolar Disorders Task Force. *Bipolar Disorders*, 17, 689–704. http://dx.doi.org/10.1111/bdi.12331

Salcedo, S., Gold, A. K., Sheikh, S., Marcus, P. H., Nierenberg, A. A., Deckersbach, T., & Sylvia, L. G. (2016). Empirically supported psychosocial interventions for bipolar disorder: Current state of the research. *Journal of Affective Disorders*, 201, 203–214. http://dx.doi.org/10.1016/j.jad.2016.05.018

Salvi, V., Fagiolini, A., Swartz, H. A., Maina, G., & Frank, E. (2008). The use of antidepressants in bipolar disorder. *The Journal of Clinical Psychiatry*, 69, 1307–1318. http://dx.doi.org/10.4088/JCP.v69n0816

Sanacora, G., Frye, M. A., McDonald, W., Mathew, S. J., Turner, M. S., Schatzberg, A. F., . . . Nemeroff, C. B., & the American Psychiatric Association (APA) Council of Research Task Force on Novel Biomarkers and Treatments. (2017). A consensus statement on the use of ketamine in the treatment of mood disorders. *JAMA Psychiatry*, 74, 399–405. http://dx.doi.org/10.1001/jamapsychiatry.2017.0080

Selle, V., Schalkwijk, S., Vázquez, G. H., & Baldessarini, R. J. (2014). Treatments for acute bipolar depression: Meta-analyses of placebo-controlled, monotherapy trials of anticonvulsants, lithium and antipsychotics. *Pharmacopsychiatry*, 47, 43–52. http://dx.doi.org/10.1055/s-0033-1363258

Seo, H. J., Wang, H. R., Jun, T. Y., Woo, Y. S., & Bahk, W. M. (2016). Factors related to suicidal behavior in patients with bipolar disorder: The effect of mixed features on suicidality. *General Hospital Psychiatry*, 39, 91–96. http://dx.doi.org/10.1016/j.genhosppsych.2015.12.005

Shorter, E. (2009). The history of lithium therapy. *Bipolar Disorders*, 11(Suppl. 2), 4–9. http://dx.doi.org/10.1111/j.1399-5618.2009.00706.x

Smith, B., & Dubovsky, S. L. (2017). Pharmacotherapy of mood disorders and psychosis in pre- and post-natal women. *Expert Opinion on Pharmacotherapy*, 18, 1703–1719. http://dx.doi.org/10.1080/14656566.2017.1391789

Solmi, M., Murru, A., Pacchiarotti, I., Undurraga, J., Veronese, N., Fornaro, M., . . . Carvalho, A. F. (2017). Safety, tolerability, and risks associated with first- and second-generation antipsychotics: A state-of-the-art clinical review. *Therapeutics and Clinical Risk*

Management, 13, 757–777. http://dx.doi.org/10.2147/TCRM.S117321

Stahl, S. M., Morrissette, D. A., Faedda, G., Fava, M., Goldberg, J. F., Keck, P. E., . . . McIntyre, R. S. (2017). Guidelines for the recognition and management of mixed depression. *CNS Spectrums, 22*, 203–219. http://dx.doi.org/10.1017/S1092852917000165

Stoll, A. L., Severus, W. E., Freeman, M. P., Rueter, S., Zboyan, H. A., Diamond, E., . . . Marangell, L. B. (1999). Omega 3 fatty acids in bipolar disorder: A preliminary double-blind, placebo-controlled trial. *Archives of General Psychiatry, 56*, 407–412. http://dx.doi.org/10.1001/archpsyc.56.5.407

Storosum, J. G., Wohlfarth, T., Schene, A., Elferink, A., van Zwieten, B. J., & van den Brink, W. (2007). Magnitude of effect of lithium in short-term efficacy studies of moderate to severe manic episode. *Bipolar Disorders, 9*, 793–798. http://dx.doi.org/10.1111/j.1399-5618.2007.00445.x

Straus, S. M., Kors, J. A., De Bruin, M. L., van der Hooft, C. S., Hofman, A., Heeringa, J., . . . Witteman, J. C. (2006). Prolonged QTc interval and risk of sudden cardiac death in a population of older adults. *Journal of the American College of Cardiology, 47*, 362–367. http://dx.doi.org/10.1016/j.jacc.2005.08.067

Temming, L. A., Cahill, A. G., & Riley, L. E. (2016). Clinical management of medications in pregnancy and lactation. *American Journal of Obstetrics and Gynecology, 214*, 698–702. http://dx.doi.org/10.1016/j.ajog.2016.01.187

Tokita, K., Yamaji, T., & Hashimoto, K. (2012). Roles of glutamate signaling in preclinical and/or mechanistic models of depression. *Pharmacology, Biochemistry, and Behavior, 100*, 688–704. http://dx.doi.org/10.1016/j.pbb.2011.04.016

Tomson, T., Battino, D., Bonizzoni, E., Craig, J., Lindhout, D., Sabers, A., . . . Vajda, F., & the EURAP study group. (2011). Dose-dependent risk of malformations with antiepileptic drugs: An analysis of data from the EURAP epilepsy and pregnancy registry. *The Lancet Neurology, 10*, 609–617. http://dx.doi.org/10.1016/S1474-4422(11)70107-7

University of South Florida, Florida Medicaid Drug Therapy Management Program. (2018). *2017–2018 Florida best practice psychotherapeutic medication guidelines for adults.* Retrieved from http://www.medicaidmentalhealth.org/_assets/file/Guidelines/2018-Psychotherapeutic%20Medication%20Guidelines%20for%20Adults%20with%20References.pdf

Valiengo, L., Stella, F., & Forlenza, O. V. (2016). Mood disorders in the elderly: Prevalence, functional impact, and management challenges. *Neuropsychiatric Disease and Treatment, 12*, 2105–2114. http://dx.doi.org/10.2147/NDT.S94643

Vieta, E., Günther, O., Locklear, J., Ekman, M., Miltenburger, C., Chatterton, M. L., . . . Paulsson, B. (2011). Effectiveness of psychotropic medications in the maintenance phase of bipolar disorder: A meta-analysis of randomized controlled trials. *International Journal of Neuropsychopharmacology, 14*, 1029–1049. http://dx.doi.org/10.1017/S1461145711000885

Viktorin, A., Lichtenstein, P., Thase, M. E., Larsson, H., Lundholm, C., Magnusson, P. K., & Landén, M. (2014). The risk of switch to mania in patients with bipolar disorder during treatment with an antidepressant alone and in combination with a mood stabilizer. *The American Journal of Psychiatry, 171*, 1067–1073. http://dx.doi.org/10.1176/appi.ajp.2014.13111501

Wald, M. F., Muzyk, A. J., & Clark, D. (2016). Bipolar depression: Pregnancy, postpartum, and lactation. *Psychiatric Clinics of North America, 39*, 57–74. http://dx.doi.org/10.1016/j.psc.2015.10.002

Wehr, T. A., & Goodwin, F. K. (1987). Can antidepressants cause mania and worsen the course of affective illness? *The American Journal of Psychiatry, 144*, 1403–1411. http://dx.doi.org/10.1176/ajp.144.11.1403

Wesseloo, R., Kamperman, A. M., Munk-Olsen, T., Pop, V. J., Kushner, S. A., & Bergink, V. (2016). Risk of postpartum relapse in bipolar disorder and postpartum psychosis: A systematic review and meta-analysis. *The American Journal of Psychiatry, 173*, 117–127. http://dx.doi.org/10.1176/appi.ajp.2015.15010124

Williams, R. S., Cheng, L., Mudge, A. W., & Harwood, A. J. (2002). A common mechanism of action for three mood-stabilizing drugs. *Nature, 417*, 292–295. http://dx.doi.org/10.1038/417292a

Woolcott, J. C., Richardson, K. J., Wiens, M. O., Patel, B., Marin, J., Khan, K. M., & Marra, C. A. (2009). Meta-analysis of the impact of 9 medication classes on falls in elderly persons. *Archives of Internal Medicine, 169*, 1952–1960. http://dx.doi.org/10.1001/archinternmed.2009.357

Yatham, L. N., Kennedy, S. H., Parikh, S. V., Schaffer, A., Beaulieu, S., Alda, M., . . . Berk, M. (2013). Canadian Network for Mood and Anxiety Treatments (CANMAT) and International Society for Bipolar Disorders (ISBD) collaborative update of CANMAT guidelines for the management of patients with bipolar disorder: Update 2013. *Bipolar Disorders, 15*, 1–44. http://dx.doi.org/10.1111/bdi.12025

Yildiz, A., Nikodem, M., Vieta, E., Correll, C. U., & Baldessarini, R. J. (2015). A network meta-analysis on comparative efficacy and all-cause discontinuation of antimanic treatments in acute bipolar mania. *Psychological Medicine, 45*, 299–317. http://dx.doi.org/10.1017/S0033291714001305

Young, A. H., & Newham, J. I. (2006). Lithium in maintenance therapy for bipolar disorder. *Journal of*

Psychopharmacology, 20, 17–22. http://dx.doi.org/
10.1177/1359786806063072

Zendjidjian, X. Y., Lodovighi, M. A., Richieri, R., Guedj, E.,
Boyer, L., Dassa, D., & Lançon, C. (2014). Resistant
bipolar depressive disorder: Case analysis of adjunctive
transcranial magnetic stimulation efficiency in medical
comorbid conditions. *Bipolar Disorders, 16,* 211–213.
http://dx.doi.org/10.1111/bdi.12170

Zhang, L., Li, H., Li, S., & Zou, X. (2016). Reproductive
and metabolic abnormalities in women taking
valproate for bipolar disorder: A meta-analysis.
*European Journal of Obstetrics, Gynecology, and
Reproductive Biology, 202,* 26–31. http://dx.doi.org/
10.1016/j.ejogrb.2016.04.038

*Zimmerman, M., Chelminski, I., Young, D., Dalrymple,
K., & Martinez, J. H. (2014). A clinically useful self-
report measure of the *DSM–5* mixed features specifier of major depressive disorder. *Journal of Affective
Disorders, 168,* 357–362. http://dx.doi.org/10.1016/
j.jad.2014.07.021

CHAPTER 9

PHARMACOLOGICAL TREATMENT OF ANXIETY DISORDERS

Allanah J. Wilson and Dan J. Stein

Anxiolytic agents have long been used to diminish symptoms of anxiety; given the ubiquity of anxiety symptoms it is not surprising that substances such as alcohol have been widely used for self-medication, and that medications such as benzodiazepines, available since the 1960s, are still widely prescribed. In recent decades, however, there have been important scientific advances in understanding the pathophysiology of anxiety disorders, and a number of medications have been registered for the treatment of these conditions. This growing evidence base has contributed to improving the outcomes of people suffering from anxiety disorders. The pathophysiology of anxiety disorders is not well understood; however, one model suggests that there is overactivity in limbic regions, such as the amygdala and insula, during processing of emotional stimuli, and aberrant functional connectivity between these regions and cortical regions, such as the medial prefrontal cortex (Craske & Stein, 2016). These networks are mediated by the neurotransmitters gamma-aminobutyric acid (GABA), glutamate, serotonin, norepinephrine, and dopamine, which may then be targets for pharmacological interventions. In this chapter, we provide a brief overview of the epidemiology and diagnosis of anxiety disorders, with particular reference to panic disorder (PD), generalized anxiety disorder (GAD), and social anxiety disorder (SAD), before discussing the efficacy of a number of pharmacological interventions,

management issues associated with such interventions, and different pharmacological approaches across the lifespan.

EPIDEMIOLOGY AND PREVALENCE

Anxiety symptoms include a range of cognitive, behavioral, and physical features, and may be adaptive within a particular context. However, when anxiety symptoms are excessive, persistent, and cause significant distress and impairment in function, they may meet the threshold for presence of an anxiety disorder. A meta-analysis of global prevalence of common mental disorders found a lifetime prevalence estimate of 12.9% for anxiety disorders (this study included GAD, PD, and SAD, as well as obsessive-compulsive disorder [OCD] and posttraumatic stress disorder [PTSD]), demonstrating that anxiety disorders are some of the most common mental disorders (Steel et al., 2014). Epidemiological studies show an increased prevalence of anxiety disorders in females, with a female to male ratio of approximately 2:1 (Steel et al., 2014; Wittchen et al., 2011).

Anxiety symptoms can be considered from both dimensional and categorical perspectives. Although there is considerable symptom overlap across the anxiety disorders, several discrete anxiety disorders have been identified based on the pattern and context in which they occur. These include social

http://dx.doi.org/10.1037/0000133-009
APA Handbook of Psychopharmacology, S. M. Evans (Editor-in-Chief)

and specific phobia, PD, agoraphobia, and GAD. The *Diagnostic and Statistical Manual of Mental Disorders* (5th ed.; *DSM–5*) included separation anxiety disorder and selective mutism, with typical childhood onset, under anxiety disorders, while OCD and related disorders and trauma- and stressor-related disorders are categorized in adjacent chapters (American Psychiatric Association [APA], 2013).

Generalized Anxiety Disorder

GAD is characterized by persistent and excessive worry, and apprehension and anxiety about a number of events and activities. Psychological and physical symptoms include difficulty concentrating, irritability, restlessness, sleep disturbances, fatigue, and muscle tension. Individuals with GAD find it difficult to control thoughts and anxieties. The clinical criterion for GAD aligns with that of other anxiety disorders in emphasizing distress and impairment associated with symptoms. GAD has a high lifetime prevalence amongst adults, with median age of onset at 30 years old, 12-month prevalence of 2.0%, and lifetime prevalence of 4.3% (Kessler, Petukhova, Sampson, Zaslavsky, & Wittchen, 2012).

Panic Disorder

PD is characterized by recurrent, unexpected panic attacks (APA, 2013). A panic attack is an acute surge of anxiety or fear coupled with at least four physical or psychological symptoms of anxiety (including palpitations/pounding heart; chest pain; shortness of breath; choking sensation; abdominal discomfort; dizziness; fear of losing control, dying, or having a heart attack). These attacks peak within 10 minutes and duration is usually less than 40 minutes. Such episodes are followed by a persistent fear of further attacks. Individuals may develop anticipatory anxiety and avoidance, and ultimately agoraphobia. PD has a median age of onset of 23 years, a 12-month prevalence of 2.4%, and lifetime prevalence of 3.8% (Kessler et al., 2012).

Social Anxiety Disorder (Social Phobia)

SAD is characterized by excessive fear and anxiety of being negatively evaluated by others in social or performance settings. The individual fears that he or she will act in a way that results in embarrassment or humiliation. This in turn results in distress, and often avoidance of social and performance related situations and activities. Median age of onset for SAD is 15 to 17 years old, and SAD has a 12-month prevalence of 7.4% and lifetime prevalence of 10.7% (Kessler et al., 2012).

Anxiety disorders are associated with impairment in quality of life, with levels of impairment similar across GAD, PD, and SAD (Barrera & Norton, 2009). Individuals with anxiety disorders frequently have more than one anxiety disorder and there is a significant increase in impairment in those with comorbid anxiety disorders (Kroenke, Spitzer, Williams, Monahan, & Lowe, 2007). Anxiety disorders also have high comorbidity with other psychiatric disorders, including major depressive disorder, bipolar disorder, somatic symptom disorder, OCD, PTSD, and substance use disorders (Kessler, Chiu, Demler, Merikangas, & Walters, 2005). Comorbid psychiatric disorders increase the probability of recurrence and contribute to lower rates of recovery (Bruce et al., 2005).

DIAGNOSING ANXIETY DISORDERS

Individuals presenting with anxiety symptoms deserve a comprehensive evaluation. This includes a history of the presenting complaint, starting with onset and duration of psychological and/or physical anxiety symptoms. Patients should also be assessed for precipitants of symptoms and their temporal relationship to the onset of symptoms, as well as for aggravating or relieving factors. Associated impairment in function and comorbid symptom clusters (e.g., depressive symptoms) should be explored. The clinician should also assess sexual functioning and the individual's weight if medication is to be considered, due to potential treatment-induced sexual dysfunction and weight gain. It is important to assess for any suicidal thoughts or behaviors, as anxiety disorders are independent risk factors for suicidal ideation and attempts, with an increased risk in individuals with comorbid anxiety and mood disorders (Nepon, Belik, Bolton, & Sareen, 2010). Structured clinical interviews are available for the diagnosis of anxiety disorders; these include the Structured Clinical Interview for DSM–5 Clinician Version (SCID-5-CV) and the Mini-International Neuropsychiatric Interview (MINI).

Past psychiatric history should include previous psychiatric symptoms, diagnoses, and hospitalizations. Previous pharmacological and psychological interventions, adherence, response to treatment, and any adverse events also require exploration. It is important to inquire in detail about past medical and surgical history, with particular attention to presentations to health services, and investigations and treatment for cardiovascular, respiratory, gastrointestinal, and neurological symptoms that have similar features to the anxiety disorders (e.g., palpitations, shortness of breath, nausea, dizziness).

A number of prescribed, over-the-counter (OTC), and recreational substances can mimic and/or aggravate anxiety symptoms, including thyroid medications (levothyroxine), asthma medications (e.g., albuterol), caffeine, and amphetamines. Anxiety symptoms also may lead to the use of certain substances in an attempt to self-medicate (Smith & Randall, 2012). Therefore, a thorough screen for substances—prescribed, OTC and recreational—should be undertaken. In addition, a family history of anxiety and other mental disorders should be obtained as well as response to treatment interventions, as a family history of anxiety disorders is associated with a more recurrent course, worse impairment, and greater service use (Milne et al., 2009).

A mental state examination, physical examination, and appropriate special investigations should also be done. The *DSM–5* diagnostic criteria may be used to make the diagnosis of an anxiety disorder (APA, 2013). A number of rating scales are available to assist with determining the severity of baseline and ongoing anxiety symptoms. These include the Panic Disorder Severity Scale (Shear et al., 1997), Liebowitz Social Anxiety Scale (LSAS; Liebowitz, 1987), Social Phobia Inventory (SPIN; Connor et al., 2000), Hamilton Anxiety Rating Scale (HAM-A; Hamilton, 1959), and Generalized Anxiety Disorder 7-Item Scale (GAD-7; Spitzer, Kroenke, Williams, & Lowe, 2006). Links to these scales are available in the Tool Kit of Resources at the end of this chapter.

EVIDENCE-BASED PHARMACOLOGICAL TREATMENTS OF ANXIETY DISORDERS

Current evidence-based guidelines recommend that prior to starting any treatment intervention, the individual should receive psychoeducation about their disorder, course of illness, treatment options (efficacy, expected time to onset of therapeutic effects, tolerance and dependence, adverse effects, treatment discontinuation), and signs of relapse. These guidelines also recommend that choice of pharmacological treatment should take into consideration patient preference (regarding side effects/tolerability), severity of anxiety symptoms, associated distress and impairment, best evidence-based approaches, previous response to pharmacological treatment (in self and family members), cost and availability of medications, concomitant medication use and subsequent drug–drug interactions, comorbid psychiatric (e.g., mood disorder) and medical conditions (e.g., cardiac disease), and availability of psychological interventions (APA, 2009; Baldwin et al., 2014; Bandelow et al., 2012; Katzman et al., 2014 [NICE], 2011, 2013).

First-line pharmacotherapy of anxiety disorders consists of therapeutic interventions that have demonstrated efficacy in randomized controlled trials (RCTs) and relative overall safety and absence of misuse potential (Craske & Stein, 2016). Initially, treatment is focused on reducing severity of the presenting anxiety symptoms and improving functioning. Over time, treatment aims to resolve symptoms, return the individual to premorbid functioning, and prevent relapse of anxiety symptoms. Table 9.1 summarizes pharmacological treatment recommendations for anxiety disorders in adults and includes adverse effects. It is important to note that not all pharmacological agents that have been shown to be efficacious in the treatment of anxiety disorders have FDA approval.

Generalized Anxiety Disorder

Guideline recommendations for first-line pharmacotherapy of GAD emphasize selective serotonin reuptake inhibitors (SSRIs), serotonin and norepinephrine reuptake inhibitors (SNRIs), and pregabalin.

TABLE 9.1

Pharmacological Treatment Recommendations for Anxiety Disorders in Adults

Medications

	Drug	Efficacy shown in RCTs for			FDA approved	Daily dose	Side effects
		PD	GAD	SAD			
SSRIs	Citalopram[1] (Celexa®)	x		x		20–40 mg	Jitteriness, nausea, restlessness, headache, fatigue, increased or decreased appetite, weight gain, weight loss, tremor, sweating, QT$_c$ prolongation, sexual dysfunction, diarrhea, constipation, and other side effects
	Escitalopram[2] (Lexapro®)		x	x	GAD	10–20 mg	
	Fluoxetine (Prozac®, Sarafem®)	x			PD	20–60 mg	
	Fluvoxamine (Luvox®, Luvox CR®)	x		x	SAD[3]	100–300 mg	
	Paroxetine (Brisdelle®, Paxil®)	x	x	x	PD, GAD, SAD	20–50 mg	
	Sertraline (Zoloft®)	x	x	x	PD, SAD	50–150 mg	
SNRIs	Duloxetine (Cymbalta®)		x		GAD	60–120 mg	Jitteriness, nausea, restlessness, headache, fatigue, increased or decreased appetite, weight gain, weight loss, tremor, sweating, QT$_c$ prolongation, sexual dysfunction, diarrhea, constipation, urination problems, and other side effects
	Venlafaxine (Effexor®, Effexor XR®)	x	x	x	PD, GAD, SAD	75–225 mg	
TCAs	Clomipramine (Anafranil®)	x			PD	25–250 mg	Anticholinergic side effects (constipation, blurred vision, dry mouth, urinary retention), somnolence, dizziness, cardiovascular side effects, weight gain, nausea, headache, sexual dysfunction, and other side effects
	Imipramine (Tofranil®)	x	x		PD	75–150 mg	
Calcium modulator	Pregabalin (Lyrica®)		x	x		150–600 mg	Dizziness, somnolence, dry mouth, edema, blurred vision, weight gain, constipation, euphoric mood, balance disorder, increased appetite, difficulty with concentration/attention, withdrawal symptoms after abrupt discontinuation, and other side effects
Azapirone	Buspirone (BuSpar®)		x		Anxiety (nonspecific)	15–60 mg	Dizziness, nausea, headache, nervousness, light-headedness, excitement, insomnia, and other side effects

Class	Drug			Indication	Dose	Side effects
RIMA	Moclobemide (Aurorix®, Manerix®)	x			300–600 mg	Restlessness, insomnia, dry mouth, headache, dizziness, gastrointestinal symptoms, nausea, and other side effects
MAOI	Phenelzine (Nardil®)	x			45–75 mg	Dizziness, sedation, fatigue, constipation, dry mouth, hypertensive crisis, and other side effects
SARI	Trazodone (Desyrel®, Oleptro™)	x			100–300 mg	Drowsiness, dizziness, blurred vision, dry mouth, GIT disturbances, hypotension, priapism, and other side effects
Melatonergic agonist	Agomelatine (Valdoxan®)	x			25–50 mg	Headache, dizziness, somnolence, fatigue, GIT disturbances, increased transaminase levels, and other side effects
Antihistamine	Hydroxyzine (Atarax®, Vistaril®)	x		Anxiety (nonspecific)	50–100 mg	Drowsiness, sedation, fatigue, dry mouth, tremor, and other side effects
Atypical antipsychotic	Quetiapine (Seroquel®)	x			50–150 mg	Metabolic syndrome, dizziness, sedation, postural hypotension, constipation, dry mouth, extrapyramidal side effects, rare neuroleptic malignant syndrome, and other side effects
Benzodiazepines	Alprazolam (Xanax®)	x	x	Anxiety (nonspecific), PD	0.5–4 mg	Sedation, fatigue, dizziness, slurred speech, ataxia, confusion, forgetfulness, dependence, falls in elderly, possible disinhibition, and other side effects
	Clonazepam (Klonopin®)	x		PD	0.5–2 mg	

Note. Not all drugs are licensed for these indications in all countries. RCT = randomized controlled study; PD = panic disorder; GAD = generalized anxiety disorder; SAD = social anxiety disorder (also known as social phobia); FDA = U.S. Food and Drug Administration; SSRI = selective serotonin reuptake inhibitor; QTc = corrected QT interval; SNRI = selective serotonin norepinephrine reuptake inhibitor; TCA = tricyclic antidepressant; RIMA = reversible monoamine oxidase A inhibitor; MAOI = monoamine oxidase inhibitor; SARI = serotonin antagonist/reuptake inhibitor; GIT = gastrointestinal tract. From "Treatment of Anxiety Disorders," by B. Bandelow, S. Michaelis, and D. Wedekind, 2017, *Dialogues in Clinical Neuroscience, 19,* p. 97. Copyright 2017 by Association La Conference Hippocrate. Adapted with permission.
[1]Do not exceed recommended dose (possible QTc interval prolongation). Maximal dose with diminished hepatic function, 30 mg/d; for older patients, 20 mg/d. [2]Do not exceed recommended dose (possible QTc interval prolongation). Maximal dose for persons over age 65, 10 mg/d. [3]Fluvoxamine Controlled Release.

Various other agents that can be used in the treatment of GAD include agomelatine and buspirone. Guidelines indicate that optimal duration of maintenance therapy is at least 6 to 18 months (Allgulander & Baldwin, 2013; Baldwin et al., 2014; Bandelow et al., 2012; Bandelow, Michaelis, & Wedekind, 2017; Katzman et al., 2014; NICE, 2011).

First-line agents in the management of generalized anxiety disorder.   SSRIs all share the core feature of selectively and potently inhibiting the reuptake of serotonin, which results in increased availability of serotonin in the synaptic cleft. SSRIs may exert their anxiolytic effect by enhancing serotonin input to limbic structures such as the amygdala. Individual SSRIs also act on other receptors, with the exception of citalopram and escitalopram, and this may contribute both to their therapeutic effects as well as to adverse reactions. In RCTs, the SSRIs escitalopram, paroxetine, and sertraline have been shown to be efficacious in the acute management of GAD (Allgulander, Dahl, et al., 2004; Baldwin, Huusom, & Maehlum, 2006; Goodman, Bose, & Wang, 2005; Rickels et al., 2003). Escitalopram and paroxetine have also been shown to be efficacious in the long-term management of GAD (Allgulander, Florea, & Huusom, 2006; Pelissolo, 2008; Stocchi et al., 2003).

The SNRIs (duloxetine, venlafaxine) inhibit both serotonin and norepinephrine reuptake. This results in increased serotonin and norepinephrine concentration in brain synapses, enhancing serotonin and norepinephrine input to the amygdala and increasing dopamine within the prefrontal cortex. Venlafaxine (extended release form) and duloxetine have both been shown to be efficacious for the acute and long-term treatment of GAD (Davidson et al., 2008; Gelenberg et al., 2000; Hartford et al., 2007).

Pregabalin, an alpha-2-delta ligand/calcium channel modulator, binds to the alpha 2 delta subunit of voltage-sensitive calcium channels, which reduces the excessive release of excitatory neurotransmitters such as glutamate. Glutamate is the major excitatory neurotransmitter of the brain, and it is postulated that these excitatory neuronal pathways are overactive in those with anxiety disorders. This agent has shown to be efficacious and tolerable in the acute and maintenance treatment of GAD (Baldwin, Ajel,

Masdrakis, Nowak, & Rafiq, 2013; Boschen, 2011; Feltner et al., 2008; Kasper et al., 2009; Mula, Pini, & Cassano, 2007). Pregabalin has no effect on cytochrome P450 (CYP450) enzymes (enzymes found predominantly in the liver that are responsible for the metabolism of medication and drugs) and this reduces potential drug–drug interactions.

Other agents used in the management of generalized anxiety disorder.   The tricyclic antidepressants (TCAs) are serotonergic and noradrenergic reuptake inhibitors, but also impact a range of other receptors. Imipramine is an efficacious agent in the treatment of GAD (Schmitt et al., 2005). However, due to its side effect profile, noted in Table 9.1, and its potentially fatal cardiac (cardiac arrhythmias and conduction disturbances) and central nervous system toxicity in overdose (Woolf et al., 2007), it is not considered a first line agent. Trazodone is a serotonin ($5HT_{2A}$ and $5HT_{2C}$) antagonist and reuptake inhibitor (SARI). At lower doses, it has more potent antagonist actions on the $5HT_{2A}$ receptor, as well as histaminic and adrenergic receptors, and has shown to be an effective anxiolytic and sedative agent. It has shown efficacy in the treatment of GAD (Rickels, Downing, Schweizer, & Hassman, 1993). Buspirone is a $5HT_{1A}$ receptor agonist and has presynaptic and postsynaptic effects at serotonergic neurons. Buspirone has been shown to be superior to placebo in the treatment of GAD in some RCTs, particularly in individuals who have not been on a benzodiazepine (Chessick et al., 2006).

Agomelatine is a melatonergic 1 and 2 receptor agonist as well as a serotonin $5HT_{2C}$ receptor antagonist. It is thought to exert its anxiolytic effect through its action on the $5HT_{2C}$ receptor. It has been shown to be efficacious in acute and longer term treatment of GAD, and is well tolerated during treatment and discontinuation (D. J. Stein, Ahokas, & de Bodinat, 2008; D. J. Stein, Ahokas, Albarran, Olivier, & Allgulander, 2012). However, this agent is currently not FDA approved for the treatment of GAD.

Studies have shown efficacy for the antihistamine hydroxyzine, which blocks histamine-1 receptors, in treating GAD. A Cochrane review noted that hydroxyzine was more efficacious than placebo in the treatment of GAD, but that recommendation as a first-line agent could not be made due to a high risk of bias of the included studies (Guaiana, Barbui, & Cipriani, 2010). Hydroxyzine has some early anxiolytic effects, but may take several weeks to become fully effective. The use of hydroxyzine has been limited by its sedative effects and its lack of efficacy in comorbid psychiatric conditions.

Evidence for atypical antipsychotic monotherapy for anxiety disorders is limited. Extended release quetiapine in GAD has been shown to be efficacious (Depping, Komossa, Kissling, & Leucht, 2010; Katzman et al., 2011; D. J. Stein et al., 2011). However, metabolic and extrapyramidal adverse effects preclude the general use of atypical antipsychotics, and they are mainly used off-label in treatment-refractory individuals (Maglione et al., 2011).

Social Anxiety Disorder

Guideline recommendations for first-line pharmacotherapy of SAD comprise the SSRIs and venlafaxine. Other agents that can be used include moclobemide (reversible inhibitor of monoamine oxidase A [RIMA]) and phenelzine (nonreversible inhibitor of monoamine oxidase A and B [MAOI]). These recommendations are based on RCTs and meta-analyses. Guidelines recommend an optimal duration of continuation therapy of at least 6 months, with longer periods considered in individual cases (Baldwin et al., 2014; Bandelow et al., 2012, 2017; Blanco, Bragdon, Schneier, & Liebowitz, 2013; Katzman et al., 2014; NICE, 2013; Williams et al., 2017).

First-line agents in the management of social anxiety disorder. Citalopram showed improvement in anxiety symptoms compared to placebo in one RCT of SAD (Furmark et al., 2005). Escitalopram, paroxetine, and sertraline are all efficacious in the acute and long-term treatment of SAD (Kasper, D. J. Stein, Loft, & Nil, 2005; Lepola, Bergtholdt, St. Lambert, Davy, & Ruggiero, 2004; Montgomery, Nil, Dürr-Pal, Loft, & Boulenger, 2005; Pelissolo, 2008; D. J. Stein, Versiani, Hair, & Kumar, 2002; Van Ameringen et al., 2001; Walker et al., 2000). Fluvoxamine and controlled release fluvoxamine have been shown to be efficacious in the acute

management of SAD (M. B. Stein, Fyer, Davidson, Pollack, & Wiita, 1999; Westenberg, Stein, Yang, Li, & Barbato, 2004), and there was continued improvement in anxiety symptoms with controlled release fluvoxamine compared to placebo in the long-term treatment of SAD (D. J. Stein, Westenberg, Yang, Li, & Barbato, 2003). The SNRI venlafaxine has been shown to be efficacious for the acute and long-term treatment of SAD (Allgulander, Mangano, et al., 2004; Davis, Smits, & Hofmann, 2014; M. B. Stein, Pollack, Bystritsky, Kelsey, & Mangano, 2005).

Other agents used in the management of social anxiety disorder. Moclobemide is a RIMA and phenelzine is an MAOI; these agents result in alterations in dopamine, norepinephrine, and serotonin neurotransmission and are efficacious in the treatment of SAD (Davis et al., 2014; Williams et al., 2017). However, due to their side effect profiles, noted in Table 9.1, potential drug–drug interactions, and phenelzine's interaction with food containing tyramine (e.g., aged cheeses) that may result in hypertensive crisis, the MAOIs are not considered first-line agents. Pregabalin has been shown to be efficacious in some studies of the acute treatment of SAD (Pande et al., 2004). Olanzapine has been shown to reduce symptom severity in SAD in one pilot study (Barnett, Kramer, Casat, Connor, & Davidson, 2002).

Panic Disorder

Guideline recommendations for first-line pharmacotherapy of PD emphasize the role of SSRIs and the SNRI venlafaxine. Other agents that can be used in PD include the TCAs. Severe panic attacks may require short-acting benzodiazepines such as alprazolam and clonazepam. Guidelines recommend an optimal duration of continuation therapy of at least 12 months (APA, 2009; Baldwin et al., 2014; Bandelow et al., 2012, 2017; Batelaan, Van Balkom, & Stein, 2012; Katzman et al., 2014; NICE, 2011).

First-line agents in the management of panic disorder. Escitalopram is efficacious in the acute management of PD (Stahl, Gergel, & Li, 2003). Citalopram, fluoxetine, fluvoxamine, paroxetine, and sertraline are all efficacious in the acute and long-term management of PD (Asnis et al., 2001;

Dannon et al., 2007; Lecrubier, Judge, & the Collaborative Paroxetine Panic Study Investigators, 1997; Lepola et al., 1998; Michelson et al., 2001; Pelissolo, 2008; Pollack et al., 2007; Pollack, Otto, Worthington, Manfro, & Wolkow, 1998; Rapaport et al., 2001; Sheehan, Burnham, Iyengar, Perera, & Paxil CR Panic Disorder Study Group, 2005; Wade, Lepola, Koponen, Pedersen, & Pedersen, 1997). The SNRI extended release venlafaxine has been shown to be efficacious for the acute and long-term treatment of PD (Ferguson, Khan, Mangano, Entsuah, & Tzanis, 2007; Pollack et al., 2007).

Other agents used in the management of panic disorder. The TCAs clomipramine and imipramine are efficacious agents in the treatment of PD (Klerman, 1992; Lecrubier, Judge, & the Collaborative Paroxetine Panic Study Investigators, 1997; Papp et al., 1997). As noted previously for other anxiety disorders, their side effect profiles and potential toxicity in overdose precludes them from being first-line agents.

Benzodiazepines act as positive allosteric modulators of GABA$_A$ receptors. When they bind to the GABA$_A$ receptor in the presence of GABA, this results in an increase in the frequency of the chloride channel opening that enhances the inhibitory effects of GABA, causing strong and rapid anxiolytic and sedative effects. A number of benzodiazepines (e.g., alprazolam, clonazepam, diazepam, lorazepam) have been shown to be efficacious for the treatment of anxiety disorders (Bandelow et al., 2012; Offidani, Guidi, Tomba, & Fava, 2013). However, benzodiazepines should be used with caution and for short duration in the treatment of anxiety disorders, due to the risk of dependence, CNS depressive effects (drowsiness, impaired psychomotor function and memory), and lack of efficacy in treating comorbid conditions such as depression (Bandelow et al., 2012, 2015; Batelaan et al., 2012; Dell'osso & Lader, 2013; Katzman et al., 2014). Benzodiazepines may be used for brief periods for acute, severe anxiety symptoms (Batelaan et al., 2012).

BEST APPROACHES FOR ASSESSING TREATMENT RESPONSE AND MANAGING SIDE EFFECTS

Patient-reported or clinician-assessed symptom severity measures are useful for monitoring symptoms. Treatment should aim to improve symptoms, with full remission of symptoms being optimal. Remission is defined as no symptoms or minimal symptoms of anxiety and no functional impairment across multiple domains of work, social, and family activity. Operationally, this would be an achievement of a prespecified low score on an appropriate disorder-specific scale (Doyle & Pollack, 2003; Katzman et al., 2014), and less than or equal to 1 on each individual item (work/school, social life, family life) on the Sheehan Disability Scale (K. H. Sheehan & D. V. Sheehan, 2008), which measures functional impairment. In GAD, a prespecified low score on disorder-specific scales would be a score of less than or equal to 5 on the GAD-7 (Spitzer et al., 2006) or a score of less than or equal to 7 to 10 on the HAM-A (Hamilton, 1959); for PD, it would be a score of less than or equal to 5 on the Panic Disorder Severity Scale (Shear et al., 1997); and for SAD, it would be a score of less than or equal to 30 on the LSAS (Liebowitz, 1987). As noted, links to these scales are available in the Tool Kit of Resources at the end of this chapter. A guideline recommendation for monitoring of individuals started on pharmacotherapy suggests that individuals should be monitored initially every 2 weeks for the first 6 weeks and then monthly thereafter for symptom improvement and any medication side effects; children, the elderly, medically ill individuals, and individuals on multiple medications may need closer monitoring (Katzman et al., 2014).

At follow-up, individuals should be encouraged to discuss any concerns that they may have with regard to the treatment, specifically exploring adverse effects. Adverse effects of antidepressants (as noted in Table 9.1), if experienced, are usually experienced early after the introduction of medication and are often transient. However, antidepressant-induced sexual dysfunction and weight gain may emerge or persist after 1 month of treatment (Hirschfeld, 2003). Psychoeducation should be provided, informing the individual about the transient nature of most side effects.

When initiating first-line anxiety treatment with SSRIs and SNRIs, there may be a period of initial worsening of anxiety and distress in GAD, PD (with an increase in panic attacks), and SAD.

Psychoeducation around increasing anxiety symptoms when starting antianxiety medication should be provided to reassure the individual that this worsening is transient. Medication should be initiated at a low dose and increased slowly ("go low and slow") to minimize treatment-emergent worsening of anxiety symptoms (Baldwin et al., 2014; Bandelow et al., 2017; Batelaan et al., 2012). However, some individuals cannot tolerate this initial worsening of anxiety, and initiation of antidepressants in conjunction with the brief and strategic use of low-dose benzodiazepines for a limited period of time may be useful (Batelaan et al., 2012; Goddard et al., 2001). SSRIs that are considered activating, such as fluoxetine, can be given in the morning, while sedating SSRIs, such as paroxetine, can be taken at night. Recommendations for the management of antidepressant-induced sexual dysfunction include antidepressant dose reduction, switching antidepressants, and the addition of other pharmacological agents to manage the dysfunction (e.g., sildenafil and tadalafil for antidepressant-induced erectile dysfunction in males, and bupropion for antidepressant-induced sexual dysfunction in females; Taylor et al., 2013). The management of antidepressant-induced weight gain includes education at the onset of treatment, appropriate dietary advice, exercise regimens, and changing to an agent with decreased potential for weight gain (see Table 9.1).

MEDICATION MANAGEMENT ISSUES

In the following section we will be addressing poor response to treatment, the switching between pharmacological agents, and the potential problems associated with discontinuing medication.

Poor Response to Treatment

If symptoms do not subside or if they reemerge on treatment, the diagnosis should be reviewed, as should medication dose and adherence. Nonadherence across the anxiety disorders ranges from 18% to 30% (Taylor, Abramowitz, & McKay, 2012). Factors that influence adherence are treatment motivation, medication adverse effects, life stressors, comorbid conditions, and logistical barriers (transport, access

to medical facilities). It is important to identify modifiable risk factors for poor adherence and implement strategies to manage these risk factors. For example, low treatment motivation may be addressed with motivational interviewing (Miller & Rollnick, 2002), and concern around medication side effects may be addressed with psychoeducation or by switching medications (Taylor et al., 2012). Comorbid psychiatric or medical disorders that may have been overlooked should be reviewed, and any concomitant medication and substance use (prescribed or recreational) should be assessed and managed appropriately. Screening for any current life stressors, work, and domestic issues that could be aggravating anxiety symptoms should be undertaken (Allgulander & Baldwin, 2013; Bandelow et al., 2017). If all these features have been considered and the individual has received an adequate dose of treatment for 4 to 6 weeks and shows no response, consideration should be given to changing the treatment (Bandelow et al., 2017).

Switching Between Pharmacological Agents

If pharmacological interventions show partial response, it is important to ensure that an adequate trial of therapy has been given; if there has been an adequate trial of the agent and it has been tolerated, increasing the dose of the initial agent may be considered. If there is a poor response or the initial agent is poorly tolerated, the next step would be to consider switching within classes (e.g., switch from one SSRI to another SSRI). If response remains poor or there is continued intolerability, current guidelines suggest switching to another first-line agent (e.g., switching from an SSRI to an SNRI with GAD, PD, and SAD; changing to pregabalin with GAD; Allgulander & Baldwin, 2013; APA, 2009; Baldwin et al., 2014; Bandelow et al., 2012, 2017; Batelaan et al., 2012; Blanco et al., 2013; Katzman et al., 2014; NICE, 2011, 2013). If first-line agents fail, changing to second-line agents can be considered, and if they show poor response, augmenting with evidence-based combinations can be considered. In GAD, an RCT showed that augmenting SSRI or SNRI pharmacotherapy with pregabalin was efficacious. Evidence for augmenting with atypical antipsychotics in GAD and SAD has been inconsistent, and due to the metabolic side effects associated with these agents, caution is required (Allgulander & Baldwin, 2013; APA, 2009; Baldwin et al., 2014; Bandelow et al., 2012, 2017; Batelaan et al., 2012; Blanco et al., 2013; Katzman et al., 2014; NICE, 2011, 2013).

Discontinuation Syndrome

When the decision is made to suspend or stop antidepressant medication, a plan should be made to discontinue gradually in order to prevent the emergence of an antidepressant discontinuation syndrome that can last between 1 to 2 weeks. An antidepressant discontinuation syndrome can occur with SSRIs, SNRIs, MAOIs, and TCAs (Shelton, 2006; Wilson & Lader, 2015). Common symptoms include headache, nausea, insomnia, irritability, restlessness, paresthesia, and dizziness (Shelton, 2006). These symptoms can be confused with reemergence of the anxiety disorder. Discontinuation symptoms are more likely to occur with medications with shorter half-lives, such as paroxetine and venlafaxine. The symptoms can be rapidly reversed by restarting the original drug at the dose prescribed immediately before the dose decrease, and then tapering slowly. To prevent discontinuation symptoms, medication can be tapered slowly over a period of several weeks or longer to minimize symptoms (Bandelow et al., 2017). Another management strategy to minimize discontinuation symptoms is to substitute a drug with a longer half-life, such as fluoxetine (Schatzberg et al., 2006).

If benzodiazepines have been used either as an anxiolytic or a hypnotic, the individual may develop dependence, and on discontinuation experience withdrawal symptoms (muscle tension and spasm, restlessness, anxiety, insomnia, and in more severe instances, hallucinations and delusions; Dell'osso & Lader, 2013). Because of these concerns, the use of benzodiazepines should be controlled from the outset and limited to brief periods. There is, however, a subset of individuals with anxiety disorders who require ongoing treatment with benzodiazepines. Such individuals should be carefully monitored and their dosage of benzodiazepines controlled (Bandelow et al., 2017). Discontinuation of benzo-

diazepines after long-term use should be done slowly, with gradual tapering of the dosage using a withdrawal schedule (a link to various withdrawal schedules is provided in the Tool Kit of Resources at the end of this chapter). In some instances when a benzodiazepine with a short half-life such as alprazolam has been used, it can be substituted with a benzodiazepine with a longer half-life, such as diazepam, prior to tapering.

EVALUATION OF PHARMACOLOGICAL APPROACHES ACROSS THE LIFESPAN

In the following section we will be address the different pharmacological approaches used in managing anxiety disorders in children and adolescents, and also the elderly.

Children and Adolescents

The diagnosis of anxiety disorders in children and adolescents is difficult at times as comorbidity with other psychiatric conditions is common. Many anxiety disorders start in childhood, so recognition is important. The treatment modalities used in childhood and adolescence are psychological interventions and pharmacological interventions, namely SSRIs and SNRIs, with the effects of SSRIs and SNRIs likely amplified by the addition of psychotherapy (Hussain, Dobson, & Strawn, 2016; Katzman et al., 2014; Mohatt, Bennett, & Walkup, 2014; Wehry, Beesdo-Baum, Hennelly, Connolly, & Strawn, 2015).

Prior to commencing pharmacological treatment, informed consent should be obtained from the individual and family. Baseline severity of symptoms and functional impairment, assessed with clinical evaluation and appropriate rating scales, should be used to monitor response to treatment. Symptom severity scales used in pediatric anxiety disorders include the Multidimensional Anxiety Scale for Children (MASC; March, Parker, Sullivan, Stallings, & Conners, 1997), Screen for Child Anxiety Related Emotional Disorders (SCARED; Birmaher et al., 1997), and Spence Children's Anxiety Scale (SCAS; Spence, 1998). Similar principles as in the pharmacological management of anxiety in adults apply; pharmacotherapy is initiated at a low dose and increased slowly. In adolescents, the maximum dose of medication is similar to that for adults. It is recommended that psychotherapy is the initial intervention in the management of anxiety disorders in children and adolescents, but if there is partial or no response or if symptoms are moderate or severe, an SSRI should be started as first-line treatment (Hussain et al., 2016; Mohatt et al., 2014; Wehry et al., 2015). In children and adolescents with GAD, RCTs show efficacy of the SSRIs fluoxetine, fluvoxamine, and sertraline and the SNRI duloxetine (Birmaher et al., 2003; Hussain et al., 2016; Katzman et al., 2014; Strawn, Prakash, et al., 2015; Walkup et al., 2008). In SAD, RCTs show efficacy of the SSRIs fluoxetine, fluvoxamine, and paroxetine and the SNRI venlafaxine XR (Hussain et al., 2016; Katzman et al., 2014). A meta-analysis of the efficacy and tolerability of antidepressants in pediatric anxiety disorders noted that there was similarity among the antidepressants, and that selection of an antidepressant is therefore governed by factors such as tolerability and half-life (Strawn, Welge, Wehry, Keeshin, & Rynn, 2015).

A meta-analysis found no differences between SSRIs and SNRIs in treatment-emergent events and serious adverse events in children and adolescents (Locher et al., 2017). However, in some work SSRIs and SNRIs have been associated with an increase in suicidal ideation, and monitoring of such symptoms is important (Ipser, Stein, Hawkridge, & Hoppe, 2009). Activating adverse effects, such as restlessness and insomnia, may also be more common in children and adolescents treated with SSRIs and SNRIs than in adults (Strawn, Welge, et al., 2015), and these symptoms should be monitored (Locher et al., 2017). As with adults, benzodiazepines should be used with caution due to limited data demonstrating efficacy and due to potential adverse effects (Katzman et al., 2014). Monotherapy is advisable as far as possible. Discontinuation syndromes should be evaluated when withdrawing medication.

Elderly

The prevalence of anxiety disorders, with the exception of GAD, decreases in the elderly population (Kessler et al., 2012). However, anxiety symptoms are common; individuals presenting for the first time with anxiety symptoms should have a thorough examination to exclude an underlying medical condition (including a neurocognitive disorder) and symptoms secondary to medication. Altered pharmacokinetics (delayed absorption, increased volume of distribution and longer duration of action, decreased excretion) need to be considered in the elderly, as these physiological changes require lower doses of medication. Drug–drug interactions also need to be considered due to high rates of polypharmacy in the elderly, who often have concurrent medical conditions. Medications that have sedation as a side effect profile should be used cautiously in elderly individuals with preexisting cognitive impairment. TCAs should generally be avoided in the elderly because of cardiac effects and increased sensitivity to anticholinergic side effects (Bandelow et al., 2012).

CONSIDERATION OF POTENTIAL SEX DIFFERENCES

There are sex differences in drug pharmacokinetics (absorption, distribution, metabolism, and excretion) and pharmacodynamics (the study of the effects of drugs on the body) due to physiological differences between males and females. There is not room in this chapter to discuss all of these differences, and here the focus will be on how particular differences may influence the pharmacological interventions used in the management of anxiety disorders.

Several factors deserve consideration, such as that females generally have reduced gastric acidity and slower gastric emptying times, which may potentially increase the absorption of TCAs and benzodiazepines (Bigos, Pollock, Stankevich, & Bies, 2009; Marazziti et al., 2013; Sramek, Murphy, & Cutler, 2016). Females generally have a higher percentage of adipose tissue, and larger proportions of body fat in women may increase the storage of lipophilic medications such as the benzodiazepine diazepam and the antidepressant trazodone, resulting in an increase in the half-life of these agents (Bigos et al., 2009; Marazziti et al., 2013; Soldin & Mattison, 2009). Some of the CYP450 enzymes involved in metabolism show clear sex differences, with higher activity of CYP2D6 and CYP3A4 in females. This increased activity may result in drug substrates being cleared faster in females. A number of SSRIs, SNRIs, TCAs, and benzodiazepines are metabolized by CYP2D6 and CYP3A4 (Bigos et al., 2009; Soldin & Mattison, 2009; Marazziti et al., 2013; Sramek et al., 2016). Females have decreased capacity for glomerular filtration (a process performed by the kidneys to filter excess fluid and waste products out of the blood), with reduced elimination of certain compounds (Marazziti et al., 2013). Pharmacodynamic differences may result in females being more responsive to SSRI antidepressants versus TCAs (Soldin & Mattison, 2009; Sramek et al., 2016). Females generally have a longer cardiac QT interval (a measurement of time between the start of the Q wave and the end of the T wave on an electrocardiogram; it reflects the time from the onset of depolarization to the onset of repolarization of the ventricles) than males, and so female sex is a predisposing risk factor when prescribing QT-prolonging medications that can lead to arrhythmias. Medications that prolong QT interval include citalopram, escitalopram, clomipramine, and imipramine (Soldin & Mattison, 2009).

In choosing interventions for the treatment of anxiety disorders in pregnant and breastfeeding women, the risk–benefit ratio should be assessed. The risk of an untreated anxiety disorder and of pharmacological interventions to the developing fetus and newborn need to be weighed against potential benefits. If possible, psychological rather than pharmacological interventions should be used during this period (Baldwin et al., 2014; Bandelow et al., 2017). Paroxetine and possibly fluoxetine use in early pregnancy may be associated with a small increased risk for cardiovascular malformations in the fetus (Ellfolk & Malm, 2010; Gao et al., 2017; Grigoriadis et al., 2013). In terms of delivery outcomes with antidepressant use, there is evidence for increased risk of preterm birth, low birth weight, or being small for gestational age, but the effects are small and scores in the exposed group are typically within normal ranges (Ross et al., 2013).

INTEGRATION OF PHARMACOTHERAPY WITH NONPHARMACOLOGICAL APPROACHES: BENEFITS AND CHALLENGES

When planning a treatment program, the individual's preferences should be considered. Psychological treatments are frequently requested, and cognitive behavior therapy (CBT) has a strong evidence base demonstrating efficacy for anxiety disorders.

In GAD, robust evidence exists for the short- and long-term efficacy of CBT (Bandelow et al., 2015; Carpenter et al., 2018; Cuijpers, Cristea, Karyotaki, Reijnders, & Huibers, 2016; Hunot, Churchill, Silva de Lima, & Teixeira, 2007; Leichsenring et al., 2009; Salzer, Winkelbach, Leweke, Leibing, & Leichsenring, 2011). There is also some evidence for the short- and long-term efficacy of short-term psychodynamic therapy and relaxation therapy (Leichsenring et al., 2009; Montero-Marin, Garcia-Campayo, Lopez-Montoyo, Zabaleta-Del-Olmo, & Cuijpers, 2017; Salzer et al., 2011). There is conflicting evidence about the benefits of combined pharmacological and psychological interventions (Katzman et al., 2014).

With PD, there is evidence for the efficacy of CBT and exposure therapy (Bandelow et al., 2015; Cuijpers et al., 2016; Hofmann & Smits, 2008). A meta-analysis of psychological interventions for PD noted that in the long term, CBT and psychodynamic psychotherapy showed the highest rate of remission among the several interventions analyzed (Pompoli et al., 2016). CBT panic disorder protocols may vary from 6 to 14 sessions, with evidence of better results with longer duration of CBT in individuals with higher baseline severity of symptoms and functional impairment. Interventions such as bibliotherapy (self-help books), telephone interventions, and Internet-based CBT may be effective options in situations with limited therapist availability (Lewis, Pearce, & Bisson, 2012). A meta-analysis suggested that due to low-quality evidence, the superiority of psychological versus pharmacological interventions cannot be established (Imai, Tajika, Chen, Pompoli, & Furukawa, 2016). However, evidence does suggest that a combination of psychotherapy and antidepressants are superior to either one alone (Cuijpers et al., 2014; Furukawa,

Watanabe, & Churchill, 2007; Hofmann, Sawyer, Korte, & Smits, 2009).

In SAD, there is good evidence to support the use of CBT (Hofmann & Smits, 2008; Mayo-Wilson et al., 2014). Evidence supports the superiority of CBT over exposure therapy for SAD in the short and long term (Ougrin, 2011). As with PD, self-help interventions and Internet-based CBT may be effective options in situations with limited therapist availability (Berger, Hohl, & Caspar, 2009; Lewis et al., 2012). As with GAD, there is conflicting evidence regarding the value of combining pharmacological and psychological interventions (Katzman et al., 2014).

INTEGRATED APPROACHES FOR ADDRESSING COMMON COMORBID DISORDERS

As noted, anxiety disorders are frequently comorbid with one another and with other psychiatric disorders; about 60% to 80% of patients with an anxiety disorder have at least one other comorbid psychiatric condition (Katzman et al., 2014). The high probability of comorbid disorders should be considered when determining treatment interventions and one should opt for interventions that are effective for both disorders.

For anxiety disorders with comorbid depressive disorder, the SSRIs and SNRIs may be useful as first-line pharmacotherapy (Baldwin et al., 2014; APA, 2010; Katzman et al., 2014). All the SSRIs and the TCA clomipramine are recommended for OCD (see Chapter 11, this volume) with anxiety disorders (Baldwin et al., 2014). With PTSD (see Chapter 13, this volume) and anxiety, the SSRIs paroxetine and sertraline and the SNRI venlafaxine are recommended (Baldwin et al., 2014). For anxiety disorders comorbid with bipolar disorder (see Chapter 8, this volume), caution in using antidepressants is required, as these agents may exacerbate bipolar symptoms, and atypical antipsychotics may have a role (Baldwin et al., 2014; Goodwin et al., 2016; Katzman et al., 2014).

Anxiety disorders are associated with increased presence of medical disorders (cardiovascular conditions, thyroid disease, migraines, allergic conditions, gastrointestinal conditions, respiratory disease, arthritis) and pain disorders (Sareen et al., 2006). When choosing a treatment intervention, the impact of anxiolytic treatment on cardiovascular and metabolic comorbidity and potential drug–drug interactions associated with concomitant psychiatric and physical medications needs to be considered.

EMERGING TRENDS

Although first-line pharmacotherapy is often efficacious, the high prevalence of anxiety disorders and the fact that not all individuals respond to treatment means that there is a need for improved treatments. In addition, current anxiolytic agents have several limitations, either related to side effects profiles, such as with TCAs, benzodiazepines, and atypical antipsychotics, or due to the delayed onset of action of the SSRIs and SNRIs. There is significant focus on translational neuroscience and personalized medicine as having the potential to provide new treatment targets and optimized management strategies over the longer term.

In the short term, a number of new agents have been introduced to the market. Vortioxetine, which inhibits the serotonin transporter and has agonistic and antagonistic actions on a number of serotonin receptors, has had equivocal results in GAD. Vilazodone, which functions as an SSRI and a $5HT_{1A}$ receptor partial agonist, has shown some benefit in the treatment of depression with anxious features, but further studies are required to assess its efficacy in the treatment of anxiety disorders. The atypical antipsychotic aripiprazole has antagonist activity at $5HT_{1A}$ and $5HT_{2A}$ receptors as well as partial agonist action at D_2 receptors, and open-label trials in GAD and PD have been encouraging, but again further studies are needed to determine its efficacy in the treatment of anxiety disorders (Murrough, Yaqubi, Sayed, & Charney, 2015).

Emphasis has also been placed on studying agents that act on the glutamate system, namely metabotropic glutamate receptor modulators, and on agents that potentiate glutamate NMDA (N-methyl-d-aspartate) receptor signaling. However, no such agents have been FDA approved. The neuropeptide and endocannabinoid systems are being targeted for study as well (Griebel & Holmes, 2013; Murrough et al., 2015). Finally, there is also growing interest in the use of specific agents such as the glutamatergic drug D-cycloserine for augmenting CBT for anxiety disorders. To date, such approaches remain at the level of proof of principle (an early stage of clinical drug development), but they provide hope for future advances.

TOOL KIT OF RESOURCES

Patient Resources

American Academy of Child and Adolescent Psychiatry, Anxiety Disorders Resource Center: https://www.aacap.org/AACAP/Families_and_Youth/Resource_Centers/Anxiety_Disorder_Resource_Center/Home.aspx

Anxiety and Depression Association of America (ADAA), Online Resources: https://adaa.org/living-with-anxiety/ask-and-learn/resources#

National Institute of Mental Health (NIMH), Health and Education, Mental Health Information: Anxiety Disorders: https://www.nimh.nih.gov/health/topics/anxiety-disorders/index.shtml

National Institute of Mental Health (NIMH), Health and Education, Publications: Generalized Anxiety Disorder: When Worry Gets Out of Control: https://www.nimh.nih.gov/health/publications/generalized-anxiety-disorder-gad/index.shtml

National Institute of Mental Health (NIMH), Health and Education, Publications: Panic Disorder: When Fear Overwhelms: https://www.nimh.nih.gov/health/publications/panic-disorder-when-fear-overwhelms/index.shtml

National Institute of Mental Health (NIMH), Health and Education, Publications: Social Anxiety Disorder: More Than Just Shyness: https://www.nimh.nih.gov/health/publications/social-anxiety-disorder-more-than-just-shyness/index.shtml

Provider Resources

Generalized Anxiety Disorder 7-Item Scale (GAD-7): https://www.mdcalc.com/gad-7-general-anxiety-disorder-7; https://psychology-tools.com/gad-7/

Hamilton Anxiety Rating Scale (HAM-A): https://www.mdcalc.com/hamilton-anxiety-scale; https://psychology-tools.com/hamilton-anxiety-rating-scale/

Panic Disorder Severity Scale: http://www.goodmedicine.org.uk/files/panic,%20assessment%20pdss.pdf

Liebowitz Social Anxiety Scale (LSAS): https://psychology-tools.com/liebowitz-social-anxiety-scale/

Social Phobia Inventory (SPIN): https://psychology-tools.com/spin/

Sheehan Disability Scale (SDS): http://www.cqaimh.org/pdf/tool_lof_sds.pdf

Benzodiazepine Withdrawal Schedules: https://www.benzo.org.uk/manual/bzsched.htm

Baldwin, D. S., Waldman, S., & Allgulander, C. (2011). Evidence-based pharmacological treatment of generalized anxiety disorder. *The International Journal of Neuropsychopharmacology, 14*, 697–710. http://dx.doi.org/10.1017/S1461145710001434

Baldwin, D. S., Anderson, I. M., Nutt, D. J., Allgulander, C., Bandelow, B., den Boer, J. A., . . . Wittchen, H. U. (2014). Evidence-based pharmacological treatment of anxiety disorders, post-traumatic stress disorder and obsessive-compulsive disorder: A revision of the 2005 guidelines from the British Association for Psychopharmacology. *Journal of Psychopharmacology (Oxford, England), 28*, 403–439. http://dx.doi.org/10.1177/0269881114525674

Bandelow, B., Sher, L., Bunevicius, R., Hollander, E., Kasper, S., Zohar, J., . . . WFSBP Task Force on Anxiety Disorders, OCD and PTSD. (2012). Guidelines for the pharmacological treatment of anxiety disorders, obsessive-compulsive disorder and post-traumatic stress disorder in primary care. *International Journal of Psychiatry in Clinical Practice, 16*, 77–84. http://dx.doi.org/10.3109/13651501.2012.667114

Bandelow, B., Michaelis, S., & Wedekind, D. (2017). Treatment of anxiety disorders. *Dialogues in Clinical Neuroscience, 19*(2), 93–107.

Batelaan, N. M., Van Balkom, A. J., & Stein, D. J. (2012). Evidence-based pharmacotherapy of panic disorder: An update. *The International Journal of Neuropsychopharmacology, 15*, 403–415. http://dx.doi.org/10.1017/S1461145711000800

Blanco, C., Bragdon, L. B., Schneier, F. R., & Liebowitz, M. R. (2013). The evidence-based pharmacotherapy of social anxiety disorder. *The International Journal of Neuropsychopharmacology, 16*, 235–249. http://dx.doi.org/10.1017/S1461145712000119

International Association for Child and Adolescent Psychiatry and Allied Professions (IACAPAP) Textbook of Child and Adolescent Mental Health: http://iacapap.org/iacapap-textbook-of-child-and-adolescent-mental-health

Katzman, M. A., Bleau, P., Blier, P., Chokka, P., Kjernisted, K., Van Ameringen, M., . . . Walker, J. R. (2014). Canadian clinical practice guidelines for the management of anxiety, posttraumatic stress and obsessive-compulsive disorders. *BMC Psychiatry, 14*(Suppl. 1), S1. http://dx.doi.org/10.1186/1471-244X-14-S1-S1

References

Allgulander, C., & Baldwin, D. S. (2013). Pharmacotherapy of generalized anxiety disorder. *Modern Trends in Pharmacopsychiatry*, *29*, 119–127. http://dx.doi.org/10.1159/000351955

Allgulander, C., Dahl, A. A., Austin, C., Morris, P. L., Sogaard, J. A., Fayyad, R., . . . Clary, C. M. (2004). Efficacy of sertraline in a 12-week trial for generalized anxiety disorder. *The American Journal of Psychiatry*, *161*, 1642–1649. http://dx.doi.org/10.1176/appi.ajp.161.9.1642

Allgulander, C., Florea, I., & Huusom, A. K. (2006). Prevention of relapse in generalized anxiety disorder by escitalopram treatment. *The International Journal of Neuropsychopharmacology*, *9*, 495–505. http://dx.doi.org/10.1017/S1461145705005973

Allgulander, C., Mangano, R., Zhang, J., Dahl, A. A., Lepola, U., Sjödin, I., Emilien, G., & the SAD 388 Study Group. (2004). Efficacy of Venlafaxine ER in patients with social anxiety disorder: A double-blind, placebo-controlled, parallel-group comparison with paroxetine. *Human Psychopharmacology: Clinical and Experimental*, *19*, 387–396. http://dx.doi.org/10.1002/hup.602

American Psychiatric Association. (2009). *Practice guideline for the treatment of patients with panic disorder*. Retrieved from https://psychiatryonline.org/pb/assets/raw/sitewide/practice_guidelines/guidelines/panicdisorder.pdf

American Psychiatric Association. (2010). *Practice guideline for the treatment of patients with major depressive disorder*. Retrieved from https://psychiatryonline.org/pb/assets/raw/sitewide/practice_guidelines/guidelines/mdd.pdf

American Psychiatric Association. (2013). *Diagnostic and statistical manual of mental disorders* (5th ed.). Arlington, VA: Author.

Asnis, G. M., Hameedi, F. A., Goddard, A. W., Potkin, S. G., Black, D., Jameel, M., . . . Woods, S. W. (2001). Fluvoxamine in the treatment of panic disorder: A multi-center, double-blind, placebo-controlled study in outpatients. *Psychiatry Research*, *103*, 1–14. http://dx.doi.org/10.1016/S0165-1781(01)00265-7

Baldwin, D. S., Ajel, K., Masdrakis, V. G., Nowak, M., & Rafiq, R. (2013). Pregabalin for the treatment of generalized anxiety disorder: An update. *Neuropsychiatric Disease and Treatment*, *9*, 883–892. http://dx.doi.org/10.2147/NDT.S36453

*Baldwin, D. S., Anderson, I. M., Nutt, D. J., Allgulander, C., Bandelow, B., den Boer, J. A., . . . Wittchen, H. U. (2014). Evidence-based pharmacological treatment of anxiety disorders, post-traumatic stress disorder and obsessive-compulsive disorder: A revision of the 2005 guidelines from the British Association for Psychopharmacology. *Journal of Psychopharmacology*, *28*, 403–439. http://dx.doi.org/10.1177/0269881114525674

Baldwin, D. S., Huusom, A. K., & Maehlum, E. (2006). Escitalopram and paroxetine in the treatment of generalised anxiety disorder: Randomised, placebo-controlled, double-blind study. *The British Journal of Psychiatry*, *189*, 264–272. http://dx.doi.org/10.1192/bjp.bp.105.012799

*Baldwin, D. S., Waldman, S., & Allgulander, C. (2011). Evidence-based pharmacological treatment of generalized anxiety disorder. *International Journal of Neuropsychopharmacology*, *14*, 697–710. http://dx.doi.org/10.1017/S1461145710001434

*Bandelow, B., Michaelis, S., & Wedekind, D. (2017). Treatment of anxiety disorders. *Dialogues in Clinical Neuroscience*, *19*(2), 93–107.

Bandelow, B., Reitt, M., Röver, C., Michaelis, S., Görlich, Y., & Wedekind, D. (2015). Efficacy of treatments for anxiety disorders: A meta-analysis. *International Clinical Psychopharmacology*, *30*, 183–192. http://dx.doi.org/10.1097/YIC.0000000000000078

*Bandelow, B., Sher, L., Bunevicius, R., Hollander, E., Kasper, S., Zohar, J., Möller, H. J., the WFSBP Task Force on Mental Disorders in Primary Care, & the WFSBP Task Force on Anxiety Disorders, OCD and PTSD. (2012). Guidelines for the pharmacological treatment of anxiety disorders, obsessive-compulsive disorder and posttraumatic stress disorder in primary care. *International Journal of Psychiatry in Clinical Practice*, *16*, 77–84. http://dx.doi.org/10.3109/13651501.2012.667114

Barnett, S. D., Kramer, M. L., Casat, C. D., Connor, K. M., & Davidson, J. R. (2002). Efficacy of olanzapine in social anxiety disorder: A pilot study. *Journal of Psychopharmacology*, *16*, 365–368. http://dx.doi.org/10.1177/026988110201600412

Barrera, T. L., & Norton, P. J. (2009). Quality of life impairment in generalized anxiety disorder, social phobia, and panic disorder. *Journal of Anxiety Disorders*, *23*, 1086–1090. http://dx.doi.org/10.1016/j.janxdis.2009.07.011

*Batelaan, N. M., Van Balkom, A. J., & Stein, D. J. (2012). Evidence-based pharmacotherapy of panic disorder: An update. *International Journal of Neuropsychopharmacology*, *15*, 403–415. http://dx.doi.org/10.1017/S1461145711000800

Berger, T., Hohl, E., & Caspar, F. (2009). Internet-based treatment for social phobia: A randomized controlled trial. *Journal of Clinical Psychology*, *65*, 1021–1035. http://dx.doi.org/10.1002/jclp.20603

Bigos, K. L., Pollock, B. G., Stankevich, B. A., & Bies, R. R. (2009). Sex differences in the pharmacokinetics and

*Asterisks indicate assessments or resources.

pharmacodynamics of antidepressants: An updated review. *Gender Medicine, 6*, 522–543. http://dx.doi.org/10.1016/j.genm.2009.12.004

Birmaher, B., Axelson, D. A., Monk, K., Kalas, C., Clark, D. B., Ehmann, M., . . . Brent, D. A. (2003). Fluoxetine for the treatment of childhood anxiety disorders. *Journal of the American Academy of Child & Adolescent Psychiatry, 42*, 415–423. http://dx.doi.org/10.1097/01.CHI.0000037049.04952.9F

Birmaher, B., Khetarpal, S., Brent, D., Cully, M., Balach, L., Kaufman, J., & Neer, S. M. (1997). The screen for child anxiety related emotional disorders (SCARED): Scale construction and psychometric characteristics. *Journal of the American Academy of Child and Adolescent Psychiatry, 36*, 545–553. http://dx.doi.org/10.1097/00004583-199704000-00018

*Blanco, C., Bragdon, L. B., Schneier, F. R., & Liebowitz, M. R. (2013). The evidence-based pharmacotherapy of social anxiety disorder. *International Journal of Neuropsychopharmacology, 16*, 235–249. http://dx.doi.org/10.1017/S1461145712000119

Boschen, M. J. (2011). A meta-analysis of the efficacy of pregabalin in the treatment of generalized anxiety disorder. *Canadian Journal of Psychiatry, 56*, 558–566. http://dx.doi.org/10.1177/070674371105600907

Bruce, S. E., Yonkers, K. A., Otto, M. W., Eisen, J. L., Weisberg, R. B., Pagano, M., . . . Keller, M. B. (2005). Influence of psychiatric comorbidity on recovery and recurrence in generalized anxiety disorder, social phobia, and panic disorder: A 12-year prospective study. *The American Journal of Psychiatry, 162*, 1179–1187. http://dx.doi.org/10.1176/appi.ajp.162.6.1179

Carpenter, J. K., Andrews, L. A., Witcraft, S. M., Powers, M. B., Smits, J. A. J., & Hofmann, S. G. (2018). Cognitive behavioral therapy for anxiety and related disorders: A meta-analysis of randomized placebo-controlled trials. *Depression and Anxiety, 35*, 502–514. http://dx.doi.org/10.1002/da.22728

Chessick, C. A., Allen, M. H., Thase, M., Batista Miralha da Cunha, A. B., Kapczinski, F. F., de Lima, M. S., & dos Santos Souza, J. J. (2006). Azapirones for generalized anxiety disorder. *Cochrane Database of Systematic Reviews, 3*, CD006115. http://dx.doi.org/10.1002/14651858.CD006115

Connor, K. M., Davidson, J. R., Churchill, L. E., Sherwood, A., Weisler, R. H., & Foa, E. (2000). Psychometric properties of the Social Phobia Inventory (SPIN). New self-rating scale. *The British Journal of Psychiatry, 176*, 379–386. http://dx.doi.org/10.1192/bjp.176.4.379

Craske, M. G., & Stein, M. B. (2016). Anxiety. *Lancet, 388*, 3048–3059. http://dx.doi.org/10.1016/S0140-6736(16)30381-6

Cuijpers, P., Cristea, I. A., Karyotaki, E., Reijnders, M., & Huibers, M. J. (2016). How effective are cognitive behavior therapies for major depression and anxiety disorders? A meta-analytic update of the evidence. *World Psychiatry, 15*, 245–258. http://dx.doi.org/10.1002/wps.20346

Cuijpers, P., Sijbrandij, M., Koole, S. L., Andersson, G., Beekman, A. T., & Reynolds, C. F., III. (2014). Adding psychotherapy to antidepressant medication in depression and anxiety disorders: A meta-analysis. *World Psychiatry, 13*, 56–67. http://dx.doi.org/10.1002/wps.20089

Dannon, P. N., Iancu, I., Lowengrub, K., Gonopolsky, Y., Musin, E., Grunhaus, L., & Kotler, M. (2007). A naturalistic long-term comparison study of selective serotonin reuptake inhibitors in the treatment of panic disorder. *Clinical Neuropharmacology, 30*, 326–334. http://dx.doi.org/10.1097/WNF.0b013e318064579f

Davidson, J. R., Wittchen, H. U., Llorca, P. M., Erickson, J., Detke, M., Ball, S. G., & Russell, J. M. (2008). Duloxetine treatment for relapse prevention in adults with generalized anxiety disorder: A double-blind placebo-controlled trial. *European Neuropsychopharmacology, 18*, 673–681. http://dx.doi.org/10.1016/j.euroneuro.2008.05.002

Davis, M. L., Smits, J. A., & Hofmann, S. G. (2014). Update on the efficacy of pharmacotherapy for social anxiety disorder: A meta-analysis. *Expert Opinion on Pharmacotherapy, 15*, 2281–2291. http://dx.doi.org/10.1517/14656566.2014.955472

Dell'osso, B., & Lader, M. (2013). Do benzodiazepines still deserve a major role in the treatment of psychiatric disorders? A critical reappraisal. *European Psychiatry, 28*, 7–20. http://dx.doi.org/10.1016/j.eurpsy.2011.11.003

Depping, A. M., Komossa, K., Kissling, W., & Leucht, S. (2010). Second-generation antipsychotics for anxiety disorders. *Cochrane Database of Systematic Reviews, 12*, CD008120. http://dx.doi.org/10.1002/14651858.CD008120.pub2

Doyle, A. C., & Pollack, M. H. (2003). Establishment of remission criteria for anxiety disorders. *The Journal of Clinical Psychiatry, 64*(Suppl. 15), 40–45.

Ellfolk, M., & Malm, H. (2010). Risks associated with in utero and lactation exposure to selective serotonin reuptake inhibitors (SSRIs). *Reproductive Toxicology, 30*, 249–260. http://dx.doi.org/10.1016/j.reprotox.2010.04.015

Feltner, D., Wittchen, H. U., Kavoussi, R., Brock, J., Baldinetti, F., & Pande, A. C. (2008). Long-term efficacy of pregabalin in generalized anxiety disorder. *International Clinical Psychopharmacology, 23*, 18–28. http://dx.doi.org/10.1097/YIC.0b013e3282f0f0d7

Ferguson, J. M., Khan, A., Mangano, R., Entsuah, R., & Tzanis, E. (2007). Relapse prevention of panic disorder in adult outpatient responders to treatment with venlafaxine extended release. *The Journal of Clinical Psychiatry, 68,* 58–68. http://dx.doi.org/10.4088/JCP.v68n0108

Furmark, T., Appel, L., Michelgard, A., Wahlstedt, K., Ahs, F., Zancan, S., . . . Fredrikson, M. (2005). Cerebral blood flow changes after treatment of social phobia with the neurokinin-1 antagonist GR205171, citalopram, or placebo. *Biological Psychiatry, 58,* 132–142. http://dx.doi.org/10.1016/j.biopsych.2005.03.029

Furukawa, T. A., Watanabe, N., & Churchill, R. (2007). Combined psychotherapy plus antidepressants for panic disorder with or without agoraphobia. *Cochrane Database of Systematic Reviews, 1,* CD004364. http://dx.doi.org/10.1002/14651858.CD004364.pub2

Gao, S. Y., Wu, Q. J., Zhang, T. N., Shen, Z. Q., Liu, C. X., Xu, X., . . . Zhao, Y. H. (2017). Fluoxetine and congenital malformations: A systematic review and meta-analysis of cohort studies. *British Journal of Clinical Pharmacology, 83,* 2134–2147. http://dx.doi.org/10.1111/bcp.13321

Gelenberg, A. J., Lydiard, R. B., Rudolph, R. L., Aguiar, L., Haskins, J. T., & Salinas, E. (2000). Efficacy of venlafaxine extended-release capsules in nondepressed outpatients with generalized anxiety disorder: A 6-month randomized controlled trial. *JAMA, 283,* 3082–3088. http://dx.doi.org/10.1001/jama.283.23.3082

Goddard, A. W., Brouette, T., Almai, A., Jetty, P., Woods, S. W., & Charney, D. (2001). Early coadministration of clonazepam with sertraline for panic disorder. *Archives of General Psychiatry, 58,* 681–686. http://dx.doi.org/10.1001/archpsyc.58.7.681

Goodman, W. K., Bose, A., & Wang, Q. (2005). Treatment of generalized anxiety disorder with escitalopram: Pooled results from double-blind, placebo-controlled trials. *Journal of Affective Disorders, 87,* 161–167. http://dx.doi.org/10.1016/j.jad.2004.11.011

Goodwin, G. M., Haddad, P. M., Ferrier, I. N., Aronson, J. K., Barnes, T., Cipriani, A., . . . Young, A. H. (2016). Evidence-based guidelines for treating bipolar disorder: Revised third edition recommendations from the British association for psychopharmacology. *Journal of Psychopharmacology, 30,* 495–553. http://dx.doi.org/10.1177/0269881116636545

Griebel, G., & Holmes, A. (2013). 50 years of hurdles and hope in anxiolytic drug discovery. *Nature Reviews. Drug Discovery, 12,* 667–687. http://dx.doi.org/10.1038/nrd4075

Grigoriadis, S., VonderPorten, E. H., Mamisashvili, L., Roerecke, M., Rehm, J., Dennis, C. L., . . . Ross, L. E. (2013). Antidepressant exposure during pregnancy and congenital malformations: Is there an association? A systematic review and meta-analysis of the best evidence. *The Journal of Clinical Psychiatry, 74,* e293–e308. http://dx.doi.org/10.4088/JCP.12r07966

Guaiana, G., Barbui, C., & Cipriani, A. (2010). Hydroxyzine for generalised anxiety disorder. *Cochrane Database of Systematic Reviews, 12,* CD006815. http://dx.doi.org/10.1002/14651858.CD006815.pub2

Hamilton, M. (1959). The assessment of anxiety states by rating. *British Journal of Medical Psychology, 32,* 50–55. http://dx.doi.org/10.1111/j.2044-8341.1959.tb00467.x

Hartford, J., Kornstein, S., Liebowitz, M., Pigott, T., Russell, J., Detke, M., . . . Erickson, J. (2007). Duloxetine as an SNRI treatment for generalized anxiety disorder: Results from a placebo and active-controlled trial. *International Clinical Psychopharmacology, 22,* 167–174. http://dx.doi.org/10.1097/YIC.0b013e32807fb1b2

Hirschfeld, R. M. (2003). Long-term side effects of SSRIs: Sexual dysfunction and weight gain. *The Journal of Clinical Psychiatry, 64*(Suppl. 18), 20–24.

Hofmann, S. G., Sawyer, A. T., Korte, K. J., & Smits, J. A. (2009). Is it beneficial to add pharmacotherapy to cognitive-behavioral therapy when treating anxiety disorders? A meta-analytic review. *International Journal of Cognitive Therapy, 2,* 160–175. http://dx.doi.org/10.1521/ijct.2009.2.2.160

Hofmann, S. G., & Smits, J. A. (2008). Cognitive-behavioral therapy for adult anxiety disorders: A meta-analysis of randomized placebo-controlled trials. *The Journal of Clinical Psychiatry, 69*(4), 621–632.

Hunot, V., Churchill, R., Silva de Lima, M., & Teixeira, V. (2007). Psychological therapies for generalised anxiety disorder. *Cochrane Database of Systematic Reviews, 1,* CD001848. http://dx.doi.org/10.1002/14651858.CD001848.pub4

Hussain, F. S., Dobson, E. T., & Strawn, J. R. (2016). Pharmacologic treatment of pediatric anxiety disorders. *Current Treatment Options in Psychiatry, 3,* 151–160. http://dx.doi.org/10.1007/s40501-016-0076-7

Imai, H., Tajika, A., Chen, P., Pompoli, A., & Furukawa, T. A. (2016). Psychological therapies versus pharmacological interventions for panic disorder with or without agoraphobia in adults. *Cochrane Database of Systematic Reviews, 10,* CD011170.

Ipser, J. C., Stein, D. J., Hawkridge, S., & Hoppe, L. (2009). Pharmacotherapy for anxiety disorders in children and adolescents. *Cochrane Database of Systematic Reviews, 3,* CD005170. http://dx.doi.org/10.1002/14651858.CD005170.pub2

Kasper, S., Herman, B., Nivoli, G., Van Ameringen, M., Petralia, A., Mandel, F. S., . . . Bandelow, B. (2009). Efficacy of pregabalin and venlafaxine-XR in generalized anxiety disorder: Results of a double-blind, placebo-controlled 8-week trial. *International Clinical Psychopharmacology, 24,* 87–96. http://dx.doi.org/10.1097/YIC.0b013e32831d7980

Kasper, S., Stein, D. J., Loft, H., & Nil, R. (2005). Escitalopram in the treatment of social anxiety disorder: Randomised, placebo-controlled, flexible-dosage study. *The British Journal of Psychiatry 186*, 222–226. http://dx.doi.org/10.1192/bjp.186.3.222

*Katzman, M. A., Bleau, P., Blier, P., Chokka, P., Kjernisted, K., Van Ameringen, M., . . . Walker, J. R. (2014). Canadian clinical practice guidelines for the management of anxiety, posttraumatic stress and obsessive-compulsive disorders. *BMC Psychiatry, 14*(Suppl. 1), S1-244X-14-S1-S1. http://dx.doi.org/10.1186/1471-244X-14-S1-S1

Katzman, M. A., Brawman-Mintzer, O., Reyes, E. B., Olausson, B., Liu, S., & Eriksson, H. (2011). Extended release quetiapine fumarate (quetiapine XR) monotherapy as maintenance treatment for generalized anxiety disorder: A long-term, randomized, placebo-controlled trial. *International Clinical Psychopharmacology, 26*, 11–24. http://dx.doi.org/10.1097/YIC.0b013e32833e34d9

Kessler, R. C., Chiu, W. T., Demler, O., Merikangas, K. R., & Walters, E. E. (2005). Prevalence, severity, and comorbidity of 12-month *DSM–IV* disorders in the national comorbidity survey replication. *Archives of General Psychiatry, 62*, 617–627. http://dx.doi.org/10.1001/archpsyc.62.6.617

Kessler, R. C., Petukhova, M., Sampson, N. A., Zaslavsky, A. M., & Wittchen, H. U. (2012). Twelve-month and lifetime prevalence and lifetime morbid risk of anxiety and mood disorders in the United States. *International Journal of Methods in Psychiatric Research, 21*, 169–184. http://dx.doi.org/10.1002/mpr.1359

Klerman, G. (1992). Drug treatment of panic disorder: Comparative efficacy of alprazolam, imipramine, and placebo: Cross-National Collaborative Panic Study, Second Phase Investigators. *The British Journal of Psychiatry, 160*, 191–202. http://dx.doi.org/10.1192/bjp.160.2.191

Kroenke, K., Spitzer, R. L., Williams, J. B., Monahan, P. O., & Lowe, B. (2007). Anxiety disorders in primary care: Prevalence, impairment, comorbidity, and detection. *Annals of Internal Medicine, 146*, 317–325. http://dx.doi.org/146/5/317

Lecrubier, Y., Judge, R., & the Collaborative Paroxetine Panic Study Investigators. (1997). Long-term evaluation of paroxetine, clomipramine and placebo in panic disorder. *Acta Psychiatrica Scandinavica, 95*, 153–160. http://dx.doi.org/10.1111/j.1600-0447.1997.tb00389.x

Leichsenring, F., Salzer, S., Jaeger, U., Kächele, H., Kreische, R., Leweke, F., . . . Leibing, E. (2009). Short-term psychodynamic psychotherapy and cognitive-behavioral therapy in generalized anxiety disorder: A randomized, controlled trial. *The American Journal of Psychiatry, 166*, 875–881. http://dx.doi.org/10.1176/appi.ajp.2009.09030441

Lepola, U., Bergholdt, B., St. Lambert, J., Davy, K. L., & Ruggiero, L. (2004). Controlled-release paroxetine in the treatment of patients with social anxiety disorder. *The Journal of Clinical Psychiatry, 65*, 222–229. http://dx.doi.org/10.4088/JCP.v65n0213

Lepola, U. M., Wade, A. G., Leinonen, E. V., Koponen, H. J., Frazer, J., Sjödin, I., . . . Lehto, H. J. (1998). A controlled, prospective, 1-year trial of citalopram in the treatment of panic disorder. *The Journal of Clinical Psychiatry, 59*, 528–534. http://dx.doi.org/10.4088/JCP.v59n1006

Lewis, C., Pearce, J., & Bisson, J. I. (2012). Efficacy, cost-effectiveness and acceptability of self-help interventions for anxiety disorders: Systematic review. *The British Journal of Psychiatry, 200*, 15–21. http://dx.doi.org/10.1192/bjp.bp.110.084756

Liebowitz, M. R. (1987). Social phobia. *Modern Problems of Pharmacopsychiatry, 22*, 141–173. http://dx.doi.org/10.1159/000414022

Locher, C., Koechlin, H., Zion, S. R., Werner, C., Pine, D. S., Kirsch, I., . . . Kossowsky, J. (2017). Efficacy and safety of selective serotonin reuptake inhibitors, serotonin-norepinephrine reuptake inhibitors, and placebo for common psychiatric disorders among children and adolescents: A systematic review and meta-analysis. *JAMA Psychiatry, 74*, 1011–1020. http://dx.doi.org/10.1001/jamapsychiatry.2017.2432

Maglione, M., Maher, A. R., Hu, J., Wang, Z., Shanman, R., Shekelle, P. G., & Perry, T. (2011). *Off-label use of atypical antipsychotics: An update*. Rockville, MD: Agency for Healthcare Research and Quality.

Marazziti, D., Baroni, S., Picchetti, M., Piccinni, A., Carlini, M., Vatteroni, E., . . . Dell'Osso, L. (2013). Pharmacokinetics and pharmacodynamics of psychotropic drugs: Effect of sex. *CNS Spectrums, 18*, 118–127. http://dx.doi.org/10.1017/S1092852912001010

March, J. S., Parker, J. D., Sullivan, K., Stallings, P., & Conners, C. K. (1997). The multidimensional anxiety scale for children (MASC): Factor structure, reliability, and validity. *Journal of the American Academy of Child and Adolescent Psychiatry, 36*, 554–565. http://dx.doi.org/10.1097/00004583-199704000-00019

Mayo-Wilson, E., Dias, S., Mavranezouli, I., Kew, K., Clark, D. M., Ades, A. E., & Pilling, S. (2014). Psychological and pharmacological interventions for social anxiety disorder in adults: A systematic review and network meta-analysis. *The Lancet Psychiatry, 1*, 368–376. http://dx.doi.org/10.1016/S2215-0366(14)70329-3

Michelson, D., Allgulander, C., Dantendorfer, K., Knezevic, A., Maierhofer, D., Micev, V., . . . Pemberton, S. C. (2001). Efficacy of usual antidepressant dosing regimens of fluoxetine in panic disorder: Randomised, placebo-controlled trial. *The British Journal of Psychiatry, 179*, 514–518. http://dx.doi.org/10.1192/bjp.179.6.514

Miller, R. W., & Rollnick, S. (2002). *Motivational interviewing: Preparing people for change*. New York, NY: Guilford Press.

Milne, B. J., Caspi, A., Harrington, H., Poulton, R., Rutter, M., & Moffitt, T. E. (2009). Predictive value of family history on severity of illness: The case for depression, anxiety, alcohol dependence, and drug dependence. *Archives of General Psychiatry, 66*, 738–747. http://dx.doi.org/10.1001/archgenpsychiatry.2009.55

Mohatt, J., Bennett, S. M., & Walkup, J. T. (2014). Treatment of separation, generalized, and social anxiety disorders in youths. *The American Journal of Psychiatry, 171*, 741–748. http://dx.doi.org/10.1176/appi.ajp.2014.13101337

Montero-Marin, J., Garcia-Campayo, J., Lopez-Montoyo, A., Zabaleta-Del-Olmo, E., & Cuijpers, P. (2017). Is cognitive-behavioural therapy more effective than relaxation therapy in the treatment of anxiety disorders? A meta-analysis. *Psychological Medicine, 48*, 1427–1436.

Montgomery, S. A., Nil, R., Dürr-Pal, N., Loft, H., & Boulenger, J. P. (2005). A 24-week randomized, double-blind, placebo-controlled study of escitalopram for the prevention of generalized social anxiety disorder. *The Journal of Clinical Psychiatry, 66*, 1270–1278. http://dx.doi.org/10.4088/JCP.v66n1009

Mula, M., Pini, S., & Cassano, G. B. (2007). The role of anticonvulsant drugs in anxiety disorders: A critical review of the evidence. *Journal of Clinical Psychopharmacology, 27*, 263–272. http://dx.doi.org/10.1097/jcp.0b013e318059361a

Murrough, J. W., Yaqubi, S., Sayed, S., & Charney, D. S. (2015). Emerging drugs for the treatment of anxiety. *Expert Opinion on Emerging Drugs, 20*, 393–406. http://dx.doi.org/10.1517/14728214.2015.1049996

National Institute for Health and Care Excellence. (2011). *Generalised anxiety disorder and panic disorder in adults: Management*. Retrieved from https://www.nice.org.uk/guidance/cg113

National Institute for Health and Care Excellence. (2013). *Social anxiety disorder: Recognition, assessment and treatment*. Retrieved from https://www.nice.org.uk/guidance/cg159

Nepon, J., Belik, S. L., Bolton, J., & Sareen, J. (2010). The relationship between anxiety disorders and suicide attempts: Findings from the National Epidemiologic Survey on Alcohol and Related Conditions. *Depression and Anxiety, 27*, 791–798. http://dx.doi.org/10.1002/da.20674

Offidani, E., Guidi, J., Tomba, E., & Fava, G. A. (2013). Efficacy and tolerability of benzodiazepines versus antidepressants in anxiety disorders: A systematic review and meta-analysis. *Psychotherapy and Psychosomatics, 82*, 355–362. http://dx.doi.org/10.1159/000353198

Ougrin, D. (2011). Efficacy of exposure versus cognitive therapy in anxiety disorders: Systematic review and meta-analysis. *BMC Psychiatry, 11*, 200. http://dx.doi.org/10.1186/1471-244X-11-200

Pande, A. C., Feltner, D. E., Jefferson, J. W., Davidson, J. R., Pollack, M., Stein, M. B., . . . Werth, J. L. (2004). Efficacy of the novel anxiolytic pregabalin in social anxiety disorder: A placebo-controlled, multicenter study. *Journal of Clinical Psychopharmacology, 24*, 141–149. http://dx.doi.org/10.1097/01.jcp.0000117423.05703.e7

Papp, L. A., Schneier, F. R., Fyer, A. J., Leibowitz, M. R., Gorman, J. M., Coplan, J. D., . . . Klein, D. F. (1997). Clomipramine treatment of panic disorder: Pros and cons. *The Journal of Clinical Psychiatry, 58*, 423–425. http://dx.doi.org/10.4088/JCP.v58n1002

Pelissolo, A. (2008). Efficacy and tolerability of escitalopram in anxiety disorders: A review. *L'Encéphale, 34*, 400–408. http://dx.doi.org/10.1016/j.encep.2008.04.004

Pollack, M. H., Lepola, U., Koponen, H., Simon, N. M., Worthington, J. J., Emilien, G., . . . Gao, B. (2007). A double-blind study of the efficacy of venlafaxine extended-release, paroxetine, and placebo in the treatment of panic disorder. *Depression and Anxiety, 24*, 1–14. http://dx.doi.org/10.1002/da.20218

Pollack, M. H., Otto, M. W., Worthington, J. J., Manfro, G. G., & Wolkow, R. (1998). Sertraline in the treatment of panic disorder: A flexible-dose multicenter trial. *Archives of General Psychiatry, 55*, 1010–1016. http://dx.doi.org/10.1001/archpsyc.55.11.1010

Pompoli, A., Furukawa, T. A., Imai, H., Tajika, A., Efthimiou, O., & Salanti, G. (2016). Psychological therapies for panic disorder with or without agoraphobia in adults: A network meta-analysis. *Cochrane Database of Systematic Reviews, 4*, CD011004.

Rapaport, M. H., Wolkow, R., Rubin, A., Hackett, E., Pollack, M., & Ota, K. Y. (2001). Sertraline treatment of panic disorder: Results of a long-term study. *Acta Psychiatrica Scandinavica, 104*, 289–298.

Rickels, K., Downing, R., Schweizer, E., & Hassman, H. (1993). Antidepressants for the treatment of generalized anxiety disorder. A placebo-controlled comparison of imipramine, trazodone, and diazepam. *Archives of General Psychiatry, 50*(11), 884–895.

Rickels, K., Zaninelli, R., McCafferty, J., Bellew, K., Iyengar, M., & Sheehan, D. (2003). Paroxetine treatment of generalized anxiety disorder: A double-blind, placebo-controlled study. *The American Journal of Psychiatry, 160*, 749–756. http://dx.doi.org/10.1176/appi.ajp.160.4.749

Ross, L. E., Grigoriadis, S., Mamisashvili, L., Vonderporten, E. H., Roerecke, M., Rehm, J., . . . Cheung, A. (2013).

Selected pregnancy and delivery outcomes after exposure to antidepressant medication: A systematic review and meta-analysis. *JAMA Psychiatry, 70*, 436–443. http://dx.doi.org/10.1001/jamapsychiatry.2013.684

Salzer, S., Winkelbach, C., Leweke, F., Leibing, E., & Leichsenring, F. (2011). Long-term effects of short-term psychodynamic psychotherapy and cognitive-behavioural therapy in generalized anxiety disorder: 12-month follow-up. *Canadian Journal of Psychiatry, 56*, 503–508. http://dx.doi.org/10.1177/070674371105600809

Sareen, J., Jacobi, F., Cox, B. J., Belik, S. L., Clara, I., & Stein, M. B. (2006). Disability and poor quality of life associated with comorbid anxiety disorders and physical conditions. *Archives of Internal Medicine, 166*, 2109–2116. http://dx.doi.org/10.1001/archinte.166.19.2109

Schatzberg, A. F., Blier, P., Delgado, P. L., Fava, M., Haddad, P. M., & Shelton, R. C. (2006). Antidepressant discontinuation syndrome: Consensus panel recommendations for clinical management and additional research. *The Journal of Clinical Psychiatry, 67*(Suppl. 4), 27–30.

Schmitt, R., Gazalle, F. K., Lima, M. S., Cunha, A., Souza, J., & Kapczinski, F. (2005). The efficacy of antidepressants for generalized anxiety disorder: A systematic review and meta-analysis. *Revista Brasileira De Psiquiatria, 27*, 18–24. http://dx.doi.org/10.1590/S1516-44462005000100007

Shear, M. K., Brown, T. A., Barlow, D. H., Money, R., Sholomskas, D. E., Woods, S. W., . . . Papp, L. A. (1997). Multicenter collaborative panic disorder severity scale. *The American Journal of Psychiatry, 154*, 1571–1575. http://dx.doi.org/10.1176/ajp.154.11.1571

Sheehan, D. V., Burnham, D. B., Iyengar, M. K., Perera, P., & the Paxil CR Panic Disorder Study Group. (2005). Efficacy and tolerability of controlled-release paroxetine in the treatment of panic disorder. *The Journal of Clinical Psychiatry, 66*, 34–40. http://dx.doi.org/10.4088/JCP.v66n0105

Sheehan, K. H., & Sheehan, D. V. (2008). Assessing treatment effects in clinical trials with the Discan metric of the Sheehan Disability Scale. *International Clinical Psychopharmacology, 23*, 70–83. http://dx.doi.org/10.1097/YIC.0b013e3282f2b4d6

Shelton, R. C. (2006). The nature of the discontinuation syndrome associated with antidepressant drugs. *The Journal of Clinical Psychiatry, 67*(Suppl. 4), 3–7.

Smith, J. P., & Randall, C. L. (2012). Anxiety and alcohol use disorders: Comorbidity and treatment considerations. *Alcohol Research: Current Reviews, 34*, 414–431.

Soldin, O. P., & Mattison, D. R. (2009). Sex differences in pharmacokinetics and pharmacodynamics. *Clinical Pharmacokinetics, 48*, 143–157. http://dx.doi.org/10.2165/00003088-200948030-00001

Spence, S. H. (1998). A measure of anxiety symptoms among children. *Behaviour Research and Therapy, 36*, 545–566. http://dx.doi.org/10.1016/S0005-7967(98)00034-5

Spitzer, R. L., Kroenke, K., Williams, J. B., & Lowe, B. (2006). A brief measure for assessing generalized anxiety disorder: The GAD-7. *Archives of Internal Medicine, 166*, 1092–1097. http://dx.doi.org/10.1001/archinte.166.10.1092

Sramek, J. J., Murphy, M. F., & Cutler, N. R. (2016). Sex differences in the psychopharmacological treatment of depression. *Dialogues in Clinical Neuroscience, 18*, 447–457.

Stahl, S. M., Gergel, I., & Li, D. (2003). Escitalopram in the treatment of panic disorder: A randomized, double-blind, placebo-controlled trial. *The Journal of Clinical Psychiatry, 64*, 1322–1327. http://dx.doi.org/10.4088/JCP.v64n1107

Steel, Z., Marnane, C., Iranpour, C., Chey, T., Jackson, J. W., Patel, V., & Silove, D. (2014). The global prevalence of common mental disorders: A systematic review and meta-analysis 1980–2013. *International Journal of Epidemiology, 43*, 476–493. http://dx.doi.org/10.1093/ije/dyu038

Stein, D. J., Ahokas, A., Albarran, C., Olivier, V., & Allgulander, C. (2012). Agomelatine prevents relapse in generalized anxiety disorder: A 6-month randomized, double-blind, placebo-controlled discontinuation study. *The Journal of Clinical Psychiatry, 73*, 1002–1008. http://dx.doi.org/10.4088/JCP.11m07493

Stein, D. J., Ahokas, A. A., & de Bodinat, C. (2008). Efficacy of agomelatine in generalized anxiety disorder: A randomized, double-blind, placebo-controlled study. *Journal of Clinical Psychopharmacology, 28*, 561–566. http://dx.doi.org/10.1097/JCP.0b013e318184ff5b

Stein, D. J., Bandelow, B., Merideth, C., Olausson, B., Szamosi, J., & Eriksson, H. (2011). Efficacy and tolerability of extended release quetiapine fumarate (quetiapine XR) monotherapy in patients with generalised anxiety disorder: An analysis of pooled data from three 8-week placebo-controlled studies. *Human Psychopharmacology: Clinical and Experimental, 26*, 614–628. http://dx.doi.org/10.1002/hup.1256

Stein, D. J., Versiani, M., Hair, T., & Kumar, R. (2002). Efficacy of paroxetine for relapse prevention in social anxiety disorder: A 24-week study. *Archives of General Psychiatry, 59*, 1111–1118. http://dx.doi.org/10.1001/archpsyc.59.12.1111

Stein, D. J., Westenberg, H. G., Yang, H., Li, D., & Barbato, L. M. (2003). Fluvoxamine CR in the long-term treatment of social anxiety disorder: The 12- to 24-week extension phase of a multicentre, randomized, placebo-controlled trial. *The International Journal of Neuropsychopharmacology, 6*, 317–323. http://dx.doi.org/10.1017/S146114570300364X

Stein, M. B., Fyer, A. J., Davidson, J. R., Pollack, M. H., & Wiita, B. (1999). Fluvoxamine treatment of social phobia (social anxiety disorder): A double-blind, placebo-controlled study. *The American Journal of Psychiatry, 156*, 756–760.

Stein, M. B., Pollack, M. H., Bystritsky, A., Kelsey, J. E., & Mangano, R. M. (2005). Efficacy of low and higher dose extended-release venlafaxine in generalized social anxiety disorder: A 6-month randomized controlled trial. *Psychopharmacology, 177*, 280–288. http://dx.doi.org/10.1007/s00213-004-1957-9

Stocchi, F., Nordera, G., Jokinen, R. H., Lepola, U. M., Hewett, K., Bryson, H., Iyengar, M. K., & the Paroxetine Generalized Anxiety Disorder Study Team. (2003). Efficacy and tolerability of paroxetine for the long-term treatment of generalized anxiety disorder. *The Journal of Clinical Psychiatry, 64*, 250–258. http://dx.doi.org/10.4088/JCP.v64n0305

Strawn, J. R., Prakash, A., Zhang, Q., Pangallo, B. A., Stroud, C. E., Cai, N., & Findling, R. L. (2015). A randomized, placebo-controlled study of duloxetine for the treatment of children and adolescents with generalized anxiety disorder. *Journal of the American Academy of Child & Adolescent Psychiatry, 54*, 283–293. http://dx.doi.org/10.1016/j.jaac.2015.01.008

Strawn, J. R., Welge, J. A., Wehry, A. M., Keeshin, B., & Rynn, M. A. (2015). Efficacy and tolerability of antidepressants in pediatric anxiety disorders: A systematic review and meta-analysis. *Depression and Anxiety, 32*, 149–157. http://dx.doi.org/10.1002/da.22329

Taylor, M. J., Rudkin, L., Bullemor-Day, P., Lubin, J., Chukwujekwu, C., & Hawton, K. (2013). Strategies for managing sexual dysfunction induced by antidepressant medication. *Cochrane Database of Systematic Reviews, 5*, CD003382. http://dx.doi.org/10.1002/14651858.CD003382.pub3

Taylor, S., Abramowitz, J. S., & McKay, D. (2012). Non-adherence and non-response in the treatment of anxiety disorders. *Journal of Anxiety Disorders, 26*, 583–589. http://dx.doi.org/10.1016/j.janxdis.2012.02.010

Van Ameringen, M. A., Lane, R. M., Walker, J. R., Bowen, R. C., Chokka, P. R., Goldner, E. M., . . . Swinson, R. P. (2001). Sertraline treatment of generalized social phobia: A 20-week, double-blind, placebo-controlled study. *The American Journal of Psychiatry, 158*, 275–281. http://dx.doi.org/10.1176/appi.ajp.158.2.275

Wade, A. G., Lepola, U., Koponen, H. J., Pedersen, V., & Pedersen, T. (1997). The effect of citalopram in panic disorder. *The British Journal of Psychiatry, 170*, 549–553. http://dx.doi.org/10.1192/bjp.170.6.549

Walker, J. R., Van Ameringen, M. A., Swinson, R., Bowen, R. C., Chokka, P. R., Goldner, E., . . . Lane, R. M. (2000). Prevention of relapse in generalized social phobia: Results of a 24-week study in responders to 20 weeks of sertraline treatment. *Journal of Clinical Psychopharmacology, 20*, 636–644. http://dx.doi.org/10.1097/00004714-200012000-00009

Walkup, J. T., Albano, A. M., Piacentini, J., Birmaher, B., Compton, S. N., Sherrill, J. T., . . . Kendall, P. C. (2008). Cognitive behavioral therapy, sertraline, or a combination in childhood anxiety. *The New England Journal of Medicine, 359*, 2753–2766. http://dx.doi.org/10.1056/NEJMoa0804633

Wehry, A. M., Beesdo-Baum, K., Hennelly, M. M., Connolly, S. D., & Strawn, J. R. (2015). Assessment and treatment of anxiety disorders in children and adolescents. *Current Psychiatry Reports, 17*, 52. http://dx.doi.org/10.1007/s11920-015-0591-z

Westenberg, H. G., Stein, D. J., Yang, H., Li, D., & Barbato, L. M. (2004). A double-blind placebo-controlled study of controlled release fluvoxamine for the treatment of generalized social anxiety disorder. *Journal of Clinical Psychopharmacology, 24*, 49–55. http://dx.doi.org/10.1097/01.jcp.0000104906.75206.8b

Williams, T., Hattingh, C. J., Kariuki, C. M., Tromp, S. A., van Balkom, A. J., Ipser, J. C., & Stein, D. J. (2017). Pharmacotherapy for social anxiety disorder (SAnD). *Cochrane Database of Systematic Reviews, 10*, CD001206.

Wilson, E., & Lader, M. (2015). A review of the management of antidepressant discontinuation symptoms. *Therapeutic Advances in Psychopharmacology, 5*, 357–368. http://dx.doi.org/10.1177/2045125315612334

Wittchen, H. U., Jacobi, F., Rehm, J., Gustavsson, A., Svensson, M., Jönsson, B., . . . Steinhausen, H. C. (2011). The size and burden of mental disorders and other disorders of the brain in Europe 2010. *European Neuropsychopharmacology, 21*, 655–679. http://dx.doi.org/10.1016/j.euroneuro.2011.07.018

Woolf, A. D., Erdman, A. R., Nelson, L. S., Caravati, E. M., Cobaugh, D. J., Booze, L. L., . . . American Association of Poison Control Centers. (2007). Tricyclic antidepressant poisoning: An evidence-based consensus guideline for out-of-hospital management. *Clinical Toxicology, 45*, 203–233. http://dx.doi.org/10.1080/15563650701226192

CHAPTER 10

PHARMACOLOGICAL TREATMENT OF SCHIZOPHRENIA AND OTHER PSYCHOTIC DISORDERS

Mark R. Serper and Karin Tong Wang

Antipsychotic drugs not only are used for the treatment of psychotic disorders, such as schizophrenia (SZ), but are frequently used to treat a wide variety of other conditions such as bipolar disorder, delirium, dementia, autistic spectrum disorders, disruptive and aggressive disorders, Tourette's disorder, and a variety of off-label conditions (e.g., Frangou & Byrne, 2000). Data indicate that use of antipsychotic medications in the United States and Europe has more than doubled in children (Cooper, Hickson, Fuchs, Arbogast, & Ray, 2004) and has increased sixfold in adults for use with nonpsychotic psychiatric conditions as well as for off-label use such as with insomnia (Olfson, Blanco, Liu, Moreno, & Laje, 2006). This increase comes despite the fact that the efficacy of antipsychotic medications for dementia, delirium, and off-label use is often not supported by the scientific evidence (e.g., Boettger & Jenewein, 2017; Kamble, Chen, Sherer, & Aparasu, 2009). In this chapter we focus on the use of antipsychotic medications used to treat SZ.

EPIDEMIOLOGY AND PREVALENCE

Despite the tremendous increase in prescriptions overall, antipsychotic medication remains underutilized for individuals with SZ (Domino & Swartz, 2008; Frank, Conti, & Goldman, 2005). Lifetime prevalence of SZ is about five per 1,000 in the general population and the incidence is about 0.2 per thousand people a year (Messias, Chen, & Eaton, 2007). The greatest risk for first psychotic SZ episode occurs in late adolescence/early adulthood (McGrath et al., 2004).

EARLY PHARMACOLOGICAL INTERVENTIONS

Before the introduction of antipsychotic medications, pharmacological interventions for psychosis were primitive and misguided. In the late 18th century, a common belief was that people with epilepsy could not be comorbid for SZ (Lieberman, 2015). Consequently, to treat SZ, physicians would induce epileptic seizures and coma via injection of insulin, camphor, or metrazol (Lieberman, 2015). Epileptic seizure therapy was practiced in the treatment of psychotic disorder starting in the 18th century to the late 19th century. In insulin shock treatment (Sakel, 1937), high doses of insulin were given to patients with acute psychosis to induce near death-state comas. In the late 19th century it was generally believed that fever-inducing illnesses such as malaria had the effect of reducing the presence of psychotic symptoms in neurosyphilis patients. Based on this observation, Austrian physician Julius Wagner von Jauregg developed "fever therapy" to treat psychotic illnesses in the 1920s (Lieberman, 2015). In fever therapy, physicians would induce fevers in their patients by

http://dx.doi.org/10.1037/0000133-010
APA Handbook of Psychopharmacology, S. M. Evans (Editor-in-Chief)

injecting sulphur or turpentine to create infections and high fevers. Ineffective nonpharmacological interventions such as castration and lobotomy were also popular treatments for SZ during this time period (Lieberman, 2015).

Given this context, it is no surprise that the advent of antipsychotic medications, with all their limitations, was a major advance in the history of psychiatry for the treatment for psychosis. The first antipsychotic, chlorpromazine, was discovered serendipitously in the 1950s. It was originally synthesized as an antiallergen and it was also used as a presurgical sedative. The effectiveness of antipsychotics was observed when patients with psychosis scheduled to undergo surgery were less psychotic after receiving the sedative. Antipsychotic medications have remained the first-line treatment for SZ and other psychotic disorders for the last 60 years (Lieberman, 2015).

DIAGNOSING SCHIZOPHRENIA AND OTHER PSYCHOTIC DISORDERS

Several diagnostic instruments have proven to be reliable for making valid diagnoses. Perhaps the best researched is the Structured Clinical Interview for DSM–5 (SCID-5; First, Williams, Karg, & Spitzer, 2015). It is administered by a trained clinician and includes an introductory overview followed by modules that include differential diagnoses for SZ, schizoaffective disorder, bipolar disorder, and psychotic depression. Using a choice decision approach, the SCID focuses on obtaining differential diagnostic information as the interview progresses. This type of decision tree approach is useful because the interviewer can evaluate diagnostic hypotheses as the interview is being conducted. The final result of the SCID is a record of the presence or absence of each of the disorders being considered, for current episode (past month) and for lifetime occurrence. In terms of pharmacological research, a modified version of the SCID, the SCID-5-CT (Clinical Trials; First et al., 2015) focuses on the diagnostic elements of the SCID-5 that are needed to determine whether a particular participant meets inclusion and exclusion criteria for a specific clinical trial.

Another diagnostic assessment instrument, developed by the National Institute of Mental Health, is a semistructured interview called the Diagnostic Interview for Genetic Studies (DIGS; Nurnberger et al., 1994). The DIGS is used for making diagnostic assessments of psychotic and major mood spectrum disorders. Like the SCID, the DIGS is administered by trained interviewers who employ clinical judgment in making choice decisions in following up on or ruling out particular diagnoses based on patient responses to questions. A final best-estimate diagnostic process using medical records, information from relatives, and algorithmic diagnoses based on clinical interview and clinician judgment confers excellent interrater reliability for SZ (Nurnberger et al., 1994). Poor to fair interrater agreement has been found for the schizo-manic type schizoaffective disorder diagnosis (Nurnberger et al., 1994).

In terms of symptom ratings, the Positive and Negative Syndrome Scale (PANSS; Kay, Fiszbein, & Opler, 1987) for SZ remains one of the most frequently used rating scales to assess symptomatology related to SZ. It contains 30 items divided into those for positive symptoms, negative symptoms, and general symptoms. While overall the PANSS is a valid and reliable instrument for assessing medication-related changes, it is generally accepted that the positive, negative, and general symptom dimensions are an oversimplification of symptom divisions in SZ and are not supported by factor analytic studies (Serper, Goldberg, & Salzinger, 2004). Various factor analytic solutions of the PANSS have yielded three to five symptom factors for SZ (Emsley, Rabinowitz, & Torreman, 2003; White, Harvey, Opler, Lindenmayer, & the PANSS Study Group, 1997). In a confirmatory factor analytic study, White et al. (1997) found the best-fit model contained five PANSS symptom factors consisting of positive, negative, dysphoric mood, activation, and autistic preoccupation symptoms. Recent clinical guidelines recommend that a reduction in symptom severity of greater than 20% represents a clinically significant treatment response (Howes et al., 2016).

EVIDENCE-BASED PHARMACOLOGICAL TREATMENTS OF SCHIZOPHRENIA

Dopamine Pathways

The dopamine (DA) hypothesis in SZ remains one of the most long-standing hypotheses in all of psychiatry (Stahl, 2008). The dopamine hypothesis proposes that hyperactivity of dopamine D2 receptor neurotransmission in subcortical and limbic brain regions contributes to positive symptoms of schizophrenia. The study of DA dysfunction presents the opportunity to examine a direct relationship between symptoms of SZ and their treatment with the DA antagonists available today, even though the DA hypothesis is incomplete in explaining the complexity of SZ.

All of the 60-plus antipsychotic compounds available to date work via DA blockade (Stahl, 2008). There are four major brain pathways involving DA, and each pathway can be affected by administration of antipsychotic medication. The four DA pathways include the:

1. *Mesolimbic pathway.* This pathway is composed of DA projections from the ventral tegmental area, which is located in the midbrain, to the nucleus accumbens and the ventral striatum (Stahl, 2008). It plays an important role in motivation, reward, and emotional expression. Overactivity of this pathway has been linked to psychosis (Seeman, 2002). All antipsychotics are believed to work by reducing the activity of the mesolimbic DA pathway (Seeman, 2002).

2. *Mesocortical pathway.* This pathway is composed of DA projections from the ventral tegmental area to the prefrontal cortex. DA hypoactivity in the mesocortical pathway is theorized to be associated with negative symptoms and cognitive dysfunction (Barbas & García-Cabezas, 2017).

3. *Nigrostriatal pathway.* This pathway is composed of DA projections from the substantia nigra to the caudate and the putamen. This pathway is involved in motor planning and smooth purposeful movement. The nigrostriatal region's extrapyramidal tract works in concert with pyramidal tract of the cerebral cortex to coordinate motor movement and contribute to fluid motion

(Stahl, 2008). DA and acetylcholine (ACH) are instrumental in coordinating smooth muscle movements in the extrapyramidal tract when there is a relatively stable ratio between these two neurotransmitters. However, neuroleptic DA blockade alters the DA to ACH as well as the DA to norepinephrine (NE) ratios and can cause extrapyramidal side effects such as parkinsonism and akathisia, respectively (Stahl, 2008).

4. *Tuberoinfundibular pathway.* This pathway consists of DA projections from the periventricular nucleus of the hypothalamus to the infundibular region of the hypothalamus and affects release of the hormone prolactin (Stahl, 2008). DA inhibits prolactin release, so low levels of DA caused by antipsychotic medication may increase prolactin levels, which can cause sexual side effects (Stahl, 2008; discussed below).

Classes of Antipsychotic Medications

Antipsychotics are generally classified into two drug classes called "conventional," "typical," or "first-generation" antipsychotic medication (FGAs) and "atypical," "novel," or "second-generation" antipsychotic medication (SGAs). However, this distinction has been viewed as too simplistic, as certain SGAs act similar to FGAs in many respects and SGAs differ from each other in many ways, defying the notion that SGAs can be conceptualized as a single class of medication (Leucht et al., 2013; see the following sections for a further discussion of this issue).

First-Generation Antipsychotics

The first antipsychotic, chlorpromazine (see Table 10.1 for a list of common FGAs and SGAs), is a low-potency FGA, meaning that it is a less potent DA receptor antagonist compared with high-potency FGAs (like haloperidol) but possesses intrinsically more anticholinergic activity (Seeman, 2002). The lower potency agents, like chlorpromazine, are less likely to produce movement disorder type side effects than higher potency agents, but have an increased likelihood of causing anticholinergic side effects such as dry mouth, blurred vision (from pupil dilation), rapid heart rate, urinary retention,

TABLE 10.1

List of Antipsychotic Drugs

Generic name	Trade name	FDA status
First-generation antipsychotics (FGAs)		
Chlorpromazine	Thorazine®	Approved in 1957
Haloperidol	Haldol®	Approved in 1967
Fluphenazine	Prolixin®	Approved in 1960
Second-generation antipsychotics (SGAs)		
Amisulpride	Solian®	Not approved by FDA
Aripiprazole	Abilify®	Approved in 2002
Asenapine	Saphris®, Sycrest®	Approved in 2009
Clozapine	Clozaril®	Approved in 1989
Iloperidone	Fanapt®, Zomaril®	Approved in 2009
Lurasidone	Latuda®	Approved in 2010
Olanzapine	Zyprexa®	Approved in 1996
Paliperidone	Invega®	Approved in 2006
Quetiapine	Seroquel®	Approved in 1997
Remoxipride	Roxiam®	Not approved by FDA
Risperidone	Risperdal®	Approved in 1993
Sertindole	Serdolect®, Serlect®	Not approved by FDA
Ziprasidone	Geodon®	Approved in 2001
Zotepine	Losizopilon®, Lodopin®, Setous®, Zoleptil®	Not approved by FDA

Note. FDA = U.S. Food and Drug Administration.

constipation, sedation, dizziness, and memory impairment (Stahl, 2008). Additionally, low potency FGAs are more likely to produce NE-blocking effects such as akathisia (discussed in more detail in the following sections).

High-potency FGAs were developed in the mid-1960s, and became widely used because they had no anticholinergic side effects (Stahl, 2008). High-potency FGAs, however, bind more tightly to DA receptors than does DA itself (Seeman, 2002), which creates a great imbalance between DA and ACH. As a result, patients are more likely to experience movement disorder side effects on high-potency FGAs compared with low-potency FGAs. In summary, the overall effect is that low-potency FGAs cause more histamine blocking, more ACH blocking, more sedation, and more NE blocking

effects, while high-potency antipsychotics are more likely to produce DA blocking side effects such as muscle rigidity and tremors.

FGAs have been examined in hundreds of double-blind studies over the years. The results unambiguously indicate that antipsychotics are superior to placebo in the treatment of acute and chronic SZ. That is, about 33% to 50% of patients are helped to some degree with FGAs (Lieberman, 2015). In addition, FGAs have also been shown to reduce negative symptoms (e.g., Goldberg, 1985) and improve cognitive functioning (e.g., Keefe et al., 2007).

Second-Generation Antipsychotics

SGAs first became available in the late 1980s and have become increasingly prescribed since the 1990s (Stahl, 2008). The introduction of SGAs was initially considered a revolutionary event in psychiatric treatment because it was thought that SGAs were more effective in treating psychosis and negative symptoms, would produce fewer side effects, and would have better treatment compliance than FGAs (Jones et al., 2006). In contrast, SGAs bind more loosely to the DA D2 receptors and release from their receptor sites at a higher rate than FGAs (Seeman, 2002), perhaps through serotonin antagonism on the DA autoreceptor for some of the SGAs (Kapur & Seeman, 2001). However, as noted above, considerable controversy exists over whether it is meaningful to classify the antipsychotic medication into FGA and SGA classes because SGAs are not a homogeneous class of medications, and have a wide range of qualitative and quantitative differences in terms of their pharmacodynamic action, clinical efficacies, and side effect profiles (e.g., Davis, Chen, & Glick, 2003; Leucht et al., 2009b, 2013). Please see the Tool Kit of Resources located at the end of the chapter for resources related to SGA medications.

Overall Treatment Effectiveness of Second-Generation Antipsychotics Versus First-Generation Antipsychotics

Evidence accumulated over the years from large-scale studies does not support contentions that, compared with FGAs, SGAs are more effective in treating psychosis, treating negative symptoms, producing less extrapyramidal symptoms (EPS), improving treatment adherence, level of patient satisfaction and quality of life, level of cognitive functioning, and ultimately lower treatment costs due to less need for rehospitalization (e.g., Caroff, Mann, Campbell, & Sullivan, 2002; Gebhardt et al., 2006; Jones et al., 2006; Potkin et al., 2003).

Instead, few significant differences exist between SGAs and FGAs in multiple outcome areas for SZ patients (Bagnall et al., 2003; Edwards & Smith, 2009; Geddes, Freemantle, Harrison, & Bebbington, 2000; Jones et al., 2006; McEvoy et al., 2005; Peluso, Lewis, Barnes, & Jones, 2012). Further, clinical trial studies have found few significant differences between FGAs and SGAs in terms of improving overall psychopathology defined by global severity ratings and/or total severity scores (e.g., Davidson et al., 2009; Geddes et al., 2000; Hartling et al., 2012; Kahn et al., 2008; Leucht et al., 2009b).

In the first meta-analysis of randomized controlled trials (RCTs) comparing the treatment effects of multiple SGAs and FGAs (Leucht, Pitschel-Walz, Abraham, & Kissling, 1999), both the FGA haloperidol and four SGAs (olanzapine, quetiapine, risperidone, and sertindole) were found to be superior to placebo in terms of their antipsychotic effectiveness, but the magnitude of their effects were only moderate. This finding was confirmed and extended by another meta-analysis based on 38 RCTs with 7,323 participants that compared nine SGAs (amisulpride, aripiprazole, clozapine, olanzapine, quetiapine, risperidone, sertindole, ziprasidone, and zotepine) and the FGA haloperidol with placebo in SZ patients. All antipsychotic drugs were found more effective than placebo, but the pooled effect size for overall symptom improvement was also only moderate (Leucht, Arbter, Engel, Kissling, & Davis, 2009a).

More recently, a multiple-treatments meta-analysis of RCTs was able to integrate both direct and indirect comparisons through a Bayesian framework (i.e., how two or more drugs compare with a common comparator) and generate a more definitive conclusion, since conventional pairwise meta-analyses were limited to direct comparisons and many antipsychotic drugs have not been compared head to head (Leucht et al., 2013). It was found that two FGAs (chlorpromazine and haloperidol) and 13 SGAs (amisulpride, aripiprazole,

asenapine, clozapine, iloperidone, lurasidone, olanzapine, paliperidone, quetiapine, risperidone, sertindole, ziprasidone, and zotepine) all were about equally effective in reducing psychosis, but had relative strengths and weakness in different outcome areas that defy a notion of a simple FGA versus SGA framework (Leucht et al., 2013).

The largest RCT sponsored by the National Institute of Mental Health (the Clinical Antipsychotic Trials of Intervention Effectiveness; CATIE) compared SGAs (olanzapine, quetiapine, risperidone, and ziprasidone) to an FGA (perphenazine), and found the SGAs were not superior to the FGA in terms of treatment efficacy (Lieberman et al., 2005). Another large scale open-label randomized clinical trial study (the European First Episode Schizophrenia Trial; EUFEST) that compared SGAs (amisulpride, olanzapine, quetiapine, and ziprasidone) with the FGA haloperidol also found that the drug efficacies in terms of symptom reductions did not significantly differ among all the antipsychotics (Kahn et al., 2008). Strikingly, Jones et al. (2006) found that older FGA drugs were associated with a trend towards better outcomes than SGA treatment.

In the Leucht et al. (1999) meta-analysis, two of the SGAs (sertindole and quetiapine) had similar efficacies as the FGA (haloperidol), whereas two other SGAs (olanzapine and risperidone) were slightly more effective than the FGA in terms of improving global schizophrenic symptoms. Another larger meta-analysis of 124 RCTs comparing FGAs and SGAs found that four of the SGAs (amisulpride, clozapine, olanzapine, and risperidone) were significantly more efficacious than the FGAs, whereas the other six SGAs (aripiprazole, quetiapine, remoxipride, sertindole, ziprasidone, and zotepine) were not significantly different from FGAs in terms of overall efficacy (Davis et al., 2003). This basic conclusion was also supported by subsequent meta-analyses (Leucht et al., 2009b, 2013).

Positive Symptoms

Meta-analyses repeatedly found that both FGAs and SGAs are significantly more effective than placebo in reducing positive symptoms, such as delusions and hallucinations, mostly with moderate pooled effect sizes (e.g., Bruijnzeel, Suryadevara, & Tandon,

2014; Buckley & Ahmed, 2013; Carpenter & Davis, 2012; Geddes et al., 2000; Leucht et al., 2009a, 2013). However, there is no consistent evidence to suggest that the FGAs and the SGAs are significantly different in their effectiveness for reducing psychotic symptoms (Geddes et al., 2000; Lehman et al., 2004; Leucht et al., 2009a). In addition, there is no consistent evidence to suggest that any individual FGA or SGA had a specific effect on either positive or negative symptoms (Geddes et al., 2000).

Similar to findings regarding overall symptom reduction, meta-analyses on randomized controlled clinical trials have revealed that the SGAs are not a homogenous group, and each compound may yield different levels of efficacy on different patients. For example, a meta-analysis on the raw data of the registrational studies of olanzapine and risperidone revealed that both of those SGAs were slightly superior to FGAs in improving positive symptoms (Davis et al., 2003). Another meta-analysis of 150 RCTs with 21,533 participants found that four SGAs (amisulpride, clozapine, olanzapine, and risperidone) were more effective than FGAs in reducing positive symptoms, whereas four other SGAs (aripiprazole, sertindole, ziprasidone, and zotepine) were just as effective as FGAs, and one SGA (quetiapine) was less effective than FGAs in reducing psychosis (Leucht et al., 2009b).

Negative Symptoms
Both FGAs and SGAs are found to be less effective in terms of treating negative symptoms than positive symptoms (Bruijnzeel et al., 2014; Carpenter & Davis, 2012; Kreyenbuhl, Buchanan, Dickerson, Dixon, & PORT 2010; Lehman et al., 2004). Though many pharmaceutical companies claimed that the SGAs are more effective in reducing negative symptoms than FGAs (see Sernyak & Rosenheck, 2007), studies reveal the two classes of medication are relatively equivalent. For example, meta-analysis has shown that all SGAs were more effective than placebo on negative symptoms, but not significantly superior to FGAs (Leucht et al., 1999), and their pooled effect size was moderate (Leucht et al., 2009a).

In addition, there is also substantial variation among SGAs in their effectiveness in improving

negative symptoms. Specifically, some studies have found that olanzapine and risperidone were slightly superior to FGAs in treating negative symptoms, whereas sertindole (used in Europe but unavailable in the United States for potentiality of sudden cardiac death) and haloperidol had similar effectiveness, and quetiapine was found to be less effective than haloperidol (Leucht et al., 1999; Lieberman et al., 2005). If pooled together as a group, the SGAs were not significantly more effective than FGAs in terms of reducing negative symptoms (Leucht et al., 1999). Another meta-analysis suggested that olanzapine and risperidone were both superior to other SGAs and FGAs in improving negative symptoms (Davis et al., 2003). A methodological issue may be that the majority of the patients recruited in clinical trials were experiencing predominant positive symptoms, suggesting that past studies involved a selection bias of patients with high positive and low negative symptoms. (Leucht et al., 2009a). Recruiting patients with primary or predominant negative symptoms would clarify if SGAs are more effective than FGAs in treating chronic patients (Leucht, Heres, Kissling, & Davis, 2011; Leucht et al., 2009a).

Overall, it can be concluded that the two classes of medications are largely equal in terms of their moderate effectiveness in improving patients' quality of life, cognitive functioning, and psychosocial functioning. Additionally, the two classes of medication are overall relatively similar in producing the development of motor side effects (Jones et al., 2006; Keefe et al., 2007; Peluso et al., 2012; Swartz et al., 2007). Along these lines, the updated Schizophrenia Patient Outcomes Research Team (PORT) recommendations advise that patients on FGAs not be switched to SGAs if they are responding and have few side effects (Stroup, McEvoy, & Lieberman, 2004; Kreyenbuhl et al., 2010).

Suicide and Aggression
SZ is associated with high rates of suicidality, with 25% to 50% of diagnosed patients making suicide attempts (Healy et al., 2006; Hor & Taylor, 2010). Clozapine has been found to be an effective agent in suicide reduction in SZ patients (Meltzer et al., 2003; Samara & Leucht, 2017). In terms of

aggression, clozapine and olanzapine have been found to be effective antiaggressive agents in schizoaffective disorder and SZ (Volavka et al., 2004). A large-scale study (Swanson et al., 2008) using data from the CATIE project examined violence reduction in 1,445 SZ patients after 6 months of treatment with one of four SGAs (olanzapine, risperidone, quetiapine or ziprasidone) or the FGA perphenazine. Results revealed that almost all the medications were associated with violence reductions and that perphenazine did not differ from olanzapine, risperidone, or ziprasidone in terms of its anti-violence efficacy. Perphenazine, however, reduced violence (dropping from 19% to 7% at follow-up) significantly more than quetiapine (dropping from 15% to 14% at follow-up; Swanson et al., 2008).

Clozapine Exception

As noted above, the use of clozapine in the treatment of SZ appears to have unique features that may set it apart from other antipsychotic medications. Several meta-regressions and systematic reviews of clozapine provide support for the notion that clozapine is significantly more effective than any other antipsychotic (McEvoy et al., 2005; Siskind, Siskind, & Kisely, 2017). Numerous large-scale studies have consistently found that clozapine resulted in greater symptom reduction and higher patient satisfaction ratings than other FGAs and SGAs (Haro et al., 2005; Lewis et al., 2006). Moreover, Tiihonen et al. (2009) conducted a long-term follow-up registry-based study involving more than 66,000 SZ patients found that clozapine treatment was also associated with reduced mortality and was the most effective antipsychotic associated with the lowest mortality in SZ patients (Tiihonen et al., 2009).

Additionally, there is evidence to indicate that clozapine treatment is more effective than other SGAs and FGAs in treating medication-refractory SZ patients (Bobo & Meltzer, 2010). Patients who fail to respond to two trials of different antipsychotics are considered treatment resistant (Kreyenbuhl et al., 2010). Up to one third of patients with SZ do not respond to two trials of antipsychotic therapy (Bobo & Meltzer, 2010). Some reports indicate that more than half of these treatment-refractory patients with SZ will improve with clozapine (Barnes et al.,

2011; Kreyenbuhl et al., 2010; Lehman et al., 2004; Meltzer, 2013; Stanton et al., 2015).

A few investigators, however, have challenged the superiority of clozapine to other SGAs in treating treatment-resistant SZ (Chakos, Lieberman, Hoffman, Bradford, & Sheitman, 2001; Samara et al., 2016). For example, Samara et al. (2016) found in their meta-analysis of 40 RCTs with 5,172 treatment-resistant patients that clozapine, olanzapine, and risperidone all showed a pattern of superiority on different measures of treatment outcomes (i.e., overall change in symptoms, change in positive and negative symptoms, response to treatment, dropout rate, and adverse events), though the results were not consistent and the effect sizes were small (Samara et al., 2016).

BEST APPROACHES FOR ASSESSING TREATMENT RESPONSE AND MANAGING SIDE EFFECTS

It has been noted that there is a lack of uniformity in defining SZ treatment response and resistance to antipsychotic therapy (Robinson, Woerner, & Schooler, 2000). Due to the lack of standardized assessment of treatment for SZ, the Treatment Response and Resistance in Psychosis (TRRIP) working group (Howes et al., 2016) has recently recommended use of a standardized, validated symptom rating scale such as the PANSS (described previously), the Scale for the Assessment of Negative Symptoms (SANS; Andreasen, 1983), and/or the Scale for the Assessment of Positive Symptoms (SAPS; Andreasen, 1984) to assess SZ patients' treatment response. The SANS assesses dimensions of negative symptoms including amotivation, alogia, and flat affect severity, while the SAPS examines dimensions of positive symptoms including severity of delusions, hallucinations, and severity of positive thought disorder.

In terms of the effects of medication on cognitive aspects of SZ illness, the Brief Assessment of Cognition in Schizophrenia (BACS; Keefe et al., 2004), the Repeatable Battery for the Assessment of Neuropsychological Status (RBANS; Wilk et al., 2004), and the Measurement and Treatment Research to Improve Cognition in Schizophrenia (MATRICS;

M. F. Green, Nuechterlein, et al., 2004) all reliably measure SZ cognitive deficits (e.g., memory, attention/vigilance, verbal learning and memory, speed of processing) and response to treatment.

Medication Side Effects

As noted above, one of the many reasons for medication noncompliance concerns the negative and disabling side effects that both FGA and SGA medications may induce in SZ patients (e.g., Caroff et al., 2002). Various antipsychotic drugs can produce a variety of undesirable physical symptoms that range from the bothersome (e.g., dry mouth, urinary retention) to severe (tardive dyskinesia [TD], memory impairment, parkinsonism, akathisia) to potentially lethal (e.g., agranulocytosis, neuroleptic malignant syndrome; see Table 10.2 for a brief description of common neuroleptic-induced side effects and syndromes).

Medication side effects play a significant role in reducing the perceived quality of life of individuals with SZ and also contribute to their medication refusal (Jones et al., 2006). Notably, few significant differences between FGA and SGA treatment groups in the development of parkinsonism, akathisia, or TD have been found in clinical trials (Peluso et al., 2012; Woods et al., 2010). Notwithstanding, some studies have reported lower rates of TD among SGAs than FGAs (e.g., Correll & Schenk, 2008).

Extrapyramidal Symptoms

One set of disabling side effects caused by antipsychotic medication exposure is extrapyramidal symptoms (EPS) resulting from the massive DA blockade in the nigrostriatal tract (Seeman, 2002). EPS include parkinsonism, akathisia, and TD. Patients suffering from parkinsonian symptoms experience muscle rigidity, resting tremor, postural instability, bradykinesia (slowed movements), and akinesia (e.g., expressionless face, monotone speech). The Simpson–Angus Extrapyramidal Side-Effect Scale (SAS; Simpson & Angus, 1970) measures various aspects of EPS in patients receiving antipsychotic treatment and has been found to be a reliable and valid instrument for assessing EPS (Janno et al., 2005).

It may be difficult to distinguish medication-induced bradykinesia and akinesia side effects

TABLE 10.2

Side Effects Associated With Various Types of Antipsychotic Medications

1. *NEUROLEPTIC MALIGNANT SYNDROME*: A rare syndrome (ranging from .02–1.4% of SZ patients; Pope, Keck, & McElroy, 1986; Ananth, Parameswaran, Gunatilake, Burgoyne, & Sidhom, 2004) that consists of mental status deterioration, generalized body rigidity, high fever, and dysautonomia. It almost invariably occurs after administration of a first- and sometimes second-generation neuroleptic medication.
2. *TARDIVE DYSKINESIA (TD)*: A disorder produced by prolonged exposure to first- or second-generation neuroleptics and characterized by involuntary, repetitive body movements including rapid jerking and slow writhing of the truck and torso, facial grimacing, tongue thrusting, and lip smacking (Stahl, 2008).
3. *EXTRAPYRAMIDAL SIDE EFFECTS*: Associated with both first-generation antipsychotics (FGAs) and second-generation antipsychotics (SGAs) and is characterized by neuroleptic induced movement disorders that include resting tremors, dystonia (continuous spasms and muscle contractions), akathisia (motor restlessness), parkinsonism (characteristic symptoms such as rigidity), and bradykinesia (slowness of movement).
4. *ANTICHOLINERGIC SIDE EFFECTS*: Associated with low potency FGAs and can include memory impairment, decreased concentration, irritability, agitation, as well as blurred vision, urinary retention, increased heart rate, dry mouth and drowsiness.
5. *METABOLIC SYNDROME*: Characterized by abdominal obesity, high blood pressure, high triglycerides, high glucose, and low high-density lipoproteins. Metabolic syndrome is due to exposure to SGAs and represents an important risk factor for the development of cardiovascular disease and diabetes.

from clinical symptoms because they appear somewhat similar in presentation (Stahl, 2008). That is, in cross-sectional evaluations it is difficult to discriminate medication side effects such as sedation and akinesia from negative symptoms and the social withdrawal that may occur in response to suspiciousness of others, and/or social withdrawal and flat affect associated with social anhedonia and/or depression (Van Putten & Marder, 1987). Careful clinical assessment may aide in distinguishing side effects from negative and positive symptoms of psychosis and depression. For example, Barnes and McPhillips (1995) recommend a thorough longitudinal observation of patients using validated rating scales that are discerning enough to operationally discriminate negative symptoms from depression and medication side effects as well in detection of symptom changes over time. For example, use of the Calgary Depression Scale for Schizophrenia (CDSS; Addington, Addington, & Maticka-Tyndale, 1993) along with measures of EPS can help distinguish depressed from nondepressed patients with SZ. As noted above, depression can be confused with negative symptoms and even EPS. The CDS has been found to be uncorrelated with both negative symptoms and severity of EPS in SZ patients (Addington et al., 1993; Barnes & McPhillips, 1995), suggesting that accurate discrimination between affective symptoms, EPS, and negative symptoms is feasible.

Akathisia is hypothesized to result from a medication-induced imbalance between DA and norepinephrine (Stahl, 2008). Its reported incidence ranges from 21% to 75% and its prevalence ranges from 20% to 35% (Halstead, Barnes, & Speller, 1994). Akathisia is best described as a subjective state of inner restlessness, feelings of anxiety, irritability, and impatience, as well as increased motor activity, inability to sit still, and repetitive movements (Halstead et al., 1994). A rating scale to assess akathisia is the Barnes Akathisia Scale (BAS; Barnes, 1989). The scale includes objective items, such as clinician ratings of severity of repetitive movements and motor activity, and subjective items, such as patient awareness of restlessness and distress related to restlessness. The BAS has demonstrated good reliability and validity (Barnes, 1989).

Antipsychotic drugs, by binding to D2 receptors in the tuberoinfundibular tract, can produce elevated serum prolactin levels (Seeman, 2002). Even moderate increases in prolactin levels can interfere with sexual function in both men and women (Stahl, 2008). Increased levels of prolactin in female patients can cause amenorrhea, or oligomenorrhea, hirsutism, vaginal dryness, and galactorrhea (i.e., spontaneous milk secretions from the breasts). In male patients, hyperprolactinemia can cause erectile dysfunction, gynecomastia (increase in breast size), and decreased muscle mass and body hair. In one large-scale study, after a year of treatment, sexual dysfunctions for both sexes were lowest for olanzapine (at 14%)

and quetiapine (at 8%), compared with patients received risperidone (23%) or haloperidol (29%; Dossenbach et al., 2006).

TD is a chronic movement disorder that is usually debilitating and long term (Stahl, 2008). TD can involve grimacing; tongue thrusting; puckering and pursing of the lips; excessive eye blinking; involuntary, grotesque repetitive and rapid jerking movements; or slow writhing movements of the legs, trunk, and torso (Baldessarini, 1988). These are frequently disabling symptoms and as many as 50% of TD patients have functional impairment as a result (Baldessarini, 1988). In severe cases, TD can involve the involuntary muscles and impair swallowing or even breathing (Stahl, 2008).

TD is most likely to occur when a patient takes high doses of antipsychotics for an extended time period, usually several years or more (Baldessarini, 1988), with some reports finding the high potency FGAs have higher TD conversion rates. For example, Correll and Schenk (2008) found that across 12 trials, the annual TD incidence rate was 3.9% for SGAs and 5.5% for FGAs. However, TD can occur with briefer exposure to high potency antipsychotics (Morgenstern & Glazer, 1993). TD is often measured using the Abnormal Involuntary Movement Scale (AIMS; Branch, 1975). The AIMS rates the severity of abnormal movements on a scale from 0 to 4. Best practices suggest that patients on antipsychotics be assessed with the AIMS every 3 to 6 months to monitor for the development of TD or movement-related side effects (Stahl, 2008).

In terms of etiology, TD is believed to be the result of chronic blockade of the D2 DA nigral-striatal receptors (Baldessarini, 1988; Morgenstern et al., 1987). The receptors become supersensitive to DA because of enduring the massive DA blockade from antipsychotic medication. A compensatory upregulation process or an increase in the number of DA receptors that are super sensitive to DA binding cause TD symptoms to develop in some patients (Morgenstern & Glazer, 1993; Seeman, 2002). Stopping the antipsychotic usually worsens the TD at least temporarily, and some patients will have symptoms of TD when their antipsychotics are rapidly decreased (Fernandez, Trieschmann, & Friedman, 2003).

Metabolic Abnormalities

Cardiometabolic abnormalities called *metabolic syndrome* can result from SGA exposure (Correll, Frederickson, Kane, & Manu, 2008). The metabolic syndrome is characterized by abdominal obesity, high blood pressure, high triglycerides, high glucose, and low high-density lipoproteins (Mitchell et al., 2013). In addition to genetic, dietary, and lifestyle practices, metabolic syndrome is attributable to exposure to SGAs and represents an important risk factor for the development of cardiovascular disease and diabetes in people with SZ (Correll et al., 2008). Individuals with SZ have a significantly increased risk for death due to cardiovascular disease relative to the general population (Carney, Jones, & Woolson, 2006). That is, cardiovascular disease is significantly overrepresented in individuals with SZ accounting for significant elevations in mortality (Carney et al., 2006). Individuals with SZ can expect a reduced life expectancy on average compared with the general population by about 20 to 25 years as a result of the emergence of early onset cardiovascular disease (Carney et al., 2006; Leucht et al., 2009b). Overall, individuals with SZ have twice the normal risk of dying from cardiovascular disease than the general population (Saha, Chant, & McGrath, 2007).

Moreover, several reports have found that even brief exposure to SGAs may result in significant cardiometabolic disturbances linked to diabetes and cardiovascular disease (e.g., Patel et al., 2009; De Hert et al., 2009; Zhai et al., 2017). In a meta-analysis and systematic review, Mitchell et al. (2013) found that 32% of SZ patients had metabolic syndrome and that clozapine exposure was associated with the highest risk for metabolic syndrome (51.9% of clozapine-prescribed patients). Olanzapine, molecularly similar to clozapine, is also associated with high rates of metabolic syndrome. Ziprasidone, in contrast, is associated with decreased risk for metabolic syndrome (Meyer et al., 2008), but has not been shown to be as clinically effective as either olanzapine or clozapine in treating psychotic symptoms (e.g., McEvoy et al., 2005).

Metabolic syndrome has a psychological effect on patients, increasing their negative symptom expression (Saddichha, Ameen, & Akhtar, 2008) and decreasing self-esteem (Leas & McCabe, 2007) and motivation to engage in exercise and health-related activities (Vancampfort et al., 2010; 2012). Along these lines, a recent study using a temporal discounting procedure has found that self-efficacy deficits and reduced reward expectancies significantly predict motivation deficits in SZ patients (Serper, Payne, Dill, Portillo, & Taliercio, 2017).

Brain Volume Loss

While neuronal loss in SZ has typically been associated with the disease process itself, a few recent studies suggest that antipsychotic medication exposure causes structural brain changes and brain volume loss (Ho, Andreasen, Ziebell, Pierson, & Magnotta, 2011; Navari & Dazzan, 2009). In the Ho et al. (2011) study, the authors examined neuro-imaging data of patients over a 14-year period and found neuronal loss across multiple brain regions was associated with increasing amounts of antipsychotic medication exposure. To date, however, available data indicate that antipsychotics appear to hold their efficacy over extended time periods, and that antipsychotic treatment is associated with better outcomes relative to withholding treatment (Goff et al., 2017). Nonetheless, neural loss associated with neuroleptic treatment is a disturbing finding, and if replicated, further advance the necessity for developing better and safer antipsychotic medications.

MEDICATION MANAGEMENT ISSUES

Despite the vast limitations and potential side effects of antipsychotic medication, for individuals experiencing psychosis related to psychiatric illness, antipsychotic medication is a necessary first-line treatment and represents a standard level of contemporary psychiatric care (Stahl, 2008). Medication noncompliance by SZ spectrum patients, however, is one of the highest for all mental illnesses, and ranges from 20% to 60% depending on the treatment setting (Lacro, Dunn, Dolder, Leckband, & Jeste, 2002). Nonadherence to psychiatric medication regimen in outpatients increases in the risk of relapse, rehospitalization, suicide attempts, and decreased functionality (Lacro et al., 2002; Novick et al., 2010).

Also, as noted previously, the noncompliance rate is fairly equivalent between FGAs and SGAs (e.g., Jones et al., 2006; Lieberman et al., 2005; Valenstein et al., 2004).

Although it is a widely held belief that patients' psychosis is the primary factor associated with medication noncompliance, studies have revealed that medication nonadherence in SZ is determined by multiple factors (Novick et al., 2010; Velligan, Sajatovic, Hatch, Kramata, & Docherty, 2017; Zhou, Rosenheck, Mohamed, Ning, & He, 2017). Some factors associated with noncompliance with neuroleptic treatment include clinical variables such as severity of symptoms, poor premorbid adjustment, lack of insight, and illness chronicity (Novick et al., 2010). Medication-related variables can also lead to noncompliance, and these factors include shorter duration of treatment, complicated polypharmacy treatment, and severity of side effects (Zhou et al., 2017). Hospital- and physician-related variables also have been linked to inadequate treatment compliance; these factors include poor hospital discharge planning, poor support systems, poor patient attitudes towards treatment, and poor therapeutic alliance between treatment team and patient (Fenton, Blyler, & Heinssen, 1997; O'Donnell et al., 2003). Additionally, person-related factors are related to medication noncompliance, including patient sociodemographics, such as ability to afford medications, preexisting cognitive deficits, and comorbidity of alcohol and/or substance abuse (Kampman & Lehtinen, 1999; Lacro et al., 2002; Velligan et al., 2017; Zhou et al., 2017).

In addition to psychosocial strategies designed to enhance treatment compliance (see the following discussion), there is some evidence that SGA long-acting injectables (LAIs) can increase compliance rates and tenure in the community compared with oral administrations (e.g., MacEwan et al., 2016). However, the findings of several large meta-analyses examining the superiority of LAI to oral administration in risk for rehospitalization have been mixed (Kishimoto, Nitta, Borenstein, Kane, & Correll, 2013). It may be the case, however, that patients receiving LAI have a more severe and chronic illness than their counterparts (Kishimoto et al., 2013), so that the lack of superiority of LAIs found in

some studies may be due to selection differences in medication treatment options. These results suggest that LAIs may be superior in increasing patients' tenure in the community. Also, SGA LAIs (particularly once-monthly paliperidone LAI and risperidone LAI) have been linked with a 30% lower all-cause mortality rate compared with other FGA and SGA oral agents, suggesting that different medications and routes of administration may have a major impact on life expectancy in SZ (Tiihonen et al., 2017).

Once a discrimination of EPS from symptoms of psychopathology is made, strategies to treat EPS may focus on attempting to reinstate the balance of DA/ACH activity in the nigrostriatal pathway (Stahl, 2008). Reducing the dose of antipsychotic medication may decrease EPS, but may cause an increase in positive symptoms. Restoring the ratio of cholinergic activity to dopamine activity is an effective way to reduce parkinsonian symptoms. That is, reducing cholinergic activity by administering anticholinergic drugs such as benztropine or trihexyphenidyl can reduce EPS (Stahl, 2008). There is some suggestion that a person experiencing untreated akathisia is at increased risk for violence directed at others and for suicidal-type behaviors (Hansen, 2001). Akathisia can be treated by reducing neuroleptic dosage and/or by administering propranolol to restore the balance between DA and NE in the nigrostriatal pathway (Stahl, 2008). In terms of managing TD, a small minority of patients may improve over time with early discontinuation of medication (e.g., Glazer, Morgenstern, Schooler, Berkman, & Moore, 1990). Other nonneuroleptic-based approaches such as the use of propranolol, vitamin B6, and ginkgo biloba and valbenazine have had preliminary success in reducing TD (Cloud, Zutshi, & Factor, 2014; Citrome, 2017).

EVALUATION OF PHARMACOLOGICAL APPROACHES ACROSS THE LIFESPAN

Examination of individuals with SZ during the early course of the illness suggests that neurocognitive and prefrontal deficits are stable and significantly less pronounced than those found in older patients (e.g., Juuhl-Langseth, Holmén, Thormodsen, Øie,

& Rund, 2014; McGorry, Killackey, & Yung, 2008). First-episode SZ patients initially show favorable response to antipsychotic treatment, but show high rates of relapse within the first 5 years (e.g., McCreadie et al., 1992). Discontinuation of maintenance antipsychotic treatment over this time, however, is associated with a fivefold increase in relapse rates (Robinson et al., 1999) Additionally, first-episode patients demonstrating poor executive and attentional deficits may portend poor long-term outcome (Bilder et al., 2000).

Young patients with SZ (and elderly patients) are much more sensitive to the effects and side-effects of neuroleptic medication compared with adults, indicating that lower doses of antipsychotic medication can be used to control hallucinations and delusions in these groups rather than standard doses used in adult patients (e.g., Armenteros & Davies, 2006; Correll et al., 2009; Sikich et al., 2008). Additionally, large-scale studies examining FGAs versus SGAs suggest fairly equal efficacy of the two types of medication when given to children and adolescents, with FGAs producing more EPS and SGAs producing more metabolic side effects (e.g., Sikich et al., 2008). A general consensus in the field indicates that the longer the duration of untreated psychosis the worse the outcome (e.g., Marshall et al., 2005; McGorry et al., 2008). In particular, individuals experiencing a recent first psychotic break who also abuse substances are more likely to have a longer duration of untreated psychosis and less favorable medication response compared with their non–substance abusing counterparts (A. I. Green, Tohen, et al., 2004).

In terms of the age, more than 35% of all public psychiatric facilities and more than 15% of all nursing homes are comprised of elderly individuals with SZ or other primary psychotic disorders (Marder et al., 2004). The use of antipsychotic medications in elderly patients with SZ requires ongoing intensive health monitoring given that SZ is related to increases in physical illness that can be exacerbated by antipsychotic medications, increasing morbidity and mortality in the elderly (Marder et al., 2004). Elderly patients are more at risk for adverse effects of antipsychotic medications than younger patients because of age-related reductions in metabolism

and increased drug sensitivity (Sera & McPherson, 2012). Monitoring of patients' health and medical comorbidities may dictate the dose and choice of antipsychotic medication. As one example, for elderly patients with increased risk for diabetes, dyslipidemia, congestive heart failure, and/or obesity, the avoidance of medications with high metabolic signatures (e.g., clozapine, olanzapine) is strongly recommended (Alexopoulos, Streim, Carpenter, & Docherty, 2004).

CONSIDERATION OF POTENTIAL SEX DIFFERENCES

Compared with women, men have a 30% to 40% higher risk for developing SZ (Aleman, Kahn, & Selten, 2003; McGrath, Saha, Chant, & Welham, 2008). Men also have a younger age of illness onset, with the highest vulnerability between ages 15 and 24, while women are more likely to develop the disorder in their late teens to mid-20s (McGrath et al., 2008). In addition, women have a higher second peak vulnerability for SZ between ages 55 and 64 (Messias et al., 2007).

There is some preliminary evidence that SGAs are more effective in reducing psychosis in women compared with men (Szymanski et al., 1995). The Schizophrenia Outpatient Health Outcomes study (SOHO; Usall et al., 2007) examined health outcomes associated with antipsychotic treatment in 4,529 men (56.68%) and 3,461 women (43.32%) over a 3-year follow-up. Findings revealed that female patients had better FGA and SGA response to treatment as measured by the Clinical Global Impression (CGI) scale. The greatest sex differences were found with women showing improved CGI on FGAs and with clozapine compared with men, with few sex differences reported for olanzapine or risperidone (Usall et al., 2007).

While men with SZ have been found to have earlier illness onset, poorer premorbid adjustment, more negative symptoms and cognitive deficits, and worse course of illness (e.g., Leung & Chue, 2000; Tang et al., 2007), women with SZ appear to have, overall, more adverse neuroleptic-induced side effects. For example, examining FGAs, women seem to be more susceptible to developing TD compared with men. Yassa and Jeste (1992) examined data from 39,187 patients, finding that women developed TD at higher rates and had more severe TD than their male counterparts. Women also appear to have higher rates of FGA induced acute dystonic reactions than men (Casey, 1991). Additionally, for both FGAs and SGAs, the risk for hyperprolactinemia appears to be twice as common in women (Smith et al., 2002), and mean prolactin levels are twice as high in women receiving FGAs or SGAs (Knegtering et al., 2004).

In terms of sex and medication side effects, the adverse metabolic risks associated with SGAs may be particularly important for female SZ patients. Several large studies have found a higher prevalence of metabolic syndrome in women compared with men (e.g., McEvoy et al., 2005; Ochoa, Usall, Cobo, Labad, & Kulkarni, 2012). More recently, a comprehensive analysis examining 287 patients (40% female) found female patients were diagnosed with metabolic disorders at higher rates than males (Kraal, Ward, & Ellingrod, 2017). Women receiving clozapine or olanzapine were at greatest risk for metabolic disturbances, particularly in BMI and weight circumference (Kraal et al., 2017). Men, however, appear to be more susceptible to neuroleptic malignant syndrome (NMS) compared with women (Gurrera, 2017).

Lastly, there is some evidence that female patients with SZ are more medication-compliant than their male counterparts. For example, the Danish OPUS trial (Thorup et al., 2005) followed 578 first break patients for more than 5 years, and the authors found that female patients had higher levels of social functioning and employment and were significantly more compliant with SGA medication than male patients (Thorup et al., 2014).

INTEGRATION OF PHARMACOTHERAPY WITH NONPHARMACOLOGICAL APPROACHES: BENEFITS AND CHALLENGES

Combined psychosocial and medication treatments can significantly enhance SZ patients' tenure in the community and improve functionality and life satisfaction (McGorry et al., 2008; Mueser, Deavers, Penn, & Cassisi, 2013; Selten, van der Ven, Rutten,

& Cantor-Graae, 2013). Employing psychosocial interventions, such as cognitive therapy, antibullying interventions, cognitive remediation, and social skills training, is crucial, because the impact of stress increases the risk for elevated psychosis, cognitive impairment, and negative symptoms in vulnerable individuals (e.g., McGorry et al., 2008; Selten et al., 2013). Individuals with SZ have an abnormal stress response (Walder, Walker, & Lewine, 2000) and stress experiences are associated with increased DA synthesis (Mizrahi et al., 2012; Vaessen, Hernaus, Myin-Germeys, & van Amelsvoort, 2015) and glutamate release (García-Bueno, Caso, & Leza, 2008).

Individuals with SZ are more likely to experience social defeat experiences (Selten et al., 2013). Social defeat is defined as a variety of stressful life experiences such as social exclusion, discrimination, and poverty, among other factors that can potentiate psychosis (Selten et al., 2013). Recent studies suggest that negative life events and stress-inducing social defeat experiences may increase risk for psychosis through sensitization of DA neurotransmission (Mizrahi et al., 2012). Psychosocial programs designed to prevent social exclusion in children at high risk for SZ may help mitigate social stress and optimize compliance with medication (e.g., Cullen, Fisher, Roberts, Pariante, & Laurens, 2014).

Psychologists have a significant role to play in mitigating medication nonadherence. For example, psychologists may help increase medication compliance by improving the therapeutic alliance. Poor rapport and communication between the prescriber and patient may be mediated by psychologists working with patients in the psychiatric inpatient setting as well as in outpatient settings. Psychologists can act as patient advocates and go-betweens for patients and physicians by helping patients recognize when they are experiencing side effects and intercede with their physicians to expedite interventions aimed at reducing potential unwanted medication side effects. If psychologists can promote an enhanced sense of subjective well-being associated with taking medication, treatment compliance can be improved (Karow et al., 2007). Clinicians who communicate uncertain attitudes toward medication have been associated with decreased rates of compliance compared with clinicians who communicated to their patients that medications were an essential part of treatment (Mitchell & Selmes, 2007; Tessier et al., 2017).

Importantly, simply disseminating information to patients about their medication does not seem to enhance compliance (Zygmunt, Olfson, Boyer, & Mechanic, 2002). That is, research examining weekly patient medication educational sessions without instruction on behavioral problem-solving strategies, self-monitoring techniques, enhancement of environmental cues to take medications, and built-in reinforcements for compliance found that they appear to have little to no impact on enhancing compliance (Zygmunt et al., 2002).

In contrast, psychological treatments that incorporate medication compliance as an explicit goal have been shown to yield significant increases in medication compliance (e.g., Kemp, David, & Hayward, 1996). Direct reinforcement strategies, for example, have been shown to enhance medication treatment compliance. In a classic study, Liberman and Davis (1975) met with patients for a monthly lunch session at an outpatient clinic. If patients were medication compliant (determined by urine screens), they were able to choose a reward (e.g., high quality toiletries or other personal items). The authors reported that rewards for compliance resulted in significantly higher levels of medication adherence. Additionally, patients reinforced for their medication compliance also reported higher levels of personal satisfaction with their medication and had better attendance at therapeutic outpatient sessions (Liberman & Davis, 1975; Ho et al., 1999).

Kemp and colleagues (1996; 1998) developed compliance therapy to enhance medication adherence in acute psychotic patients. The treatment is a brief (five sessions lasting 30–60 minutes) cognitive behavioral intervention combined with psycho-education and motivational interviewing strategies. Kemp et al. (1996; 1998) found that the cognitive-based program increased medication compliance that was maintained over an 18-month follow-up period compared with a nonspecific counseling control group. However, a follow-up study failed to show any advantage of compliance therapy over nonspecific counseling in improving medication

adherence in SZ patients (O'Donnell et al., 2003; Donohoe, 2006).

Eckman, Liberman, Phipps, and Blair (1990) reported that medication skills training could significantly impact medication treatment compliance. Teaching patients assertion skills to question and evaluate the benefits of their medication as well as to identify and communicate any side effects they may be experiencing may result in patients experiencing a greater sense of control over their treatment. It has long been found that increasing patients' sense of control over their treatment regimens enhances their medication compliance (e.g., Nelson, Gold, Hutchinson, & Benezra, 1975; Williams, Rodin, Ryan, Grolnick, & Deci, 1998).

Lastly, family warmth may play an important role in patients' antipsychotic medication adherence. Studies have found that family households high in expressed emotion (EE; hostility, criticism, emotional over-involvement) directed at a patient with SZ was a potent predictor of relapse, partially because patients in this environment were less likely to adhere to their medication (Brown, Birley, & Wing, 1972). However, patients in high EE households who remained medication compliant were protected from relapse (Leff, Kuipers, Berkowitz, Vaughn, & Sturgeon, 1983). SZ patients in the community who are medication noncompliant and who experience a negative life event or experience chronic stress as a result of living with a high EE relative are significantly more likely to relapse (Sellwood, Tarrier, Quinn, & Barrowclough, 2003). It may be the case that patients in low EE environments require lower maintenance medication doses than patients discharged to high EE environments (Hogarty et al., 1988). Psychologists helping to reduce household EE may result in lower incidence of side effects associated with higher dosage antipsychotic treatment. The role of the psychologists in providing SZ patients with psychosocial treatments such as family psychoeducation, cognitive behavioral therapy (CBT), and assertive community treatment all may play a significant role in medication adherence and relapse prevention (Bustillo, Lauriello, Horan, & Keith, 2001).

Psychologists can play a role in recognition of EPS and akathisia and alert medical staff when a patient is experiencing subtle signs of EPS. Akathisia, for example, can be mistaken as a worsening of psychosis rather than a medication side effect, which may result in increased dose of the medication that is causing the symptom in the first place (Hansen, 2001). Psychologists can play a role in discriminating akathisia from psychosis as well as providing psychosocial interventions to help reduce a patient's subjective anxiety stemming from the stress caused by akathisia (Kane et al., 2009). For example, clinicians should discuss and educate patients about the nature of akathisia so patients themselves can recognize this symptom as a medication-induced side effect rather than a new psychiatric symptom (Kane et al., 2009). The psychologist also can help provide comfort and encouragement to patients by listening to their daily living experiences in dealing with akathisia.

In terms of metabolic syndrome, psychologists, working with physicians and physical therapists on the treatment team, can be instrumental in increasing patients' engagement in physical activity. Psychologists can aide physical therapists in designing activity programs by taking into account the severity of patients' negative symptoms, self-esteem, self-efficacy, reward expectancies, and life stress factors that may impact their willingness to participate and continued adherence to a physical activity regimen (Vancampfort et al., 2010). Psychologists also can provide reinforcement schedules that are incremental and tangible for patients in return for engaging in physical activities and for problem-solving psychological impediments that might interfere with an exercise regimen. Engagement in physical exercise can improve physical health as well as negative symptoms and self-esteem, resulting in reductions in SGA dosages (Beebe et al., 2005; Birt, 2003) that may potentially contribute to a reduction in diabetes, obesity, and cardiovascular illness severity (Birt, 2003).

INTEGRATED APPROACHES FOR ADDRESSING COMMON COMORBID DISORDERS

Comorbidities in SZ remain among the highest for all psychiatric disorders. Antisocial personality disorder appears to be more common in individuals

with SZ than it is in the general population (Moran & Hodgins, 2004). Anxiety and depression are very common throughout the course of schizophrenic illness. About 15% of SZ patients receive comorbid diagnoses for panic disorder, 29% for posttraumatic stress disorder, and 25% for obsessive-compulsive disorder. Comorbidity with depression occurs in about 50% of patients (Buckley, Miller, Lehrer, & Castle, 2009). While the use of SSRIs as an add-on therapy to improve negative symptoms in SZ has not been shown to be very effective (e.g., Sepehry, Potvin, Élie, & Stip, 2007), SSRIs are effective in reducing anxiety, obsessive-compulsive symptoms, and some aspects of depressive symptoms in SZ patients (Buoli, Serati, Ciappolino, & Altamura, 2016).

The high prevalence of substance abuse comorbidity for SZ has been well documented, with as many as 50% of patients comorbid for cannabis, alcohol, and/or drug dependence (Buckley et al., 2009), and more than 75% of patients addicted to nicotine (Hartz et al., 2014; Maremmani et al., 2017). In particular, heavy cannabis abuse may be associated with an SZ first break as well as an increased risk for relapse in SZ (Leweke & Koethe, 2008).

The high comorbidity of substance use in SZ has been linked to increased morbidity and mortality in part because substance use reduces compliance and efficacy of psychiatric medications relative to that of nonabusing counterparts (A. I. Green, Tohen, et al., 2004; Wilkins, 1997). Additionally, abuse of alcohol and cocaine compounds cognitive deficits exhibited by SZ patients (Bowie, Serper, Riggio, & Harvey, 2005; Serper et al., 2000) as well as potentially increasing the risk for EPS (Potvin et al., 2006).

Treatment of comorbid substance use disorder in SZ involves judicious use of pharmacotherapy along with evidence-based psychosocial approaches with multidisciplinary trained personnel (Horsfall, Cleary, Hunt, & Walter, 2009). Effective interventions include a wide range of programs, with 24-hour access to patients and long-term follow-up as key components in successful outcomes (Horsfall et al., 2009). Effective psychological interventions include contingency management, social skills training, family therapy, and CBT (e.g., Dixon et al., 2009; Horsfall et al., 2009) to compliment SGAs. All approaches share a common emphasis of increasing medication compliance and drug abstinence. Studies also suggest that naltrexone and disulfiram treatment of comorbid alcohol abuse (see Chapter 22, this volume) and bupropion for tobacco use termination (see Chapter 27, this volume) can be effective in SZ (Bennett, Bradshaw, & Catalano, 2017; Petrakis et al., 2005).

EMERGING TRENDS

While dopaminergic abnormalities herald the onset of psychosis (Howes & Kapur, 2009), glutamatergic abnormalities appear to be associated with the development of psychotic symptoms and social and cognitive deficits in SZ (Pocklington et al., 2015; Schmidt & Mirnics, 2015; Guidotti et al., 2000). Glutamate-modifying compounds such as D-serine and the NMDA receptor partial agonist D-cycloserine may be available treatment options for SZ in the future. To date, however, D-serine and D-cycloserine have yielded mixed results at best in the treatment of symptoms and in reducing cognitive deficits in SZ (Iwata et al., 2015; van Berckel et al., 1999; Weiser et al., 2012). Yet, some glutamate-modifying agents still represent a possible avenue for further study in SZ (Sommer et al., 2016). Another possible pharmacological intervention for SZ may be to improve cognition in high-risk patients by altering GABAergic pathways. Two types of GABAergic drugs, $\alpha5$-selective inverse $GABA_A$ receptor agonists and $\alpha2/3$-selective $GABA_A$ receptor agonists, may show some possibilities for SZ (Benes & Berretta, 2001; Guidotti et al., 2000; Vinkers, Mirza, Olivier, & Kahn, 2010).

Increasing cholinergic transmission also has the potential to improve cognitive functioning in SZ (Meck & Williams, 1999). There is some evidence that using cholinesterase inhibitors may improve SZ patients' cognitive and symptom functioning, particularly if combined with glutamate agonists (Friedman, 2004). Consequently, future medications may include a variety of compounds working on different systems to achieve gains in various symptom domains.

TOOL KIT OF RESOURCES

Publications

Gardner, D. M., & Teehan, M. D. (2010). *Antipsychotics and their side effects.* Cambridge, United Kingdom: Cambridge University Press.

This book provides a comprehensive review of the adverse effects antipsychotic drugs, covering all commonly used conventional and atypical agents. In the first section, each chapter provides background information about an adverse effect, reviews the evidence linking the effect to various antipsychotics, and provides specific detection and monitoring recommendations. The second section provides unique monitoring guides for each antipsychotic. The third section provides the clinician with a program to monitor patients over the long term.

Kerner, J., & McCoy, B. (2017). *Antipsychotics: History, science, and issues.* Santa Barbara, CA: ABC-CLIO.

This book offers a robust explanation of antipsychotic medications that covers the historical, ethical, medical, legal, and scientific dimensions of antipsychotics.

Rothschild, A. J. (Ed.). (2010). *The evidence-based guide to antipsychotic medications.* Washington, DC: American Psychiatric Publishing.

This book is designed to provide both clinicians and residents with focused, comprehensive, and clinically relevant information regarding the use of antipsychotic medications to treat a broad range of psychiatric conditions—from mood and anxiety disorders to substance abuse, personality disorders, and SZ.

Stahl, S. M., & Mignon, L. (2010). *Stahl's illustrated antipsychotics: Treating psychosis, mania and depression.* Cambridge, United Kingdom: Cambridge University Press.

This book is user-friendly and designed to be fun, as all of the titles in the Stahl's Illustrated series. Concepts are illustrated by full-color images that will be familiar to all readers of Stahl's Essential Psychopharmacology. The visual learner will find that these books make psychopharmacology concepts easy to master, while the nonvisual learner will enjoy a shortened text version of complex psychopharmacology concepts. Novices may want to approach it by first looking through all the graphics and gaining a feel for the visual vocabulary. Readers more familiar with these topics should find that going back and forth between images and text provides an interaction with which to vividly conceptualize complex pharmacologies. And, to help guide the reader toward more in-depth learning about particular concepts, each book ends with a Suggested Reading section.

Online Resources

Antipsychotic Medicines for Children and Teens: A Review of the Research for Parents and Caregivers

This summary discusses using antipsychotic medicines to treat psychiatric conditions in children. It explains what medical research says about the benefits and possible side effects of these medicines when taken by children.

https://www.ncbi.nlm.nih.gov/books/NBK109556/

Antipsychotics: Taking the Long View

Post by former National Institute of Mental Health Director Thomas Insel, MD.

https://www.nimh.nih.gov/about/directors/
thomas-insel/blog/2013/antipsychotics-taking-
the-long-view.shtml

Clinical Antipsychotic Trials of Intervention Effectiveness (CATIE)

The National Institute of Mental Health-funded Clinical Antipsychotic Trials of Intervention Effectiveness (CATIE) Study was a nationwide public health-focused clinical trial that compared the effectiveness of older (first available in the 1950s) and newer (available since the 1990s) antipsychotic medications used to treat SZ. This page provides information about the study.

https://www.nimh.nih.gov/funding/clinical-research/
practical/catie/index.shtml

DailyMed

The website provides trustworthy information about marketed drugs. DailyMed is the official provider of U.S. Food and Drug Administration label information (package inserts). This website provides a standard, comprehensive, up-to-date, look-up and download resource of medication content and labeling found in medication package inserts.

https://dailymed.nlm.nih.gov/dailymed/
about-dailymed.cfm

MedlinePlus Drugs, Herbs and Supplements

MedlinePlus is the National Institutes of Health's website for patients and their families and friends. Produced by the National Library of Medicine, the world's largest medical library, it provides information about diseases, conditions, and wellness.

https://medlineplus.gov/druginformation.html

National Institute of Mental Health Medications Web Page on Antipsychotics

https://www.nimh.nih.gov/health/topics/
mental-health-medications/index.shtml#part_149866

Publication Bias Favoring Newer Antipsychotics

Post by Phillip W. Long, MD, a retired psychiatrist in Vancouver, BC, Canada, and founder of Internet Mental Health, a free encyclopedia of mental health information. Dr. Long received the Canadian Psychiatric Association's Special Recognition Award for 1995.

http://www.mentalhealth.com/mag/p53-publication-bias.htm

Schizophrenia: Sticking with Treatment (Video)

John M. Kane, MD, chairman of psychiatry at The Zucker Hillside Hospital and Hofstra Northwell School of Medicine, talks about SZ, treatment options, medications and medication adherence, relapse, and recovery.

http://molmed.org/video/118

U.S. Food and Drug Administration (FDA)

The website (http://www.fda.gov/) provides the latest information on warnings, patient medication guides, and newly approved medications.

Information on Conventional Antipsychotics

https://www.fda.gov/Drugs/DrugSafety/Postmarket
DrugSafetyInformationforPatientsandProviders/
ucm107211.htm

Atypical Antipsychotic Drugs Information

https://www.fda.gov/Drugs/DrugSafety/Postmarket
DrugSafetyInformationforPatientsandProviders/
ucm094303.htm

References

*Addington, D., Addington, J., & Maticka-Tyndale, E. (1993). Assessing depression in schizophrenia: The Calgary Depression Scale. *The British Journal of Psychiatry, 163*, 39–44. http://dx.doi.org/10.1192/S0007125000292581

Aleman, A., Kahn, R. S., & Selten, J. P. (2003). Sex differences in the risk of schizophrenia: Evidence from meta-analysis. *Archives of General Psychiatry, 60*, 565–571. http://dx.doi.org/10.1001/archpsyc.60.6.565

Alexopoulos, G. S., Streim, J., Carpenter, D., Docherty, J. P., & the Expert Consensus Panel for Using Antipsychotic Drugs in Older Patients. (2004). Using antipsychotic agents in older patients. *The Journal of Clinical Psychiatry, 65*(Suppl. 2), 5–99.

Ananth, J., Parameswaran, S., Gunatilake, S., Burgoyne, K., & Sidhom, T. (2004). Neuroleptic malignant syndrome and atypical antipsychotic drugs. *The Journal of Clinical Psychiatry, 65*, 464–470. http://dx.doi.org/10.4088/JCP.v65n0403

*Andreasen, N. C. (1983). *Scale for the Assessment of Negative Symptoms (SANS)*. Iowa City, IA: University of Iowa.

*Andreasen, N. C. (1984). *Schedule for the Assessment of Positive Symptoms (SAPS)*. Iowa City, IA: University of Iowa.

Armenteros, J. L., & Davies, M. (2006). Antipsychotics in early onset Schizophrenia: Systematic review and meta-analysis. *European Child & Adolescent Psychiatry, 15*, 141–148. http://dx.doi.org/10.1007/s00787-005-0515-2

*Asterisks indicate assessments or resources.

Bagnall, A. M., Jones, L., Ginnelly, L., Lewis, R., Glanville, J., Gilbody, S., . . . Kleijnen, J. (2003). A systematic review of atypical antipsychotic drugs in schizophrenia. *Health Technology Assessment, 7*, 171–193. http://dx.doi.org/10.3310/hta7130

Baldessarini, R. J. (1988). A summary of current knowledge of tardive dyskinesia. *L'Encéphale: Revue de psychiatrie clinique biologique et thérapeutique, 14*, 263–268.

Barbas, H., & García-Cabezas, M. Á. (2017). Prefrontal Cortex Integration of Emotion and Cognition. In M. Watanabe (Ed.), *The Prefrontal Cortex as an Executive, Emotional, and Social Brain* (pp. 51–76). New York, NY: Springer. http://dx.doi.org/10.1007/978-4-431-56508-6_4

*Barnes, T. R., & the Schizophrenia Consensus Group of British Association for Psychopharmacology. (2011). Evidence-based guidelines for the pharmacological treatment of schizophrenia: Recommendations from the British Association for Psychopharmacology. *Journal of Psychopharmacology, 25*, 567–620. http://dx.doi.org/10.1177/0269881110391123

*Barnes, T. R. E. (1989). A rating scale for drug-induced akathisia. *The British Journal of Psychiatry, 154*, 672–676. http://dx.doi.org/10.1192/bjp.154.5.672

Barnes, T. R. E., & McPhillips, M. A. (1995). How to distinguish between the neuroleptic-induced deficit syndrome, depression and disease-related negative symptoms in schizophrenia. *International Clinical Psychopharmacology, 10*(Suppl. 3), 115–121.

Beebe, L. H., Tian, L., Morris, N., Goodwin, A., Allen, S. S., & Kuldau, J. (2005). Effects of exercise on mental and physical health parameters of persons with schizophrenia. *Issues in Mental Health Nursing, 26*, 661–676. http://dx.doi.org/10.1080/01612840590959551

Benes, F. M., & Berretta, S. (2001). GABAergic interneurons: Implications for understanding schizophrenia and bipolar disorder. *Neuropsychopharmacology, 25*, 1–27. http://dx.doi.org/10.1016/S0893-133X(01)00225-1

Bennett, M. E., Bradshaw, K. R., & Catalano, L. T. (2017). Treatment of substance use disorders in schizophrenia. *The American Journal of Drug and Alcohol Abuse, 43*, 377–390. http://dx.doi.org/10.1080/00952990.2016.1200592

Bilder, R. M., Goldman, R. S., Robinson, D., Reiter, G., Bell, L., Bates, J. A., . . . Lieberman, J. A. (2000). Neuropsychology of first-episode schizophrenia: Initial characterization and clinical correlates. *The American Journal of Psychiatry, 157*, 549–559. http://dx.doi.org/10.1176/appi.ajp.157.4.549

Birt, J. (2003). Management of weight gain associated with antipsychotics. *Annals of Clinical Psychology, 15,* 49–58. http://dx.doi.org/10.3109/10401230309085669

Bobo, W. V., & Meltzer, H. Y. (2010). Duration of untreated psychosis and premorbid functioning: Relationship with treatment response and treatment-resistant schizophrenia. *Therapy-Resistant Schizophrenia, 26,* 74–86. http://dx.doi.org/10.1159/000319810

Boettger, S., & Jenewein, J. (2017). Placebo might be superior to antipsychotics in management of delirium in the palliative care setting. *Evidence-Based Medicine, 22,* 152–153. http://dx.doi.org/10.1136/ebmed-2017-110723

Bowie, C. R., Serper, M. R., Riggio, S., & Harvey, P. D. (2005). Neurocognition, symptomatology, and functional skills in older alcohol-abusing schizophrenia patients. *Schizophrenia Bulletin, 31,* 175–182. http://dx.doi.org/10.1093/jschbul/sbi001

*Branch, P. R. (1975). Abnormal involuntary movement scale (AIMS). *Early Clinical Drug Evaluation Unit Intercom, 4,* 3–6.

Brown, G., Birley, J. L. T., & Wing, J. K. (1972). Influence of family life on the course of schizophrenia. *The British Journal of Psychiatry, 121,* 241–258. http://dx.doi.org/10.1192/bjp.121.3.241

Bruijnzeel, D., Suryadevara, U., & Tandon, R. (2014). Antipsychotic treatment of schizophrenia: An update. *Asian Journal of Psychiatry, 11,* 3–7. http://dx.doi.org/10.1016/j.ajp.2014.08.002

Buckley, P. F., & Ahmed, A. O. (2013). Principles and practices of medication management for people with schizophrenia. *Modern Community Mental Health: An Interdisciplinary Approach,* 337.

Buckley, P. F., Miller, B. J., Lehrer, D. S., & Castle, D. J. (2009). Psychiatric comorbidities and schizophrenia. *Schizophrenia Bulletin, 35,* 383–402. http://dx.doi.org/10.1093/schbul/sbn135

Buoli, M., Serati, M., Ciappolino, V., & Altamura, A. C. (2016). May selective serotonin reuptake inhibitors (SSRIs) provide some benefit for the treatment of schizophrenia? *Expert Opinion on Pharmacotherapy, 17,* 1375–1385. http://dx.doi.org/10.1080/14656566.2016.1186646

Bustillo, J., Lauriello, J., Horan, W., & Keith, S. (2001). The psychosocial treatment of schizophrenia: An update. *The American Journal of Psychiatry, 158,* 163–175. http://dx.doi.org/10.1176/appi.ajp.158.2.163

Carney, C. P., Jones, L., & Woolson, R. F. (2006). Medical comorbidity in women and men with schizophrenia: A population-based controlled study. *Journal of General Internal Medicine, 21,* 1133–1137. http://dx.doi.org/10.1111/j.1525-1497.2006.00563.x

Caroff, S. N., Mann, S. C., Campbell, E. C., & Sullivan, K. A. (2002). Movement disorders associated with atypical antipsychotic drugs. *The Journal of Clinical Psychiatry, 63*(Suppl. 4), 12–19.

Carpenter, W. T., Jr., & Davis, J. M. (2012). Another view of the history of antipsychotic drug discovery and development. *Molecular Psychiatry, 17,* 1168–1173. http://dx.doi.org/10.1038/mp.2012.121

Casey, D. E. (1991). Neuroleptic drug-induced extrapyramidal syndromes and tardive dyskinesia. *Schizophrenia Research, 4,* 109–120. http://dx.doi.org/10.1016/0920-9964(91)90029-Q

Chakos, M., Lieberman, J., Hoffman, E., Bradford, D., & Sheitman, B. (2001). Effectiveness of second-generation antipsychotics in patients with treatment-resistant schizophrenia: A review and meta-analysis of randomized trials. *The American Journal of Psychiatry, 158,* 518–526. http://dx.doi.org/10.1176/appi.ajp.158.4.518

Citrome, L. (2017). Valbenazine for tardive dyskinesia: A systematic review of the efficacy and safety profile for this newly approved novel medication—What is the number needed to treat, number needed to harm and likelihood to be helped or harmed? *International Journal of Clinical Practice, 71,* e12964.

Cloud, L. J., Zutshi, D., & Factor, S. A. (2014). Tardive dyskinesia: Therapeutic options for an increasingly common disorder. *Neurotherapeutics, 11,* 166–176. http://dx.doi.org/10.1007/s13311-013-0222-5

Cooper, W. O., Hickson, G. B., Fuchs, C., Arbogast, P. G., & Ray, W. A. (2004). New users of antipsychotic medications among children enrolled in TennCare. *Archives of Pediatrics & Adolescent Medicine, 158,* 753–759. http://dx.doi.org/10.1001/archpedi.158.8.753

Correll, C. U., Frederickson, A. M., Kane, J. M., & Manu, P. (2008). Equally increased risk for metabolic syndrome in patients with bipolar disorder and schizophrenia treated with second-generation antipsychotics. *Bipolar Disorders, 10,* 788–797. http://dx.doi.org/10.1111/j.1399-5618.2008.00625.x

Correll, C. U., Manu, P., Olshanskiy, V., Napolitano, B., Kane, J. M., & Malhotra, A. K. (2009). Cardiometabolic risk of second-generation antipsychotic medications during first-time use in children and adolescents. *JAMA, 302,* 1765–1773. http://dx.doi.org/10.1001/jama.2009.1549

Correll, C. U., & Schenk, E. M. (2008). Tardive dyskinesia and new antipsychotics. *Current Opinion in Psychiatry, 21,* 151–156. http://dx.doi.org/10.1097/YCO.0b013e3282f53132

Cullen, A. E., Fisher, H. L., Roberts, R. E., Pariante, C. M., & Laurens, K. R. (2014). Daily stressors and negative life events in children at elevated risk of developing schizophrenia. *The British Journal of*

Psychiatry, 204, 354–360. http://dx.doi.org/10.1192/
bjp.bp.113.127001

Davidson, M., Galderisi, S., Weiser, M., Werbeloff, N.,
Fleischhacker, W. W., Keefe, R. S., . . . Kahn, R. S.
(2009). Cognitive effects of antipsychotic drugs in
first-episode schizophrenia and schizophreniform
disorder: A randomized, open-label clinical trial
(EUFEST). *The American Journal of Psychiatry,
166*, 675–682. http://dx.doi.org/10.1176/
appi.ajp.2008.08060806

Davis, J. M., Chen, N., & Glick, I. D. (2003). A meta-
analysis of the efficacy of second-generation antipsychotics. *Archives of General Psychiatry, 60*, 553–564.
http://dx.doi.org/10.1001/archpsyc.60.6.553

De Hert, M., Dekker, J. M., Wood, D., Kahl, K. G., Holt,
R. I. G., & Möller, H. J. (2009). Cardiovascular
disease and diabetes in people with severe mental
illness position statement from the European
Psychiatric Association (EPA), supported by the
European Association for the Study of Diabetes
(EASD) and the European Society of Cardiology
(ESC). *European Psychiatry, 24*, 412–424.
http://dx.doi.org/10.1016/j.eurpsy.2009.01.005

*Dixon, L. B., Dickerson, F., Bellack, A. S., Bennett, M.,
Dickinson, D., Goldberg, R. W., . . . Kreyenbuhl, J.,
& the Schizophrenia Patient Outcomes Research
Team (PORT). (2009). The 2009 schizophrenia
PORT psychosocial treatment recommendations
and summary statements. *Schizophrenia Bulletin, 36*,
48–70. http://dx.doi.org/10.1093/schbul/sbp115

Domino, M. E., & Swartz, M. S. (2008). Who are the
new users of antipsychotic medications? *Psychiatric
Services, 59*, 507–514. http://dx.doi.org/10.1176/
ps.2008.59.5.507

Donohoe, G. (2006). Adherence to antipsychotic
treatment in schizophrenia. *Disease Management
& Health Outcomes, 14*, 207–214. http://dx.doi.org/
10.2165/00115677-200614040-00003

Dossenbach, M., Dyachkova, Y., Pirildar, S., Anders, M.,
Khalil, A., Araszkiewicz, A., . . . Treuer, T. (2006).
Effects of atypical and typical antipsychotic treat-
ments on sexual function in patients with schizo-
phrenia: 12-month results from the Intercontinental
Schizophrenia Outpatient Health Outcomes
(IC-SOHO) study. *European Psychiatry, 21*, 251–258.
http://dx.doi.org/10.1016/j.eurpsy.2005.12.005

Eckman, T. A., Liberman, R. P., Phipps, C. C., & Blair,
K. E. (1990). Teaching medication management
skills to schizophrenic patients. *Journal of Clinical
Psychopharmacology, 10*, 33–38. http://dx.doi.org/
10.1097/00004714-199002000-00006

Edwards, S. J., & Smith, C. J. (2009). Tolerability of
atypical antipsychotics in the treatment of adults
with schizophrenia or bipolar disorder: A mixed
treatment comparison of randomized controlled

trials. *Clinical Therapeutics, 31*, 1345–1359.
http://dx.doi.org/10.1016/j.clinthera.2009.07.004

Emsley, R., Rabinowitz, J., Torreman, M., & the
RIS-INT-35 Early Psychosis Global Working Group.
(2003). The factor structure for the Positive and
Negative Syndrome Scale (PANSS) in recent-onset
psychosis. *Schizophrenia Research, 61*, 47–57.
http://dx.doi.org/10.1016/S0920-9964(02)00302-X

Fenton, W. S., Blyler, C. R., & Heinssen, R. K. (1997).
Determinants of medication compliance in
schizophrenia: Empirical and clinical findings.
Schizophrenia Bulletin, 23, 637–651. http://dx.doi.org/
10.1093/schbul/23.4.637

Fernandez, H. H., Trieschmann, M. E., & Friedman, J. H.
(2003). Treatment of psychosis in Parkinson's disease:
Safety considerations. *Drug Safety, 26*, 643–659.
http://dx.doi.org/10.2165/00002018-200326090-00004

First, M. B., Williams, J. B. W., Karg, R. S., & Spitzer,
R. L. (2015). *Structured Clinical Interview for DSM 5
Disorders, Clinical Trials Version (SCID-5-CT)*.
Arlington, VA: American Psychiatric Association
Press.

Frangou, S., & Byrne, P. (2000). How to manage the
first episode of schizophrenia. *BMJ: British Medical
Journal, 321*, 522–523. http://dx.doi.org/10.1136/
bmj.321.7260.522

Frank, R. G., Conti, R. M., & Goldman, H. H. (2005).
Mental health policy and psychotropic drugs.
Milbank Quarterly, 83, 271–298. http://dx.doi.org/
10.1111/j.1468-0009.2005.00347.x

Friedman, J. I. (2004). Cholinergic targets for cognitive enhancement in schizophrenia: Focus on
cholinesterase inhibitors and muscarinic agonists.
Psychopharmacology, 174, 45–53. http://dx.doi.org/
10.1007/s00213-004-1794-x

García-Bueno, B., Caso, J. R., & Leza, J. C. (2008).
Stress as a neuroinflammatory condition in brain:
Damaging and protective mechanisms. *Neuroscience
and Biobehavioral Reviews, 32*, 1136–1151.
http://dx.doi.org/10.1016/j.neubiorev.2008.04.001

Gebhardt, S., Härtling, F., Hanke, M., Mittendorf, M.,
Theisen, F. M., Wolf-Ostermann, K., . . .
Remschmidt, H. (2006). Prevalence of movement
disorders in adolescent patients with schizophrenia
and in relationship to predominantly atypical antipsychotic treatment. *European Child & Adolescent
Psychiatry, 15*, 371–382. http://dx.doi.org/10.1007/
s00787-006-0544-5

Geddes, J., Freemantle, N., Harrison, P., & Bebbington, P.
(2000). Atypical antipsychotics in the treatment
of schizophrenia: Systematic overview and meta-
regression analysis. *BMJ: British Medical Journal,
321*, 1371–1376. http://dx.doi.org/10.1136/
bmj.321.7273.1371

Glazer, W. M., Morgenstern, H., Schooler, N., Berkman, C. S., & Moore, D. C. (1990). Predictors of improvement in tardive dyskinesia following discontinuation of neuroleptic medication. *The British Journal of Psychiatry, 157*, 585–592. http://dx.doi.org/10.1192/bjp.157.4.585

Goff, D. C., Falkai, P., Fleischhacker, W. W., Girgis, R. R., Kahn, R. M., Uchida, H., . . . Lieberman, J. A. (2017). The long-term effects of antipsychotic medication on clinical course in schizophrenia. *The American Journal of Psychiatry, 174*, 840–849. http://dx.doi.org/10.1176/appi.ajp.2017.16091016

Goldberg, S. C. (1985). Negative and deficit symptoms in schizophrenia do respond to neuroleptics. *Schizophrenia Bulletin, 11*, 453–456. http://dx.doi.org/10.1093/schbul/11.3.453

Green, A. I., Tohen, M. F., Hamer, R. M., Strakowski, S. M., Lieberman, J. A., Glick, I., . . . the HGDH Research Group. (2004). First episode schizophrenia-related psychosis and substance use disorders: Acute response to olanzapine and haloperidol. *Schizophrenia Research, 66*, 125–135. http://dx.doi.org/10.1016/j.schres.2003.08.001

*Green, M. F., Nuechterlein, K. H., Gold, J. M., Barch, D. M., Cohen, J., Essock, S., . . . Marder, S. R. (2004). Approaching a consensus cognitive battery for clinical trials in schizophrenia: The NIMH-MATRICS conference to select cognitive domains and test criteria. *Biological Psychiatry, 56*, 301–307. http://dx.doi.org/10.1016/j.biopsych.2004.06.023

Guidotti, A., Auta, J., Davis, J. M., DiGiorgi Gerevini, V., Dwivedi, Y., Grayson, D. R., . . . Costa, E. (2000). Decrease in reelin and glutamic acid decarboxylase67 (GAD67) expression in schizophrenia and bipolar disorder: A postmortem brain study. *Archives of General Psychiatry, 57*, 1061–1069. http://dx.doi.org/10.1001/archpsyc.57.11.1061

Gurrera, R. J. (2017). A systematic review of sex and age factors in neuroleptic malignant syndrome diagnosis frequency. *Acta Psychiatrica Scandinavica, 135*, 398–408. http://dx.doi.org/10.1111/acps.12694

Halstead, S. M., Barnes, T. R. E., & Speller, J. C. (1994). Akathisia: Prevalence and associated dysphoria in an in-patient population with chronic schizophrenia. *The British Journal of Psychiatry, 164*, 177–183. http://dx.doi.org/10.1192/bjp.164.2.177

Hansen, L. (2001). A critical review of akathisia, and its possible association with suicidal behaviour. *Human Psychopharmacology: Clinical and Experimental, 16*, 495–505. http://dx.doi.org/10.1002/hup.325

Hartling, L., Abou-Setta, A. M., Dursun, S., Mousavi, S. S., Pasichnyk, D., & Newton, A. S. (2012). Antipsychotics in adults with schizophrenia: Comparative effectiveness of first-generation versus second-generation medications: A systematic review and meta-analysis. *Annals of Internal Medicine,*

157, 498–511. http://dx.doi.org/10.7326/0003-4819-157-7-201210020-00525

Haro, J. M., Edgell, E. T., Novick, D., Alonso, J., Kennedy, L., Jones, P. B., . . . Breier, A., & the SOHO advisory board. (2005). Effectiveness of antipsychotic treatment for schizophrenia: 6-month results of the Pan-European Schizophrenia Outpatient Health Outcomes (SOHO) study. *Acta Psychiatrica Scandinavica, 111*, 220–231. http://dx.doi.org/10.1111/j.1600-0447.2004.00450.x

Hartz, S. M., Pato, C. N., Medeiros, H., Cavazos-Rehg, P., Sobell, J. L., Knowles, J. A., . . . Pato, M. T., & the Genomic Psychiatry Cohort Consortium. (2014). Comorbidity of severe psychotic disorders with measures of substance use. *JAMA Psychiatry, 71*, 248–254. http://dx.doi.org/10.1001/jamapsychiatry.2013.3726

Healy, D., Harris, M., Tranter, R., Gutting, P., Austin, R., Jones-Edwards, G., & Roberts, A. P. (2006). Lifetime suicide rates in treated schizophrenia: 1875–1924 and 1994–1998 cohorts compared. *The British Journal of Psychiatry, 188*, 223–228. http://dx.doi.org/10.1192/bjp.188.3.223

Ho, A. P., Tsuang, J. W., Liberman, R. P., Wang, R., Wilkins, J. N., Eckman, T. A., & Shaner, A. L. (1999). Achieving effective treatment of patients with chronic psychotic illness and comorbid substance dependence. *The American Journal of Psychiatry, 156*, 1765–1770.

Ho, B. C., Andreasen, N. C., Ziebell, S., Pierson, R., & Magnotta, V. (2011). Long-term antipsychotic treatment and brain volumes: A longitudinal study of first-episode schizophrenia. *Archives of General Psychiatry, 68*, 128–137. http://dx.doi.org/10.1001/archgenpsychiatry.2010.199

Hogarty, G. E., McEvoy, J. P., Munetz, M., DiBarry, A. L., Bartone, P., Cather, R., . . . Madonia, M. J. (1988). Dose of fluphenazine, familial expressed emotion, and outcome in schizophrenia. Results of a two-year controlled study. *Archives of General Psychiatry, 45*, 797–805. http://dx.doi.org/10.1001/archpsyc.1988.01800330021002

Hor, K., & Taylor, M. (2010). Suicide and schizophrenia: A systematic review of rates and risk factors. *Journal of Psychopharmacology, 24*(Suppl.), 81–90. http://dx.doi.org/10.1177/1359786810385490

Horsfall, J., Cleary, M., Hunt, G. E., & Walter, G. (2009). Psychosocial treatments for people with co-occurring severe mental illnesses and substance use disorders (dual diagnosis): A review of empirical evidence. *Harvard Review of Psychiatry, 17*, 24–34. http://dx.doi.org/10.1080/10673220902724599

Howes, O. D., & Kapur, S. (2009). The dopamine hypothesis of schizophrenia: Version III—the final common pathway. *Schizophrenia Bulletin, 35,* 549–562. http://dx.doi.org/10.1093/schbul/sbp006

*Howes, O. D., McCutcheon, R., Agid, O., de Bartolomeis, A., van Beveren, N. J., Birnbaum, M. L., . . . Correll, C. U. (2016). Treatment-resistant schizophrenia: Treatment Response and Resistance in Psychosis (TRRIP) working group consensus guidelines on diagnosis and terminology. *The American Journal of Psychiatry, 174,* 216–229. http://dx.doi.org/10.1176/appi.ajp.2016.16050503

Iwata, Y., Nakajima, S., Suzuki, T., Keefe, R. S. E., Plitman, E., Chung, J. K., . . . Uchida, H. (2015). Effects of glutamate positive modulators on cognitive deficits in schizophrenia: A systematic review and meta-analysis of double-blind randomized controlled trials. *Molecular Psychiatry, 20,* 1151–1160. http://dx.doi.org/10.1038/mp.2015.68

Janno, S., Holi, M. M., Tuisku, K., & Wahlbeck, K. (2005). Validity of Simpson-Angus Scale (SAS) in a naturalistic schizophrenia population. *BMC Neurology, 5,* 5–11. http://dx.doi.org/10.1186/1471-2377-5-5

Jones, P. B., Barnes, T. R., Davies, L., Dunn, G., Lloyd, H., Hayhurst, K. P., . . . Lewis, S. W. (2006). Randomized controlled trial of the effect on quality of life of second- vs first-generation antipsychotic drugs in schizophrenia: Cost Utility of the Latest Antipsychotic Drugs in Schizophrenia Study (CUtLASS 1). *Archives of General Psychiatry, 63,* 1079–1087. http://dx.doi.org/10.1001/archpsyc.63.10.1079

Juuhl-Langseth, M., Holmén, A., Thormodsen, R., Øie, M., & Rund, B. R. (2014). Relative stability of neurocognitive deficits in early onset schizophrenia spectrum patients. *Schizophrenia Research, 156,* 241–247. http://dx.doi.org/10.1016/j.schres.2014.04.014

Kahn, R. S., Fleischhacker, W. W., Boter, H., Davidson, M., Vergouwe, Y., Keet, I. P., . . . Grobbee, D. E., & the EUFEST study group. (2008). Effectiveness of antipsychotic drugs in first-episode schizophrenia and schizophreniform disorder: An open randomised clinical trial. *The Lancet, 371,* 1085–1097. http://dx.doi.org/10.1016/S0140-6736(08)60486-9

Kamble, P., Chen, H., Sherer, J. T., & Aparasu, R. R. (2009). Use of antipsychotics among elderly nursing home residents with dementia in the US: An analysis of National Survey data. *Drugs & Aging, 26,* 483–492. http://dx.doi.org/10.2165/00002512-200926060-00005

Kampman, O., & Lehtinen, K. (1999). Compliance in psychoses. *Acta Psychiatrica Scandinavica, 100,* 167–175. http://dx.doi.org/10.1111/j.1600-0447.1999.tb10842.x

Kane, J. M., Fleischhacker, W. W., Hansen, L., Perlis, R., Pikalov, A., III, & Assunção-Talbott, S. (2009). Akathisia: An updated review focusing on second-generation antipsychotics. *The Journal of Clinical Psychiatry, 70,* 627–643. http://dx.doi.org/10.4088/JCP.08r04210

Kapur, S., & Seeman, P. (2001). Does fast dissociation from the dopamine d(2) receptor explain the action of atypical antipsychotics? A new hypothesis. *The American Journal of Psychiatry, 158,* 360–369. http://dx.doi.org/10.1176/appi.ajp.158.3.360

Karow, A., Czekalla, J., Dittmann, R. W., Schacht, A., Wagner, T., Lambert, M., . . . Naber, D. (2007). Association of subjective well-being, symptoms, and side effects with compliance after 12 months of treatment in schizophrenia. *The Journal of Clinical Psychiatry, 68,* 75–80. http://dx.doi.org/10.4088/JCP.v68n0110

*Kay, S. R., Fiszbein, A., & Opler, L. A. (1987). The positive and negative syndrome scale (PANSS) for schizophrenia. *Schizophrenia Bulletin, 13,* 261–276. http://dx.doi.org/10.1093/schbul/13.2.261

Keefe, R. S., Bilder, R. M., Davis, S. M., Harvey, P. D., Palmer, B. W., Gold, J. M., . . . Lieberman, J. A., & the CATIE Investigators, & the Neurocognitive Working Group. (2007). Neurocognitive effects of antipsychotic medications in patients with chronic schizophrenia in the CATIE Trial. *Archives of General Psychiatry, 64,* 633–647. http://dx.doi.org/10.1001/archpsyc.64.6.633

*Keefe, R. S., Goldberg, T. E., Harvey, P. D., Gold, J. M., Poe, M. P., & Coughenour, L. (2004). The Brief Assessment of Cognition in Schizophrenia: Reliability, sensitivity, and comparison with a standard neurocognitive battery. *Schizophrenia Research, 68,* 283–297. http://dx.doi.org/10.1016/j.schres.2003.09.011

Kemp, R., David, A., & Hayward, P. (1996). Compliance therapy: An intervention targeting insight and treatment adherence in psychotic patients. *Behavioural and Cognitive Psychotherapy, 24,* 331–350. http://dx.doi.org/10.1017/S135246580001523X

Kemp, R., Kirov, G., Everitt, B., Hayward, P., & David, A. (1998). Randomised controlled trial of compliance therapy. 18-month follow-up. *The British Journal of Psychiatry, 172,* 413–419. http://dx.doi.org/10.1192/bjp.172.5.413

Kishimoto, T., Nitta, M., Borenstein, M., Kane, J. M., & Correll, C. U. (2013). Long-acting injectable versus oral antipsychotics in schizophrenia: A systematic review and meta-analysis of mirror-image studies. *The Journal of Clinical Psychiatry, 74,* 957–965. http://dx.doi.org/10.4088/JCP.13r08440

Knegtering, R., Castelein, S., Bous, H., Van Der Linde, J., Bruggeman, R., Kluiter, H., & van den Bosch, R. J. (2004). A randomized open-label study of the impact of quetiapine versus risperidone on sexual functioning. *Journal of Clinical Psychopharmacology, 24,* 56–61. http://dx.doi.org/10.1097/01.jcp.0000106220.36344.04

Kraal, A. Z., Ward, K. M., & Ellingrod, V. L. (2017). Sex differences in antipsychotic related metabolic functioning in schizophrenia spectrum disorders. *Psychopharmacology Bulletin, 47,* 8–21.

*Kreyenbuhl, J., Buchanan, R. W., Dickerson, F. B., Dixon, L. B., & the Schizophrenia Patient Outcomes Research Team (PORT). (2010). The schizophrenia patient outcomes research team (PORT): Updated treatment recommendations 2009. *Schizophrenia Bulletin, 36,* 94–103. http://dx.doi.org/10.1093/schbul/sbp130

Lacro, J. P., Dunn, L. B., Dolder, C. R., Leckband, S. G., & Jeste, D. V. (2002). Prevalence of and risk factors for medication nonadherence in patients with schizophrenia: A comprehensive review of recent literature. *The Journal of Clinical Psychiatry, 63,* 892–909. http://dx.doi.org/10.4088/JCP.v63n1007

Leas, L., & McCabe, M. (2007). Health behaviors among individuals with schizophrenia and depression. *Journal of Health Psychology, 12,* 563–579. http://dx.doi.org/10.1177/1359105307078162

*Leff, J., Kuipers, L., Berkowitz, R., Vaughn, C., & Sturgeon, D. (1983). Life events, relatives' expressed emotion and maintenance neuroleptics in schizophrenic relapse. *Psychological Medicine, 13,* 799–806. http://dx.doi.org/10.1017/S0033291700051503

*Lehman, A. F., Kreyenbuhl, J., Buchanan, R. W., Dickerson, F. B., Dixon, L. B., Goldberg, R., . . . Steinwachs, D. M. (2004). The schizophrenia patient outcomes research team (PORT): Updated treatment recommendations 2003. *Schizophrenia Bulletin, 30,* 193–217. http://dx.doi.org/10.1093/oxfordjournals.schbul.a007071

Leucht, S., Arbter, D., Engel, R. R., Kissling, W., & Davis, J. M. (2009a). How effective are second-generation antipsychotic drugs? A meta-analysis of placebo-controlled trials. *Molecular Psychiatry, 14,* 429–447. http://dx.doi.org/10.1038/sj.mp.4002136

Leucht, S., Cipriani, A., Spineli, L., Mavridis, D., Örey, D., Richter, F., . . . Davis, J. M. (2013). Comparative efficacy and tolerability of 15 antipsychotic drugs in schizophrenia: A multiple-treatments meta-analysis. *The Lancet, 382,* 951–962. http://dx.doi.org/10.1016/S0140-6736(13)60733-3

Leucht, S., Corves, C., Arbter, D., Engel, R. R., Li, C., & Davis, J. M. (2009b). Second-generation versus first-generation antipsychotic drugs for schizophrenia: A meta-analysis. *Lancet, 373,* 31–41. http://dx.doi.org/10.1016/S0140-6736(08)61764-X

Leucht, S., Heres, S., Kissling, W., & Davis, J. M. (2011). Evidence-based pharmacotherapy of schizophrenia. *International Journal of Neuropsychopharmacology, 14,* 269–284. http://dx.doi.org/10.1017/S1461145710001380

Leucht, S., Pitschel-Walz, G., Abraham, D., & Kissling, W. (1999). Efficacy and extrapyramidal side-effects of the new antipsychotics olanzapine, quetiapine, risperidone, and sertindole compared to conventional antipsychotics and placebo. A meta-analysis of randomized controlled trials. *Schizophrenia Research, 35,* 51–68. http://dx.doi.org/10.1016/S0920-9964(98)00105-4

Leung, A., & Chue, P. (2000). Sex differences in schizophrenia, a review of the literature. *Acta Psychiatrica Scandinavica, 101,* 3–38. http://dx.doi.org/10.1111/j.0065-1591.2000.0ap25.x

Leweke, F. M., & Koethe, D. (2008). Cannabis and psychiatric disorders: It is not only addiction. *Addiction Biology, 13,* 264–275. http://dx.doi.org/10.1111/j.1369-1600.2008.00106.x

Lewis, S. W., Barnes, T. R., Davies, L., Murray, R. M., Dunn, G., Hayhurst, K. P., . . . Jones, P. B. (2006). Randomized controlled trial of effect of prescription of clozapine versus other second-generation antipsychotic drugs in resistant schizophrenia. *Schizophrenia Bulletin, 32,* 715–723. http://dx.doi.org/10.1093/schbul/sbj067

Lieberman, J. A. (2015). *Shrinks: The Untold Story.* New York, NY: Little Brown.

Lieberman, J. A., Stroup, T. S., McEvoy, J. P., Swartz, M. S., Rosenheck, R. A., Perkins, D. O., . . . Hsiao, J. K., & the Clinical Antipsychotic Trials of Intervention Effectiveness (CATIE) Investigators. (2005). Effectiveness of antipsychotic drugs in patients with chronic schizophrenia. *The New England Journal of Medicine, 353,* 1209–1223. http://dx.doi.org/10.1056/NEJMoa051688

Liberman, R. P., & Davis, J. (1975). Drugs and behavior analysis. *Progress in Behavior Modification, 1,* 307–330. http://dx.doi.org/10.1016/B978-0-12-535601-5.50015-9

MacEwan, J. P., Kamat, S. A., Duffy, R. A., Seabury, S., Chou, J. W., Legacy, S. N., . . . Karson, C. (2016). Hospital readmission rates among patients with schizophrenia treated with long-acting injectables or oral antipsychotics. *Psychiatric Services, 67,* 1183–1188. http://dx.doi.org/10.1176/appi.ps.201500455

Marder, S. R., Essock, S. M., Miller, A. L., Buchanan, R. W., Casey, D. E., Davis, J. M., . . . Shon, S. (2004). Physical health monitoring of patients with schizophrenia. *The American Journal of Psychiatry, 161,* 1334–1349. http://dx.doi.org/10.1176/appi.ajp.161.8.1334

Maremmani, A. G., Bacciardi, S., Gehring, N. D., Cambioli, L., Schütz, C., Jang, K., & Krausz, M. (2017). Substance use among homeless individuals with schizophrenia and bipolar disorder. *Journal of Nervous and Mental Disease, 205,* 173–177. http://dx.doi.org/10.1097/NMD.0000000000000462

Marshall, M., Lewis, S., Lockwood, A., Drake, R., Jones, P., & Croudace, T. (2005). Association between duration of untreated psychosis and outcome in cohorts of first-episode patients: A systematic review. *Archives of General Psychiatry, 62*, 975–983. http://dx.doi.org/10.1001/archpsyc.62.9.975

McCreadie, R. G., Wiles, D. H., Livingston, M. G., Watt, J. A., Greene, J. G., Kershaw, P. W., Loudon, J., & The Scottish Schizophrenia Research Group. (1992). The Scottish first episode schizophrenia study: VIII. Five-year follow-up: Clinical and psychosocial findings. *The British Journal of Psychiatry, 161*, 496–500. http://dx.doi.org/10.1192/bjp.161.4.496

McEvoy, J. P., Meyer, J. M., Goff, D. C., Nasrallah, H. A., Davis, S. M., Sullivan, L., . . . Lieberman, J. A. (2005). Prevalence of the metabolic syndrome in patients with schizophrenia: Baseline results from the Clinical Antipsychotic Trials of Intervention Effectiveness (CATIE) schizophrenia trial and comparison with national estimates from NHANES III. *Schizophrenia Research, 80*, 19–32. http://dx.doi.org/10.1016/j.schres.2005.07.014

McGrath, J., Saha, S., Chant, D., & Welham, J. (2008). Schizophrenia: A concise overview of incidence, prevalence, and mortality. *Epidemiologic Reviews, 30*, 67–76. http://dx.doi.org/10.1093/epirev/mxn001

McGrath, J., Saha, S., Welham, J., El Saadi, O., MacCauley, C., & Chant, D. (2004). A systematic review of the incidence of schizophrenia: The distribution of rates and the influence of sex, urbanicity, migrant status and methodology. *BMC Medicine, 2*, 13. http://dx.doi.org/10.1186/1741-7015-2-13

McGorry, P. D., Killackey, E., & Yung, A. (2008). Early intervention in psychosis: Concepts, evidence and future directions. *World Psychiatry, 7*, 148–156. http://dx.doi.org/10.1002/j.2051-5545.2008.tb00182.x

Meck, W. H., & Williams, C. L. (1999). Choline supplementation during prenatal development reduces proactive interference in spatial memory. *Developmental Brain Research, 118*, 51–59. http://dx.doi.org/10.1016/S0165-3806(99)00105-4

Meltzer, H. Y. (2013). Update on typical and atypical antipsychotic drugs. *Annual Review of Medicine, 64*, 393–406. http://dx.doi.org/10.1146/annurev-med-050911-161504

Meltzer, H. Y., Alphs, L., Green, A. I., Altamura, A. C., Anand, R., Bertoldi, A., . . . Potkin, S., & the International Suicide Prevention Trial Study Group. (2003). Clozapine treatment for suicidality in schizophrenia: International Suicide Prevention Trial (InterSePT). *Archives of General Psychiatry, 60*, 82–91. http://dx.doi.org/10.1001/archpsyc.60.1.82

Messias, E. L., Chen, C. Y., & Eaton, W. W. (2007). Epidemiology of schizophrenia: Review of findings and myths. *Psychiatric Clinics of North America, 30*, 323–338. http://dx.doi.org/10.1016/j.psc.2007.04.007

Meyer, J. M., Davis, V. G., Goff, D. C., McEvoy, J. P., Nasrallah, H. A., Davis, S. M., . . . Lieberman, J. A.

(2008). Change in metabolic syndrome parameters with antipsychotic treatment in the CATIE Schizophrenia Trial: Prospective data from phase 1. *Schizophrenia Research, 101*, 273–286. http://dx.doi.org/10.1016/j.schres.2007.12.487

Mitchell, A. J., & Selmes, T. (2007). Why don't patients take their medicine? Reasons and solutions in psychiatry. *Advances in Psychiatric Treatment, 13*, 336–346. http://dx.doi.org/10.1192/apt.bp.106.003194

Mitchell, A. J., Vancampfort, D., Sweers, K., van Winkel, R., Yu, W., & De Hert, M. (2013). Prevalence of metabolic syndrome and metabolic abnormalities in schizophrenia and related disorders—a systematic review and meta-analysis. *Schizophrenia Bulletin, 39*, 306–318. http://dx.doi.org/10.1093/schbul/sbr148

Mizrahi, R., Addington, J., Rusjan, P. M., Suridjan, I., Ng, A., Boileau, I., . . . Wilson, A. A. (2012). Increased stress-induced dopamine release in psychosis. *Biological Psychiatry, 71*, 561–567. http://dx.doi.org/10.1016/j.biopsych.2011.10.009

Moran, P., & Hodgins, S. (2004). The correlates of comorbid antisocial personality disorder in schizophrenia. *Schizophrenia Bulletin, 30*(4), 791–802.

Morgenstern, H., & Glazer, W. M. (1993). Identifying risk factors for tardive dyskinesia among long-term outpatients maintained with neuroleptic medications. Results of the Yale Tardive Dyskinesia Study. *Archives of General Psychiatry, 50*, 723–733. http://dx.doi.org/10.1001/archpsyc.1993.01820210057007

Morgenstern, H., Glazer, W. M., Gibowski, L. D., & Holmberg, S. (1987). Predictors of tardive dyskinesia: Results of a cross-sectional study in an outpatient population. *Journal of Chronic Diseases, 40*, 319–327. http://dx.doi.org/10.1016/0021-9681(87)90047-6

Mueser, K. T., Deavers, F., Penn, D. L., & Cassisi, J. E. (2013). Psychosocial treatments for schizophrenia. *Annual Review of Clinical Psychology, 9*, 465–497. http://dx.doi.org/10.1146/annurev-clinpsy-050212-185620

Navari, S., & Dazzan, P. (2009). Do antipsychotic drugs affect brain structure? A systematic and critical review of MRI findings. *Psychological Medicine, 39*, 1763–1777. http://dx.doi.org/10.1017/S0033291709005315

Nelson, A. A., Jr., Gold, B. H., Hutchinson, R. A., & Benezra, E. (1975). Drug default among schizophrenic patients. *American Journal of Hospital Pharmacy, 32*, 1237–1242.

Novick, D., Haro, J. M., Suarez, D., Perez, V., Dittmann, R. W., & Haddad, P. M. (2010). Predictors and clinical consequences of non-adherence with antipsychotic medication in the outpatient treatment of schizophrenia. *Psychiatry Research, 176*, 109–113. http://dx.doi.org/10.1016/j.psychres.2009.05.004

*Nurnberger, J. I., Jr., Blehar, M. C., Kaufmann, C. A., York-Cooler, C., Simpson, S. G., Harkavy-

Friedman, J., . . . Reich, T., & the NIMH Genetics Initiative. (1994). Diagnostic interview for genetic studies. Rationale, unique features, and training. *Archives of General Psychiatry, 51*, 849–859. http://dx.doi.org/10.1001/archpsyc.1994.03950110009002

Ochoa, S., Usall, J., Cobo, J., Labad, X., & Kulkarni, J. (2012). Gender differences in schizophrenia and first-episode psychosis: A comprehensive literature review. *Schizophrenia Research and Treatment, 2012*, 916198. http://dx.doi.org/10.1155/2012/916198

O'Donnell, C., Donohoe, G., Sharkey, L., Owens, N., Migone, M., Harries, R., . . . O'Callaghan, E. (2003). Compliance therapy: A randomised controlled trial in schizophrenia. *BMJ: British Medical Journal, 327*, 834–837. http://dx.doi.org/10.1136/bmj.327.7419.834

Olfson, M., Blanco, C., Liu, L., Moreno, C., & Laje, G. (2006). National trends in the outpatient treatment of children and adolescents with antipsychotic drugs. *Archives of General Psychiatry, 63*, 679–685. http://dx.doi.org/10.1001/archpsyc.63.6.679

Patel, J. K., Buckley, P. F., Woolson, S., Hamer, R. M., McEvoy, J. P., Perkins, D. O., Lieberman, J. A., & for the CAFE Investigators. (2009). Metabolic profiles of second-generation antipsychotics in early psychosis: Findings from the CAFE study. *Schizophrenia Research, 111*, 9–16. http://dx.doi.org/10.1016/j.schres.2009.03.025

Peluso, M. J., Lewis, S. W., Barnes, T. R. E., & Jones, P. B. (2012). Extrapyramidal motor side-effects of first- and second-generation antipsychotic drugs. *The British Journal of Psychiatry, 200*, 387–392. http://dx.doi.org/10.1192/bjp.bp.111.101485

Petrakis, I. L., Poling, J., Levinson, C., Nich, C., Carroll, K., Rounsaville, B., & the VA New England VISN I MIRECC Study Group. (2005). Naltrexone and disulfiram in patients with alcohol dependence and comorbid psychiatric disorders. *Biological Psychiatry, 57*, 1128–1137. http://dx.doi.org/10.1016/j.biopsych.2005.02.016

Pocklington, A. J., Rees, E., Walters, J. T., Han, J., Kavanagh, D. H., Chambert, K. D., . . . Owen, M. J. (2015). Novel findings from CNVs implicate inhibitory and excitatory signaling complexes in schizophrenia. *Neuron, 86*, 1203–1214. http://dx.doi.org/10.1016/j.neuron.2015.04.022

Pope, H. G., Jr., Keck, P. E., Jr., & McElroy, S. L. (1986). Frequency and presentation of neuroleptic malignant syndrome in a large psychiatric hospital. *The American Journal of Psychiatry, 143*, 1227–1233. http://dx.doi.org/10.1176/ajp.143.10.1227

Potkin, S. G., Saha, A. R., Kujawa, M. J., Carson, W. H., Ali, M., Stock, E., . . . Marder, S. R. (2003). Aripiprazole, an antipsychotic with a novel mechanism of action, and risperidone vs placebo in patients with schizophrenia and schizoaffective disorder.

Archives of General Psychiatry, 60, 681–690. http://dx.doi.org/10.1001/archpsyc.60.7.681

Potvin, S., Pampoulova, T., Mancini-Marië, A., Lipp, O., Bouchard, R. H., & Stip, E. (2006). Increased extrapyramidal symptoms in patients with schizophrenia and a comorbid substance use disorder. *Journal of Neurology, Neurosurgery, & Psychiatry, 77*, 796–798. http://dx.doi.org/10.1136/jnnp.2005.079228

Robinson, D., Woerner, M., & Schooler, N. (2000). Intervention research in psychosis: Issues related to clinical assessment. *Schizophrenia Bulletin, 26*, 551–556. http://dx.doi.org/10.1093/oxfordjournals.schbul.a033476

Robinson, D., Woerner, M. G., Alvir, J. M. J., Bilder, R., Goldman, R., Geisler, S., . . . Lieberman, J. A. (1999). Predictors of relapse following response from a first episode of schizophrenia or schizoaffective disorder. *Archives of General Psychiatry, 56*, 241–247. http://dx.doi.org/10.1001/archpsyc.56.3.241

Saddichha, S., Ameen, S., & Akhtar, S. (2008). Predictors of antipsychotic-induced weight gain in first-episode psychosis: Conclusions from a randomized, double-blind, controlled prospective study of olanzapine, risperidone, and haloperidol. *Journal of Clinical Psychopharmacology, 28*, 27–31. http://dx.doi.org/10.1097/jcp.0b013e3181602fe6

Saha, S., Chant, D., & McGrath, J. (2007). A systematic review of mortality in schizophrenia: Is the differential mortality gap worsening over time? *Archives of General Psychiatry, 64*, 1123–1131. http://dx.doi.org/10.1001/archpsyc.64.10.1123

Sakel, M. (1937). A new treatment of schizophrenia. *The American Journal of Psychiatry, 93*, 829–841. http://dx.doi.org/10.1176/ajp.93.4.829

Samara, M., & Leucht, S. (2017). Clozapine in treatment-resistant schizophrenia. *The British Journal of Psychiatry, 210*, 299–299. http://dx.doi.org/10.1192/bjp.210.4.299

Samara, M. T., Dold, M., Gianatsi, M., Nikolakopoulou, A., Helfer, B., Salanti, G., & Leucht, S. (2016). Efficacy, acceptability, and tolerability of antipsychotics in treatment-resistant schizophrenia: A network meta-analysis. *JAMA Psychiatry, 73*, 199–210. http://dx.doi.org/10.1001/jamapsychiatry.2015.2955

Schmidt, M. J., & Mirnics, K. (2015). Neurodevelopment, GABA system dysfunction, and schizophrenia. *Neuropsychopharmacology, 40*, 190–206. http://dx.doi.org/10.1038/npp.2014.95

Seeman, P. (2002). Atypical antipsychotics: Mechanism of action. *The Canadian Journal of Psychiatry, 47*, 29–38. http://dx.doi.org/10.1177/070674370204700106

Sellwood, W., Tarrier, N., Quinn, J., & Barrowclough, C. (2003). The family and compliance in schizophrenia: The influence of clinical variables, relatives' knowledge and expressed emotion. *Psychological Medicine, 33*, 91–96. http://dx.doi.org/10.1017/S0033291702006888

Selten, J. P., van der Ven, E., Rutten, B. P., & Cantor-Graae, E. (2013). The social defeat hypothesis of schizophrenia: An update. *Schizophrenia Bulletin, 39*, 1180–1186. http://dx.doi.org/10.1093/schbul/sbt134

Sepehry, A. A., Potvin, S., Élie, R., & Stip, E. (2007). Selective serotonin reuptake inhibitor (SSRI) add-on therapy for the negative symptoms of schizophrenia: A meta-analysis. *The Journal of Clinical Psychiatry, 68*, 604–610. http://dx.doi.org/10.4088/JCP.v68n0417

Sera, L. C., & McPherson, M. L. (2012). Pharmaco-kinetics and pharmacodynamic changes associated with aging and implications for drug therapy. *Clinics in Geriatric Medicine, 28*, 273–286. http://dx.doi.org/10.1016/j.cger.2012.01.007

Sernyak, M., & Rosenheck, R. (2007). Experience of VA psychiatrists with pharmaceutical detailing of antipsychotic medications. *Psychiatric Services, 58*, 1292–1296. http://dx.doi.org/10.1176/ps.2007.58.10.1292

Serper, M., Goldberg, B., & Salzinger, K. (2004). Behavioral assessment of psychiatric patients in restrictive settings. In E. Heiby & M. Hersen (Eds.), *Comprehensive handbook of psychological assessment: Behavioral assessment* (Vol. 3, pp. 320–345). New York, NY: Wiley.

Serper, M., Payne, E., Dill, C., Portillo, C., & Taliercio, J. (2017). Allocating effort and anticipating pleasure in schizophrenia: Relationship with real world functioning. *European Psychiatry, 46*, 57–64. http://dx.doi.org/10.1016/j.eurpsy.2017.07.008

Serper, M. R., Bergman, A., Copersino, M. L., Chou, J. C., Richarme, D., & Cancro, R. (2000). Learning and memory impairment in cocaine-dependent and comorbid schizophrenic patients. *Psychiatry Research, 93*, 21–32. http://dx.doi.org/10.1016/S0165-1781(99)00122-5

Sikich, L., Frazier, J. A., McClellan, J., Findling, R. L., Vitiello, B., Ritz, L., . . . Lieberman, J. A. (2008). Double-blind comparison of first- and second-generation antipsychotics in early-onset schizophrenia and schizo-affective disorder: Findings from the treatment of early-onset schizophrenia spectrum disorders (TEOSS) study. *The American Journal of Psychiatry, 165*, 1420–1431. http://dx.doi.org/10.1176/appi.ajp.2008.08050756

*Simpson, G. M., & Angus, J. W. S. (1970). A rating scale for extrapyramidal side effects. *Acta Psychiatrica Scandinavica, 45*(S212), 11–19. http://dx.doi.org/10.1111/j.1600-0447.1970.tb02066.x

Siskind, D., Siskind, V., & Kisely, S. (2017). Clozapine response rates among people with treatment-resistant schizophrenia: Data from a systematic review and meta-analysis. *The Canadian Journal of Psychiatry, 62*, 772–777. http://dx.doi.org/10.1177/0706743717718167

Smith, S., Wheeler, M. J., Murray, R., & O'Keane, V. (2002). The effects of antipsychotic-induced hyperprolacti-naemia on the hypothalamic-pituitary-gonadal axis. *Journal of Clinical Psychopharmacology, 22*, 109–114. http://dx.doi.org/10.1097/00004714-200204000-00002

Sommer, I. E., Bearden, C. E., van Dellen, E., Breetvelt, E. J., Duijff, S. N., Maijer, K., . . . Vorstman, J. A. (2016). Early interventions in risk groups for schizophrenia: What are we waiting for? *NPJ Schizophrenia, 2*, 16003. http://dx.doi.org/10.1038/npjschz.2016.3

Stahl, S. M. (2008). *Stahl's essential psychopharmacology.* New York, NY: Cambridge University Press.

Stanton, R. J., Paxos, C., Geldenhuys, W. J., Pharm, B., Boss, J. L., Munetz, M., . . . Pharm, M. (2015). Clozapine underutilization in treatment-resistant schizophrenia. *Mental Health Clinician, 5*(2), 63–67.

Stroup, T. S., McEvoy, J. P., & Lieberman, J. A. (2004). Revised PORT recommendations. *Schizophrenia Bulletin, 30*, 609–611. http://dx.doi.org/10.1093/oxfordjournals.schbul.a007106

Swanson, J. W., Swartz, M. S., Van Dorn, R. A., Volavka, J., Monahan, J., Stroup, T. S., . . . Lieberman, J. A., & the CATIE investigators. (2008). Comparison of antipsychotic medication effects on reducing violence in people with schizophrenia. *The British Journal of Psychiatry, 193*, 37–43. http://dx.doi.org/10.1192/bjp.bp.107.042630

Swartz, M. S., Perkins, D. O., Stroup, T. S., Davis, S. M., Capuano, G., Rosenheck, R. A., . . . Lieberman, J. A., & the CATIE Investigators. (2007). Effects of anti-psychotic medications on psychosocial functioning in patients with chronic schizophrenia: Findings from the NIMH CATIE study. *The American Journal of Psychiatry, 164*, 428–436. http://dx.doi.org/10.1176/ajp.2007.164.3.428

Szymanski, S., Lieberman, J. A., Alvir, J. M., Mayerhoff, D., Loebel, A., Geisler, S., . . . Woerner, M. (1995). Gender differences in onset of illness, treatment response, course, and biologic indexes in first-episode schizophrenic patients. *The American Journal of Psychiatry, 152*, 698–703. http://dx.doi.org/10.1176/ajp.152.5.698

Tang, Y. L., Gillespie, C. F., Epstein, M. P., Mao, P. X., Jiang, F., Chen, Q., . . . Mitchell, P. B. (2007). Gender differences in 542 Chinese inpatients with schizophrenia. *Schizophrenia Research, 97*, 88–96. http://dx.doi.org/10.1016/j.schres.2007.05.025

Tessier, A., Boyer, L., Husky, M., Baylé, F., Llorca, P. M., & Misdrahi, D. (2017). Medication adherence in schizophrenia: The role of insight, therapeutic alliance and perceived trauma associated with psychiatric care. *Psychiatry Research*, 257, 315–321. http://dx.doi.org/10.1016/j.psychres.2017.07.063

Thorup, A., Albert, N., Bertelsen, M., Petersen, L., Jeppesen, P., Le Quack, P., . . . Nordentoft, M. (2014). Gender differences in first-episode psychosis at 5-year follow-up—two different courses of disease? Results from the OPUS study at 5-year follow-up. *European Psychiatry*, 29, 44–51. http://dx.doi.org/10.1016/j.eurpsy.2012.11.005

Thorup, A., Petersen, L., Jeppesen, P., Øhlenschlæger, J., Christensen, T., Krarup, G., . . . Nordentoft, M. (2005). Integrated treatment ameliorates negative symptoms in first episode psychosis—Results from the Danish OPUS trial. *Schizophrenia Research*, 79, 95–105. http://dx.doi.org/10.1016/j.schres.2004.12.020

Tiihonen, J., Lönnqvist, J., Wahlbeck, K., Klaukka, T., Niskanen, L., Tanskanen, A., & Haukka, J. (2009). 11-year follow-up of mortality in patients with schizophrenia: A population-based cohort study (FIN11 study). *The Lancet*, 374(9690), 620–627.

Tiihonen, J., Mittendorfer-Rutz, E., Alexanderson, K., Majak, M., Mehtälä, J., Hoti, F., . . . Tanskanen, A. (2017). Antipsychotics and mortality in a nation-wide cohort of 29,823 patients with schizophrenia. *European Neuropsychopharmacology*, 27, S937–S938.

Usall, J., Suarez, D., Haro, J. M., & the SOHO Study Group. (2007). Gender differences in response to anti-psychotic treatment in outpatients with schizophrenia. *Psychiatry Research*, 153, 225–231. http://dx.doi.org/10.1016/j.psychres.2006.09.016

Vaessen, T., Hernaus, D., Myin-Germeys, I., & van Amelsvoort, T. (2015). The dopaminergic response to acute stress in health and psycho-pathology: A systematic review. *Neuroscience and Biobehavioral Reviews*, 56, 241–251. http://dx.doi.org/10.1016/j.neubiorev.2015.07.008

Valenstein, M., Blow, F. C., Copeland, L. A., McCarthy, J. F., Zeber, J. E., Gillon, L., . . . Stavenger, T. (2004). Poor antipsychotic adherence among patients with schizophrenia: Medication and patient factors. *Schizophrenia Bulletin*, 30, 255–264. http://dx.doi.org/10.1093/oxfordjournals.schbul.a007076

Vancampfort, D., Knapen, J., Probst, M., Scheewe, T., Remans, S., & De Hert, M. (2012). A systematic review of correlates of physical activity in patients with schizophrenia. *Acta Psychiatrica Scandinavica*, 125, 352–362. http://dx.doi.org/10.1111/j.1600-0447.2011.01814.x

Vancampfort, D., Knapen, J., Probst, M., van Winkel, R., Deckx, S., Maurissen, K., . . . De Hert, M. (2010). Considering a frame of reference for physical activity research related to the cardiometabolic risk profile in schizophrenia. *Psychiatry Research*, 177, 271–279. http://dx.doi.org/10.1016/j.psychres.2010.03.011

van Berckel, B. N. M., Evenblij, C. N., van Loon, B. J. A. M., Maas, M. F., van der Geld, M. A., Wynne, H. J., . . . Kahn, R. S. (1999). D-cycloserine increases positive symptoms in chronic schizophrenic patients when administered in addition to antipsychotics: A double-blind, parallel, placebo-controlled study. *Neuropsychopharmacology*, 21, 203–210. http://dx.doi.org/10.1016/S0893-133X(99)00014-7

Van Putten, T., & Marder, S. R. (1987). Behavioral toxicity of antipsychotic drugs. *The Journal of Clinical Psychiatry*, 48(Suppl.), 13–19.

Velligan, D. I., Sajatovic, M., Hatch, A., Kramata, P., & Docherty, J. P. (2017). Why do psychiatric patients stop antipsychotic medication? A systematic review of reasons for nonadherence to medication in patients with serious mental illness. *Patient Preference and Adherence*, 11, 449–468. http://dx.doi.org/10.2147/PPA.S124658

Vinkers, C. H., Mirza, N. R., Olivier, B., & Kahn, R. S. (2010). The inhibitory GABA system as a therapeutic target for cognitive symptoms in schizophrenia: Investigational agents in the pipeline. *Expert Opinion on Investigational Drugs*, 19, 1217–1233. http://dx.doi.org/10.1517/13543784.2010.513382

Volavka, J., Czobor, P., Nolan, K., Sheitman, B., Lindenmayer, J. P., Citrome, L., . . . Lieberman, J. A. (2004). Overt aggression and psychotic symptoms in patients with schizophrenia treated with clozapine, olanzapine, risperidone, or haloperidol. *Journal of Clinical Psychopharmacology*, 24, 225–228. http://dx.doi.org/10.1097/01.jcp.0000117424.05703.29

Walder, D. J., Walker, E. F., & Lewine, R. J. (2000). Cognitive functioning, cortisol release, and symptom severity in patients with schizophrenia. *Biological Psychiatry*, 48, 1121–1132. http://dx.doi.org/10.1016/S0006-3223(00)01052-0

Weiser, M., Heresco-Levy, U., Davidson, M., Javitt, D. C., Werbeloff, N., Gershon, A. A., . . . Zimmerman, Y. (2012). A multicenter, add-on randomized controlled trial of low-dose d-serine for negative and cognitive symptoms of schizophrenia. *The Journal of Clinical Psychiatry*, 73, e728–e734. http://dx.doi.org/10.4088/JCP.11m07031

*White, L., Harvey, P. D., Opler, L., Lindenmayer, J. P., & the PANSS Study Group. (1997). Empirical assessment of the factorial structure of clinical symptoms in schizophrenia. A multisite, multimodel evaluation of the factorial structure of the Positive and Negative Syndrome Scale. *Psychopathology*, 30, 263–274. http://dx.doi.org/10.1159/000285058

*Wilk, C. M., Gold, J. M., Humber, K., Dickerson, F., Fenton, W. S., & Buchanan, R. W. (2004). Brief cognitive assessment in schizophrenia: Normative data for the Repeatable Battery for the Assessment of Neuropsychological Status. *Schizophrenia Research*, 70, 175–186. http://dx.doi.org/10.1016/j.schres.2003.10.009

Wilkins, J. N. (1997). Pharmacotherapy of schizophrenia patients with comorbid substance abuse. *Schizophrenia Bulletin, 23*, 215–228. http://dx.doi.org/10.1093/schbul/23.2.215

Williams, G. C., Rodin, G. C., Ryan, R. M., Grolnick, W. S., & Deci, E. L. (1998). Autonomous regulation and long-term medication adherence in adult outpatients. *Health Psychology, 17*, 269–276. http://dx.doi.org/10.1037/0278-6133.17.3.269

Woods, S. W., Morgenstern, H., Saksa, J. R., Walsh, B. C., Sullivan, M. C., Money, R., . . . Glazer, W. M. (2010). Incidence of tardive dyskinesia with atypical versus conventional antipsychotic medications: A prospective cohort study. *The Journal of Clinical Psychiatry, 71*, 463–474. http://dx.doi.org/10.4088/JCP.07m03890yel

Yassa, R., & Jeste, D. V. (1992). Gender differences in tardive dyskinesia: A critical review of the literature. *Schizophrenia Bulletin, 18*, 701–715. http://dx.doi.org/10.1093/schbul/18.4.701

Zhai, D., Cui, T., Xu, Y., Feng, Y., Wang, X., Yang, Y., . . . Zhang, R. (2017). Cardiometabolic risk in first-episode schizophrenia (FES) patients with the earliest stages of both illness and antipsychotic treatment. *Schizophrenia Research, 179*, 41–49. http://dx.doi.org/10.1016/j.schres.2016.09.001

Zhou, Y., Rosenheck, R., Mohamed, S., Ning, Y., & He, H. (2017). Factors associated with complete discontinuation of medication among patients with schizophrenia in the year after hospital discharge. *Psychiatry Research, 250*, 129–135. http://dx.doi.org/10.1016/j.psychres.2017.01.036

Zygmunt, A., Olfson, M., Boyer, C. A., & Mechanic, D. (2002). Interventions to improve medication adherence in schizophrenia. *The American Journal of Psychiatry, 159*, 1653–1664. http://dx.doi.org/10.1176/appi.ajp.159.10.1653

PHARMACOLOGICAL TREATMENT OF OBSESSIVE-COMPULSIVE DISORDER AND RELATED DISORDERS

Dean McKay

Obsessive-compulsive disorder (OCD) is marked by intrusive and unwanted images, ideas, and thoughts that may or may not have corresponding ritualistic behavior designed to alleviate them (American Psychiatric Association, 2013). In the current edition of the *Diagnostic and Statistical Manual of Mental Disorders* (5th ed.; *DSM–5*), OCD is the reference condition in a separate category, the obsessive-compulsive and related disorders (OCRDs). The disorders that make up the OCRDs are OCD, hoarding disorder (HD), body dysmorphic disorder (BDD), trichotillomania (TM), and excoriation (skin picking) disorder (ED). In the current edition of the *DSM*, there is also the diagnostic specifier for OCD related to insight or with co-occurring tic disorders. These disorders could be classified as being more compulsive in nature or more impulsive in nature. This compulsive-impulsive dimension had been previously considered a basis for a spectrum of obsessive-compulsive disorders (i.e., McElroy, Phillips, & Keck, 1994).

In the prior editions of the *DSM*, OCD was a member of the anxiety disorders category, and it included hoarding as a symptom of the disorder. In the *DSM–IV*, the specifier "with poor insight" was added to the diagnosis of OCD. This feature of the condition is also known as "overvalued ideation" (Kozak & Foa, 1994) or "fixity of beliefs" (Foa et al., 1995). In the *DSM–5*, this specifier has been expanded slightly to include good or fair insight,

poor insight, or absent insight/delusional obsessive-compulsive disorder beliefs. It should be noted that there have been no investigations into the reliability or validity of these specifiers. There are, however, several measures of overvalued ideation available (Fixity of Belief Scale, used in the *DSM–IV* field trial, Foa et al., 1995; Brown Assessment of Beliefs, Eisen et al., 1998; Overvalued Ideas Scale, Neziroglu, McKay, Yaryura-Tobias, Stevens, & Todaro, 1999).

Before proceeding, an important caveat is necessary. The development of the OCRD category is premised on a basic shared underlying pathophysiology among these disorders. Starting from the basic assumption that repetitive problematic behaviors represent the shared component of the OCRDs, it had been suggested that a wide range of psychopathology was part of a broad category of conditions that had obsessionality and/or compulsivity associated with them (i.e., Hollander, Braun, & Simeon, 2008). Methodological critiques pointed out that many of the studies purporting to support the assertion that a disorder shared its pathology with OCD were faulty on grounds of attempting to prove the null hypothesis by predicting no significant differences, or that they failed to identify taxonic components that suggest that two or more disorders were part of the same syndrome (discussed in McKay & Neziroglu, 2009). In addition, the premise that each of the conditions in the OCRDs share common features would suggest similar

http://dx.doi.org/10.1037/0000133-011
APA Handbook of Psychopharmacology, S. M. Evans (Editor-in-Chief)

brain circuitry, neurotransmitter abnormalities, comorbid psychopathology, and treatment response with topographically comparable interventions. For each of these, however, the evidence is limited to nonexistent (Abramowitz, Storch, McKay, Taylor, & Asmundson, 2009), and the aforementioned premise that these conditions rest along a continuum from compulsive to impulsive is likewise not supported (McKay, Abramowitz, & Taylor, 2008; see Figure 11.1). One condition, ED, is the end result of a proposal to include nonsuicidal self-injury in the OCRDs, given the ritual-like process many individuals who deliberately self-harm exhibit. Briefly, ED is characterized by repetitive and compulsive skin picking that leads to tissue damage. It can include damaging the skin with sharp objects, and can be localized to specific areas or be widespread across the body. While ED is part of the OCRDs, it has been argued that this problem is better described as an impulse disorder or one associated with ruminative problems associated with depression rather than OCD (McKay & Andover, 2012). Accordingly, while the remainder of this chapter covers the OCRDs as though they conformed to the philosophical principles that guide valid formation of broad psychiatric taxometric categories (i.e., Zachar, 2008), it is essential to keep in mind that the sorting of disorders into the OCRD is conceptually driven rather than empirically determined.

EPIDEMIOLOGY AND PREVALENCE

The available epidemiology and prevalence data on the OCRDs is highly variable. In the *DSM–5*, one disorder was formerly a symptom with OCD (hoarding), and the other is a new condition (ED). In addition to these two new disorders, BDD is now a member of this group (formerly part of the somatoform disorders), as is trichotillomania, formerly an impulse control disorder.

Obsessive-Compulsive Disorder

OCD is a highly prevalent disorder. Estimates of the lifetime prevalence are approximately 2.7%, with a 12-month prevalence of 1.3% (Beesdo-Baum & Knappe, 2014). However, OCD is also highly comorbid with other severe psychopathologies.

Pierre Janet provided an early and comprehensive description of OCD (discussed in Taylor et al., 2014). Following from Janet's description, OCD was considered rare and generally unresponsive to both psychosocial and medical interventions (Kringlen, 1965). The following year, the first series of cases were documented that involved application of exposure with response prevention (ERP; Meyer, 1966), which remains the psychosocial treatment of choice for OCD (McKay et al., 2015). Efficacious psychopharmacological approaches for OCD were not widely available until 1989, with the approval by the U.S. Food and Drug Administration (FDA) of the tricyclic antidepressant (TCA) clomipramine (trade name Anafranil®; discussed in Zohar, 2012). Since that time the broader classes of serotonin reuptake inhibitors (SRIs) and serotonin norepinephrine reuptake inhibitors (SNRIs) have been evaluated in their efficacy for treating OCD, but clomipramine remains the only medication specifically FDA approved for OCD.

Hoarding Disorder

Hoarding is a common problem, and one that becomes increasingly prevalent with age. Research suggests that the rate of hoarding in adults over age 70 is 6% (Ayers, 2017). As this condition is relatively new as a stand-alone diagnosis, there is

Obsessive-Compulsive Disorder
Body Dysmorphic Disorder
Hoarding Disorder
Trichotillomania
Excoriation Disorder

FIGURE 11.1.   Obsessive-compulsive related disorders: compulsivity to impulsivity.

limited available data on its prevalence across all ages. Previously it was considered part of OCD, but this symptom was specifically unlike other symptoms in the disorder, and individuals presenting with hoarding had significantly different clinical characteristics and response to treatment (Pertusa et al., 2010).

At the present time, there are no agreed-upon psychopharmacological interventions for HD. There have been case illustrations of treatment response using the full range of medications prescribed for OCD (Saxena, 2011), but none have been demonstrated effective in controlled clinical trials. In addition to SRI and SNRI treatments, case illustrations suggest potential treatment relief with stimulant medication such as that used for attention deficit with or without hyperactivity (Rodriguez, Bender et al., 2013). However, as noted, there is no agreed-upon psycho-pharmacological treatment for HD at this time.

Body Dysmorphic Disorder

The prevalence rates for BDD are widely variable, owing to cultural values about attractiveness and social comparison (Myers & Crowther, 2009). Morselli (1891) first described the condition, termed dysmorphophobia at the time and referring to an exaggerated level of concern that one or more body part is malformed. The current definition of the disorder is ruled out if the individual has an eating disorder or other global body image disturbance. Due to the cultural constraints and variations in social pressures regarding specific physical appearances, prevalence rates are highly variable, ranging from 2.2% to 15% (discussed in Hartmann & Lyons, 2017). Further, the rates of BDD decline with age, and age of onset is estimated to be in late adolescence.

Trichotillomania

Subclinical levels of TM have been reported to be quite common in college age adults (between 11% and 22%) and clinical levels of the condition are approximately 3.4% for women and 1.5% for men (Houghton & Woods, 2017). TM has a long history in the medical literature. In some instances, the practice has been condoned and even encouraged by some religious orders as part of "mortification of the flesh," a way of demonstrating devotion or self-

denial of pleasure, with the first documented case reported by Hippocrates (discussed in Kim, 2014).

While the condition has been described in the clinical literature for centuries, treatment options have only recently emerged, primarily in the form of structured behavioral interventions (Francazio, Murphy, & Flessner, 2017). Medication treatments have been tested, with moderate effects when SRI pharmacotherapy is used (McGuire et al., 2014).

Excoriation Disorder

A newly defined disorder in the *DSM–5*, there is limited research on ED. The criteria for the diagnosis are considered liberal, covering a broad range of deliberate self-harm behaviors. Specifically, the criteria involve recurrent skin picking that results in lesions; clinically significant distress due to the skin picking; and that the skin picking is not better accounted for by substance use, a medical condition, or another psychological condition. This means that anything from severe nail and cuticle biting to nonsuicidal self-injury (i.e., deliberate self-inflicted cuts and burns) would be potential behaviors suitable for a diagnosis of ED.

Excoriation has been defined throughout history in relation to self-inflicted punishments (i.e., self-flagellation), as part of religious practices, and in other cultural rituals (i.e., Favazza & Favazza, 1987; Shaw, 2002). Reliability estimates for ED from the *DSM–5* field trials were not reported and estimates of prevalence range from 1.4% to 5.4% (Selles, McGuire, Small, & Storch, 2016). Treatments have been primarily psychosocial in nature. However, any evaluation of treatment of excoriation necessarily leads to overlap with other disorders associated with deliberate self-harm, notably borderline personality disorder. SRI medication has been used in alleviating ED, but as with conditions other than OCD per se, these instances have been limited in scope and primarily uncontrolled case series (i.e., Arnold, Auchenbach, & McElroy, 2001).

DIAGNOSING OBSESSIVE-COMPULSIVE AND RELATED DISORDERS

Structured clinical interviews are available to diagnose each of the OCRDs. It should be noted that in the field trials for the *DSM–5*, the reliability of diagnosis for many of the disorders was lower than in the prior editions (Freedman et al., 2013). In the case of the OCRDs, the field trial reliability data was not reported in the published literature. However, the field trials relied on a combination of diagnostic checklists and clinician interviews to determine diagnoses (Regier et al., 2013). The structured interviews developed based on the *DSM–5* criteria have reliability data separate from the field trials. Methods of assessing symptom severity are discussed later in this chapter in the section titled Best Approaches for Assessing Treatment Response and Managing Side Effects.

Structured Clinical Interview for *DSM–5*

The Structured Clinical Interview for *DSM–5* (SCID-5) covers all of the diagnoses in the *DSM–5* and includes supplemental ratings to assess modifiers to each diagnosis. In the case of the OCRDs, the modifiers are, "with good or fair insight," "poor insight," or "absent insight/delusional obsessive-compulsive disorder beliefs." These modifiers stem from the observation that some sufferers of OCD can fail to recognize the senselessness of their rituals or the reasonableness of the intrusive ideas (see Kozak & Foa, 1994, for a conceptual discussion). Data on the SCID-5 suggest that the interview schedule has good reliability across trained raters for all diagnoses (Shankman et al., 2017). However, it should be noted that administration of the SCID-5 is often time intensive, typically requiring approximately 90 minutes or more, depending on the number of areas endorsed in the preinterview screening.

Anxiety Disorder Interview Schedule for *DSM–5*

The Anxiety Disorder Interview Schedule for *DSM–5* (ADIS-5; Brown & Barlow, 2014) covers all the anxiety disorders, OCD and related disorders, posttraumatic stress disorder, and major depression. Reliability data have not been published as of this writing, but prior editions of this interview schedule have been reliable (see Taylor, Abramowitz, & McKay, 2010). As with the SCID-5, the ADIS-5 typically requires about 90 minutes of administration time.

Diagnostic Interview for *DSM–5* Anxiety, Mood, and Obsessive-Compulsive and Related Neuropsychiatric Disorders

The Diagnostic Interview for *DSM–5* Anxiety, Mood, and Obsessive-Compulsive and Related Neuropsychiatric Disorders (DIAMOND; Tolin et al., 2018) is a new measure available for free from the authors (https://giving.harthosp.org/tolin-diamond-training-video) that covers all the diagnoses in the *DSM–5*. The authors report an administration time of just over 1 hour. It is also the only published scale with reliability data on all of the *DSM–5* OCRDs, with kappa values in the good to excellent range for this class of disorders.

EVIDENCE-BASED PHARMACOLOGICAL TREATMENTS OF OBSESSIVE-COMPULSIVE AND RELATED DISORDERS

The majority of research on the OCRDs centers on the use of SRI medications. Among the OCRDs, OCD has been by far the most extensively studied for medication treatment response, with the other OCRDs having only limited research evaluating psychopharmacological interventions. The medications evaluated and routinely prescribed for the OCRDs include: SNRIs, second-generation neuroleptics, and first-generation neuroleptics, with some additional compounds depending on the specific disorder. Additional psychoactive agents have been examined in small investigations, and recent work on cognitive modifiers in conjunction with cognitive behavioral therapy (CBT) has been conducted.

In recent years, there has been increased use of second-generation neuroleptics as either augmentation strategies for antidepressant medication or as a monotherapy for the OCRDs. The rationale for this approach is based on the dual action of targeting dopaminergic systems involved in reward sensitivity and indirect effects on serotonergic pathways that have been hypothesized as involved in OCD (Jacobsen, 1995). This strategy has been considered especially appealing for individuals who are refractory to treatment with SRIs, or who have comorbid complicating pathology such as schizotypal personality, highly atypical symptoms (e.g., beliefs that contact with certain people will cause physical transformation), or overvalued ideation. Small trials have been conducted to examine the benefits of augmenting SRI treatment with second-generation neuroleptics, with only modest benefits. For example, McDougle, Epperson, Pelton, Wasylink, and Price (2000) added risperidone (trade name Risperdal®) to SRI in a sample of treatment-refractory ($n = 70$) patients in a double-blind trial, with no added benefit. In a small trial ($n = 26$), olanzapine (trade name Zyprexa®) was administered to SRI-refractory individuals, with half of the individuals receiving olanzapine improving by 25% on the Yale-Brown Obsessive Compulsive Scale (Y-BOCS; Bystritsky et al., 2004; Goodman et al., 1989b). Overall, research has suggested that there are benefits to inclusion of second-generation neuroleptics, although these benefits are modest, and that treatment with SRI monotherapy should be considered for at least 3 months before considering additional medication augmentation strategies (Bloch et al., 2006).

Obsessive-Compulsive Disorder

The group of medications most commonly prescribed for OCD is antidepressants. One group of these medications, SRIs, shows variations in selectivity in targeting serotonin. Those with lower selectivity are prescribed at higher doses for OCD than for depression (see Leonard, 2004). This led some investigators to assume that OCD was a result of serotonergic dysfunction; however, medications with greater serotonin selectivity show no greater efficacy, and has thus allowed investigators to conclude that the diffuse targeting of other neurotransmitters (i.e., acetylcholine, dopamine) is also necessary to produce benefits from medications (also discussed in Leonard, 2004).

The first medication with demonstrated efficacy in reducing OCD symptoms was the TCA clomipramine. In numerous meta-analyses, this medication has been found superior to placebo in randomized controlled trials (see Piccinelli, Pini, Bellantuono, & Wilkinson, 1995). In more recent analyses, clomipramine shows superiority in symptom reduction compared with other medications, with a mean reduction on the Y-BOCS of 4.72 points over the course of the trial (Skapinakis et al., 2016). However, the side

effects are difficult for many patients to tolerate (see the section in this chapter titled Best Approaches for Assessing Treatment Response and Managing Side Effects).

Several SRI medications have been examined for efficacy for OCD. While these medications have somewhat lower efficacy compared with clomipramine, these medications as a class are better tolerated. For example, Jenike, Baer, and Greist (1990) conducted a clinical trial comparing clomipramine to fluoxetine (trade name Prozac®), with the latter better tolerated even at high doses. In another investigation, it was found that dropout rates with clomipramine were double the rate for sertraline (trade name Zoloft®), another SRI medication, and that there was generally poor tolerance for clomipramine (Flament & Bisserbe, 1997). Similar to the findings for fluoxetine and sertraline, research has shown that fluvoxamine (trade name Luvox®) is also better tolerated than clomipramine (Pigott & Seay, 1999).

Other more highly selective SRIs have also been evaluated. These medications are generally considered better tolerated, but have lower efficacy in alleviating symptoms. Paroxetine (trade name Paxil®), for example, has been shown to have a modest effect size ($d = 0.41$; Kobak et al., 1998). Newer SRI compounds show similarly modest effects. For instance, escitalopram (trade name Lexapro®) was evaluated in several doses, and regardless of dosage there was a one- to two-point change in the Clinical Global Impression scale (CGI; Kadouri, Corruble, & Falissard, 2007; Shim et al., 2011). Other newer compounds have been examined to a limited extent, such as in uncontrolled case series. Insight, or overvalued ideation, has also been shown responsive to SRI medication (Alonso et al., 2008).

The other class of medications commonly prescribed for OCD is the SNRIs. However, this class of medications is considered a second- or third-line option following clomipramine and SRIs. Research has suggested that these compounds have lower efficacy than SRI medications but comparable tolerability (Dell'Osso, Nestadt, Allen, & Hollander, 2006).

Hoarding Disorder

Prior to the *DSM–5*, hoarding was a symptom within the diagnosis of OCD. However, extensive research has shown that it is syndromally unique (Pertusa et al., 2010), leading to the development of a separate diagnosis. There are few investigations into medication for HD alone. In a summary of the limited available research on medication response, there was a medium effect size associated with pharmacological treatments (Brakoulias, Eslick, & Starcevic, 2015) that included research involving SRI, SNRI, second-generation neuroleptic, second-generation neuroleptic augmented SRI, and stimulant medication trials (in a sample of $n = 7$ studies). These authors reported no substantial heterogeneity of effect size among this series of open label trials, and the assessments employed were generally unstandardized scales (i.e., a modified Y-BOCS for hoarding). Aside from this meta-analysis, there have been examinations into the efficacy of other medications in case series, with no compound emerging as a recommended therapeutic strategy.

Body Dysmorphic Disorder

BDD is associated with high levels of depressed mood, suicide risk, and poor insight. Treatment trials employing SRI medication show medium effect sizes (Williams, Hadjistavropoulos, & Sharpe, 2006), but with high dropout (ranging from 16.25% to 38%). Early treatment recommendations for BDD included augmentation of SRI medication with neuroleptic medication (i.e., Phillips, 1996), but as of this writing there has been only one controlled study employing pimozide (a first-generation neuroleptic; trade name Orap®) augmentation of fluoxetine treatment. Pimozide did not incrementally improve outcome, although the sample was small ($n = 28$), and with or without augmentation only $n = 5$ patients were rated improved or much improved at the end of the trial (Phillips, 2005). More recently, Phillipou, Rossell, Wilding, and Castle (2016) reviewed the available research, and similarly found that SRI medication provided modest relief from symptoms, but also noted that there were few systematic evaluations ($n = 3$ controlled trials). As a result, there are no clear medication recommendations for BDD.

Trichotillomania

In the limited controlled research investigating medications for TM, fluoxetine has not been shown

effective in substantially alleviating symptoms, but clomipramine, olanzapine, and the dietary supplement (and glutamate modulator) N-acetylcysteine have large effect sizes in alleviating symptoms (Slikboer, Nedeljkovic, Bowe, & Moulding, 2017). In a summary of all SRI investigations of TM treatment, a modest effect size ($d = 0.41$) was observed (McGuire et al., 2014). At the present time, medication management of TM should be considered exploratory.

Excoriation Disorder

While ED is a comparably new diagnosis, there have been several trials of SRI medication for the disorder, with a large effect size for symptom reduction (Selles et al., 2016). In addition to these trials, treatment with the anticonvulsant lamotrigine (trade name Lamictal®) has demonstrated efficacy ($d = 0.98$; Selles et al., 2016). In a search of the literature, there were no additional studies of medication for excoriation, self-injury, or self-mutilation.

Summary of Evidence-Based Medication for Obsessive-Compulsive and Related Disorders

In general, SRI medication is the most effective intervention for OCRDs, but with notable exceptions. Specifically, HD has not been shown to be particularly responsive to medications generally. Research on BDD shows that there are comparably high dropout rates, and special additional attention needs to be paid to suicide risk, particularly if SRIs are administered to adolescents with this condition owing to the black box warning on this class of medications. TM appears more responsive to a dietary supplement than to marketed medication compounds. Although augmentation with second-generation neuroleptics was hypothesized to be beneficial and widely prescribed (Verdoux, Tournier, & Bégaud, 2010), the incremental gain from this class of medications is modest, and as will be discussed in this chapter, the side effects are considerable. Therefore, if medication is the preferred approach, the best evidence is for monotherapy—typically SRIs except in the case of TM.

BEST APPROACHES FOR ASSESSING TREATMENT RESPONSE AND MANAGING SIDE EFFECTS

Numerous measures are available to assess symptom severity for the OCRDs. In this section, a brief survey of measures is provided. More detailed information on severity rating scales for the full range of OCRDs and complicating symptoms can be found in Abramowitz, McKay, and Storch (2017) and Storch, Abramowitz, and McKay (2017). Separately, side effect management is an essential component of any psychopharmacological course of treatment, and in consideration of the dosages involved in medications for OCD, considerable clinical energy should be devoted to this part of patient care.

Assessment Instruments

Most of the major assessment tools for the OCRDs are interview or client self-report scales. There are several reliable and valid measures available for each of the member disorders that are widely available to clinicians at no cost. Before proceeding, however, it is important to note that many measures used to assess severity and improvement in medication trials rely on the CGI severity and CGI improvement (CGImp) scales (for discussion, see Kadouri et al., 2007), both single-item clinician-rated assessments. Psychometric theory (Nunnally & Bernstein, 1994) would suggest that such single-item assessments are incomplete for the purposes of evaluating the diversity of dimensions in psychopathology, and so the material that follows highlights measures that are multidimensional in scope and possessing of adequate psychometric qualities.

Obsessive-compulsive disorder.   OCD is a heterogeneous condition that is marked by symptom subtypes. Broadly, there are three major subtypes: obsessions (sexual, religious, or somatic) and checking rituals; symmetry obsessions and counting, ordering, and repeating rituals; and contamination obsessions and cleaning rituals (Abramowitz, McKay, & Taylor, 2005; McKay et al., 2004).[1] The Y-BOCS (Goodman et al., 1989a, 1989b) is a widely used

clinician-administered rating scale. The scale is comprised of a symptom checklist that is later used as the basis for evaluation of symptom severity. The severity-rating portion of the scale is comprised of five items for compulsions and another five for obsessions, each item assessing frequency, distress, interference, resistance, and control. There are additional supplemental items assessing insight, avoidance, indecisiveness, responsibility, slowness, and doubting. The measure has demonstrated validity and treatment sensitivity (Taylor, Abramowitz, & McKay, 2010).

There are several widely used self-report measures, but in everyday clinical practice the Obsessive-Compulsive Inventory-Revised (OCI-R; Foa et al., 2002) would likely be most appealing given its brevity (18 items), coverage of multiple symptom domains, and easily computed total score. In the development of the measure, statistical analyses showed that a clinical cutoff of 21 distinguished individuals diagnosed with OCD from other anxiety disorders. Anecdotally, that cutoff score for OCD may be overly liberal, with analogue community samples for this author's lab showing more than 30% scoring above the cutoff score (i.e., Taylor et al., 2014). The OCI-R is generally considered a good measure for evaluating the extent that there are changes in symptoms as a result of treatment (Taylor, Abramowitz, & McKay, 2010).

More recently, the Dimensional Obsessive-Compulsive Scale (DOCS) was developed to assess four dimensions of OCD—contamination, inflated responsibility, unacceptable thoughts, and symmetry (Abramowitz et al., 2010). Comprised of 20 items, the measure is brief, has good psychometric properties, has convergent and discriminant validity, and detects changes resulting from treatment.

Hoarding disorder.   Hoarding is characterized by disability due to excessive clutter around one's living environment, and due to excessive drive to acquire and save possessions. One well validated measure of acquisition and saving is the Saving Inventory—

---

[1] Prior research included hoarding as a separate symptom subtype given its presence as a criterion for OCD. This has been dropped in this discussion given that hoarding is now a separate disorder in the *DSM–5*.

Revised (Frost, Steketee, & Grisham, 2004). The sensitivity to treatment for the measure has not been established.

An objective rating scale for environmental clutter has been developed, the Clutter Image Rating (Frost, Steketee, Tolin, & Renaud, 2008). The scale is comprised of photos of three rooms in a typical home, each with nine photos depicting increasing levels of clutter; respondents choose the photo that most represents the appearance of the corresponding room in their home. The measure is brief and possesses good psychometric properties. The extent that this measure detects changes due to treatment is not yet established.

Body dysmorphic disorder. As noted earlier, BDD is considered to be associated with high overvalued ideas. Therefore, it is more likely that individuals with this condition will not recognize the presence of exaggerated concerns with specific body areas. Therefore, the best assessments for this condition are interview/clinician rated scales. Two major measures have been validated for this purpose. The Body Dysmorphic Disorder Examination (Rosen & Reiter, 1996) is comprehensive in scope, possesses good reliability and validity, and is related to assessments of body image disturbance. The measure has been widely used for baseline assessment of symptom severity, but treatment sensitivity evaluations have not yet been conducted.

The Y-BOCS has been modified for use in BDD (BDD-YBOCS; Phillips, Hart, & Menard, 2014). The measure has adequate psychometric properties and has demonstrated sensitivity to treatment effects with SRI medication and in CBT with adolescents diagnosed with the condition (Krebs et al., 2017).

Trichotillomania. There are few measures of TM, although one self-report scale was developed, titled the Milwaukee Inventory for Subtypes of Trichotillomania-Adult Version, comprised of 24 self-report items that cover two broad domains—focused and automatic hair pulling (Flessner et al., 2008). The measure has good psychometric properties and forms the two factors (obsessions, compulsions) based on the initial conceptualizations of the scale. No treatment data with the scale has yet been published, although it has been used in clinical case series.

Excoriation disorder. One self-report measure was identified that shows good psychometric properties, the Skin Picking Scale-Revised (Snorrason et al., 2012). The scale is comprised of eight items, with four items each on two subscales titled impairment and symptom severity. Treatment sensitivity is not yet established, but the scale has been utilized in published case series.

Side Effect Management

There are several classes of medications commonly prescribed for the OCRDs. While clomipramine remains the most efficacious treatment for OCD, it also has the greatest number of side effects, leading to lower compliance and adherence and increased risk of dropout when employed. Most of the side effects that are found intolerable are anticholinergic, such as dry mouth, blurry vision, sweating, dizziness, drowsiness, restlessness, constipation, weight gain, and urinary retention. In the case of clomipramine specifically, sexual side effects are prominent, particularly in males experiencing impotence and difficulty achieving orgasm. These side effects are sufficiently prominent that some investigators suggest starting treatment with SRIs and resorting to clomipramine only should other medications fail to provide sufficient relief (i.e., Fineberg & Craig, 2010).

Clinical guidelines have been developed to manage anticholinergic side effects. The first and most prominent guideline is to lower the medication dose to the lowest one while retaining beneficial effects (Lieberman, 2004). Other strategies include changing the time of day that medication is taken (to manage drowsiness) and use of lozenges and mouthwash (for dry mouth; Leonard, 2004). Some side effects fade with continued administration, although most persist throughout the course of treatment.

As clomipramine has the most difficult side effects to manage, the SRIs are the current first-line medication class (Fineberg & Craig, 2010). These also have common side effects. Many are similar to the ones associated with TCAs, but to a milder degree (Ferguson, 2001), particularly with medications that target acetylcholine as well as serotonin, such as the older SRI medications. An important additional side effect common among the SRIs in treatment of OCRDs is increased anxiety and several symptoms on discontinuation, including dizziness, nausea, agitation, and headache (Ferguson, 2001). Regarding headache, one SRI, paroxetine, stands out for severe headache on discontinuation. These withdrawal effects are sufficiently severe that the FDA issued a warning about this problem to alert consumers before initiating treatment with the medication (Tonks, 2002).

The other highly significant side effect associated with SRIs involves suicide risk in adolescents. The risk was so great that in 2004 the FDA issued a black box warning, which is the strictest warning that the agency can assign to a medication. In the lead up to the FDA issuance of this warning, it was found that the rate of suicidal ideation with the medication was double the rate for those receiving placebo, after a review of 372 studies and more than 100,000 participants (discussed in Friedman, 2014).[2] It is essential for prescribers to warn prospective patients about this risk, and critical for psychologists working with patients taking these medications to be aware of and to monitor if any change in suicidal ideation should occur.

After SRI medications, SNRI medications are often prescribed for management of OCRD symptoms. This class of medications has similar side effects to SRIs, but there is no black box warning associated with them. Unique to this class of medications are potential increased blood pressure and exacerbation of preexisting liver problems (Stahl, Grady, Moret, & Briley, 2005).

As noted previously, second-generation neuroleptics are commonly prescribed as augmentation agents for other medication treatments for OCRDs. This class of medications has significant side effects. These include most of the side effects listed for the TCAs, including anticholinergic effects. The notable additional side effect is weight gain and concomitant risk of developing diabetes (Üçok & Gaebel, 2008). These side effects arise due to metabolic effects associated with second-generation neuroleptics. Specifically, as a class, second-generation neuroleptics increase endocrine secretion that

stimulates appetite, stimulate endocrine secretion that prompts fat storage, and inhibit endocrine secretion of gastric satiety, with these effects worsened with higher doses (Simon, van Winkel, & De Hert, 2009).

Serotonin toxicity, also referred to as "serotonin syndrome," has been observed in some SRI medications and other compounds that target the serotonergic system. Prescribers conceptualize it as "a form of poisoning, not an idiosyncratic reaction" (Gillman, 2006, p. 1046). Patients are at higher risk when administered two or more serotonergic agents, but it can result from monotherapy. Symptoms include increased heart rate, shivering, sweating, involuntary twitching of limbs (myoclonus), and hypothermia. Citalopram and escitalopram, which are newer and far more selective of targeting serotonin, are more likely to lead to serotonin toxicity compared with older and less selective medications (Kelly et al., 2004). Management of serotonin toxicity primarily entails stopping administration of the medication, and potentially administering serotonin antagonists. Since a large proportion of serotonin receptors are in the gastrointestinal track, oral administration of activated charcoal can serve to absorb excess medication to further alleviate symptoms. In extreme cases hospitalization with medical sedation and administration of other pharmacological agents to manage symptoms of hyperthermia and agitation are necessary (discussed in Gillman, 2006).

MEDICATION MANAGEMENT ISSUES

SRIs have emerged as the first-line medication approach for the OCRDs. This is due to the comparably mild side effect profile and generally good compliance and adherence when prescribed (Bandelow et al., 2012). However, as noted earlier, particularly when prescribed to younger patients, this class of medications requires significantly greater levels of risk management due to its black box warning of higher suicide risk. This includes patients with no prior suicidal ideation. Clinicians need to be acutely aware of this risk and conduct

---

[2] The research documenting the increased risk of suicidal ideation and attempts in SRI medication for youth may have led to a black box warning sooner were it not for problematic reporting of suicide events in several treatment trials. This was uncovered in Bass (2008).

regular risk assessments—more than might be typical for ongoing clinical care.

While producing greater symptom reduction, clomipramine, like other TCA medications, has a side effect profile that is more difficult to tolerate and has lower compliance. Second-generation neuroleptics are also commonly prescribed, especially for nonresponsive patients. These medications have substantial side effects, including metabolic changes that increase medical liability and morbidity. These compounds should be considered only after other treatment options have been exhausted, particularly given the modest benefits and significant side effects. Careful attention to dosing to minimize these side effects is required given their impact on quality of life (Naber, 2008).

Relapse

Systematic reviews show that symptom remission is not expected with medication management alone. Indeed, continued administration of SRI medication resulted in limited relapse (based on a five-or-more point increase on the Y-BOCS; Fineberg, Pampaloni, Pallanti, Ipser, & Stein, 2007). In combined treatment trials (medication plus CBT, specifically ERP), relapse rates were lower with ERP, whether with or without medication (i.e., Simpson et al., 2004).

Discontinuation

Among the SRIs, there is a general risk on discontinuation of antidepressant discontinuation syndrome, which is marked by flu-like symptoms, affective disturbance, and tardive akathisia (Warner, Bobo, Warner, Reid, & Rachal, 2006). In some patients these symptoms can persist for months, and there are documented cases with symptoms persisting for several years, although symptoms can also resolve spontaneously after a short period and typically also resolve with readministration of antidepressant medication (Haddad & Anderson, 2007). As noted earlier, among the SRI medications, paroxetine stands out for difficulties during discontinuation due to severe headaches (Tonks, 2002), and discontinuation has also been suggested to result in the more general antidepressant discontinuation syndrome (Black, Shea, Dursun, & Kutcher, 2000).

EVALUATION OF PHARMACOLOGICAL APPROACHES ACROSS THE LIFESPAN

Pharmacotherapy for OCRDs requires consideration of developmental stage. The compounds used for these disorders have different effects based on the age of the patient that are well documented.

Youth

As discussed previously, one of the major developmental considerations in medication management for OCRDs is the black box warning regarding suicide risk with SRI medications, especially in younger patients. A review of risk–benefit analyses of SRI medications for youth (ages 5–18) showed that fluoxetine had a generally favorable risk–benefit analysis, but when considering all available data (published and unpublished), it was the only SRI for which benefits outweighed the risks, with published data skewed toward a favorable risk–benefit analysis across SRIs (Whittington et al., 2004). That is, there is a significant file-drawer problem in assessing the risk–benefit ratio for SRI medications. Given that dose administration of less-selective SRI medications is higher for OCRDs than for depression, these risk–benefit analyses would be comparable or worse in the case of OCRDs. There are no specific methods for mitigating these risks except careful monitoring throughout the course of treatment. Should these risks emerge, it may be necessary to change medication.

Older Adults

Analyses with samples of adults ages 50 and older who were administered SRI medication shows an increased risk of falls and bone fractures, particularly in female patients (Richards et al., 2007). It has been suggested that these adverse outcomes are due to the impact of SRI medication on reduced bone density, given that there is a high density of serotonin receptors in the osteopathic system, as well as to serotonin's role in modulating parathyroid functioning (Bliziotes, Eshleman, Zhang, & Wiren, 2001). Serotonin is also implicated in cardiovascular functioning, and SRI medications can lead to hypotension (Cherin, Colvez, Deville de Periere, & Sereni, 1997). As a result, there is an approximately twofold increased risk of falls and fractures in older adults who are administered SRI medications (Richards et al., 2007). At this point there are no identified mitigating factors or specific methods for managing this potential side effect. Accordingly, it is recommended that close monitoring be conducted with older adults who are prescribed SRI medication, with regularly scheduled bone scans to detect possible bone density loss.

CONSIDERATION OF POTENTIAL SEX DIFFERENCES

Research has shown that females are more often diagnosed with anxiety disorders and OCD than males (discussed in Craske, 2003). Although it is hypothesized that androgens in women interfere with response to SRI medication, data have not borne this out (Lochner & Stein, 2001). More recent analyses continue to show that there are no sex differences for pharmacotherapy for OCD, but that sex did moderate other psychosocial treatments (Maher et al., 2010). It should be noted that although research generally suggests that there are no differences in outcome for females or males, the research on this is limited. Indeed, over a 30-year period, only eight studies specifically considered sex differences in medication response among OCRDs. This represents a significant gap in the research literature that requires careful study.

INTEGRATION OF PHARMACOTHERAPY WITH NONPHARMACOLOGICAL APPROACHES: BENEFITS AND CHALLENGES

As discussed throughout this chapter, psychopharmacotherapy for OCRDs primarily involves SRIs, SNRIs, and in the case of TM, *N*-acetylcysteine. Extensive examination of psychosocial research suggests that CBT is highly efficacious in reducing symptoms and improving functioning.

Figure 11.1 highlights the placement on the continuum from compulsive to impulsive for the OCRDs. This dimension figures prominently in determining the nature of psychosocial interventions. For the compulsive side, exposure to situations that provoke obsessional experiences with blockage of associated compulsive behaviors (ERP)

has demonstrated efficacy in OCD, with large effect sizes in adults (McKay et al., 2015) and children (Franklin et al., 2015). In the case of BDD, ERP has been shown to alleviate symptoms when part of a comprehensive program of CBT (Harrison, Fernández de la Cruz, Enander, Radua, & Mataix-Cols, 2016). HD interventions are based on improving organizational strategies rather than exposure (Tolin, Frost, Steketee, & Muroff, 2015). TM has been shown responsive to habit reversal, which focuses on training people in engaging in competing behaviors when the urge to pull hair arises (McGuire et al., 2014). Ostensibly this approach would be useful for ED, but the research is as yet limited for any treatments for this newly defined disorder. However, given the broad nature of the diagnosis, prior research on other body-focused behaviors (i.e., nail biting) suggests that habit reversal is efficacious (Bate, Malouff, Thorsteinsson, & Bhullar, 2011).

Obsessive-Compulsive Disorder

Many treatment guidelines for OCRDs recommend combined CBT and SRI medication as the most efficacious method of treatment. This could be a reasonable conclusion if one were to consider just the largest effect size for treatment (see Skapinakis et al., 2016). However, the incremental gain for combined treatment is very slight, particularly in light of the risk–benefit analysis described earlier for pharmacotherapy. Indeed, other researchers, including medical professionals, have instead recommended that treatment begin with CBT in lieu of medication (psychosocial monotherapy) because of the risks associated with medication and the comparably small gain in treatment outcome (Wheaton, DeSantis, & Simpson, 2016). In some circumstances medication may be recommended, such as for patients who reside in remote areas with limited access to qualified CBT providers, or for patients who cannot tolerate or are not receptive to the demands of CBT treatment. In these instances, it is important to discuss the full range of benefits and risks associated with medication as compared with undergoing a course of CBT or undergoing CBT in conjunction with medication. Specifically, it has been acknowledged that many individuals who suffer from OCRDs lack good access to sound, expert-driven CBT. McKay et al. (2015) and Franklin et al. (2015), in laying out the efficacy of CBT for OCD in adults and children respectively, pointedly note that there are specific criteria for individuals to claim expert knowledge in delivering evidence-based psychosocial treatment. It is not within the scope of this chapter to cover, but dissemination remains a significant problem given hesitations among practitioners to deliver ERP (discussed in Garner, Steinberg, & McKay, in press).

Hoarding Disorder

It is important to note that CBT alone is associated with symptom reduction effect sizes that are considerably lower than those obtained for OCD. There are, however, no controlled or uncontrolled investigations of combined treatment for HD. It was noted previously that medication management for HD has been underexamined and that SRIs have limited benefits. This has not prevented investigators from recommending combined treatment for the condition (i.e., Saxena, 2011).

Body Dysmorphic Disorder

There is comparably less research evaluating combined treatment for BDD. In light of the complexity of the disorder, clinical wisdom has suggested reliance on multiple treatment approaches (exposure-based behavioral interventions, mindfulness-based CBT, behavioral activation to address depressed mood), and outcome with medication in combination with CBT is generally efficacious (i.e., Rashid, Khan, & Fineberg, 2015).

Trichotillomania and Excoriation Disorder

As with HD, there is limited controlled research evaluating the combined treatment of TM with medication. One study started all TM patients with sertraline, and nonresponders were then offered habit reversal (Dougherty, Loh, Jenike, & Keuthen, 2006). Those administered both habit reversal and sertraline were more likely to achieve symptom remission following 22 weeks of treatment. This study, while encouraging, does not answer the question of whether habit reversal as a monotherapy is of comparable efficacy to medication or combined treatment. No studies examining combined treatment for ED were identified. However, as with OCD,

the added challenge facing sufferers of TM and ED is that habit reversal is not well known among practitioners. Further, misconceptions exist, such as that suppression of the urge to pull hair leads to rebound worsening and that habit reversal will result in symptom substitution (van de Griendt, Verdellen, van Dijk, & Verbraak, 2013). Accordingly, some people with these disorders may request medication even in recognition that the outcomes will be limited.

The Problem of Overvalued Ideation

Overvalued ideas (poor insight in *DSM–5*, or fixity of beliefs in the *DSM–IV* field trials) have been conceptualized as being closer in kind to delusional processes than frank recognition of the senselessness of intrusive ideas, or that the behavioral symptoms (i.e., compulsions) are unnecessary. This feature of OCRDs has been infrequently evaluated in a systematic manner. In one trial, it was shown that risperidone, when added to SRI and ERP treatment, produced better outcomes including improvement specifically in overvalued ideas (Simpson et al., 2013).

Summary

Combined pharmacotherapy and CBT has been primarily examined in OCD, but not systematically in other disorders in the broader OCRDs. While clinical practice guidelines generally suggest providing combined interventions (i.e., Koran et al., 2007), the available evidence suggests that the incremental gain from adding medication is slight, and in a cost–benefit analysis is associated with higher medical liability. Accordingly, it appears that initial treatment should focus on psychosocial interventions before considering medical interventions. Patients and clinicians can find a wide range of online resources to assist further in clinical decision making by referring to the Tool Kit of Resources included at the end of this chapter.

INTEGRATED APPROACHES FOR ADDRESSING COMMON COMORBID DISORDERS

The OCRDs typically present with comorbid psychopathology (Keeley et al., 2008). The majority of research examining treatment for common comorbid conditions with OCRDs involves uncontrolled case research; studies evaluating symptom dimensions from these comorbid symptoms have been evaluated as moderators of outcome in psychopharmacology research. It should be noted, however, that contrary to prevailing assumptions, controlled research in psychopathology generally is characterized by samples with comorbid conditions (discussed in Pilecki & McKay, 2013, p. 544). Accordingly, the previously described research is generalizable to the majority of cases of OCRDs. Nonetheless, there are some particularly common clinical presentations whereby additional management with medication can be considered.

One of the most common co-occurring conditions with OCD is major depression (Keeley et al., 2008), and for which additional research findings on treatment have accumulated. The prevailing assumption has been that comorbid major depression complicates treatment with ERP. Recent research has suggested that treatment outcome for CBT can be improved with the addition of SRI medication in OCD with comorbid depression (Maher et al., 2010). In more recent experimental research, riluzole (trade name Rilutek®) has been used to augment SRI medication in individuals with refractory OCD (individuals who suffer from clinically disabling residual symptoms posttreatment; Pittenger et al., 2015). This small trial ($n = 38$) showed improvement, but not to the point of statistical significance. Nonetheless, in this sample with difficult-to-treat symptoms, the majority achieved at least 25% symptom improvement.

Aside from comorbid depression, overvalued ideation represents an important clinical challenge with OCRDs. Although the literature on this is limited, individuals with overvalued ideas are sometimes grouped with the larger "treatment resistant"[3] group of patients. However, in one trial, $n = 39$ adolescents with treatment-resistant OCD, including a group identified by the investigators as having overvalued ideas, had significant symptom reduction when SRI medication was augmented with the second-generation antipsychotic medication aripiprazole (trade name Abilify®; Masi,

Pfanner, Millepiedi, & Berloffa, 2010). This is an area requiring additional investigation.

EMERGING TRENDS

Biomedical interventions remain a significant area of research investigation. As a result, several new treatments for OCRDs are being investigated. It should be noted that there are few new pharmacological treatments in development for treating OCRDs, and a range of approaches that are intended solely for use in conjunction with CBT.

Transcranial Direct Current Stimulation

Transcranial direct current stimulation (tDCS; see Chapter 32, this volume) involves placing electrodes on the scalp in locations that correspond with brain areas considered potentially involved in OCD, stimulating those areas, with CBT following shortly after. In order to conduct this approach properly, magnetic resonance imaging (MRI) is necessary to locate the brain area within an individual participant to ensure proper electrode placement. At the current time this approach is purely experimental, with limited data on outcome aside from case examples (Kekic et al., 2016).

Transcranial Magnetic Stimulation

Stimulation of brain areas with magnetic waves as a monotherapy has been tested in OCD. As with tDCS, exact electrode placement is necessary, with target brain areas identified through MRI. Acute symptom reduction has been found for this approach (Zhou, Wang, Wang, Li, & Kuang, 2017), but small effect sizes over long-term administration (Trevizol et al., 2016).

Deep Brain Stimulation

As a treatment for refractory OCD, deep brain stimulation (DBS) involves surgically implanting electrodes in hypothesized affected brain areas (i.e., basal ganglia) that provide a regular pulse to stimulate the area in order to alleviate symptoms.

---

[3]As of this writing, there is no consensus on what constitutes treatment resistance in the OCRDs (discussed briefly in McKay et al., 2015).

It is a treatment of last resort after other noninvasive approaches have been exhausted. Data are relatively limited on the approach, with preliminary suggestions that DBS can be helpful with people who have refractory OCD (Kisely et al., 2014; Naesström, Blomstedt, & Bodlund, 2016). However, Kisely et al. (2014) showed that more than a third of DBS patients suffered significant adverse events (e.g., seizure, headache).

Ketamine

Ketamine has as its site of action the *N*-methyl-D-aspartate receptor system, which research has suggested is involved in anxiety disorder pathology. Ketamine produces a "glutamate surge" (Abdallah et al., 2016) that results in stimulation of the prefrontal cortex and alleviates depressive affect. There has been recent interest in ketamine as a medical intervention for depression, with acute benefits of approximately a week, but without lasting benefits (i.e., Xu et al., 2016). In a small randomized controlled trial ($n = 15$), significant decreases in obsessions were observed with ketamine compared with placebo, with benefits lasting for 1 week (Rodriguez, Kegeles et al., 2013). At the present time, ketamine's benefits are restricted to acute effects lasting no more than a week.

CONCLUSION

There are numerous medications available for the treatment of OCD, in several different classes. The common feature among all the medications is that they target serotonin, either directly (TCAs, SRIs, SNRIs) or indirectly (second-generation antipsychotics). For OCRDs on the impulsive side of the spectrum, serotonergic medications have been demonstrated as beneficial, but newer compounds targeting glutamate (i.e., *N*-acetylcysteine) may prove more effective.

Although there are a wide range of psychopharmacological options available, cost–benefit analysis does not lead to a clear recommendation for medication as a first-line treatment choice, nor does it suggest that medication should be included in a course of evidence-based psychosocial treatment relying on CBT (either ERP or habit reversal, depending on the OCRD). This is an important point that is not captured in existing clinical guidelines, which generally recommend combined treatments (i.e., Koran et al., 2007). Instead, as noted, each class of medications has significant side effects, risks associated with withdrawal, and potential medical liabilities for toxicity.

As a result of this review, and in line with the recommendations of Wheaton, DeSantis, and Simpson (2016), psychosocial treatment should be the first-line intervention recommended for OCRDs. Medications, when added, should be recommended with caution. Polypharmacy approaches should also be approached with caution given the significant liabilities associated with each medication and the limited added benefit of additional compounds.

TOOL KIT OF RESOURCES

Obsessive-Compulsive Disorder

Patient Resources

International Obsessive-Compulsive Disorder Foundation: http://www.iocdf.org

National Institute of Mental Health Fact Sheets: https://www.nimh.nih.gov/health/topics/obsessive-compulsive-disorder-ocd/index.shtml

American Psychiatric Association OCD Help: https://www.psychiatry.org/patients-families/ocd

American Academy of Child and Adolescent Psychiatry OCD Help page: https://www.aacap.org/aacap/Families_and_Youth/Resource_Centers/Obsessive_Compulsive_Disorder_Resource_Center/OCD_Resource_Center.aspx

National Alliance on Mental Illness: https://www.nami.org/Learn-More/Mental-Health-Conditions/Obsessive-compulsive-Disorder/Support

Mental Health America: http://www.mentalhealthamerica.net/conditions/ocd

Provider Resources

International Obsessive-Compulsive Disorder Foundation Training materials: https://iocdf.org/professionals/training-institute/

Anxiety & Depression Association of America Clinical Practice Guidelines: https://adaa.org/resources-professionals/practice-guidelines-ocd#

Storch, E. A., McGuire, J., & McKay, D. (Eds.). (2018). *Clinicians' guide to cognitive-behavioral therapy for childhood obsessive-compulsive disorder.* Amsterdam, the Netherlands: Academic Press.

Hoarding Disorder

Patient Resources

American Psychiatric Association Hoarding Help: https://www.psychiatry.org/patients-families/hoarding-disorder

Anxiety & Depression Association of America, Hoarding: The Basics: https://adaa.org/understanding-anxiety/obsessive-compulsive-disorder-ocd/hoarding-basics#

Tolin, D. F., Frost, R. O., & Steketee, G. (2013). *Buried in treasures* (2nd ed.). New York, NY: Oxford.

Provider Resources

Tolin, D. F., Frost, R. O., & Steketee, G. (2013). *Buried in treasures* (2nd ed.). New York, NY: Oxford.

Pertusa, A., Frost, R. O., Fullana, M. A., Samuels, J., Steketee, G., Tolin, D., . . . Mataix-Cols, D. (2010). Refining the diagnostic boundaries of compulsive hoarding: A critical review. *Clinical Psychology Review, 30,* 371–386.

Body Dysmorphic Disorder

Patient Resources

BDD Foundation Resources: https://bddfoundation.org/resources/

Anxiety & Depression Association of America, Understand the Facts of BDD: https://adaa.org/understanding-anxiety/related-illnesses/other-related-conditions/body-dysmorphic-disorder-bdd#

BDD Resources, International OCD Foundation: https://bdd.iocdf.org

Provider Resources

International Obsessive-Compulsive Disorder Foundation, Diagnosing and Treating BDD: https://bdd.iocdf.org/professionals/diagnosis/

Wilhelm, S., Phillips, K. A., & Steketee, G. (2013). *A cognitive behavioral treatment manual for body dysmorphic disorder.* New York, NY: Guilford Press.

Trichotillomania

Patient Resources

Trichotillomania Learning Center: https://www.bfrb.org/

Mental Health America, Trichotillomania: http://www.mentalhealthamerica.net/conditions/trichotillomania-hair-pulling

Provider Resources

Franklin, M. E., Zagrabbe, K., & Benavides, K. L. (2011). Trichotillomania and its treatment: A review and recommendations. *Expert Review of Neurotherapeutics, 11,* 1165–1174.

Morris, S. H., Zickgraf, H. F., Dingfelder, H. E., & Franklin, M. E. (2013). Habit reversal training in trichotillomania: Guide for the clinician. *Expert Review of Neurotherapeutics, 13,* 1069–1077.

Excoriation Disorder

Patient Resources

Trichotillomania Learning Center, What Is Excoriation?: http://www.bfrb.org/learn-about-bfrbs/skin-picking-disorder

Mental Health America, Skin Picking: http://www.mentalhealthamerica.net/conditions/excoriation-disorder-skin-picking-or-dermatillomania

Provider Resources

Arnold, L., Auchenbach, M. B., & McElroy, S. L. (2001). Psychogenic excoriation. *CNS Drugs, 15,* 351–359.

Phillips, K. A., & Stein, D. J. (2015). *Handbook on obsessive-compulsive and related disorders.* Washington, DC: American Psychiatric Association.

References

Abdallah, C. G., Adams, T. G., Kelmendi, B., Esterlis, I., Sanacora, G., & Krystal, J. H. (2016). Ketamine's mechanism of action: A path to rapid-acting antidepressants. *Depression and Anxiety, 33,* 689–697. http://dx.doi.org/10.1002/da.22501

*Abramowitz, J. S., Deacon, B. J., Olatunji, B. O., Wheaton, M. G., Berman, N. C., Losardo, D., . . . Hale, L. R. (2010). Assessment of obsessive-compulsive symptom dimensions: Development and evaluation of the Dimensional Obsessive-Compulsive Scale.

*Asterisks indicate assessments or resources.

Psychological Assessment, 22, 180–198. http://dx.doi.org/10.1037/a0018260

Abramowitz, J. S., McKay, D., & Storch, E. A. (Eds.). (2017). *The Wiley handbook of obsessive compulsive disorders: Vol. I. Obsessive-compulsive disorder across the lifespan.* Chichester, UK: Wiley.

Abramowitz, J., McKay, D., & Taylor, S. (2005). Special series: Subtypes of obsessive-compulsive disorder. *Behavior Therapy, 36*, 367–369. http://dx.doi.org/10.1016/S0005-7894(05)80118-2

Abramowitz, J. S., Storch, E. A., McKay, D., Taylor, S., & Asmundson, G. J. G. (2009). The obsessive-compulsive spectrum: A critical review. In D. McKay, J. S. Abramowitz, S. Taylor, & G. J. G. Asmundson (Eds.), *Current perspectives on anxiety disorders: Implications for DSM–V and beyond* (pp. 329–352). New York, NY: Springer.

Alonso, P., Menchón, J. M., Segalàs, C., Jaurrieta, N., Jiménez-Murcia, S., Cardoner, N., . . . Vallejo, J. (2008). Clinical implications of insight assessment in obsessive-compulsive disorder. *Comprehensive Psychiatry, 49*, 305–312. http://dx.doi.org/10.1016/j.comppsych.2007.09.005

American Psychiatric Association. (2013). *Diagnostic and statistical manual of mental disorders* (5th ed.). Washington, DC: Author.

Arnold, L. M., Auchenbach, M. B., & McElroy, S. L. (2001). Psychogenic excoriation: Clinical features, proposed diagnostic criteria, epidemiology and approaches to treatment. *CNS Drugs, 15*, 351–359. http://dx.doi.org/10.2165/00023210-200115050-00002

Ayers, C. R. (2017). Age-specific prevalence of hoarding and obsessive-compulsive disorder: A population-based study. *The American Journal of Geriatric Psychiatry, 25*, 256–257. http://dx.doi.org/10.1016/j.jagp.2016.12.001

Bandelow, B., Sher, L., Bunevicius, R., Hollander, E., Kasper, S., Zohar, J., Möller, H. J., the WFSBP Task Force on Mental Disorders in Primary Care, & the WFSBP Task Force on Anxiety Disorders, OCD and PTSD. (2012). Guidelines for the pharmacological treatment of anxiety disorders, obsessive-compulsive disorder and posttraumatic stress disorder in primary care. *International Journal of Psychiatry in Clinical Practice, 16*, 77–84. http://dx.doi.org/10.3109/13651501.2012.667114

Bass, A. (2008). *Side effects: A prosecutor, a whistleblower, and a bestselling antidepressant on trial.* Chapel Hill, NC: Algonquin Books.

Bate, K. S., Malouff, J. M., Thorsteinsson, E. T., & Bhullar, N. (2011). The efficacy of habit reversal therapy for tics, habit disorders, and stuttering: A meta-analytic review. *Clinical Psychology Review, 31*, 865–871. http://dx.doi.org/10.1016/j.cpr.2011.03.013

Brakoulias, V., Eslick, G. D., & Starcevic, V. (2015). A meta-analysis of the response of pathological hoarding to pharmacotherapy. *Psychiatry Research, 229*, 272–276. http://dx.doi.org/10.1016/j.psychres.2015.07.019

Beesdo-Baum, K., & Knappe, S. (2014). Epidemiology and natural course. In P. M. G. Emmelkamp & T. Ehring (Eds.), *The Wiley handbook of anxiety disorders: Vol. 1. Theory and research* (pp. 26–46). Chichester, UK: Wiley. http://dx.doi.org/10.1002/9781118775349.ch3

Black, K., Shea, C., Dursun, S., & Kutcher, S. (2000). Selective serotonin reuptake inhibitor discontinuation syndrome: Proposed diagnostic criteria. *Journal of Psychiatry & Neuroscience, 25*, 255–261.

Bliziotes, M. M., Eshleman, A. J., Zhang, X. W., & Wiren, K. M. (2001). Neurotransmitter action in osteoblasts: Expression of a functional system for serotonin receptor activation and reuptake. *Bone, 29*, 477–486. http://dx.doi.org/10.1016/S8756-3282(01)00593-2

Bloch, M. H., Landeros-Weisenberger, A., Kelmendi, B., Coric, V., Bracken, M. B., & Leckman, J. F. (2006). A systematic review: Antipsychotic augmentation with treatment refractory obsessive-compulsive disorder. *Molecular Psychiatry, 11*, 622–632. http://dx.doi.org/10.1038/sj.mp.4001823

Brown, T. A., & Barlow, D. H. (2014). *Anxiety and related disorders interview schedule for DSM–5 (ADIS-5L): Lifetime version, client interview schedule.* New York, NY: Oxford University Press.

Bystritsky, A., Ackerman, D. L., Rosen, R. M., Vapnik, T., Gorbis, E., Maidment, K. M., & Saxena, S. (2004). Augmentation of serotonin reuptake inhibitors in refractory obsessive-compulsive disorder using adjunctive olanzapine: A placebo-controlled trial. *The Journal of Clinical Psychiatry, 65*, 565–568. http://dx.doi.org/10.4088/JCP.v65n0418

Cherin, P., Colvez, A., Deville de Periere, G., & Sereni, D. (1997). Risk of syncope in the elderly and consumption of drugs: A case-control study. *Journal of Clinical Epidemiology, 50*, 313–320. http://dx.doi.org/10.1016/S0895-4356(96)00385-X

Craske, M. G. (2003). *Origins of phobias and anxiety: Why more women than men?* Amsterdam, Netherlands: Elsevier.

Dell'Osso, B., Nestadt, G., Allen, A., & Hollander, E. (2006). Serotonin-norepinephrine reuptake inhibitors in the treatment of obsessive-compulsive disorder: A critical review. *The Journal of Clinical Psychiatry, 67*, 600–610. http://dx.doi.org/10.4088/JCP.v67n0411

Dougherty, D. D., Loh, R., Jenike, M. A., & Keuthen, N. J. (2006). Single modality versus dual modality treatment for trichotillomania: Sertraline, behavioral therapy, or both? *The Journal of Clinical Psychiatry, 67*, 1086–1092. http://dx.doi.org/10.4088/JCP.v67n0711

Eisen, J. L., Phillips, K. A., Baer, L., Beer, D. A., Atala, K. D., & Rasmussen, S. A. (1998). The Brown Assessment of Beliefs Scale: Reliability and validity. *The American Journal of Psychiatry, 155*, 102–108. http://dx.doi.org/10.1176/ajp.155.1.102

Favazza, A. R., & Favazza, B. (1987). *Bodies under siege: Self-mutilation in culture and psychiatry*. Baltimore, MD: Johns Hopkins University Press.

Ferguson, J. M. (2001). SSRI antidepressant medications: Adverse effects and tolerability. *Primary Care Companion to the Journal of Clinical Psychiatry, 3,* 22–27. http://dx.doi.org/10.4088/PCC.v03n0105

Fineberg, N. A., & Craig, K. J. (2010). Pharmacotherapy for obsessive-compulsive disorder. In D. J. Stein, E. Hollander, & B. O. Rothbaum (Eds.), *Textbook of Anxiety Disorders* (2nd ed., pp. 311–337). Washington, DC: American Psychiatric Association.

Fineberg, N. A., Pampaloni, I., Pallanti, S., Ipser, J., & Stein, D. J. (2007). Sustained response versus relapse: The pharmacotherapeutic goal for obsessive-compulsive disorder. *International Clinical Psychopharmacology, 22,* 313–322. http://dx.doi.org/10.1097/YIC.0b013e32825ea312

Flament, M. F., & Bisserbe, J. C. (1997). Pharmacologic treatment of obsessive-compulsive disorder: Comparative studies. *The Journal of Clinical Psychiatry, 58*(Suppl. 12), 18–22.

*Flessner, C. A., Woods, D. W., Franklin, M. E., Cashin, S. E., & Keuthen, N. J. (2008). The Milwaukee Inventory for Subtypes of Trichotillomania-Adult Version (MIST-A): Development of an instrument for the assessment of "focused" and "automatic" hair pulling. *Journal of Psychopathology and Behavioral Assessment, 30,* 20–30. http://dx.doi.org/10.1007/s10862-007-9073-x

*Foa, E. B., Huppert, J. D., Leiberg, S., Langner, R., Kichic, R., Hajcak, G., & Salkovskis, P. M. (2002). The Obsessive-Compulsive Inventory: Development and validation of a short version. *Psychological Assessment, 14,* 485–496. http://dx.doi.org/10.1037/1040-3590.14.4.485

Foa, E. B., Kozak, M. J., Goodman, W. K., Hollander, E., Jenike, M. A., & Rasmussen, S. A. (1995). *DSM–IV* field trial: Obsessive-compulsive disorder. *The American Journal of Psychiatry, 152,* 90–96.

Francazio, S. K., Murphy, Y. E., & Flessner, C. A. (2017). Psychological treatment of trichotillomania. In E. A. Storch, J. S. Abramowitz, & D. McKay (Eds.), *The Wiley handbook of obsessive-compulsive disorders* (Vol. II, pp. 1009–1022). Chichester, United Kingdom: Wiley. http://dx.doi.org/10.1002/9781118890233.ch57

Franklin, M. E., Kratz, H. E., Freeman, J. B., Ivarsson, T., Heyman, I., Sookman, D., . . . March, J., & the Accreditation Task Force of The Canadian Institute for Obsessive Compulsive Disorders. (2015). Cognitive-behavioral therapy for pediatric obsessive-compulsive disorder: Empirical review and clinical recommendations. *Psychiatry Research, 227,* 78–92. http://dx.doi.org/10.1016/j.psychres.2015.02.009

Freedman, R., Lewis, D. A., Michels, R., Pine, D. S., Schultz, S. K., Tamminga, C. A., . . . Yager, J. (2013). The initial field trials of *DSM–5*: New blooms and old thorns. *The American Journal of Psychiatry, 170,* 1–5. http://dx.doi.org/10.1176/appi.ajp.2012.12091189

Friedman, R. A. (2014). Antidepressants' black-box warning—10 years later. *The New England Journal of Medicine, 371,* 1666–1668. http://dx.doi.org/10.1056/NEJMp1408480

*Frost, R. O., Steketee, G., & Grisham, J. (2004). Measurement of compulsive hoarding: Saving inventory-revised. *Behaviour Research and Therapy, 42,* 1163–1182. http://dx.doi.org/10.1016/j.brat.2003.07.006

*Frost, R. O., Steketee, G., Tolin, D. F., & Renaud, S. (2008). Development and validation of the clutter image rating. *Journal of Psychopathology and Behavioral Assessment, 30,* 193–203. http://dx.doi.org/10.1007/s10862-007-9068-7

Garner, L., Steinberg, E., & McKay, D. (in press). Exposure therapy. In A. Wenzel (Ed.), *Handbook of Cognitive Behavioral Therapy*. Washington, DC: American Psychological Association.

Gillman, P. K. (2006). A review of serotonin toxicity data: Implications for the mechanisms of antidepressant drug action. *Biological Psychiatry, 59,* 1046–1051. http://dx.doi.org/10.1016/j.biopsych.2005.11.016

*Goodman, W. K., Price, L. H., Rasmussen, S. A., Mazure, C., Delgado, P., Heninger, G. R., & Charney, D. S. (1989a). The Yale-Brown Obsessive Compulsive Scale: II. Validity. *Archives of General Psychiatry, 46,* 1012–1016. http://dx.doi.org/10.1001/archpsyc.1989.01810110054008

*Goodman, W. K., Price, L. H., Rasmussen, S. A., Mazure, C., Fleischmann, R. L., Hill, C. L., . . . Charney, D. S. (1989b). The Yale-Brown Obsessive Compulsive Scale: I. Development, use, and reliability. *Archives of General Psychiatry, 46,* 1006–1011. http://dx.doi.org/10.1001/archpsyc.1989.01810110048007

Haddad, P. M., & Anderson, I. M. (2007). Recognising and managing antidepressant discontinuation symptoms. *Advances in Psychiatric Treatment, 13,* 447–457. http://dx.doi.org/10.1192/apt.bp.105.001966

Harrison, A., Fernández de la Cruz, L., Enander, J., Radua, J., & Mataix-Cols, D. (2016). Cognitive-behavioral therapy for body dysmorphic disorder: A systematic review and meta-analysis of randomized controlled trials. *Clinical Psychology Review, 48,* 43–51. http://dx.doi.org/10.1016/j.cpr.2016.05.007

Hartmann, A. S., & Lyons, N. (2017). Body dysmorphic disorder. In E. A. Storch, J. S. Abramowitz, & D. McKay (Eds.), *The Wiley handbook of obsessive compulsive disorders* (Vol. II, pp. 774–789). Chichester, UK: Wiley. http://dx.doi.org/10.1002/9781118890233.ch43

Hollander, E., Braun, A., & Simeon, D. (2008). Should OCD leave the anxiety disorders in *DSM–V*? The case for obsessive compulsive-related disorders. *Depression and Anxiety, 25,* 317–329. http://dx.doi.org/10.1002/da.20500

Houghton, D. C., & Woods, D. W. (2017). Phenomenology of trichotillomania. In E. A. Storch, J. S. Abramowitz, & D. McKay (Eds.), *The Wiley handbook of obsessive compulsive disorders* (Vol. II, pp. 817–831). Chichester, UK: Wiley. http://dx.doi.org/10.1002/9781118890233.ch46

Jacobsen, F. M. (1995). Risperidone in the treatment of affective illness and obsessive-compulsive disorder. *The Journal of Clinical Psychiatry, 56,* 423–429.

Jenike, M. A., Baer, L., & Greist, J. H. (1990). Clomipramine versus fluoxetine in obsessive-compulsive disorder: A retrospective comparison of side effects and efficacy. *Journal of Clinical Psychopharmacology, 10,* 122–124. http://dx.doi.org/10.1097/00004714-199004000-00008

*Kadouri, A., Corruble, E., & Falissard, B. (2007). The improved Clinical Global Impression Scale (iCGI): Development and validation in depression. *BMC Psychiatry, 7,* 7. http://dx.doi.org/10.1186/1471-244X-7-7

Keeley, M. L., Storch, E. A., Merlo, L. J., & Geffken, G. R. (2008). Clinical predictors of response to cognitive-behavioral therapy for obsessive-compulsive disorder. *Clinical Psychology Review, 28,* 118–130. http://dx.doi.org/10.1016/j.cpr.2007.04.003

Kekic, M., Boysen, E., Campbell, I. C., & Schmidt, U. (2016). A systematic review of the clinical efficacy of transcranial direct current stimulation (tDCS) in psychiatric disorders. *Journal of Psychiatric Research, 74,* 70–86. http://dx.doi.org/10.1016/j.jpsychires.2015.12.018

Kelly, C. A., Dhaun, N., Laing, W. J., Strachan, F. E., Good, A. M., & Bateman, D. N. (2004). Comparative toxicity of citalopram and the newer antidepressants after overdose. *Journal of Toxicology. Clinical Toxicology, 42,* 67–71. http://dx.doi.org/10.1081/CLT-120028747

Kim, W. B. (2014). On trichotillomania and its hairy history. *JAMA Dermatology, 150,* 1179. In E. A. Storch, J. S. Abramowitz, & D. McKay (Eds.), *The Wiley handbook of obsessive compulsive disorders* (Vol. II, pp. 1009–1022). Chichester, UK: Wiley.

Kisely, S., Hall, K., Siskind, D., Frater, J., Olson, S., & Crompton, D. (2014). Deep brain stimulation for obsessive-compulsive disorder: A systematic review and meta-analysis. *Psychological Medicine, 44,* 3533–3542. http://dx.doi.org/10.1017/S0033291714000981

Kobak, K. A., Greist, J. H., Jefferson, J. W., Katzelnick, D. J., & Henk, H. J. (1998). Behavioral versus pharmacological treatments of obsessive compulsive disorder: A meta-analysis. *Psychopharmacology, 136,* 205–216. http://dx.doi.org/10.1007/s002130050558

Koran, L. M., Hanna, G. L., Hollander, E., Nestadt, G., & Simpson, H. B. (2007). *Practice guideline for the treatment of patients with obsessive-compulsive disorder.* Washington, DC: American Psychiatric Association.

Kozak, M. J., & Foa, E. B. (1994). Obsessions, overvalued ideas, and delusions in obsessive-compulsive disorder. *Behaviour Research and Therapy, 32,* 343–353. http://dx.doi.org/10.1016/0005-7967(94)90132-5

Krebs, G., de la Cruz, L. F., Monzani, B., Bowyer, L., Anson, M., Cadman, J., . . . Mataix-Cols, D. (2017). Long-term outcomes of cognitive-behavioral therapy for adolescent body dysmorphic disorder. *Behavior Therapy, 48,* 462–473. http://dx.doi.org/10.1016/j.beth.2017.01.001

Kringlen, E. (1965). Obsessional neurotics: Long-term follow-up. *The British Journal of Psychiatry, 111,* 709–722. http://dx.doi.org/10.1192/bjp.111.477.709

Leonard, B. E. (2004). *Fundamentals of psychopharmacology* (3rd ed.). Chichester, UK: Wiley.

Lieberman, J. A., III. (2004). Managing anticholinergic side effects. *Primary Care Companion to the Journal of Clinical Psychiatry, 6*(Suppl. 2), 20–23.

Lochner, C., & Stein, D. J. (2001). Gender in obsessive-compulsive disorder and obsessive-compulsive spectrum disorders. *Archives of Women's Mental Health, 4,* 19–26. http://dx.doi.org/10.1007/s007370170004

Maher, M. J., Huppert, J. D., Chen, H., Duan, N., Foa, E. B., Liebowitz, M. R., & Simpson, H. B. (2010). Moderators and predictors of response to cognitive-behavioral therapy augmentation of pharmacotherapy in obsessive-compulsive disorder. *Psychological Medicine, 40,* 2013–2023. http://dx.doi.org/10.1017/S0033291710000620

Masi, G., Pfanner, C., Millepiedi, S., & Berloffa, S. (2010). Aripiprazole augmentation in 39 adolescents with medication-resistant obsessive-compulsive disorder. *Journal of Clinical Psychopharmacology, 30,* 688–693. http://dx.doi.org/10.1097/JCP.0b013e3181fab7b1

McDougle, C. J., Epperson, C. N., Pelton, G. H., Wasylink, S., & Price, L. H. (2000). A double-blind, placebo-controlled study of risperidone addition in serotonin reuptake inhibitor-refractory obsessive-compulsive disorder. *Archives of General Psychiatry, 57,* 794–801. http://dx.doi.org/10.1001/archpsyc.57.8.794

McElroy, S. L., Phillips, K. A., & Keck, P. E., Jr. (1994). Obsessive compulsive spectrum disorder. *The Journal of Clinical Psychiatry, 55*(Suppl.), 33–51.

McGuire, J. F., Ung, D., Selles, R. R., Rahman, O., Lewin, A. B., Murphy, T. K., & Storch, E. A. (2014). Treating trichotillomania: A meta-analysis of treatment effects and moderators for behavior therapy and serotonin reuptake inhibitors. *Journal of Psychiatric*

Research, *58*, 76–83. http://dx.doi.org/10.1016/ j.jpsychires.2014.07.015

McKay, D., Abramowitz, J. S., Calamari, J. E., Kyrios, M., Radomsky, A., Sookman, D., . . . Wilhelm, S. (2004). A critical evaluation of obsessive-compulsive disorder subtypes: Symptoms versus mechanisms. *Clinical Psychology Review*, *24*, 283–313. http://dx.doi.org/ 10.1016/j.cpr.2004.04.003

McKay, D., Abramowitz, J. S., & Taylor, S. (2008). How should we conceptualize the obsessive-compulsive spectrum? In J. S. Abramowitz, D. McKay, & S. Taylor (Eds.), *Obsessive-compulsive disorder: Subtypes and spectrum conditions* (pp. 287–300). Oxford, UK: Elsevier.

McKay, D., & Andover, M. (2012). Should nonsuicidal self-injury be a putative obsessive-compulsive-related condition? A critical appraisal. *Behavior Modification*, *36*, 3–17. http://dx.doi.org/10.1177/ 0145445511417707

McKay, D., & Neziroglu, F. (2009). Methodological issues in the obsessive-compulsive spectrum. *Psychiatry Research*, *170*, 61–65. http://dx.doi.org/10.1016/j. psychres.2009.01.004

McKay, D., Sookman, D., Neziroglu, F., Wilhelm, S., Stein, D. J., Kyrios, M., . . . Veale, D. (2015). Efficacy of cognitive-behavioral therapy for obsessive-compulsive disorder. *Psychiatry Research*, *225*, 236–246. http://dx.doi.org/10.1016/j.psychres.2014.11.058

Meyer, V. (1966). Modification of expectations in cases with obsessional rituals. *Behaviour Research and Therapy*, *4*, 273–280. http://dx.doi.org/10.1016/ 0005-7967(66)90023-4

Morselli, E. (1891). Sulla dismorfofobia e sulla tafefobia [On dysmorphophobia and tafefobia]. *Bolletino della R academia di Genova*, *6*, 110–119.

Myers, T. A., & Crowther, J. H. (2009). Social comparison as a predictor of body dissatisfaction: A meta-analytic review. *Journal of Abnormal Psychology*, *118*, 683–698. http://dx.doi.org/10.1037/a0016763

Naber, D. (2008). Subjective effects of antipsychotic drugs and their relevance for compliance and remission. *Epidemiologia e Psichiatria Sociale*, *17*, 174–176. http://dx.doi.org/10.1017/S1121189X00001238

Naesström, M., Blomstedt, P., & Bodlund, O. (2016). A systematic review of psychiatric indications for deep brain stimulation, with focus on major depressive and obsessive-compulsive disorder. *Nordic Journal of Psychiatry*, *70*, 483–491. http://dx.doi.org/10.3109/ 08039488.2016.1162846

Neziroglu, F., McKay, D., Yaryura-Tobias, J. A., Stevens, K. P., & Todaro, J. (1999). The Overvalued Ideas Scale: Development, reliability and validity in obsessive-compulsive disorder. *Behaviour Research and Therapy*, *37*, 881–902. http://dx.doi.org/10.1016/ S0005-7967(98)00191-0

Nunnally, J., & Bernstein, I. H. (1994). *Psychometric theory* (3rd ed.). New York, NY: McGraw-Hill.

Pertusa, A., Frost, R. O., Fullana, M. A., Samuels, J., Steketee, G., Tolin, D., . . . Mataix-Cols, D. (2010). Refining the diagnostic boundaries of compulsive hoarding: A critical review. *Clinical Psychology Review*, *30*, 371–386. http://dx.doi.org/10.1016/ j.cpr.2010.01.007

Phillipou, A., Rossell, S. L., Wilding, H. E., & Castle, D. J. (2016). Randomised controlled trials of psychological and pharmacological treatments for body dysmorphic disorder: A systematic review. *Psychiatry Research*, *245*, 179–185.

Phillips, K. A. (1996). Pharmacologic treatment of body dysmorphic disorder. *Psychopharmacology Bulletin*, *32*, 597–605.

Phillips, K. A. (2005). Placebo-controlled study of pimozide augmentation of fluoxetine in body dysmorphic disorder. *The American Journal of Psychiatry*, *162*, 377–379. http://dx.doi.org/10.1176/appi.ajp.162.2.377

*Phillips, K. A., Hart, A. S., & Menard, W. (2014). Psychometric evaluation of the Yale-Brown Obsessive-Compulsive Scale modified for Body Dysmorphic Disorder (BDD-YBOCS). *Journal of Obsessive-Compulsive and Related Disorders*, *3*, 205–208. http://dx.doi.org/10.1016/j.jocrd.2014.04.004

Piccinelli, M., Pini, S., Bellantuono, C., & Wilkinson, G. (1995). Efficacy of drug treatment in obsessive-compulsive disorder. A meta-analytic review. *The British Journal of Psychiatry*, *166*, 424–443. http://dx.doi.org/10.1192/bjp.166.4.424

Pigott, T. A., & Seay, S. M. (1999). A review of the efficacy of selective serotonin reuptake inhibitors in obsessive-compulsive disorder. *The Journal of Clinical Psychiatry*, *60*, 101–106. http://dx.doi.org/10.4088/ JCP.v60n0206

Pilecki, B., & McKay, D. (2013). The theory-practice gap in cognitive-behavior therapy. *Behavior Therapy*, *44*, 541–547. http://dx.doi.org/10.1016/j.beth.2013.03.004

Pittenger, C., Bloch, M. H., Wasylink, S., Billingslea, E., Simpson, R., Jakubovski, E., . . . Coric, V. (2015). Riluzole augmentation in treatment-refractory obsessive-compulsive disorder: A pilot randomized placebo-controlled trial. *The Journal of Clinical Psychiatry*, *76*, 1075–1084. http://dx.doi.org/10.4088/ JCP.14m09123

Rashid, H., Khan, A. A., & Fineberg, N. A. (2015). Adjunctive antipsychotic in the treatment of body dysmorphic disorder—A retrospective naturalistic case note study. *International Journal of Psychiatry in Clinical Practice*, *19*, 84–89. http://dx.doi.org/ 10.3109/13651501.2014.981546

*Regier, D. A., Narrow, W. E., Clarke, D. E., Kraemer, H. C., Kuramoto, S. J., Kuhl, E. A., & Kupfer, D. J. (2013). *DSM–5* field trials in the United States and

Canada, Part II: Test-retest reliability of selected categorical diagnoses. *The American Journal of Psychiatry, 170*, 59–70. http://dx.doi.org/10.1176/appi.ajp.2012.12070999

Richards, J. B., Papaioannou, A., Adachi, J. D., Joseph, L., Whitson, H. E., Prior, J. C., Goltzman, D., & the Canadian Multicentre Osteoporosis Study Research Group. (2007). Effect of selective serotonin reuptake inhibitors on the risk of fracture. *Archives of Internal Medicine, 167*, 188–194. http://dx.doi.org/10.1001/archinte.167.2.188

Rodriguez, C. I., Bender, J., Jr., Morrison, S., Mehendru, R., Tolin, D., & Simpson, H. B. (2013). Does extended release methylphenidate help adults with hoarding disorder?: A case series. *Journal of Clinical Psychopharmacology, 33*, 444–447. http://dx.doi.org/10.1097/JCP.0b013e318290115e

Rodriguez, C. I., Kegeles, L. S., Levinson, A., Feng, T., Marcus, S. M., Vermes, D., . . . Simpson, H. B. (2013). Randomized controlled crossover trial of ketamine in obsessive-compulsive disorder: Proof-of-concept. *Neuropsychopharmacology, 38*, 2475–2483. http://dx.doi.org/10.1038/npp.2013.150

*Rosen, J. C., & Reiter, J. (1996). Development of the body dysmorphic disorder examination. *Behaviour Research and Therapy, 34*, 755–766. http://dx.doi.org/10.1016/0005-7967(96)00024-1

Saxena, S. (2011). Pharmacotherapy of compulsive hoarding. *Journal of Clinical Psychology, 67*, 477–484. http://dx.doi.org/10.1002/jclp.20792

Selles, R. R., McGuire, J. F., Small, B. J., & Storch, E. A. (2016). A systematic review and meta-analysis of psychiatric treatments for excoriation (skin-picking) disorder. *General Hospital Psychiatry, 41*, 29–37. http://dx.doi.org/10.1016/j.genhosppsych.2016.04.001

*Shankman, S. A., Funkhouser, C. J., Klein, D. N., Davila, J., Lerner, D., & Hee, D. (2017). Reliability and validity of severity dimensions of psychopathology assessed using the Structured Clinical Interview for DSM–5 (SCID). *International Journal of Methods in Psychiatric Research, 27*, e1590.

Shaw, S. N. (2002). Shifting conversations on girls' and women's self-injury: An analysis of the clinical literature in historical context. *Feminism & Psychology, 12*, 191–219.

Shim, G., Park, H. Y., Jang, J. H., Kim, E., Park, H. Y., Hwang, J. Y., . . . Kwon, J. S. (2011). What is the optimal dose of escitalopram for the treatment of obsessive-compulsive disorder? A naturalistic open-label study. *International Clinical Psychopharmacology, 26*, 284–290. http://dx.doi.org/10.1097/YIC.0b013e32834a5c09

Simon, V., van Winkel, R., & De Hert, M. (2009). Are weight gain and metabolic side effects of atypical antipsychotics dose dependent? A literature review. *The Journal of Clinical Psychiatry, 70*, 1041–1050. http://dx.doi.org/10.4088/JCP.08r04392

Simpson, H. B., Foa, E. B., Liebowitz, M. R., Huppert, J. D., Cahill, S., Maher, M. J., . . . Campeas, R. (2013). Cognitive-behavioral therapy vs risperidone for augmenting serotonin reuptake inhibitors in obsessive-compulsive disorder: A randomized clinical trial. *JAMA Psychiatry, 70*, 1190–1199. http://dx.doi.org/10.1001/jamapsychiatry.2013.1932

Simpson, H. B., Liebowitz, M. R., Foa, E. B., Kozak, M. J., Schmidt, A. B., Rowan, V., . . . Campeas, R. (2004). Post-treatment effects of exposure therapy and clomipramine in obsessive-compulsive disorder. *Depression and Anxiety, 19*, 225–233. http://dx.doi.org/10.1002/da.20003

Skapinakis, P., Caldwell, D. M., Hollingworth, W., Bryden, P., Fineberg, N. A., Salkovskis, P., . . . Lewis, G. (2016). Pharmacological and psychotherapeutic interventions for management of obsessive-compulsive disorder in adults: A systematic review and network meta-analysis. *The Lancet Psychiatry, 3*, 730–739. http://dx.doi.org/10.1016/S2215-0366(16)30069-4

Slikboer, R., Nedeljkovic, M., Bowe, S. J., & Moulding, R. (2017). A systematic review and meta-analysis of behaviourally-based psychological interventions and pharmacological interventions for trichotillomania. *Clinical Psychologist, 21*, 20–32. http://dx.doi.org/10.1111/cp.12074

*Snorrason, I., Olafsson, R. P., Flessner, C. A., Keuthen, N. J., Franklin, M. E., & Woods, D. W. (2012). The Skin Picking Scale-Revised: Factor structure and psychometric properties. *Journal of Obsessive-Compulsive and Related Disorders, 1*, 133–137. http://dx.doi.org/10.1016/j.jocrd.2012.03.001

Stahl, S. M., Grady, M. M., Moret, C., & Briley, M. (2005). SNRIs: The pharmacology, clinical efficacy, and tolerability in comparison with other classes of antidepressants. *CNS Spectrums, 10*, 732–747. http://dx.doi.org/10.1017/S1092852900019726

Storch, E. A., Abramowitz, J. S., & McKay, D. (Eds.). (2017). *The Wiley handbook of obsessive compulsive disorders: Vol. II. Obsessive-compulsive related disorders.* Chichester, UK: Wiley.

Taylor, S., Abramowitz, J. S., & McKay, D. (2010). Obsessive-compulsive disorder. In M. M. Antony & D. H. Barlow (Eds.), *Handbook of assessment and treatment planning for psychological disorders* (2nd ed., pp. 267–300). New York, NY: Guilford.

Taylor, S., McKay, D., Crowe, K. B., Abramowitz, J. S., Conelea, C. A., Calamari, J. E., & Sica, C. (2014). The sense of incompleteness as a motivator of obsessive-compulsive symptoms: An empirical analysis of concepts and correlates. *Behavior Therapy, 45*, 254–262. http://dx.doi.org/10.1016/j.beth.2013.11.004

Tolin, D. F., Frost, R. O., Steketee, G., & Muroff, J. (2015). Cognitive behavioral therapy for hoarding disorder: A meta-analysis. *Depression and Anxiety, 32*, 158–166. http://dx.doi.org/10.1002/da.22327

*Tolin, D. F., Gilliam, C., Wootton, B. M., Bowe, W., Bragdon, L. B., Davis, E., . . . Hallion, L. S. (2018). Psychometric properties of a structured diagnostic interview for *DSM–5* anxiety, mood, and obsessive-compulsive and related disorders. *Assessment, 25,* 3–13. http://dx.doi.org/10.1177/1073191116638410

Tonks, A. (2002). Withdrawal from paroxetine can be severe, warns FDA. *British Medical Journal, 324,* 260. http://dx.doi.org/10.1136/bmj.324.7332.260

Trevizol, A. P., Shiozawa, P., Cook, I. A., Sato, I. A., Kaku, C. B., Guimarães, F. B. S., . . . Cordeiro, Q. (2016). Transcranial magnetic stimulation for obsessive-compulsive disorder: An updated systematic review and meta-analysis. *The Journal of ECT, 32,* 262–266. http://dx.doi.org/10.1097/YCT.0000000000000335

Üçok, A., & Gaebel, W. (2008). Side effects of atypical antipsychotics: A brief overview. *World Psychiatry, 7,* 58–62. http://dx.doi.org/10.1002/j.2051-5545.2008.tb00154.x

van de Griendt, J. M. T. M., Verdellen, C. W. J., van Dijk, M. K., & Verbraak, M. J. P. M. (2013). Behavioural treatment of tics: Habit reversal and exposure with response prevention. *Neuroscience and Biobehavioral Reviews, 37,* 1172–1177. http://dx.doi.org/10.1016/j.neubiorev.2012.10.007

Warner, C. H., Bobo, W., Warner, C., Reid, S., & Rachal, J. (2006). Antidepressant discontinuation syndrome. *American Family Physician, 74,* 449–456.

Wheaton, M. G., DeSantis, S. M., & Simpson, H. B. (2016). Network meta-analyses and treatment recommendations for obsessive-compulsive disorder. *The Lancet Psychiatry, 3,* 920. http://dx.doi.org/10.1016/S2215-0366(16)30280-2

Whittington, C. J., Kendall, T., Fonagy, P., Cottrell, D., Cotgrove, A., & Boddington, E. (2004). Selective serotonin reuptake inhibitors in childhood depression: A systematic review of published versus unpublished data. *Lancet, 363,* 1341–1345.

Williams, J., Hadjistavropoulos, T., & Sharpe, D. (2006). A meta-analysis of psychological and pharmacological treatments for body dysmorphic disorder. *Behaviour Research and Therapy, 44,* 99–111. http://dx.doi.org/10.1016/j.brat.2004.12.006

Verdoux, H., Tournier, M., & Bégaud, B. (2010). Antipsychotic prescribing trends: A review of pharmaco-epidemiological studies. *Acta Psychiatrica Scandinavica, 121,* 4–10. http://dx.doi.org/10.1111/j.1600-0447.2009.01425.x

Xu, Y., Hackett, M., Carter, G., Loo, C., Gálvez, V., Glozier, N., . . . Rodgers, A. (2016). Effects of low-dose and very low-dose ketamine among patients with major depression: A systematic review and meta-analysis. *International Journal of Neuropsychopharmacology, 19,* pyv124. http://dx.doi.org/10.1093/ijnp/pyv124

Zachar, P. (2008). Real kinds but no true taxonomy: An essay in psychiatric semantics. In K. S. Kendler & J. Parnas (Eds.), *Philosophical issues in psychiatry: Explanation, phenomenology, and nosology* (pp. 327–355). Baltimore, MD: Johns Hopkins Press.

Zhou, D. D., Wang, W., Wang, G. M., Li, D. Q., & Kuang, L. (2017). An updated meta-analysis: Short-term therapeutic effects of repeated transcranial magnetic stimulation in treating obsessive-compulsive disorder. *Journal of Affective Disorders, 215,* 187–196. http://dx.doi.org/10.1016/j.jad.2017.03.033

Zohar, J. (Ed.). (2012). *Obsessive-compulsive disorder: Current science and clinical practice.* New York, NY: Wiley. http://dx.doi.org/10.1002/9781119941125

CHAPTER 12

PHARMACOLOGICAL TREATMENT OF IMPULSE CONTROL DISORDERS

Emil F. Coccaro and Jon E. Grant

The inclusion of impulse control disorders (ICD) in the *Diagnostic and Statistical Manual of Mental Disorders* (*DSM*) has varied over the years. Beginning with *DSM–III*, the ICD group of disorders included intermittent explosive disorder (IED), pyromania, kleptomania, trichotillomania, and pathological gambling. At the time, such disorders were defined by a failure to resist acting upon impulses to be aggressive, set fires, steal merchandise, pull one's own hair, or to gamble, associated with distress and/or psychosocial impairment.

As research continued over the next 3 decades, it became clear that trichotillomania and pathological gambling belonged to other diagnostic groupings. For *DSM–5*, trichotillomania was moved to the section on Obsessive-Compulsive and Related Disorders and pathological gambling was moved to the section on Substance-Related and Addictive Disorders. This left IED, kleptomania, and pyromania as ICDs in *DSM–5*. At the same time, *DSM–5* moved conduct disorder and oppositional defiant disorder to the section titled Disruptive, Impulse-Control, and Conduct Disorders. These latter two disorders will not be discussed in this chapter because, historically, these disorders have not been conceptualized as impulse control disorders, and because they are typically discussed in the context of disorders that begin in childhood.

Finally, while the degree to which *DSM–5* ICDs may share clinical, genetic, phenomenological, and biological features is not fully known, common features include repetitive engagement in problematic behaviors despite consequences and impaired control in inhibiting problematic behavior. That said, IED differs from pyromania and kleptomania in that individuals with IED do not have an appetitive urge or craving state prior to engagement in their problematic behavior and do not experience a hedonic reward in the context of acting out their problematic behavior (Grant, Brewer, & Potenza, 2006).

EPIDEMIOLOGY AND PREVALENCE

The first thing to know about any disorder is how prevalent it is in the general population. For most of the impulse control disorders, however, there is little data on this topic, with the exception of IED, for which data do exist from large community surveys. See also the Tool Kit of Resources at the end of the chapter.

Intermittent Explosive Disorder

Human aggression constitutes a behavioral act that results in physical (or verbal) injury to self, others, or objects. It may be defensive, premeditated (e.g., predatory), or impulsive (e.g., nonpremeditated) in nature. While the latter two forms may appear in the same individual at different times, the underpinnings of the two forms are different (Barratt, Stanford, Felthous, & Kent, 1997; Raine et al., 1998). Specifically, acts of impulsive aggression represent a quick, typically angry, response to social threat or

http://dx.doi.org/10.1037/0000133-012
APA Handbook of Psychopharmacology, S. M. Evans (Editor-in-Chief)

frustration that is out of proportion to the situation, while premeditated aggressive acts are planned in advance and are carried out to achieve a tangible objective. Impulsive aggressive acts may include verbal arguments, temper tantrums (with or without property damage or harm to others), property assault, or assault to other living beings including animals. Most importantly, the impulsive aggressive acts cause distress to the individual or impairment in the psychosocial function of the individual, and are not due to another disorder (i.e., do not occur exclusively during that other disorder).

There are no epidemiologic data regarding DSM–5 IED available at this time. All such data exists from community surveys of individuals interviewed before the publication of the DSM–5. DSM–IV criteria for IED differ in many ways from those in DSM–5 and the primary source of epidemiological data on IED, from the National Comorbidity Survey Replication (NCS-R), only queried interviewees about the frequency of "anger attacks" that largely dovetail with the A.2. criteria for DSM–5 IED. One difference, however, is that threats of aggression are not part of current A.2. IED criteria (they would likely meet A.1. IED criteria), though they are included in the NCS-R definition of "anger attack." This means that translations of the prevalence of IED by DSM–IV criteria to DSM–5 criteria are imprecise, though still worthwhile until more contemporary community survey data is available. According to the NCS-R study, the prevalence of DSM–IV IED by "narrow" criteria (which require aggressive outbursts at least three times in a single year) was 5.4% lifetime and 2.7% in the past year (Kessler et al., 2006). Recently, we revisited these data and have estimated that lifetime and past year prevalence of IED, applying the A.2. (and B–F) DSM–5 criteria, is about 3.6% and 2.2%, respectively (Coccaro, Fanning, & Lee, 2017). Studies of adolescents estimate the lifetime and past year prevalence for the "narrow" definition of DSM–IV IED at 5.3% and 1.7%, respectively (McLaughlin et al., 2012). IED appears as early as childhood (e.g., prepubertal) and peaks in midadolescence with a mean age of onset ranging from about 13 to 18 years in adult samples (Coccaro, Posternak, & Zimmerman, 2005; Kessler et al., 2006) and younger in adolescent samples (McLaughlin et al., 2012).

The duration of active IED ranges from nearly 12 years to 20 years to almost the whole lifetime.

Kleptomania

Kleptomania is characterized by repetitive stealing behavior precipitated by significant and uncontrollable urges to steal items not needed for personal use (American Psychiatric Association, 2013). The DSM–5 sets forth diagnostic criteria for kleptomania, including: impulsive stealing of unneeded items, building tension before the act and satisfaction or relief when doing it, that the stealing is not done antagonistically, and that the stealing is not better accounted for by another disorder (American Psychiatric Association, 2013).

The National Epidemiologic Survey on Alcohol and Related Conditions (NESARC) assessed rates of stealing (not a formal diagnosis of kleptomania) among 43,000 adults. The lifetime prevalence of shoplifting in the U.S. population was 11.3% (Blanco et al., 2008). Although no large-scale epidemiologic studies have been conducted to assess the prevalence of kleptomania in the general population, a survey of college students ($N = 791$) found that three (0.38%) met criteria for kleptomania (Odlaug & Grant, 2010). Kleptomania is also experienced by a broad range of psychiatric patient populations, including 3.7% of depressed patients ($n = 107$; Lejoyeux, Arbaretaz, McLoughlin, & Ades, 2002) and 24% of those with bulimia (Hudson, Pope, Jonas, & Yurgelun-Todd, 1983). A recent study of psychiatric inpatients ($n = 204$) with a range of admitting disorders revealed that 7.8% ($n = 16$) endorsed current kleptomania and 9.3% ($n = 19$) met lifetime criteria (Grant, Levine, Kim, & Potenza, 2005). Approximately two thirds of individuals with kleptomania in clinical samples are women.

Pyromania

Pyromania is characterized by a preoccupation with fire setting. The DSM–5 criteria for the diagnosis of pyromania include intentional setting of fires (more than once), tension or arousal before fire setting and satisfaction or relief when setting fires or watching/taking part in the aftermath, and interest in fire (American Psychiatric Association, 2013).

The NESARC assessed rates of fire setting (not a formal diagnosis of pyromania) among 43,000 adults (Blanco et al., 2010). The prevalence of lifetime fire setting in the U.S. population was 1.13% (95% confidence interval [CI] 1.0, 1.3; Blanco et al., 2010). Being male, never married, U.S.-born, and having a yearly income of more than $70,000 were risk factors for lifetime fire setting, while being Asian or Hispanic and older than 30 years were protective factors for lifetime fire setting. The strongest associations with fire-setting were with disorders often associated with deficits in impulse control, such as antisocial personality disorder (odds ratio [OR] = 21.8; 95% CI 6.6, 28.5), substance use disorders (OR = 7.6; 95% CI 5.2, 10.9), bipolar disorder (OR = 5.6; 95% CI 4.0–7.9), and pathological gambling (OR = 4.8; 95% CI 2.4, 9.5).

Although no large-scale epidemiologic studies have assessed pyromania, a survey of college students (*N* = 791) found that eight (1.01%) met criteria for pyromania (Odlaug & Grant, 2010). One study of 107 patients with depression found that three (2.8%) met current criteria for pyromania (Lejoyeux, Arbaretaz, McLoughlin, & Ades, 2002), and a study of 204 psychiatric inpatients revealed that 3.4% (*n* = 7) endorsed current symptoms and 5.9% (*n* = 12) had lifetime symptoms of pyromania (Grant et al., 2005).

DIAGNOSING IMPULSE CONTROL DISORDERS

Intermittent Explosive Disorder

The A criteria for IED in *DSM–5* now defines the frequency and temporal nature of applicable aggressive behavior. The A.1. criteria require verbally aggressive and/or nonassaultive and nondestructive physically aggressive outbursts occurring at an average of twice weekly for at least 3 months, while the A.2. criteria require assaultive and/or destructive, aggressive outbursts occurring at least three times a year. About 70% of those meeting criteria for *DSM–5* IED meet both the A.1. and A.2. criteria, while 20% meet the A.2. criteria only and 10% meet the A.1. only (Coccaro, 2011). Empiric studies have shown that those meeting the A.1. criteria only do not differ from those meeting only the A.2. criteria

or those meeting both A.1. and A.2. (Coccaro, Lee, & McCloskey, 2014). While the B criterion for *DSM–5* does not differ from that in *DSM–IV* and continues to require that the aggressive behavior be out of proportion to the situation, the remaining criteria have all been revised.

The C criteria require that most of the aggressive outbursts be impulsive in nature, so that IED may not be given to someone who predominately engages in premeditated aggressive behavior. The D criteria require that the aggressive outbursts cause distress and/or impairment for the individual so that the IED diagnosis is not made in the absence of clinically significant consequences. The E criteria require that the individual is at least 6 years of age before a diagnosis of IED is given, so that typical aggressive behaviors seen in children younger than 6 years of age are not considered pathological. The last criteria (F) were revised so that the diagnosis of IED can be given as long as the aggressive outbursts do not occur only during the course of another disorder or exogenous factor known to be associated with aggression. With these changes the exclusion of selected disorders was removed, such as borderline personality disorder and/or antisocial personality disorder. This was added because individuals with these disorders were frequently not particularly aggressive compared with those with only IED (Coccaro, 2012).

IED can be diagnosed using the Scheduled Clinical Interview for DSM–5 disorders (SCID), which includes a module for IED (First, Williams, Karg, & Spitzer, 2015). A self-report assessment for the diagnosis has been published and is also available for use for screening for the presence of IED (Coccaro, Berman, & McCloskey, 2017).

Kleptomania

The Structured Clinical Interview for Kleptomania (SCI-K) is the only available validated clinician-administered instrument to assess for a current diagnosis of kleptomania (Grant, Brewer, & Potenza, 2006). The SCI-K has demonstrated excellent test–retest (phi coefficient = 0.956 [95% CI = 0.937, 0.970]) and interrater reliability (phi coefficient = 0.718 [95% CI = 0.506, 0.848]) in the diagnosis of kleptomania. Concurrent validity was observed with a self-report measure using kleptomania criteria (phi coefficient = 0.769 [95% CI = 0.653, 0.850]), and discriminant validity was observed with a measure of depression (point biserial coefficient = −0.020 [95% CI = −0.205, 0.166]). The SCI-K has demonstrated both high sensitivity and specificity based on longitudinal assessment.

Pyromania

The Minnesota Impulsive Disorders Interview (MIDI), a semistructured clinical interview assessing pyromania along with other impulse control disorders, is the only validated diagnostic instrument to assess for pyromania (Grant, 2008). The pyromania module has shown excellent sensitivity and specificity compared with self-report using the *DSM* criteria (Grant et al., 2005).

EVIDENCE-BASED PHARMACOLOGICAL TREATMENTS OF IMPULSE CONTROL DISORDERS

Intermittent Explosive Disorder

Understanding the role of neurotransmitters in aggression is critical to developing pharmacotherapy to reduce impulsive aggressive behavior. To date, individuals with IED are reported to have altered serotonin (5-HT) function compared with individuals without IED, or healthy controls (Coccaro, Lee, & Kavoussi, 2010a, 2010b; New et al., 2004). Overall, most psychobiological studies of aggression report an association with anomalies of 5-HT, including reduced levels of cerebrospinal fluid metabolites of 5-HT, reduced responsiveness of 5-HT receptors to stimulation, and reduced numbers of 5-HT transporter sites both on circulating platelets and on neurons in the brain (Duke, Bègue, Bell, & Eisenlohr-Moul, 2013). In addition, reduction of 5-HT levels after tryptophan depletion is associated with increased aggression on laboratory aggression tasks in "aggressive" human volunteers and is associated with greater ratings of anger in IED compared with healthy individuals (Lee, Gill, Chen, McCloskey, & Coccaro, 2012). Notably, successful treatment with the selective serotonin reuptake inhibitor (SSRI), fluoxetine (Prozac®), is associated with having more, rather than less,

functional presynaptic serotonin transporters (Coccaro, Kavoussi, & Hauger, 1997; Silva et al., 2010). While several other neurotransmitter/modulators have been found to correlate with measures of aggression (Fanning & Coccaro, 2018), none of these have led to a specific double-blind, placebo-controlled, clinical trial in impulsively aggressive individuals. In addition to neurochemistry, functional magnetic resonance imaging (fMRI) studies report greater amygdala response to exposure to angry faces in those with IED compared with healthy controls. This finding is true for implicit (Coccaro, McCloskey, Fitzgerald, & Phan, 2007; McCloskey et al., 2016) and explicit emotional processing. Notably, successful treatment with fluoxetine or the anticonvulsant/mood stabilizer divalproex (Depakote®) suppresses the fMRI blood oxygenation level-dependent (BOLD) amygdala response to anger faces, and the extent of anti-aggressive response appears to correlate with the degree of amygdala suppression (Coccaro, Fanning, Phan, & Lee, 2015).

Thus, these two findings underlie the current pharmacologic treatment of impulsive aggression in those with IED with serotonergic agents. Initial studies reported a reduction in impulsive aggressive behavior by the serotonin-activating antidepressant fluoxetine in impulsive aggressive individuals with personality disorders (Coccaro & Kavoussi, 1997; Salzman et al., 1995) and this has been replicated in two other studies (George et al., 2011; Silva et al., 2010) and in a study with individuals with IED (Coccaro, Lee, & Kavoussi, 2010b). Most individuals with IED respond to fluoxetine in daily doses from 20 mg to 40 mg orally. The antiaggressive response becomes significant by the end of the first 4 weeks of treatment and tends to continue through the length of 12-week trials. Clinical data suggests that fluoxetine suppresses aggressive responding and that within 4 weeks after discontinuance impulsive aggressive behavior begins to return to baseline levels.

Other classes of agents shown to have anti-aggressive effects in double-blind, placebo-controlled trials of individuals with *primary* aggression (i.e., not secondary to psychosis, severe mood disorder, or organic brain syndromes) include mood stabilizers (lithium; Sheard, Marini, Bridges, & Wagner, 1976) and anticonvulsants (phenytoin [Dilantin®], Barratt, Stanford, Felthous, & Kent, 1997; carbamazepine [Tegretol®], Gardner & Cowdry, 1986; oxcarbazepine [Trileptal®], Mattes, 2005; divalproex [Depakote®], Hollander et al., 2003). While norepinephrine beta-blockers (e.g., propranolol [Inderal®], nadolol [Corgard®]; Mattes, 1990; Ratey et al., 1992) have also been shown to reduce aggression, these agents have been exclusively tested in patient populations with *secondary* aggression (e.g., aggression in those with intellectual disability, organic brain syndromes, etc.). Classes of agents that may have "proaggressive" effects include tricyclic antidepressants (amitriptyline [Elavil®]; Soloff, George, Nathan, Schulz, & Perel, 1986), benzodiazepines (Gardner & Cowdry, 1985), and stimulant and hallucinatory drugs of abuse (amphetamines, cocaine, phencyclidine; Fishbein & Tarter, 2009). Findings from double-blind, placebo-controlled clinical trials suggest that anti-aggressive efficacy is specific to impulsive, rather than nonimpulsive, aggression (Barratt et al., 1997).

Kleptomania

There have been only two controlled pharmacological trials for kleptomania. One study examined escitalopram (Lexapro®) treatment with every individual being given the medication, and then those who responded were randomized to either continue on escitalopram or be switched to placebo (Koran, Aboujaoude, & Gamel, 2007). When the responders were randomized, 43% of those on escitalopram relapsed compared with 50% on placebo, indicating that escitalopram was no more effective than placebo.

The only other formal trial of medication for kleptomania examined naltrexone (Vivatrol®) in a placebo-controlled, double-blind study. In that study, 25 adults with kleptomania were randomized in a 1:1 fashion to either naltrexone or placebo for 8 weeks. By the study end point, 66.7% of those assigned to naltrexone compared with 7.7% on placebo (p < .001) reported symptom remission. The mean effective dose of naltrexone was 116.7 mg/day (Grant, Kim, & Odlaug, 2009). Although the double-blind study of naltrexone did not report any elevations of liver enzymes, opioid antagonists, particularly at

doses higher than 50 mg/day, have been associated with hepatotoxicity.

Memantine (Namenda®), an N-methyl-D-aspartate (NMDA) receptor antagonist approved by the U.S. Food and Drug Administration (FDA) for the treatment of dementia, has shown promising results in the treatment of behavioral and substance addictions (Olive, Cleva, Kalivas, & Malcolm, 2012). Based on this extent literature, 12 individuals with kleptomania were treated with memantine (10 mg/day, titrated to 30 mg/day) in an open-label, 8-week trial. The kleptomania severity scores decreased using the Kleptomania Symptom Assessment Scale (K-SAS; Grant, Kim, & McCabe, 2006) and Yale-Brown Obsessive-Compulsive Scale Modified for Kleptomania (see Assessments in Grant, Kim, & Odlaug, 2009), and 11 (91.7%) of the participants met the responder criteria. Although these results need to be interpreted cautiously since it was an open-label study in a very small sample, significant improvements were observed in terms of cognitive deficits (i.e., improvement in stop-signal response inhibition; Grant, Schreiber, & Odlaug, 2013).

Thus, these findings underlie the current pharmacologic treatment of individuals with kleptomania using naltrexone or possibly memantine. Naltrexone appears to reduce urges to steal, while memantine appears to reduce the behavior via improved motor impulsivity. Either medication seems to produce effects within the first 4 weeks of treatment. Adverse events for individuals with kleptomania taking these medications (mild headache and dizziness being the most common) are similar in frequency and severity to those that occur when the medications are used in either alcohol use disorders or dementia cases, respectively.

Pyromania

There are no randomized controlled clinical trials of pharmacotherapy for the treatment of pyromania and there are no FDA-approved medications for the treatment of pyromania. Medications described in case reports that have shown benefit in the treatment of pyromania include topiramate (Topamax®), escitalopram (Lexapro), sertraline (Zoloft®), fluoxetine (Prozac), lithium, and a combination of olanzapine (Zyprexa®) and sodium valproate

(Depakote). A number of medications have also shown no benefit in the treatment of pyromania in case reports: fluoxetine, valproic acid, lithium, sertraline, olanzapine, escitalopram, citalopram (Celexa®), and clonazepam (Klonopin®; Grant, Schreiber, & Odlaug, 2013).

These findings suggest that there is little guidance in the pharmacological treatment of pyromania. In our clinical experience, we tend to use medications that reduce reward sensitivity, such as those used in alcohol and related addictive disorders (e.g., topiramate, naltrexone).

BEST APPROACHES FOR ASSESSING TREATMENT RESPONSE AND MANAGING SIDE EFFECTS

Intermittent Explosive Disorder

Treatment response in double-blind placebo-controlled trials in patients with impulsive aggression has been assessed using the Overt Aggression Scale Modified (OAS-M; Coccaro, Harvey, Kupsaw-Lawrence, Herbert, & Bernstein, 1991) for outpatient use. The OAS-M has two scores: First, a "total aggression" score representing a frequency/severity weighted assessment of actual impulsive aggressive behaviors in the past week; second, a "global anger and aggression" score (formerly referred to as "irritability") assessed by the interviewer. Additional outcome measures include a clinical global impression of improvement rated on a 7-point scale in which score of 1 ("very much improved") and 2 ("much improved") represent a good clinical response. Adverse events for individuals with IED treated with fluoxetine are similar in frequency and severity to those for individuals treated with fluoxetine for depression or anxiety, and the management of these adverse events is the same regardless of therapeutic indication—for example, reduction of dose for most adverse events and/or the addition of bupropion (Wellbutrin XL®; 150 mg to 300 mg daily of the extended-release formulation) for sexual side effects such as anorgasmia.

Kleptomania

Treatment response in patients with kleptomania has been assessed using the K-SAS (Grant, Kim, & McCabe, 2006) and Yale-Brown Obsessive-Compulsive Scale Modified for Kleptomania (Grant et al., 2009). The K-SAS is a brief self-report questionnaire adapted from the Gambling Symptom Assessment Scale. The psychometric properties of the K-SAS have been evaluated with a Cronbach's alpha value of 0.93 and a positive correlation with the Clinical Global Impressions scale ($r = 0.85$, $p < 0.02$) as well as with the Global Assessment of Functioning ($r = 0.81$, $p < 0.05$).

Pyromania

Treatment response in patients with pyromania is usually assessed by tracking intensity of urges to set fires and by the number of fires set. There are no severity instruments validated for the purpose of assessing treatment response in pyromania. We have developed the Pyromania Symptom Assessment Scale (P-SAS; unpublished and available upon request) but this instrument lacks psychometric data.

MEDICATION MANAGEMENT ISSUES

Intermittent Explosive Disorder

While most individuals with IED respond to fluoxetine in daily doses from 20 mg to 40 mg orally, about half of those with impulsive aggression enrolled in clinical trials drop out of treatment before 3 months of therapy. Analysis of our own data (Coccaro, Lee, & Kavoussi, 2009) reveals that study completers in our study tended to be older by a modest degree (39.5 ± 9.0 vs. 33.7 ± 7.3 years; $p = 0.001$), White (93% vs. 76%; $p = 0.026$), and have lower trait aggression scores (Buss-Durkee Aggression Questionnaire score 30.6 ± 7.4 vs. 35.4 ± 4.1; $p = 0.001$). These differences, however, are relatively modest in size and it remains to be seen if they are clinically significant.

We advise that individuals with IED be started on the typical starting dose for the drug in question, and then be given increases in dose depending on response and type of agent. For example, fluoxetine could be started at 20 mg daily and increased to 40 mg daily after 4 weeks. If response is not adequate at that point (e.g., there is only a minimal change from baseline in the Clinical Global Impression of improvement assessment, less than a 50% reduction in aggressive behavior), fluoxetine could be switched to escitalopram at 10 mg daily, increased to 20 mg daily within a week, and then increased to 30 mg daily after another 4 weeks. In the end, a trial of at least 3 months with an SSRI should be tried before switching to another agent. If one began patient treatment on an SSRI, one could try another SSRI before trying a different agent, as described above. Given some evidence for the antiaggressive effects of mood stabilizers, one could then move to lithium (e.g., 300 mg orally three times per day [p.o. t.i.d.]) or divalproex extended release (e.g., 750 mg orally twice per day [p.o. b.i.d.]), aiming for the same dose and blood levels (0.8 mg/ml for lithium and 0.8 microgram/ml for divalproex) typically used with mood disordered individuals.

Kleptomania

Due to the rewarding qualities of stealing (i.e., getting something for nothing and the excitement of the behavior), many people drop out of treatment and never receive a full trial of medication. Combining medication with psychotherapy often improves compliance with medication treatment. In terms of treatment with naltrexone, nausea tends to be the reason for medication noncompliance. Starting at 25 mg daily for a week or so allows for better tolerance. In some cases, adding the 5-HT$_3$ receptor antagonist ondansetron (Zofran®) at 4 mg twice a day for the first week also addresses the nausea side effect. If naltrexone is ineffective or cannot be tolerated, then patients can be switched to memantine 10 mg daily and increased to 20 mg daily after 4 weeks if the medication is ineffective or only partially effective at the lower dose (Grant, Odlaug, Schreiber, Chamberlain, & Won Kim, 2013).

Pyromania

Urges to set fires are common in individuals with this disorder, and the fire setting is almost always pleasurable (Grant & Kim, 2007). Thus, many people drop out of treatment and never receive a full trial of medication. Based on the authors' experience, combining medication with psychotherapy often improves compliance with medication treatment.

EVALUATION OF PHARMACOLOGICAL APPROACHES ACROSS THE LIFESPAN

Intermittent Explosive Disorder

Analysis of our own data (Coccaro et al., 2009) reveals no difference in antiaggressive response to fluoxetine as a function of age (median split: 18–35 years vs. 36–56 years). To our knowledge there is no other data regarding pharmacologic approaches or response as a function of age.

Kleptomania

There are no data regarding the pharmacologic approach to kleptomania as a function of age. We have found that naltrexone is generally well tolerated and seems to be equally effective across the lifespan (from adolescence to older adults).

Pyromania

There are no data regarding the pharmacologic approach to kleptomania as a function of age.

CONSIDERATION OF POTENTIAL SEX DIFFERENCES

Intermittent Explosive Disorder

Early clinical studies suggested that IED is more prevalent in males than females by a ratio of 2:1 to 3:1 (American Psychiatric Association, 1994). However, recent community surveys suggest that the male to female ratio is likely closer to 1.50:1.00 (Kessler et al., 2006). This is because earlier clinical studies of IED focused on serious physical assault rather than on less serious physical assault and/or verbal aggression, both of which are clearly present in females with recurrent, problematic, impulsive aggressive behavior. In addition, there is no difference in antiaggressive response as a function of sex (Coccaro et al., 2009).

Kleptomania

Clinical samples suggest that most people seeking treatment for kleptomania are female. In terms of clinical presentation, one study found that men with kleptomania are more likely to have a history of birth trauma (Presta et al., 2002). Men with kleptomania appear less likely to suffer from a co-occurring eating disorder or bipolar disorder, but appear to have higher rates of co-occurring paraphilias (McElroy, Pope, Hudson, Keck, & White, 1991). Women with kleptomania were more likely to be a later age at shoplifting onset, steal household items, and hoard stolen items, and were less likely to have another impulse-control disorder (Grant & Potenza, 2008). These clinical sex differences do not appear to have associations with treatment response. The only difference we have found, based on clinical experience, is that females with kleptomania often respond well to a lower dose of naltrexone (even 25 mg daily) compared with men. This clinical observation, however, may not hold up to research scrutiny given that efficacy and tolerability differences with naltrexone based on gender in other addictive disorders such as alcoholism are somewhat equivocal on this point (see O'Malley, Krishnan-Sarin, Farren, & O'Connor, 2000; Greenfield, Pettinati, O'Malley, Randall, & Randall, 2010; Yoon, Kim, Petrakis, & Westermeyer, 2016).

Pyromania

Although pyromania has long been thought to be a disorder primarily affecting men, recent research suggests that the male/female ratio is equal in adults and may be slightly higher among females in adolescence (Grant & Kim, 2007). These clinical sex differences do not appear to have associations with treatment response based on clinical experience. Finally, there are no data regarding pharmacologic approaches for pyromania as a function of age.

INTEGRATION OF PHARMACOTHERAPY WITH NONPHARMACOLOGICAL APPROACHES: BENEFITS AND CHALLENGES

Intermittent Explosive Disorder

A variety of cognitive behavioral treatments have been found to be moderately effective in the treatment of anger and/or aggression. Specifically, some cognitive behavioral techniques have demonstrated a reduction in anger or the aggressive behaviors of children in the classroom, juvenile delinquents,

residentially placed adolescents, college students, drivers, abusive parents and spouses, and prison inmates (Beck & Fernandez, 1998; Deffenbacher, Huff, Lynch, Oetting, & Salvatore, 2000; Edmondson & Conger, 1996; Novaco, 1977). Many psychosocial treatments have been found to be effective at follow-up of up to 15 months, often with additional improvement gains noted at follow-up relative to posttreatment (e.g., Deffenbacher, Oetting, Huff, & Thwaites, 1995; Hazaleus & Deffenbacher, 1986). Specific treatments have included relaxation training, social skills training, skill assembly, social skills training, problem-solving, negative thought reduction, self-instruction, cognitive therapy, and combined cognitive relaxation or cognitive behavioral treatment. Notably, however, the anger treatment literature does not discriminate between clinical anger problems without aggression and pathological aggression, and so these findings may not generalize to more severely aggressive individuals with IED (McCloskey, Noblett, Deffenbacher, Gollan, & Coccaro, 2008). That said, the first and only study of cognitive behavioral therapy (CBT; CBT vs. wait-list control) with *DSM–5* IED demonstrated that impulsive aggression, anger, and hostile thoughts were significantly reduced by a CBT package including relaxation training, cognitive restructuring, and coping skills training (McCloskey et al., 2008).

While fluoxetine and CBT appear to affect similar therapeutic responses despite likely working through different mechanisms, the combination of the two has not been tested. However, based on work with other disorders, we expect that these two treatments will be more effective than either one alone.

Kleptomania

There are no controlled studies of psychological treatments for kleptomania. Case reports suggest that cognitive and behavioral therapies may be effective in treating kleptomania, often when used in combination with pharmacotherapy (Grant, Schreiber, & Odlaug, 2013). Covert sensitization, in which a person is instructed to imagine stealing as well as the negative consequences of stealing (e.g., being handcuffed, feeling embarrassed), has been successful in reducing kleptomania symptoms.

Imaginal desensitization (i.e., recording a client's "typical" stealing episode) in brief sessions over 5 days resulted in complete remission of symptoms for a 2-year period for two patients (Hodgins & Peden, 2008). Case reports also support the use of CBT with imaginal desensitization and motivational interviewing (Grant, Odlaug, & Donahue, 2012).

Pyromania

There are no controlled studies of psychological treatments for pyromania. The only documented case of psychotherapy involved an 18-year-old male with pyromania who was successfully treated using a combination of topiramate with 3 weeks of daily CBT (Grant, 2006). The daily therapy consisted of 15 sessions of CBT using imaginal desensitization plus motivational interviewing. The client was instructed to listen to a recording several times each day that included his urges to set fires, a negative mood induction element, and how to deal with the urges (Grant & Odlaug, 2011).

INTEGRATED APPROACHES FOR ADDRESSING COMMON COMORBID DISORDERS

Intermittent Explosive Disorder

Impulsive aggressive behavior is manifest in all humans and, when problematic, typically begins early in life before the onset of other psychiatric disorders. Clinical studies suggest significant co-occurrence of IED with mood disorders, anxiety disorders, and substance use disorders. As noted, in most cases the age of onset of IED is earlier than the co-occurring disorder, suggesting the independence of IED or suggesting that IED is a risk factor for the co-occurring disorder (Coccaro, 2012). The presence of another disorder does not impact the treatment of aggression except in cases in which the comorbid disorder responds better to another agent than an SSRI, for example.

Kleptomania

Kleptomania is associated with lifetime psychiatric comorbidity with other impulse-control (20–46%), substance use (23–50%), and mood (45–100%) disorders (Grant, 2006; McElroy et al., 1991).

Personality disorders are also common in kleptomania. A study involving 28 individuals with kleptomania revealed that 12 (42.9%) met criteria for at least one personality disorder, and two (14.3%) met criteria for two personality disorders. Paranoid (17.9%), borderline (10.3%), and schizoid (10.7%) personality disorders were the most common (Grant, 2004). Suicide attempts are common among these patients (Grant, Odlaug, Medeiros, Christianine, & Tavares, 2015). In one study of 107 adolescents and adults with kleptomania, 24.3% reported a history of suicide attempts, of which 92.3% were attributed specifically to kleptomania (Odlaug, Grant, & Kim, 2012). Among these individuals, suicide attempts were more frequent for those with current and lifetime bipolar disorder and lifetime personality disorder (Odlaug et al., 2012).

Pyromania

Pyromania is associated with high lifetime rates of psychiatric comorbidity, such as affective (61.9%), anxiety (33.3%), substance use (33.3%), and impulse-control (66.7%) disorders (Grant & Kim, 2007). There are no data regarding how or to what extent the presence of another disorder impacts the treatment of pyromania. In general, when mood symptoms are present, an antidepressant, lithium, or antiepileptic may need to be used in combination with medications focusing on the pyromania. Also, therapy focusing on co-occurring disorders may be necessary when treating pyromania.

EMERGING TRENDS

Intermittent Explosive Disorder

Clinical psychopharmacology for impulsive aggression in IED is still in early development. Empirical studies only show support for SSRIs and mood stabilizers in the treatment of impulsive aggression. While nonserotonergic mechanisms may well be associated with aggression, clinical trials targeting nonserotonergic systems have not been performed, limiting the pharmacologic armamentarium to only a few agents. In addition, recent data focusing on social cognition (Coccaro, Fanning, Keedy, & Lee, 2016) suggests that it is possible to reduce impulsive aggression by reducing hostile attribution through the use of cognitive training by computer, which trains individuals to view faces as less emotionally hostile (Stoddard et al., 2016).

Kleptomania

Data regarding the psychopharmacology of kleptomania is sparse. Understanding the cognitive domains and associated neurobiology that underpin addictive disorders, however, may offer the greatest future benefit for developing pharmacological agents for this seemingly reward-driven behavior.

Pyromania

The systematic study of treatment of pyromania is also sparse. With few studies published, it is not possible to make treatment recommendations with a substantial degree of confidence. No drugs are currently approved by the FDA for the treatment of pyromania. Nonetheless, specific drug and behavioral therapies offer promise for the effective treatment of pyromania.

TOOL KIT OF RESOURCES

Intermittent Explosive Disorder

Patient Resources

https://www.psychologytoday.com/us/conditions/intermittent-explosive-disorder

https://www.drugs.com/mcd/intermittent-explosive-disorder

Provider Resources

Coccaro, E. F. (2012). Intermittent explosive disorder as a disorder of impulsive aggression for *DSM–5*. *American Journal of Psychiatry, 169*, 577–588. http://dx.doi.org/10.1176/appi.ajp.2012.11081259

McCloskey, M. S., Noblett, K. L., Deffenbacher, J. L., Gollan, J. K., & Coccaro, E. F. (2008). Cognitive-behavioral therapy for intermittent explosive disorder: A pilot randomized clinical trial. *Journal of Consulting and Clinical Psychology, 76*, 876–886. http://dx.doi.org/10.1037/0022-006X.76.5.876

Coccaro, E. F., Berman, M. E., & McCloskey, M. S. (2017). Development of a screening questionnaire for *DSM–5* intermittent explosive disorder (IED-SQ). *Comprehensive Psychiatry, 74*, 21–26. http://dx.doi.org/10.1016/j.comppsych.2016.12.004

Kleptomania

Patient Resources

https://www.psychologytoday.com/us/conditions/kleptomania

https://www.mayoclinic.org/diseases-conditions/kleptomania/symptoms-causes/syc-20364732

Provider Resources

Grant, J. E., Correia, S., & Brennan-Krohn, T. (2006). White matter integrity in kleptomania: A pilot study. *Psychiatry Research, 147*(2–3), 233–237. http://dx.doi.org/10.1016/j.pscychresns.2006.03.003

Grant, J. E., Kim, S. W., & Odlaug, B. L. (2009). A double-blind, placebo-controlled study of the opiate antagonist, naltrexone, in the treatment of kleptomania. *Biological Psychiatry, 65*, 600–606. http://dx.doi.org/10.1016/j.biopsych.2008.11.022

Pyromania

Patient Resources

https://www.psychologytoday.com/us/conditions/pyromania

https://www.allaboutcounseling.com/library/pyromania/

Provider Resources

Grant, J. E., & Kim, S. W. (2007). Clinical characteristics and psychiatric comorbidity of pyromania. *Journal of Clinical Psychiatry, 68*, 1717–22.

Grant, J. E. (2009). SPECT imaging and treatment of pyromania. *Journal of Clinical Psychiatry, 67*, 998–998.

References

American Psychiatric Association. (1994). *Diagnostic and Statistical Manual of Mental Disorders* (4th ed.). Washington, DC: Author.

*Asterisks indicate assessments or resources.

American Psychiatric Association. (2013). *Diagnostic and Statistical Manual of Mental Disorders* (5th ed.). Washington, DC: Author.

Barratt, E. S., Stanford, M. S., Felthous, A. R., & Kent, T. A. (1997). The effects of phenytoin on impulsive and premeditated aggression: A controlled study. *Journal of Clinical Psychopharmacology, 17,* 341–349. http://dx.doi.org/10.1097/00004714-199710000-00002

Beck, R., & Fernandez, E. (1998). Cognitive-behavioral therapy in the treatment of anger: A meta-analysis. *Cognitive Therapy and Research, 1,* 2263–2274.

Blanco, C., Alegria, A. A., Petry, N. M., Grant, J. E., Simpson, H. B., Liu, S. M., . . . Hasin, D. S. (2010). Prevalence and correlates of fire-setting in the United States: Results from the National Epidemiologic Survey on Alcohol and Related Conditions (NESARC). *The Journal of Clinical Psychiatry, 71,* 1218–1225. http://dx.doi.org/10.4088/JCP.08m04812gry

Blanco, C., Grant, J., Petry, N. M., Simpson, H. B., Alegria, A., Liu, S. M., & Hasin, D. (2008). Prevalence and correlates of shoplifting in the United States: Results from the National Epidemiologic Survey on Alcohol and Related Conditions (NESARC). *The American Journal of Psychiatry, 165,* 905–913. http://dx.doi.org/10.1176/appi.ajp.2008.07101660

Coccaro, E. F. (2011). Intermittent explosive disorder: Development of integrated research criteria for *Diagnostic and Statistical Manual of Mental Disorders* (5th ed.). *Comprehensive Psychiatry, 52,* 119–125. http://dx.doi.org/10.1016/j.comppsych.2010.05.006

Coccaro, E. F. (2012). Intermittent explosive disorder as a disorder of impulsive aggression for *DSM–5. The American Journal of Psychiatry, 169,* 577–588. http://dx.doi.org/10.1176/appi.ajp.2012.11081259

*Coccaro, E. F., Berman, M. E., & McCloskey, M. S. (2017). Development of a screening questionnaire for *DSM–5* intermittent explosive disorder (IED-SQ). *Comprehensive Psychiatry, 74,* 21–26. http://dx.doi.org/10.1016/j.comppsych.2016.12.004

Coccaro, E. F., Fanning, J. R., Keedy, S. K., & Lee, R. J. (2016). Social cognition in Intermittent Explosive Disorder and aggression. *Journal of Psychiatric Research, 83,* 140–150. http://dx.doi.org/10.1016/j.jpsychires.2016.07.010

Coccaro, E. F., Fanning, J. R., & Lee, R. (2017). Intermittent explosive disorder and substance use disorder: Analysis of the National Comorbidity Survey Replication sample. *The Journal of Clinical Psychiatry, 78,* 697–702. http://dx.doi.org/10.4088/JCP.15m10306

Coccaro, E. F., Fanning, J. R., Phan, K. L., & Lee, R. (2015). Serotonin and impulsive aggression. *CNS Spectrums, 20,* 295–302. http://dx.doi.org/10.1017/S1092852915000310

*Coccaro, E. F., Harvey, P. D., Kupsaw-Lawrence, E., Herbert, J. L., & Bernstein, D. P. (1991). Development of neuropharmacologically based behavioral assessments of impulsive aggressive behavior. *The Journal of Neuropsychiatry and Clinical Neurosciences, 3,* S44–S51.

Coccaro, E. F., & Kavoussi, R. J. (1997). Fluoxetine and impulsive aggressive behavior in personality-disordered subjects. *Archives of General Psychiatry, 54,* 1081–1088. http://dx.doi.org/10.1001/archpsyc.1997.01830240035005

Coccaro, E. F., Kavoussi, R. J., & Hauger, R. L. (1997). Serotonin function and antiaggressive response to fluoxetine: A pilot study. *Biological Psychiatry, 42,* 546–552. http://dx.doi.org/10.1016/S0006-3223(97)00309-0

Coccaro, E. F., Lee, R., & Kavoussi, R. J. (2010a). Aggression, suicidality, and intermittent explosive disorder: Serotonergic correlates in personality disorder and healthy control subjects. *Neuropsychopharmacology, 35,* 435–444. http://dx.doi.org/10.1038/npp.2009.148

Coccaro, E. F., Lee, R., & Kavoussi, R. J. (2010b). Inverse relationship between numbers of 5-HT transporter binding sites and life history of aggression and intermittent explosive disorder. *Journal of Psychiatric Research, 44,* 137–142. http://dx.doi.org/10.1016/j.jpsychires.2009.07.004

Coccaro, E. F., Lee, R., & McCloskey, M. S. (2014). Validity of the new A1 and A2 criteria for *DSM–5* intermittent explosive disorder. *Comprehensive Psychiatry, 55,* 260–267. http://dx.doi.org/10.1016/j.comppsych.2013.09.007

Coccaro, E. F., Lee, R. J., Kavoussi, R. J. (2009). A double-blind, randomized, placebo-controlled trial of fluoxetine in patients with intermittent explosive disorder. *Journal of Clinical Psychiatry, 70,* 653–662. http://dx.doi.org/10.4088/JCP.08m04150

Coccaro, E. F., McCloskey, M. S., Fitzgerald, D. A., & Phan, K. L. (2007). Amygdala and orbitofrontal reactivity to social threat in individuals with impulsive aggression. *Biological Psychiatry, 62,* 168–178. http://dx.doi.org/10.1016/j.biopsych.2006.08.024

Coccaro, E. F., Posternak, M. A., & Zimmerman, M. (2005). Prevalence and features of intermittent explosive disorder in a clinical setting. *The Journal of Clinical Psychiatry, 66,* 1221–1227. http://dx.doi.org/10.4088/JCP.v66n1003

Deffenbacher, J. L., Huff, M. E., Lynch, R. S., Oetting, E. R., & Salvatore, N. F. (2000). Characteristics and treatment of high-anger drivers. *Journal of Counseling Psychology, 47,* 5–17. http://dx.doi.org/10.1037/0022-0167.47.1.5

Deffenbacher, J. L., Oetting, E. R., Huff, M. E., & Thwaites, G. A. (1995). Fifteen-month follow-up of social skills and cognitive-relaxation approaches to general anger reduction. *Journal of Counseling*

Psychology, 42, 400–405. http://dx.doi.org/10.1037/ 0022-0167.42.3.400

Duke, A. A., Bègue, L., Bell, R., & Eisenlohr-Moul, T. (2013). Revisiting the serotonin-aggression relation in humans: A meta-analysis. *Psychological Bulletin, 139,* 1148–1172. http://dx.doi.org/10.1037/a0031544

Edmondson, C. B., & Conger, J. C. (1996). A review of treatment efficacy for individuals with anger problems: Conceptual, assessment, and methodological issues. *Clinical Psychology Review, 16,* 251–275. http://dx.doi.org/10.1016/S0272-7358(96)90003-3

Fanning, J. R., & Coccaro, E. F. (2018). Neurobiology of personality disorder. In J. W. Livesley & R. Larstone (Eds.), *Handbook of Personality Disorders* (pp. 251–270). New York, NY: Guilford Publishing.

*First, M. B., Williams, J. B. W., Karg, R. S., & Spitzer, R. L. (2015). *Structured Clinical Interview for DSM–5 Disorders, Clinician Version (SCID-5-CV).* Arlington, VA: American Psychiatric Association.

Fishbein, D., & Tarter, R. (2009). Infusing neuroscience into the study and prevention of drug misuse and co-occurring aggressive behavior. *Substance Use & Misuse, 44*(9–10), 1204–1235. http://dx.doi.org/ 10.1080/10826080902959975

Gardner, D. L., & Cowdry, R. W. (1985). Alprazolam-induced dyscontrol in borderline personality disorder. *The American Journal of Psychiatry, 142,* 98–100. http://dx.doi.org/10.1176/ajp.142.1.98

Gardner, D. L., & Cowdry, R. W. (1986). Positive effects of carbamazepine on behavioral dyscontrol in borderline personality disorder. *The American Journal of Psychiatry, 143,* 519–522. http://dx.doi.org/ 10.1176/ajp.143.4.519

George, D. T., Phillips, M. J., Lifshitz, M., Lionetti, T. A., Spero, D. E., Ghassemzedeh, N., . . . Rawlings, R. R. (2011). Fluoxetine treatment of alcoholic perpetrators of domestic violence: A 12-week, double-blind, randomized, placebo-controlled intervention study. *The Journal of Clinical Psychiatry, 72,* 60–65. http://dx.doi.org/10.4088/JCP.09m05256gry

Grant, J. E. (2004). Co-occurrence of personality disorders in persons with kleptomania: A preliminary investigation. *Journal of the American Academy of Psychiatry and the Law, 32,* 395–398.

Grant, J. E. (2006). SPECT imaging and treatment of pyromania. *The Journal of Clinical Psychiatry, 67,* 998–998. http://dx.doi.org/10.4088/JCP.v67n0619f

*Grant, J. E. (2008). *Impulse control disorders: A clinician's guide to understanding and treating behavioral addictions.* New York, NY: Norton Press.

Grant, J. E., Brewer, J. A., & Potenza, M. N. (2006). The neurobiology of substance and behavioral addictions.

CNS Spectrums, 11, 924–930. http://dx.doi.org/ 10.1017/S109285290001511X

Grant, J. E., & Kim, S. W. (2007). Clinical characteristics and psychiatric comorbidity of pyromania. *The Journal of Clinical Psychiatry, 68,* 1717–1722. http://dx.doi.org/ 10.4088/JCP.v68n1111

*Grant, J. E., Kim, S. W., & McCabe, J. S. (2006). A Structured Clinical Interview for Kleptomania (SCI-K): Preliminary validity and reliability testing. *International Journal of Methods in Psychiatric Research, 15,* 83–94. http://dx.doi.org/10.1002/ mpr.24

Grant, J. E., Kim, S. W., & Odlaug, B. L. (2009). A double-blind, placebo-controlled study of the opiate antagonist, naltrexone, in the treatment of kleptomania. *Biological Psychiatry, 65,* 600–606. http://dx.doi.org/ 10.1016/j.biopsych.2008.11.022

Grant, J. E., Levine, L., Kim, D., & Potenza, M. N. (2005). Impulse control disorders in adult psychiatric inpatients. *American Journal of Psychiatry, 162*(11), 2184–2188.

*Grant, J. E., & Odlaug, B. L. (2011). Assessment and treatment of pyromania. In J. E. Grant and M. N. Potenza (Eds.), *The Oxford library of psychology: Oxford handbook of impulse control disorders* (pp. 353–359). Oxford, United Kingdom: Oxford University Press.

Grant, J. E., Odlaug, B. L., & Donahue, C. B. (2012). Adolescent stealing treated with motivational interviewing and imaginal desensitization: Case report. *Journal of Behavioral Addictions, 1,* 191–192. http://dx.doi.org/10.1556/JBA.1.2012.4.7

Grant, J. E., Odlaug, B. L., Medeiros, G., Christianine, A. R., & Tavares, H. (2015). Cross-cultural comparison of compulsive stealing (kleptomania). *Annals of Clinical Psychiatry, 27,* 150–151.

Grant, J. E., Odlaug, B. L., Schreiber, L. R., Chamberlain, S. R., & Won Kim, S. (2013). Memantine reduces stealing behavior and impulsivity in kleptomania: A pilot study. *International Clinical Psychopharmacology, 28,* 106–111. http://dx.doi.org/ 10.1097/YIC.0b013e32835c8c8c

Grant, J. E., & Potenza, M. N. (2008). Gender-related differences in individuals seeking treatment for kleptomania. *CNS Spectrums, 13,* 235–245. http://dx.doi.org/10.1017/S1092852900028492

Grant, J. E., Schreiber, L. R., & Odlaug, B. L. (2013). Phenomenology and treatment of behavioural addictions. *The Canadian Journal of Psychiatry, 58,* 252–259. http://dx.doi.org/10.1177/070674371305800502

Greenfield, S. F., Pettinati, H. M., O'Malley, S., Randall, P. K., & Randall, C. L. (2010). Gender differences in alcohol treatment: An analysis of outcome from the COMBINE study. *Alcoholism: Clinical and Experi-*

mental Research, 34, 1803–1812. http://dx.doi.org/ 10.1111/j.1530-0277.2010.01267.x

Hazaleus, S. L., & Deffenbacher, J. L. (1986). Relaxation and cognitive treatments of anger. *Journal of Consulting and Clinical Psychology, 54,* 222–226. http://dx.doi.org/10.1037/0022-006X.54.2.222

Hodgins, D. C., & Peden, N. (2008). Cognitive-behavioral treatment for impulse control disorders. *Revista Brasileira de Psiquiatria, 30*(Suppl. 1), S31–S40. http://dx.doi.org/10.1590/S1516-44462006005000055

Hollander, E., Tracy, K. A., Swann, A. C., Coccaro, E. F., McElroy, S. L., Wozniak, P., . . . Nemeroff, C. B. (2003). Divalproex in the treatment of impulsive aggression: Efficacy in cluster B personality disorders. *Neuropsychopharmacology, 28,* 1186–1197. http://dx.doi.org/10.1038/sj.npp.1300153

Hudson, J. I., Pope, H. G., Jonas, J. M., & Yurgelun-Todd, D. (1983). Phenomenologic relationship of eating disorders to major affective disorder. *Psychiatry Research, 9,* 345–354.

Kessler, R. C., Coccaro, E. F., Fava, M., Jaeger, S., Jin, R., & Walters, E. (2006). The prevalence and correlates of *DSM–IV* intermittent explosive disorder in the National Comorbidity Survey Replication. *Archives of General Psychiatry, 63,* 669–678. http://dx.doi.org/10.1001/archpsyc.63.6.669

Koran, L. M., Aboujaoude, E. N., & Gamel, N. N. (2007). Escitalopram treatment of kleptomania: An open-label trial followed by double-blind discontinuation. *Journal of Clinical Psychiatry, 68,* 422–427.

Lee, R. J., Gill, A., Chen, B., McCloskey, M., & Coccaro, E. F. (2012). Modulation of central serotonin affects emotional information processing in impulsive aggressive personality disorder. *Journal of Clinical Psychopharmacology, 32,* 329–335. http://dx.doi.org/10.1097/JCP.0b013e31825368b7

Lejoyeux, M., Arbaretaz, M., McLoughlin, M., & Ades, J. (2002). Impulse control disorders and depression. *Journal of Nervous and Mental Disease, 190,* 310–314.

Mattes, J. A. (1990). Comparative effectiveness of carbamazepine and propranolol for rage outbursts. *The Journal of Neuropsychiatry and Clinical Neurosciences, 2,* 159–164. http://dx.doi.org/10.1176/jnp.2.2.159

Mattes, J. A. (2005). Oxcarbazepine in patients with impulsive aggression: A double-blind, placebo-controlled trial. *Journal of Clinical Psychopharmacology, 25,* 575–579. http://dx.doi.org/10.1097/01.jcp.0000186739.22395.6b

McCloskey, M. S., Noblett, K. L., Deffenbacher, J. L., Gollan, J. K., & Coccaro, E. F. (2008). Cognitive-behavioral therapy for intermittent explosive disorder: A pilot randomized clinical trial. *Journal of Consulting and Clinical Psychology, 76,* 876–886. http://dx.doi.org/10.1037/0022-006X.76.5.876

McCloskey, M. S., Phan, K. L., Angstadt, M., Fettich, K. C., Keedy, S., & Coccaro, E. F. (2016). Amygdala hyperactivation to angry faces in intermittent explosive disorder. *Journal of Psychiatric Research, 79,* 34–41. http://dx.doi.org/10.1016/j.jpsychires.2016.04.006

McElroy, S. L., Pope, H. G., Jr., Hudson, J. I., Keck, P. E., Jr., & White, K. L. (1991). Kleptomania: A report of 20 cases. *The American Journal of Psychiatry, 148,* 652–657. http://dx.doi.org/10.1176/ajp.148.5.652

McLaughlin, K. A., Green, J. G., Hwang, I., Sampson, N. A., Zaslavsky, A. M., & Kessler, R. C. (2012). Intermittent explosive disorder in the National Comorbidity Survey Replication Adolescent Supplement. *JAMA Psychiatry, 69,* 1131–1139. http://dx.doi.org/10.1001/archgenpsychiatry.2012.592

New, A. S., Trestman, R. F., Mitropoulou, V., Goodman, M., Koenigsberg, H. H., Silverman, J., & Siever, L. J. (2004). Low prolactin response to fenfluramine in impulsive aggression. *Journal of Psychiatric Research, 38,* 223–230. http://dx.doi.org/10.1016/j.jpsychires.2003.09.001

Novaco, R. W. (1977). Stress inoculation: A cognitive therapy for anger and its application to a case of depression. *Journal of Consulting and Clinical Psychology, 45,* 600–608. http://dx.doi.org/10.1037/0022-006X.45.4.600

Odlaug, B. L., & Grant, J. E. (2010). Impulse-control disorders in a college sample: Results from the self-administered Minnesota Impulse Disorders Interview (MIDI). *Primary Care Companion for CNS Disorders, 12*(2), e1–e5.

Odlaug, B. L., Grant, J. E., & Kim, S. W. (2012). Suicide attempts in 107 adolescents and adults with kleptomania. *Archives of Suicide Research, 16,* 348–359. http://dx.doi.org/10.1080/13811118.2013.722058

Olive, M. F., Cleva, R. M., Kalivas, P. W., & Malcolm, R. J. (2012). Glutamatergic medications for the treatment of drug and behavioral addictions. *Pharmacology: Biochemistry, and Behavior, 100,* 801–810. http://dx.doi.org/10.1016/j.pbb.2011.04.015

O'Malley, S. S., Krishnan-Sarin, S., Farren, C., & O'Connor, P. G. (2000). Naltrexone-induced nausea in patients treated for alcohol dependence: Clinical predictors and evidence for opioid-mediated effects. *Journal of Clinical Psychopharmacology, 20,* 69–76. http://dx.doi.org/10.1097/00004714-200002000-00012

Presta, S., Marazziti, D., Dell'Osso, L., Pfanner, C., Pallanti, S., & Cassano, G. B. (2002). Kleptomania: Clinical features and comorbidity in an Italian sample. *Comprehensive Psychiatry, 43,* 7–12. http://dx.doi.org/10.1053/comp.2002.29851

Raine, A., Meloy, J. R., Bihrle, S., Stoddard, J., LaCasse, L., & Buchsbaum, M. S. (1998). Reduced prefrontal and increased subcortical brain functioning assessed using positron emission tomography in predatory and affective murderers. *Behavioral Sciences & the Law, 16*, 319–332. http://dx.doi.org/10.1002/(SICI)1099-0798(199822)16:3<319::AID-BSL311>3.0.CO;2-G

Ratey, J. J., Sorgi, P., O'Driscoll, G. A., Sands, S., Daehler, M. L., Fletcher, J. R., . . . Lindem, K. J. (1992). Nadolol to treat aggression and psychiatric symptomatology in chronic psychiatric inpatients: A double-blind, placebo-controlled study. *The Journal of Clinical Psychiatry, 53*, 41–46.

Salzman, C., Wolfson, A. N., Schatzberg, A., Looper, J., Henke, R., Albanese, M., . . . Miyawaki, E. (1995). Effect of fluoxetine on anger in symptomatic volunteers with borderline personality disorder. *Journal of Clinical Psychopharmacology, 15*, 23–29. http://dx.doi.org/10.1097/00004714-199502000-00005

Sheard, M. H., Marini, J. L., Bridges, C. I., & Wagner, E. (1976). The effect of lithium on impulsive aggressive behavior in man. *The American Journal of Psychiatry, 133*, 1409–1413. http://dx.doi.org/10.1176/ajp.133.12.1409

Silva, H., Iturra, P., Solari, A., Villarroel, J., Jerez, S., Jiménez, M., . . . Bustamante, M. L. (2010). Fluoxetine response in impulsive-aggressive behavior and serotonin transporter polymorphism in personality disorder. *Psychiatric Genetics, 20*, 25–30. http://dx.doi.org/10.1097/YPG.0b013e328335125d

Soloff, P. H., George, A., Nathan, R. S., Schulz, P. M., & Perel, J. M. (1986). Paradoxical effects of amitriptyline on borderline patients. *The American Journal of Psychiatry, 143*, 1603–1605. http://dx.doi.org/10.1176/ajp.143.12.1603

Stoddard, J., Sharif-Askary, B., Harkins, E. A., Frank, H. R., Brotman, M. A., Penton-Voak, I. S., . . . Leibenluft, E. (2016). An open pilot study of training hostile interpretation bias to treat disruptive mood dysregulation disorder. *Journal of Child and Adolescent Psychopharmacology, 26*, 49–57. http://dx.doi.org/10.1089/cap.2015.0100

Yoon, G., Kim, S. W., Petrakis, I. L., & Westermeyer, J. (2016). High-dose naltrexone treatment and gender in alcohol dependence. *Clinical Neuropharmacology, 39*, 165–168. http://dx.doi.org/10.1097/WNF.0000000000000152

CHAPTER 13

PHARMACOLOGICAL TREATMENT OF TRAUMA AND STRESSOR-RELATED DISORDERS

Lesia M. Ruglass, Kathryn Z. Smith, Therese K. Killeen, and Denise A. Hien

Posttraumatic stress disorder (PTSD) first emerged in the third edition of the *Diagnostic and Statistical Manual of Mental Disorders* (*DSM*) as an anxiety disorder (American Psychiatric Association, 1980). Previously, there was recognition with various disorders (e.g., neuroses, adjustment reactions; American Psychiatric Association, 1963) that stressful life experiences can have an influence on psychopathology and functioning, but there was no disorder whereby specific traumatic events were considered key etiological factors in the development of a specific syndrome (Breslau, 2009). Although PTSD is the most well studied and understood trauma- and stressor-related disorder, the *DSM–5* also includes two additional trauma- and stressor-related diagnoses that are not limited to any specific developmental period: acute stress disorder (ASD) and adjustment disorders. Given that literature on the epidemiology, course, and psychopharmacological treatment of adjustment disorders is sparse (for a review, see Carta, Balestrieri, Murru, & Hardoy, 2009), the focus of this chapter will be on PTSD and ASD.

EPIDEMIOLOGY AND PREVALENCE

This section provides a brief overview of epidemiological findings on prevalence rates of trauma exposure and PTSD. In this section, we also discuss sex and racial/ethnic differences in exposure and response to trauma.

Trauma Exposure

Data from epidemiological studies suggest that the vast majority of U.S. adults (up to 90%) will experience one or more potentially traumatic events in their lifetime (Breslau, 2009). Most individuals with trauma exposure report experiencing events categorized as interpersonal traumas. For example, in the Detroit Area Survey of Trauma, Breslau and colleagues (1998) found that the most prevalent forms of trauma all had an interpersonal component: 60% reported unexpected death of a loved one, 62.4% reported learning about trauma that occurred to others, and 37.7% reported experiencing assaultive violence. Exposure to traumatic events typically peaks between adolescence and emerging adulthood, and then declines as individuals transition into early adulthood, with the steepest decline occurring for assaultive violence (Breslau, 2009).

Studies have found that overall, men experience significantly more traumas than women, including more assaultive violence (Breslau, 2009). However, specific traumas, such as rape, that carry a high conditional probability of the development of PTSD are higher among women (Breslau, 2009).

Differences in trauma exposure have also been reported based on race/ethnicity. In the Detroit Area Survey of Trauma, Breslau and colleagues (1998) found that being non-White was associated with 97% greater odds of exposure to assaultive violence, 39% greater odds of exposure to learning about

http://dx.doi.org/10.1037/0000133-013
APA Handbook of Psychopharmacology, S. M. Evans (Editor-in-Chief)

others' trauma, and 31% higher odds of other injury/shock, even after controlling for place of residence. Using a nationally representative sample of adolescents, López and colleagues (2017) reported that non-White adolescents were more likely to be victims of multiple traumas than non-Hispanic Whites, after controlling for sex and other demographic variables.

Posttraumatic Stress Disorder

Over the last 20 years several nationally representative surveys have provided information regarding the prevalence of PTSD. Estimates of the lifetime prevalence of PTSD in the general population range between 6.1% (Goldstein et al., 2016) and 7.8% (Kessler et al., 1995). Estimates of past-year prevalence range between 4.7% (Goldstein et al., 2016) and 6.5% (McLaughlin, Conron, Koenen, & Gilman, 2010). Prevalence of PTSD varies across the lifespan. Kessler and colleagues (2005) found a small but steady increase in PTSD prevalence from emerging adulthood (6.3%) to middle adulthood (9.2%), but the prevalence in those aged 60 and older was significantly lower (2.5%).

Sex and racial/ethnic differences. Although men are more likely to be exposed to trauma, studies have consistently found that women have nearly two times greater odds than men of developing PTSD in their lifetime, even after controlling for type of traumatic event exposure (Breslau, 2009). Similar results were found in the second wave of the National Epidemiologic Survey on Alcohol and Related Conditions (NESARC) for both full and subthreshold PTSD (Pietrzak, Goldstein, Southwick, & Grant, 2011) and in the National Comorbidity Survey (Kessler et al., 1995).

Findings regarding differences in risk for a lifetime PTSD diagnosis based on race or ethnicity have been mixed. For example, the Detroit Area Survey of Trauma, which surveyed a representative sample in the metro Detroit area, found that even after accounting for geographic area (city vs. suburbs), being non-White was associated with 52% greater odds of a PTSD diagnosis (Breslau et al., 1998). Similarly, using the second wave of the NESARC, after controlling for exposure to traumatic events, Pietrzak et al. (2011) found that being Black was

associated with 22% higher odds of a lifetime PTSD diagnosis, while being of Asian/Hawaiian/Pacific Islander descent was associated with 33% lower odds of a lifetime PTSD diagnosis.

Comorbidities. One of the most significant complicating factors in treating PTSD is the high prevalence of comorbid conditions and associated problems. Using the second wave of the NESARC, Pietrzak and colleagues (2011) examined the odds of having another psychiatric condition associated with a lifetime diagnosis of PTSD after controlling for the presence of all other psychiatric conditions. They found that a lifetime PTSD diagnosis was associated with 2.6 greater odds of having a diagnosis of a mood disorder, 2.3 greater odds of having a diagnosis of an anxiety disorder, 1.3 greater odds of a drug use disorder, 1.3 greater odds of nicotine dependence, and 2.0 greater odds of reporting a suicide attempt (Pietrzak et al., 2011).

Data from the NESARC also indicate that PTSD is associated with a higher risk for violence perpetration, even after controlling for a number of covariates, including alcohol use disorder (AUD) and antisocial personality disorder (Smith, Smith, Violanti, Bartone, & Homish, 2015).

Acute Stress Disorder

Given the nature of ASD—a transient, acute stress reaction to a trauma lasting 1 month or less—large, nationally representative studies have not examined the prevalence of this disorder (Bryant, 2017). However, in a review, Bryant (2017) stated that the incidence is estimated to be between 12% and 37%, depending on the nature of trauma. ASD was initially thought to predict the development of PTSD, but data has indicated that the diagnosis of ASD is a better predictor of the development of any psychiatric disorder, rather than a specific predictor for the development of PTSD (Bryant, Creamer, O'Donnell, Silove, & McFarlane, 2012).

HISTORICAL PERSPECTIVE ON PHARMACOLOGICAL TREATMENTS

Research on treatment efficacy for PTSD began in the 1980s, after PTSD was included in the *DSM–III*. Most treatment research for PTSD has focused on psychosocial approaches (Friedman, 2016), but pharmacotherapy has also been an important focus. In 2004, the U.S. Department of Veterans Affairs (VA) and the U.S. Department of Defense (DoD) reviewed the literature on interventions for acute trauma reactions and PTSD in order to establish clinical guidelines for both behavioral and pharmacological treatments (U.S. VA & U.S. DoD, 2004). These guidelines have since been updated (VA & DoD, 2017) and are reflective of trends in pharmacotherapy.

The current 2017 guidelines have no recommendations for pharmacotherapy for early intervention, and state that there is a need for more research on early pharmacological treatments for trauma- and stressor-related disorders, as well as potential agents to prevent PTSD.

Clinical guidelines in 2004 recommended that selective serotonin reuptake inhibitors (SSRIs) be the first-line pharmacological treatment for PTSD and recommended against benzodiazepines, antipsychotics, and atypical antipsychotics. Updated guidelines in 2010 added serotonin and norepinephrine reuptake inhibitors (SNRIs) as another first-line treatment and indicated that the specific drugs with the most evidence were paroxetine (Paxil®), sertraline (Zoloft®), fluoxetine (Prozac®), and venlafaxine (Effexor®). The latest 2017 guidelines maintained the same list for first-line medications for overall PTSD symptoms, and indicate that nefazodone (Serzone®), imipramine (Tofranil®), and phenelzine (Nardil®) can be considered only if other medications have proven ineffective, along with other behavioral interventions. They further indicate that there is mixed evidence that prazosin has a benefit for treating nightmares/sleep disturbance but recommend against its use as monotherapy. See Table 13.1 for a list of U.S. Food and Drug Administration (FDA) approved and VA/DoD-recommended pharmacotherapies for PTSD.

DIAGNOSING TRAUMA AND STRESS-RELATED DISORDERS

This section provides a brief overview of standard screening and assessment measures for trauma exposure, PTSD, and ASD. Please also see the Tool Kit of Resources at the end of this chapter for more assessment resources.

Assessment of Trauma Exposure

A thorough assessment of trauma exposure is important to understand the potential for traumatic experiences to engender dysfunction. The Life Events Checklist (LEC; Gray, Litz, Hsu, & Lombardo, 2004) is a widely used measure to assess trauma exposure and was designed alongside the Clinician Administered PTSD Scale (CAPS), which is the gold-standard measure for the diagnosis of PTSD (Gray et al., 2004). Research on the LEC has indicated that it has good psychometric properties (Gray et al., 2004) and is a good predictor of future PTSD diagnosis (Wilker et al., 2015). The LEC was recently updated to match the *DSM–5* criteria (Weathers et al., 2013b).

Assessment of Posttraumatic Stress Disorder

Screening. The Posttraumatic Stress Disorder Checklist for DSM–5 (PCL-5; Blevins, Weathers, Davis, Witte, & Domino, 2015) is the measure recommended and most widely used by the VA and DoD (Department of Veterans Affairs, 2017) to both screen for PTSD and to measure change during treatment. The PCL-5 consists of 20 items rated on a 5-point Likert-type scale and has demonstrated excellent internal consistency ($r = .94$), good test–retest reliability at 1 week ($r = .82$), and good convergent and discriminant validity (Blevins et al., 2015). The VA/DoD clinical guidelines (Department of Veterans Affairs, 2017) recommend a cutoff score of 33 to 38 for a positive screen for PTSD, depending on the level of specificity desired and the prevalence of PTSD in the setting.

The other screening instrument recommended by the VA/DoD (Department of Veterans Affairs, 2017) clinical guidelines is the Primary Care PTSD Screen for DSM–5 (PC-PTSD-5; Prins et al., 2016). This measure is a brief screening tool administered by a physician consisting of one question to assess past trauma exposure and five questions to screen for PTSD symptoms (Prins et al., 2016). The PC-PTSD-5 has been shown to have strong diagnostic

TABLE 13.1

U.S. Department of Veterans Affairs Guidelines for Monotherapy for Posttraumatic Stress Disorder

Drug	Brand	Recommendation	Evidence quality rating	FDA approved for PTSD	Initial dose	Dose range	Toxicity concern
Antidepressants							
SSRIs							
Sertraline	Zoloft®	Recommend for	Moderate	Yes	25–60 mg daily	50–200 mg daily	No
Paroxetine	Paxil®	Recommend for	Moderate	Yes	10–20 mg daily	20–50 mg daily	No
Fluoxetine	Prozac®	Recommend for	Moderate	No	10–20 mg daily	20–80 mg daily	No
Citalopram	Celexa®	Suggest against	Low	No	—	—	No
SNRIs							
Venlafaxine	Effexor®	Recommend for	Moderate	No	IR: 25 mg 2–3 times daily; ER: 37.5 mg daily	IR: 75–375 mg in 2–3 divided doses; ER: 75–225 mg once daily	No
TCAs							
Imipramine	Tofranil®	Suggest for	Very low	No	25–75 mg daily	100–300 mg in 1–2 divided doses	No
Amitriptyline	Elavil®	Suggest against	Low	No	—	—	No
MAOIs							
Phenelzine	Nardil®	Suggest for	Very low	No	15 mg 3 times daily	15 mg daily; 90 mg in divided doses	Yes
Other ADs							
Nefazodone	Serzone®	Suggest for	Low	No	25–100 mg 2 times daily	150–600 mg in divided doses	Yes

Mood Stabilizers						
Topiramate	Topamax®	No	—	No	Very low	Suggest against
divalproex	Depakote®	No	—	No	Low	Recommend against
lamotrigine	Lamictal®	No	—	No	Very low	Suggest against
Tiagabine	Gabitril®	No	—	No	Low	Recommend against
Atypical APs						
Risperidone	Risperdal®	No	—	No	Very low	Recommend against
Olanzapine	Zyprexa®	No	—	No	Low	Suggest against
quetiapine	Seroquel®	No	—	No	Low	Suggest against
Benzodiazepines	Xanax®, Klonopin®, etc.	No	—	No	Very low	Recommend against
Other Drugs						
guanfacine	Intuniv® ER	No	—	No	Low	Recommend against
prazosin	Minipress®	No	—	No	Moderate	Recommend against
ketamine	Not applicable	No	—	No	Very low	Recommend against
d-cycloserine	Seromycin®	No	—	No	Very low	Recommend against
hydrocortisone	Cortef®	No	—	No	Very low	Recommend against

Note. Information about initial dose and dose ranges provided for medications listed as "recommend for" and "suggest for." FDA = U.S. Food and Drug Administration; PTSD = posttraumatic stress disorder; SSRIs = selective serotonin reuptake inhibitors; SNRIs = serotonin and norepinephrine reuptake inhibitors; TCAs = tricyclic antidepressants; IR = immediate release; ER = extended release; MAOIs = monoamine oxidase inhibitors; ADs = antidepressants; APs = antipsychotics. Recommendation categories: recommend for = first-line pharmacotherapy; suggest for = pharmacotherapy to be tried only after first-line behavioral and pharmacological treatments have failed; suggest against = not recommended, caution in prescribing; recommend against = not recommended, extreme caution in prescribing. Adapted from *VA/DoD Clinical Practice Guideline for the Management of Posttraumatic Stress Disorder and Acute Stress Disorder, Version 3.0* (pp. 51–65), by the U.S. Department of Veterans Affairs and U.S. Department of Defense, 2017, Washington, DC: Authors. In the public domain.

accuracy, and recommendations for cutoffs range between 3 and 5, depending on the sensitivity, specificity, and prevalence of PTSD in the setting (Prins et al., 2016). For those who screen positive for probable PTSD, further assessment is indicated with a structured or semistructured clinical interview to confirm a diagnosis of PTSD.

Diagnosis. The CAPS (Blake et al., 1995) is considered the gold-standard measure for the diagnosis of PTSD (Department of Veterans Affairs, 2017). Data on the psychometric properties were established for the version that corresponds with *DSM–IV*, and 10 years of research on the measure indicated that it had excellent interrater reliability, convergent validity, and discriminant validity (Weathers, Keane, & Davidson, 2001). The CAPS has recently been updated to correspond with *DSM–5* (Weathers et al., 2013a) and training for the interview is available for free from the VA website: https://www.ptsd.va.gov/professional/continuing_ed/caps5_clinician_training.asp

Assessment of Acute Stress Disorder

The VA (Gibson, 2016) recommends two measures for the assessment of ASD: the Acute Stress Disorder Scale (ASDS; Bryant, Moulds, & Guthrie, 2000) and the Acute Stress Disorder Interview (ASDI; Bryant, Harvey, Dang, & Sackville, 1998). The ASDS is self-report scale, appropriate as a screening tool for ASD that has demonstrated good psychometric properties (Bryant et al., 2000). The ASDI is a semistructured clinician-led interview that was developed to assess *DSM–IV* criteria for ASD and has also demonstrated good psychometric properties (Bryant et al., 1998).

Assessment of Comorbid Conditions and Problems

Common comorbid conditions, such as alcohol or substance use disorders, mood disorders, anxiety disorders, suicide risk, and violence risk should be included as part of a thorough assessment. A review of assessment of substance use disorders and comorbid PTSD suggests that an assessment include screening for substance use problems, follow-up with urinalysis, formal diagnosis with a semistructured interview (e.g., the Structured Clinical Interview for DSM), and continued monitoring using urinalysis and measures of frequency and quantity of use (McCauley, Killeen, Gros, Brady, & Back, 2012). Screening of mood and anxiety disorders can be assessed with brief measures, such as the Hamilton Depression Rating Scale (Hamilton, 1960), and the Hamilton Anxiety Rating Scale (Hamilton, 1959). The Columbia-Suicide Severity Rating Scale (C-SSRS; Posner et al., 2011) is a comprehensive measure of suicide ideation, suicide behaviors, and the severity of both that is useful for the assessment of lifetime suicide risk as well as ongoing monitoring. With regard to violence risk, the VA recommends that broad measures of violence risk be used, as well measures that help understand current and past violent behaviors in intimate and nonintimate relationships (Elbogen, Norman, Schnurr, & Matteo, 2016; see the Tool Kit of Resources).

EVIDENCE-BASED PHARMACOLOGICAL TREATMENTS OF POSTTRAUMATIC STRESS DISORDER

Although the best approaches for the treatment of PTSD are trauma-focused psychotherapies, pharmacotherapy can be an effective adjunct to enhance treatment outcomes. Medications are typically not a first-line treatment for PTSD, but may be used when psychotherapies are not available or are ineffective, when patients present with comorbid disorders, or when patients are not interested in psychotherapy.

The neurobiology of PTSD is complex, but proposed dysfunctions involve abnormalities in the neural circuitry between the prefrontal cortex (PFC), hippocampus, amygdala, hypothalamic–pituitary–adrenal axis (HPA axis), and other neural pathways that control stress reactivity, emotions, fear learning and memory encoding, and fear conditioning (Åhs, Frick, Furmark, & Fredrikson, 2015; Steckler & Risbrough, 2012). Neuroendocrine and neurotransmitter systems such as glucocorticoid, serotonin, norepinephrine/noradrenergic, gamma-aminobutyric acid (GABA), and glutamate are directly or indirectly involved in maintaining normal neural circuitry (Åhs et al., 2015; Steckler & Risbrough, 2012). The pathology of PTSD results largely from failure of the stress response system to recover from traumatic events. During a stressful experience norepinephrine is released from the locus coeruleus in the brainstem into brain areas involved in emotion, memory, and stress response. In PTSD, a hyperactive norepinephrine system results in abnormalities in these adaptive functions. Norepinephrine exerts an activating effect on the amygdala, which modulates emotional memory formation in the hippocampus (Krystal & Neumeister, 2009). Fear acquisition and conditioning result from emotionally intense memories formed and stored in the hippocampus, coupled with decreased PFC inhibitory control over the amygdala (Nash, Galatzer-Levy, Krystal, Duman, & Neumeister, 2014).

Selective Serotonin Reuptake Inhibitors

SSRIs work by blocking the presynaptic reuptake of serotonin, thereby increasing the availability of serotonin in the neural pathways (Abdallah, Southwick, & Krystal, 2017). Serotonin has also been shown to normalize HPA axis response to stress and enhance hippocampal neurogenesis (Steckler & Risbrough, 2012). Currently, the SSRIs sertraline and paroxetine are the only medications that have been approved for PTSD treatment by the FDA (Ipser & Stein, 2012). The dosage of sertraline for PTSD (50–200 mg per day titrated as tolerated) is higher than that used for the treatment of depression (Brady et al., 2000). Two large double-blind randomized controlled trials (RCTs) of sertraline versus placebo in adults with PTSD demonstrated a significantly higher response rate, defined as greater than 30% reduction in CAPS from baseline to end of treatment. Adverse effects more common in the sertraline group included insomnia, diarrhea, nausea, and fatigue (Brady et al., 2000; Davidson et al., 2003). In another large RCT, Marshall, Beebe, Oldham, and Zaninelli (2001) found that paroxetine in doses of 20 and 40 mg per day had higher rates of PTSD symptom severity improvement than placebo in adults with chronic PTSD, although a dose–response relationship was not detected. Abrupt discontinuation of paroxetine can result in a withdrawal syndrome including headache, fatigue, nausea, dizziness, agitation, and worsened mood (Sugarman, Loree, Baltes, Grekin, & Kirsch, 2014).

Other Antidepressants

Other antidepressants have also been explored less extensively for the treatment of PTSD. Recently, the American Psychological Association developed clinical practice guidelines for the treatment of PTSD that included four medications that had "moderate evidence of a small magnitude" (APA, 2017) in reducing PTSD symptom severity. The guidelines gave a conditional recommendation for using either venlafaxine extended release (ER; an SNRI) or sertraline, when both are considered compared with no intervention. In a large multisite RCT comparing venlafaxine ER, sertraline, and placebo, venlafaxine ER (37.5–300 mg/day with average dose of 164 mg daily) was comparable to sertraline (average dose of 110 mg), and both were more effective in reducing PTSD symptoms than placebo. In addition, significantly more participants receiving venlafaxine ER versus placebo achieved remission, defined as scores of less than 20 on the CAPS (Davidson et al., 2006). Treatment-emergent adverse events reported more often in the venlafaxine ER group (although not significantly different in all three groups) included headache, nausea, dry mouth, dizziness, insomnia, constipation, and decreased appetite.

Other antidepressants with histamine (H_1) and serotonin (5-HT_1, 5-HT_2, and 5-HT_3) receptor blockade such as mirtazapine (7.5–45 mg) and trazodone (50–200 mg) have been used as adjunctives with other medications for their sedation properties (Friedman & Davidson, 2014). A 24-week study comparing mirtazapine plus sertraline to sertraline plus placebo showed some preliminary efficacy in PTSD remission and depression severity scores in the combined medication group (Schneier et al., 2015). Both of these medications can cause drowsiness and hypotension, and there is a risk of priapism (i.e., prolonged erection of the penis) with trazodone.

Antiadrenergic Medications

The fear response elicited by exposure to traumatic stress is accompanied by perceptual, sensory, cognitive, and affective information that is stored in memory during an aroused state. Activation of the amygdala, hippocampus, and PFC by noradrenergic hyperactivity results in consolidation of the trauma memory, with associated emotional and physiologic responses (Kolassa et al., 2015). Consolidation involves the process of forming, encoding, and storage of memories in the hippocampus. The intensity of the emotion and level of arousal at the time of the traumatic stimulus affect the memory consolidation process. In PTSD, memories can be reactivated by associated contextual cues (LaLumiere, McGaugh, & McIntyre, 2017). Prophylactic prevention of PTSD involves addressing the adrenergic and HPA axis dysregulation posttrauma. As such, the beta-adrenergic antagonist propranolol has been proposed to prevent memory consolidation following trauma. However, the use of propranolol has had mixed results when studied as a prophylactic medication following trauma (Friedman & Davidson, 2014). This may be due to variations in the timing of the initiation of the medication posttrauma, the dosage administered, and duration of treatment (Argolo, Cavalcanti-Ribeiro, Netto, & Quarantini, 2015).

Alpha$_1$-noradrenergic antagonist prazosin, in doses titrated from 3 to 10 mg, has been explored for PTSD and was shown to reduce nightmares, improve sleep quality and duration, reduce daytime hyperarousal symptoms, and improve overall PTSD symptom severity (Khachatryan, Groll, Booij, Sepehry, & Schütz, 2016; Raskind, 2015). In a small pilot study with veterans, a longer acting alpha$_1$-noradrenergic antagonist, doxazosin ER, at doses titrated from 4 to 16 mg over 12 days with 4 days at 16 mg, was shown to reduce self-report PTSD symptom severity (Rodgman et al., 2016). Antiadrenergic drugs may produce hypotension and bradycardia, and thus should be used cautiously.

Glucocorticoid Medications

Adrenal stress hormones may also play a role in modulation of memory consolidation (LaLumiere et al., 2017). Individuals at risk for PTSD have been shown to have low cortisol levels after experiencing trauma, which can prolong the adrenergic response posttrauma, thus enhancing the consolidation of the traumatic memory. Administering glucocorticoids within 6 hours after trauma may stabilize the HPA axis and impair trauma memory consolidation and

recall. Hydrocortisone, a corticosteroid, was studied as a prophylactic medication to prevent development of PTSD following trauma by disrupting trauma memory retrieval. Individuals receiving hydrocortisone (20 mg twice daily for 10 days) initiated within 12 hours posttrauma reported less PTSD symptoms at 1- and 3-month follow-ups than those receiving placebo. A meta-analysis of pharmacologic prevention interventions for PTSD found a large effect for use of hydrocortisone following trauma. However, the use of hydrocortisone even briefly may cause adverse effects such as mood instability, irritability, aggression, and irregular heartbeat. In addition, individuals may be reluctant to take such a preventative medication when they are not symptomatic (Sijbrandij, Kleiboer, Bisson, Barbui, & Cuijpers, 2015).

Atypical Antipsychotics

Atypical antipsychotics have been explored for the treatment of PTSD either alone as monotherapy or as an adjunct to other medications. However, small early phase studies have shown only modest efficacy or inconsistent outcomes. In a recent study, quetiapine (Seroquel®), a serotonin 5-HT$_{2A}$ and dopamine D2 receptor antagonist, was explored in combat veterans with PTSD. Mechanisms that may account for the efficacy of quetiapine in PTSD include increasing neuropeptide Y, which lowers corticotropin releasing hormone in the cerebral spinal fluid and has alpha$_1$-adrenergic antagonist and antihistaminergic effects. Specifically, quetiapine in doses of 25 mg to 800 mg (average 258 mg) versus placebo was explored as a monotherapy in a group of veterans with PTSD. Those in the quetiapine group had significantly greater reduction in total CAPS scores, including the reexperiencing and hyperarousal subscale scores, compared with those in the placebo group (Villarreal et al., 2016). Although side effects were not significantly different between the two groups, atypical antipsychotics are associated with higher risk for weight gain, metabolic syndrome, and tardive dyskinesia. In the VA, atypical antipsychotic medications are commonly prescribed as an adjunct for the treatment of PTSD, but use as monotherapy is not recommended (Bauer et al., 2014).

Anticonvulsants/Mood Stabilizers

Topiramate, an anticonvulsant, has been explored in individuals with PTSD. The mechanism of action may be activation of GABA and inhibition of glutamate neurotransmission. A small randomized trial using topiramate (103 mg average dose) or placebo for 12 weeks (Yeh et al., 2011) did not find significant between-group differences in PTSD symptom severity at the end of treatment. However, for those who were retained and completed all 12 weeks of treatment, there was a significant 82% reduction in CAPS scores in the topiramate group (Yeh et al., 2011). There is also some evidence that topiramate was significantly more effective in reducing PTSD symptom severity than placebo (–57.8 vs. –32.4 reduction in total CAPS score, respectively). Batki et al. (2014) explored topiramate versus placebo in a 12-week RCT in veterans with comorbid PTSD and AUD. In addition to a significantly greater reduction in frequency and amount of alcohol use, there was a trend for greater improvement in PTSD symptom severity in the topiramate group versus the placebo group. Although this medication looks promising, the transient learning and memory deficits observed in the veterans taking topiramate may interfere with certain psychosocial interventions such as prolonged exposure or cognitive processing therapy (Batki et al., 2014).

Anxiolytics/Sedative-Hypnotics

Benzodiazepines are generally not prescribed for patients with PTSD and may actually interfere with the fear activation associated with beneficial effects of prolonged exposure therapy (Friedman & Davidson, 2014). Given their abuse potential, benzodiazepines should be carefully monitored in patients with comorbid substance use disorder (SUD). The nonbenzodiazepine GABA-A receptor agonist eszopiclone has been investigated in a small sample of individuals with PTSD. In a double-blind randomized crossover-designed study, participants received either 3 mg eszopiclone or placebo for 7 weeks (Pollack et al., 2011). Participants in the eszopiclone versus the placebo group had significantly better sleep and a greater reduction in PTSD symptom severity that was independent of sleep improvement. Adverse events were mild to moderate

and included unpleasant taste, sedation, and headache (see Table 13.1).

BEST APPROACHES FOR ASSESSING TREATMENT RESPONSE AND MANAGING SIDE EFFECTS

Assessing PTSD symptom severity pretreatment and posttreatment with self-report or interviewer rating scales can best determine treatment response and/or remission. Rates of PTSD remission using the CAPS (*DSM–IV* version) in the early sertraline trials were 23% to 26%. Remission was defined as a CAPS score of less than 20 and a self-report Davidson Trauma Scale score of less than 18 (Davidson et al., 1997). Treatment response has been defined as a 30% or more reduction in CAPS score from pretreatment to posttreatment (Londborg et al., 2001). The efficacy of sustained treatment response with sertraline beyond a 12-week RCT was explored in an open-label continuation phase in which participants who completed the 12-week acute phase received sertraline for an additional 24 weeks. At the end of the continuation phase 92% percent maintained their treatment response and 54% of nonresponders converted to responders (Londborg et al., 2001). In the paroxetine study, treatment response was defined as "much improved" and "very much improved" on the Clinician Global Impression (CGI) improvement scale. The proportion of patients with a treatment response was higher for the group receiving paroxetine (62%) versus the group receiving placebo (37%; Marshall et al., 2001). Although remission rates were not reported in this study, the average CAPS score for the paroxetine groups after 12 weeks of treatment was in the mild/moderate range, between 35 and 40.

For nonresponders, increasing the medication dose within the therapeutic range and the patient's tolerance level may improve effectiveness. Other choices include augmenting with another medication or switching medications. Patients may need to be switched to another class of medication with a different mechanism of action (D. L. Taylor & Laraia, 2009).

The goals of medication management include maximizing therapeutic benefits while minimizing adverse effects. With some medications, such as the

SSRIs, patients may experience adverse reactions soon after initiation of a medication and before the desired effects of the medication take effect. SSRIs typically take 4 to 6 weeks to reach steady state. Patients need to be aware of the time it will take to achieve desired effects. Upon initiating treatment, titrating and adjusting the dosage of medications as tolerated may minimize adverse effects. Dosage adjustments need to be made for medications that are metabolized by the same liver enzyme systems. For example, SSRI antidepressants are potent cytochrome enzyme P450 inhibitors and may result in increased drug levels of certain other medications a patient may be taking. Clinicians need to monitor all medications to avoid harmful drug interactions (Madhusoodanan, Velama, Parmar, Goia, & Brenner, 2014).

Patients should be educated on the adverse events associated with the medications they are taking. Patients taking medications with sedative properties, such as certain SSRIs, SNRIs, benzodiazepines, nonbenzodiazepine sedatives, and atypical antipsychotics, need to avoid hazardous activities such as driving or operating machinery. These medications may need to be taken at bedtime. Alternately, medications that cause insomnia are best taken in the morning. For those medications that cause gastrointestinal upset, patients can be instructed to take the medication with food. Undesirable adverse events such as weight gain and sexual dysfunction are associated with certain antidepressants and atypical antipsychotics. Increasing exercise, making dietary changes, and lowering caloric intake may help with the weight gain. Certain medications may be contraindicated in patients with certain medical conditions. For example, venlafaxine should not be used in patients with hypertension. A good initial history and physical, including medication history, is important when making safe medication choices. If adverse events become intolerable or interfere with functioning and activities, clinicians can consider a different medication (D. L. Taylor & Laraia, 2009).

MEDICATION MANAGEMENT ISSUES

An important component of pharmacotherapy outcome involves adherence to prescribed medications. Patients prescribed psychotropic medication have the highest rates of nonadherence, averaging about 40% to 50% (Farooq & Naeem, 2014). A study in veterans found that 66% of patients with PTSD were nonadherent during the 12 months post-discharge (Lockwood, Steinke, & Botts, 2009).

Nonadherence generally includes discontinuation of medication, missed doses, or not taking the medication as prescribed, all of which adversely affect treatment efficacy. Some of the most common barriers to medication adherence include costs, multiple dosing regimens, polypharmacy, adverse events, beliefs about medication efficacy, concerns about the medication, stigma, and lack of knowledge about the medication (Brown & Bussell, 2011; van Servellen, Heise, & Ellis, 2011). Treatment motivation, social factors, and life stressors also play a role in whether an individual will adhere to prescribed treatment. Understanding patients' beliefs regarding treatment preference is an important consideration, and patients should be offered a menu of options if feasible. Many adherence barriers can be addressed with a patient-centered approach to treatment. Clinicians should assess patient characteristics that may put them at risk for nonadherence. Furthermore, nonadherence should be a signal for reevaluation of treatment options (S. Taylor, Abramowitz, & McKay, 2012). Actively involving patients in treatment decisions can improve adherence rates. Many adherence enhancement interventions use motivational interviewing to engage patients in their treatment (Farooq & Naeem, 2014).

Certain comorbid disorders that impair cognition, such as SUD and traumatic brain injury, may also interfere with medication adherence. Identifying and including a supportive significant other in the patient's treatment may be necessary in certain cases. Complicated medication regimens can be inconvenient and constraining, and require memory aids to assist with adherence. Prescriptions of multiple medications and frequency of daily dosing have been associated with higher risk of nonadherence. Use of extended release formulations and the minimization of complex treatment regimens can reduce missed doses. Working with patients on dosing regimens that fit in with routine daily activities can also enhance adherence. Several tools, such as reminder apps on cellphones or pill dispensing trays with reminder signals, have been developed to assist with medication adherence.

Patients who have been on medication for a period of time and are feeling better often may discontinue the medication on their own. The decision to discontinue a medication should be a collaborative decision between the patient and provider so that benefits and risks associated with discontinuation are discussed. Patients should be informed that for certain psychotropic medications, such as antidepressants, benzodiazepines, and atypical antipsychotics, abrupt discontinuation may result in a recurrence of original symptoms, uncomfortable physical and psychological symptoms, or physiologic withdrawal. A gradual taper and careful monitoring can minimize uncomfortable discontinuation symptoms.

EVALUATION OF PHARMACOLOGICAL APPROACHES ACROSS THE LIFESPAN

Children and Adolescents

A recent meta-analysis of 43 independent samples of children revealed that approximately 16% of children and adolescents developed PTSD after trauma exposure (Alisic et al., 2014). PTSD in children and adolescents is a heterogeneous disorder often coexisting with other psychiatric symptoms and comorbid conditions such as depression, anxiety, and internalizing and externalizing disorders (Alisic et al., 2014). Given the neurobiological differences between children/adolescents and adults in response to trauma and the resulting clinical symptoms, empirical findings relevant to pharmacological treatment of PTSD in adults may not be generalizable to the treatment of children/adolescents (Huemer, Erhart, & Steiner, 2010).

There has been a dearth of high-quality RCTs testing the efficacy of medications for childhood and adolescent PTSD, thus rendering the benefit of pharmacological approaches inconclusive. Nevertheless, several evidence-based practice and treatment planning guidelines exist that provide clinicians with recommendations on how to assess and pharmacologically treat PTSD in children and adolescents (Cohen et al., 2010; National Collaborating Centre for Mental Health, 2005). Treatment planning

necessarily entails a comprehensive and multimodal approach that takes into consideration the symptom severity and level of impairment in functioning of the child or adolescent (Cohen et al., 2010; National Collaborating Centre for Mental Health, 2005). A variety of pharmacological agents have been examined and utilized in the treatment of PTSD in children and adolescents, including SSRIs, tricyclic antidepressants, adrenergic agents, benzodiazepines, antipsychotics, and anticonvulsants. The overall efficacy and/or superiority of any of these medications over psychosocial approaches alone, however, has yet to be demonstrated.

Reviews by Strawn, Keeshin, DelBello, Geracioti, and Putnam (2010) and Keeshin and Strawn (2014) identified only three RCTs of SSRIs and one RCT of a tricyclic antidepressant with child and adolescent samples. Cohen, Mannarino, Perel, and Staron (2007) conducted a 12-week pilot RCT comparing trauma-focused cognitive behavioral therapy (TF-CBT) with sertraline to TF-CBT with placebo in a sample of 24 children and adolescents aged 10 to 17. At end of treatment, both groups demonstrated comparable reductions in PTSD symptoms. Since sertraline did not confer additional benefits above and beyond the psychosocial intervention, the authors recommended that a trial of trauma-focused psychotherapy should be implemented first before adding medications (Cohen et al., 2007). In a 10-week double-blind, placebo-controlled trial of sertraline with 129 children and adolescents age 6 to 17, there was no statistically significant difference between sertraline and placebo in PTSD symptoms at posttreatment. Despite lack of superiority to placebo, sertraline was found to be generally safe (Robb, Cueva, Sporn, Yang, & Vanderburg, 2010). Robert et al. (2008) conducted a 1-week double-blind RCT of imipramine and fluoxetine compared with placebo in a sample of 60 thermally-injured children and adolescents aged 4 to 18 with ASD and found no statistically significant differences among the three treatment groups. The evidence thus far has not supported the utilization of SSRIs as a front-line treatment for PTSD in children and adolescents (Keeshin & Strawn, 2014). There are no or limited data to support the utilization of benzodiazepines, antipsychotics, or anticonvulsants to treat PTSD symptoms in children and adolescents (Cohen et al., 2010; Keeshin & Strawn, 2014). More recently, a large meta-analysis of studies published up to 2015 examining psychological and pharmacological treatments for child and adolescent PTSD (Morina, Koerssen, & Pollet, 2016) found only two RCTs that met stringent inclusion criteria and based on null findings, the authors advised that "psychopharmacological interventions should be used cautiously and only after determining that the child or adolescent with PTSD may not benefit from psychotherapeutic interventions such as TF-CBT" (p. 51).

Despite the lack of RCT support for their utilization in treating PTSD symptoms in children and adolescents, anecdotal reports and case studies show that, in practice, pharmacological agents are being utilized by psychiatrists to treat reexperiencing and hyperarousal symptoms, chronic anxiety, aggression, depression, and other comorbid conditions in children and adolescents with PTSD (Cohen et al., 2010). Experts recommend that TF-CBT should be considered the front-line treatment for child/adolescent PTSD, and adjunctive pharmacological treatments, in particular SSRIs, may be considered when PTSD symptoms are severe, comorbid conditions are prevalent, and/or response to trauma-focused psychotherapy is suboptimal (Cohen et al., 2010; Keeshin & Strawn, 2014). Note, however, that compared with placebo, antidepressant usage is associated with increased risk for suicidality in children and adolescents (Department of Veterans Affairs, 2017).

Elderly

Prevalence rates of PTSD are typically lower in older adults (age 65 and older) than younger adults (Pietrzak, Goldstein, Southwick, & Grant, 2012). Studies suggest older adults are also more likely to evidence subthreshold PTSD (Chopra et al., 2014). Lower rates of PTSD are often attributed to lower admission of psychiatric distress by older adults due to stigma, prior negative experiences with trauma disclosures resulting in lower likelihood of admitting distress, and/or reduction of perception of problems due to age-related processes such as loss of hearing and vision (Cook, Simiola, & Brown, 2017). In older adults, PTSD symptoms are often comorbid

with certain medical conditions (e.g., cancer, cardiovascular disease, dementia, Alzheimer's disease) and age-related decline in physical and cognitive functioning. Stressors associated with aging, such as loss of a spouse and cognitive, physical, or financial decline, may lead to resurfacing of or worsening of PTSD symptoms associated with earlier traumatic events (Cook et al., 2017; Moye & Rouse, 2014). Most of the RCTs on pharmacological interventions for PTSD, to date, however, have been conducted with younger adults. Thus, findings may not be generalizable to older adults whose needs are distinct. Age-related neurophysiological changes may influence the pharmacodynamics and pharmacokinetics of psychotropic medications, contributing to lower metabolism, increased half-life, and reduced drug clearance. Moreover, older adults have been found to be more susceptible to adverse drug-related side effects, and certain medications can worsen health problems and increase older adults' risk for falls and other accidents (Moye & Rouse, 2014).

There is a dearth of RCTs testing the safety and efficacy of pharmacotherapies for PTSD and other stressor-related disorders among older adults. In a chart review study of drug classes prescribed for older veterans with PTSD in the VA health and mental health system, Mohamed and Rosenheck (2008) found that 88.3% of older veterans were prescribed antidepressants, 61.2% were prescribed anxiolytics/sedative hypnotics, and 32.9% were prescribed antipsychotics. Moreover, they found that psychotropic medication utilization declined with age, particularly among older veterans utilizing specialty mental health clinics, suggesting either a cautious approach due to age-related medical comorbidities, decline in PTSD symptomatology, or undertreatment of older veterans in these settings (Mohamed & Rosenheck, 2008).

Experts advise against the utilization of benzodiazepines to treat PTSD among older adults for various reasons, including risk for adverse negative effects secondary to medical conditions (e.g., cancer, dementia, vascular disorders) that may contribute to confusion and falls, and risk of developing tolerance and eventual dependence (Moye & Rouse, 2014). Moye and Rouse (2014) recommend a stepwise approach for the pharmacological treatment of older adults with PTSD, with the utilization of prazosin and trazodone (a tetracyclic antidepressant) for nightmares and sleep problems. However, risk for hypotension and dizziness should be monitored closely and may be prevented by starting at the lowest dose possible and titrating up very slowly (Moye & Rouse, 2014). A trial of SSRIs is also recommended if prazosin or trazodone has not resolved the sleep problems or nightmares. Low-dose antipsychotics (quetiapine, risperidone, and aripiprazole) can also be considered when psychotic symptoms are comorbid with PTSD (Moye & Rouse, 2014). Psychotic symptoms may be associated with dementia, which, as noted earlier, can contribute to a resurgence of PTSD symptoms from many years earlier (Moye & Rouse, 2014). A recent cross-sectional study of veterans 65 years old and older receiving treatment in inpatient or outpatient VA settings during the years 2004 to 2009 found that older veterans with PTSD plus dementia were twice as likely to be prescribed a second-generation antipsychotic (SGA; i.e., atypical antipsychotic medications developed in the 1980s; e.g., aripiprazole, olanzapine, quetiapine, risperidone, ziprasidone) with less neurological side-effects than older veterans with PTSD alone (Semla et al., 2017). Although the authors noted that the prescribing of SGAs decreased during the years assessed, they argued that greater prescribing of SGAs to older veterans with PTSD and comorbid dementia is problematic, given the high level of medical comorbidities among older veterans and lack of empirical support for the use of SGAs among those with dementia (Semla et al., 2017). Indeed, the VA/DoD (Department of Veterans Affairs, 2017) practice guidelines for PTSD strongly recommend against the use of antipsychotics for PTSD. Thus, the risk of adverse effects from the utilization of antipsychotics must be weighed against their benefits for older adults with PTSD (Moye & Rouse, 2014). In summary, the empirical research on the treatment and management of PTSD in older adults is sparse. Although the literature on pharmacotherapy for younger adults with PTSD can be utilized for insights into the general treatment of trauma-related disorders, the unique needs and concerns of older adults must be taken into consideration during treatment planning and monitoring.

CONSIDERATION OF POTENTIAL SEX DIFFERENCES

This section provides an overview of sex differences in the risk factors associated with the development of PTSD. This section also provides an overview of sex differences in the pharmacodynamics and pharmacokinetics of various medications for PTSD.

Risk

Various theories have been put forth to explain the differential sex risk for developing PTSD, including the *situational vulnerability theory* and the *female vulnerability theory*. Those adhering to the situational vulnerability theory (Pimlott-Kubiak & Cortina, 2003) argue that the greater rates of PTSD found among women may be due to the type or severity of trauma women are exposed to. Despite lower rates of trauma exposure in general, women are more likely to be exposed to chronic high-impact traumas such as childhood sexual abuse and rape, increasing their risk for PTSD (Olff, Langeland, Draijer, & Gersons, 2007; Tolin & Foa, 2006). The female vulnerability hypothesis argues that women may be more likely to develop PTSD because of specific psychological or biological vulnerabilities that place them at greater risk than men (Olff et al., 2007). Research has found sex differences in the cognitive appraisals of traumatic events and in the acute psychological and biological reactions to stress, with women experiencing more intense fear, helplessness, horror, and dissociative reactions (Felmingham et al., 2010; Inslicht et al., 2014; Irish et al., 2011). Nevertheless, once PTSD has been diagnosed, studies suggest men and women display similar types and levels of PTSD symptoms with comparable clinical profiles (Christiansen & Elklit, 2012) and are equally likely to benefit from psychosocial treatments for PTSD (Blain, Galovski, & Robinson, 2010).

Pharmacodynamics and Pharmacokinetics

Studies have shown there are sex differences in the pharmacodynamics and pharmacokinetics of psychotropic medications (Bergiannaki & Kostaras, 2016). For example, given women's lower body mass index and greater body fat, the distribution and absorption of medications may differ substantially compared with men. Sex differences have also been found in the metabolism and clearance of psychotropic medications, with premenopausal women demonstrating slower elimination and greater bioavailability of the drugs, contributing to higher rates of adverse drug reactions. Additional physiological differences between men and women, including hormonal fluctuations (e.g., of estrogen and progesterone) during the menstrual cycle, pregnancy, and utilization of hormonal contraceptives, may influence the dosing of, efficacy of, and response to certain psychotropic medications (Bergiannaki & Kostaras, 2016).

In one of the few studies examining sex differences, Rothbaum et al. (2008) pooled data from two flexible-dose, randomized, double-blind, placebo controlled trials (one trial of 12 weeks duration; the second of 24 weeks duration) of the SNRI venlafaxine (extended release [ER]; 37.5 mg/day–300 mg/day). Participants included 271 males and 416 females aged 18 or older with a primary diagnosis of PTSD. They found a significant treatment effect of venlafaxine ER on posttreatment PTSD symptoms compared with placebo. However, sex was not found to be a moderator of treatment outcomes, even after examining effects by menopausal status (women younger than 40 versus women older than 54) suggesting that the efficacy of venlafaxine ER cut across sex. Bernardy and Friedman (2016) highlighted that many of the RCTs that led to the FDA approval of SSRIs/SNRIs consisted of samples that included a high proportion of women (ranging from 19% to 91% of the total sample) and that sex did not appear to be an influential factor in treatment outcomes, suggesting equivalent benefits from approved medications.

In terms of treatment engagement, a study of returning veterans seeking treatment for PTSD found no sex differences in type of treatment utilized (psychotherapy only, pharmacotherapy only, or psychotherapy and pharmacotherapy; Haller, Myers, McKnight, Angkaw, & Norman, 2016). In private outpatient settings, however, women with PTSD are more likely to be prescribed psychotropic medications than their male counterparts (Bernardy & Friedman, 2016). Likewise, Bernardy, Lund,

Alexander, and Friedman (2012) found that, compared with male veterans, female veterans with PTSD receiving care in the VA health system during the years 1999 to 2009 were more likely to be prescribed all drug classes (except prazosin). They also found an increase in the prescribing of first-line SSRIs/SRNIs for female veterans with PTSD, which the authors speculated may "reflect a positive shift towards evidence-based pharmacological care" (Bernardy et al., 2013, p. S545).

Findings to date suggest women are equally likely to engage in and benefit from pharmacotherapy for PTSD (particularly SRNIs). However, given the finding that women with PTSD are more likely to be prescribed psychotropic medication in both private settings and the VA health systems, and given the sex differences in pharmacodynamics and pharmacokinetics, it is imperative that more studies are conducted to understand and improve pharmacotherapy for PTSD for women (see the Tool Kit of Resources).

INTEGRATION OF PHARMACOTHERAPY WITH NONPHARMACOLOGICAL APPROACHES: BENEFITS AND CHALLENGES

A number of multimodal behavioral interventions remain the gold standard for treating PTSD. Few studies have examined combination pharmacotherapy with trauma-specific approaches; nonetheless, integrating medication treatment with nonpharmacologic approaches is the clinical norm. There are a number of psychotherapy approaches to address traumatic stress disorders and reactions. Broadly, they can be divided into two types of psychotherapy: stabilization-focused approaches and trauma processing therapies (Ford & Courtois, 2009). The stabilization treatments provide psychoeducation and build coping strategies and other social skills to facilitate symptom management for patients who may be severely ill or have significant psychosocial stressors (i.e., social support, housing, medical, and relationship deficits). Trauma processing approaches, in contrast, seek to assist the patient to reexperience the emotions, cognitions, and behaviors that are directly linked to the traumatic exposure in order to achieve a diminishment in symptoms (Hien, Litt, Cohen, Miele, & Campbell, 2009b; Najavits, Hyman, Ruglass, Hien, & Read, 2017). One example of a stabilization behavioral intervention is dialectical behavior therapy (DBT; Linehan, 2015). DBT teaches patients a broad range of cognitive and behavioral strategies, such as identification of emotional states and distress tolerance, to help trauma survivors develop emotional regulation skills.

Examples of trauma processing cognitive behavioral techniques include exposure-based therapy, or prolonged exposure (Foa, 2011), and cognitive processing therapy (Nishith, Resick, & Griffin, 2002). These two evidence-based treatments are recommended by the International Society for Traumatic Stress Studies treatment guidelines for PTSD (Foa, Keane, & Friedman, 2003) and have been shown to be highly efficacious for the treatment of PTSD and acute stress disorders. Whereas prolonged exposure targets fear and avoidance through progressive exposure to fearful situations and narratives that lead to habituation of intense affects, cognitive processing therapy employs cognitive therapy to address faulty cognitions that reinforce avoidance behavior.

Notably, since the existing behavioral treatments for PTSD still leave many patients with less than optimal clinical benefits (Bomyea & Lang, 2012), there is a need for more study on medication combinations typically used in clinical practice. Clinical trials of combined medication and trauma-focused CBT have typically focused on the use of prolonged exposure techniques in combination with SSRI treatments for augmenting prolonged exposure outcomes (Jun, Zoellner, & Feeny, 2013; Sonne, Carlsson, Elklit, Mortensen, & Ekstrøm, 2013).

INTEGRATED APPROACHES FOR ADDRESSING COMMON COMORBID DISORDERS

Research has identified a number of shared mechanisms that increase the risk of developing comorbid disorders among those with PTSD/ASD, such as dysregulations in anatomical structures, circuitry, and neurotransmitters; noradrenergic sensitivities including HPA axis hyperresponsiveness; and

genetic factors (Neigh, Gillespie, & Nemeroff, 2009; Norman et al., 2012). Thus, in many patients with PTSD/ASD, comorbidities appear to be more the norm than the exception (Kessler et al., 1995). Given the known overlap in many of the neurobiological underpinnings of traumatic stress and other comorbid disorders, considerations regarding specific targets for pharmacologic intervention are complex, with as much evidence arising from anecdotal clinical practice and studies as from clinical trials supporting directions for providing comprehensive care that can most parsimoniously address all existing symptoms (e.g., McCauley et al., 2012; Norman et al., 2012).

Multiple pathways of disorder onset and maintenance must be considered in order to develop meaningful treatment plans. All evidence points to a complex, reciprocal, and reinforcing relationship between traumatic stress-related disorders and other comorbidities, such as SUDs (López-Castro, Hu, Papini, Ruglass, & Hien, 2015). In an influential analysis of the association between trauma and the development of SUD, no direct relationship was observed between traumatic stress exposure and development of addictions (Chilcoat & Breslau, 1998). However, in this large-scale study and in many others like it (e.g., Back, Brady, Sonne, & Verduin, 2006; Hien et al., 2010), a prior diagnosis of PTSD did predict the later appearance of a substance problem, supporting a model whereby early stress exposure leading to PTSD increases the vulnerability to develop SUDs (Kendler et al., 2000). More recent longitudinal studies with large data sets have revealed that childhood exposures to traumatic life events have been shown to increase the likelihood of adulthood disorders, from single to multiple comorbidities (including, but not limited to alcohol and drug use disorders; Young-Wolff, Kendler, Ericson, & Prescott, 2011).

Treatment decisions should take into account the kind of clinical presentation of the comorbidity. For example, some individuals presenting with PTSD have preexisting psychological problems prior to trauma exposure, while others develop additional disorders secondary to the onset of PTSD. For those whose related psychiatric conditions developed simultaneously at the time of trauma exposure, treatment considerations may include both targets at the same time (Hien, Litt, Cohen, Miele, & Campbell, 2009a). When addressing significant comorbid symptoms and syndromes, pharmacotherapy is often an essential component of treatment. Personalized medicine warrants considering each case and its details individually. Although many different types of medications exist for different types of symptoms and disorders, clients may need to try more than one type of medication before finding one that is most effective. Given the nature of the co-occurring problems, questions regarding course of treatment have been studied in the literature (Hien, Litt, Cohen, Miele, & Campbell, 2009a). Prevailing clinical concerns have led providers to adopt either a sequential or parallel treatment approach, whereby individuals with both disorders would be sent to segregated treatment programs (i.e., for mental health only or for substance abuse only) for staged care (Najavits et al., 2017). Even when treating both disorders simultaneously, the sequencing of a treatment plan will vary depending upon substance use severity. If PTSD is determined to have developed before the onset of substance abuse, it may be clinically appropriate to address the "root" symptoms of PTSD directly as a way to also address substance use. Alternately, if a traumatic event and subsequent PTSD occur after the onset of a SUD, a clinician might choose to focus on the substance abuse first. Either of these two models may be considered sequential or parallel in nature.

In most situations, however, causality may be difficult to untangle, including cases in which someone experiences a childhood trauma but does not start using substances until much later in life. Compounding the ambiguity of causal associations, clients with PTSD and SUDs often have more severe clinical profiles, including abusing more serious substances such as cocaine and opioids and experiencing interpersonal and medical problems (e.g., Morrison, Berenz, & Coffey, 2014). Attempting to treat only one disorder in sequence may lead to a worsening of symptoms (e.g., Ouimette, Read, Wade, & Tirone, 2010). In line with these needs, the research evidence base (van Dam, Vedel, Ehring, & Emmelkamp, 2012) on behavioral treatment for the combined disorders supports addressing trauma and substance use in rapid sequence or simultaneously (i.e., integrated treatment), as opposed to postponing treatment of one set of problems until the other has been resolved.

Pharmacotherapy for Co-Occurring Alcohol/Substance Use and Trauma-Related Disorders

There are currently few RCTs that have tested the efficacy of pharmacologic agents to treat PTSD and comorbid alcohol or substance use disorders (Petrakis & Simpson, 2017; Sofuoglu, Rosenheck, & Petrakis, 2014). In the extant literature base, strategic decisions about treatment targets tend to favor symptom reduction in one or both conditions. Examples would include use of SSRIs to target PTSD symptoms alone (de Kleine, Rothbaum, & van Minnen, 2013; Shad, Suris, & North, 2011) or as an agent that would impact alcohol use outcomes as well as PTSD (Brady et al., 2005; Hien, Levin, Ruglass, & Lopez-Castro, 2015). Other studies have attempted to address substance craving through the use of agents such as naltrexone, an antagonist for blocking the effects of opioids that has also been shown to reduce craving in alcohol users (e.g., Foa et al., 2013; Kaczkurkin, Asnaani, Alpert, & Foa, 2016). Strategies for intervention using medications with substance-dependent individuals target their primary substance of abuse. Agonist (methadone) and partial agonist (buprenorphine) medications are used as maintenance therapy in individuals with opioid use disorders to promote stabilization and harm reduction (Nielsen et al., 2016). Medications such as disulfiram (Antabuse®) that produce a severe noxious physical reaction when combined with alcohol are used to create a form of aversive conditioning that aims to prevent use and relapse (e.g., Petrakis et al., 2006). Finally, medications (typically agonist agents such as clonidine and benzodiazepines) that can help patients manage withdrawal symptoms are employed, but none has been studied directly in an RCT solely for the purpose of examining outcomes on withdrawal in comorbid populations.

From clinical trials focusing on AUDs (with or without drug use), four medications are currently approved by the FDA to treat AUD: disulfiram, naltrexone, an intramuscular form of naltrexone (Vivitrol®), and acamprosate (Petrakis & Simpson, 2017; see Chapter 22, this volume, for more details). Six studies have evaluated pharmacotherapies for patients with PTSD and comorbid AUD (Ralevski, Olivera-Figueroa, & Petrakis, 2014). Whereas these medications had positive indications for drinking outcomes across all studies (open trials and RCTs), only half revealed superiority of medications for PTSD outcomes when compared with placebo. A systematic review by Petrakis and Simpson (2017) identified nine RCTs for individuals with PTSD and AUD. Of those RCTs, three targeted PTSD symptom reduction alone, four targeted alcohol use symptoms alone, and another three targeted both disorders (one study tested both a medication for PTSD and one for AUD, and thus was counted twice in this breakdown). Their review concluded that the majority of evidence pointed to significant reductions in both PTSD and AUD outcomes, despite failing to provide support for any one medication approach. Conclusions about best practices for targeting PTSD in this comorbid group were not available. Despite some contradictory findings, importantly, the authors concluded that there was no evidence *against* using medications that have been found efficacious in noncomorbid populations.

Pharmacotherapy for Co-Occurring Mood and Trauma-Related Disorders

The SSRIs have been a critical component of pharmacotherapy for PTSD and traumatic stress. Given the high comorbidity of PTSD with mood disorders, the same agents (e.g., citalopram, escitalopram, sertraline, paroxetine) that can decrease problematic symptoms and help regulate sleeping and eating patterns, energy levels, and overall mood should be used for those with significant depressive symptoms. As with comorbid SUDs, those with comorbid mood disorders typically evidence higher severity of symptoms, lower quality of life, and less positive treatment responses to medications alone (e.g., Steiner et al., 2017). Mood stabilizers may also be used, as comorbid bipolar II disorder is a frequent presentation that aligns with the emotional dysregulation underpinning

PTSD. The newer generation lamotrigine (Reid, Gitlin, & Altshuler, 2013) and gabapentin (Berlin, Butler, & Perloff, 2015) are more commonly used in clinical practice. One study examined the impact of combining two medication treatments targeting depression in those with PTSD and found improvements in the combined group that received sertraline plus mirtazapine, in comparison with sertraline alone, on depression symptoms (Schneier et al., 2015).

Pharmacotherapy for Co-Occurring Anxiety and Trauma-Related Disorders

Pharmacotherapy for anxiety is typically aimed at the primary symptoms of these disorders. Because the SSRIs have also been approved for use with both trauma-related and anxiety disorders (e.g., panic disorders, generalized anxiety), typically their selection would be a parsimonious, first-line treatment for individuals with comorbid anxiety and PTSD. Findings of a secondary anxiety disorder (in addition to PTSD and SUDs) do not suggest that treatment responses to sertraline are diminished because of the presence of the anxiety disorder per se (e.g., Labbate, Sonne, Randal, Anton, & Brady, 2004), although teasing out which comorbidity is most responsive to a specific pharmacologic agent is a research design challenge.

Although short acting antianxiety agents such as benzodiazepines (clonazepam, alprazolam, diazepam, and lorazepam) may also be employed, because of the abuse liability, caution about dosing and longer term use should be exercised (e.g., Bandelow et al., 2012). One large effectiveness study demonstrated significant benefits for anxiety and comorbid PTSD with an adaptive design intervention called Coordinated Anxiety Learning and Management, or CALM, which combined medication with CBT, and used a computer-assisted technology to facilitate delivery of CBT by health care managers who promoted adherence with medications collaterally with primary care practitioners (Roy-Byrne et al., 2010). Other avenues have included efforts to target the memory consolidation process in the immediate aftermath of acute exposure to a traumatic event with the beta blocker propranolol; while this seemed a promising pharmacologic target theoretically, it ultimately was not confirmed in clinical trials (Hoge et al., 2012). Similarly, efforts to impact fear conditioning and fear learning through administration of glutaminergic agents (d-cycloserine) with and without behavior therapy have had mixed results (e.g., de Kleine, Rothbaum, & van Minnen, 2013; Rothbaum et al., 2014). Overall, the past decade of findings suggest that the combined treatment of anxiety, trauma, and other comorbidities (such as SUDs) is clinically warranted and beneficial (Ruglass, Lopez-Castro, Cheref, Papini, & Hien, 2014). However, results of both psychotherapy and medication trials have been limited by the lack of clearly identified and understood mechanisms underlying this comorbidity (Baillie et al., 2010) and the documented heterogeneity of this population.

Based on the evidence to date, treatments should include a multimodal, problem-oriented approach focusing attention on individualized needs in the timing and sequencing of treatment services and the application of relevant treatment models.

Pharmacotherapy for Posttraumatic Stress Disorder and Psychotic Features

A recent systematic review of 24 published studies identified that rates of psychosis-related PTSD ranged from 11% to 67% (Berry, Ford, Jellicoe-Jones, & Haddock, 2013). If psychotic features are present, they may often appear in the context of a comorbid mood disorder, but may also be part of a severe persistent illness or even part of a paranoid personality disorder continuum (Grubaugh, Zinzow, Paul, Egede, & Frueh, 2011). Interventions with an atypical antipsychotic medication, such as risperidone, aripiprazole, quetiapine, or olanzapine, might be used along with other antidepressants or mood stabilizers. These "newer generation" antipsychotic medications can be particularly useful in treating the hyperarousal symptoms of PTSD that overlap with other disorders (Hien et al., 2009a). Used judiciously, antipsychotic medications can exert a nonaddictive, tranquilizing effect that clients report helps with sleeplessness, anxiety, and other symptoms. Long-term reliance on these medications should be cautioned, as the effects on health over time remain unknown.

Pharmacotherapy for Posttraumatic Stress Disorder and Sleep Disturbances

Many of the hallmark symptom clusters of PTSD impact sleep, leading to one of the more frequently discussed problems in the consulting room with patients who have trauma histories. Several of the symptom clusters of PTSD may interfere with sleep, including nightmares, night terrors, and autonomic hyperarousal, which is associated with a dysregulated HPA axis and manifested in symptoms of sympathetic arousal, irritability, and sensitivity to startle (Germain, 2013). In a secondary analysis of women in community treatment for PTSD and SUD, McHugh et al. (2014) reported results of high rates of residual sleep disorders, suggesting a need for targeted sleep interventions in this population. At present, most of the treatments in the area of sleep disturbances and trauma-related disorders are pharmacologic. Nonaddictive sleeping medications could be used to aid insomnia and should be considered carefully for short-term usage (Greenbaum, Neylan, & Rosen, 2017). Combining prazosin to address nightmares and insomnia with propranolol for emotional intensity of symptoms is another possible avenue of intervention for sleep disorders related to PTSD (Shad et al., 2011). Notably, sleep problems are one of the most reported reasons for nighttime cannabis use in those with PTSD (Bonn-Miller, Babson, & Vandrey, 2014), but although many patients with PTSD anecdotally may turn to medical cannabis to treat this aspect of their PTSD, there are currently mixed findings from the animal and human literatures (Babson, Sottile, & Morabito, 2017; Papini, Sullivan, Hien, Shvil, & Neria, 2015) to empirically support this form of self-medication.

We have reviewed a number of suggested treatment modalities that encompass behavioral/psychosocial intervention approaches in combination with medication for symptom reductions. In treating patients with PTSD and other comorbidities, clinicians must be vigilant in identifying and providing treatment for additional symptoms that often arise. Existing clinical trials and anecdotal reports provide agreement among clinicians that multimodal approaches, with clear symptom and syndrome targets and goals that take into consideration the full scope of problems faced by such clients, must be implemented for successful outcomes.

EMERGING TRENDS

Novel medication development for PTSD is evolving as more research accumulates on the complex psychopathology of PTSD, and neurobiological targets are identified in both preventative and treatment areas. Neurobiologic salient features of PTSD that are the target for several medications include HPA axis and locus coeruleus noradrenergic system (stress response system) dysfunction (Baker et al., 1999; Bremner et al., 1997). Novel medications that act on serotonergic, adrenergic, glutamatergic, GABAergic, and other mechanisms implicated in traumatic stress response, particularly pathways involved in fear learning and extinction, are important targets being investigated (Kolassa, Illek, Wilker, Karabatsiakis, & Elbert, 2015).

Glutamate transmission disruption, specifically NMDA receptor activity that affects learning and memory, has been implicated in PTSD. Several glutamate modulating compounds are currently being explored for the treatment of PTSD. N-acetylcysteine, an amino acid derivative supplement used for acetaminophen toxicity and as a mucolytic for chronic pulmonary conditions, restores drug-induced glutamatergic dysregulation and has shown some modest efficacy in reducing PTSD symptom severity in comorbid PTSD and SUD (Back et al., 2016). Ketamine, a glutamate NMDA receptor antagonist, has been explored as a rapid treatment for PTSD. In a preliminary proof of concept RCT, a single intravenous (IV) ketamine infusion (.5 mg/kg) versus IV midazolam (.045 mg/kg) administered to individuals with chronic PTSD resulted in a significant reduction in PTSD symptom severity at 24 hours and 7 days post infusion (Feder et al., 2014). Mild transient dissociative symptoms occurred in patients receiving the ketamine infusion. More well-designed research studies with larger sample sizes are needed to develop and validate new medications that can prevent development of PTSD, help understand mechanisms of action, and improve treatment outcomes.

Although pharmacological treatments for PTSD have been relatively well investigated, the evidence for treatment with comorbid SUDs and other mental health conditions is still emerging. Some clinical trials of novel agents currently underway at the time of this writing include (see www.clinicaltrials.gov for details, using the NCT numbers listed) combining prolonged exposure therapy with (a) oxytocin for PTSD (Flanagan, NCT03238924), (b) ketamine to promote rapid treatment for PTSD (Harpaz-Rotem, NCT02727998), and (c) d-cycloserine (a broad-spectrum antibiotic) as a cognitive enhancer (Difede, NCT00875342). Another trauma-focused therapy trial uses cognitive processing therapy combined with zonisamide (an anticonvulsant) for veterans with comorbid PTSD and alcohol or other drug use disorders (see Ralevski, Olivera-Figueroa, & Petrakis, 2014; Petrakis, NCT01847469). Finally, a study on the efficacy of brexpiprazole (an atypical antipsychotic) for monotherapy or combined with sertraline for PTSD (Otsuka Pharmaceutical Development, NCT03033069) is underway.

TOOL KIT OF RESOURCES

Acute Stress Disorder and Posttraumatic Stress Disorder

Provider Resources

American Psychological Association, Clinical Practice Guideline for the Treatment of PTSD: http://www.apa.org/ptsd-guideline/index.aspx

Assessment resources: https://www.ptsd.va.gov/professional/assessment/overview/index.asp

Cognitive Processing Therapy: https://cptforptsd.com

National Child Traumatic Stress Network: http://www.nctsn.org/

Pharmacotherapy for children and adolescents: https://www.uptodate.com/contents/pharmacotherapy-for-posttraumatic-stress-disorder-in-children-and-adolescents

Pharmacological treatment of acute stress reactions: https://www.ptsd.va.gov/professional/treatment/overview/pharmacological-treatment-stress.asp

Prolonged Exposure Therapy: http://pe.musc.edu/introduction

Published International Literature on Traumatic Stress (PILOTS Database): https://search.proquest.com/pilots/index?accountid=28179

Sign-up for Clinician's trauma update online: https://www.ptsd.va.gov/professional/publications/ctu-online.asp

Skills Training in Affect and Interpersonal Regulation (STAIR), Online Training: https://www.ptsd.va.gov/professional/continuing_ed/STAIR_online_training.asp

U.S. Department of Veteran's Affairs, National Center for PTSD: https://www.ptsd.va.gov/

VA/DoD Clinical Practice Guidelines for the Management of PTSD and Acute Stress Disorder: https://www.healthquality.va.gov/guidelines/MH/ptsd/

Patient Resources

American Psychiatric Association, What Is PTSD?: https://www.psychiatry.org/patients-families/ptsd/what-is-ptsd

American Psychological Association: http://www.apa.org/ptsd-guideline/patients-and-families/index.aspx

Mayo Clinic, What Is PTSD?: https://www.mayoclinic.org/diseases-conditions/post-traumatic-stress-disorder/diagnosis-treatment/drc-20355973

National Center for PTSD (for veterans, general public, family, and friends): https://www.ptsd.va.gov/public/index.asp

National Institute of Mental Health, What Is PTSD?: https://www.nimh.nih.gov/health/topics/post-traumatic-stress-disorder-ptsd/index.shtml

National Center for PTSD, Acute Stress Disorder: https://www.ptsd.va.gov/professional/treatment/early/acute-stress-disorder.asp

References

Abdallah, C. G., Southwick, S. M., & Krystal, J. H. (2017). Neurobiology of posttraumatic stress disorder (PTSD): A path from novel pathophysiology to innovative therapeutics. *Neuroscience Letters*, 649, 130–132. http://dx.doi.org/10.1016/j.neulet.2017.04.046

Åhs, F., Frick, A., Furmark, T., & Fredrikson, M. (2015). Human serotonin transporter availability predicts fear conditioning. *International Journal of Psychophysiology*, 98(3 Pt. 2), 515–519. http://dx.doi.org/10.1016/j.ijpsycho.2014.12.002

Alisic, E., Zalta, A. K., van Wesel, F., Larsen, S. E., Hafstad, G. S., Hassanpour, K., & Smid, G. E. (2014). Rates of post-traumatic stress disorder in trauma-exposed children and adolescents: Meta-analysis. *The British Journal of Psychiatry*, 204, 335–340. http://dx.doi.org/10.1192/bjp.bp.113.131227

American Psychiatric Association. (1963). *Diagnostic and statistical manual of mental disorders* (2nd ed.). Washington, DC: Author.

American Psychiatric Association. (1980). *Diagnostic and statistical manual of mental disorders* (3rd ed.). Washington, DC: Author.

*American Psychological Association. (2017). *Clinical practice guideline for the treatment of posttraumatic stress disorder (PTSD) in adults*. Retrieved from http://www.apa.org/ptsd-guideline/

Argolo, F. C., Cavalcanti-Ribeiro, P., Netto, L. R., & Quarantini, L. C. (2015). Prevention of posttraumatic stress disorder with propranolol: A meta-analytic review. *Journal of Psychosomatic Research*, 79, 89–93. http://dx.doi.org/10.1016/j.jpsychores.2015.04.006

Babson, K. A., Sottile, J., & Morabito, D. (2017). Cannabis, cannabinoids, and sleep: A review of the literature. *Current Psychiatry Reports*, 19, 23. http://dx.doi.org/10.1007/s11920-017-0775-9

Back, S. E., Brady, K. T., Sonne, S. C., & Verduin, M. L. (2006). Symptom improvement in co-occurring PTSD and alcohol dependence. *Journal of Nervous and Mental Disease*, 194, 690–696. http://dx.doi.org/10.1097/01.nmd.0000235794.12794.8a

Back, S. E., McCauley, J. L., Korte, K. J., Gros, D. F., Leavitt, V., Gray, K. M., . . . Brady, K. T. (2016). A double-blind, randomized, controlled pilot trial of N-Acetylcysteine in veterans with posttraumatic stress disorder and substance use disorders. *The Journal of Clinical Psychiatry*, 77, e1439. http://dx.doi.org/10.4088/JCP.15m10239

Baillie, A. J., Stapinski, L., Crome, E., Morley, K., Sannibale, C., Haber, P., & Teesson, M. (2010). Some new directions for research on psychological interventions for comorbid anxiety and substance use disorders. *Drug and Alcohol Review*, 29, 518–524. http://dx.doi.org/10.1111/j.1465-3362.2010.00206.x

Baker, D. G., West, S. A., Nicholson, W. E., Ekhator, N. N., Kasckow, J. W., Hill, K. K., . . . Geracioti, T. D., Jr. (1999). Serial CSF corticotropin-releasing hormone levels and adrenocortical activity in combat veterans with posttraumatic stress disorder. *The American Journal of Psychiatry*, 156(4), 585–588.

Bandelow, B., Sher, L., Bunevicius, R., Hollander, E., Kasper, S., Zohar, J., Möller, H.-J., the WFSBP Task Force on Mental Disorders in Primary Care, & the

*Asterisks indicate assessments or resources.

WFSBP Task Force on Anxiety Disorders, OCD and PTSD. (2012). Guidelines for the pharmacological treatment of anxiety disorders, obsessive-compulsive disorder and posttraumatic stress disorder in primary care. *International Journal of Psychiatry in Clinical Practice, 16*, 77–84. http://dx.doi.org/10.3109/13651501.2012.667114

Batki, S. L., Pennington, D. L., Lasher, B., Neylan, T. C., Metzler, T., Waldrop, A., . . . Herbst, E. (2014). Topiramate treatment of alcohol use disorder in veterans with posttraumatic stress disorder: A randomized controlled pilot trial. *Alcoholism: Clinical and Experimental Research, 38*, 2169–2177. http://dx.doi.org/10.1111/acer.12496

Bauer, M. S., Lee, A., Li, M., Bajor, L., Rasmusson, A., & Kazis, L. E. (2014). Off-label use of second generation antipsychotics for post-traumatic stress disorder in the Department of Veterans Affairs: Time trends and sociodemographic, comorbidity, and regional correlates. *Pharmacoepidemiology and Drug Safety, 23*, 77–86. http://dx.doi.org/10.1002/pds.3507

Bergiannaki, J. D., & Kostaras, P. (2016). Pharmacokinetic and pharmacodynamic effects of psychotropic medications: Differences between sexes. *Psychiatrike = Psychiatriki, 27*(2), 118–126.

Berlin, R. K., Butler, P. M., & Perloff, M. D. (2015). Gabapentin therapy in psychiatric disorders: A systematic review. *The Primary Care Companion for CNS Disorders, 17*(5). http://dx.doi.org/10.4088/PCC.15r01821

Bernardy, N. C., & Friedman, M. J. (2016). How and why does the pharmaceutical management of PTSD differ between men and women? *Expert Opinion on Pharmacotherapy, 17*, 1449–1451. http://dx.doi.org/10.1080/14656566.2016.1199686

Bernardy, N. C., Lund, B. C., Alexander, B., & Friedman, M. J. (2012). Prescribing trends in veterans with posttraumatic stress disorder. *The Journal of Clinical Psychiatry, 73*, 297–303. http://dx.doi.org/10.4088/JCP.11m07311

Bernardy, N. C., Lund, B. C., Alexander, B., Jenkyn, A. B., Schnurr, P. P., & Friedman, M. J. (2013). Gender differences in prescribing among veterans diagnosed with posttraumatic stress disorder. *Journal of General Internal Medicine, 28*(Suppl. 2), S542–S548. http://dx.doi.org/10.1007/s11606-012-2260-9

Berry, K., Ford, S., Jellicoe-Jones, L., & Haddock, G. (2013). PTSD symptoms associated with the experiences of psychosis and hospitalisation: A review of the literature. *Clinical Psychology Review, 33*, 526–538. http://dx.doi.org/10.1016/j.cpr.2013.01.011

Blain, L. M., Galovski, T. E., & Robinson, T. (2010). Gender differences in recovery from posttraumatic stress disorder: A critical review. *Aggression and Violent Behavior, 15*, 463–474. http://dx.doi.org/10.1016/j.avb.2010.09.001

*Blake, D. D., Weathers, F. W., Nagy, L. M., Kaloupek, D. G., Gusman, F. D., Charney, D. S., & Keane, T. M. (1995). The development of a clinician-administered PTSD scale. *Journal of Traumatic Stress, 8*, 75–90. http://dx.doi.org/10.1002/jts.2490080106

Blevins, C. A., Weathers, F. W., Davis, M. T., Witte, T. K., & Domino, J. L. (2015). The Posttraumatic Stress Disorder Checklist for DSM-5 (PCL-5): Development and initial psychometric evaluation. *Journal of Traumatic Stress, 28*, 489–498. http://dx.doi.org/10.1002/jts.22059

Bomyea, J., & Lang, A. J. (2012). Emerging interventions for PTSD: Future directions for clinical care and research. *Neuropharmacology, 62*, 607–616. http://dx.doi.org/10.1016/j.neuropharm.2011.05.028

Bonn-Miller, M. O., Babson, K. A., & Vandrey, R. (2014). Using cannabis to help you sleep: Heightened frequency of medical cannabis use among those with PTSD. *Drug and Alcohol Dependence, 136*, 162–165. http://dx.doi.org/10.1016/j.drugalcdep.2013.12.008

Brady, K., Pearlstein, T., Asnis, G. M., Baker, D., Rothbaum, B., Sikes, C. R., & Farfel, G. M. (2000). Efficacy and safety of sertraline treatment of posttraumatic stress disorder: A randomized controlled trial. *JAMA, 283*, 1837–1844. http://dx.doi.org/10.1001/jama.283.14.1837

Brady, K. T., Sonne, S., Anton, R. F., Randall, C. L., Back, S. E., & Simpson, K. (2005). Sertraline in the treatment of co-occurring alcohol dependence and posttraumatic stress disorder. *Alcoholism: Clinical and Experimental Research, 29*, 395–401. http://dx.doi.org/10.1097/01.ALC.0000156129.98265.57

Bremner, J. D., Licinio, J., Darnell, A., Krystal, J. H., Owens, M. J., Southwick, S. M., . . . Charney, D. S. (1997). Elevated CSF corticotropin-releasing factor concentrations in posttraumatic stress disorder. *The American Journal of Psychiatry, 154*, 624–629. http://dx.doi.org/10.1176/ajp.154.5.624

Breslau, N. (2009). The epidemiology of trauma, PTSD, and other posttrauma disorders. *Trauma, Violence, & Abuse, 10*, 198–210. http://dx.doi.org/10.1177/1524838009334448

Breslau, N., Kessler, R. C., Chilcoat, H. D., Schultz, L. R., Davis, G. C., & Andreski, P. (1998). Trauma and posttraumatic stress disorder in the community: The 1996 Detroit Area Survey of Trauma. *Archives of General Psychiatry, 55*, 626–632. http://dx.doi.org/10.1001/archpsyc.55.7.626

Brown, M. T., & Bussell, J. K. (2011). Medication adherence: WHO cares? *Mayo Clinic Proceedings, 86*, 304–314. http://dx.doi.org/10.4065/mcp.2010.0575

Bryant, R. A. (2017). Acute stress disorder. *Current Opinion in Psychology, 14*, 127–131. http://dx.doi.org/10.1016/j.copsyc.2017.01.005

Bryant, R. A., Creamer, M., O'Donnell, M., Silove, D., & McFarlane, A. C. (2012). The capacity of acute stress disorder to predict posttraumatic psychiatric disorders. *Journal of Psychiatric Research, 46*, 168–173. http://dx.doi.org/10.1016/j.jpsychires.2011.10.007

*Bryant, R. A., Harvey, A. G., Dang, S. T., & Sackville, T. (1998). Assessing acute stress disorder: Psychometric properties of a structured clinical interview. *Psychological Assessment, 10*, 215–220. http://dx.doi.org/10.1037/1040-3590.10.3.215

*Bryant, R. A., Moulds, M. L., & Guthrie, R. M. (2000). Acute Stress Disorder Scale: A self-report measure of acute stress disorder. *Psychological Assessment, 12*, 61–68. http://dx.doi.org/10.1037/1040-3590.12.1.61

Carta, M. G., Balestrieri, M., Murru, A., & Hardoy, M. C. (2009). Adjustment Disorder: Epidemiology, diagnosis and treatment. *Clinical Practice and Epidemiology in Mental Health, 5*, 15. http://dx.doi.org/10.1186/1745-0179-5-15

Chilcoat, H. D., & Breslau, N. (1998). Investigations of causal pathways between PTSD and drug use disorders. *Addictive Behaviors, 23*, 827–840. http://dx.doi.org/10.1016/S0306-4603(98)00069-0

Chopra, M. P., Zhang, H., Pless Kaiser, A., Moye, J. A., Llorente, M. D., Oslin, D. W., & Spiro, A., III. (2014). PTSD is a chronic, fluctuating disorder affecting the mental quality of life in older adults. *The American Journal of Geriatric Psychiatry, 22*, 86–97. http://dx.doi.org/10.1016/j.jagp.2013.01.064

Christiansen, D., & Elklit, A. (2012). *Sex Differences in PTSD*. London, United Kingdom: IntechOpen. http://dx.doi.org/10.5772/28363

Cohen, J. A., Bukstein, O., Walter, H., Benson, S. R., Chrisman, A., Farchione, T. R., . . . Medicus, J., & the AACAP Work Group On Quality Issues. (2010). Practice parameter for the assessment and treatment of children and adolescents with posttraumatic stress disorder. *Journal of the American Academy of Child & Adolescent Psychiatry, 49*, 414–430.

Cohen, J. A., Mannarino, A. P., Perel, J. M., & Staron, V. (2007). A pilot randomized controlled trial of combined trauma-focused CBT and sertraline for childhood PTSD symptoms. *Journal of the American Academy of Child & Adolescent Psychiatry, 46*, 811–819. http://dx.doi.org/10.1097/chi.0b013e3180547105

Cook, J., Simiola, V., & Brown, L. (2017). *Trauma and Posttraumatic Stress Disorder in Older Adults Fact Sheet*. Retrieved from https://www.apatraumadivision.org/633/resources-on-underserved-populations.html

Davidson, J., Pearlstein, T., Londborg, P., Brady, K. T., Rothbaum, B., Bell, J., . . . Farfel, G. (2003). Efficacy of sertraline in preventing relapse of posttraumatic stress disorder: Results of a 28-week double-blind, placebo-controlled study. *Focus (San Francisco, Calif.), 1*, 273–281.

Davidson, J., Rothbaum, B. O., Tucker, P., Asnis, G., Benattia, I., & Musgnung, J. J. (2006). Venlafaxine extended release in posttraumatic stress disorder: A sertraline- and placebo-controlled study. *Journal of Clinical Psychopharmacology, 26*, 259–267. http://dx.doi.org/10.1097/01.jcp.0000222514.71390.c1

Davidson, J. R. T., Book, S. W., Colket, J. T., Tupler, L. A., Roth, S., David, D., . . . Feldman, M. (1997). Assessment of a new self-rating scale for posttraumatic stress disorder. *Psychological Medicine, 27*, 153–160. Cambridge, England: Cambridge University Press.

de Kleine, R. A., Rothbaum, B. O., & van Minnen, A. (2013). Pharmacological enhancement of exposure-based treatment in PTSD: A qualitative review. *European Journal of Psychotraumatology, 4*, 21626. http://dx.doi.org/10.3402/ejpt.v4i0.21626

*Department of Veterans Affairs. (2017). *VA/DoD clinical practice guideline for the management of posttraumatic stress disorder and acute stress disorder*. Retrieved from https://www.healthquality.va.gov/guidelines/MH/ptsd/VADoDPTSDCPGFinal.pdf.

Elbogen, E. B., Norman, S., Schnurr, P. P., & Matteo, R. A. (2016). *Assessing risk of violence in individuals with PTSD*. Retrieved from https://www.ptsd.va.gov/professional/co-occurring/assessing_risk_violence_ptsd.asp

Farooq, S., & Naeem, F. (2014). Tackling nonadherence in psychiatric disorders: Current opinion. *Neuropsychiatric Disease and Treatment, 10*, 1069–1077. http://dx.doi.org/10.2147/NDT.S40777

Feder, A., Parides, M. K., Murrough, J. W., Perez, A. M., Morgan, J. E., Saxena, S., . . . Charney, D. S. (2014). Efficacy of intravenous ketamine for treatment of chronic posttraumatic stress disorder: A randomized clinical trial. *JAMA Psychiatry, 71*, 681–688. http://dx.doi.org/10.1001/jamapsychiatry.2014.62

Felmingham, K., Williams, L. M., Kemp, A. H., Liddell, B., Falconer, E., Peduto, A., & Bryant, R. (2010). Neural responses to masked fear faces: Sex differences and trauma exposure in posttraumatic stress disorder. *Journal of Abnormal Psychology, 119*, 241–247. http://dx.doi.org/10.1037/a0017551

Foa, E. B. (2011). Prolonged exposure therapy: Past, present, and future. *Depression and Anxiety, 28*(12), 1043–1047. http://dx.doi.org/10.1002/da.20907

Foa, E. B., Keane, T. M., & Friedman, M. J. (2003). Effective treatments for PTSD: Practice guidelines from the International Society for Traumatic Stress Studies. *Psycho-Oncology, 12*(1), 99–100.

Foa, E. B., Yusko, D. A., McLean, C. P., Suvak, M. K., Bux, D. A., Jr., Oslin, D., . . . Volpicelli, J. (2013). Concurrent naltrexone and prolonged exposure therapy for patients with comorbid alcohol dependence and PTSD: A randomized clinical trial. *JAMA, 310*, 488–495. http://dx.doi.org/10.1001/jama.2013.8268

Ford, J. D., & Courtois, C. A. (2009). Defining and understanding complex trauma and complex traumatic stress disorders. In C. A. Courtois & J. D. Ford (Eds.), *Treating complex traumatic stress disorders: An evidence-based guide* (pp. 13–30). New York, NY: Guilford Press.

*Friedman, M., & Davidson, J. (2014). Pharmacotherapy for PTSD. In M. Friedman, T. M. Keane, & P. Resnick (Eds.), *Handbook of PTSD: Science and practice* (2nd ed., pp. 482–501). New York, NY: Guilford Press.

Friedman, M. J. (2016). PTSD History and Overview. Retrieved from https://www.ptsd.va.gov/professional/PTSD-overview/ptsd-overview.asp

Germain, A. (2013). Sleep disturbances as the hallmark of PTSD: Where are we now? *The American Journal of Psychiatry*, *170*, 372–382. http://dx.doi.org/10.1176/appi.ajp.2012.12040432

Gibson, L. E. (2016). Acute Stress Disorder. Retrieved from https://www.ptsd.va.gov/professional/treatment/early/acute-stress-disorder.asp

Goldstein, R. B., Smith, S. M., Chou, S. P., Saha, T. D., Jung, J., Zhang, H., . . . Grant, B. F. (2016). The epidemiology of *DSM–5* posttraumatic stress disorder in the United States: Results from the National Epidemiologic Survey on Alcohol and Related Conditions-III. *Social Psychiatry and Psychiatric Epidemiology*, *51*, 1137–1148. http://dx.doi.org/10.1007/s00127-016-1208-5

Gray, M. J., Litz, B. T., Hsu, J. L., & Lombardo, T. W. (2004). Psychometric properties of the life events checklist. *Assessment*, *11*, 330–341. http://dx.doi.org/10.1177/1073191104269954

Greenbaum, M. A., Neylan, T. C., & Rosen, C. S. (2017). Symptom presentation and prescription of sleep medications for veterans with posttraumatic stress disorder. *Journal of Nervous and Mental Disease*, *205*(2), 112–118.

Grubaugh, A. L., Zinzow, H. M., Paul, L., Egede, L. E., & Frueh, B. C. (2011). Trauma exposure and post-traumatic stress disorder in adults with severe mental illness: A critical review. *Clinical Psychology Review*, *31*, 883–899. http://dx.doi.org/10.1016/j.cpr.2011.04.003

Haller, M., Myers, U. S., McKnight, A., Angkaw, A. C., & Norman, S. B. (2016). Predicting engagement in psychotherapy, pharmacotherapy, or both psycho-therapy and pharmacotherapy among returning veterans seeking PTSD treatment. *Psychological Services*, *13*, 341–348. http://dx.doi.org/10.1037/ser0000093

Hamilton, M. (1959). The assessment of anxiety states by rating. *British Journal of Medical Psychology*, *32*, 50–55. http://dx.doi.org/10.1111/j.2044-8341.1959.tb00467.x

Hamilton, M. (1960). A rating scale for depression. *Journal of Neurology, Neurosurgery, & Psychiatry*, *23*, 56–62. http://dx.doi.org/10.1136/jnnp.23.1.56

Hien, D. A., Jiang, H., Campbell, A. N. C., Hu, M. C., Miele, G. M., Cohen, L. R., . . . Nunes, E. V. (2010). Do treatment improvements in PTSD severity affect substance use outcomes? A secondary analysis from a randomized clinical trial in NIDA's Clinical Trials Network. *The American Journal of Psychiatry*, *167*, 95–101. http://dx.doi.org/10.1176/appi.ajp.2009.09091261

Hien, D. A., Levin, F. R., Ruglass, L., & Lopez-Castro, T. (2015). Enhancing the effects of cognitive behavioral therapy for PTSD and alcohol use disorders with antidepressant medication: A randomized clinical trial. *Drug and Alcohol Dependence*, *146*, e142. http://dx.doi.org/10.1016/j.drugalcdep.2014.09.303

Hien, D. A., Litt, L. C., Cohen, L. R., Miele, G. M., & Campbell, A. (2009a). *Trauma Services for Women in Substance Abuse Treatment: An Integrated Approach*. Washington, DC: American Psychological Association. http://dx.doi.org/10.1037/11864-000

Hien, D. A., Litt, L. C., Cohen, L. R., Miele, G. M., & Campbell, A. (2009b). Psychotherapy models and treatment considerations. In D. Hien, L. C. Litt, L. R. Cohen, G. M. Miele, & A. Campbell, *Trauma services for women in substance abuse treatment: An integrated approach* (pp. 19–35). Washington, DC: American Psychological Association. http://dx.doi.org/10.1037/11864-002

Hoge, E. A., Worthington, J. J., Nagurney, J. T., Chang, Y., Kay, E. B., Feterowski, C. M., . . . Pitman, R. K. (2012). Effect of acute posttrauma propranolol on PTSD outcome and physiological responses during script-driven imagery. *CNS Neuroscience & Therapeutics*, *18*, 21–27. http://dx.doi.org/10.1111/j.1755-5949.2010.00227.x

Huemer, J., Erhart, F., & Steiner, H. (2010). Posttraumatic stress disorder in children and adolescents: A review of psychopharmacological treatment. *Child Psychiatry and Human Development*, *41*, 624–640. http://dx.doi.org/10.1007/s10578-010-0192-3

Inslicht, S. S., Richards, A., Madden, E., Rao, M. N., O'Donovan, A., Talbot, L. S., . . . Neylan, T. C. (2014). Sex differences in neurosteroid and hormonal responses to metyrapone in posttraumatic stress disorder. *Psychopharmacology*, *231*, 3581–3595. http://dx.doi.org/10.1007/s00213-014-3621-3

Ipser, J. C., & Stein, D. J. (2012). Evidence-based pharmacotherapy of post-traumatic stress disorder (PTSD). *International Journal of Neuropsycho-pharmacology*, *15*, 825–840. http://dx.doi.org/10.1017/S1461145711001209

Irish, L. A., Fischer, B., Fallon, W., Spoonster, E., Sledjeski, E. M., & Delahanty, D. L. (2011). Gender differences in PTSD symptoms: An exploration of peritraumatic mechanisms. *Journal of Anxiety Disorders*, *25*, 209–216. http://dx.doi.org/10.1016/j.janxdis.2010.09.004

Jun, J. J., Zoellner, L. A., & Feeny, N. C. (2013). Sudden gains in prolonged exposure and sertraline for chronic PTSD. *Depression and Anxiety, 30*, 607–613. http://dx.doi.org/10.1002/da.22119

Kaczkurkin, A. N., Asnaani, A., Alpert, E., & Foa, E. B. (2016). The impact of treatment condition and the lagged effects of PTSD symptom severity and alcohol use on changes in alcohol craving. *Behaviour Research and Therapy, 79*, 7–14. http://dx.doi.org/10.1016/j.brat.2016.02.001

Keeshin, B. R., & Strawn, J. R. (2014). Psychological and pharmacologic treatment of youth with post-traumatic stress disorder: An evidence-based review. *Child and Adolescent Psychiatric Clinics of North America, 23*, 399–411, x. http://dx.doi.org/10.1016/j.chc.2013.12.002

Kendler, K. S., Bulik, C. M., Silberg, J., Hettema, J. M., Myers, J., & Prescott, C. A. (2000). Childhood sexual abuse and adult psychiatric and substance use disorders in women: An epidemiological and cotwin control analysis. *Archives of General Psychiatry, 57*, 953–959. http://dx.doi.org/10.1001/archpsyc.57.10.953

Kessler, R. C., Berglund, P., Demler, O., Jin, R., Merikangas, K. R., & Walters, E. E. (2005). Lifetime prevalence and age-of-onset distributions of *DSM–IV* disorders in the National Comorbidity Survey Replication. *Archives of General Psychiatry, 62*, 593–602. http://dx.doi.org/10.1001/archpsyc.62.6.593

Kessler, R. C., Sonnega, A., Bromet, E., Hughes, M., & Nelson, C. B. (1995). Posttraumatic stress disorder in the national comorbidity survey. *Archives of General Psychiatry, 52*, 1048–1060. http://dx.doi.org/10.1001/archpsyc.1995.03950240066012

Khachatryan, D., Groll, D., Booij, L., Sepehry, A. A., & Schütz, C. G. (2016). Prazosin for treating sleep disturbances in adults with posttraumatic stress disorder: A systematic review and meta-analysis of randomized controlled trials. *General Hospital Psychiatry, 39*, 46–52. http://dx.doi.org/10.1016/j.genhosppsych.2015.10.007

Kolassa, I. T., Illek, S., Wilker, S., Karabatsiakis, A., & Elbert, T. (2015). Neurobiological findings in post-traumatic stress disorder. In U. Schnyder & M. Cloitre (Eds.), *Evidence based treatments for trauma-related psychological disorders* (pp. 63–86). New York, NY: Springer.

Krystal, J. H., & Neumeister, A. (2009). Noradrenergic and serotonergic mechanisms in the neurobiology of posttraumatic stress disorder and resilience. *Brain Research, 1293*, 13–23. http://dx.doi.org/10.1016/j.brainres.2009.03.044

Labbate, L. A., Sonne, S. C., Randal, C. L., Anton, R. F., & Brady, K. T. (2004). Does comorbid anxiety or depression affect clinical outcomes in patients with post-traumatic stress disorder and alcohol use disorders? *Comprehensive Psychiatry, 45*, 304–310. http://dx.doi.org/10.1016/j.comppsych.2004.03.015

LaLumiere, R. T., McGaugh, J. L., & McIntyre, C. K. (2017). Emotional modulation of learning and memory: Pharmacological implications. *Pharmacological Reviews, 69*, 236–255. http://dx.doi.org/10.1124/pr.116.013474

Linehan, M. M. (2015). *DBT skills training manual.* New York, NY: Guilford Press.

Lockwood, A., Steinke, D. T., & Botts, S. R. (2009). Medication adherence and its effect on relapse among patients discharged from a Veterans Affairs posttraumatic stress disorder treatment program. *The Annals of Pharmacotherapy, 43*, 1227–1232. http://dx.doi.org/10.1345/aph.1M017

Londborg, P. D., Hegel, M. T., Goldstein, S., Goldstein, D., Himmelhoch, J. M., Maddock, R., . . . Farfel, G. M. (2001). Sertraline treatment of posttraumatic stress disorder: Results of 24 weeks of open-label continuation treatment. *The Journal of Clinical Psychiatry, 62*, 325–331. http://dx.doi.org/10.4088/JCP.v62n0503

López, C. M., Andrews, A. R., Chisolm, A. M., de Arellano, M. A., Saunders, B., & Kilpatrick, D. G. (2017). Racial/ethnic differences in trauma exposure and mental health disorders in adolescents. *Cultural Diversity and Ethnic Minority Psychology, 23*, 382–387. http://dx.doi.org/10.1037/cdp0000126

López-Castro, T., Hu, M. C., Papini, S., Ruglass, L. M., & Hien, D. A. (2015). Pathways to change: Use trajectories following trauma-informed treatment of women with co-occurring post-traumatic stress disorder and substance use disorders. *Drug and Alcohol Review, 34*, 242–251. http://dx.doi.org/10.1111/dar.12230

Madhusoodanan, S., Velama, U., Parmar, J., Goia, D., & Brenner, R. (2014). A current review of cytochrome P450 interactions of psychotropic drugs. *Annals of Clinical Psychiatry, 26*, 120–138.

Marshall, R. D., Beebe, K. L., Oldham, M., & Zaninelli, R. (2001). Efficacy and safety of paroxetine treatment for chronic PTSD: A fixed-dose, placebo-controlled study. *The American Journal of Psychiatry, 158*, 1982–1988. http://dx.doi.org/10.1176/appi.ajp.158.12.1982

McCauley, J. L., Killeen, T., Gros, D. F., Brady, K. T., & Back, S. E. (2012). Posttraumatic stress disorder and co-occurring substance use disorders: Advances in assessment and treatment. *Clinical Psychology: Science and Practice, 19*, 283–304. http://dx.doi.org/10.1111/cpsp.12006

McHugh, R. K., Hu, M.-C., Campbell, A. N. C., Hilario, E. Y., Weiss, R. D., & Hien, D. A. (2014). Changes in sleep disruption in the treatment of co-occurring posttraumatic stress disorder and substance use disorders. *Journal of Traumatic Stress, 27*, 82–89. http://dx.doi.org/10.1002/jts.21878

McLaughlin, K. A., Conron, K. J., Koenen, K. C., & Gilman, S. E. (2010). Childhood adversity, adult stressful life events, and risk of past-year psychiatric disorder: A test of the stress sensitization hypothesis in a population-based sample of adults. *Psychological Medicine, 40*, 1647–1658. http://dx.doi.org/10.1017/S0033291709992121

Mohamed, S., & Rosenheck, R. (2008). Pharmacotherapy for older veterans diagnosed with posttraumatic stress disorder in Veterans Administration. *The American Journal of Geriatric Psychiatry, 16*, 804–812. http://dx.doi.org/10.1097/JGP.0b013e318173f617

Morina, N., Koerssen, R., & Pollet, T. V. (2016). Interventions for children and adolescents with posttraumatic stress disorder: A meta-analysis of comparative outcome studies. *Clinical Psychology Review, 47*, 41–54. http://dx.doi.org/10.1016/j.cpr.2016.05.006

Morrison, J. A., Berenz, E. C., & Coffey, S. F. (2014). Exposure-based, trauma-focused treatment for comorbid PTSD-SUD. In P. Ouimette & J. P. Read (Eds.), *Trauma and substance abuse: Causes, consequences, and treatment of comorbid disorders* (pp. 253–279). Washington, DC: American Psychological Association. http://dx.doi.org/10.1037/14273-013

Moye, J., & Rouse, S. J. (2014). Posttraumatic stress in older adults: When medical diagnoses or treatments cause traumatic stress. *Clinics in Geriatric Medicine, 30*, 577–589. http://dx.doi.org/10.1016/j.cger.2014.04.006

Najavits, L. M., Hyman, S. M., Ruglass, L. M., Hien, D. A., & Read, J. P. (2017). Substance use disorder and trauma. In S. N. Gold (Ed.), *APA handbook of trauma psychology: Vol. 1. Foundations in knowledge* (pp. 195–213). Washington, DC: American Psychological Association. http://dx.doi.org/10.1037/0000019-012

Nash, M., Galatzer-Levy, I. R., Krystal, J. H., Duman, R., & Neumeister, A. (2014). Neurocircuitry and neuroplasticity in PTSD. In M. J. Freidman, T. M. Keane, & P. Resick (Eds.), *Handbook of PTSD: Science and practice* (2nd ed., pp. 251–274). New York, NY: Guilford Press.

National Collaborating Centre for Mental Health. (2005). *Post-traumatic stress disorder: The management of PTSD in adults and children in primary and secondary care.* Leicester, United Kingdom: Gaskell.

Neigh, G. N., Gillespie, C. F., & Nemeroff, C. B. (2009). The neurobiological toll of child abuse and neglect. *Trauma, Violence, & Abuse, 10*, 389–410. http://dx.doi.org/10.1177/1524838009339758

Nielsen, S., Larance, B., Degenhardt, L., Gowing, L., Kehler, C., & Lintzeris, N. (2016). Opioid agonist treatment for pharmaceutical opioid dependent people. *Cochrane Database of Systematic Reviews, 9*, CD011117. http://dx.doi.org/10.1002/14651858.CD011117.pub2

Nishith, P., Resick, P. A., & Griffin, M. G. (2002). Pattern of change in prolonged exposure and cognitive-processing therapy for female rape victims with posttraumatic stress disorder. *Journal of Consulting and Clinical Psychology, 70*, 880–886. http://dx.doi.org/10.1037/0022-006X.70.4.880

Norman, S. B., Myers, U. S., Wilkins, K. C., Goldsmith, A. A., Hristova, V., Huang, Z., . . . Robinson, S. K. (2012). Review of biological mechanisms and pharmacological treatments of comorbid PTSD and substance use disorder. *Neuropharmacology, 62*, 542–551. http://dx.doi.org/10.1016/j.neuropharm.2011.04.032

Olff, M., Langeland, W., Draijer, N., & Gersons, B. P. R. (2007). Gender differences in posttraumatic stress disorder. *Psychological Bulletin, 133*, 183–204. http://dx.doi.org/10.1037/0033-2909.133.2.183

Ouimette, P., Read, J. P., Wade, M., & Tirone, V. (2010). Modeling associations between posttraumatic stress symptoms and substance use. *Addictive Behaviors, 35*, 64–67. http://dx.doi.org/10.1016/j.addbeh.2009.08.009

Papini, S., Sullivan, G. M., Hien, D. A., Shvil, E., & Neria, Y. (2015). Toward a translational approach to targeting the endocannabinoid system in posttraumatic stress disorder: A critical review of preclinical research. *Biological Psychology, 104*, 8–18. http://dx.doi.org/10.1016/j.biopsycho.2014.10.010

Petrakis, I. L., Poling, J., Levinson, C., Nich, C., Carroll, K., Ralevski, E., & Rounsaville, B. (2006). Naltrexone and disulfiram in patients with alcohol dependence and comorbid post-traumatic stress disorder. *Biological Psychiatry, 60*, 777–783. http://dx.doi.org/10.1016/j.biopsych.2006.03.074

Petrakis, I. L., & Simpson, T. L. (2017). Posttraumatic stress disorder and alcohol use disorder: A critical review of pharmacologic treatments. *Alcoholism: Clinical and Experimental Research, 41*, 226–237. http://dx.doi.org/10.1111/acer.13297

Pietrzak, R. H., Goldstein, R. B., Southwick, S. M., & Grant, B. F. (2011). Prevalence and Axis I comorbidity of full and partial posttraumatic stress disorder in the United States: Results from Wave 2 of the National Epidemiologic Survey on Alcohol and Related Conditions. *Journal of Anxiety Disorders, 25*, 456–465. http://dx.doi.org/10.1016/j.janxdis.2010.11.010

Pietrzak, R. H., Goldstein, R. B., Southwick, S. M., & Grant, B. F. (2012). Psychiatric comorbidity of full and partial posttraumatic stress disorder among older adults in the United States: Results from wave 2 of the National Epidemiologic Survey on Alcohol and Related Conditions. *The American Journal of Geriatric Psychiatry, 20*, 380–390. http://dx.doi.org/10.1097/JGP.0b013e31820d92e7

Pimlott-Kubiak, S., & Cortina, L. M. (2003). Gender, victimization, and outcomes: Reconceptualizing risk. *Journal of Consulting and Clinical Psychology*, *71*, 528–539. http://dx.doi.org/10.1037/0022-006X.71.3.528

Pollack, M. H., Hoge, E. A., Worthington, J. J., Moshier, S. J., Wechsler, R. S., Brandes, M., & Simon, N. M. (2011). Eszopiclone for the treatment of posttraumatic stress disorder and associated insomnia: A randomized, double-blind, placebo-controlled trial. *The Journal of Clinical Psychiatry*, *72*, 892–897. http://dx.doi.org/10.4088/JCP.09m05607gry

Posner, K., Brown, G. K., Stanley, B., Brent, D. A., Yershova, K. V., Oquendo, M. A., . . . Mann, J. J. (2011). The Columbia-Suicide Severity Rating Scale: Initial validity and internal consistency findings from three multisite studies with adolescents and adults. *The American Journal of Psychiatry*, *168*, 1266–1277. http://dx.doi.org/10.1176/appi.ajp.2011.10111704

Prins, A., Bovin, M. J., Smolenski, D. J., Marx, B. P., Kimerling, R., Jenkins-Guarnieri, M. A., . . . Tiet, Q. Q. (2016). The Primary Care PTSD Screen for DSM–5 (PC-PTSD-5): Development and evaluation within a veteran primary care sample. *Journal of General Internal Medicine*, *31*, 1206–1211. http://dx.doi.org/10.1007/s11606-016-3703-5

Ralevski, E., Olivera-Figueroa, L. A., & Petrakis, I. (2014). PTSD and comorbid AUD: A review of pharmacological and alternative treatment options. *Substance Abuse and Rehabilitation*, *5*, 25–36.

Raskind, M. A. (2015). Prazosin for the treatment of PTSD. *Current Treatment Options in Psychiatry*, *2*, 192–203. http://dx.doi.org/10.1007/s40501-015-0040-y

Reid, J. G., Gitlin, M. J., & Altshuler, L. L. (2013). Lamotrigine in psychiatric disorders. *The Journal of Clinical Psychiatry*, *74*, 675–684. http://dx.doi.org/10.4088/JCP.12r08046

Robb, A. S., Cueva, J. E., Sporn, J., Yang, R., & Vanderburg, D. G. (2010). Sertraline treatment of children and adolescents with posttraumatic stress disorder: A double-blind, placebo-controlled trial. *Journal of Child and Adolescent Psychopharmacology*, *20*, 463–471. http://dx.doi.org/10.1089/cap.2009.0115

Robert, R., Tcheung, W. J., Rosenberg, L., Rosenberg, M., Mitchell, C., Villarreal, C., . . . Meyer, W. J., III. (2008). Treating thermally injured children suffering symptoms of acute stress with imipramine and fluoxetine: A randomized, double-blind study. *Burns*, *34*, 919–928. http://dx.doi.org/10.1016/j.burns.2008.04.009

Rodgman, C., Verrico, C. D., Holst, M., Thompson-Lake, D., Haile, C. N., De La Garza, R., II, . . . Newton, T. F. (2016). Doxazosin XL reduces symptoms of posttraumatic stress disorder in veterans with PTSD: A pilot clinical trial. *The Journal of Clinical Psychiatry*, *77*, e561–e565. http://dx.doi.org/10.4088/JCP.14m09681

Rothbaum, B. O., Davidson, J. R. T., Stein, D. J., Pedersen, R., Musgnung, J., Tian, X. W., . . . Baldwin, D. S. (2008). A pooled analysis of gender and trauma-type effects on responsiveness to treatment of PTSD with venlafaxine extended release or placebo. *The Journal of Clinical Psychiatry*, *69*, 1529–1539. http://dx.doi.org/10.4088/JCP.v69n1002

Rothbaum, B. O., Price, M., Jovanovic, T., Norrholm, S. D., Gerardi, M., Dunlop, B., . . . Ressler, K. J. (2014). A randomized, double-blind evaluation of D-cycloserine or alprazolam combined with virtual reality exposure therapy for posttraumatic stress disorder in Iraq and Afghanistan War veterans. *The American Journal of Psychiatry*, *171*, 640–648. http://dx.doi.org/10.1176/appi.ajp.2014.13121625

Roy-Byrne, P., Craske, M. G., Sullivan, G., Rose, R. D., Edlund, M. J., & Lang, A. J., . . . Stein, M. B. (2010). Delivery of evidence-based treatment for multiple anxiety disorders in primary care: A randomized controlled trial. *JAMA*, *303*, 1921–1928. http://dx.doi.org/10.1001/jama.2010.608

Ruglass, L. M., Lopez-Castro, T., Cheref, S., Papini, S., & Hien, D. A. (2014). At the crossroads: The intersection of substance use disorders, anxiety disorders, and posttraumatic stress disorder. *Current Psychiatry Reports*, *16*, 505. http://dx.doi.org/10.1007/s11920-014-0505-5

Schneier, F. R., Campeas, R., Carcamo, J., Glass, A., Lewis-Fernandez, R., Neria, Y., . . . Wall, M. M. (2015). Combined mirtazapine and SSRI treatment of PTSD: A placebo-controlled trial. *Depression and Anxiety*, *32*, 570–579. http://dx.doi.org/10.1002/da.22384

Semla, T. P., Lee, A., Gurrera, R., Bajor, L., Li, M., Miller, D. R., . . . Bauer, M. S. (2017). Off-label prescribing of second-generation antipsychotics to elderly veterans with posttraumatic stress disorder and dementia. *Journal of the American Geriatrics Society*, *65*, 1789–1795. http://dx.doi.org/10.1111/jgs.14897

Shad, M. U., Suris, A. M., & North, C. S. (2011). Novel combination strategy to optimize treatment for PTSD. *Human Psychopharmacology: Clinical and Experimental*, *26*, 4–11. http://dx.doi.org/10.1002/hup.1171

Sijbrandij, M., Kleiboer, A., Bisson, J. I., Barbui, C., & Cuijpers, P. (2015). Pharmacological prevention of post-traumatic stress disorder and acute stress disorder: A systematic review and meta-analysis. *The Lancet Psychiatry*, *2*, 413–421. http://dx.doi.org/10.1016/S2215-0366(14)00121-7

Smith, K. Z., Smith, P. H., Violanti, J. M., Bartone, P. T., & Homish, G. G. (2015). Posttraumatic stress disorder symptom clusters and perpetration of intimate partner violence: Findings from a U.S. nationally representative sample. *Journal of Traumatic Stress*, *28*, 469–474. http://dx.doi.org/10.1002/jts.22048

Sofuoglu, M., Rosenheck, R., & Petrakis, I. (2014). Pharmacological treatment of comorbid PTSD and substance use disorder: Recent progress. *Addictive Behaviors, 39*, 428–433. http://dx.doi.org/10.1016/j.addbeh.2013.08.014

Sonne, C., Carlsson, J., Elklit, A., Mortensen, E. L., & Ekstrøm, M. (2013). Treatment of traumatized refugees with sertraline versus venlafaxine in combination with psychotherapy: Study protocol for a randomized clinical trial. *Trials, 14*, 137. http://dx.doi.org/10.1186/1745-6215-14-137

Steckler, T., & Risbrough, V. (2012). Pharmacological treatment of PTSD: Established and new approaches. *Neuropharmacology, 62*, 617–627. http://dx.doi.org/10.1016/j.neuropharm.2011.06.012

Steiner, A. J., Boulos, N., Mirocha, J., Wright, S. M., Collison, K. L., & IsHak, W. W. (2017). Quality of life and functioning in comorbid posttraumatic stress disorder and major depressive disorder after treatment with citalopram monotherapy. *Clinical Neuropharmacology, 40*, 16–23.

Strawn, J. R., Keeshin, B. R., DelBello, M. P., Geracioti, T. D., Jr., & Putnam, F. W. (2010). Psychopharmacologic treatment of posttraumatic stress disorder in children and adolescents: A review. *The Journal of Clinical Psychiatry, 71*, 932–941. http://dx.doi.org/10.4088/JCP.09r05446blu

Sugarman, M. A., Loree, A. M., Baltes, B. B., Grekin, E. R., & Kirsch, I. (2014). The efficacy of paroxetine and placebo in treating anxiety and depression: A meta-analysis of change on the Hamilton Rating Scales. *PLoS One, 9*, e106337. http://dx.doi.org/10.1371/journal.pone.0106337

Taylor, D. L., & Laraia, M. T. (2009). Psychopharmacology. In G. W. Stuart (Ed.), *Principles and practices of psychiatric nursing* (9th ed., pp. 500–534). St. Louis, Missouri: Mosby.

Taylor, S., Abramowitz, J. S., & McKay, D. (2012). Non-adherence and non-response in the treatment of anxiety disorders. *Journal of Anxiety Disorders, 26*, 583–589. http://dx.doi.org/10.1016/j.janxdis.2012.02.010

Tolin, D. F., & Foa, E. B. (2006). Sex differences in trauma and posttraumatic stress disorder: A quantitative review of 25 years of research. *Psychological Bulletin, 132*, 959–992. http://dx.doi.org/10.1037/0033-2909.132.6.959

U.S. Department of Veterans Affairs & U.S. Department of Defense. (2004). *VA/DoD clinical practice guideline for the management of post-traumatic stress, 1.0.* Washington, DC: Authors.

U.S. Department of Veterans Affairs & U.S. Department of Defense. (2017). *VA/DoD clinical practice guideline for the management of posttraumatic stress disorder and acute stress disorder, version 3.0.* Washington, DC: Authors. Retrieved from https://www.healthquality.va.gov/guidelines/MH/ptsd/VADoDPTSDCPGFinal012418.pdf

van Dam, D., Vedel, E., Ehring, T., & Emmelkamp, P. M. G. (2012). Psychological treatments for concurrent posttraumatic stress disorder and substance use disorder: A systematic review. *Clinical Psychology Review, 32*, 202–214. http://dx.doi.org/10.1016/j.cpr.2012.01.004

van Servellen, G., Heise, B. A., & Ellis, R. (2011). Factors associated with antidepressant medication adherence and adherence-enhancement programmes: A systematic literature review. *Mental Health in Family Medicine, 8*(4), 255–271.

Villarreal, G., Hamner, M. B., Cañive, J. M., Robert, S., Calais, L. A., Durklaski, V., . . . Qualls, C. (2016). Efficacy of quetiapine monotherapy in posttraumatic stress disorder: A randomized, placebo-controlled trial. *The American Journal of Psychiatry, 173*, 1205–1212. http://dx.doi.org/10.1176/appi.ajp.2016.15070967

*Weathers, F. W., Blake, D. D., Schnurr, P. P., Kaloupek, D. G., Marx, B. P., & Keane, T. M. (2013a). *The Clinician-Administered PTSD Scale for DSM–5 (CAPS-5).* Retrieved from https://www.ptsd.va.gov/professional/assessment/adult-int/caps.asp

*Weathers, F. W., Blake, D. D., Schnurr, P. P., Kaloupek, D. G., Marx, B. P., & Keane, T. M. (2013b). *The Life Events Checklist for DSM–5 (LEC-5).* Retrieved from https://www.ptsd.va.gov/professional/assessment/te-measures/life_events_checklist.asp

Weathers, F. W., Keane, T. M., & Davidson, J. R. T. (2001). Clinician-administered PTSD scale: A review of the first ten years of research. *Depression and Anxiety, 13*, 132–156. http://dx.doi.org/10.1002/da.1029

Wilker, S., Pfeiffer, A., Kolassa, S., Koslowski, D., Elbert, T., & Kolassa, I.-T. (2015). How to quantify exposure to traumatic stress? Reliability and predictive validity of measures for cumulative trauma exposure in a post-conflict population. *European Journal of Psychotraumatology, 6*, 28306. http://dx.doi.org/10.3402/ejpt.v6.28306

Yeh, M. S. L., Mari, J. J., Costa, M. C. P., Andreoli, S. B., Bressan, R. A., & Mello, M. F. (2011). A double-blind randomized controlled trial to study the efficacy of topiramate in a civilian sample of PTSD. *CNS Neuroscience & Therapeutics, 17*, 305–310. http://dx.doi.org/10.1111/j.1755-5949.2010.00188.x

Young-Wolff, K. C., Kendler, K. S., Ericson, M. L., & Prescott, C. A. (2011). Accounting for the association between childhood maltreatment and alcohol-use disorders in males: A twin study. *Psychological Medicine, 41*, 59–70. http://dx.doi.org/10.1017/S0033291710000425

CHAPTER 14

PHARMACOLOGICAL TREATMENT OF SLEEP–WAKE DISORDERS

Emmanuel H. During and Clete A. Kushida

Per the *International Classification of Sleep Disorders* (3rd ed.; ICSD–3), sleep–wake disorders encompass more than 90 classified sleep disorders organized in six broad categories: insomnias, hypersomnias (including narcolepsy), sleep-related breathing disorders (including obstructive sleep apnea [OSA]), circadian rhythm sleep–wake disorders (e.g., advanced sleep phase, delayed sleep phase, jet lag disorder), parasomnias (including sleepwalking, nightmare disorder, and rapid eye movement sleep behavior disorder [RBD]), and sleep-related movement disorders (including restless-legs syndrome [RLS]; American Academy of Sleep Medicine, 2014). The *Diagnostic and Statistical Manual of Mental Disorders* (5th ed.; *DSM–5*), in turn, lists 10 disorders or disorder groups: insomnia disorder, hypersomnolence disorder, narcolepsy, breathing-related sleep disorders, circadian rhythm sleep–wake disorders, non–rapid eye movement (NREM) sleep arousal disorders, nightmare disorder, RBD, RLS, and substance/medication-induced sleep disorder (American Psychiatric Association, 2013). These disorders have heterogeneous pathophysiology and treatments, many of which are nonpharmacological. In addition, some of these disorders, such as hypersomnia disorders, are rarely encountered outside a sleep medicine clinic. Discussing the management of all sleep–wake disorders is beyond the scope of this chapter; instead, we focus on the pharmacological treatment of insomnia, a common sleep disorder that is often associated with psychiatric disorders. However, we begin by reviewing the main characteristics and treatments of other sleep–wake disorders, directing the interested reader to previously published work and online references.

Hypersomnia disorders, including narcolepsy, are a heterogeneous group of disorders in which the core symptom is excessive daytime sleepiness (abnormal propensity to fall asleep), as measured by the Epworth Sleepiness Scale (Johns, 1991) and objectively demonstrated during the multiple sleep latency test (MSLT). During the MSLT, a participant is given the opportunity to nap every 2 hours during daytime in the laboratory setting; an average latency to sleep onset of less than 8 minutes is considered abnormally short. Among disorders of hypersomnia, narcolepsy is the best understood, resulting from the selective loss of hypocretin (also called orexin) neurons in the hypothalamus. Hypocretin/orexin is a major wake-promoting neurotransmitter and also a modulator of rapid eye movement (REM) sleep. This explains why sleepiness is a major symptom of narcolepsy, and most other symptoms result from the disinhibition and intrusion of REM sleep features into wakefulness: cataplexy attacks (sudden loss of muscle tone triggered by laughter or other strong emotions), scary dream-like hallucinations before falling sleep (hypnagogic hallucinations) or after waking up (hypnopompic hallucinations), and distressful episodes of sleep paralysis (transient

http://dx.doi.org/10.1037/0000133-014
APA Handbook of Psychopharmacology, S. M. Evans (Editor-in-Chief)

state of complete muscle paralysis although a person is fully awake). REM sleep propensity is also demonstrated on the MSLT and even on overnight polysomnography, showing rapid onset of REM sleep during any sleep period. Other than sodium oxybate (or γ-hydroxybutyric acid [GHB], marketed in the United States as Xyrem®), a potent central nervous system (CNS) depressant and promoter of deep slow-wave sleep specifically used in narcolepsy, pharmacological treatment of hypersomnias relies on wake-promoting and CNS stimulants, including drugs such as modafinil (Provigil®)—a mild dopamine reuptake antagonist—methylphenidate (e.g., Ritalin®), and various combinations of amphetamine salts (e.g., Adderall®, Dexedrine®, Desoxyn®), causing release of dopamine and noradrenaline in the synaptic cleft. The interested reader is invited to find further information in a recent review (Malhotra & Kushida, 2013).

Sleep-related breathing disorders include various disorders with different pathophysiology, implications, and treatments. The most common of them is OSA, a condition resulting in periodic upper airway obstruction during sleep, causing sleep disruption and decreases in oxygen blood levels (hypoxia). Although OSA is suspected based on body habitus and a history of snoring, witnessed apnea, and excessive daytime sleepiness—which can be conveniently screened by nonspecialists with the STOP-Bang Questionnaire and the Berlin Questionnaire (Ahmadi, Chung, Gibbs, & Shapiro, 2008; Chung et al., 2008)—the diagnosis requires a polysomnography recording, which can be done either in the ambulatory or laboratory setting. The treatment of OSA generally involves a device delivering continuous positive airway pressure (CPAP) during sleep via a nasal mask. Alternative treatments include custom-made oral appliances and specific surgeries of the upper airway. We refer the interested reader to a recent review for an overview of this condition (Foldvary-Schaefer & Waters, 2017).

Circadian rhythm sleep disorders result from the misalignment between actual sleep and wake phases and either one's internal clock (i.e., endogenous circadian rhythm, regulated by the suprachiasmatic nucleus of the hypothalamus) or external cues (i.e., exogenous rhythms, or *zeitgebers* ["time givers"],

imposed by light, work schedule, or social demand). The treatment of circadian rhythm sleep disorders frequently hinges on the *entrainment* of a person's endogenous rhythm using bright light or melatonin at specific times of the day or night. For instance, light exposure early during the wake phase results in advancing the sleep phase, as opposed to light exposure late in the wake phase up to bedtime, which delays the sleep phase. Pharmacotherapy of circadian rhythm sleep disorders is nearly limited to melatonin, which, when administered several hours before desired bedtime, can advance the sleep phase. We refer the reader to a comprehensive review and recent guidelines for further information on circadian rhythm sleep disorders (Auger et al., 2015; Zee, Attarian, & Videnovic, 2013).

Parasomnias are defined as undesirable physical events or experiences during entry into sleep, within sleep, or during arousal from sleep. They have a wide range of manifestations and medical implications. NREM parasomnias manifest as episodes of confusion and inappropriate behaviors arising from deep sleep lasting seconds to minutes, more often occurring in the first third of the night. These episodes can take the form of simple confusional arousals, sudden panic-like incoherent spells in the case of sleep terrors, or more elaborate and prolonged behaviors leading to ambulation (in the case of sleepwalking, also known as somnambulism) or eating during sleep (in sleep-related eating disorder). They are generally followed by rapid return to sleep with subsequent partial or complete amnesia. NREM parasomnias are very common (especially in childhood) and tend to cluster in genetically predisposed families, but can also be triggered or aggravated by an underlying sleep disorder such as OSA or RLS. In most cases, these parasomnias remain benign, are relatively infrequent, do not result in injuries, and improve or resolve with nonpharmacological measures emphasizing a consistent sleep hygiene and avoidance of precipitants such as alcohol or sedative drugs. RBD, in turn, consists of abnormal dream enactment potentially leading to serious injuries to self or bed partner. RBD often presages neurodegenerative disorders such as Parkinson's disease or dementia with Lewy bodies by several years. RBD can also be precipitated by antidepressants. RBD requires the implementation of effective safety measures, and violent behaviors generally reduce with melatonin or clonazepam (Klonopin®). Nightmares are vivid dreams provoking fear or anxiety. Although they are part of the spectrum of normal human experience and usually benign, nightmares, when they become excessively frequent or disturbing, can result in significant distress and impaired function. A number of prescription drugs can provoke nightmares, including antidepressants. Other than prazosin, which can be effective in the treatment of posttraumatic stress disorder–related nightmares (see Chapter 13, this volume), no treatment has shown consistent effectiveness. We direct the reader to recent reviews on parasomnias (Iranzo, Santamaria, & Tolosa, 2016; Irfan, Schenck, & Howell, 2017).

Sleep-related movement disorders are exemplified by RLS, which is defined as an unpleasant, often "creepy," "crawly" sensation and, in particular, an urge to move the legs, which is worse at rest or occurs exclusively at night, interfering with sleep or daytime function, and is temporarily relieved by movement. The diagnosis of RLS is based on history alone, and scales such as the 10-item International Restless Legs Scale (Walters et al., 2003) can be used to grade and monitor symptom severity. RLS is a very common disorder commonly misdiagnosed as insomnia. Symptoms of RLS tend to manifest or worsen when a person's iron stores are low, and tend to be aggravated by most psychotropic drugs. First-line pharmacotherapy of RLS consists of $\alpha_2\delta$ calcium channel agents such as gabapentin, pregabalin, or gabapentin enacarbil (sold under the brand names Neurontin®, Lyrica®, and Horizant®, respectively), while, preferably, dopaminergic agonists (e.g., pramipexole [Mirapex®]) should be used intermittently. Opioid analgesics (e.g., oxycodone and methadone) remain the treatment of choice in chronic refractory cases. We direct the reader to a recent review and some guidelines for the diagnosis and treatment of RLS (Garcia-Borreguero et al., 2016; Trenkwalder, Winkelmann, Inoue, & Paulus, 2015).

EPIDEMIOLOGY AND PREVALENCE

Insomnia is defined by the *DSM–5* as dissatisfaction with one's sleep quantity or quality that results in clinically significant distress or impairment in social, occupational, or other important areas of functioning. Depending on the timing of difficulty sleeping, insomnia is divided into three subtypes: initiation (difficulty falling asleep), maintenance (undesirable periods of arousals in the middle of the night), or late insomnia (awakening earlier than desired wake time with inability to fall back asleep). Maintenance insomnia is the most common subtype, although in practice, patients often have a combination of them (Winkelman, 2015). In children and the elderly requiring a caretaker, insomnia may present with resistance to going to bed on an appropriate schedule. Chronic insomnia, defined as occurring at least 3 days a week for more than 3 months, is estimated to affect up to 22.1% of the U.S. population, or 70.7 million individuals (Roth et al., 2011), with one third of adults in Western countries experiencing weekly difficulties with sleep initiation, maintenance, or nonrestorative sleep (LeBlanc et al., 2009; Morphy, Dunn, Lewis, Boardman, & Croft, 2007; Stein, Belik, Jacobi, & Sareen, 2008). Insomnia has a crippling impact on U.S. work productivity, with estimated annual losses in work performance of 252.7 million days and $63.2 billion (Kessler et al., 2011). Insomnia has been shown to be more prevalent in women (sex ratio 1.4:1) and in the elderly, affecting between 40% and 50% of the elderly population (Bloom et al., 2009; Budhiraja, Roth, Hudgel, Budhiraja, & Drake, 2011; Mellinger, Balter, & Uhlenhuth, 1985).

Although formalized cognitive behavior therapy for insomnia (CBT-I) has in the last 10 years become the standard of care in the management of chronic insomnia (Espie, Inglis, Tessier, & Harvey, 2001; Trauer, Qian, Doyle, Rajaratnam, & Cunnington, 2015), pharmacological treatments have been used for decades and continue to be widely prescribed alone or in conjunction with CBT-I. Opioids, alcohol, and various herbal preparations have been used as sedatives for centuries; in the early 20th century barbiturates and related compounds were the first sleep-inducing drugs manufactured. Strongly binding to the gamma-aminobutyric acid class A ($GABA_A$) receptors, a major sleep-inducing pathway, barbiturates have fallen out of favor over the past century due to their narrow therapeutic index and serious side effects, including potential for abuse and fatal overdoses. The first benzodiazepines (BZs) were introduced on the U.S. market in 1963. This new class of sedatives and anxiolytics also binds to the GABA$_A$ receptor, but at a different site. They started to be widely used in various indications, including for anxiety, seizures, alcohol withdrawal states, and other states of psychomotor agitation, in addition to insomnia. After an acceleration of benzodiazepine prescriptions in the 1960s and 1970s, prescriptions significantly declined until the 1990s due to growing concerns over their potential for tolerance and dependence. Physicians started to prescribe sedating antidepressants off-label, particularly trazodone (Desyrel®). Zolpidem (Ambien®) became available in 1992, and was the first so-called nonbenzodiazepine GABA$_A$ receptor agonist (nBZ), soon followed by two other "Z-drugs," zaleplon (Sonata®) and zopiclone, manufactured in the United States as its enantiomer eszopiclone (Lunesta®). While the Z-drugs have continued to be widely used, several new classes of hypnotics have become available in the last decade, including the melatonin receptor agonist ramelteon (Rozerem®) and the dual hypocretin/orexin receptor antagonist suvorexant (Belsomra®; see Table 14.1).

DIAGNOSING INSOMNIA

The diagnosis of insomnia requires a thorough clinical interview. Additionally, self-administered sleep logs and diaries will provide information about a person's insomnia based on their own estimation of sleep latency (time elapsed before falling asleep), wake time during the middle or end of the night, total sleep time, and rating of overall sleep quality. The Structured Clinical Interview for DSM–5 Sleep Disorders (SCISD; Taylor et al., 2018), the Insomnia Severity Index (ISI; Bastien, Vallières, & Morin, 2001), or standardized sleep questionnaires such as the Pittsburgh Sleep Quality Index (Buysse et al., 1989) are also useful tools for diagnosing and evaluating the severity of insomnia, its impact on someone's daytime functioning, and treatment response over time (Edinger et al., 2015).

The history should include the identification of possible psychological and environmental triggers precipitating and perpetuating insomnia in addition to past and current pharmacological and

nonpharmacological treatments, including their efficacy and side effects. It is important to note that the diagnosis of insomnia should only be made if conditions for achieving adequate sleep quality and quantity are met, such as sufficient time allotted for sleep and a comfortable sleep environment. Daytime functioning is affected by insomnia, and should be systematically assessed pretreatment and posttreatment; symptoms include fatigue; subjective sleepiness; impaired attention, concentration, and memory; mood and somatic complaints; and impairment in professional and social functioning. Insomnia can mimic or be comorbid with other sleep disorders. OSA is highly prevalent and can mimic or contribute to the complaint of insomnia, particularly in women (Subramanian et al., 2011), in whom it often presents without snoring and can be aggravated by BZs. RLS also contributes to or mimics insomnia and should therefore be recognized, as hypnotic treatments can worsen or complicate RLS, as discussed later in this chapter.

EVIDENCE-BASED PHARMACOLOGICAL TREATMENTS OF INSOMNIA

The pharmacological approach to insomnia relies on two sets of pathways: inhibition of the arousal circuits—mediated by histamine, dopamine, norepinephrine, and serotonin (5-HT), known as the monoaminergic system, in addition to acetylcholine, hypocretin/orexin, and glutamate—or activation of sleep-inducing circuits, mostly GABAergic and melatonergic pathways.

Pharmacological agents currently approved by the U.S. Food and Drug Administration (FDA) include five classes: BZs, nBZs (GABAergic drugs), melatonin receptor agonists, doxepin (antihistaminic), and suvorexant (hypocretin/orexin antagonist). Many off-label drugs are prescribed for insomnia, with the same level of evidence as FDA-approved drugs, per the American Academy of Sleep Medicine (AASM) Clinical Practice Guidelines (Schutte-Rodin, Broch, Buysse, Dorsey, & Sateia, 2008): these include various BZs (e.g., lorazepam [Ativan®], clonazepam [Klonopin]), sedating antidepressants (e.g., trazodone, mirtazapine [Remeron®], amitriptyline [Elavil®]), antipsychotics (olanzapine [Zyprexa®],

TABLE 14.1

U.S. FDA-Approved Hypnotic Agents for the Treatment of Chronic Initiation and/or Maintenance Insomnia

Drug	Common brand name (U.S.)	Dosage	Onset of action	Elimination half-life	Common side effects	U.S. Drug Enforcement Administration schedule	U.S. FDA pregnancy category
Nonbenzodiazepine GABA_A receptor agonists							
zaleplon	Sonata®	5–10 mg	very rapid	1 h	headache, paresthesia, nausea	IV	C
zolpidem (sublingual)	Intermezzo®	1.75–3.52 mg	very rapid	2–3 h	amnesia, headache, nausea	IV	C
zolpidem	Ambien®	5–10 mg	rapid	2–3 h	NREM parasomnias, amnesia, headache, nausea	IV	C
zolpidem (extended release)	Ambien CR	6.25–12.5 mg	rapid	3 h	NREM parasomnias, amnesia, headache, nausea	IV	C
eszopiclone	Lunesta®	1–3 mg	rapid	6 h	unpleasant (metallic) taste, headache	IV	C
Benzodiazepine GABA_A receptor agonists							
triazolam	Halcion®	0.125–0.25 mg	very rapid	2–4 h	headache, nausea	IV	X
temazepam	Restoril®	7.5–30 mg	rapid	4–20 h	hangover effect	IV	X
estazolam	ProSom®	1–2 mg	intermediate	10–24 h	hangover effect	IV	X
quazepam	Doral®	7.5–15 mg	rapid	40–70 h	daytime sedation, headache	IV	X
flurazepam	Dalmane®	15–30 mg	rapid	48–120 h	daytime sedation	IV	X
Melatonin receptor agonist							
ramelteon	Rozerem®	8 mg	very rapid	1–2.6 h	well tolerated	none	C
H_1 receptor antagonist tricyclic antidepressant							
doxepin	Silenor®	3–6 mg	intermediate	15 h	nausea, upper respiratory infections	none	C
Orexin/hypocretin receptor antagonist							
suvorexant	Belsomra®	5–20 mg	rapid	12 h	hypnagogic/hypnopompic hallucinations, headache	IV	C

Note. Drugs are organized by pharmacological class/mechanism of action, and for each class by shorter to longer elimination half-life and duration of action. All hypnotics can result in side effects of excessive sedation and daytime grogginess and dizziness; these generic side effects have not been listed in this table. Instead, specific or other common side effects are listed for each agent, when shown to occur significantly more often than with placebo. CR = controlled (extended) release; Drug Enforcement Administration schedule IV = low potential for abuse; GABA_A = gamma-aminobutyric acid class A; NREM = non–rapid eye movement; pregnancy category C = risk not ruled out: animal reproduction studies have shown an adverse effect on the fetus and there are no adequate and well-controlled studies in humans, but potential benefits may warrant use of the drug in pregnant women despite potential risks; pregnancy category X = contraindicated in pregnancy: studies in animals or humans have demonstrated fetal abnormalities and/or there is positive evidence of human fetal risk; U.S. FDA = U.S. Food and Drug Administration.

quetiapine [Seroquel®]), and the $\alpha_2\delta$ ligands of the calcium channel gabapentin (Neurontin). In addition, many patients self-medicate with over-the-counter melatonin and antihistaminic agents, such as diphenhydramine (Benadryl®, also contained in Tylenol® PM) and doxylamine succinate (Unisom®). Given the wide use of these off-label and over-the-counter treatments, in this chapter we attempt to cover the most common ones and some specific issues related to their use. Important aspects in the choice of an agent include desired onset of action, elimination half-life, and differences in metabolic clearance, in addition to the particular characteristics of a patient's insomnia (see Table 14.1). For a comprehensive review of the literature on the evidence for sedative-hypnotic drugs, we refer the reader to the Practice Guidelines recently published by the AASM (Sateia, Buysse, Krystal, Neubauer, & Heald, 2017).

Benzodiazepine and Nonbenzodiazepine GABA$_A$ Receptor Agonists

BZ and nBZ GABA$_A$ receptor agonists are among the most prescribed drugs for insomnia (Gottesmann, 2002; Sanger, 2004). Their efficacy relies on the potent inhibitory effect of GABAergic neurons projecting from the median ventrolateral preoptic nucleus of the hypothalamus to all wake-promoting structures, resulting in a relative "switch off" of the arousal system (Suntsova, Szymusiak, Alam, Guzman-Marin, & McGinty, 2002; Takahashi, Lin, & Sakai, 2009). Due to their higher pharmacological selectivity, nBZs are often preferred over BZs as first-line agents. Certain nBZs are available in fast (sublingual) or sustained release (controlled release [CR] or extended release [ER]) formulations, when rapid onset of action (for pure initiation insomnia or occasional middle of the night use) or prolonged duration of action is desired, respectively (see Table 14.1). By default, prescribers should first consider a short- to intermediate-acting BZ or nBZ agent, which is less likely to cause daytime adverse effects.

Doxepin

Doxepin is a tricyclic antidepressant (TCA). At the low dose recommended for insomnia (6 mg and less),

doxepin induces sleep via selective histamine-1 (H$_1$) receptor blockade, with four times the potency of amitriptyline and 800 times the potency of diphenhydramine. Its long elimination half-life of 15 hours makes it an appropriate treatment for maintenance insomnia; however, its slow onset of action is not suited for treating initiation insomnia (see Table 14.1; Atkin, Comai, & Gobbi, 2018; Yeung, Chung, Yung, & Ng, 2015).

Ramelteon

Ramelteon is a melatonin-1 and -2 (MT$_1$ and MT$_2$) receptor agonist. It has higher affinity than melatonin itself for these receptors that control various aspects of NREM and REM sleep. Ramelteon, like melatonin, inhibits the arousal-promoting effect of the suprachiasmatic nucleus—a purposeful arousal effect in the evening hours when accumulated fatigue and subsequent sleep drive reach their maximum. Its effect on the MT$_1$ receptor facilitates sleep initiation; the MT$_2$ receptor is more involved in circadian regulation. Ramelteon has shown to decrease sleep latency by a few minutes, although it does not appear to significantly increase total sleep time (Kuriyama, Honda, & Hayashino, 2014). This modest net effect on sleep parameters may result from partially opposing effects of MT$_1$ and MT$_2$ on sleep (Atkin et al., 2018). With a relatively short elimination half-life (1–2.6 hours), ramelteon remains a suitable agent for initiation insomnia.

Suvorexant

Suvorexant is an orexin-1 and -2 (OX$_1$ and OX$_2$) receptor antagonist. It induces sedation via the inhibition of the wake-promoting neurotransmitter hypocretin/orexin, which inhibits REM sleep and is also a potent enhancer of the arousal system (de Lecea et al., 1998). Hypocretin/orexin deficiency is implicated in the pathogenesis of narcolepsy. Inhibition of OX$_2$ receptors may have the most important role in promoting sleep, while inhibition of OX$_1$ may only produce a mild additive effect. With an intermediate half-life elimination of 12 hours, suvorexant is an appropriate treatment for both initiation and maintenance insomnia. Suvorexant is contraindicated in narcolepsy, as it may worsen preexisting symptoms (e.g., sleep paralyses, sleep-related hallucinations).

Off-label Sedating Prescription Drugs

Off-label sedating prescription drugs are often used as hypnotics. These include antidepressants (trazodone, mirtazapine, amitriptyline), gabapentin, and certain antipsychotics (quetiapine, olanzapine).

The most widely prescribed antidepressant for treating insomnia is trazodone, a serotonin antagonist and reuptake inhibitor (SARI), which at low doses (25–150 mg) induces sleep via selective H_1, noradrenergic α_1, and $5\text{-}HT_{2A}$ blockade; inhibition of serotonin reuptake is only achieved at higher doses (Stahl, 2013). The $5\text{-}HT_{2A}$ receptors are present in the GABAergic cells of the thalamus that promote sleep over wakefulness (RodríGuez, Noristani, Hoover, Linley, & Vertes, 2011). Mirtazapine is another antidepressant used at low doses at bedtime to induce sleepiness via H_1 and $5\text{-}HT_{2A}$ blockade. Finally, low doses of sedative TCAs such as amitriptyline are also commonly used to treat insomnia in selected patients, such as those with chronic pain or those requiring migraine prevention treatment. TCAs induce sleepiness via H_1, M_1 muscarinic, and $5\text{-}HT_{2A}$ receptor blockade. For more information on the effectiveness of TCAs for insomnia, we refer the reader to a recent meta-analysis by Liu and colleagues (Liu, Xu, Dong, Jia, & Wei, 2017).

Gabapentin (Neurontin) is a commonly used antiepileptic, antinociceptive, and psychotropic drug, used off-label in the treatment of maintenance insomnia (Lo et al., 2010); it enhances deep sleep and shortens sleep latency. Binding at the $\alpha_2\delta$ subunit of the presynaptic voltage-gated calcium channel, gabapentin modulates the synthesis of GABA and glutamate and reduces the action of excitatory neurotransmitters overall.

Various antipsychotics such as quetiapine (Seroquel) and olanzapine (Zyprexa) have been used in selected cases of refractory insomnia, due to their sedative properties via H_1, M_1 muscarinic, and α_1 blockade (Tassniyom, Paholpak, Tassniyom, & Kiewyoo, 2010). Quetiapine has primarily sleep-inducing properties at low doses of 50 mg and less,

whereas it has mood and antipsychotic properties at moderate and higher doses, respectively.

BEST APPROACHES FOR ASSESSING TREATMENT RESPONSE AND MANAGING SIDE EFFECTS

Treatment effectiveness and ongoing indication should be reevaluated on a regular basis via clinical interviews, supported by quantitative longitudinal measures (sleep logs/diaries, the ISI, Pittsburgh Sleep Quality Index) at each visit. Each follow-up evaluation should include the assessment of daytime functioning, and monitor for the emergence of side effects (Edinger et al., 2015). A number of side effects can occur with any hypnotic and thus need to be watched for systematically: residual morning sedation, dizziness and impaired balance, nausea or other gastrointestinal symptoms, headaches, nightmares or unpleasant dreams, amnesia, confusion, and occasionally depression.

Residual morning grogginess is more likely to occur with agents with a long elimination half-life, such as long-acting BZs or nBZs (eszopiclone) or antidepressant agents (doxepin, trazodone, miratazapine, amitriptyline), but can usually be mitigated by reducing the dose of the hypnotic used or by slightly advancing the nighttime dosing. Due to the longer duration of action of eszopiclone (*S* enantiomer of zopiclone, available outside the United States) potentially resulting in driving hazard the next morning, the FDA issued a safety communication recommending that the lowest (1 mg) dose be tried first. Conversely, insufficient clinical efficacy toward the end of the night can result in excessively early morning awakenings, which may resolve after switching to an agent with a longer duration of action.

Z-drugs and BZ agents considered as a class can result in complex nocturnal behaviors with subsequent amnesia: sleepwalking, eating behaviors, or complex episodes with medicolegal complications (Gunja, 2013; Pressman, 2011). It has been shown that this risk is particularly high in patients with undiagnosed or untreated RLS (Howell & Schenck, 2012; Provini et al., 2009).

Ramelteon is metabolized via the hepatic CYP1A2 enzymatic pathway, which is inhibited by fluvoxamine

(Luvox®), a selective serotonin reuptake inhibitor (SSRI) antidepressant; therefore these drugs should not be prescribed together.

Although suvorexant is more effective at higher doses, due to safety concerns over residual morning sedation, the maximum FDA approved dose is 20 mg (Patel, Aspesi, & Evoy, 2015; Vermeeren et al., 2015). Other potential side effects with suvorexant may include sleep-related hallucinations. The risk of sleep paralyses or cataplexy is low, although this remains a potential concern with suvorexant.

Due to their usually long half-life, antihistaminic drugs (doxepin, mirtazapine, olanzapine) can cause nausea and weight gain with prolonged use, in addition to residual sedation (hangover feeling). Although the underlying mechanism is not elucidated, olanzapine significantly increases cardiovascular risk via insulin resistance and hypertriglyceridemia.

Anticholinergic (antimuscarinic) side effects associated with TCAs (particularly amitriptyline) and over-the-counter sleeping aids (diphenhydramine and doxylamine) include confusion, memory loss, blurry vision, urinary retention, and constipation. Although doxepin is a TCA, it has antimuscarinic effects only at the high doses used for depression (100–150 mg), not at the low dose approved for insomnia (3–6 mg). Trazodone increases the risk of priapism (Rhodes, 2001).

Gabapentin can result in weight gain and extremity edema. The initial concern over risk of iatrogenic depression has been challenged by some higher quality evidence that gabapentin may have a neutral or favorable effect on mood (Gibbons, Hur, Brown, & Mann, 2010).

MEDICATION MANAGEMENT ISSUES

Current guidelines favor short-term over long-term use of hypnotics for insomnia, emphasizing the importance of addressing all comorbid conditions and factors that may perpetuate insomnia. Long-term hypnotic treatments should be reserved for refractory cases, including those for which CBT-I was not effective (Schutte-Rodin et al., 2008). Although most patients report continuing benefit after several weeks, there is currently insufficient evidence to determine and compare the long-term effective-

ness of pharmacotherapies for insomnia (Wilt et al., 2016). In practice, however, all hypnotic drugs, when used on a daily basis, may lead to pharmacological tolerance due to receptor adaptation, inclining some prescribers and patients to rotate hypnotics according to a weekly or daily schedule or to limit their use to 3 or 4 nights weekly (Buysse, Rush, & Reynolds, 2017).

Among hypnotics, risk of tolerance may be higher with BZs compared with nBZs (Vinkers & Olivier, 2012; Zammit, McNabb, Caron, Amato, & Roth, 2004), as well as with antihistamine sedatives (Richardson, Roehrs, Rosenthal, Koshorek, & Roth, 2002). BZs and to some extent nBZs hypnotics also present a higher risk of abuse compared with other pharmacotherapies (Griffiths & Johnson, 2005). In this regard, they are both U.S. Drug Enforcement Administration Schedule IV controlled substances. Abrupt cessation of BZ can result in withdrawal anxiety and seizures, while discontinuation of any hypnotic can result in transient rebound insomnia, and more commonly to a return of prior insomnia (Schutte-Rodin et al., 2008). In this respect, the remission rate of insomnia is particularly low when insomnia is comorbid to a medical or psychiatric condition (Pillai et al., 2016). Although there may be less concern over tolerance, risk of abuse potential, and dependence compared with BZ, suvorexant is also a Schedule IV substance. In contrast, ramelteon and doxepin are not known to present any abuse potential.

EVALUATION OF PHARMACOLOGICAL APPROACHES ACROSS THE LIFESPAN

The FDA recommends lower doses in the elderly than in the younger adult population, due to the risk of excessive sedation, falls, and confusion. Although CBT-I is recommended as the standard of care in all adults with chronic insomnia (Qaseem et al., 2016; Schutte-Rodin et al., 2008), including in the elderly (Bloom et al., 2009; Gooneratne & Vitiello, 2014), CBT-I may not be an appropriate choice for individuals with dementia. Hypnotic drugs are therefore often needed to improve sleep in the elderly.

The overall evidence and guidelines on sedative hypnotics in the elderly are somewhat scarce and conflicting. The American Geriatrics Society (AGS) recommends a limited course of nBZ or melatonin receptor agonists but advises against most other options, including antihistaminic and anticholinergic agents (Bloom et al., 2009; Gooneratne & Vitiello, 2014). In this regard, melatonin receptor agonists may provide further benefit in the case of insomnia associated with an abnormal sleep–wake cycle, as commonly seen in the elderly. The American College of Physicians (ACP), in turn, suggests that there is overall higher quality evidence regarding suvorexant and low-dose doxepin (6 mg and below) compared with other drugs in the elderly. A pooled analysis from five double-blind trials using suvorexant against placebo in the elderly showed that when given for 3 consecutive months, suvorexant had no additional risk of falls, a minimally increased rate of reported somnolence (5.4% vs. 3.2% for 15 mg suvorexant dose and placebo, respectively), and no effect on early morning psychomotor performance (Herring et al., 2017). Highest level of concern in the elderly arises from the potential harm of anticholinergic drugs. A systematic review and meta-analysis including more than 124,000 elderly individuals demonstrated an increase in the odds of cognitive impairment with anticholinergic agents, while olanzapine and trazodone were associated with an increased risk of falls (Ruxton, Woodman, & Mangoni, 2015). In contrast, according to the 2015 Beers Criteria issued by the AGS, low-dose doxepin is deemed to not result in such anticholinergic effects (The American Geriatrics Society 2015 Beers Criteria Update Expert Panel, 2015). The use of BZ and nBZ drugs in the elderly is also associated with an important safety concern due to the risk of falls and the possible long-term worsening of cognitive outcomes. A study in young healthy adults demonstrated that zolpidem was associated with imbalance during middle of the night awakenings, while no differences were detected between doxepin and placebo (Drake et al., 2017), a finding that raises even further concern in the elderly population. Although the exact mechanism needs to be understood, evidence suggests that prolonged regular use of BZs and possibly nBZs may be associated with an increased risk of dementia with a cumulative dose-dependent relationship (Billioti de Gage et al.,

2014; Gallacher et al., 2012; Wu, Wang, Chang, & Lin, 2009). Despite a possible increased risk of falls based on one study (Ruxton et al., 2015), trazodone could be an acceptable option in patients with Alzheimer's dementia and insomnia. In a study including 36 elderly participants receiving either 50 mg of trazodone or placebo, Camargos et al. demonstrated that trazodone improved subjective and objective sleep parameters without causing cognitive side effects (Camargos et al., 2014).

Altogether, based on the previously presented evidence and guidelines, we would favor the use of non-GABAergic and nonanticholinergic drugs in the elderly population when chronic sedative treatments are needed, while the choice of a specific agent should depend on a patient's individual characteristics.

There are no FDA-approved hypnotics and no guidelines for the pharmacotherapy of pediatric insomnia, which highlights the importance of developing clinical trials and recommendations (Mindell et al., 2006). Off-label drugs commonly used in children have included melatonin and over-the-counter antihistaminic agents (Owens & Moturi, 2009). Melatonin was shown to be effective in children with autism and attention-deficit/hyperactivity disorder (ADHD; Andersen, Kaczmarska, McGrew, & Malow, 2008; Van der Heijden, Smits, Van Someren, Ridderinkhof, & Gunning, 2007), while guanfacin (Tenex®), a noradrenergic α_2 agonist, may also be considered in those with ADHD (Biederman et al., 2008).

CONSIDERATION OF POTENTIAL SEX DIFFERENCES

In 2013, the FDA recommended that women be prescribed lower doses of zolpidem compared with men, based on reports of increased residual morning sedation (U.S. Food and Drug Administration, 2013). In fact, zolpidem metabolism results in slower clearance in women compared with men for the same dose, which warrants using lower doses in women (typically 5 mg instead of 10 mg). The FDA warning was issued almost 20 years after zolpidem came on the market, demonstrating that in general, little is known regarding sex differences in pharmacokinetics and bioavailability of hypnotics. It should be noted that, except for benzodiazepines, which are all FDA pregnancy Category X (contraindicated in pregnancy), all FDA-approved hypnotics are pregnancy Category C (potential risk of malformation; see Table 14.1).

INTEGRATION OF PHARMACOTHERAPY WITH NONPHARMACOLOGICAL APPROACHES: BENEFITS AND CHALLENGES

The ACP and the AASM emphasize behavioral interventions or comprehensive CBT-I as the standard of care and first-line therapy in the treatment of chronic insomnia for all adult age groups, including in patients using hypnotics (Qaseem et al., 2016; Schutte-Rodin et al., 2008). CBT-I provides reliable and durable benefits in about 70% to 80% of patients (Trauer et al., 2015). It has been shown that short-term nBZ, CBT-I, or a combination of both yield equivalent efficacy; however CBT-I alone and maintenance CBT-I may provide better long-term benefit (Beaulieu-Bonneau, Ivers, Guay, & Morin, 2017; Morin et al., 2009; Morin, Colecchi, Stone, Sood, & Brink, 1999). Limitations of in-person CBT-I include patient adherence and access to providers. For those without access to a provider in their area, online self-guided automated programs present convenient and effective alternatives (Gosling et al., 2014; Lancee, Eisma, van Straten, & Kamphuis, 2015; Van der Zweerde et al., 2016). For a few examples of these online CBT-I programs, we refer the reader to the Tool Kit of Resources at the end of this chapter.

INTEGRATED APPROACHES FOR ADDRESSING COMMON COMORBID DISORDERS

Fifty percent to 80% of adult patients with a psychiatric disorder, particularly those with depression and general anxiety disorder, experience symptoms of insomnia (Krystal, 2012; Ohayon, 2002; Seow et al., 2018). On the other hand, most medications used for the treatment of depression or anxiety disorders (notably SSRIs) can have deleterious effects on sleep, more often in the form of insomnia and

disturbed dreams (DeMartinis & Winokur, 2007). When comorbid with major depressive disorder (see Chapter 7, this volume), insomnia may herald other depressive symptoms (Perlis, Giles, Buysse, Tu, & Kupfer, 1997). Insomnia may also persist as a residual symptom of otherwise treated depression, increasing risk for suicide and relapse (Ağargün, Kara, & Solmaz, 1997). Psychiatric disorders have been known to have a bidirectional relationship with insomnia, as illustrated by the fact that treatment of insomnia independently improves psychiatric treatment outcomes (Fava et al., 2011). As a result, the *DSM–5* abolished the distinction between "primary" and "secondary" insomnia, calling for the independent clinical importance of insomnia regardless of a coexisting mental condition.

In addition to their indication in insomnia, BZs have been used in a wide range of clinical settings for their anxiolytic, antiepileptic, and even myorelaxant properties. This contrasts with nBZs although BZ and nBZ drugs bind at the same receptors between the γ and α subunits; nBZs such as zolpidem (Ambien) and zaleplon (Sonata) have greater selectivity for the $\alpha 1$ subunit, and eszopiclone (Lunesta) for the $\alpha 3$ subunit, of the $GABA_A$ receptor, neither of which are known to result in anxiolytic or myorelaxant effects.

As discussed above, OSA is commonly associated with insomnia (Krakow, Ulibarri, Romero, & McIver, 2013). In such cases, outcomes are optimized when both conditions are addressed and treated effectively (Guilleminault, Davis, & Huynh, 2008).

Chronic pain (see Chapter 19, this volume) and insomnia are commonly associated as they, too, have a bidirectional relationship. A number of drugs can improve pain control while reducing symptoms of insomnia. These include gabapentin and some TCAs (amitriptyline, nortriptyline [Pamelor™]). Gabapentin has additional benefit with regard to anxiety and RLS symptoms (Berlin, Butler, & Perloff, 2015).

EMERGING TRENDS

As mentioned, online self-guided automated CBT-I programs present convenient and effective alternatives to face-to-face sessions with behavioral sleep medicine specialists, especially since the number of such specialists do not, at the present time, meet the demand (Edinger, 2009; Manber et al., 2012).

With respect to pharmacotherapies, several unexplored pharmacological pathways hold promises for the development of new drugs, such as adenosine receptor inhibitors and casein kinase inhibitors (for review, see Atkin et al., 2018). In addition, several compounds binding to specific sets of receptors, or receptor subtypes, are under investigation. These include drugs specifically binding to the MT_1 receptor thought to be less likely to alter sleep architecture while promoting sleep onset. Complementing the currently available drug suvorexant, several selective (OX_2) or dual (OX_1 and OX_2) orexin receptor antagonists such as almorexant are under development, and may soon become additional options for the elderly with insomnia (Roth et al., 2017). Piromelatin, owing to a unique mechanism of action, agonist at the MT_1 and MT_2 and $5\text{-}HT_{1A}$ and $5\text{-}HT_{1D}$ receptors, was shown to improve sleep parameters in Phase I and II trials and is currently being investigated in patients with mild Alzheimer's disease. Finally, a novel antipsychotic agent, lumateperone, due to a strong and selective $5\text{-}HT_{2A}$-blocking property at low dose, may become an interesting new hypnotic agent (Atkin et al., 2018).

Transcranial magnetic stimulation (Jiang, Zhang, Yue, Yi, & Gao, 2013) and frontal cerebral thermal therapy (Roth et al., 2018) also have recently shown promising results, although further data is needed to confirm the effectiveness of these interventions.

TOOL KIT OF RESOURCES

Insomnia Disorders

Patient Resources

American Academy of Sleep Medicine, Sleep Education: Insomnias: http://sleepeducation.org/ sleep-disorders-by-category/insomnias

National Sleep Foundation, Insomnia: https:// sleepfoundation.org/sleep-disorders-problems

World Sleep Foundation, About: Insomnia: http://worldsleepfoundation.org/insomnia

Online Cognitive Behavioral Therapy for Insomnia, SHUTi: http://www.myshuti.com/

Online Cognitive Behavioral Therapy for Insomnia, Sleepio: https://www.sleepio.com/

Provider Resources

Clinical Practice Guideline for the Pharmacologic Treatment of Chronic Insomnia in Adults: An American Academy of Sleep Medicine Clinical Practice Guideline: http://jcsm.aasm.org/ ViewAbstract.aspx?pid=30954

Clinical Guideline for the Evaluation and Management of Chronic Insomnia in Adults: http:// jcsm.aasm.org/viewabstract.aspx?pid=27286

Agency for Healthcare Research and Quality, Effective Health Care Program, Management of Insomnia Disorder: https://www.effectivehealthcare.ahrq.gov/ topics/insomnia/research

Hypersomnolence and Narcolepsy Disorder

Patient Resources

Narcolepsy Network: https://narcolepsynetwork.org/

Hypersomnia Foundation: http://www.hypersomnia-foundation.org/

American Academy of Sleep Medicine, Sleep Education: Narcolepsy: http://sleepeducation.org/ essentials-in-sleep/narcolepsy

National Sleep Foundation, Excessive Daytime Sleepiness Disorder: https://sleepfoundation.org/ category/excessive-daytime-sleepiness-disorders

World Sleep Foundation, About: Excessive Sleep Disorder: http://worldsleepfoundation.org/ excessive-sleep-disorder

Provider Resources

Practice Parameters for the Treatment of Narcolepsy and Other Hypersomnias of Central Origin: https://aasm.org/clinical-resources/ practice-standards/practice-guidelines/

Circadian Rhythm Sleep–Wake Disorder

Patient Resources

American Academy of Sleep Medicine, Sleep Education: Circadian Rhythm Disorders: http:// sleepeducation.org/sleep-disorders-by-category/ circadian-rhythm-disorders

National Sleep Foundation, Circadian Rhythm Sleep
Disorders: https://sleepfoundation.org/category/
circadian-rhythm-disorders

Provider Resources

Clinical Practice Guideline for the Treatment of
Intrinsic Circadian Rhythm Sleep–Wake Disorders:
An Update for 2015: http://jcsm.aasm.org/
ViewAbstract.aspx?pid=30219

Clinical Practice Guideline for the Treatment
of Extrinsic Circadian Rhythm Sleep–Wake
Disorders: https://aasm.org/clinical-resources/
practice-standards/practice-guidelines/

Non–Rapid Eye Movement Sleep Arousal Disorders

Patient Resources

American Academy of Sleep Medicine, Sleep
Education: Parasomnias: http://sleepeducation.org/
sleep-disorders-by-category/parasomnias

National Sleep Foundation, Abnormal Sleep Behavior
Disorders: https://sleepfoundation.org/category/
abnormal-sleep-behavior

Provider Resources

Irfan, M., Schenck, C. H., & Howell, M. J. (2017).
Non–rapid eye movement sleep and overlap
parasomnias. *Continuum: Lifelong Learning in
Neurology, 23,* 1035–1050. http://dx.doi.org/
10.1212/CON.0000000000000503

Nightmare Disorder

Provider Resources

Best Practice Guide for the Treatment of Nightmare
Disorder in Adults (2010): http://jcsm.aasm.org/
viewabstract.aspx?pid=27883

Rapid Eye Movement (REM) Sleep Behavior Disorders

Patient Resources

American Academy of Sleep Medicine, Sleep
Education: REM Sleep Behavior Disorder: http://
sleepeducation.org/sleep-disorders-by-category/
parasomnias/rem-sleep-behavior-disorder

National Sleep Foundation, Abnormal Sleep Behavior
Disorder: https://sleepfoundation.org/category/
abnormal-sleep-behavior

Provider Resources

Best Practice Guide for the Treatment of REM Sleep
Behavior Disorder: http://jcsm.aasm.org/
viewabstract.aspx?pid=27717

Restless Legs Syndrome

Patient Resources

Restless Legs Syndrome Foundation: https://www.rls.org/

National Sleep Foundation—Abnormal Sleep
Behavior Disorders: https://sleepfoundation.org/
sleep-disorders-problems/restless-legs-syndrome

Provider Resources

Garcia-Borreguero, D., Silber M. H., Winkelman J. W.,
Högl, B., Bainbridge, J., Buchfuhrer, M., . . . Allen, R. P.
(2016). Guidelines for the first-line treatment of restless legs syndrome/Willis–Ekbom disease, prevention and treatment of dopaminergic augmentation:
A combined task force of the IRLSSG, EURLSSG,
and the RLS-foundation. *Sleep Medicine, 21,* 1–11.
http://dx.doi.org/10.1016/j.sleep.2016.01.017

Winkelman, J. W., Armstrong, M. J., Allen, R. P.,
Chaudhuri, K. R., Ondo, W., Trenkwalder, C., . . .
Zesiewicz, T. (2016). Practice guideline summary:
Treatment of restless legs syndrome in adults—
Report of the Guideline Development, Dissemination,
and Implementation Subcommittee of the
American Academy of Neurology. *Neurology,
87,* 2585–2593. http://dx.doi.org/10.1212/
WNL.0000000000003388

References

Ağargün, M. Y., Kara, H., & Solmaz, M. (1997). Sleep
disturbances and suicidal behavior in patients with
major depression. *The Journal of clinical psychiatry, 58,* 249–51. http://www.ncbi.nlm.nih.gov/
pubmed/9228889

Ahmadi, N., Chung, S. A., Gibbs, A., & Shapiro, C. M.
(2008). The Berlin Questionnaire for Sleep Apnea in
a sleep clinic population: Relationship to polysomnographic measurement of respiratory disturbance. *Sleep
and Breathing, 12,* 39–45. http://dx.doi.org/10.1007/
s11325-007-0125-y

American Academy of Sleep Medicine. (2014). *International
Classification of Sleep Disorders (ICSD-3): Diagnostic*

*Asterisks indicate assessments or resources.

and Coding Manual (3rd ed). Westchester, IL: American Academy of Sleep Medicine.

American Psychiatric Association. (2013). *Diagnostic and statistical manual of mental disorders* (5th ed.). Washington, DC: Author.

Andersen, I. M., Kaczmarska, J., McGrew, S. G., & Malow, B. A. (2008). Melatonin for insomnia in children with autism spectrum disorders. *Journal of Child Neurology, 23*, 482–485. http://dx.doi.org/10.1177/0883073807309783

Atkin, T., Comai, S., & Gobbi, G. (2018). Drugs for insomnia beyond benzodiazepines: Pharmacology, clinical applications, and discovery. *Pharmacological Reviews, 70*, 197–245. http://dx.doi.org/10.1124/pr.117.014381

Auger, R. R., Burgess, H. J., Emens, J. S., Deriy, L. V., Thomas, S. M., & Sharkey, K. M. (2015). Clinical Practice Guideline for the Treatment of Intrinsic Circadian Rhythm Sleep–Wake Disorders. *Journal of Clinical Sleep Medicine, 11*, 1199–1236. http://dx.doi.org/10.5664/jcsm.5100

*Bastien, C. H., Vallières, A., & Morin, C. M. (2001). Validation of the Insomnia Severity Index as an outcome measure for insomnia research. *Sleep Medicine, 2*, 297–307. http://dx.doi.org/10.1016/S1389-9457(00)00065-4

Beaulieu-Bonneau, S., Ivers, H., Guay, B., & Morin, C. M. (2017). Long-term maintenance of therapeutic gains associated with cognitive-behavioral therapy for insomnia delivered alone or combined with zolpidem. *Sleep, 40*, zsx002. http://dx.doi.org/10.1093/sleep/zsx002

Berlin, R. K., Butler, P. M., & Perloff, M. D. (2015). Gabapentin therapy in psychiatric disorders: A systematic review. *The Primary Care Companion for CNS Disorders, 17*, 1–27.

Biederman, J., Melmed, R. D., Patel, A., McBurnett, K., Konow, J., Lyne, A., Scherer, N., & the SPD503 Study Group. (2008). A randomized, double-blind, placebo-controlled study of guanfacine extended release in children and adolescents with attention-deficit/hyperactivity disorder. *Pediatrics, 121*, e73–e84. http://dx.doi.org/10.1542/peds.2006-3695

Billioti de Gage, S., Moride, Y., Ducruet, T., Kurth, T., Verdoux, H., Tournier, M., . . . Begaud, B. (2014). Benzodiazepine use and risk of Alzheimer's disease: Case-control study. *BMJ, 349*, g5205. http://dx.doi.org/10.1136/bmj.g5205

Bloom, H. G., Ahmed, I., Alessi, C. A., Ancoli-Israel, S., Buysse, D. J., Kryger, M. H., . . . Zee, P. C. (2009). Evidence-based recommendations for the assessment and management of sleep disorders in older persons. *Journal of the American Geriatrics Society, 57*, 761–789. http://dx.doi.org/10.1111/j.1532-5415.2009.02220.x

Budhiraja, R., Roth, T., Hudgel, D. W., Budhiraja, P., & Drake, C. L. (2011). Prevalence and polysomnographic correlates of insomnia comorbid with medical disorders. *Sleep, 34*, 859–867. http://dx.doi.org/10.5665/SLEEP.1114

*Buysse, D. J., Reynolds, C. F., III, Monk, T. H., Berman, S. R., & Kupfer, D. J., III. (1989). The Pittsburgh Sleep Quality Index: A new instrument for psychiatric practice and research. *Psychiatry Research, 28*, 193–213. http://dx.doi.org/10.1016/0165-1781(89)90047-4

*Buysse, D. J., Rush, A. J., & Reynolds, C. F., III. (2017). Clinical management of insomnia disorder. *JAMA, 318*, 1973–1974. http://dx.doi.org/10.1001/jama.2017.15683

Camargos, E. F., Louzada, L. L., Quintas, J. L., Naves, J. O. S., Louzada, F. M., & Nobrega, O. T. (2014). Trazodone improves sleep parameters in Alzheimer disease patients: A randomized, double-blind, and placebo-controlled study. *The American Journal of Geriatric Psychiatry, 22*, 1565–1574. http://dx.doi.org/10.1016/j.jagp.2013.12.174

*Chung, F., Yegneswaran, B., Liao, P., Chung, S. A., Vairavanathan, S., Islam, S., . . . Shapiro, C. M. (2008). STOP Questionnaire: A tool to screen patients for obstructive sleep apnea. *Anesthesiology, 108*, 812–821. http://dx.doi.org/10.1097/ALN.0b013e31816d83e4

de Lecea, L., Kilduff, T. S., Peyron, C., Gao, X.-B., Foye, P. E., Danielson, P. E., . . . Sutcliffe, J. G. (1998). The hypocretins: Hypothalamus-specific peptides with neuroexcitatory activity. *Proceedings of the National Academy of Sciences, 95*, 322–327. http://dx.doi.org/10.1073/pnas.95.1.322

DeMartinis, N. A., & Winokur, A. (2007). Effects of psychiatric medications on sleep and sleep disorders. *CNS & Neurological Disorders - Drug Targets, 6*, 17–29. http://dx.doi.org/10.2174/187152707779940835

Drake, C. L., Durrence, H., Cheng, P., Roth, T., Pillai, V., Peterson, E. L., . . . Tran, K. M. (2017). Arousability and fall risk during forced awakenings from nocturnal sleep among healthy males following administration of zolpidem 10 mg and doxepin 6 mg: A randomized, placebo-controlled, four-way crossover trial. *Sleep, 40*. http://dx.doi.org/10.1093/sleep/zsx086

Edinger, J. D. (2009). Is it time to step up to stepped care with our cognitive-behavioral insomnia therapies? *Sleep, 32*, 1539–1541. http://dx.doi.org/10.1093/sleep/32.12.1539

*Edinger, J. D., Buysse, D. J., Deriy, L., Germain, A., Lewin, D. S., Ong, J. C., & Morgenthaler, T. I. (2015). Quality measures for the care of patients with insomnia. *Journal of Clinical Sleep Medicine, 11*, 311–334.

Espie, C. A., Inglis, S. J., Tessier, S., & Harvey, L. (2001). The clinical effectiveness of cognitive behaviour therapy for chronic insomnia: Implementation and evaluation of a sleep clinic in general medical practice. *Behaviour Research and Therapy, 39*, 45–60. http://dx.doi.org/10.1016/S0005-7967(99)00157-6

Fava, M., Schaefer, K., Huang, H., Wilson, A., Iosifescu, D. V., Mischoulon, D., & Wessel, T. C. (2011). A post hoc analysis of the effect of nightly administration of eszopiclone and a selective serotonin reuptake inhibitor in patients with insomnia and anxious depression. *The Journal of Clinical Psychiatry, 72*, 473–479. http://dx.doi.org/10.4088/JCP.09m05131gry

Foldvary-Schaefer, N. R., & Waters, T. E. (2017). Sleep-disordered breathing. *CONTINUUM: Lifelong Learning in Neurology, 23*, 1093–1116. http://dx.doi.org/10.1212/01.CON.0000522245.13784.f6

Gallacher, J., Elwood, P., Pickering, J., Bayer, A., Fish, M., & Ben-Shlomo, Y. (2012). Benzodiazepine use and risk of dementia: Evidence from the Caerphilly Prospective Study (CaPS). *Journal of Epidemiology and Community Health, 66*, 869–873. http://dx.doi.org/10.1136/jech-2011-200314

*Garcia-Borreguero, D., Silber, M. H., Winkelman, J. W., Högl, B., Bainbridge, J., Buchfuhrer, M., . . . Allen, R. P. (2016). Guidelines for the first-line treatment of restless legs syndrome/Willis-Ekbom disease, prevention and treatment of dopaminergic augmentation: A combined task force of the IRLSSG, EURLSSG, and the RLS-foundation. *Sleep Medicine, 21*, 1–11. http://dx.doi.org/10.1016/j.sleep.2016.01.017

Gibbons, R. D., Hur, K., Brown, C. H., & Mann, J. J. (2010). Gabapentin and suicide attempts. *Pharmacoepidemiology and Drug Safety, 19*, 1241–1247. http://dx.doi.org/10.1002/pds.2036

Gooneratne, N. S., & Vitiello, M. V. (2014). Sleep in older adults: Normative changes, sleep disorders, and treatment options. *Clinics in Geriatric Medicine, 30*, 591–627. http://dx.doi.org/10.1016/j.cger.2014.04.007

Gosling, J. A., Glozier, N., Griffiths, K., Ritterband, L., Thorndike, F., Mackinnon, A., . . . Christensen, H. (2014). The GoodNight study—online CBT for insomnia for the indicated prevention of depression: Study protocol for a randomised controlled trial. *Trials, 15*, 56. http://dx.doi.org/10.1186/1745-6215-15-56

Gottesmann, C. (2002). GABA mechanisms and sleep. *Neuroscience, 111*, 231–239. http://dx.doi.org/10.1016/S0306-4522(02)00034-9

Griffiths, R. R., & Johnson, M. W. (2005). Relative abuse liability of hypnotic drugs: A conceptual framework and algorithm for differentiating among compounds. *The Journal of Clinical Psychiatry, 66*(Suppl. 9), 31–41.

Guilleminault, C., Davis, K., & Huynh, N. T. (2008). Prospective randomized study of patients with insomnia and mild sleep disordered breathing. *Sleep, 31*, 1527–1533. http://dx.doi.org/10.1093/sleep/31.11.1527

Gunja, N. (2013). In the Zzz zone: The effects of Z-drugs on human performance and driving. *Journal of Medical Toxicology, 9*, 163–171. http://dx.doi.org/10.1007/s13181-013-0294-y

Herring, W. J., Connor, K. M., Snyder, E., Snavely, D. B., Zhang, Y., Hutzelmann, J., . . . Michelson, D. (2017). Suvorexant in elderly patients with insomnia: Pooled analyses of data from Phase III randomized controlled clinical trials. *The American Journal of Geriatric Psychiatry, 25*, 791–802. http://dx.doi.org/10.1016/j.jagp.2017.03.004

Howell, M. J., & Schenck, C. H. (2012). Restless nocturnal eating: A common feature of Willis-Ekbom syndrome (RLS). *Journal of Clinical Sleep Medicine, 8*, 413–419.

Iranzo, A., Santamaria, J., & Tolosa, E. (2016). Idiopathic rapid eye movement sleep behaviour disorder: Diagnosis, management, and the need for neuroprotective interventions. *The Lancet Neurology, 15*, 405–419. http://dx.doi.org/10.1016/S1474-4422(16)00057-0

Irfan, M., Schenck, C. H., & Howell, M. J. (2017). Non-rapid eye movement sleep and overlap parasomnias. *CONTINUUM: Lifelong Learning in Neurology, 23*, 1035–1050. http://dx.doi.org/10.1212/CON.0000000000000503

Jiang, C. G., Zhang, T., Yue, F. G., Yi, M. L., & Gao, D. (2013). Efficacy of repetitive transcranial magnetic stimulation in the treatment of patients with chronic primary insomnia. *Cell Biochemistry and Biophysics, 67*, 169–173. http://dx.doi.org/10.1007/s12013-013-9529-4

Johns, M. W. (1991). A new method for measuring daytime sleepiness: The Epworth sleepiness scale. *Sleep, 14*, 540–545. http://dx.doi.org/10.1093/sleep/14.6.540

Kessler, R. C., Berglund, P. A., Coulouvrat, C., Hajak, G., Roth, T., Shahly, V., . . . Walsh, J. K. (2011). Insomnia and the performance of US workers: Results from the America insomnia survey. *Sleep, 34*, 1161–1171. http://dx.doi.org/10.5665/SLEEP.1230

Krakow, B., Ulibarri, V. A., Romero, E. A., & McIver, N. D. (2013). A two-year prospective study on the frequency and co-occurrence of insomnia and sleep-disordered breathing symptoms in a primary care population. *Sleep Medicine, 14*, 814–823. http://dx.doi.org/10.1016/j.sleep.2013.02.015

Krystal, A. D. (2012). Psychiatric disorders and sleep. *Neurologic Clinics, 30*, 1389–1413. http://dx.doi.org/10.1016/j.ncl.2012.08.018

Kuriyama, A., Honda, M., & Hayashino, Y. (2014). Ramelteon for the treatment of insomnia in adults: A systematic review and meta-analysis. *Sleep Medicine, 15*, 385–392. http://dx.doi.org/10.1016/j.sleep.2013.11.788

Lancee, J., Eisma, M. C., van Straten, A., & Kamphuis, J. H. (2015). Sleep-related safety behaviors and dysfunctional beliefs mediate the efficacy of online CBT for insomnia: A randomized controlled trial. *Cognitive Behaviour Therapy, 44*, 406–422. http://dx.doi.org/10.1080/16506073.2015.1026386

LeBlanc, M., Mérette, C., Savard, J., Ivers, H., Baillargeon, L., & Morin, C. M. (2009). Incidence and risk factors of insomnia in a population-based sample. *Sleep, 32*, 1027–1037. http://dx.doi.org/10.1093/sleep/32.8.1027

Liu, Y., Xu, X., Dong, M., Jia, S., & Wei, Y. (2017). Treatment of insomnia with tricyclic antidepressants: A meta-analysis of polysomnographic randomized controlled trials. *Sleep Medicine, 34*, 126–133. http://dx.doi.org/10.1016/j.sleep.2017.03.007

Lo, H.-S., Yang, C.-M., Lo, H. G., Lee, C.-Y., Ting, H., & Tzang, B.-S. (2010). Treatment effects of gabapentin for primary insomnia. *Clinical Neuropharmacology, 33*, 84–90. http://dx.doi.org/10.1097/WNF.0b013e3181cda242

Malhotra, S., & Kushida, C. A. (2013). Primary hypersomnias of central origin. *CONTINUUM: Lifelong Learning in Neurology, 19*, 67–85. http://dx.doi.org/10.1212/01.CON.0000427212.05930.c4

Manber, R., Carney, C., Edinger, J., Epstein, D., Friedman, L., Haynes, P. L., . . . Trockel, M. (2012). Dissemination of CBTI to the non-sleep specialist: Protocol development and training issues. *Journal of Clinical Sleep Medicine, 8*, 209–218. http://dx.doi.org/10.5664/jcsm.1786

Mellinger, G. D., Balter, M. B., & Uhlenhuth, E. H. (1985). Insomnia and its treatment. Prevalence and correlates. *Archives of General Psychiatry, 42*, 225–232. http://dx.doi.org/10.1001/archpsyc.1985.01790260019002

Mindell, J. A., Emslie, G., Blumer, J., Genel, M., Glaze, D., Ivanenko, A., . . . Banas, B. (2006). Pharmacologic management of insomnia in children and adolescents: Consensus statement. *Pediatrics, 117*, e1223–e1232. http://dx.doi.org/10.1542/peds.2005-1693

Morin, C. M., Colecchi, C., Stone, J., Sood, R., & Brink, D. (1999). Behavioral and pharmacological therapies for late-life insomnia: A randomized controlled trial. *JAMA, 281*, 991–999. http://dx.doi.org/10.1001/jama.281.11.991

Morin, C. M., Vallières, A., Guay, B., Ivers, H., Savard, J., Mérette, C., . . . Baillargeon, L. (2009). . . . Cognitive behavioral therapy, singly and combined with medication, for persistent insomnia. *JAMA, 301*, 2005–2015. http://dx.doi.org/10.1001/jama.2009.682

Morphy, H., Dunn, K. M., Lewis, M., Boardman, H. F., & Croft, P. R. (2007). Epidemiology of insomnia: A longitudinal study in a UK population. *Sleep, 30*, 274–280.

Ohayon, M. M. (2002). Epidemiology of insomnia: What we know and what we still need to learn. *Sleep Medicine Reviews, 6*, 97–111. http://dx.doi.org/10.1053/smrv.2002.0186

Owens, J. A., & Moturi, S. (2009). Pharmacologic treatment of pediatric insomnia. *Child and Adolescent Psychiatric Clinics of North America, 18*, 1001–1016. http://dx.doi.org/10.1016/j.chc.2009.04.009

Patel, K. V., Aspesi, A. V., & Evoy, K. E. (2015). Suvorexant: A dual orexin receptor antagonist for the treatment of sleep onset and sleep maintenance insomnia. *The Annals of Pharmacotherapy, 49*, 477–483. http://dx.doi.org/10.1177/1060028015570467

Perlis, M. L., Giles, D. E., Buysse, D. J., Tu, X., & Kupfer, D. J. (1997). Self-reported sleep disturbance as a prodromal symptom in recurrent depression. *Journal of Affective Disorders, 42*, 209–212. http://dx.doi.org/10.1016/S0165-0327(96)01411-5

Pillai, V., Roth, T., Roehrs, T., Moss, K., Peterson, E. L., & Drake, C. L. (2016). Effectiveness of benzodiazepine receptor agonists in the treatment of insomnia: An examination of response and remission rates. *Sleep, 40*, zsw044. http://dx.doi.org/10.1093/sleep/zsw044

Pressman, M. R. (2011). Sleep driving: Sleepwalking variant or misuse of z-drugs? *Sleep Medicine Reviews, 15*, 285–292. http://dx.doi.org/10.1016/j.smrv.2010.12.004

Provini, F., Antelmi, E., Vignatelli, L., Zaniboni, A., Naldi, G., Calandra-Buonaura, G., . . . Montagna, P. (2009). Association of restless legs syndrome with nocturnal eating: A case-control study. *Movement Disorders, 24*, 871–877. http://dx.doi.org/10.1002/mds.22460

Qaseem, A., Kansagara, D., Forciea, M. A., Cooke, M., Denberg, T. D., . . . Wilt, T., & the Clinical Guidelines Committee of the American College of Physicians. (2016). Management of chronic insomnia disorder in adults: A clinical practice guideline from the American college of physicians. *Annals of Internal Medicine, 165*, 125–133. http://dx.doi.org/10.7326/M15-2175

Rhodes, C. T. (2001). Trazodone and priapism: Implications for responses to adverse events. *Clinical Research and Regulatory Affairs, 18*, 47–52. http://dx.doi.org/10.1081/CRP-100104930

Richardson, G. S., Roehrs, T. A., Rosenthal, L., Koshorek, G., & Roth, T. (2002). Tolerance to daytime sedative effects of H1 antihistamines. *Journal of Clinical Psychopharmacology, 22*, 511–515. http://dx.doi.org/10.1097/00004714-200210000-00012

RodríGuez, J. J., Noristani, H. N., Hoover, W. B., Linley, S. B., & Vertes, R. P. (2011). Serotonergic projections and serotonin receptor expression in the reticular nucleus of the thalamus in the rat. *Synapse, 65*, 919–928. http://dx.doi.org/10.1002/syn.20920

Roth, T., Black, J., Cluydts, R., Charef, P., Cavallaro, M., Kramer, F., . . . Walsh, J. (2017). Dual orexin receptor antagonist, almorexant, in elderly patients with primary insomnia: A randomized, controlled study. *Sleep, 40*. http://dx.doi.org/10.1093/sleep/zsw034

Roth, T., Coulouvrat, C., Hajak, G., Lakoma, M. D., Sampson, N. A., Shahly, V., . . . Kessler, R. C. (2011). Prevalence and perceived health associated with insomnia based on *DSM–IV–TR*; International Statistical Classification of Diseases and Related Health Problems, tenth revision; and research diagnostic criteria/international classification of sleep disorders. *Biological Psychiatry, 69*, 592–600. http://dx.doi.org/10.1016/j.biopsych.2010.10.023

Roth, T., Mayleben, D., Feldman, N., Lankford, A., Grant, T., & Nofzinger, E. (2018). A novel forehead temperature-regulating device for insomnia: A randomized clinical trial. *Sleep, 41*, zsy045. http://dx.doi.org/10.1093/sleep/zsy045

Ruxton, K., Woodman, R. J., & Mangoni, A. A. (2015). Drugs with anticholinergic effects and cognitive impairment, falls and all-cause mortality in older adults: A systematic review and meta-analysis. *British Journal of Clinical Pharmacology, 80*, 209–220. http://dx.doi.org/10.1111/bcp.12617

Sanger, D. J. (2004). The pharmacology and mechanisms of action of new generation, non-benzodiazepine hypnotic agents. *CNS Drugs, 18*(Suppl. 1), 9–15. http://dx.doi.org/10.2165/00023210-200418001-00004

*Sateia, M. J., Buysse, D. J., Krystal, A. D., Neubauer, D. N., & Heald, J. L. (2017). Clinical Practice Guideline for the Pharmacologic Treatment of Chronic Insomnia in Adults: An American Academy of Sleep Medicine clinical practice guideline. *Journal of Clinical Sleep Medicine, 13*, 307–349. http://dx.doi.org/10.5664/jcsm.6470

Schutte-Rodin, S., Broch, L., Buysse, D., Dorsey, C., & Sateia, M. (2008). Clinical guideline for the evaluation and management of chronic insomnia in adults. *Journal of Clinical Sleep Medicine, 4*, 487–504.

Seow, L. S. E., Verma, S. K., Mok, Y. M., Kumar, S., Chang, S., Satghare, P., . . . Subramaniam, M. (2018). Evaluating *DSM–5* insomnia disorder and the treatment of sleep problems in a psychiatric population. *Journal of Clinical Sleep Medicine, 14*, 237–244. http://dx.doi.org/10.5664/jcsm.6942

Stahl, S. M. (2013). *Stahl's essential psychopharmacology neuroscientific basis and practical applications* (4th ed.). Cambridge, UK: Cambridge University Press.

Stein, M. B., Belik, S.-L., Jacobi, F., & Sareen, J. (2008). Impairment associated with sleep problems in the community: Relationship to physical and mental health comorbidity. *Psychosomatic Medicine, 70*, 913–919. http://dx.doi.org/10.1097/PSY.0b013e3181871405

Subramanian, S., Guntupalli, B., Murugan, T., Bopparaju, S., Chanamolu, S., Casturi, L., & Surani, S. (2011). Gender and ethnic differences in prevalence of self-reported insomnia among patients with obstructive sleep apnea. *Sleep and Breathing, 15*, 711–715. http://dx.doi.org/10.1007/s11325-010-0426-4

Suntsova, N., Szymusiak, R., Alam, M. N., Guzman-Marin, R., & McGinty, D. (2002). Sleep-waking discharge patterns of median preoptic nucleus neurons in rats. *The Journal of Physiology, 543*, 665–677. http://dx.doi.org/10.1113/jphysiol.2002.023085

Takahashi, K., Lin, J. S., & Sakai, K. (2009). Characterization and mapping of sleep-waking specific neurons in the basal forebrain and preoptic hypothalamus in mice. *Neuroscience, 161*, 269–292. http://dx.doi.org/10.1016/j.neuroscience.2009.02.075

Tassniyom, K., Paholpak, S., Tassniyom, S., & Kiewyoo, J. (2010). Quetiapine for primary insomnia: A double blind, randomized controlled trial. *Journal of the Medical Association of Thailand, 93*, 729–734.

*Taylor, D., Wilkerson, A., Pruiksma, K., Williams, J., Ruggero, C., Hale, W., . . . Peterson, A. L. (2018). Reliability of the Structured Clinical Interview for DSM-5 Sleep Disorders Module. *J Clinical Sleep Medicine, 14*, 459–464. http://dx.doi.org/10.5664/jcsm.7000

The American Geriatrics Society 2015 Beers Criteria Update Expert Panel. (2015). American Geriatrics Society 2015 updated Beers criteria for potentially inappropriate medication use in older adults. *Journal of the American Geriatrics Society, 63*, 2227–2246. http://dx.doi.org/10.1111/jgs.13702

Trauer, J. M., Qian, M. Y., Doyle, J. S., Rajaratnam, S. M. W., & Cunnington, D. (2015). Cognitive behavioral therapy for chronic insomnia: A systematic review and meta-analysis. *Annals of Internal Medicine, 163*, 191–204. http://dx.doi.org/10.7326/M14-2841

Trenkwalder, C., Winkelmann, J., Inoue, Y., & Paulus, W. (2015). Restless legs syndrome-current therapies and management of augmentation. *Nature Reviews. Neurology, 11*, 434–445. http://dx.doi.org/10.1038/nrneurol.2015.122

U.S. Food and Drug Administration. (2013, January 10). *Risk of next-morning impairment after use of insomnia drugs; FDA requires lower recommended doses for certain drugs containing zolpidem (Ambien, Ambien CR, Edluar, and Zolpimist)* [Safety Announcement]. Retrieved from https://www.fda.gov/downloads/Drugs/DrugSafety/UCM335007.pdf

Van der Heijden, K. B., Smits, M. G., Van Someren, E. J. W., Ridderinkhof, K. R., & Gunning, W. B. (2007). Effect of melatonin on sleep, behavior, and cognition in ADHD and chronic sleep-onset insomnia. *Journal of the American Academy of Child & Adolescent Psychiatry, 46*, 233–241. http://dx.doi.org/10.1097/01.chi.0000246055.76167.0d

Van der Zweerde, T., Lancee, J., Slottje, P., Bosmans, J., Van Someren, E., Reynolds, C., III, . . . van Straten, A. (2016). Cost-effectiveness of i-Sleep, a guided online CBT intervention, for patients with insomnia in general practice: Protocol of a pragmatic randomized controlled trial. *BMC Psychiatry, 16*, 85. http://dx.doi.org/10.1186/s12888-016-0783-z

Vermeeren, A., Sun, H., Vuurman, E. F. P. M., Jongen, S., Van Leeuwen, C. J., Van Oers, A. C. M., . . . McCrea, J. (2015). On-the-road driving performance the morning after bedtime use of suvorexant 20 and 40 mg: A study in non-elderly healthy volunteers. *Sleep, 38*, 1803–1813. http://dx.doi.org/10.5665/sleep.5168

Vinkers, C. H., & Olivier, B. (2012). Mechanisms underlying tolerance after long-term benzodiazepine use: A future for subtype-selective GABA$_A$ receptor modulators? *Advances in Pharmacological Sciences, 2012*, 416864. http://dx.doi.org/10.1155/2012/416864

Walters, A. S., LeBrocq, C., Dhar, A., Hening, W., Rosen, R., Allen, R. P., & Trenkwalder, C., & the International Restless Legs Syndrome Study Group. (2003). Validation of the International Restless Legs Syndrome Study Group rating scale for restless legs syndrome. *Sleep Medicine, 4*, 121–132. http://dx.doi.org/10.1016/S1389-9457(02)00258-7

*Wilt, T. J., MacDonald, R., Brasure, M., Olson, C. M., Carlyle, M., Fuchs, E., . . . Kane, R. L. (2016). Pharmacologic treatment of insomnia disorder: An evidence report for a clinical practice guideline by the American College of Physicians. *Annals of Internal Medicine, 165*, 103–112. http://dx.doi.org/10.7326/M15-1781

Winkelman, J. W. (2015). Insomnia disorder. *The New England Journal of Medicine, 373*(15), 1437–1444. http://dx.doi.org/10.1056/NEJMcp1412740

Wu, C.-S., Wang, S.-C., Chang, I.-S., & Lin, K.-M. (2009). The association between dementia and long-term use of benzodiazepine in the elderly: Nested case-control study using claims data. *The American Journal of Geriatric Psychiatry, 17*, 614–620. http://dx.doi.org/10.1097/JGP.0b013e3181a65210

Yeung, W.-F., Chung, K.-F., Yung, K.-P., & Ng, T. H.-Y. (2015). Doxepin for insomnia: A systematic review of randomized placebo-controlled trials. *Sleep Medicine Reviews, 19*, 75–83. http://dx.doi.org/10.1016/j.smrv.2014.06.001

Zammit, G. K., McNabb, L. J., Caron, J., Amato, D. A., & Roth, T. (2004). Efficacy and safety of eszopiclone across 6-weeks of treatment for primary insomnia. *Current Medical Research and Opinion, 20*, 1979–1991. http://dx.doi.org/10.1185/174234304X15174

Zee, P. C., Attarian, H., & Videnovic, A. (2013). Circadian rhythm abnormalities. *CONTINUUM: Lifelong Learning in Neurology, 19*, 132–147. http://dx.doi.org/10.1212/01.CON.0000427209.21177.a

CHAPTER 15

PHARMACOLOGICAL TREATMENT OF EATING DISORDERS

Robyn Sysko, Tom Hildebrandt, and B. Timothy Walsh

Eating disorders are commonly defined by the diagnoses presented in the *Diagnostic and Statistical Manual of Mental Disorders* (5th ed; *DSM–5*; American Psychiatric Association, 2013). In this classification scheme, conditions previously listed in the Eating Disorders and the Feeding and Eating Disorders of Infancy or Early Childhood sections of the *DSM–IV* have been combined into a single section of Feeding and Eating Disorders, to include pica, rumination disorder, and the newly added avoidant/restrictive food intake disorder. As the focus of this chapter is on eating disorders, and limited research has been devoted to pharmacological treatments of feeding disorders, we describe criteria for the primary *DSM–5* eating disorders and give information about their prevalence and pharmacologic interventions.

Anorexia nervosa (AN) is characterized by the presence of a significantly low body weight, and clinicians are expected to determine whether an individual's weight is low given factors including age, sex, and developmental trajectory. To receive this diagnosis, individuals must also demonstrate a fear of gaining weight or show overt behavior (e.g., avoidance of high calorie foods, reluctance to consume a range of foods) consistent with such fear. A disturbance in the evaluation of one's shape or weight is also required. Individuals with AN who do not regularly engage in binge eating or purging behaviors (i.e., self-induced vomiting and laxative or diuretic abuse) are classified with AN restricting

type (AN-R), and patients reporting binge eating or purging are diagnosed with AN binge-eating/purging type (AN-B/P).

The diagnosis of bulimia nervosa (BN) in *DSM–5* requires recurrent episodes of binge eating and inappropriate compensatory behavior (e.g., self-induced vomiting, fasting, excessive exercise). An episode of binge eating is characterized by consuming a large amount of food and the experience of a loss of control over eating. These behaviors (binge eating/inappropriate compensation) must occur at least once weekly over a 3-month period, and patients with BN are required to experience an undue influence of shape and weight on their self-evaluation. A subtyping scheme from prior versions of the *DSM*, whereby individuals with BN were further classified with either the purging or non-purging BN, was eliminated in the *DSM–5*.

The most significant change in eating disorder classification in the *DSM–5* was the formal inclusion of binge eating disorder (BED) as a diagnosis. The diagnosis of BED requires recurrent episodes of binge eating at least once weekly over a 3-month period, defined in an identical manner to the binge eating and frequency aforementioned in BN, but in the absence of compensatory behaviors. Patients must also report distress over binge eating episodes, as well as three of the following: eating until feeling uncomfortably full; eating large amounts of food when not physically hungry; eating much faster

http://dx.doi.org/10.1037/0000133-015
APA Handbook of Psychopharmacology, S. M. Evans (Editor-in-Chief)

than normal; eating alone because of embarrassment; or feeling disgusted, depressed, or guilty after overeating. Although individuals with BED may also be overweight or obese, the presence of excess body fat is a general medical condition and not an eating disorder within the *DSM–5* system.

Along with revised diagnostic criteria for eating disorders, the *DSM–5* also added specifiers intended to help clinicians characterize severity of the eating disorders with a dimensional measure. The severity specifiers are based on body mass index (BMI; kg/m²) for AN, frequency of inappropriate compensatory behaviors (e.g., self-induced vomiting) for BN, and frequency of binge eating episodes for BED. In addition to these behavioral features, the *DSM–5* encourages clinicians to also consider the intensity of other symptoms, degree of functional impairment, and the requirement for medical or clinical supervision (American Psychiatric Association, 2013). Emerging empirical research suggests that the *DSM–5* severity ratings for AN may provide information about both low body weight required and the use of more psychiatric services (e.g., number of hospitalizations; Gianini et al., 2017), but may not distinguish based on cross-sectional measures of eating pathology or frequency of binge eating or purging (Machado, Grilo, & Crosby, 2017). Some statistically significant associations with cross-sectional measures of psychopathology and *DSM–5* severity measures for BN and BED have also been noted in several studies (Gianini et al., 2017; Grilo, Ivezaj, & White, 2015a, 2015b, 2015c). Although there is the potential for utility in these subcategorizations, more consistent patterns of statistically significant relationships with cross-sectional measures of psychological symptoms have been noted in alternative severity classifications for BN (based on number of purging methods; Eddy et al., 2009; Edler, Haedt, & Keel, 2007; Favaro & Santonastaso, 1996) and BED (based on overvaluation of shape and weight; Grilo et al., 2008).

Individuals experiencing a clinically significant problem with eating but not meeting criteria for AN, BN, or BED are classified with a residual category in *DSM–5*, specifically, either other specified feeding and eating disorder (OSFED) or unspecified feeding and eating disorder (USFED). The OSFED category includes five example presentations (atypical anorexia nervosa, subthreshold binge eating disorder, subthreshold bulimia nervosa, purging disorder, and night eating syndrome). All other individuals not grouped into another category are classified within USFED. Severity specifiers are not included for OSFED or USFED.

EPIDEMIOLOGY AND PREVALENCE

Eating disorders are relatively uncommon in the general population, particularly when compared with psychiatric diagnoses such as major depression or substance use disorders. Some data suggest an increasing prevalence of eating disorders; however, this may be the result of broadened diagnostic criteria in the *DSM–5* (Lindvall Dahlgren & Wisting, 2016; Qian et al., 2013). For example, one retrospective study noted an increase of 14% in diagnoses of AN in a clinical sample after applying *DSM–5* criteria and a 2.4% increase in the rate of BN diagnoses (Gualandi et al., 2016), which appear related to the shifting of cases in the residual not otherwise specified category in the *DSM–IV* to a formal category under the *DSM–5*. Other studies examining changes in post-*DSM–5* prevalence of residual diagnoses noted that rates of residual diagnoses are substantially reduced (Caudle et al., 2015; Keel et al., 2011; Machado et al., 2013; Mustelin et al., 2016, Ornstein et al., 2013).

A meta-analysis of 15 studies of the general population using the *DSM–IV* scheme indicated lifetime prevalence for eating disorders was highest for BED (2.2%), followed by BN (0.81%) and AN (0.21%; Qian et al., 2013). These data parallel other research indicating a 12-month BED prevalence estimate of 1.6% using *DSM–5* (2.0% and 1.2% in women and men, respectively). If considering only adolescents, eating disorders are more common, with the highest incidence rate of 109.2 per 100,000 per year in females ages 15 to 19, or about 40% of all cases of AN (Smink, van Hoeken, & Hoek, 2012). The point prevalence of BED is highest among adolescents (3.7% females, 0.5% males), followed by AN (1.2% females, 0.1% males) and BN (0.6% females, 0.1% males; Smink, van Hoeken, Oldehinkel, & Hoek, 2014).

Eating disorders are often assumed to be culturally bound and Western syndromes, but AN has been documented in every region of the world, with a similar prevalence in Western and non-Western countries (Keel & Klump, 2003). BN occurs outside of Western countries, but Western cultural influences appear be more significant than for AN, with an overall greater variation in prevalence, and an increase in the incidence of BN found during the latter half of the 20th century (Keel & Klump, 2003). Cultural influences, such as the media, are found to result in increases in body dissatisfaction and problem eating (Becker, Burwell, Gilman, Herzog, & Hamburg, 2002), suggesting the potential for different etiologies in the development of AN, BN, and other body image disturbances.

A range of biological, environmental, and psychological variables appear to contribute to the complex etiology of eating disorders. Cascading psychosocial and biological (e.g., hormonal) changes in adolescence are thought to affect eating disorder onset, both with an onset typically around puberty and because of the more common presentation of females with these disorders. Peer influences also affect beliefs about shape and weight or dieting (Jones & Crawford, 2006), and genetic factors are hypothesized to predispose individuals to the development of eating disorders. There are currently no models for particular forms of peer influence or genes that are consistently identified as specific to people with eating disorders (Duncan et al., 2017). It is therefore not known whether different biological, social, or genetic factors are responsible for the development of these disorders and maintenance of symptoms, or if eating disorders occur as a result of some interaction between these variables.

The use of pharmacological treatments, and of antidepressants in particular, was a logical outgrowth of observations regarding comorbid psychiatric diagnoses among treatment-seeking patients with eating disorders (Zhu & Walsh, 2002). Lifetime major depressive disorder is observed in 9.5% to 64.7% of patients with AN-R, 50% to 71.3% of those with AN-B/P, 20% to 80% of patients with BN (Godart et al., 2007), and 58% of those with BED (Wilfley et al., 2000). Similar lifetime prevalence rates are documented for anxiety disorders, with a range from approximately 33% to 72% of patients with AN-R, 55% of patients with AN-B/P, 41% to 75% of patients with BN (Godart, Flament, Perdereau, & Jeammet, 2002), and 29% of patients with BED (Wilfley et al., 2000). A large body of research has accumulated in the last several decades to guide treatment decisions around the use of medications to address eating disorder symptoms; however, many clinical recommendations are derived from data on specific eating disorder diagnoses. Thus, obtaining an accurate *DSM–5* diagnosis is an appropriate first step when considering pharmacological interventions.

DIAGNOSING EATING DISORDERS

Assigning an eating disorder diagnosis requires information about specific symptoms, as only the presence of eating disorder symptoms can justify *DSM–5* diagnoses. Research evaluating pharmacological interventions primarily categorizes patients on the basis of *DSM* diagnoses, and therefore an assessment grouping individuals into these categories is more likely to allow clinicians to use empirically supported treatments in routine practice. Regardless of the chosen assessment method, the measurement of body weight is crucial in determining whether an individual should receive a diagnosis of AN-B/P versus BN, as similar bulimic symptoms are present in both disorders. After weighing the patient, clinicians can use a calculation of BMI (weight in kg/height in m^2) or BMI percentile for youth (see https://www.cdc.gov/healthyweight/bmi/calculator.html).

As detailed elsewhere (e.g., Sysko & Alavi, 2018), diagnosis can be assigned by either semistructured interview or self-report questionnaires. In research settings, the Eating Disorder Examination (EDE; current version 17.0D; Fairburn, Cooper, & O'Connor, 2008) is a commonly used semistructured interview that measures the psychopathology associated with AN, BN, and BED along with assigning *DSM–5* eating disorder diagnoses. To administer the EDE, comprehensive training is required, which can limit the utility of the instrument outside of specialty clinics. A version of the EDE suitable for children and adolescents (child EDE; ChEDE) is also available (Bryant-Waugh, Cooper, Taylor, & Lask, 1996). While the EDE commonly diagnoses patients enrolled in treatment studies, relatively limited information is available about the psychometrics of diagnoses generated by EDE (for a review, see Berg et al., 2012). Updated questions corresponding to the diagnostic criteria for AN, BN, BED, and OSFED appear in the Structured Clinical Interview for DSM–5 (SCID; First, Williams, Karg, & Spitzer, 2015). Psychometric data are not currently available for *DSM–5* eating disorders from the SCID. The SCID-IV (First, Spitzer, Gibbon, & Williams, 2002) provided eating disorder diagnoses in a number of studies (e.g., Engel et al., 2005; Grilo & Masheb, 2005), but limited data evaluate the psychometric properties of *DSM–IV* diagnoses. Interrater reliability of *DSM–IV* eating disorder diagnoses had a good κ value (= 0.77), and the SCID-IV has appropriate norms and construct validity; however, the test–retest reliability (correlation = 0.64) is less than acceptable. Like the EDE, the SCID requires interviewer training and can be time-consuming, but also only assesses diagnostic criteria and not other eating disorder pathology, which provides flexibility for utilizing the instrument in routine clinical practice to consider a broader range of symptoms. Most recently, the Eating Disorder Assessment for DSM–5 (EDA-5), an electronically-guided assessment, was developed to comprehensively measure all *DSM–5* feeding and eating disorders. The EDA-5 can be administered with limited training and in a brief time to reduce participant burden (Glasofer, Sysko, & Walsh, 2016). Two studies administering the EDA-5 in treatment-seeking adults across multiple sites found the measure to have utility for diagnosis (for details, see Sysko et al., 2015). Additional information about these instruments can be found in the Tool Kit of Resources at the end of this chapter.

Several self-report questionnaires are also available to offer eating disorder diagnoses, but data on updated versions of these assessments for *DSM–5* are sparse. The most frequently used self-report measures attempt to avoid costly or time-consuming interviews (Stice, Telch, & Rizvi, 2000); however, clinicians may need to obtain scoring algorithms and, in some cases, pay for the questionnaires (Peterson & Mitchell, 2005). The Eating Disorder Examination Questionnaire (EDE-Q, current version 6.0; Fairburn & Beglin, 2008) is a self-report version of the EDE. Clinicians should be aware that the EDE-Q does not evaluate several of the diagnostic criteria for *DSM–5* (e.g., lack of recognition of the seriousness of low body weight; Mancuso et al., 2015), and only moderate diagnostic concordance has been found between the EDE and EDE-Q (Berg et al., 2012), which limits the utility of this measure for diagnosis.

The Eating Disorder Diagnostic Scale (EDDS; Stice et al., 2000) was developed to diagnose eating disorders in etiological research, studies requiring frequent measurements, or to classify individuals with eating disorders in clinical practice (e.g., primary care; Stice et al., 2000). Extant research suggests that the EDDS is appropriate psychometrically for *DSM–IV* eating disorders (Stice et al., 2000; Stice, Fisher, & Martinez, 2004; Stice, Orjada, & Tristan, 2006; Stice & Ragan, 2002) and can be completed quickly, and therefore has potential applicability for nonspecialists. A revised EDDS fits the *DSM–5* diagnostic changes, but has not yet been validated.

EVIDENCE-BASED PHARMACOLOGICAL TREATMENTS OF EATING DISORDERS

Research on the neurobiology of eating disorders has existed for decades; however, the results have not led to the selection of medication treatments or specific neurobiological hypotheses. Thus, although the treatments described in this section influence neural circuits of the brain central to the eating disorders, the vast majority of extant studies on pharmacological treatments have selected medications based on core eating disorder symptoms (e.g., agents that increase appetite or cause weight gain in other populations for AN), data on efficacy in other psychiatric conditions with overlapping presentations (e.g., antidepressant medications for BN where patients commonly report low mood or meet criteria for a depressive episode), and/or documented efficacy in another eating disorder (e.g., fluoxetine for BED after an indication in BN). A recent expert review by Himmerich and Treasure (2018) suggested using the results of neurobiological research to inform future studies of psychopharmacology, including targeting molecules and receptors that show disturbances in eating disorders (e.g., serotonin, norepinephrine, acetylcholine, glutamate, opioids, cannabinoids, and dopamine, histamine, ghrelin, leptin, insulin, glucagon-like peptide-1) or medications that influence the immune or metabolic systems.

Pharmacological Treatments for Anorexia Nervosa

Significant variability is noted in prognosis for individuals with eating disorders across diagnostic categories. AN has the highest mortality rate of all psychiatric disorders, and interventions are of limited benefit, as the majority of treatments (psychological or pharmacological) have no demonstrable effect (Zipfel et al., 2015). Over time, 27.5% of patients with AN are shown to have a good outcome, 25.3% have an intermediate outcome, 39.6% have a poor outcome, and 7.7% die (Fichter, Quadflieg, & Hedlund, 2006). In theory, pharmacological treatments seem an appropriate option in light of the depressive symptoms (e.g., depressed mood, low energy, anhedonia, social isolation) reported by many patients with AN in the context of acute illness. Further, clinicians hoped to capitalize on the weight gain side effects of many antidepressants to augment antidepressant effects and potentially spur greater improvements (Zhu & Walsh, 2002).

However, as described in this chapter and consistently in reviews of the topic over time (e.g., Bulik et al., 2007; Frank & Shott, 2016), there are no robust empirically supported medication interventions for AN. Table 15.1 presents information on several promising trials described in the sections that follow, and detailed information about the entire range of psychopharmacological studies of patients with AN can be found in Frank and Shott (2016).

Antidepressant medications. In four available placebo-controlled trials of antidepressants for underweight patients with AN (Attia, Haiman, Walsh, & Flater, 1998; Biederman et al., 1985; Halmi, Eckert, LaDu, & Cohen, 1986; Lacey & Crisp, 1980), no more than a small effect was noted. Antidepressant medications are useful in the treatment of major depressive disorder and BN, disorders with notable similarities to AN, which makes the consistent failure to detect significant effects in this diagnostic category unexpected. It is possible that the consequences of malnutrition or other physiological disturbances present in AN (e.g., alterations in serotonin pathways; Kaye, Fudge, & Paulus, 2009) interfere with the action of antidepressant medications.

Atypical antipsychotic medications. Although data from two early small placebo-controlled trials of antipsychotic medication were not promising (Vandereycken, 1984; Vandereycken & Pierloot, 1982), atypical antipsychotics have more recently

TABLE 15.1

Published Randomized Controlled Pharmacological Treatment Studies for Eating Disorders With Empirical Support for Medication Utilization for Anorexia Nervosa

Author	Medication (class) and dose	Duration	Sample size	Sample characteristics	Primary outcome
Attia et al., 2011	Olanzapine (antipsychotic) flexibly dosed 2.5–10 mg, or placebo	8 weeks	33	32 female, 1 male	Olanzapine was associated with a greater increase in body mass index in comparison with placebo; no differences were noted in psychological symptoms
Bissada, Tasca, Barber, and Bradwejn, 2008	Olanzapine (antipsychotic) flexibly dosed 2.5–10 mg, or placebo	10 weeks	34	All female	Medication produced greater and more rapid weight gain in conjunction with day hospital treatment

become a focus of novel pharmacological research for the treatment of AN because of notable weight gain side effects observed in other psychiatric conditions. While research is not uniformly positive (e.g., with quetiapine; Powers, Klabunde, & Kaye, 2012), the outcome of placebo-controlled randomized controlled trials indicate that olanzapine may be useful for adults with AN, with two studies observing reduced obsessionality among patients receiving adjunctive olanzapine (Bissada et al., 2008; Brambilla et al., 2007), three studies noting that olanzapine produced a greater rate of weight gain (Attia, 2016; Attia et al., 2011; Bissada et al., 2008), and one study indicating that earlier achievement of target BMI occurred in the group randomized to olanzapine (Bissada et al., 2008).

Other medications. Reports of zinc deficiency in AN, in combination with the association of zinc deficiency with symptoms commonly noted among these patients (e.g., weight loss, a decrease in appetite, changes in taste perception, amenorrhea, depression) led to several trials of zinc supplementation, and one controlled study in adults noted an increased rate of weight gain with zinc (Birmingham, Goldner, & Bakan, 1994). As with antipsychotic medications, lithium usage is associated with weight gain, and a single controlled trial of lithium among inpatients with AN was conducted, although little support was found for the utility of this intervention (Gross et al., 1981). A randomized controlled crossover add-on study of dronabinol, which has orexigenic (appetite stimulating) properties including treating nausea and vomiting and increasing appetite, observed a small effect among women with long-standing AN (0.73 kg weight gain above placebo), suggesting the potential utility of synthetic cannabinoid agonists. Several studies have also examined other agents to address symptoms related to AN, including oxytocin for either social emotional stimuli (Kim, Kim, Park, Pyo, & Treasure, 2014), or attention to eating, shape, and weight stimuli (Kim, Kim, Cardi, Eom, Seong, & Treasure, 2014), and alprazolam for anxiety during meal intake, none of which suggested therapeutic effects for weight gain (Steinglass, Kaplan, Liu, Wang, & Walsh, 2014).

Pharmacological Treatments for Bulimia Nervosa

In the following sections, we describe research examining pharmacological treatments for BN, including antidepressant and other medication treatments.

Antidepressant medications. In contrast to the limited benefits of interventions for individuals with AN, both cognitive behavior therapy (CBT) and antidepressant medications are of documented benefit in the treatment of BN. As described generally in this chapter and in detail in published reviews (e.g., Shapiro et al., 2007), antidepressant medications are consistently superior to placebo in pharmacological treatment studies for BN, and median reductions of up to 70% have been observed for symptoms of binge eating and vomiting (Agras, 1997). Despite the availability of effective treatments, binge eating and purging can be chronic for some patients, with about 30% of patients experiencing recurrent symptoms more than a decade after presentation for their disorder (Keel, Mitchell, Miller, Davis, & Crow, 1999).

Most classes of antidepressant medications have been examined in placebo-controlled double-blind studies of adults with BN. Both tricyclic antidepressants (TCAs) and selective serotonin reuptake inhibitors (SSRIs) seem equally efficacious for BN, but SSRI antidepressants are considered the medication treatment of choice for these patients because these treatments are typically better tolerated and have fewer side effects (Golden & Attia, 2011). Further, fluoxetine, an SSRI, is the only drug approved by the U.S. Food and Drug Administration (FDA) for the treatment of BN. Data from the studies of fluoxetine supporting the indication for patients with BN are presented in Table 15.2. A dose of 20 mg per day, typical for major depression, is significantly less effective for BN than 60 mg per day (Fluoxetine Bulimia Nervosa Collaborative Study Group, 1992), and no pretreatment characteristics have been found to predict response to medication among patients with BN. However, by the third week of treatment, it is possible to reliably identify eventual nonresponders to fluoxetine, which allows clinicians to use early response to guide clinical decisions (Sysko et al., 2010). Despite the observed benefits of fluoxetine,

TABLE 15.2

Published Randomized Controlled Pharmacological Treatment Studies for Eating Disorders
With Empirical Support for Medication Utilization for Bulimia Nervosa

Author	Medication (class) and dose	Duration	Sample size	Sample characteristics	Primary outcome
Fluoxetine Bulimia Nervosa Collaborative Study Group, 1992	Fluoxetine (antidepressant) 20 and 60 mg, or placebo	8 weeks medication or placebo	387	All female	Fluoxetine 60 mg was superior to placebo in decreasing episodes of binge eating and vomiting; fluoxetine 20 mg was not different from placebo
Goldstein et al., 1995	Fluoxetine (antidepressant)60 mg, or placebo	16 weeks medication or placebo	398	382 female, 16 male	Fluoxetine associated with greater reduction in binge eating and vomiting

limited controlled data on other SSRIs are available, with some of the extant data indicating positive results (fluvoxamine: Milano, Siano, Putrella, & Capasso, 2005; sertraline: Milano, Petrella, Sabatino, & Capasso, 2004) and others not observing significant reductions in binge eating and vomiting (fluvoxamine: Schmidt et al., 2004; citalopram: Sundblad, Landén, Eriksson, Bergman, & Eriksson, 2005).

Across randomized controlled studies, reductions in binge eating and vomiting from medications vary widely, with an average of about 70% and complete abstinence in less than 20% of individuals (Bacaltchuk & Hay, 2003). Response to antidepressants occurs independent of mood, as depressed and nondepressed patients with BN show equivalent improvements in symptoms, suggesting that the mechanism of action may be different than in depression (Hughes, Wells, & Cunningham, 1986; Walsh, Hadigan, Devlin, Gladis, & Roose, 1991).

Other medications. Other medications may also have utility for bulimic symptoms. Specifically, two placebo-controlled studies observed superior effects of the anticonvulsant topiramate compared with placebo (Hoopes et al., 2003; Nickel et al., 2005). Ondansetron, a serotonin antagonist used for the treatment of chemotherapy-induced nausea and vomiting, was helpful for adults with refractory BN (Faris et al., 2000), and baclofen, a $GABA_B$ agonist shown to decrease craving and use of alcohol and drugs in the treatment of alcohol, cocaine, and opiate use, decreased binge eating episodes in an open trial (Broft et al., 2007). Finally, zonisamide, an antiepileptic drug, produced a significant decrease in binge eating and purging in an open trial, but only 50% of the patients completed the 12 weeks of medication treatment (Guerdjikova et al., 2013). Additional research is needed to confirm any of these preliminary findings.

Pharmacological Treatments for Binge Eating Disorder

A more positive treatment outcome is generally found for patients with BED than the other previously described eating disorders. Pharmacological treatment is not considered the first choice for BED. Research on adults with BED has examined treatment response to antidepressants (fluoxetine, fluvoxamine, escitalopram, citalopram, sertraline), the serotonin and norepinephrine inhibitor duloxetine, the selective norepinephrine reuptake inhibitor atomoxetine, the anticonvulsant topiramate, the antiobesity medication orlistat, and the psychostimulant lisdexamfetamine (Sysko & Devlin, 2010–2017). These trials are detailed in prior reviews, including Brownley and colleagues (2007). Lisdexamfetamine is the only FDA-approved medication for the treatment of BED, and the studies supporting this indication are summarized in Table 15.3. Most psychopharmacology trials for BED are of limited duration (typically 12 weeks

TABLE 15.3

Published Randomized Controlled Pharmacological Treatment Studies for Eating Disorders With Empirical Support for Medication Utilization in Binge Eating Disorder

Author	Medication (class) and dose	Duration	Sample size	Sample characteristics	Primary outcome
McElroy et al., 2015	Lisdexamfetamine (stimulant) 30, 50, 70 mg, or placebo	11 weeks	271	202 female, 69 male	Significant effect on binge eating in comparison with placebo for 50 and 70 mg doses, but not for 30 mg
McElroy et al., 2016	Lisdexamfetamine (stimulant) 50, 70 mg, or placebo	12 weeks	383	328 female, 55 male	Significant effect on binge eating in comparison with placebo for 50 and 70 mg doses
McElroy et al., 2016	Lisdexamfetamine (stimulant) 50, 70 mg, or placebo	12 weeks	390	312 female, 78 male	Significant effect on binge eating in comparison with placebo for 50 and 70 mg doses

or less), which limits generalization of the data to longer term effects (Brownley et al., 2016; Reas & Grilo, 2008), particularly in light of findings for binge eating outcomes in psychotherapy trials, which observe significant differences between symptoms at 6 months and 2-year follow-ups (e.g., Wilson et al., 2010). All of the pharmacologic treatments utilized in studies of BED are efficacious for reducing binge eating episodes (Flament, Bissada, & Spettigue, 2012; Golden & Attia, 2011; McElroy et al., 2016). Similar to the data on psychosocial interventions, medications successfully treat the core psychopathology of BED, but observed weight losses in randomized controlled studies are generally modest, at most.

BEST APPROACHES FOR ASSESSING TREATMENT RESPONSE AND MANAGING SIDE EFFECTS

Assessments of treatment response for medication should focus on the primary symptoms in each diagnostic group; body weight in AN, binge eating and purging in BN, and binge eating episodes in BED. In addition to these core disturbances in patients with eating disorders, there are a wide range of other symptoms experienced by patients with AN, BN, and BED, and residual forms of eating disorders, including cognitive restraint over eating; concerns about shape and weight; and obsessions and compulsions about food, eating, shape, and weight. Instruments

like the EDE and EDE-Q (aforementioned) measure a wide range of symptoms, which can allow the clinician to determine whether related psychopathology is persisting even if the primary behavioral disturbances improve (Sysko & Alavi, 2018). In addition, as a large proportion of patients with eating disorders meet criteria for a comorbid Axis I or Axis II disorders, screening assessments for depression, anxiety, and substance use could also be considered.

The side effects associated with pharmacological treatment of eating disorders are similar to those described in the treatment of other conditions, as the primary interventions occur with antidepressant or antipsychotic medications. However, the physical problems often associated with eating disorders (e.g., starvation in AN, electrolyte disturbances in BN, overweight/obesity in BED) may increase the risks and severity of side effects (e.g., sleep changes, gastrointestinal disturbance). Further, adherence to medications because of side effects (e.g., cognitive problems with topiramate, weight gain with olanzapine) can also be an important factor in clinical management.

MEDICATION MANAGEMENT ISSUES

A surprising number of challenges have arisen in the course of attempting to identify effective pharmacological treatments for AN, including challenges in simply executing medication trials for both adults and adolescents (Halmi et al., 2005; Lock et al., 2012; Norris et al., 2007). Further, the use of medications with individuals with AN is often directed by data from literature on mood disorders or schizophrenia, which may not be appropriate for an eating disordered population, with the potential for increased side effects given the interaction between medication and starvation (Frank & Shott, 2016). It has thus been difficult to gather sufficient information on adherence or discontinuation. However, there are no pharmacologic treatments with a potent therapeutic effect in AN, and therefore medication is not typically recommended as a first-line option or for the prevention of relapse (Walsh et al., 2006).

Many patients with BN are reluctant to take medication and discontinue antidepressants prematurely in clinical practice, which is reflected in notable attrition rates in most studies of medications for BN (Hay & Claudino, 2012). Clinicians may consider discussing the early response phenomenon noted with fluoxetine with their patients with BN (e.g., Sysko et al., 2010), which may allow patients to feel more comfortable with a medication option, as it is possible to evaluate whether an antidepressant can be helpful with bulimic symptoms in a relatively short period of time.

Although several medications are effective for the treatment of BED, as noted above, substantial weight change is generally not observed, which is often a goal of treatment for many patients. It is therefore important for clinicians to discuss the likely outcomes related to a pharmacological intervention (e.g., reduction in binge eating episodes) and how weight will be addressed (e.g., with a behavioral intervention, weight loss surgery) to ensure shared goals and increase the likelihood of adherence to the medication.

EVALUATION OF PHARMACOLOGICAL APPROACHES ACROSS THE LIFESPAN

As eating disorders most commonly emerge during adolescence, data on pharmacologic treatment in children are very limited. Further, there is no evidence that adolescents and adults differ in ways that would alter prescribing decisions. Pharmacological treatment of adolescents must be derived from the adult literature, as with few exceptions (e.g., Biederman et al., 1985), there are no published randomized controlled trials focusing on adolescents. Little is known about the use of medications in older adults with AN or BN, as many studies restrict the age range of participants to younger than 45; however, eating disorder symptoms are notable in population studies of older women (Gagne et al., 2012), suggesting that it will be important to ensure additional work and evaluate the necessity of age-appropriate adaptations to pharmacologic treatments.

In AN, the best prognosis is found among individuals who are younger or receive treatment after a short duration of illness, particularly in comparison to adults with a longer course of illness (Forsberg & Lock, 2015; Herpertz-Dahlmann et al., 2001). In a pilot retrospective study of adolescents during inpatient treatment or following discharge, adjunctive SSRIs (fluoxetine, fluvoxamine, or sertraline) demonstrated a lack of improvement similar to adults with AN (Holtkamp et al., 2005). Adjunctive antipsychotics were found to produce improvements for children, adolescents, and adults with AN in several open and a few controlled studies, including for olanzapine (Barbarich et al., 2004; Boachie, Goldfield, & Spettigue, 2003; Dennis, Le Grange, & Bremer, 2006; Hansen, 1999; Jensen & Mejlhede, 2000; La Via, Gray, & Kaye, 2000; Leggero et al., 2010; Mehler et al., 2001; Mondraty et al., 2005; Powers, Santana, & Bannon, 2002), aripiprazole (Frank, 2016; Frank et al., 2017; Trunko, Schwartz, Duvvuri, & Kaye, 2011), quetiapine (alone: Bosanac et al., 2007; Powers, Bannon, Eubanks, & McCormick, 2007; adjunctive: Mehler-Wex, Romanos, Kirchheiner, & Schulze, 2008), and risperidone (Fisman, Steele, Short, Byrne, & Lavallee, 1996; Newman-Toker, 2000). Other studies show more limited promise for antipsychotic medications, with one pilot placebo-controlled trial of adjunctive olanzapine failing to identify improvements beyond those found with standard eating disorders treatment (Kafantaris et al., 2011), and no significant benefit from risperidone versus placebo in a similar study (Hagman et al., 2011). In comparison with the data in adults, two studies of adolescents showed no effect of zinc on weight gain (Katz et al., 1987; Lask, Fosson, Rolfe, & Thomas, 1993).

In BN, fluoxetine at 60 mg is well tolerated and potentially useful based on a small open trial (Kotler, Devlin, Davies, & Walsh, 2003), and although the trials were conducted with adults, topiramate is approved for the treatment of seizure disorders with individuals as young as 2 years old. No research provides insight into the use of medication with adolescents with BED.

There are several issues to consider in treating adolescents with medications, which are reviewed in greater detail in recent publications (Eating Disorders Commission, 2017), particularly given that the pharmacokinetics and pharmacodynamics in children and adolescents are not well studied. In brief, differences in the metabolism and/or the effects of medications in adolescents with eating disorders may be present, which could require changes to dosage or result in different responses to pharmacology treatment. Potential safety concerns related to medical instability should also be taken into account. For example, although TCAs and mood stabilizers are used less frequently at this time, these medications were associated with sudden death among adolescents without eating disorders (Geller, Reising, Leonard, Riddle, & Walsh, 1999), and risks from tricyclics theoretically increase the cardiac abnormalities related to AN. Further, a black box warning was issued by the FDA in 2004 warning of the potential for some SSRIs to increase suicidal ideation among adolescents (U.S. Food and Drug Administration, 2004). Clinicians should monitor for potential suicidal ideation when starting an SSRI, particularly with younger patients.

CONSIDERATION OF POTENTIAL SEX DIFFERENCES

Sex differences in prevalence rates for BED are less significant than for AN and BN, with several studies showing that BED occurs in about as many men and women (Lewinsohn et al., 2002; Mond & Hay, 2007; Striegel-Moore et al., 2009). In contrast, research on other eating disorders note a much more prominent difference, with a range from a 10:1 ratio of women to men (Götestam et al., 1998; Hoek et al.,

1995; Lucas, Beard, O'Fallon, & Kurland, 1991) to a 3:1 ratio of women to men (Hudson et al., 2007). There are several possible reasons for the range of observed sex differences in prevalence for AN and BN. From earlier studies demonstrating a 10:1 ratio and the Hudson and colleagues (2007) study, there may have been an actual rise in the numbers of male cases with eating disorders, or a reduction in gender bias in more revisions to the diagnostic criteria, or clinicians having a greater awareness of eating disorders in males (Hildebrandt & Craigen, 2016). There are no data suggesting sex-specific pharmacological treatment effects or pharmacokinetic differences in eating disorders; however, it should be noted that most randomized controlled trials in AN (e.g., Bissada et al., 2008; Walsh et al., 2006) and BN (e.g., Fluoxetine Bulimia Nervosa Collaborative Study Group, 1992) have enrolled only women. Even studies of BED are not evenly distributed across the sexes, with Reas and Grilo (2015) observing that a total of 85.2% ($n = 1,705$ of 2,001) of participants enrolled in 22 randomized controlled trials were women. Future studies should evaluate potential sex-specific differences in treatment response to pharmacologic agents.

INTEGRATION OF PHARMACOTHERAPY WITH NONPHARMACOLOGICAL APPROACHES: BENEFITS AND CHALLENGES

There are no controlled trials examining the combination of psychological and pharmacological treatment for underweight individuals with AN. As research to date does not suggest substantial utility of psychiatric medications for AN, any potential benefits from combined treatments are not known.

Patients with BN treated with CBT typically evidence reductions in binge eating and purging of 80% or more, and at the end of treatment, approximately 30% of patients are abstinent from binge eating and purging (National Institute of Clinical Excellence, 2004). Some studies (e.g., Walsh et al., 1997) and meta-analyses of studies that combine treatments for adults with BN, primarily antidepressants and psychotherapy (e.g., CBT; Bacaltchuk, Hay, & Trefiglio, 2001; Nakash-Eisikovits, Dierberger, &

Westen, 2002), indicate an advantage for combined treatments. However, the available research may not be sufficient to determine whether combination therapy or psychotherapy alone are superior to antidepressant treatment (Bacaltchuk et al., 2001), and there are no controlled studies of combined treatments in adolescents with BN.

Reductions in binge eating among individuals with BED occur in response to a variety of treatments (CBT, interpersonal psychotherapy, behavioral weight loss [BWL]; Wilson et al., 2010), and are usually maintained for at least 1 year following the intervention (Ricca et al., 2001; Wilson et al., 2010). CBT is currently considered to be the treatment of first choice for BED. Psychological treatments for BED have been shown to successfully reduce binge eating and associated psychological symptoms, but for individuals with BED, a majority of whom are overweight or obese, psychotherapies are not associated with any significant weight loss in the short or long term (Wilson et al., 2010; Wonderlich, de Zwaan, Mitchell, Peterson, & Crow, 2003), which is independently associated with morbidity and mortality (National Task Force on the Prevention and Treatment of Obesity, 2000). As with BN, a dearth of research exists for combined psychological and pharmacological treatments for BED. A recent review (Grilo, Reas, & Mitchell, 2016) indicated that the combination of pharmacological treatment with CBT or BWL leads to better outcomes in comparison to medication alone; however, superior outcomes are not observed for those with CBT or BWL alone. With regard to weight change, orlistat produced minimally improved weight losses with CBT or BWL, and topiramate was the only medication showing enhanced reductions in binge eating and weight in combination with CBT (Grilo et al., 2016).

INTEGRATED APPROACHES FOR ADDRESSING COMMON COMORBID DISORDERS

Comorbid psychiatric diagnoses are expected among treatment-seeking patients with eating disorders. Frequencies of lifetime anxiety disorders are reported to range from approximately 33% to 72% of patients with AN-R, 55% of patients with AN-B/P, 41% to 75% of patients with BN (Godart, Flament, Perdereau, & Jeammet, 2002), and 29% of patients with BED (Wilfley, Friedman, et al., 2000). Similarly wide ranges of lifetime major depressive disorder have been noted, including 9.5% to 64.7% in AN-R, 50% to 71.3% in AN-B/P, 20% to 80% of patients with BN (Godart et al., 2007), and 58% in BED (Wilfley, Friedman, et al., 2000). The most rigorous and well-conducted population-based study reported a 33.7% comorbidity between eating and alcohol use disorders, yielding a prevalence of approximately 4.85 million people in the United States (Hudson et al., 2007). In clinical samples, patients with binge eating behavior reported a higher prevalence of alcohol or drug problems (Braun et al., 1994; Bulik et al., 2004; Herzog et al., 1992; Wiederman & Pryor, 1996a, 1996b), with approximately 45% of patients consuming alcohol regularly (mean of 12 drinks/week; Bulik, 1992), 34.8% using alcohol weekly (Wiederman & Pryor, 1996a), and a median prevalence of 22.9% (Holderness et al., 1994).

In general, improvements in concurrent symptoms are not noted among individuals with AN receiving medication treatment (e.g., Attia et al., 1998). As previously mentioned, it is possible that the effects of starvation interfere with the antidepressant effects in patients with acute AN, as significant improvements in concurrent mood and anxiety symptoms have been observed as a consequence of weight restoration via behavioral means in these individuals (Meehan, Loeb, Roberto, & Attia, 2006). Further, the assessment of depressive symptoms could result in inconsistent results, with some research using continuous self-report measures (e.g., Beck Depression Inventory) and other work examining a diagnosis of major depressive disorder (Frank & Shott, 2016). Assigning a diagnosis of major depression is also complicated when an individual is experiencing acute AN, where some symptoms (e.g., sleep disturbance, low energy, trouble concentrating) could originate from starvation or an underlying mood problem. Statistically significant improvements have been found for mood symptoms among inpatients with AN when nutritional rehabilitation and psychotherapy is provided (Meehan et al., 2006). Successful medication treatment also appears to alleviate comorbid depressive symptoms for BN (e.g., Fluoxetine Bulimia Nervosa Collaborative Study Group, 1992) and BED (e.g., Devlin et al., 2005).

Decisions to initiate a psychopharmacological intervention are influenced by a number of factors, including psychiatric comorbidity. Although as described above, some data from studies of the effects of medications on eating disorders have also measured improvements in co-occurring symptoms, there are no empirical studies that focused solely on comorbid samples. It is therefore possible that a clinician might decide to prescribe fluoxetine at a 60 mg dosage to an individual with BN because of empirical support suggesting effects on binge eating and purging, and wait to see whether benefits are observed for comorbid OCD, or to initiate fluoxetine at a higher dosage in the range typically used for OCD treatment.

Co-occurring medical conditions can affect the safety of using a medication for eating disorder treatment. For example, the consequences of starvation in AN and the possibility of electrolyte disturbances in BN may influence the risk associated with taking a medication. Further, medical status appears to impact the potential for side effects, including the example of an increased prevalence of grand mal seizures among patients with BN taking bupropion.

EMERGING TRENDS

Outside of the increasing use of antipsychotic medications for the treatment of AN, as described previously, and the recent FDA approval of lisdexamfetamine for the treatment of BED, little has changed significantly in the last decade with regard to empirical data on pharmacological treatments for eating disorders. As lisdexamfetamine is a U.S. Drug Enforcement Administration Schedule II controlled stimulant with a potential for abuse or physiological dependence and has cardiovascular side effects, there are concerns about wider usage of this medication in the population of individuals with BED when other effective psychological and pharmacological treatments are available.

The study of pharmacologic treatment and application of medications to eating disorders has resulted in dissimilar outcomes across conditions. In AN, despite decades of work, medication options do not offer robust effects on the core psychopathology of this diagnosis (low body weight). Data from studies of patients with BN and BED have found contrasting results, with two medications (BN: fluoxetine; BED: lisdexamfetamine) currently approved by the FDA for the treatment of these conditions. Although the pharmaceutical industry has moved away from the development of compounds intended to target psychiatric symptoms, it is possible that novel methods for studying the human brain could lead to a better understanding of the mechanisms maintaining AN in particular, which would allow for the development of specific medication treatments (Frank & Shott, 2016).

TOOL KIT OF RESOURCES

Eating Disorders

Assessment Measures

Eating Disorder Examination (17.0D): http://www.credo-oxford.com/pdfs/EDE_17.0D.pdf

Eating Disorder Assessment for DSM–5: http://www.eda5.org

Eating Disorder Diagnostic Scale: http://www.ori.org/sticemeasures

Patient Resources

National Eating Disorders Association Handouts: http://www.nationaleatingdisorders.org/learn

American Psychiatric Association: https://www.psychiatry.org/patients-families/eating-disorders/what-are-eating-disorders

National Institute of Mental Health: https://www.nimh.nih.gov/health/topics/eating-disorders/index.shtml

Provider Resources

PhenX Toolkit for resources on eating disorder assessment: https://www.phenxtoolkit.org/index.php

Academy for Eating Disorders, Medical Guidelines: https://www.aedweb.org/learn/publications/medical-care-standards

Walsh, B. T., Attia, E. A., Glasofer, D. R., & Sysko, R. (Eds.). (2016). *Handbook of assessment and treatment of eating disorders*. Washington, DC: American Psychiatric Association.

References

American Psychiatric Association. (2013). *Diagnostic and statistical manual of mental disorders* (5th ed.). Washington, DC: American Psychiatric Association.

Agras, W. S. (1997). Pharmacotherapy of bulimia nervosa and binge eating disorder: Longer-term outcomes. *Psychopharmacology Bulletin, 33*, 433–436.

Attia, E. (October, 2016). Who is willing to take olanzapine and why? An initial look at outpatient participants in an olanzapine vs placebo trial for anorexia nervosa. Presented at the XXII Annual Meeting of the Eating Disorders Research Society, New York, NY.

Attia, E., Haiman, C., Walsh, B. T., & Flater, S. R. (1998). Does fluoxetine augment the inpatient treatment of anorexia nervosa? *The American Journal of Psychiatry, 155*, 548–551. http://dx.doi.org/10.1176/ajp.155.4.548

Attia, E., Kaplan, A. S., Walsh, B. T., Gershkovich, M., Yilmaz, Z., Musante, D., & Wang, Y. (2011). Olanzapine versus placebo for out-patients with anorexia nervosa. *Psychological Medicine, 41*, 2177–2182. http://dx.doi.org/10.1017/S0033291711000390

Bacaltchuk, J., & Hay, P. (2003). Antidepressants versus placebo for people with bulimia nervosa. *Cochrane Database of Systematic Reviews, 2003*(4), CD003391.

Bacaltchuk, J., Hay, P., & Trefiglio, R. (2001). Antidepressants versus psychological treatments and their combination for bulimia nervosa. *Cochrane Database of Systematic Reviews, 2001*(4), CD003385.

Barbarich, N. C., McConaha, C. W., Gaskill, J., La Via, M., Frank, G. K., Achenbach, S., . . . Kaye, W. H. (2004). An open trial of olanzapine in anorexia nervosa. *The Journal of Clinical Psychiatry, 65*, 1480–1482. http://dx.doi.org/10.4088/JCP.v65n1106

Becker, A. E., Burwell, R. A., Gilman, S. E., Herzog, D. B., & Hamburg, P. (2002). Eating behaviours and attitudes following prolonged television exposure among ethnic Fijian adolescent girls. *The British Journal of Psychiatry, 180*, 509–514. http://dx.doi.org/10.1192/bjp.180.6.509

Berg, K. C., Peterson, C. B., Frazier, P., & Crow, S. J. (2012). Psychometric evaluation of the eating disorder examination and eating disorder examination-questionnaire: A systematic review of the literature. *International Journal of Eating Disorders, 45*, 428–438. http://dx.doi.org/10.1002/eat.20931

Biederman, J., Herzog, D. B., Rivinus, T. M., Harper, G. P., Ferber, R. A., Rosenbaum, J. F., . . . Schildkraut, J. J. (1985). Amitriptyline in the treatment of anorexia nervosa: A double-blind, placebo-controlled study. *Journal of Clinical Psychopharmacology, 5*, 10–16. http://dx.doi.org/10.1097/00004714-198502000-00003

Birmingham, C. L., Goldner, E. M., & Bakan, R. (1994). Controlled trial of zinc supplementation in anorexia nervosa. *International Journal of Eating Disorders, 15*, 251–255.

Bissada, H., Tasca, G. A., Barber, A. M., & Bradwejn, J. (2008). Olanzapine in the treatment of low body weight and obsessive thinking in women with anorexia nervosa: A randomized, double-blind, placebo-controlled trial. *The American Journal of Psychiatry, 165*, 1281–1288. http://dx.doi.org/10.1176/appi.ajp.2008.07121900

Boachie, A., Goldfield, G. S., & Spettigue, W. (2003). Olanzapine use as an adjunctive treatment for hospitalized children with anorexia nervosa: Case reports. *International Journal of Eating Disorders, 33*, 98–103. http://dx.doi.org/10.1002/eat.10115

Bosanac, P., Kurlender, S., Norman, T., Hallam, K., Wesnes, K., Manktelow, T., & Burrows, G. (2007). An open-label study of quetiapine in anorexia nervosa. *Human Psychopharmacology: Clinical and Experimental, 22*, 223–230. http://dx.doi.org/10.1002/hup.845

Brambilla, F., Garcia, C. S., Fassino, S., Daga, G. A., Favaro, A., Santonastaso, P., . . . Monteleone, P. (2007). Olanzapine therapy in anorexia nervosa: Psychobiological effects. *International Clinical Psychopharmacology, 22*, 197–204. http://dx.doi.org/10.1097/YIC.0b013e328080ca31

Braun, D. L., Sunday, S. R., & Halmi, K. A. (1994). Psychiatric comorbidity in patients with eating disorders. *Psychological Medicine, 24*, 859–867. http://dx.doi.org/10.1017/S0033291700028956

Broft, A. I., Spanos, A., Corwin, R. L., Mayer, L., Steinglass, J., Devlin, M. J., . . . Walsh, B. T. (2007). Baclofen for binge eating: An open-label trial. *International Journal of Eating Disorders, 40*, 687–691. http://dx.doi.org/10.1002/eat.20434

Brownley, K. A., Berkman, N. D., Peat, C. M., Lohr, K. N., Cullen, K. E., Bann, C. M., & Bulik, C. M. (2016). Binge-eating disorder in adults: A systematic review and meta-analysis. *Annals of Internal Medicine, 165*, 409–420. http://dx.doi.org/10.7326/M15-2455

Brownley, K. A., Berkman, N. D., Sedway, J. A., Lohr, K. N., & Bulik, C. M. (2007). Binge eating disorder treatment: A systematic review of randomized controlled trials. *International Journal of Eating Disorders, 40*, 337–348. http://dx.doi.org/10.1002/eat.20370

Bryant-Waugh, R. J., Cooper, P. J., Taylor, C. L., & Lask, B. D. (1996). The use of the eating disorder examination with children: A pilot study. *International Journal of Eating Disorders, 19*, 391–397. http://dx.doi.org/10.1002/(SICI)1098-108X(199605)19:4<391::AID-EAT6>3.0.CO;2-G

Bulik, C. M. (1992). Abuse of drugs associated with eating disorders. *Journal of Substance Abuse, 4*, 69–90. http://dx.doi.org/10.1016/0899-3289(92)90029-W

*Asterisks indicate assessments or resources.

Bulik, C. M., Berkman, N. D., Brownley, K. A., Sedway, J. A., & Lohr, K. N. (2007). Anorexia nervosa treatment: A systematic review of randomized controlled trials. *International Journal of Eating Disorders, 40*, 310–320. http://dx.doi.org/10.1002/eat.20367

Bulik, C. M., Klump, K. L., Thornton, L., Kaplan, A. S., Devlin, B., Fichter, M. M., . . . Kaye, W. H. (2004). Alcohol use disorder comorbidity in eating disorders: A multicenter study. *The Journal of Clinical Psychiatry, 65*, 1000–1006. http://dx.doi.org/10.4088/JCP.v65n0718

Caudle, H., Pang, C., Mancuso, S., Castle, D., & Newton, R. (2015). A retrospective study of the impact of *DSM–5* on the diagnosis of eating disorders in Victoria, Australia. *Journal of Eating Disorders, 3*, 35. http://dx.doi.org/10.1186/s40337-015-0072-0

Dennis, K., Le Grange, D., & Bremer, J. (2006). Olanzapine use in adolescent anorexia nervosa. *Eating and Weight Disorders, 11*, e53–e56. http://dx.doi.org/10.1007/BF03327760

Devlin, M. J., Goldfein, J. A., Petkova, E., Jiang, H., Raizman, P. S., Wolk, S., . . . Walsh, B. T. (2005). Cognitive behavioral therapy and fluoxetine as adjuncts to group behavioral therapy for binge eating disorder. *Obesity Research, 13*, 1077–1088. http://dx.doi.org/10.1038/oby.2005.126

Duncan, L., Yilmaz, Z., Gaspar, H., Walters, R., Goldstein, J., Anttila, V., . . . Bulik, C. M., & the Eating Disorders Working Group of the Psychiatric Genomics Consortium. (2017). Significant locus and metabolic genetic correlations revealed in genome-wide association study of anorexia nervosa. *The American Journal of Psychiatry, 174*, 850–858. http://dx.doi.org/10.1176/appi.ajp.2017.16121402

Eating Disorders Commission. (2017). Part IV: Eating disorders. In D. L. Evans, E. Foa, R. Gur, H. Hendin, C. P. O'Brien, M. E. P. Seligman, & B. T. Walsh (Eds.), *Treating and preventing adolescent mental health disorders: What we know and what we don't know* (pp. 13–16). Oxford, UK: Oxford University Press.

Eddy, K. T., Crosby, R. D., Keel, P. K., Wonderlich, S. A., le Grange, D., Hill, L., . . . Mitchell, J. E. (2009). Empirical identification and validation of eating disorder phenotypes in a multisite clinical sample. *Journal of Nervous and Mental Disease, 197*, 41–49. http://dx.doi.org/10.1097/NMD.0b013e3181927389

Edler, C., Haedt, A. A., & Keel, P. K. (2007). The use of multiple purging methods as an indicator of eating disorder severity. *International Journal of Eating Disorders, 40*, 515–520. http://dx.doi.org/10.1002/eat.20416

Engel, S. G., Corneliussen, S. J., Wonderlich, S. A., Crosby, R. D., le Grange, D., Crow, S., . . . Steiger, H. (2005). Impulsivity and compulsivity in bulimia

nervosa. *International Journal of Eating Disorders, 38*, 244–251. http://dx.doi.org/10.1002/eat.20169

Fairburn, C. G., & Beglin, S. J. (2008). Eating Disorder Examination Questionnaire (6.0). In C. G. Fairburn (Ed.), *Cognitive behavior therapy and eating disorders* (pp. 309–314). New York, NY: Guilford Press.

Fairburn, C. G., Cooper, Z., & O'Connor, M. (2008). Eating Disorder Examination (16.0D). In C. G. Fairburn (Ed.), *Cognitive behavior therapy and eating disorders* (pp. 265–308). New York, NY: Guilford Press.

Faris, P. L., Kim, S. W., Meller, W. H., Goodale, R. L., Oakman, S. A., Hofbauer, R. D., . . . Hartman, B. K. (2000). Effect of decreasing afferent vagal activity with ondansetron on symptoms of bulimia nervosa: A randomised, double-blind trial. *Lancet, 355*, 792–797. http://dx.doi.org/10.1016/S0140-6736(99)09062-5

Favaro, A., & Santonastaso, P. (1996). Purging behaviors, suicide attempts, and psychiatric symptoms in 398 eating disordered subjects. *International Journal of Eating Disorders, 20*, 99–103. http://dx.doi.org/10.1002/(SICI)1098-108X(199607)20:1<99::AID-EAT11>3.0.CO;2-E

Fichter, M. M., Quadflieg, N., & Hedlund, S. (2006). Twelve-year course and outcome predictors of anorexia nervosa. *International Journal of Eating Disorders, 39*, 87–100. http://dx.doi.org/10.1002/eat.20215

First, M. B., Spitzer, R. L., Gibbon, M., & Williams, J. B. W. (2002). *Structured Clinical Interview for DSM–IV Axis I Disorders, Research Version, Patient Edition.* (SCID-I/P). New York, NY: Biometrics Research, New York State Psychiatric Institute.

First, M. B., Williams, J. B. W., Karg, R. S., & Spitzer, R. L. (2015). *Structured Clinical Interview for DSM–5—Research Version (SCID-5 for DSM–5, Research Version; SCID-5-RV).* Washington, DC: American Psychiatric Association.

Fisman, S., Steele, M., Short, J., Byrne, T., & Lavallee, C. (1996). Case study: Anorexia nervosa and autistic disorder in an adolescent girl. *Journal of the American Academy of Child & Adolescent Psychiatry, 35*, 937–940. http://dx.doi.org/10.1097/00004583-199607000-00021

Flament, M. F., Bissada, H., & Spettigue, W. (2012). Evidence-based pharmacotherapy of eating disorders. *International Journal of Neuropsychopharmacology, 15*, 189–207. http://dx.doi.org/10.1017/S1461145711000381

*Fluoxetine Bulimia Nervosa Collaborative Study Group. (1992). Fluoxetine in the treatment of bulimia nervosa. A multicenter, placebo-controlled, double-blind trial. *Archives of General Psychiatry, 49*, 139–147. http://dx.doi.org/10.1001/archpsyc.1992.01820020059008

Forsberg, S., & Lock, J. (2015). Family-based treatment of child and adolescent eating disorders. *Child and Adolescent Psychiatric Clinics of North America, 24*, 617–629. http://dx.doi.org/10.1016/j.chc.2015.02.012

Frank, G. K. (2016). Aripiprazole, a partial dopamine agonist to improve adolescent anorexia nervosa-A case series. *International Journal of Eating Disorders, 49*, 529–533. http://dx.doi.org/10.1002/eat.22485

Frank, G. K., & Shott, M. E. (2016). The role of psychotropic medications in the management of anorexia nervosa: Rationale, evidence and future prospects. *CNS Drugs, 30*, 419–442. http://dx.doi.org/10.1007/s40263-016-0335-6

Frank, G. K., Shott, M. E., Hagman, J. O., Schiel, M. A., DeGuzman, M. C., & Rossi, B. (2017). The partial dopamine D2 receptor agonist aripiprazole is associated with weight gain in adolescent anorexia nervosa. *International Journal of Eating Disorders, 50*, 447–450. http://dx.doi.org/10.1002/eat.22704

Gagne, D. A., Von Holle, A., Brownley, K. A., Runfola, C. D., Hofmeier, S., Branch, K. E., & Bulik, C. M. (2012). Eating disorder symptoms and weight and shape concerns in a large web-based convenience sample of women ages 50 and above: Results of the Gender and Body Image (GABI) study. *International Journal of Eating Disorders, 45*, 832–844. http://dx.doi.org/10.1002/eat.22030

Geller, B., Reising, D., Leonard, H. L., Riddle, M. A., & Walsh, B. T. (1999). Critical review of tricyclic antidepressant use in children and adolescents. *Journal of the American Academy of Child & Adolescent Psychiatry, 38*, 513–516. http://dx.doi.org/10.1097/00004583-199905000-00012

Gianini, L., Roberto, C. A., Attia, E., Walsh, B. T., Thomas, J. J., Eddy, K. T., . . . Sysko, R. (2017). Mild, moderate, meaningful? Examining the psychological and functioning correlates of *DSM–5* eating disorder severity specifiers. *International Journal of Eating Disorders, 50*, 906–916. http://dx.doi.org/10.1002/eat.22728

Glasofer, D. R., Sysko, R., & Walsh, B. T. (2016). The use of the EDA-5. In B. T. Walsh, E. A. Attia, D. R. Glasofer, & R. Sysko (Eds.), *Handbook of assessment and treatment of eating disorders* (pp. 175–205). Washington, DC: American Psychiatric Association.

Godart, N. T., Flament, M. F., Perdereau, F., & Jeammet, P. (2002). Comorbidity between eating disorders and anxiety disorders: A review. *International Journal of Eating Disorders, 32*, 253–270. http://dx.doi.org/10.1002/eat.10096

Godart, N. T., Perdereau, F., Rein, Z., Berthoz, S., Wallier, J., Jeammet, P., & Flament, M. F. (2007). Comorbidity studies of eating disorders and mood disorders. Critical review of the literature. *Journal of Affective Disorders, 97*, 37–49. http://dx.doi.org/10.1016/j.jad.2006.06.023

*Golden, N. H., & Attia, E. (2011). Psychopharmacology of eating disorders in children and adolescents. *Pediatric Clinics of North America, 58*, 121–138, xi. http://dx.doi.org/10.1016/j.pcl.2010.11.001

Goldstein, D. J., Wilson, M. G., Thompson, V. L., Potvin, J. H., Rampey, A. H., Jr., & the Fluoxetine Bulimia Nervosa Research Group. (1995). Long-term fluoxetine treatment of bulimia nervosa. *The British Journal of Psychiatry, 166*, 660–666. http://dx.doi.org/10.1192/bjp.166.5.660

Götestam, K. G., Eriksen, L., Heggestad, T., & Nielsen, S. (1998). Prevalence of eating disorders in Norwegian general hospitals 1990–1994: Admissions per year and seasonality. *International Journal of Eating Disorders, 23*, 57–64. http://dx.doi.org/10.1002/(SICI)1098-108X(199801)23:1<57::AID-EAT7>3.0.CO;2-0

Grilo, C. M., Hrabosky, J. I., White, M. A., Allison, K. C., Stunkard, A. J., & Masheb, R. M. (2008). Overvaluation of shape and weight in binge eating disorder and overweight controls: Refinement of a diagnostic construct. *Journal of Abnormal Psychology, 117*, 414–419. http://dx.doi.org/10.1037/0021-843X.117.2.414

Grilo, C. M., Ivezaj, V., & White, M. A. (2015a). Evaluation of the *DSM–5* severity indicator for bulimia nervosa. *Behaviour Research and Therapy, 67*, 41–44. http://dx.doi.org/10.1016/j.brat.2015.02.002

Grilo, C. M., Ivezaj, V., & White, M. A. (2015b). Evaluation of the *DSM–5* severity indicator for binge eating disorder in a community sample. *Behaviour Research and Therapy, 66*, 72–76. http://dx.doi.org/10.1016/j.brat.2015.01.004

Grilo, C. M., Ivezaj, V., & White, M. A. (2015c). Evaluation of the *DSM–5* severity indicator for binge eating disorder in a clinical sample. *Behaviour Research and Therapy, 71*, 110–114. http://dx.doi.org/10.1016/j.brat.2015.05.003

Grilo, C. M., & Masheb, R. M. (2005). A randomized controlled comparison of guided self-help cognitive behavioral therapy and behavioral weight loss for binge eating disorder. *Behaviour Research and Therapy, 43*, 1509–1525. http://dx.doi.org/10.1016/j.brat.2004.11.010

Grilo, C. M., Reas, D. L., & Mitchell, J. E. (2016). Combining pharmacological and psychological treatments for binge eating disorder: Current status, limitations, and future directions. *Current Psychiatry Reports, 18*, 55. http://dx.doi.org/10.1007/s11920-016-0696-z

Gross, H. A., Ebert, M. H., Faden, V. B., Goldberg, S. C., Nee, L. E., & Kaye, W. H. (1981). A double-blind controlled trial of lithium carbonate primary anorexia nervosa. *Journal of Clinical Psychopharmacology, 1*, 376–381. http://dx.doi.org/10.1097/00004714-198111000-00005

Gualandi, M., Simoni, M., Manzato, E., & Scanelli, G. (2016). Reassessment of patients with Eating Disorders after moving from *DSM–IV* towards *DSM–5*: A retrospective study in a clinical sample. *Eating and Weight Disorders, 21*, 617–624. http://dx.doi.org/10.1007/s40519-016-0314-4

Guerdjikova, A. I., Blom, T. J., Martens, B. E., Keck, P. E., Jr., & McElroy, S. L. (2013). Zonisamide in the treatment of bulimia nervosa: An open-label, pilot, prospective study. *International Journal of Eating Disorders, 46*, 747–750. http://dx.doi.org/10.1002/eat.22159

Hagman, J., Gralla, J., Sigel, E., Ellert, S., Dodge, M., Gardner, R., . . . Wamboldt, M. Z. (2011). A double-blind, placebo-controlled study of risperidone for the treatment of adolescents and young adults with anorexia nervosa: A pilot study. *Journal of the American Academy of Child & Adolescent Psychiatry, 50*, 915–924. http://dx.doi.org/10.1016/j.jaac.2011.06.009

Halmi, K. A., Agras, W. S., Crow, S., Mitchell, J., Wilson, G. T., Bryson, S. W., & Kraemer, H. C. (2005). Predictors of treatment acceptance and completion in anorexia nervosa: Implications for future study designs. *Archives of General Psychiatry, 62*, 776–781. http://dx.doi.org/10.1001/archpsyc.62.7.776

Halmi, K. A., Eckert, E., LaDu, T. J., & Cohen, J. (1986). Anorexia nervosa: Treatment efficacy of cyproheptadine and amitriptyline. *Archives of General Psychiatry, 43*, 177–181. http://dx.doi.org/10.1001/archpsyc.1986.01800020087011

Hansen, L. (1999). Olanzapine in the treatment of anorexia nervosa. *The British Journal of Psychiatry, 175*, 592. http://dx.doi.org/10.1192/S000712500026354X

Hay, P. J., & Claudino, A. M. (2012). Clinical psychopharmacology of eating disorders: A research update. *International Journal of Neuropsychopharmacology, 15*, 209–222. http://dx.doi.org/10.1017/S1461145711000460

Herpertz-Dahlmann, B., Müller, B., Herpertz, S., Heussen, N., Hebebrand, J., & Remschmidt, H. (2001). Prospective 10-year follow-up in adolescent anorexia nervosa—Course, outcome, psychiatric comorbidity, and psychosocial adaptation. *Journal of Child Psychology and Psychiatry, 42*, 603–612. http://dx.doi.org/10.1111/1469-7610.00756

Herzog, D. B., Keller, M. B., Sacks, N. R., Yeh, C. J., & Lavori, P. W. (1992). Psychiatric comorbidity in treatment-seeking anorexics and bulimics. *Journal of the American Academy of Child & Adolescent Psychiatry, 31*, 810–818. http://dx.doi.org/10.1097/00004583-199209000-00006

Hildebrandt, T., & Craigen, K. (2016). Eating-related pathology in men and boys. In B. T. Walsh, E. A. Attia, D. R. Glasofer, & R. Sysko (Eds.), *Handbook of assessment and treatment of eating disorders*. Washington, DC: American Psychiatric Association.

*Himmerich, H., & Treasure, J. (2018). Psychopharmacological advances in eating disorders. *Expert Review of Clinical Pharmacology, 11*, 95–108. http://dx.doi.org/10.1080/17512433.2018.1383895

Hoek, H. W., Bartelds, A. I., Bosveld, J. J., van der Graaf, Y., Limpens, V. E., Maiwald, M., & Spaaij, C. J. (1995). Impact of urbanization on detection rates of eating disorders. *The American Journal of Psychiatry, 152*, 1272–1278. http://dx.doi.org/10.1176/ajp.152.9.1272

Holderness, C. C., Brooks-Gunn, J., & Warren, M. P. (1994). Co-morbidity of eating disorders and substance abuse review of the literature. *International Journal of Eating Disorders, 16*, 1–34. http://dx.doi.org/10.1002/1098-108X(199407)16:1<1::AID-EAT2260160102>3.0.CO;2-T

Holtkamp, K., Konrad, K., Kaiser, N., Ploenes, Y., Heussen, N., Grzella, I., & Herpertz-Dahlmann, B. (2005). A retrospective study of SSRI treatment in adolescent anorexia nervosa: Insufficient evidence for efficacy. *Journal of Psychiatric Research, 39*, 303–310. http://dx.doi.org/10.1016/j.jpsychires.2004.08.001

Hoopes, S. P., Reimherr, F. W., Hedges, D. W., Rosenthal, N. R., Kamin, M., Karim, R., . . . Karvois, D. (2003). Treatment of bulimia nervosa with topiramate in a randomized, double-blind, placebo-controlled trial, part 1: Improvement in binge and purge measures. *The Journal of Clinical Psychiatry, 64*, 1335–1341. http://dx.doi.org/10.4088/JCP.v64n1109

*Hudson, J. I., Hiripi, E., Pope, H. G., Jr., & Kessler, R. C. (2007). The prevalence and correlates of eating disorders in the National Comorbidity Survey Replication. *Biological Psychiatry, 61*, 348–358. http://dx.doi.org/10.1016/j.biopsych.2006.03.040

Hughes, P. L., Wells, L. A., & Cunningham, C. J. (1986). The dexamethasone suppression test in bulimia before and after successful treatment with desipramine. *The Journal of Clinical Psychiatry, 47*, 515–517.

Jensen, V. S., & Mejlhede, A. (2000). Anorexia nervosa: Treatment with olanzapine. *The British Journal of Psychiatry, 177*, 87. http://dx.doi.org/10.1192/bjp.177.1.87

Jones, D. C., & Crawford, J. K. (2006). The peer appearance culture during adolescence: Gender and body mass variations. *Journal of Youth and Adolescence, 35*, 243–255. http://dx.doi.org/10.1007/s10964-005-9006-5

Kafantaris, V., Leigh, E., Hertz, S., Berest, A., Schebendach, J., Sterling, W. M., . . . Malhotra, A. K. (2011). A placebo-controlled pilot study of adjunctive olanzapine for adolescents with anorexia nervosa. *Journal of Child and Adolescent Psychopharmacology, 21*, 207–212. http://dx.doi.org/10.1089/cap.2010.0139

Katz, R. L., Keen, C. L., Litt, I. F., Hurley, L. S., Kellams-Harrison, K. M., & Glader, L. J. (1987). Zinc deficiency in anorexia nervosa. *Journal of Adolescent Health*

Care, 8, 400–406. http://dx.doi.org/10.1016/0197-0070(87)90227-0

Kaye, W. H., Fudge, J. L., & Paulus, M. (2009). New insights into symptoms and neurocircuit function of anorexia nervosa. *Nature Reviews Neuroscience, 10,* 573–584. http://dx.doi.org/10.1038/nrn2682

Keel, P. K., Brown, T. A., Holm-Denoma, J., & Bodell, L. P. (2011). Comparison of *DSM–IV* versus proposed *DSM–5* diagnostic criteria for eating disorders: Reduction of eating disorder not otherwise specified and validity. *International Journal of Eating Disorders, 44,* 553–560. http://dx.doi.org/10.1002/eat.20892

Keel, P. K., & Klump, K. L. (2003). Are eating disorders culture-bound syndromes? Implications for conceptualizing their etiology. *Psychological Bulletin, 129,* 747–769. http://dx.doi.org/10.1037/0033-2909.129.5.747

Keel, P. K., Mitchell, J. E., Miller, K. B., Davis, T. L., & Crow, S. J. (1999). Long-term outcome of bulimia nervosa. *Archives of General Psychiatry, 56,* 63–69. http://dx.doi.org/10.1001/archpsyc.56.1.63

Kim, Y. R., Kim, C. H., Cardi, V., Eom, J. S., Seong, Y., & Treasure, J. (2014). Intranasal oxytocin attenuates attentional bias for eating and fat shape stimuli in patients with anorexia nervosa. *Psychoneuroendocrinology, 44,* 133–142. http://dx.doi.org/10.1016/j.psyneuen.2014.02.019

Kim, Y. R., Kim, C. H., Park, J. H., Pyo, J., & Treasure, J. (2014). The impact of intranasal oxytocin on attention to social emotional stimuli in patients with anorexia nervosa: A double blind within-subject cross-over experiment. *PLoS ONE, 9,* e90721. http://dx.doi.org/10.1371/journal.pone.0090721

Kotler, L. A., Devlin, M. J., Davies, M., & Walsh, B. T. (2003). An open trial of fluoxetine for adolescents with bulimia nervosa. *Journal of Child and Adolescent Psychopharmacology, 13,* 329–335. http://dx.doi.org/10.1089/104454603322572660

Lacey, J. H., & Crisp, A. H. (1980). Hunger, food intake and weight: The impact of clomipramine on a refeeding anorexia nervosa population. *Postgraduate Medical Journal, 56*(Suppl. 1), 79–85.

Lask, B., Fosson, A., Rolfe, U., & Thomas, S. (1993). Zinc deficiency and childhood-onset anorexia nervosa. *The Journal of Clinical Psychiatry, 54,* 63–66.

La Via, M. C., Gray, N., & Kaye, W. H. (2000). Case reports of olanzapine treatment of anorexia nervosa. *International Journal of Eating Disorders, 27,* 363–366. http://dx.doi.org/10.1002/(SICI)1098-108X(200004)27:3<363::AID-EAT16>3.0.CO;2-5

Leggero, C., Masi, G., Brunori, E., Calderoni, S., Carissimo, R., Maestro, S., & Muratori, F. (2010). Low-dose olanzapine monotherapy in girls with anorexia nervosa, restricting subtype: Focus on

hyperactivity. *Journal of Child and Adolescent Psychopharmacology, 20,* 127–133. http://dx.doi.org/10.1089/cap.2009.0072

Lewinsohn, P. M., Seeley, J. R., Moerk, K. C., & Striegel-Moore, R. H. (2002). Gender differences in eating disorder symptoms in young adults. *International Journal of Eating Disorders, 32,* 426–440. http://dx.doi.org/10.1002/eat.10103

Lindvall Dahlgren, C., & Wisting, L. (2016). Transitioning from *DSM–IV* to *DSM–5:* A systematic review of eating disorder prevalence assessment. *International Journal of Eating Disorders, 49,* 975–997. http://dx.doi.org/10.1002/eat.22596

Lock, J., Brandt, H., Woodside, B., Agras, W. S., Halmi, K., Johnson, C., . . . Wilfley, D. (2012). Challenges in conducting a multi-site randomized clinical trial comparing treatments for adolescent anorexia nervosa. *International Journal of Eating Disorders, 45,* 202–213. http://dx.doi.org/10.1002/eat.20923

Lucas, A. R., Beard, C. M., O'Fallon, W. M., & Kurland, L. T. (1991). 50-year trends in the incidence of anorexia nervosa in Rochester, Minn.: A population-based study. *The American Journal of Psychiatry, 148,* 917–922. http://dx.doi.org/10.1176/ajp.148.7.917

Machado, P. P., Gonçalves, S., & Hoek, H. W. (2013). *DSM–5* reduces the proportion of EDNOS cases: Evidence from community samples. *International Journal of Eating Disorders, 46,* 60–65. http://dx.doi.org/10.1002/eat.22040

Machado, P. P., Grilo, C. M., & Crosby, R. D. (2017). Evaluation of the *DSM–5* severity indicator for anorexia nervosa. *European Eating Disorders Review, 25,* 221–223. http://dx.doi.org/10.1002/erv.2508

Mancuso, S. G., Newton, J. R., Bosanac, P., Rossell, S. L., Nesci, J. B., & Castle, D. J. (2015). Classification of eating disorders: Comparison of relative prevalence rates using *DSM–IV* and *DSM–5* criteria. *The British Journal of Psychiatry, 206,* 519–520. http://dx.doi.org/10.1192/bjp.bp.113.143461

McElroy, S. L., Hudson, J., Ferreira-Cornwell, M. C., Radewonuk, J., Whitaker, T., & Gasior, M. (2016). Lisdexamfetamine dimesylate for adults with moderate to severe binge eating disorder: Results of two pivotal phase 3 randomized controlled trials. *Neuropsychopharmacology, 41,* 1251–1260. http://dx.doi.org/10.1038/npp.2015.275

McElroy, S. L., Hudson, J. I., Mitchell, J. E., Wilfley, D., Ferreira-Cornwell, M. C., Gao, J., . . . Gasior, M. (2015). Efficacy and safety of lisdexamfetamine for treatment of adults with moderate to severe binge-eating disorder: A randomized clinical trial. *JAMA Psychiatry, 72,* 235–246. http://dx.doi.org/10.1001/jamapsychiatry.2014.2162

Meehan, K. G., Loeb, K. L., Roberto, C. A., & Attia, E. (2006). Mood change during weight restoration in patients with anorexia nervosa. *International Journal of Eating Disorders, 39,* 587–589. http://dx.doi.org/10.1002/eat.20337

Mehler, C., Wewetzer, C., Schulze, U., Warnke, A., Theisen, F., & Dittmann, R. W. (2001). Olanzapine in children and adolescents with chronic anorexia nervosa. A study of five cases. *European Child & Adolescent Psychiatry, 10,* 151–157. http://dx.doi.org/10.1007/s007870170039

Mehler-Wex, C., Romanos, M., Kirchheiner, J., & Schulze, U. M. (2008). Atypical antipsychotics in severe anorexia nervosa in children and adolescents— Review and case reports. *European Eating Disorders Review, 16,* 100–108. http://dx.doi.org/10.1002/erv.843

Milano, W., Petrella, C., Sabatino, C., & Capasso, A. (2004). Treatment of bulimia nervosa with sertraline: A randomized controlled trial. *Advances in Therapy, 21,* 232–237. http://dx.doi.org/10.1007/BF02850155

Milano, W., Siano, C., Putrella, C., & Capasso, A. (2005). Treatment of bulimia nervosa with fluvoxamine: A randomized controlled trial. *Advances in Therapy, 22,* 278–283. http://dx.doi.org/10.1007/BF02849936

Mond, J. M., & Hay, P. J. (2007). Functional impairment associated with bulimic behaviors in a community sample of men and women. *International Journal of Eating Disorders, 40,* 391–398. http://dx.doi.org/10.1002/eat.20380

Mondraty, N., Birmingham, C. L., Touyz, S., Sundakov, V., Chapman, L., & Beumont, P. (2005). Randomized controlled trial of olanzapine in the treatment of cognitions in anorexia nervosa. *Australasian Psychiatry, 13,* 72–75. http://dx.doi.org/10.1080/j.1440-1665.2004.02154.x

Mustelin, L., Silén, Y., Raevuori, A., Hoek, H. W., Kaprio, J., & Keski-Rahkonen, A. (2016). The *DSM–5* diagnostic criteria for anorexia nervosa may change its population prevalence and prognostic value. *Journal of Psychiatric Research, 77,* 85–91. http://dx.doi.org/10.1016/j.jpsychires.2016.03.003

Nakash-Eisikovits, O., Dierberger, A., & Westen, D. (2002). A multidimensional meta-analysis of pharmacotherapy for bulimia nervosa: Summarizing the range of outcomes in controlled clinical trials. *Harvard Review of Psychiatry, 10,* 193–211.

National Institute for Clinical Excellence. (2004). *Eating disorders. Core interventions in the treatment and management of eating disorders in primary and secondary care.* London, UK: Author.

National Task Force on the Prevention and Treatment of Obesity. (2000). Dieting and the development of eating disorders in overweight and obese adults. *Archives of Internal Medicine, 160,* 2581–2589. http://dx.doi.org/10.1001/archinte.160.17.2581

Newman-Toker, J. (2000). Risperidone in anorexia nervosa. *Journal of the American Academy of Child & Adolescent Psychiatry, 39,* 941–942. http://dx.doi.org/10.1097/00004583-200008000-00002

Nickel, C., Tritt, K., Muehlbacher, M., Pedrosa Gil, F., Mitterlehner, F. O., Kaplan, P., . . . Nickel, M. K. (2005). Topiramate treatment in bulimia nervosa patients: A randomized, double-blind, placebo-controlled trial. *International Journal of Eating Disorders, 38,* 295–300. http://dx.doi.org/10.1002/eat.20202

Norris, M. L., Spettigue, W., Buchholz, A., & Henderson, K. A. (2007). Challenges associated with controlled psychopharmacological research trials in adolescents with eating disorders. *Journal of the Canadian Academy of Child and Adolescent Psychiatry, 16,* 167–172.

Ornstein, R. M., Rosen, D. S., Mammel, K. A., Callahan, S. T., Forman, S., Jay, M. S., . . . Walsh, B. T. (2013). Distribution of eating disorders in children and adolescents using the proposed *DSM–5* criteria for feeding and eating disorders. *Journal of Adolescent Health, 53,* 303–305. http://dx.doi.org/10.1016/j.jadohealth.2013.03.025

Peterson, C. B., & Mitchell, J. E. (2005). Self-report measures. In J. E. Mitchell & C. B. Peterson (Eds.), *Assessment of eating disorders* (pp. 98–119). New York, NY: Guilford Press.

Powers, P. S., Bannon, Y., Eubanks, R., & McCormick, T. (2007). Quetiapine in anorexia nervosa patients: An open label outpatient pilot study. *International Journal of Eating Disorders, 40,* 21–26. http://dx.doi.org/10.1002/eat.20325

Powers, P. S., Klabunde, M., & Kaye, W. (2012). Double-blind placebo-controlled trial of quetiapine in anorexia nervosa. *European Eating Disorders Review, 20,* 331–334. http://dx.doi.org/10.1002/erv.2169

Powers, P. S., Santana, C. A., & Bannon, Y. S. (2002). Olanzapine in the treatment of anorexia nervosa: An open label trial. *International Journal of Eating Disorders, 32,* 146–154. http://dx.doi.org/10.1002/eat.10084

Qian, J., Hu, Q., Wan, Y., Li, T., Wu, M., Ren, Z., & Yu, D. (2013). Prevalence of eating disorders in the general population: A systematic review. *Shanghai Archives of Psychiatry, 25,* 212–223.

Reas, D. L., & Grilo, C. M. (2008). Review and meta-analysis of pharmacotherapy for binge-eating disorder. *Obesity, 16,* 2024–2038. http://dx.doi.org/10.1038/oby.2008.333

*Reas, D. L., & Grilo, C. M. (2015). Pharmacological treatment of binge eating disorder: Update review and synthesis. *Expert Opinion in Pharmacotherapy, 16,* 1463–1478. http://dx.doi.org/10.1517/14656566.2015.1053465

Ricca, V., Mannucci, E., Mezzani, B., Di Bernardo, M., Zucchi, T., Paionni, A., . . . Faravelli, C. (2001).

Psychopathological and clinical features of outpatients with an eating disorder not otherwise specified. *Eating and Weight Disorders, 6*, 157–165. http://dx.doi.org/10.1007/BF03339765

Schmidt, U., Cooper, P. J., Essers, H., Freeman, C. P., Holland, R. L., Palmer, R. L., . . . Webster, J. (2004). Fluvoxamine and graded psychotherapy in the treatment of bulimia nervosa: A randomized, double-blind, placebo-controlled, multicenter study of short-term and long-term pharmacotherapy combined with a stepped care approach to psychotherapy. *Journal of Clinical Psychopharmacology, 24*, 549–552. http://dx.doi.org/10.1097/01.jcp.0000138776.32891.3e

Shapiro, J. R., Berkman, N. D., Brownley, K. A., Sedway, J. A., Lohr, K. N., & Bulik, C. M. (2007). Bulimia nervosa treatment: A systematic review of randomized controlled trials. *International Journal of Eating Disorders, 40*, 321–336. http://dx.doi.org/10.1002/eat.20372

Smink, F. R., van Hoeken, D., & Hoek, H. W. (2012). Epidemiology of eating disorders: Incidence, prevalence and mortality rates. *Current Psychiatry Reports, 14*, 406–414. http://dx.doi.org/10.1007/s11920-012-0282-y

Smink, F. R., van Hoeken, D., Oldehinkel, A. J., & Hoek, H. W. (2014). Prevalence and severity of *DSM–5* eating disorders in a community cohort of adolescents. *International Journal of Eating Disorders, 47*, 610–619. http://dx.doi.org/10.1002/eat.22316

Steinglass, J. E., Kaplan, S. C., Liu, Y., Wang, Y., & Walsh, B. T. (2014). The (lack of) effect of alprazolam on eating behavior in anorexia nervosa: A preliminary report. *International Journal of Eating Disorders, 47*, 901–904. http://dx.doi.org/10.1002/eat.22343

Stice, E., Fisher, M., & Martinez, E. (2004). Eating Disorder Diagnostic Scale: Additional evidence of reliability and validity. *Psychological Assessment, 16*, 60–71. http://dx.doi.org/10.1037/1040-3590.16.1.60

Stice, E., Orjada, K., & Tristan, J. (2006). Trial of a psychoeducational eating disturbance intervention for college women: A replication and extension. *International Journal of Eating Disorders, 39*, 233–239. http://dx.doi.org/10.1002/eat.20252

Stice, E., & Ragan, J. (2002). A preliminary controlled evaluation of an eating disturbance psycho-educational intervention for college students. *International Journal of Eating Disorders, 31*, 159–171. http://dx.doi.org/10.1002/eat.10018

Stice, E., Telch, C. F., & Rizvi, S. L. (2000). Development and validation of the Eating Disorder Diagnostic Scale: A brief self-report measure of anorexia, bulimia, and binge-eating disorder. *Psychological Assessment, 12*, 123–131. http://dx.doi.org/10.1037/1040-3590.12.2.123

Striegel-Moore, R. H., Rosselli, F., Perrin, N., DeBar, L., Wilson, G. T., May, A., & Kraemer, H. C. (2009). Gender difference in the prevalence of eating disorder symptoms. *International Journal of Eating Disorders, 42*, 471–474. http://dx.doi.org/10.1002/eat.20625

Sundblad, C., Landén, M., Eriksson, T., Bergman, L., & Eriksson, E. (2005). Effects of the androgen antagonist flutamide and the serotonin reuptake inhibitor citalopram in bulimia nervosa: A placebo-controlled pilot study. *Journal of Clinical Psychopharmacology, 25*, 85–88. http://dx.doi.org/10.1097/01.jcp.0000150222.31007.a9

*Sysko, R., & Alavi, S. (2018). Eating disorders. In J. Hunsley & E. J. Mash (Eds.), *A guide to assessments that work* (2nd ed., pp. 541–562). New York, NY: Oxford University Press.

Sysko, R., & Devlin, M. J. (2010–2017). Binge eating disorder: Cognitive-behavioral therapy (CBT). In Yager, J. (Ed.), *UpToDate*. Waltham, MA: UpToDate. Retrieved from http://www.uptodate.com/contents/binge-eating-disorder-cognitive-behavioral-therapy-cbt

*Sysko, R., Glasofer, D. R., Hildebrandt, T., Klimek, P., Mitchell, J. E., Berg, K. C., & Walsh, B. T. (2015). The Eating Disorder Assessment for DSM–5 (EDA–5): Development and validation of a structured interview for feeding and eating disorders. *International Journal of Eating Disorders, 48*, 452–463. http://dx.doi.org/10.1002/eat.22388

Sysko, R., Sha, N., Wang, Y., Duan, N., & Walsh, B. T. (2010). Early response to antidepressant treatment in bulimia nervosa. *Psychological Medicine, 40*, 999–1005. http://dx.doi.org/10.1017/S0033291709991218

Trunko, M. E., Schwartz, T. A., Duvvuri, V., & Kaye, W. H. (2011). Aripiprazole in anorexia nervosa and low-weight bulimia nervosa: Case reports. *International Journal of Eating Disorders, 44*, 269–275. http://dx.doi.org/10.1002/eat.20807

U.S. Food and Drug Administration. (2004). *Labeling change request letter for antidepressant medications.* Rockville, MD: Author. Retrieved from http://wayback.archive-it.org/7993/20170723172451/https://www.fda.gov/Drugs/DrugSafety/InformationbyDrugClass/ucm096352.htm

Vandereycken, W. (1984). Neuroleptics in the short-term treatment of anorexia nervosa. A double-blind placebo-controlled study with sulpiride. *The British Journal of Psychiatry, 144*, 288–292. http://dx.doi.org/10.1192/bjp.144.3.288

Vandereycken, W., & Pierloot, R. (1982). Pimozide combined with behavior therapy in the short-term treatment of anorexia nervosa. A double-blind placebo-controlled cross-over study. *Acta Psychiatrica Scandinavica, 66*, 445–450. http://dx.doi.org/10.1111/j.1600-0447.1982.tb04501.x

Walsh, B. T., Attia, E. A., Glasofer, D. R., & Sysko, R. (Eds.). (2016). *Handbook of assessment and treatment of eating disorders.* Washington, DC: American Psychiatric Association.

Walsh, B. T., Hadigan, C. M., Devlin, M. J., Gladis, M., & Roose, S. P. (1991). Long-term outcome of antidepressant treatment for bulimia nervosa. *The American Journal of Psychiatry, 148,* 1206–1212. http://dx.doi.org/10.1176/ajp.148.9.1206

*Walsh, B. T., Kaplan, A. S., Attia, E., Olmsted, M., Parides, M., Carter, J. C., . . . Rockert, W. (2006). Fluoxetine after weight restoration in anorexia nervosa: A randomized controlled trial. *JAMA, 295,* 2605–2612. http://dx.doi.org/10.1001/jama.295.22.2605

Walsh, B. T., Wilson, G. T., Loeb, K. L., Devlin, M. J., Pike, K. M., Roose, S. P., . . . Waternaux, C. (1997). Medication and psychotherapy in the treatment of bulimia nervosa. *American Journal of Psychiatry, 154,* 523–531.

Wiederman, M. W., & Pryor, T. (1996a). Substance use among women with eating disorders. *International Journal of Eating Disorders, 20,* 163–168. http://dx.doi.org/10.1002/(SICI)1098-108X(199609)20:2<163::AID-EAT6>3.0.CO;2-E

Wiederman, M. W., & Pryor, T. (1996b). Substance use and impulsive behaviors among adolescents with eating disorders. *Addictive Behaviors, 21,* 269–272. http://dx.doi.org/10.1016/0306-4603(95)00062-3

Wilfley, D. E., Friedman, M. A., Dounchis, J. Z., Stein, R. I., Welch, R. R., & Ball, S. A. (2000). Comorbid psychopathology in binge eating disorder: Relation to eating disorder severity at baseline and following treatment. *Journal of Consulting and Clinical Psychology, 68,* 641–649. http://dx.doi.org/10.1037/0022-006X.68.4.641

*Wilson, G. T., Wilfley, D. E., Agras, W. S., & Bryson, S. W. (2010). Psychological treatments of binge eating disorder. *Archives of General Psychiatry, 67,* 94–101. http://dx.doi.org/10.1001/archgenpsychiatry.2009.170

Wonderlich, S. A., de Zwaan, M., Mitchell, J. E., Peterson, C., & Crow, S. (2003). Psychological and dietary treatments of binge eating disorder: Conceptual implications. *International Journal of Eating Disorders, 34*(Suppl.), S58–S73. http://dx.doi.org/10.1002/eat.10206

*Zhu, A. J., & Walsh, B. T. (2002). Pharmacologic treatment of eating disorders. *The Canadian Journal of Psychiatry, 47,* 227–234. http://dx.doi.org/10.1177/070674370204700302

Zipfel, S., Giel, K. E., Bulik, C. M., Hay, P., & Schmidt, U. (2015). Anorexia nervosa: Aetiology, assessment, and treatment. *The Lancet Psychiatry, 2,* 1099–1111. http://dx.doi.org/10.1016/S2215-0366(15)00356-9

PHARMACOLOGICAL TREATMENT OF ATTENTION-DEFICIT/ HYPERACTIVITY DISORDER

Bradley H. Smith, Erin K. Reid, Patrick Sajovec, and Lisa Namerow

Attention-deficit/hyperactivity disorder (ADHD) is a neurodevelopmental disorder characterized by deficits in attention and impulse control. First observed in childhood, it causes significant social and academic impairment (American Psychiatric Association, 2013). The term *ADHD* was formally adopted in the mid-1980s, but the concept of ADHD can be traced back at least 2 centuries in the pediatric literature (Barkley, 2015b). Studies consistently show that ADHD is a prevalent, persistent, and highly impairing disorder that nonetheless can be effectively treated.

In this chapter, we describe the most effective treatment approaches for ADHD across the lifespan, with a focus on pharmacological treatment in the context of psychosocial or behavioral treatment. The research suggests that low doses of medication combined with low levels of multimodal behavioral intervention is the most effective and cost-efficient treatment for ADHD, at least for children and adolescents. We preface our review of treatment with a review of the epidemiology and prevalence of ADHD, as well as best practices for diagnosing ADHD.

EPIDEMIOLOGY AND PREVALENCE

According to the *Diagnostic and Statistical Manual of Mental Health Disorders* (5th ed.; *DSM–5*), the prevalence rate of ADHD in children is about 5% (American Psychiatric Association, 2013).

This estimated rate is supported by a review of 102 international studies, which found the worldwide prevalence is about 5.29% (Roberts, Milich, & Barkley, 2015). Sampling and research methods, however, impact the prevalence estimates of ADHD. For instance, one review found ADHD rates ranging from 1.6% to 16% (Roberts et al., 2015). Rates vary depending on methodological factors, particularly how much emphasis is placed on interrater agreement, measuring impairment, and ruling out alternative disorders. Furthermore, geographic, contextual, and demographic considerations are very important when assessing ADHD. For instance, the rate of ADHD is much higher in clinical and special education settings than in the general population (Roberts et al., 2015).

There are big sex and age effects on the rate of ADHD as well (Roberts et al., 2015). The prevalence of ADHD is about two times higher for boys than for girls in the general population, and this disparity is even larger in clinical settings. Age-related influence follows an inverted U-shaped function across school years and the lifespan. Specifically, there are relatively low rates of ADHD in preschool (about 2%), relatively high rates in elementary school (around 7%), and declining rates through adolescence and adulthood, from 5% in adolescence to 2.5% in adulthood (Roberts et al., 2015).

The prevalence of ADHD has increased in the past 20 years. A recent meta-analysis found a pooled estimate of 7.2% for persons aged 18 and under

http://dx.doi.org/10.1037/0000133-016
APA Handbook of Psychopharmacology, S. M. Evans (Editor-in-Chief)

(Thomas, Sanders, Doust, Beller, & Glasziou, 2015), which is about 2% higher than estimates from studies published before 2000. The reasons for this increase are unclear, controversial, and beyond the scope of this chapter to address. Yet, the important clinical consideration is that a diagnosis of ADHD should account for many factors that impact prevalence estimates, such as setting, diagnostic procedures, age, and sex.

There was a time when ADHD was thought to be a self-limiting disorder of childhood. Contemporary research shows this belief to be mistaken: The majority of persons diagnosed with ADHD in childhood continue to meet diagnostic criteria for ADHD through adolescence and into adulthood (Barkley, 2015b). Adjustments have been made in *DSM–5* to make it easier to get a diagnosis of ADHD in adulthood, such as lowering the symptom count for adults from six to five (American Psychiatric Association, 2013).

According to *DSM–5*, the base rate for ADHD in adults is about 2.5%. This may be a low estimate, owing to limitations in self-report of ADHD symptoms (Roberts et al., 2015). Numerous studies converge on the finding that persons with ADHD are not the best sources of information about ADHD symptoms. For example, in a longitudinal study of children with ADHD followed into adulthood, only 5% of persons previously diagnosed with ADHD self-reported sufficient symptoms for a diagnosis of ADHD, whereas 66% met criteria based on parent report (Barkley, Fischer, Smallish, & Fletcher, 2002). This and many other studies show that collateral reports are essential for diagnosing ADHD. Unfortunately, the usual sources of collateral report, such as parents and teachers, become increasing less available or less dependable as persons mature. As a consequence, the putative drop in prevalence of ADHD across the lifespan may be a methodological artifact. The clinical implication is that ADHD should be treated as a chronic disorder and be measured with the assistance of collateral report (Roberts et al., 2015).

Impairments related to ADHD often emerge at an early age and become more problematic across the lifespan. Compared to parents of typically developing children, parents of toddlers with ADHD report more problems such as tantrums, disobedience,

and difficulty sleeping. Furthermore, toddlers with ADHD often have difficulty adjusting to educational or peer activities. Preschoolers with ADHD are discharged from day care or summer camps because of behavior problems at a much higher rate than their peers (Dupaul & Langberg, 2015). The tasks and expectations of contemporary elementary schools are very difficult for children with ADHD, and the peak for referrals for ADHD is in the third grade. Problems in elementary school usually consist of poor academic performance, not following rules in the classroom, and conflict with peers that gets worse with decreasing structure (Dupaul & Langberg, 2015).

In middle school, the problems that started earlier tend to persist, and they become more consequential (Dupaul & Langberg, 2015). Poor academic performance results in failing classes, low test scores, and repeating years of school. Behavior problems lead to suspensions or expulsions, or referral to special education or the juvenile justice system. In high school, risky sexual behaviors and substance use can result in serious personal consequences. High school students with ADHD are more likely to be truant and less likely to graduate (Dupaul & Langberg, 2015). Teens with ADHD have an elevated risk for involvement with traffic accidents and involvement with the criminal justice and mental health systems (Barkley, 2015a). Young adults with ADHD have disproportionately high rates of problems at work and have trouble maintaining positive personal and professional relationships (Barkley, 2015a).

Taken together, ADHD causes a lifetime of disability. Even persons who no longer meet diagnostic criteria for ADHD tend to have significant impairment relative to persons who were never diagnosed with ADHD. In addition to the previously noted functional problems, issues related to poor diet and self-care start to emerge, such as poor dental health, obesity and diabetes, substance use, risky sexual behavior, sleep problems, and Internet abuse (Barkley, 2015a). The financial consequences of untreated or unsuccessfully treated ADHD include increased health care costs (e.g., from accidents, risky sexual behavior, and substance use), higher educational costs (e.g., for special education or repeated grades), lower work productivity and income, higher use of social services (e.g., welfare, child support services), crime and criminal justice costs (i.e., policing, court, and incarceration), and costs related to automobile accidents. Some have argued that the costs of untreated ADHD are the highest of any mental health disorder (Barkley, 2015a). At the very least, the costs of untreated ADHD far outweigh the costs that would have been incurred for effective treatment (Barkley, 2015a).

DIAGNOSING ATTENTION-DEFICIT/ HYPERACTIVITY DISORDER

Assessing ADHD is a complicated process with different expectations, procedures, and measures across settings. Practitioners operate under different laws, guidelines, traditions, and constraints that impact their approaches to assessment of ADHD. For example, a school psychologist can observe a child at school and talk directly with teachers, whereas a psychologist in a medical or psychiatric practice may rely on teacher ratings or teacher observations relayed by parents. Perhaps a bigger consideration is that physician guidelines emphasize diagnosis based on a medical model (e.g., *DSM* criteria), whereas school-based practitioners must follow special education law, which does not formally incorporate *DSM* criteria.

In recognition of the unique considerations involved, in this section we present community- and school-based assessments as distinct activities even though there is overlap between the two. Because incorporating *DSM* criteria promotes consistency of diagnoses and improved communication between health care providers (American Academy of Pediatrics, 2011), we include an overview of the *DSM* criteria pertinent to ADHD. Also, owing to the high rate of comorbidity between ADHD and several other *DSM* disorders, and the need to rule out plausible alternatives to ADHD, we detail how consideration of *DSM* disorders and other medical conditions is an essential component of ADHD assessment.

DSM–5–Based Assessment of Attention-Deficit/Hyperactivity Disorder

The merits and limitations of *DSM* are hotly debated in the literature. Nevertheless, the *DSM* criteria, or the related *International Classification of Disorders*

criteria (World Health Organization, 2015), are accepted by the large majority of mental health professionals as the consensus source for diagnostic criteria based on current knowledge (American Psychiatric Association, 2013). ADHD is an excellent example of a *DSM* disorder that has developed iteratively based on careful consideration of theory, practice, and research (Barkley, 2015b). With each revision of the *DSM*—from the second edition to the fourth edition (which includes four iterations)—the conceptualization of ADHD changed substantially; between *DSM–IV* and *DSM–5* there were relatively subtle changes. *DSM–II*, published in 1952, included *hyperkinetic reaction of childhood*, which is far removed from the current concept of ADHD. The third edition of *DSM* made attention deficits the core symptoms and introduced the enduring term *ADD*, based on the diagnostic categories of attention-deficit disorder (ADD) with or without hyperactivity. A revision of *DSM–III* in 1987 put inattention and impulsivity on equal footing, as well as introduced the contemporary diagnostic term attention-deficit/ hyperactivity disorder. However, the meaning of ADHD changed in subsequent revisions. In 1994, *DSM–IV* distinguished inattention and hyperactivity/ impulsivity as separate domains, giving three disorder subtypes: predominately inattentive, predominately hyperactive/impulsive, and combined. *DSM–5*, published in 2013, kept most of the *DSM–IV* criteria but demoted the concept of subtypes of ADHD to *presentations*, a change that recognizes the considerable overlap and fluidity of the symptom cluster expression.

Diagnostic Procedures in Community or Medical Settings

Clinical practice guidelines by the American Academy of Pediatrics (2011) and the American Academy of Child and Adolescent Psychiatry (Pliszka & AACAP Work Group on Quality Issues, 2007) detail best practices for health care providers diagnosing ADHD. Many of the guidelines for physicians mirror those outlined in this chapter for psychologists and school-based practitioners, including screening for risk, gathering interviews and rating scales from multiple informants across multiple settings, collecting family and medical histories, and considering differential diagnoses as well as potential comorbid disorders.

Screening.   The American Academy of Child and Adolescent Psychiatry guidelines state that as part of routine medical exams, pediatricians should ask parents whether children present symptoms in the domains of ADHD (i.e., hyperactivity, impulsivity, inattention) and whether those symptoms cause functional impairment. If a child presents with symptoms that are clinically significant and cause impairment, the health care provider should conduct a full evaluation for ADHD.

Brief rating scales are excellent screening tools for ADHD. A number of these scales are available at no cost and are easy to score (see the Tool Kit of Resources at the end of this chapter for some examples). We recommend pairing the Impairment Rating Scale (Fabiano et al., 2006) with a brief rating scale. The Vanderbilt ADHD Diagnostic Rating Scale (Wolraich et al., 2003) has a slightly broader scope than ADHD, including items on internalizing and externalizing problems that are often comorbid with ADHD.

Norm-referenced rating scales.   If there is a positive screen for ADHD symptoms and impairment, we recommend following up with standardized rating scales that provide norm-referenced scores that allow for age and gender comparisons, as well as insight into other possible comorbid concerns. Two very well established broadband scales that cover symptoms of many emotional and behavioral disorders in addition to ADHD are the Behavior Assessment System for Children (3rd ed.; BASC-3; Reynolds & Kamphaus, 2015) and the Child Behavior Checklist (CBCL; Achenbach & Rescorla, 2001).

Narrowband scales specific to ADHD measure core symptoms and related problems of the disorder in a more detailed and comprehensive manner than the previously mentioned broadband scales. Several psychometrically sound narrowband measures align with the ADHD criteria in *DSM*, including the Conners–3 (Conners, 2008) and the ADHD Rating Scale–V (DuPaul et al., 2016). To avoid false negatives with adult cases, it may be worthwhile to collect data using the Barkley Adult ADHD Rating Scale–IV (Barkley, 2011).

It cannot be stressed strongly enough that collateral report is essential for assessing ADHD, and ratings should be completed by multiple sources, with the least weight given to self-report. Disagreement among raters often occurs during ADHD evaluations and may arise from cultural differences, parenting styles, setting-dependent behavior, or personal biases (Nass, 2005). Discussing disagreement as a common phenomenon without criticizing informants' viewpoints can lead to a deeper understanding of influential environmental and interpersonal factors that impact the expression of ADHD symptoms and related problems. Clarifying interrater disagreements is often one of the most enlightening aspects of the diagnostic interview.

Family histories and diagnostic interviews.   After a positive screening and the collection of follow-up ratings, the next step in the assessment process is an interview with parents, other collateral informants, and the person thought to have ADHD. Interviews take into consideration family and medical history, functional impairment, treatment history, and other details about the individual that are not captured through observations and ratings. Owing to high heritability of ADHD among first-degree relatives (American Psychiatric Association, 2013), family histories should be routinely collected during ADHD evaluations. Information regarding developmental milestones, such as walking and talking, is particularly helpful in differentiating attention problems from developmental or language disorders when assessing preschool children. Family medical history, such as the presence of mental health disorders (e.g., tic disorders, anxiety, mood disorders), helps inform decisions regarding treatment and comorbid conditions (Pliszka & AACAP Work Group on Quality Issues, 2007). Most treatments rely on parent or other adult support, so evaluation of the ability of families, schools, and other social structures (e.g., religious institutions, the workplace) to provide support and structure is critically important.

Interviews of younger children can be conducted only with parents and teachers present. Starting in adolescence, interviews may be administered to individuals with suspected ADHD separately as well as together with additional informants (e.g., parents, teachers). It is also advisable to gather information from multiple informants who interact with the individual in different settings (e.g., school, work, home) because environmental differences such as routines, structure, and rewards can greatly impact the manifestation of ADHD symptoms. For a formal diagnosis, ADHD must be shown to be pervasive across multiple settings.

When deciding what type of interview to implement, it is unclear whether highly structured interviews are better in clinical settings than semistructured interviews (Nass, 2005). A structured, psychometrically sound child-and-parent interview that captures symptoms and psychosocial impairment associated with ADHD and other mental health disorders is the Child and Adolescent Psychiatric Assessment (CAPA; Angold & Costello, 2000). Structured measures like the CAPA have better reliability and specificity than semistructured or informal interviews, and structured interviews are superior at ruling out plausible alternative diagnoses. However, structured interviews often require substantial time to administer, and they tend to focus narrowly on diagnostic considerations, so some important contextual or historical information may be missed if only the structured interview is used.

Differential diagnoses and comorbidities. In addition to assessing for ADHD, it is essential to consider several other disorders that are plausible or are likely comorbid conditions (Pliszka, 2015). Some health conditions, such as a metabolic disorder (e.g., hyperthyroidism), substance use, infections, and neurological conditions (e.g., seizures), might present with symptoms that resemble ADHD or are important considerations when treating ADHD (Barkley, 2015a). Thus, a first step in assessing ADHD is a thorough physical examination, preferably conducted by a behavioral pediatrician or psychiatrist who is astute at differentiating between ADHD and physical symptoms that resemble ADHD.

Some presentations of anxiety can resemble ADHD. Similarly, children exposed to recent trauma or abuse often present with agitation, restlessness, and behavioral disturbances that resemble ADHD. Cases of posttraumatic stress disorder are often mistakenly thought to be ADHD (Pliszka, 2015). To differentiate between these concerns, tracking the onset of anxiety symptoms and screening for traumatic events during ADHD assessment is essential.

It is also critical to assess for mood disorders (Pliszka, 2015). This can be done through interviews and rating scales, as discussed previously in this chapter. The cognitive symptoms of major depressive disorder may resemble the inattention attributed to ADHD, and mania can be confused with hyperactivity. Differential diagnosis of mood disorders from ADHD has major treatment implications.

Chronic sleep deprivation or other sleep disorders may appear to be ADHD (Barkley, 2015a). Short sleep duration in healthy children is associated with inattention and poor academic performance. Teacher ratings of the classroom behavior and academic performance of sleep-deprived children often resemble the inattention and cognitive impairments seen in ADHD. Most cases of sleep deprivation are related to lifestyle factors; however, conditions such as sleep apnea and restless leg syndrome should be considered. Self-report of sleep is notoriously poor, so sleep studies or the use of activity trackers might be needed to thoroughly address sleep deprivation or other sleep problems that could masquerade as ADHD.

Laboratory measures. Evaluations conducted in medical settings often include laboratory measures, which directly measure the core symptoms of ADHD. For example, in the Continuous Performance Test (CPT), participants complete an intentionally boring task in which they press a button when they view one stimulus and inhibit a response when they see another stimulus. Some laboratory measures have demonstrated high discriminant validity between groups of individuals with and without ADHD; however they lack sufficient research on their diagnostic accuracy (i.e., sensitivity, specificity; Rapport, Chung, Shore, Denney, & Isaacs, 2000). Moreover, the measures have low ecological validity, as indicated by low to moderate correlations with teacher ratings (Smith, Barkley, & Shapiro, 2007). Although laboratory measures may be appropriate in research comparing group means or testing ideas about the presentation of ADHD, their use in diagnosing ADHD and related treatment evaluation is questionable. Laboratory tests, such as the CPT, should not be used to titrate doses of medication.

Diagnostic Procedures in School Settings

Schools are ideal settings for the assessment of ADHD, as school mental health professionals (e.g., diagnosticians, school psychologists) have relatively easy access to students, families, and teachers to conduct a multi-informant, multimethod evaluation. One benefit of this accessibility is the opportunity to conduct observations of student behavior in a naturalistic setting.

Observation. Informal observations provide school-based examples of student behaviors that are reflective of ADHD symptoms (i.e., requiring individual prompts to follow instructions, gazing off, moving around the room at inappropriate times). Several formal observation coding schemes reviewed by Volpe, DiPerna, Hintze, and Shapiro (2005) demonstrate adequate interobserver reliability, discriminant validity, and treatment sensitivity among students with ADHD. The Behavior Observation of Students in Schools (BOSS; Shapiro, 2013) is an easy-to-use momentary time-sampling observation schedule available in paper and phone application formats. From a 15-minute observation, the BOSS provides quantitative data on academic engagement (active and passive) and off-task behavior (motor, verbal, and passive), as well as peer comparison data. Recommended best practice is to conduct observations across settings (e.g., math, reading, lunch, gym class) and types of instruction (e.g., independent work, group projects, lecture) to capture environmental effects on behavior. In addition to observational data, there are other unique sources of information at schools, such as progress monitoring data collected through *response to intervention* (RTI).

Response to intervention. A growing number of schools are using RTI, which is an innovative means through which students with ADHD may receive supports in the general education setting. RTI is a prevention-focused service delivery model in which universal screening identifies students at risk for academic issues or behavior problems. Universal behavior screening is a well established method to identify students who need extra behavior support (Kamphaus, Reynolds, & Dever, 2014). Although universal screening specifically for ADHD is not indicated, many comprehensive behavior screeners probe for attention problems (e.g., Social, Academic,

and Emotional Behavior Screener; Behavioral and Emotional Screening System). Ongoing progress monitoring is conducted for students identified as at risk through measures such as curriculum-based measurement or a daily behavior score. These data are excellent for assessing ADHD, as they provide consistent information that can be compared with other students' and the target student's baseline and response to treatment. RTI data also can be an excellent source of response to pharmacological treatment when titrating new medications or adjusting doses of medication.

In the context of RTI, schools implement tiered services according to individual need and assess effectiveness by progress monitoring (Fletcher & Vaughn, 2009). As its foundation, RTI includes universal (i.e., school-wide) supports called *Tier 1 interventions* that are used to create a safe and engaging environment that encourages student learning and positive behaviors. Students with ADHD are often more sensitive to behavior supports (e.g., explicitly taught expectations, contingent social reinforcement for good behavior) than are students without ADHD, so universal behavioral interventions can be very helpful in promoting positive school adjustment in students with ADHD.

Despite the benefits of universal school supports, many students with ADHD may receive academic or behavioral screening scores indicative of problems. When this occurs, a problem-solving team will select a *Tier 2 intervention* to provide additional behavior support (e.g., Check-In-Check-Out, daily report card). In response to progress-monitoring data, the team will alter the Tier 2 intervention or recommend a more intensive intervention (e.g., behavior modification with a school psychologist) as needed. If functional impairments persist after intensive intervention, the team will consider making a referral for special education services.

Response to intervention and special education. If Tier 1 and 2 interventions are not sufficient, schools are required to provide additional services. Under the Individuals With Disabilities Education Improvement Act of 2004 (IDEIA), if parents or guardians think that their child has ADHD and that the ADHD is causing significant impairments in school, they can request an evaluation by the school. Likewise, teachers or other school personnel can refer students for evaluation for special education services under the eligibility category of other health impairment (OHI). Full individual evaluations in the schools include review of RTI academic and behavioral data, interviews, history taking, rating scales, and observations. The evaluation should determine if the child meets criteria for development of an individual education plan (IEP), which must be approved by parents and appropriate school personnel. The least restrictive intervention should be provided whenever possible, with every effort made to include the student in regular education classrooms. However, in some cases, the student may spend all or part of the school day in highly controlled special education classrooms. Many of these students will be receiving medication during the school day.

EVIDENCE-BASED PHARMACOLOGICAL TREATMENTS OF ATTENTION-DEFICIT/ HYPERACTIVITY DISORDER

In this section, we review research on the pharmacological treatment of ADHD and various treatment guidelines for pharmacotherapy of ADHD promulgated by leading experts and professional organizations. We also briefly review the mechanism of action of the drugs approved by the U.S. Food and Drug Administration (FDA) for ADHD treatment. Although very strong recommendations can be derived from the extant research literature, these recommendations address group-level trends in response to pharmacological treatment of ADHD. In practice, response to treatment can vary widely from person to person. Therefore, careful attention to individual titration is needed for successful treatment of ADHD.

There are many options for the pharmacological treatment of ADHD (see Table 16.1). There are four broad classes of FDA-approved drugs, and there are various methods for delivering the drugs within each class. For example, methylphenidate (MPH) is one of the most commonly prescribed drugs. It is available in immediate-release form (i.e., the original form that acts for about 4 hours); transdermal form (i.e., an MPH patch); and several extended-release forms, including OROS MPH (osmotically controlled–release oral delivery system), diffucaps MPH (30% immediate release and 70% extended

TABLE 16.1

FDA-Approved Drugs for Treating Attention-Deficit/Hyperactivity Disorder

Drug classification	Chemical name	Trade name	Common side effects
Stimulant	dextroamphetamine	Dexedrine®, ProCentra®, Zensedi®	Decreased appetite, headache, stomachache, trouble sleeping, weight loss, dry mouth, nervousness, mood swings, dizziness, fast heart beat
	amphetamine and dextroamphetamine	Adderall®, Adderall XR	
	dexmethylphenidate	Focalin®, Focalin XR	Dry mouth, dyspepsia, headache, anxiety
	lisdexamfetamine	Vyvanse®	Upper abdominal pain, diarrhea, nausea, fatigue, feeling jittery, irritability, decreased appetite, headaches, insomnia
	methylphenidate	Concerta®, Daytrana®, Metadate® CD, Metadate XR, Methylin®, Methylin ER, Ritalin®, Ritalin SR, Ritalin LA, Quillivant® XR	Decreased appetite, headache, nausea, insomnia, weight loss, dry mouth, nervousness, irritability, dizziness, hyperhidrosis
Nonstimulant	atomoxetine	Strattera®	Decreased appetite, abdominal pain, nausea, sleepiness, suicidal ideation
	clonidine	Kapvay®	Decreased appetite, abdominal pain, nausea, sleepiness
	guanfacine	Intuniv®	Decreased appetite, abdominal pain, nausea, sleepiness

Note. FDA = U.S. Food and Drug Administration.

time-release capsules), and SODAS MPH (spheroidal oral drug absorption system, with 50% immediate release and 50% extended release). Thus, when discussing MPH, one needs to be very specific about which form of MPH is being used. This is true as well for all other FDA-approved medications used to treat ADHD.

The four major drug categories approved by the FDA to treat ADHD are stimulants, atomoxetine, guanfacine, and clonidine. There is robust research on each of these pharmacological agents, including good information supporting favorable risk-to-benefit ratios, with the caveat that there can be considerable individual differences in response. There also are several common *off-label medications* used to treat ADHD. Owing to limited information, in this chapter we do not make any recommendations regarding drugs that are not FDA approved to treat ADHD.

Mechanism of Action of FDA-Approved Pharmacotherapy for Attention-Deficit/ Hyperactivity Disorder

The mechanisms of action of the drugs used to treat ADHD are not completely understood. A common theme among all of the drugs is that they act as catecholamine agonists, with different drugs having unique effects on dopamine and norepinephrine systems. We now discuss some of the pertinent differences.

Stimulants. There are a variety of stimulant medications available to treat ADHD, the most popular being MPH and amphetamine (AMP). The prevailing hypothesis is that MPH and AMP have three main effects. They work primarily as dopamine agonists, increasing underactive dopamine system functioning in the frontal lobes of persons with ADHD (Heal, Cheetham, & Smith, 2009). They also work as norepinephrine agonists in the frontal lobes (Solanto, 1998). There are also indications that subcortical areas, such as the basal ganglia, are involved in the therapeutic effects of stimulants on ADHD (Volkow, Fowler, Wang, Ding, & Gatley, 2002).

Both MPH and AMP inhibit catecholamine reuptake by blocking the dopamine and norepi-nephrine transporter, leading to increased concentrations of dopamine and norepinephrine within the synaptic cleft. Furthermore, amphetamine also facilitates release of dopamine by presynaptic neurons independent of firing rates (Heal et al., 2009), which might help to account for the slightly higher efficacy of AMP relative to MPH in treating ADHD. The most common adverse side effects from stimulants are also seen with other catecholamine agonists, and these include gastrointestinal symptoms (e.g., nausea, stomachache, appetite suppression), nervousness, headache, and insomnia. Stimulants also increase dopamine in the mesolimbic dopamine system associated with reward, thus contributing to the abuse potential of stimulants.

Atomoxetine. The mechanism of action of atom-oxetine (ATX) is presumably related to its ability to increase norepinephrine levels in the frontocortico subsystems (Solanto, 1998). ATX has a high affin-ity and selectivity for norepinephrine transporters, and it increases norepinephrine levels by selectively blocking reuptake of this catecholamine. ATX does not have a big impact on other catecholamines, most notably dopamine. This might account for the lower abuse potential of ATX relative to the stimulants. Side effects associated with ATX tend to be mild to moderate. Common adverse events include head-ache, abdominal pain, decreased appetite, vomiting, somnolence, and nausea.

Guanfacine and clonidine. These drugs appear to work as norepinephrine agonists that strengthen neuron activity in the prefrontal cortex by stimulat-ing specific postsynaptic alpha receptors (Sallee, 2010). There may be an indirect effect of these drugs, as stimulation of alpha 2a receptors with guanfacine or clonidine ultimately strengthens glutamatergic stimulation of cells in the prefrontal cortex, resulting in greater control over attention and behavior. These drugs are usually well toler-ated, but there are significant issues with sedation or fatigue. The rate of sedation in studies ranged from 16% to 35%, and fatigue was reported by 12% to 60% of students. This could be a significant problem for individuals, as daytime fatigue is a major threat to school performance (Perfect & Smith, 2016). Other common side effects of guanfacine and clonidine include dry mouth, headache, stomachache, sleep disturbance, and irritability.

Research on Pharmacological Treatment of Attention-Deficit/Hyperactivity Disorder

Hundreds of studies have examined the efficacy of the FDA-approved pharmacological treatments of ADHD. Most of these studies compare one medication against baseline, placebo, or treatment as usual. Taken together, these studies have firmly established the efficacy and safety of these medications. However, in this chapter, we are interested in examining the relative efficacy of these medications compared with other medications and treatments. Meta-analysis is a method for comparing results quantitatively across multiple studies, and it is one of the best ways to examine the relative efficacy of different drugs.

Faraone and Buitelaar (2010) compared the influence of MPH and AMP on core symptoms of ADHD (hyperactivity, impulsivity, and inattention). After reviewing 23 double-blind, placebo-controlled studies of stimulant medication for youth and adolescents with ADHD, they concluded that AMP was moderately more effective than MPH in treating ADHD. Although not a meta-analytic review, Arnold (2000) provided an important systematic comparison of MPH and AMP. Among 174 patients in six crossover studies reviewed by Arnold, 48 responded better to AMP, 27 to MPH, and at least 72 responded well to either MPH or AMP. Thus, there is a trend for a slight advantage of AMP over MPH. A more recent review found no differences between the various types of stimulants, including dextroamphetamine, lisdexamfetamine, and mixed amphetamine salts (Punja et al., 2016). This study also found no credible evidence of differences in response to short-acting verses longer acting versions of stimulants.

A meta-analysis comparing ATX and MPH found them to be equally efficacious in the reduction of ADHD symptoms and in treatment acceptability to families (Hanwella, Senanayake, & de Silva, 2011). However, a more recent meta-analysis of 11 randomized controlled trials that directly compared ATX and MPH found higher response rates for MPH on clinical symptoms (Liu, Zhang, Fang, & Qin, 2017). Furthermore, there was a lower risk with MPH for some side effects, including drowsiness, nausea, and vomiting. There was a higher risk of insomnia with

MPH than ATX. Consistent with many treatment guidelines, Liu et al.'s data support the notion that MPH should be tried prior to a trial of ATX.

A meta-analysis that focused exclusively on the effects of medication treatment on school behavior and academic achievement examined 43 randomized controlled trials of MPH, AMP, and ATX with children ages 4 to 16 (Prasad et al., 2013). There was an overall significant impact for medication treatment on seatwork completion and observed time on task with MPH and AMP formulations but not with ATX. Additionally, there was no impact for any of these drugs on the accuracy of academic performance. Thus, stimulant medications can make small but measurable improvements (approximately 15%) in academic behavior with school-aged children, but the quality of academic work was not improved by medication.

A meta-analysis of 34 studies of randomized placebo-controlled trials of approved medications found effect sizes for stimulants were typically higher than for nonstimulants on symptoms of ADHD (Hennissen et al., 2017). Importantly, this study showed that the benefits of medication treatment for ADHD extend beyond symptom control. The positive effects included improvements in functional impairments and quality of life. The effects on impairment and quality of life were higher for stimulants than nonstimulants, and much higher for children and adolescents than adults. The available meta-analytic studies do not provide firm conclusions about the relative efficacy of the nonstimulant medications compared with other nonstimulant drugs (Faraone et al., 2006).

In conclusion, in terms of efficacy assessed by meta-analytic reviews, the research suggests that stimulants (i.e., MPH, AMP, dextroamphetamine, the combination of AMP and dextroamphetamine, dexmethylphenidate, and lisdexamfetamine) are more effective than nonstimulants (i.e., ATX, guanfacine, and clonidine). There seems to be a slight advantage of AMP over MPH in clinical response. Moreover, there is a sequencing effect, such that the response rate of an initial trial of a stimulant (e.g., AMP) is about 70%, but if a second stimulant is tried (e.g., MPH), then the response rate to stimulants climbs to about 90% (Arnold, 2000). This suggests that two stimulants should be tried prior to attempting pharmacological treatment of ADHD with a nonstimulant.

Treatment Guidelines

Several influential treatment guidelines have been published (American Academy of Pediatrics, 2011; Pliszka & AACAP Work Group on Quality Issues, 2007). Consistent with the meta-analytic studies described earlier, when medication is used, all of the guidelines or medication algorithms (i.e., clinical decision trees) recommend beginning with a trial of a stimulant. We should note that it is usually recommended to start with a psychosocial intervention prior to trial of a pharmacological treatment. This critically important issue is addressed in greater detail in the subsequent section of this chapter on the Integration of Pharmacotherapy With Nonpharmacological Approaches.

Our review of meta-analytic studies suggests that AMP should be tried prior to MPH. However, most of the algorithms do not distinguish between MPH and AMP. About 30% of children and adolescents have adverse side effects (e.g., severe headaches) or inadequate functional improvement from stimulants (Pliszka & AACAP Work Group on Quality Issues, 2007). Thus, a substantial minority of patients can be expected to try at least two different stimulant medications, as well as a variety of doses of such stimulants, prior to trying a nonstimulant medication.

Although the vast majority of patients respond to stimulants, about 10% may not respond or their response is compromised by intolerable side effects. If a stimulant does not work or is intolerable, then the majority of guidelines recommend trying ATX. ATX is recommended primarily because of the relatively low risk of side effects compared with guanfacine and clonidine. If ATX does not work, it is not clear from the literature if guanfacine or clonidine should be used next. Indeed, some might try ATX plus a stimulant prior to a trial of guanfacine or clonidine (Childress, 2016). Guanfacine and clonidine can be used as monotherapies for ADHD, and they often are used in conjunction with stimulants.

BEST APPROACHES FOR ASSESSING TREATMENT RESPONSE AND MANAGING SIDE EFFECTS

Treatment response may fall into four broad categories: recovered, improved, unchanged, and worse. Recovery is achieved when normalization has occurred. A commonly used index of normalization is whether the person no longer meets diagnostic criteria, such as symptom counts dropping below cutoffs. Alternatively, some of the measures used to diagnose ADHD can be used to assess treatment response. Using appropriately normed measures, students may have normal scores on RTI or measures of child psychopathology (e.g., the CBCL). Many normed measures use 2 standard deviations above the mean to define the clinical range, and 1 standard deviation above as the at-risk range. On such measures, movement from the clinical range to the at-risk range would be considered improvement, and movement from the clinical or at-risk range to the normal range (i.e., within 1 standard deviation of the mean) is defined as recovered.

In some cases, standardized measures may not fully capture the presenting problems. In such cases, daily report cards may be used to provide frequent feedback to students and parents on targeted behaviors of interest (Fabiano et al., 2010). Teachers can document progress on target behaviors each day on a personalized form, and the document can be shared with family members and school personnel to coordinate treatment. Graphing progress on each target behavior over time can provide important feedback about treatment efficacy.

Whatever measure is used, when assessing response to treatment the clinician should consider changes from baseline and determine if the treatment is associated with recovery, improvement, no response, or worsening. Given that ADHD tends to be a chronic disorder, it is not realistic to expect full recovery, particularly in the domain of ADHD symptoms. Thus, assessments of response to medication may focus on other areas of functioning or impairment. Even in these areas, it may be unrealistic to expect full recovery. Thus, in many cases, the standard of care is improvement. If there is no improvement, it is hard to justify the effort, cost, and risk of treatment (e.g., side effects). However, when there is improvement or recovery, side effects might be tolerable if they are not too severe and result in a favorable risk-to-benefit ratio. Clinicians should look for worsening and should make sure the deterioration is not caused by treatment. Physicians, parents, and patients should consider the benefits and costs of increasing dosages, such as reduced ADHD symptoms but worsened side effects (McVoy & Findling, 2017).

The common side effects of the FDA-approved drugs for treating ADHD are presented in Table 16.1 and in the section of this chapter on Mechanism of Action. As stated earlier, these side effects tend to be mild to moderate, and they usually can be managed by titration and habituation. The common side effects of stimulants tend to diminish over time, be dose dependent, and disappear when the drug is discontinued (McVoy & Findling, 2017). For students with severe impairments, moderate-severity side effects may be worth the degree of functional improvement provided by medication. As discussed later in this chapter, if the dose of stimulant medication needs to be reduced, the dose of psychosocial intervention can be increased to maintain the therapeutic effect. Also, some medication side effects can be addressed with other medications. For example, a person having insomnia from a stimulant may be given a sedating drug, such as guanfacine or clonidine, in the evening. However, in most cases, lowering the daytime dose or taking the last dose earlier in the day will be sufficient to manage insomnia.

When taken as prescribed, MPH and AMP are some of the safest drugs for children and adolescents. Millions of persons have been taking these drugs for decades, but few serious adverse effects have been reported. While several safety concerns have been raised by the popular media about the use of stimulants, follow-up on these concerns has not found any clear problems related to stimulant treatment of ADHD. For example, one concern about stimulants is the growth slowdown in weight and height that has been documented in some studies (MTA Cooperative Group, 2004; Spencer et al., 1996), but long-term effects are minimal and there is insufficient evidence to show whether ADHD itself or treatment with stimulants leads to growth changes. Some have raised concerns regarding sudden death related to stimulants, but later evidence has revealed

that rates of sudden death among individuals taking stimulants in fact is less than the rate in the general population (Pliszka & AACAP Work Group on Quality Issues, 2007). Taken together, the negative consequences of untreated ADHD clearly outweigh the risks of the stimulant medicines when these are used in an appropriate and careful manner (Merkel, 2010).

The FDA has a black box warning for potential increased risk of suicidal ideation among adolescents taking ATX. A meta-analysis by Bangs and colleagues (2008) found that suicidal ideation was significantly more common among individuals taking ATX, compared with those taking MPH, although there was no difference found in suicide attempts between the groups. Thus, clinicians should monitor suicidal ideation when adolescents are first prescribed ATX. If there is increased suicidal ideation or significant nausea or abdominal pain, then ATX should be discontinued.

The most concerning side effect with clonidine and guanfacine is sedation or sleepiness, and the impact of this side effect on performance, especially learning, should be carefully monitored. Nausea and vomiting may be a treatment-emergent side effect with these drugs. If there is severe impairment from these side effects, these drugs should be discontinued. Clonidine and guanfacine interact with a number of other drugs, so the possibility of adverse combinations of drugs should be considered. Finally, unlike stimulants and ATX, which are only dangerous at extreme overdose, a small overdose of clonidine or guanfacine could be life-threatening and requires immediate medical attention.

Certain populations (e.g., preschoolers, individuals with autism spectrum disorders, individuals with intellectual disabilities) appear to experience increased side effects from medications (Research Units on Pediatric Psychopharmacology Autism Network, 2005). For example, compared with outcomes from the Multimodal Treatment of ADHD Study (MTA study; i.e., the largest clinical trial to date studying treatment for children with ADHD), children with comorbid autism spectrum disorder and ADHD were nearly 13 times as likely to discontinue treatment due to side effects than were children with a wide range of other comorbid conditions (MTA Cooperative Group, 1999). Individuals in special populations associated with increased sensitivity to pharmacological treatments should be monitored closely to discern whether discomfort from the medication outweighs its benefits.

Some debate exists around the use of stimulants to treat ADHD in children with comorbid tic disorders. A recent meta-analysis revealed that stimulant medications at various dosages and durations of treatment did not exacerbate preexisting tic disorder symptoms (Cohen et al., 2015). Because prior studies have documented that stimulants may increase symptoms of tic disorders, families should discuss with their doctors the severity of ADHD and tic symptoms, as well as possible side effects, when selecting types and dosages of medication to treat ADHD.

MEDICATION MANAGEMENT ISSUES

It cannot be stressed strongly enough that effective pharmacological treatment of ADHD involves much more than prescribing pills. Essential components of effective pharmacological treatment of ADHD include rapport building, psychoeducation, dose titration, and monitoring for treatment-emergent side effects. Taken together, these activities fall under the broader concept of *medication management*. The MTA study found that systematic medication management produced a greater reduction in symptoms compared with treatment as usual in the community (MTA Cooperative Group, 1999). The MTA result is consistent with many other studies showing that pharmacological treatment should be part of an intervention package that includes medication management.

Published guidelines for pharmacological treatment of ADHD suggest that patients should attend weekly doctor visits for monitoring of treatment-emergent side effects at the start of treatment (Pliszka & AACAP Work Group on Quality Issues, 2007). This often includes starting with a lower dose than expected for maintenance, so that patients can get used to or develop tolerance for treatment-emergent side effects. Subsequently, monthly visits are suggested, during which doctors monitor dose-response, schedule of administration, and side effects and determine whether a different dose or prescription

schedule is needed. Medication management via phone or e-mail may replace office visits, depending on family need.

Compliance with pharmacological treatment recommendations varies among different age groups. Young children and adolescents typically have high adherence and compliance with their medication because their parents and school nurses assist in the delivery process. As younger adolescents move toward later adolescence and young adulthood, they are given more autonomy in multiple facets of life, including in adherence (or lack thereof) to a treatment program. Once adolescents have left the home for college or employment, parents are no longer involved in daily adherence and compliance.

There are a number of family factors that predict increased (or decreased) adherence to medication regimens. Parents' perceptions about medication, types of family structure, and other family factors can influence adherence. For example, children from two-parent families and children from families with high socioeconomic status are more likely to adhere to medication protocols (Charach & Gajaria, 2008). Parental beliefs about the safety of medications in general can lead to both increased and decreased adherence in children (Bussing et al., 2012). Insurance coverage for medication is associated with increased adherence, while overall cost of the medication is associated with decreased adherence (Fiks, Mayne, Localio, Alessandrini, & Guevara, 2012).

In children, prior history of medication treatment and a positive relationship with the prescribing doctor are associated with increased adherence. For adolescents, academic success and the presence of relatively few adverse effects have been associated with increased adherence. Adolescents are also more likely to express concerns about treatment dependence, which has a negative influence on their adherence.

Characteristics related to the medication itself and the treatment plan affect the likelihood for medication adherence. Long-acting or extended-release formulations are associated with the highest adherence. Alternatively, multiple daily doses can be seen as a barrier to adherence (Gau et al., 2006). General ineffectiveness of the medication, whether perceived or actual, is associated with decreased adherence. Medication recipients also cite difficulties in adjusting and readjusting medication dosage as a barrier to adherence (Bussing et al., 2012).

EVALUATION OF PHARMACOLOGICAL APPROACHES ACROSS THE LIFESPAN

Although in this chapter we focus on pharmacological treatments for children and adolescents with ADHD, the disorder continues past these developmental stages into adulthood. While most impairments in children and adolescents are noticed in school and social environments, these and similar impairments are evident in adults in the workplace, in personal relationships, and in postsecondary education. There are currently five medications approved by the FDA to treat ADHD in adults: Adderall XR®, Concerta®, Focalin XR®, Strattera®, and Vyvanse®. Further research on these medications, and nonpharmacological treatments for adults, is needed.

Of note, there has been debate regarding the possibility of adult-onset or late-onset ADHD. While ADHD is typically diagnosed between ages 5 and 12, some researchers have argued that a separate form of ADHD emerges in late adolescence or early adulthood (Agnew-Blais et al., 2016). Opponents of this assertion contend that late-onset ADHD is a late identification rather than a late onset (Castellanos, 2015). Others have posited that individuals seeking treatment for late-onset ADHD more likely have a different comorbid disorder or a substance use problem (Sibley et al., 2018). Furthermore, given that the *DSM–5* classifies ADHD as a neurodevelopmental disorder, so-called late-onset ADHD could be qualitatively different. No information on treatment of late-onset ADHD is available.

CONSIDERATION OF POTENTIAL SEX DIFFERENCES

Research suggests that efficacy of treatment for ADHD does not differ according to sex. In a review of 14 studies of stimulant treatments, 10 studies found no sex differences in functional, neuropsychological, or symptom reduction outcomes,

and the remaining four studies produced conflicting results (Williamson & Johnston, 2015). For AMP formulations of stimulants, studies have also failed to demonstrate a sex-by-treatment interaction (Wigal, Kollins, Childress, & Adeyi, 2010). However, the lack of sex differences may be attributable to underreporting in the literature (Williamson & Johnston, 2015) or limitations in study designs (Sonuga-Barke et al., 2007). For instance, studies often recruit too few females with ADHD to conduct an adequately powered sex-by-treatment comparison. Furthermore, few studies of persons with ADHD have looked at sex differences in how medications move through the body (i.e., pharmacokinetics) or how they work at the site of action (i.e., pharmacodynamics). This work could be important, considering that in a synthesis of 163 drug reviews by the FDA, one fifth found significant sex differences in pharmacokinetics, and about 7% of the drugs had differences exceeding 40% (Anderson, 2008). The few available studies of sex differences in MPH pharmacokinetics have found mixed evidence concerning pharmacokinetics among adult men and women with ADHD (Sonuga-Barke et al., 2007). To date, no dosing recommendations have been made according to sex.

INTEGRATION OF PHARMACOTHERAPY WITH NONPHARMACOLOGICAL APPROACHES: BENEFITS AND CHALLENGES

For the purposes of this chapter, we define *combined treatments* as those that integrate psychosocial interventions with pharmacological interventions. We define *multimodal approaches* as those that combine multiple psychosocial approaches (e.g., parent training and classroom interventions). *Polypharmacy* is when multiple medications are provided during the course of the day. Studies such as the MTA have compared intensive multimodal psychosocial treatments separately and in combination with intensive pharmacological treatment (MTA Cooperative Group, 1999). Several other studies also have compared pharmacotherapy separately and in combination with multimodal treatment (Smith & Shapiro, 2004). In this section, we examine the separate and combined effects of stimulant treatment and multimodal behavior therapy packages. We begin by discussing the many reasons to use stimulants and multimodal psychosocial therapies together.

Rationale for Combined Treatments

One of the reasons for using combined treatments is because there are complementary effects of pharmacological and psychological interventions that may overcome the limitations of either of these interventions delivered alone. For instance, stimulant treatment cannot be used 24 hours a day because there must be breaks to allow for sleeping. Consequently, persons with ADHD who rely on stimulant monotherapy are essentially untreated in the evening when the medication wears off and in the morning before medication takes effect. A type of combined treatment is to provide behavioral interventions in the morning and evening only, when stimulant medication is not a viable intervention. One might call this phenomenon a *sequential combined-treatment effect*.

A second reason for using combined treatments is that biological and behavioral interventions might interact to create a sum that is greater than the individual parts. For example, medication alone does not teach persons the skills necessary for more competent functioning. Likewise, behavioral treatment alone may not encourage sufficiently focused attention for a person to benefit from instruction. It is possible that medication and behavior therapy provided simultaneously can create a unique combination of therapeutic benefits that are more likely to help the person than is either intervention alone. If the sum of the therapeutic effects is greater than the individual effects of the therapies, this is a *synergistic combined-treatment effect*.

Summary of the Multimodal Treatment of ADHD Study. The most robust study to date regarding combined treatment for ADHD is the MTA study (MTA Cooperative Group, 1999), which examined four conditions: medication management (MedMgt), multimodal psychosocial interventions (BehMod), combined MedMgt and BehMod (COMB), and community control (CC). A description of MedMgt was given previously in the section of this chapter on Best Approaches for Assessing Treatment Response and Managing Side Effects. The BehMod in the MTA

consisted of an 8-week summer camp running 5 days per week, up to 28 parent training sessions, an aide in the classroom, and consultation with teachers. The CC condition comprised community care as usual, and about 70% of these participants received medication, mostly stimulant monotherapy.

Although some of the initial reports of the MTA study suggested that there was little additional benefit from adding BehMod to MedMgt (MTA Cooperative Group, 1999), subsequent analyses have painted a different picture (Smith & Shapiro, 2004). For example, when the MTA Cooperative Group rank ordered treatments based on the number of times each group had the largest treatment effect compared with the other groups, the results were as follows: COMB (12), MedMgt (4), BehMod (2), and CC (1). The four times that MedMgt was superior were for parent ratings of symptoms of inattention and hyperactivity and for classroom observations of hyperactivity and impulsivity (MTA Cooperative Group, 1999). Furthermore, satisfaction scores given by parents for the COMB and BehMod conditions were equal to each other and significantly higher than were parent satisfaction scores for the MedMgt condition (MTA Cooperative Group, 1999). This is important because satisfaction and compliance with intervention were correlated in the MTA study. For instance, the MedMgt group had the highest attrition and the COMB group had the best participation in treatment. In terms of effect sizes, COMB outperformed MedMgt, with an incremental effect size of 0.28, which is a small to moderate difference. The differences between COMB and other treatments were moderate to large in size, with an effect size of .54 between COMB and BehMod and an effect size of .63 between COMB and CC.

Meta-analytic studies. Majewicz-Hefley and Carlson (2007) found 26 rigorous studies of combined treatment relative to pharmacology-only treatments. Unfortunately, most of the studies of combined treatments (18 of 26) had to be excluded from analysis by Majewicz-Hefley and Carlson because data needed to calculate effect sizes were missing. Based on the eight studies with appropriate data, combined treatment had the largest and most significant impact on core symptoms of ADHD and on improving social skills. The impact on academic functioning was small.

A meta-analysis by Van der Oord, Prins, Oosterlaan, and Emmelkamp (2008) reviewed 26 studies of short-acting MPH, behavioral or cognitive behavior interventions, and combined treatment for school-age children (6–12 years old). These authors concluded that for ADHD symptoms, both MPH and combined interventions were equally effective (with large effect sizes) and behavioral/cognitive behavior interventions were somewhat less effective (with moderate to large effect sizes). They found that all three treatments resulted in moderate to large improvements in oppositional defiant disorder and conduct disorder symptoms and social behavior. In the limited number of studies on educational outcomes ($n = 7$), medication had no appreciable impact on academic functioning and behavioral therapy had a small positive effect (effect size = .19).

Of note, the mean weighted effect sizes in Van der Oord et al. (2008) were largest for combined treatment approaches in all domains. However, owing to the limited number of studies and resultant low statistical power, the difference in effect size between combined treatment and medication alone was not statistically significant. Rather than viewing this statistical conclusion as a potential Type 2 validity error (i.e., missing an effect because of low power), Van der Oord and colleagues concluded there was no advantage of combined treatments. This potentially erroneous statistical reasoning (i.e., low power leading to a Type 2 error) was also seen in the early reporting on the MTA study. Conversely, one might argue that the advantage of combined treatments over medication is small, and thus an appropriate question about combined treatments is whether the incremental benefit is clinically meaningful. In the following section, we review evidence that medication effects are highly context dependent, and that psychosocial treatment is an important determinant of overall treatment effect sizes.

Synergistic Effects of Combined Treatments

In a groundbreaking study, Fabiano and colleagues (2007) tested the hypothesis that combining low doses of stimulant medication with low doses of behavior modification could achieve the same effect as high doses of either of these interventions delivered individually. This hypothesis was based on clinical observations and published reports about the phenomenon of a synergy from two low doses of medication and behavior therapy (Smith & Shapiro, 2004). However, prior to Fabiano et al. (2007), researchers had not systematically varied the dose of medication or behavioral therapies when looking for potential synergistic combined-treatment effects.

To address the ambiguity regarding the strength of the behavioral interventions, Fabiano and colleagues (2007) operationalized three ecologically valid levels of school behavior support, which might be called Tier 0, Tier 1.5, and Tier 3 in an RTI framework (Sugai & Horner, 2009). The doses of medication chosen by Fabiano and colleagues extended the range of doses of the stimulant medication MPH to lower doses than were typically used in previous studies. In many previous studies, the so-called low dose was 0.3 mg/kg of MPH. There were indications from some prior studies that, in the context of strong behavioral treatments, doses of MPH less than 0.3 mg/kg could result in sufficient therapeutic gain. Therefore, Fabiano and colleagues chose the low dose of 0.15 mg/kg MPH, which they compared with 0.3 and 0.6 mg/kg doses of MPH. The average doses in the study were about 5 mg, about 11 mg, and about 21 mg of MPH, administered three times a day.

Fabiano et al. (2007) randomized doses of medication and behavioral support in the context of a counterbalanced 3×4 within-subject factorial design (three levels of behavioral support and three levels of medication plus placebo). Data were collected on 48 children ages 6 to 12 years who were diagnosed with ADHD and participated in the 9-week Summer Treatment Program. The overall pattern of results from the Fabiano and colleagues (2007) study showed a synergistic effect of combining treatments. In the presence of the lowest dose of behavioral treatment, the lowest dose of MPH resulted in similar effects to large doses of either behavior modification or medication. In other words, the overall effect of the low dose, or the "whole" combined effect, was greater than the sum of the parts.

Documentation by Fabiano et al. (2007) that combining treatments for synergistic effect has important implications for the practicality and sustainability of treatment. Most negative stimulant medication side effects are dose dependent, so using lower doses of medication in the context of low doses of behavior therapy should result in a safer, more tolerable, and more sustainable treatment. Also of note, a major limitation of intensive psychosocial treatments is that they are not feasible or sustainable by most parents and schools. For instance, the Tier 3 intensity in Fabiano et al. was similar to what is implemented in high-quality special education classrooms and might not be feasible for implementation by most parents and classroom teachers, including special education teachers. Fortunately, lower level behavior management can be effective when it is concurrent with stimulant treatment.

Sequencing Effects of Combined Treatments

Studies have shown that when pharmacological and psychosocial treatments are started may influence efficacy and costs. Pelham and colleagues (2016) conducted a year-long adaptive treatment study with 146 students aged 5 to 12 years and found that students who began with behavioral treatment first then added medication later had significantly better outcomes than students who started with medication first then had behavioral treatment added later. A cost-effectiveness analysis of the Pelham et al. study, which examined costs arising from physician time, clinician time, paraprofessional time, teacher time, parent time, medication, and gasoline, found that starting with a behavioral intervention prior to medication was about half as expensive compared with starting medication prior to behavioral intervention (Page et al., 2016).

INTEGRATED APPROACHES FOR ADDRESSING COMMON COMORBID DISORDERS

Comorbid disorders frequently occur among individuals with ADHD, and the type of comorbidity often depends on ADHD presentation (American Psychiatric Association, 2013). Individuals with ADHD are more likely than not to have a comorbid condition; about 30% of children are diagnosed with ADHD only. Oppositional defiant disorder co-occurs with ADHD for about one third of children with ADHD. Conduct disorder co-occurs in approximately 25% of cases (American Psychiatric Association, 2013). About 30% of children with ADHD meet criteria for a specific learning disability (Massetti et al., 2008). Other disorders, such as speech language disorders, autism spectrum disorders, bipolar disorder, intellectual disability, anxiety, and depression, all co-occur with ADHD at a rate much higher than expected in the general population.

Co-occurring disorders with ADHD often add associated impairment beyond that incurred from ADHD symptoms, and treatment should focus on these unique considerations (Pelham et al., 2016). For most disorders that co-occur with ADHD, it is appropriate to prescribe the same stimulant medications and behavior therapy as typically would be used to treat ADHD. However, some conditions are associated with reduced effectiveness of stimulants or with adverse reactions, and other conditions benefit from additional psychosocial interventions (Fonagy, Target, Cottrell, Phillips, & Kurtz, 2015). Some of these specific disorders are considered in the subsequent paragraphs.

Oppositional Defiant Disorder and Conduct Disorder

Multiple studies converge on the notion that stimulant treatment is effective for children and adolescents with comorbid oppositional defiant disorder and conduct disorder. A meta-analysis found that stimulants produce improvements in aggression and oppositionality with effect sizes of similar magnitude to improvements in ADHD symptoms (Connor, Glatt, Lopez, Jackson, & Melloni, 2002). In addition, the MTA study found that MedMgt, BehMod, and COMB reduced aggression and oppositionality, with the biggest effects for COMB (MTA Cooperative Group, 1999).

Conduct disorder often is associated with substance use disorder, and parents and mental health practitioners have worried that prescribing stimulants to adolescents with behavior and attention problems could lead to stimulant abuse or exacerbation of other substance use. To the contrary, the literature indicates that stimulants may serve as a protective factor for later substance use disorders, as children treated with stimulants have lower prevalence of substance use disorder than non-treated children (Wilens, Faraone, Biederman, & Gunawardene, 2003). Thus, stimulants are a well-supported and safe treatment to reduce symptoms of conduct problems comorbid with ADHD.

Aggression is a common problem for children with ADHD and comorbid oppositional defiant disorder or conduct disorder. Treatment with stimulants reduces aggression in children with ADHD, an approach that is safe and FDA approved. Some atypical antipsychotics, particularly risperidone, have been shown to reduce aggression. However, the literature is limited and has focused largely on individuals with lower cognitive abilities or autism spectrum disorders (see Chapter 17, this volume; McVoy & Findling, 2017). Given the lack of research and concern about side effects, use of atypical antipsychotics for aggressive children with ADHD should be limited.

Research clearly shows that the most effective interventions for conduct problems are supervision and structure. Effective psychosocial interventions include family/parent-based, child-oriented, and school-based treatments. A meta-analysis by Epstein and colleagues (2015) found similar effect sizes for parent interventions and multicomponent interventions consisting of parent and child elements, suggesting that parent interventions are most influential in addressing disruptive behavior. Child-oriented interventions produced superior effects compared with control conditions; however, an insufficient number of child-focused intervention studies met criteria to make comparisons with parent and multi-component treatments (Epstein, Fonnesbeck, Potter, Rizzone, & McPheeters, 2015).

Parent management training is a well-supported behavioral intervention that can be delivered in group or individual formats. Strong parent management training programs include The Incredible Years®, Triple P—Positive Parenting Program, Oregon Social Learning Center Programs, Parent–Child Interaction Therapy, and Families and Schools Together, among others. Child programs include problem-solving skills training and cognitive behavior therapy with a focus on social information processing. Such programs should be delivered as adjunct treatments to parent

training to produce meaningful outcomes (McCart, Priester, Davies, & Azen, 2006). Before delivering a child-focused intervention, a clinician should determine whether a child's developmental level matches the cognitive demands of the selected intervention.

Universal supports delivered in schools as part of Tier I RTI provide two key elements for addressing disruptive behaviors: structure and monitoring. School-wide positive behavioral interventions and supports build structure through clear rules, established procedures, and positive reinforcement for desired behavior. Universal screening of child behavior and academic achievement identifies at-risk students, monitors their progress, and determines whether additional supports are required (Fletcher & Vaughn, 2009).

Problem-solving consultation is an evidence-based model that can be undertaken both within the context of RTI to address concerns about individual students and at the classroom or school level to address system-level concerns. Problem-solving consultation is a service-delivery model through which behavioral and instructional principles are chosen, implemented, and monitored to address problem behaviors (Kratochwill, 2008). Conjoint behavioral consultation is another evidence-based model that includes a consultant and a parent and teacher as consultees (Sheridan & Kratochwill, 2007). A benefit of consultation is that mental health professionals such as school psychologists equip teachers with tools to serve many students, thus reducing the burden of a traditional, one-on-one service delivery model.

Learning Disabilities

While there is no pharmacological treatment to improve the cognitive processing difficulties that contribute to learning disabilities, stimulants for comorbid ADHD often provide short-term improvements in academic achievement (Carlson & Bunner, 1993). Stimulants may improve students' abilities to attend to instructions, complete multistep tasks, and sustain attention. Some studies have noted concerns about high doses of stimulants producing zombie-like behaviors in students, which may reduce academic engagement rather than enhance it (Swanson, Cantwell, Lerner, McBurnett, & Hanna, 1991). With appropriate dosing, achieved through regular monitoring, stimulants should produce positive effects in the classroom for most children. Combined pharmacological and psychosocial interventions, which were reviewed earlier in this chapter, are also beneficial for children with learning disabilities and ADHD.

In addition to behavioral supports, educational interventions are needed to address the academic components of a learning disability, such as problems with word recognition, computation, and spelling (Fletcher, Lyon, Fuchs, & Barnes, 2006). An RTI framework for intervention enables educators to identify students who need help and support them before their academic difficulties become intractable, and to remediate existing problems using evidence-based interventions (Fletcher & Vaughn, 2009). Students with comorbid learning disabilities and ADHD should also be monitored for internalizing disorders that may emerge as a result of repeated academic and behavior difficulties in school.

Anxiety Disorders

The MTA study suggests that psychosocial interventions and stimulants together produced positive effects for ADHD and internalizing symptoms among individuals with anxiety disorders (March et al., 2000). Findings from other research have raised concerns about a lack of response and the adverse effects of stimulants among this population (DuPaul, Barkley, & McMurray, 1994). Yet, in each of these other studies, a proportion of individuals has responded positively to stimulant medication, which warrants their continued use to treat comorbid anxiety disorders, provided that concurrent cognitive behavior treatment and medication monitoring is provided.

In the first controlled trial of polypharmacy for childhood ADHD and anxiety using stimulants and selective serotonin reuptake inhibitors, researchers found that children with the comorbid disorders responded as well to stimulant medications as children with ADHD only, and selective serotonin reuptake inhibitors did not demonstrate any noticeable added therapeutic benefit (Abikoff et al., 2005). As in the MTA study, a few children demonstrated a reduction in internalizing symptoms, and stimulant medication did not worsen existing anxiety. Abikoff et al. noted that while selective serotonin reuptake inhibitors did not significantly improve functional

outcomes, results were in the desired direction, so it is possible that a study with greater power may be able to detect effects of selective serotonin reuptake inhibitors among this population.

Epilepsy

An estimated 12% to 39% of children with epilepsy have ADHD symptoms, predominantly of the inattentive presentation (Dunn, Austin, & Harezlak, 2003). Two concerns arise regarding whether stimulants are an appropriate solution to ADHD symptoms comorbid with epilepsy. First, it is unclear whether symptoms are a side effect of antiepileptic drugs or a separate disorder; second, stimulants may increase seizure frequency (Fonagy et al., 2015). In a review of pharmacological treatments for comorbid ADHD and epilepsy, MPH emerged as the best supported treatment for safe use with antiepileptic drugs (Torres, Whitney, & Gonzalez-Heydrich, 2008). Trials with MPH did not demonstrate a seizure-promoting effect, and 70% of participants experienced improvement in ADHD symptoms. It appears safe to prescribe stimulants for ADHD and antiepileptic drugs simultaneously without harmful effects.

Tic Disorders

For a review of stimulant use with comorbid tic disorders, see the earlier section of this chapter on Best Approaches for Assessing Treatment Response and Managing Side Effects.

EMERGING TRENDS

Phillips et al. (2001) reported that up to 43% of the variability in the way an individual tolerates or responds to medication is due to genetic contributions. Given that medication nonresponse or adverse medication reactions are an issue for anyone being treated with psychiatric medications, the discovery of clinically meaningful genetic markers that can help guide medication selection and predict treatment response is a very exciting prospect. *Pharmacogenomics*, the field of genetic testing that focuses on genes involved in either medication metabolism or how medication acts on targets, is not yet part of standard practice, but it certainly qualifies as an emerging trend. Because affordable genetic testing is leading the transition into the age of personalized medicine, clinicians treating ADHD should pay attention to developments in pharmacogenomics.

Proper interpretation of pharmacogenomic testing requires an understanding of which genes are being tested, why the genes pertain to the condition being treated, and what information testing provides about the potential medications that might be used. One category of genes considered highly relevant to pharmacogenomics are those that code for the enzymes that metabolize medications. These are the *pharmacokinetic genes*. Another important category of relevant genes are the *pharmacodynamic genes*, which code for the target of medications, such as the receptors to which the medication might bind, the neurotransmitter transporter proteins, or the enzymes related to the synthesis or degradation of the neurotransmitters influenced by the drug.

The critical information about genes that is obtained from pharmacogenomic testing is whether there are two functional alleles or there are single nucleotide polymorphisms present that will interfere with the product made by those genes. If there are two functional alleles, the gene will make functional products (e.g., enzymes). If there is a single nucleotide polymorphism, the gene product will be deficient or abnormal in its functioning. For the pharmacokinetic genes, a problematic allele may mean that the enzyme will have unusually low activity or high activity. For the pharmacodynamic genes, a single nucleotide polymorphism may cause receptors, transporter proteins, or enzymes along the neurotransmitter cascade to not work properly, which in turn changes the ability of a medication to impact its target site. Although there is research to suggest that certain polymorphisms may reduce the impact of distinct medications or classes of medications, the research on the application of these results remain mixed. It is also extremely important for the ADHD practitioner to understand that pharmacogenomic testing, like most genetic testing, is about detecting vulnerability and risk, which is important but cannot alone be used to predict outcome. With that caveat in mind, certain genes seem highly relevant to the pharmacotherapy of ADHD.

Perhaps the most relevant pharmacokinetic gene for ADHD is the one that codes for the 2D6 enzyme, which is within the P450 pathway and is involved in the metabolism of ATX and the AMP class of ADHD medications. This gene product is so crucial to ATX that the FDA requires the medication label include a warning about 2D6 "poor" metabolizers and the Clinical Pharmacogenomics Implementation Consortium is developing specific guidelines for linking gene findings to dosing strategies (Hicks et al., 2015). Regarding pharmacodynamic genes, there are no current actionable pairings between these and medications used for ADHD. However, there is some research to suggest that certain polymorphisms within the *COMT* gene and the *ADRA2A* gene may impact responsiveness of an individual to stimulant medication (da Silva et al., 2008).

In light of these gene findings and their potential impact on the treatment of ADHD, some providers might be tempted to use commercially available pharmacogenomic ADHD panels. These panels provide the clinician with the specific gene results, and some provide a guide that lists relevant ADHD medications in categories of green (safe to use), yellow (proceed with caution), and red (to be avoided). Although there is research to support the utilization of pharmacogenomic panels in enhancing the treatment of depression, such studies have been criticized for their design and potential conflict of interest in being industry sponsored. There are no such studies yet on the panels for the treatment of ADHD.

Given the cost of pharmacogenomic testing and the lack of research on its clinical utility, this testing is not yet recommended as part of routine pharmacologic treatment. However, for individuals who have unusual side effects from common ADHD medications, genetic testing may be helpful in directing medication trials. As long as the clinician provides accurate information to the patient and family about the cost–benefit ratio for genetic testing, including stating that it is about determining general vulnerability rather than certainty about individual clinical outcome, pharmacogenomic testing may provide additional information that, when combined with evidence-based guidelines regarding the treatment of ADHD, can help to reduce the trial-and-error strategy of pharmacotherapy, which is often so disconcerting for many patients and families.

OVERALL SUMMARY AND CONCLUSION

There is considerable evidence that the FDA-approved drugs for treating ADHD are safe and effective (see Table 16.1). Moreover, multiple lines of research indicate there are many advantages to combining pharmacological and nonpharmacological treatment of ADHD. The research, and many treatment guidelines now available, indicate that treatment for ADHD should begin with a behavioral intervention. If mild to moderate behavioral treatment is not sufficient or sustainable, then medication can be added. When using stimulants, 90% of children and adolescents are expected to respond positively after two complete trials of the medication, which may include titration over several weeks or months. For people who respond to stimulants, strong behavior therapy may be needed in the morning and evening when stimulants are not active in the system. During the day, low doses of behavior therapy can be combined with stimulants to produce strong behavioral effects. If minimally sufficient behavior therapy is not available during the day (e.g., during a play date at a friend's house, Sunday school, sports practice), then temporarily higher doses of medication may be advisable.

Research on treatment of adults with ADHD is limited, and the efficacy, safety, and practicality of psychosocial and pharmacological treatments have not been robustly investigated. Individual attention and intensive case management, supported by collateral report, is needed to manage treatment of ADHD across the lifespan. The time, effort, and cost of treatment should far offset the costs incurred from untreated ADHD. In the future, genetic testing may reduce the amount of trial and error needed to find the best medication and dose for treating ADHD.

TOOL KIT OF RESOURCES

Attention-Deficit/Hyperactivity Disorder (ADHD): Patient Resources

National Institute of Mental Health: Authoritative source of state-of-the-art, peer-reviewed information about ADHD: http://www.nimh.nih.gov/health/topics/attention-deficit-hyperactivity-disorder-adhd/index.shtml

Children and Adults With Attention-Deficit/Hyperactivity Disorder: Information from the largest national advocacy group for persons with ADHD: http://www.chadd.org

Florida International University Center for Children and Families: A variety of parent- and teacher-friendly resources for the assessment and treatment of ADHD in multiple settings: https://ccf.fiu.edu/about/resources/index.html

Recommended Assessment Measures

Observation

Behavior Observation of Students in Schools (Shapiro, 2013): http://downloads.pearsonclinical.com/images/Assets/BOSS/BOSSLandingPage.pdf

Interview

Child and Adolescent Psychiatric Assessment–V (Angold & Costello, 2000): http://devepi.duhs.duke.edu/capa.html

Broadband Rating Scales (select one)

Behavior Assessment System for Children–3 (Reynolds & Kamphaus, 2015): https://www.pearsonclinical.com/education/products/100001402/behavior-assessment-system-for-children-third-edition-basc-3.html

Child Behavior Checklist (Achenbach & Rescorla, 2001): http://www.aseba.org/schoolage.html

Conners Comprehensive Behavior Rating Scales (Conners, 2008): https://www.mhs.com/MHS-Assessment?prodname=cbrs

Narrowband Rating Scales (select one)

ADHD Rating Scale–V (DuPaul et al., 2016): https://www.guilford.com/books/ADHD-Rating-Scale-5-for-Children-and-Adolescents/DuPaul-Power-Anastopoulos-Reid/9781462524877

Barkley Adult ADHD Rating Scale–IV (BAARS-IV; Barkley, 2011): https://www.guilford.com/books/Barkley-Adult-ADHD-Rating-Scale-IV-BAARS-IV/Russell-Barkley/9781609182038

Vanderbilt Rating Scale (Wolraich et al., 2003): https://www.nichq.org/resource/nichq-vanderbilt-assessment-scales

Impairment Rating Scale (Fabiano et al., 2006): https://ccf.fiu.edu/research/publications/articles-2000-2009/impairment-in-children.pdf

Useful Information Related to Pharmacogenomics

Pharmacogenomics: Overview of the Genomics and Targeted Therapy Group: Provides information about drug development and labeling, including genomics guidance, relevant publications, lists of biomarkers and related evidence, and more: https://www.fda.gov/Drugs/ScienceResearch/ucm572617.htm

References

Abikoff, H., McGough, J., Vitiello, B., McCracken, J., Dames, M., Walkup, J., . . . Ritz, L. (2005). Sequential pharmacotherapy for children with comorbid attention-deficit/hyperactivity and anxiety disorders. *Journal of the American Academy of Child and Adolescent Psychiatry, 44,* 418–427. http://dx.doi.org/10.1097/01.chi.0000155320.52322.37

*Achenbach, T. M., & Rescorla, L. A. (2001). *Manual for the ASEBA School-Age Forms and Profiles: An integrated system of multi-informant assessment.* Burlington, VT: University of Vermont.

Agnew-Blais, J. C., Polanczyk, G. V., Danese, A., Wertz, J., Moffitt, T. E., & Arseneault, L. (2016). Evaluation of the persistence, remission, and emergence of attention-deficit/hyperactivity disorder in young adulthood. *JAMA Psychiatry, 73,* 713–720. http://dx.doi.org/10.1001/jamapsychiatry.2016.0465

American Academy of Pediatrics, Subcommittee on Attention-Deficit/Hyperactivity Disorder. (2011). ADHD: Clinical practice guideline for the diagnosis, evaluation, and treatment of attention-deficit/hyperactivity disorder in children and adolescents. *Pediatrics, 128,* 1007–1022. http://dx.doi.org/10.1542/peds.2011-2654

American Psychiatric Association. (2013). *Diagnostic and statistical manual of mental disorders* (5th ed.). Washington, DC: Author.

Anderson, G. D. (2008). Gender differences in pharmacological response. *International Review of Neurobiology, 83,* 1–10. http://dx.doi.org/10.1016/S0074-7742(08)00001-9

*Angold, A., & Costello, E. J. (2000). The Child and Adolescent Psychiatric Assessment (CAPA). *Journal of the American Academy of Child & Adolescent Psychiatry, 39,* 39–48. http://dx.doi.org/10.1097/00004583-200001000-00015

Arnold, L. E. (2000). Methylphenidate vs. amphetamine: Comparative review. *Journal of Attention Disorders, 3,* 200–211. http://dx.doi.org/10.1177/108705470000300403

Bangs, M. E., Tauscher-Wisniewski, S., Polzer, J., Zhang, S., Acharya, N., Desaiah, D., . . . Allen, A. J. (2008). Meta-analysis of suicide-related behavior events in patients treated with atomoxetine. *Journal of the American Academy of Child & Adolescent Psychiatry, 47,* 209–218. http://dx.doi.org/10.1097/chi.0b013e31815d88b2

*Barkley, R. A. (2011). *Barkley Adult ADHD Rating Scale–IV (BAARS-IV).* New York, NY: Guilford.

Barkley, R. A. (2015a). Health problems and related impairments in children and adults with ADHD. In R. A. Barkley (Ed.), *Attention-deficit hyperactivity disorder: A handbook for diagnosis and treatment* (4th ed., pp. 267–313). New York, NY: Guilford.

Barkley, R. A. (2015b). History of ADHD. In R. A. Barkley (Ed.), *Attention-deficit hyperactivity disorder: A handbook for diagnosis and treatment* (4th ed., pp. 3–50). New York, NY: Guilford.

Barkley, R. A., Fischer, M., Smallish, L., & Fletcher, K. (2002). The persistence of attention-deficit/hyperactivity disorder into young adulthood as a function of reporting source and definition of disorder. *Journal of Abnormal Psychology, 111,* 279–289. http://dx.doi.org/10.1037/0021-843X.111.2.279

Bussing, R., Zima, B. T., Mason, D. M., Meyer, J. M., White, K., & Garvan, C. W. (2012). ADHD knowledge, perceptions, and information sources: Perspectives from a community sample of adolescents and their parents. *Journal of Adolescent Health, 51,* 593–600. http://dx.doi.org/10.1016/j.jadohealth.2012.03.004

Carlson, C. L., & Bunner, M. R. (1993). Effects of methylphenidate on the academic performance of children with attention-deficit hyperactivity disorder and learning disabilities. *School Psychology Review, 22,* 184–198.

Castellanos, F. X. (2015). Is adult-onset ADHD a distinct entity? *The American Journal of Psychiatry, 172,* 929–931. http://dx.doi.org/10.1176/appi.ajp.2015.15070988

Charach, A., & Gajaria, A. (2008). Improving psychostimulant adherence in children with ADHD. *Expert Review of Neurotherapeutics, 8,* 1563–1571. http://dx.doi.org/10.1586/14737175.8.10.1563

Childress, A. C. (2016). A critical appraisal of atomoxetine in the management of ADHD. *Therapeutics and Clinical*

---

*Asterisks indicate assessments or resources.

Risk Management, 12, 27–39. http://dx.doi.org/10.2147/tcrm.s59270

Cohen, S. C., Mulqueen, J. M., Ferracioli-Oda, E., Stuckelman, Z. D., Coughlin, C. G., Leckman, J. F., & Bloch, M. H. (2015). Meta-analysis: Risk of tics associated with psychostimulant use in randomized, placebo-controlled trials. *Journal of the American Academy of Child & Adolescent Psychiatry, 54*, 728–736. http://dx.doi.org/10.1016/j.jaac.2015.06.011

Conners, C. K. (2008). *Conners Comprehensive Behavior Rating Scales*. Toronto, Canada: Multi-Health Systems.

Connor, D. F., Glatt, S. J., Lopez, I. D., Jackson, D., & Melloni, R. H., Jr. (2002). Psychopharmacology and aggression. I: A meta-analysis of stimulant effects on overt/covert aggression-related behaviors in ADHD. *Journal of the American Academy of Child & Adolescent Psychiatry, 41*, 253–261. http://dx.doi.org/10.1097/00004583-200203000-00004

da Silva, T. L., Pianca, T. G., Roman, T., Hutz, M. H., Faraone, S. V., Schmitz, M., & Rohde, L. A. (2008). Adrenergic α2A receptor gene and response to methylphenidate in attention-deficit/hyperactivity disorder-predominantly inattentive type. *Journal of Neural Transmission, 115*, 341–345. http://dx.doi.org/10.1007/s00702-007-0835-0

Dunn, D. W., Austin, J. K., & Harezlak, J. (2003). ADHD and epilepsy in childhood. *Developmental Medicine & Child Neurology, 45*, 50–54. http://dx.doi.org/10.1111/j.1469-8749.2003.tb00859.x

DuPaul, G. J., Barkley, R. A., & McMurray, M. B. (1994). Response of children with ADHD to methylphenidate: Interaction with internalizing symptoms. *Journal of the American Academy of Child & Adolescent Psychiatry, 33*, 894–903. http://dx.doi.org/10.1097/00004583-199407000-00016

DuPaul, G. J., & Langberg, J. M. (2015). Educational impairments in children with ADHD. In R. A. Barkley (Ed.), *Attention-deficit hyperactivity disorder: A handbook for diagnosis and treatment* (4th ed., pp. 169–190). New York, NY: Guilford.

*DuPaul, G. J., Power, T. J., Anastopoulos, A. D., & Reid, R. (2016). *ADHD Rating Scale–5 for Children and Adolescents: Checklists, norms, and clinical interpretation*. New York, NY: Guilford.

Epstein, R. A., Fonnesbeck, C., Potter, S., Rizzone, K. H., & McPheeters, M. (2015). Psychosocial interventions for child disruptive behaviors: A meta-analysis. *Pediatrics, 136*, 947–960. http://dx.doi.org/10.1542/peds.2015-2577

Fabiano, G. A., Pelham, W. E., Jr., Gnagy, E. M., & Burrows-MacLean, L. (2007). The single and combined effects of multiple intensities of behavior modification and methylphenidate for children with attention deficit hyperactivity disorder in a classroom setting. *School Psychology Review, 36*, 195–216.

*Fabiano, G. A., Pelham, W. E. P., Jr., Waschbusch, D. A., Gnagy, E. M., Lahey, B. B., Chronis, A. M., . . . Burrows-Maclean, L. (2006). A practical measure of impairment: Psychometric properties of the impairment rating scale in samples of children with attention deficit hyperactivity disorder and two school-based samples. *Journal of Clinical Child and Adolescent Psychology, 35*, 369–385. http://dx.doi.org/10.1207/s15374424jccp3503_3

Fabiano, G. A., Vujnovic, R. K., Pelham, W. E., Waschbusch, D. A., Massetti, G. M., Pariseau, M. E., . . . Volker, M. (2010). Enhancing the effectiveness of special education programming for children with attention deficit hyperactivity disorder using a daily report card. *School Psychology Review, 39*, 219–239.

Faraone, S. V., Biederman, J., Spencer, T. J., & Aleardi, M. (2006). Comparing the efficacy of medications for ADHD using meta-analysis. *Medscape General Medicine, 8*(4), 4.

Faraone, S. V., & Buitelaar, J. (2010). Comparing the efficacy of stimulants for ADHD in children and adolescents using meta-analysis. *European Child & Adolescent Psychiatry, 19*, 353–364. http://dx.doi.org/10.1007/s00787-009-0054-3

Fiks, A., Mayne, S., Localio, A., Alessandrini, E., & Guevara, J. (2012). Shared decision-making and health care expenditures among children with special health care needs. *Pediatrics, 129*, 99–107. http://dx.doi.org/10.1542/peds.2011-1352

Fletcher, J. M., Lyon, G. R., Fuchs, L. S., & Barnes, M. A. (2006). *Learning disabilities: From identification to intervention*. New York, NY: Guilford.

Fletcher, J. M., & Vaughn, S. (2009). Response to intervention: Preventing and remediating academic difficulties. *Child Development Perspectives, 3*, 30–37. http://dx.doi.org/10.1111/j.1750-8606.2008.00072.x

Fonagy, P., Target, M., Cottrell, D., Phillips, J., & Kurtz, Z. (2015). *What works for whom? A critical review of treatments for children and adolescents* (2nd ed.). New York, NY: Guilford.

Gau, S. S., Shen, H. Y., Chou, M. C., Tang, C. S., Chiu, Y. N., & Gau, C. S. (2006). Determinants of adherence to methylphenidate and the impact of poor adherence on maternal and family measures. *Journal of Child and Adolescent Psychopharmacology, 16*, 286–297. http://dx.doi.org/10.1089/cap.2006.16.286

Hanwella, R., Senanayake, M., & de Silva, V. (2011). Comparative efficacy and acceptability of methylphenidate and atomoxetine in treatment of attention deficit hyperactivity disorder in children and adolescents: A meta-analysis. *BMC Psychiatry, 11*, 176. http://dx.doi.org/10.1186/1471-244X-11-176

Heal, D. J., Cheetham, S. C., & Smith, S. L. (2009). The neuropharmacology of ADHD drugs in vivo: Insights on efficacy and safety. *Neuropharmacology, 57,* 608–618. http://dx.doi.org/10.1016/j.neuropharm.2009.08.020

Hennissen, L., Bakker, M. J., Banaschewski, T., Carucci, S., Coghill, D., Danckaerts, M., . . . Buitelaar, J. K. (2017). Cardiovascular effects of stimulant and non-stimulant medication for children and adolescents with ADHD: A systematic review and meta-analysis of trials of methylphenidate, amphetamines and atomoxetine. *CNS Drugs, 31,* 199–215. http://dx.doi.org/10.1007/s40263-017-0410-7

Hicks, J. K., Bishop, J. R., Sangkuhl, K., Müller, D. J., Ji, Y., Leckband, S. G., . . . Gaedigk, A. (2015). Clinical Pharmacogenetics Implementation Consortium (CPIC) guideline for *CYP2D6* and *CYP2C19* genotypes and dosing of selective serotonin reuptake inhibitors. *Clinical Pharmacology and Therapeutics, 98,* 127–134. http://dx.doi.org/10.1002/cpt.147

Kamphaus, R. W., Reynolds, C. R., & Dever, B. V. (2014). Behavioral and mental health screening. In R. J. Kettler, T. A. Glover, C. A. Albers, & K. A. Feeney-Kettler (Eds.), *Universal screening in educational settings: Evidence-based decision making for schools* (pp. 249–273). Washington, DC: American Psychological Association. http://dx.doi.org/10.1037/14316-010

Kratochwill, T. R. (2008). Best practices in school-based consultation: Applications in prevention and interventions systems. In A. Thomas & J. Grimes (Eds.), *Best practices in school psychology* (Vol. 5, pp. 1673–1688). Washington, DC: National Association of School Psychologists.

Liu, Q., Zhang, H., Fang, Q., & Qin, L. (2017). Comparative efficacy and safety of methylphenidate and atomoxetine for attention-deficit hyperactivity disorder in children and adolescents: Meta-analysis based on head-to-head trials. *Journal of Clinical and Experimental Neuropsychology, 39,* 854–865. http://dx.doi.org/10.1080/13803395.2016.1273320

Majewicz-Hefley, A., & Carlson, J. S. (2007). A meta-analysis of combined treatments for children diagnosed with ADHD. *Journal of Attention Disorders, 10,* 239–250. http://dx.doi.org/10.1177/1087054706289934

March, J. S., Swanson, J. M., Arnold, L. E., Hoza, B., Conners, C. K., Hinshaw, S. P., . . . Pelham, W. E. (2000). Anxiety as a predictor and outcome variable in the Multimodal Treatment Study of Children With ADHD (MTA). *Journal of Abnormal Child Psychology, 28,* 527–541. http://dx.doi.org/10.1023/A:1005179014321

Massetti, G. M., Lahey, B. B., Pelham, W. E., Loney, J., Ehrhardt, A., Lee, S. S., & Kipp, H. (2008). Academic achievement over 8 years among children who met modified criteria for attention-deficit/hyperactivity disorder at 4–6 years of age. *Journal of Abnormal Child Psychology, 36,* 399–410. http://dx.doi.org/10.1007/s10802-007-9186-4

McCart, M. R., Priester, P. E., Davies, W. H., & Azen, R. (2006). Differential effectiveness of behavioral parent-training and cognitive-behavioral therapy for antisocial youth: A meta-analysis. *Journal of Abnormal Child Psychology, 34,* 525–541. http://dx.doi.org/10.1007/s10802-006-9031-1

McVoy, M., & Findling, R. (Eds.). (2017). *Clinical manual of child and adolescent psychopharmacology* (3rd ed.). Arlington, VA: American Psychiatric Publishing. http://dx.doi.org/10.1176/appi.books.9781615371266

Merkel, R. L. (2010). Safety of stimulant treatment in attention deficit hyperactivity disorder: Part II. *Expert Opinion on Drug Safety, 9,* 917–935. http://dx.doi.org/10.1517/14740338.2010.503238

MTA Cooperative Group. (1999). A 14-month randomized clinical trial of treatment strategies for attention-deficit/hyperactivity disorder. *Archives of General Psychiatry, 56,* 1073–1086. http://dx.doi.org/10.1001/archpsyc.56.12.1073

MTA Cooperative Group. (2004). National Institute of Mental Health Multimodal Treatment Study of ADHD follow-up: Changes in effectiveness and growth after the end of treatment. *Pediatrics, 113,* 762–769. http://dx.doi.org/10.1542/peds.113.4.762

Nass, R. D. (2005). Evaluation and assessment issues in the diagnosis of attention deficit hyperactivity disorder. *Seminars in Pediatric Neurology, 12,* 200–216. http://dx.doi.org/10.1016/j.spen.2005.12.002

Page, T. F., Pelham, W. E., III, Fabiano, G. A., Greiner, A. R., Gnagy, E. M., Hart, K. C., . . . Pelham, W. E., Jr. (2016). Comparative cost analysis of sequential, adaptive, behavioral, pharmacological, and combined treatments for childhood ADHD. *Journal of Clinical Child and Adolescent Psychology, 45,* 416–427. http://dx.doi.org/10.1080/15374416.2015.1055859

Perfect, M., & Smith, B. H. (2016). Hypnotic relaxation and yoga to improve sleep and school functioning. *International Journal of School and Educational Psychology, 41,* 43–51. http://dx.doi.org/10.1080/21683603.2016.113055

Pelham, W. E., Jr., Fabiano, G. A., Waxmonsky, J. G., Greiner, A. R., Gnagy, E. M., Pelham, W. E., III, . . . Murphy, S. A. (2016). Treatment sequencing for childhood ADHD: A multiple-randomization study of adaptive medication and behavioral interventions. *Journal of Clinical Child and Adolescent Psychology, 45,* 396–415. http://dx.doi.org/10.1080/15374416.2015.1105138

Phillips, K. A., Veenstra, D. L., Oren, E., Lee, J. K., & Sadee, W. (2001). Potential role of pharmacogenomics in reducing adverse drug reactions: A systematic review. *Journal of the American Medical Association, 286,* 2270–2279. http://dx.doi.org/10.1001/jama.286.18.2270

Pliszka, S., & the AACAP Work Group on Quality Issues. (2007). Practice parameter for the assessment and treatment of children and adolescents with attention-deficit/hyperactivity disorder. *Journal of the American Academy of Child & Adolescent Psychiatry, 46,* 894–921. http://dx.doi.org/10.1097/chi.0b013e318054e724

Pliszka, S. R. (2015). Comorbid psychiatric disorders in children with ADHD. In R. A. Barkley (Ed.), *Attention-deficit hyperactivity disorder: A handbook for diagnosis and treatment* (4th ed. pp. 140–168). New York, NY: Guilford.

Prasad, V., Brogan, E., Mulvaney, C., Grainge, M., Stanton, W., & Sayal, K. (2013). How effective are drug treatments for children with ADHD at improving on-task behaviour and academic achievement in the school classroom? A systematic review and meta-analysis. *European Child & Adolescent Psychiatry, 22,* 203–216. http://dx.doi.org/10.1007/s00787-012-0346-x

Punja, S., Xu, D., Schmid, C. H., Hartling, L., Urichuk, L., Nikles, C. J., & Vohra, S. (2016). N-of-1 trials can be aggregated to generate group mean treatment effects: A systematic review and meta-analysis. *Journal of Clinical Epidemiology, 76,* 65–75. http://dx.doi.org/10.1016/j.jclinepi.2016.03.026

Rapport, M. D., Chung, K.-M., Shore, G., Denney, C. B., & Isaacs, P. (2000). Upgrading the science and technology of assessment and diagnosis: Laboratory and clinic-based assessment of children with ADHD. *Journal of Clinical Child Psychology, 29,* 555–568. http://dx.doi.org/10.1207/S15374424JCCP2904_8

Research Units on Pediatric Psychopharmacology Autism Network. (2005). Randomized, controlled, crossover trial of methylphenidate in pervasive developmental disorders with hyperactivity. *Archives of General Psychiatry, 62,* 1266–1274. http://dx.doi.org/10.1001/archpsyc.62.11.1266

*Reynolds, C. R., & Kamphaus, R. W. (2015). *BASC-3 Behavioral and Emotional Screening System.* Bloomington, MN: Pearson.

Roberts, W., Milich, R., & Barkley, R. A. (2015). Primary symptoms, diagnostic criteria, and prevalence of ADHD. In R. A. Barkley (Ed.), *Attention-deficit hyperactivity disorder: A handbook for diagnosis and treatment* (4th ed., pp. 51–80). New York, NY: Guilford.

Sallee, F. R. (2010). The role of alpha2-adrenergic agonists in attention-deficit/hyperactivity disorder. *Postgraduate Medicine, 122,* 78–87. http://dx.doi.org/10.3810/pgm.2010.09.2204

*Shapiro, E. S. (2013). *Behavioral Observation of Students in Schools* [Computer software]. Bloomington, MN: Pearson.

Sheridan, S. M., & Kratochwill, T. R. (2007). *Conjoint behavioral consultation: Promoting family-school connections and interventions.* Berlin, Germany: Springer Science & Business Media.

Sibley, M. H., Rohde, L. A., Swanson, J. M., Hechtman, L. T., Molina, B. S. G., Mitchell, J. T., . . . Stehli, A. (2018). Late-onset ADHD reconsidered with comprehensive repeated assessments between ages 10 and 25. *The American Journal of Psychiatry, 175,* 140–149. http://dx.doi.org/10.1176/appi.ajp.2017.17030298

Smith, B., Barkley, R., & Shapiro, C. (2007). Attention-deficit/hyperactivity disorder. In E. Mash & R. Barkley (Eds.), *Assessment of childhood disorders* (pp. 53–123). New York, NY: Guilford.

Smith, B. H., & Shapiro, C. J. (2004). Combined treatments for ADHD. In R. A. Barkley (Ed.), *Attention-deficit/hyperactivity disorder: A handbook for diagnosis and treatment* (4th ed., pp. 686–704). New York, NY: Guilford.

Solanto, M. V. (1998). Neuropsychopharmacological mechanisms of stimulant drug action in attention-deficit hyperactivity disorder: A review and integration. *Behavioural Brain Research, 94,* 127–152. http://dx.doi.org/10.1016/S0166-4328(97)00175-7

Sonuga-Barke, E. J., Coghill, D., Markowitz, J. S., Swanson, J. M., Vandenberghe, M., & Hatch, S. J. (2007). Sex differences in the response of children with ADHD to once-daily formulations of methylphenidate. *Journal of the American Academy of Child & Adolescent Psychiatry, 46,* 701–710. http://dx.doi.org/10.1097/chi.0b013e31804659f1

Spencer, T. J., Biederman, J., Harding, M., O'Donnell, D., Faraone, S. V., & Wilens, T. E. (1996). Growth deficits in ADHD children revisited: Evidence for disorder-associated growth delays. *Journal of the American Academy of Child and Adolescent Psychiatry, 35,* 1460–1469. http://dx.doi.org/10.1097/00004583-199611000-00014

Sugai, G., & Horner, R. H. (2009). Responsiveness-to-intervention and school-wide positive behavior supports: Integration of multi-tiered system approaches. *Exceptionality, 17,* 223–237. http://dx.doi.org/10.1080/09362830903235375

Swanson, J. M., Cantwell, D., Lerner, M., McBurnett, K., & Hanna, G. (1991). Effects of stimulant medication on learning in children with ADHD. *Journal of Learning Disabilities, 24,* 219–230, 255. http://dx.doi.org/10.1177/002221949102400406

Thomas, R., Sanders, S., Doust, J., Beller, E., & Glasziou, P. (2015). Prevalence of attention-deficit/hyperactivity disorder: A systematic review and meta-analysis. *Pediatrics, 135,* e994–e1001. http://dx.doi.org/10.1542/peds.2014-3482

Torres, A. R., Whitney, J., & Gonzalez-Heydrich, J. (2008). Attention-deficit/hyperactivity disorder in pediatric patients with epilepsy: Review of pharmacological treatment. *Epilepsy & Behavior, 12,* 217–233. http://dx.doi.org/10.1016/j.yebeh.2007.08.001

Van der Oord, S., Prins, P. J., Oosterlaan, J., & Emmelkamp, P. M. (2008). Efficacy of methylphenidate, psychosocial treatments and their combination in school-aged children with ADHD: A meta-analysis. *Clinical Psychology Review, 28*, 783–800. http://dx.doi.org/10.1016/j.cpr.2007.10.007

Volkow, N. D., Fowler, J. S., Wang, G., Ding, Y., & Gatley, S. J. (2002). Mechanism of action of methylphenidate: Insight from PET imaging studies. *Journal of Attention Disorders, 6*(Suppl. 1), s31–s43.

Volpe, R. J., DiPerna, J. C., Hintze, J. M., & Shapiro, E. S. (2005). Observing students in classroom settings: A review of seven coding schemes. *School Psychology Review, 34*(4), 454–474.

Wigal, S. B., Kollins, S. H., Childress, A. C., & Adeyi, B. (2010). Efficacy and tolerability of lisdexamfetamine dimesylate in children with attention-deficit/ hyperactivity disorder: Sex and age effects and effect size across the day. *Child and Adolescent Psychiatry and Mental Health, 4*, 32. http://dx.doi.org/10.1186/ 1753-2000-4-32

Wilens, T. E., Faraone, S. V., Biederman, J., & Gunawardene, S. (2003). Does stimulant therapy of attention-deficit/hyperactivity disorder beget later substance abuse? A meta-analytic review of the literature. *Pediatrics, 111*, 179–185. http://dx.doi.org/10.1542/peds.111.1.179

Williamson, D., & Johnston, C. (2015). Gender differences in adults with attention-deficit/hyperactivity disorder: A narrative review. *Clinical Psychology Review, 40*, 15–27. http://dx.doi.org/10.1016/ j.cpr.2015.05.005

*Wolraich, M. L., Lambert, W., Doffing, M. A., Bickman, L., Simmons, T., & Worley, K. (2003). Psychometric properties of the Vanderbilt ADHD Diagnostic Parent Rating Scale in a referred population. *Journal of Pediatric Psychology, 28*, 559–568. http://dx.doi.org/ 10.1093/jpepsy/jsg046

World Health Organization. (2015). *International statistical classification of diseases and related health problems* (10th rev.). Geneva, Switzerland: Author.

CHAPTER 17

PHARMACOLOGICAL TREATMENT OF AUTISM SPECTRUM DISORDER

Johnny L. Matson and Claire O. Burns

Autism spectrum disorder (ASD) is a neuro-developmental disorder whose core symptoms include difficulties with social communication and interactions and restricted, repetitive behaviors, interests, and activities (American Psychiatric Association, 2013; Tidmarsh & Volkmar, 2003). ASD is a disorder that has been the subject of much controversy over recent years, from its etiological basis to diagnostic practices to effective treatments. Current best-practice approaches to treatment involve behavioral interventions, specifically applied behavior analysis (ABA), which has been shown to be effective in increasing socialization, adaptive skills, and communication (Virués-Ortega, 2010). There are currently no approved medications that are considered evidence based in addressing core autism symptomology, such as deficits in social communication (Baribeau & Anagnostou, 2014; Mohiuddin & Ghaziuddin, 2013; Poling, Ehrhardt, & Li, 2017; Siegel, 2012). Rather, pharmacological interventions in this population target common comorbid psychopathologies and/or behavioral difficulties, such as hyperactivity, depression, aggression, and irritability (Baribeau & Anagnostou, 2014; Mohiuddin & Ghaziuddin, 2013). This distinction between core symptoms associated with the ASD diagnosis and comorbid concerns of practitioners prescribing medications is related to effective treatment, and consideration of medication management concerns, such as potential side effects and assessing effectiveness, is essential to apply best-practice approaches to treatment. Given the extreme heterogeneity in symptom expression across individuals and the limited evidence for certain types of medication in its management, ASD is a condition that warrants extremely careful consideration when approaching potential psycho-pharmacological treatments.

EPIDEMIOLOGY AND PREVALENCE

Once considered a relatively rare disorder, the prevalence of ASD has increased dramatically in recent years (Howlin, 2006). The most recent survey conducted by the Autism and Developmental Disabilities Monitoring (ADDM) Network of the Centers for Disease Control and Prevention (CDC) estimated that ASD occurs in 1 in 59 children (Baio et al., 2018). Explanations for this recent rise in prevalence rates include changes in diagnostic criteria, greater public awareness, better assessment practices, and more robust research methodologies (Fombonne, 2009; Matson & Kozlowski, 2011; Volkmar, Lord, Bailey, Schultz, & Klin, 2004).

The ADDM study also found differences in prevalence across demographic variables. Robust sex differences were evident, with ASD reportedly occurring 4 to 5 times more often in males than females. There were also discrepancies in prevalence across race and ethnicity, as non-Hispanic White

http://dx.doi.org/10.1037/0000133-017
APA Handbook of Psychopharmacology, S. M. Evans (Editor-in-Chief)

children were significantly more likely to have an ASD diagnosis than non-Hispanic Black children and Hispanic children (Baio et al., 2018). However, many researchers have posited that differences in rates of diagnosis across race and ethnicities are likely due to factors related to socioeconomic status (Daniels & Mandell, 2013; Thomas et al., 2012), such as access to quality health care (Magaña, Parish, Rose, Timberlake, & Swaine, 2012). This is further supported by findings by Mandell and colleagues (2009) that White children on average receive a diagnosis at a younger age than Black or Hispanic children.

A great deal of controversy has existed regarding the cause of autism. Incorrect theories, which have spanned from demonic possession to "refrigerator mothers" to vaccinations (Miles, 2011; Richdale & Schreck, 2011), can have extremely detrimental effects, as they can lead to ineffective or even harmful treatments. The potential role of vaccines has been refuted time and again by a multitude of studies (Hviid, Stellfeld, Wohlfahrt, & Melbye, 2003; Jain et al., 2015; Kaye, del Mar Melero-Montes, & Jick, 2001; Taylor et al., 1999), and the original study on its veracity has been retracted by *The Lancet*. Yet the connection continues to have far-reaching societal impacts and public health implications, as many parents still express concern (Bazzano, Zeldin, Schuster, Barrett, & Lehrer, 2012). Additionally, the refrigerator mother theory, which holds that children with autism develop social difficulties due to cold and unloving dispositions and attitudes of their mothers, resulted in recommendations of "parentectomy," or removal of a child from his or her parents' care and placement in a residential institution (Bettelheim, 1967). Current research is now trending toward understanding potential genetic etiologies, as recent studies indicate that for approximately 25% of individuals with ASD, there is an identifiable genetic factor (Miles, 2011). Studies have established that there is a genetic component to the disorder, though the mechanism and specific genes implicated are still under investigation (Zafeiriou, Ververi, & Vargiami, 2007). Despite a long history of controversy regarding etiology, ASD is considered a behavioral disorder, and the only treatment that currently meets

evidence-based criteria is ABA (Richdale & Schreck, 2011).

DIAGNOSING AUTISM SPECTRUM DISORDER

Autism is a relatively recent diagnostic category in the mental health and medical field, and treatments have changed correspondingly as the perception of ASD has shifted. The etiology of ASD has long been a topic that has received a great deal of attention from researchers, policymakers, and families alike. The disorder was originally thought to be indicative of early-onset schizophrenia or childhood psychosis. Psychiatrist Eugen Bleuler first coined the term "autism" for patients who seemed to withdraw into themselves and away from others. Several years later, psychiatrist Leo Kanner described "infantile autism" in young children who isolated themselves and demonstrated rigidity and the need for sameness. Pediatrician Hans Asperger began similar work to Kanner's in Austria, though his research did not reach the United States for many years (Achkova & Manolova, 2014). The *Diagnostic and Statistical Manual of Mental Disorders* (*DSM*), published by the American Psychiatric Association, first recognized infantile autism in the third edition; prior to this publication, these symptoms had fallen under psychosis or schizophrenic reactions (Achkova & Manolova, 2014). The criteria have since been revised in each new edition to reflect advances in research on the disorder. The current *DSM–5* criteria fall into two domains: social communication deficits and restricted, repetitive behaviors (RRBs) and interests (American Psychiatric Association, 2013), which are described in more detail in this chapter.

As awareness of the heterogeneity of ASD has increased, the approach to diagnosis has been adapted to reflect the complexity of the disorder. Huerta and Lord (2012) recommend a multidisciplinary method, which they specify should involve assessment of multiple areas of functioning. Current best-practice approaches to diagnosis involves a multimethod approach that includes interview of multiple informants (e.g., parents, caregivers, teachers), review of developmental history, observation, and standardized assessment measures. This approach involves integration of the information acquired throughout the assessment by trained professionals with experience in the field to aid in their clinical judgement.

The *DSM–5* (American Psychiatric Association, 2013) outlines the current criteria for ASD. The International Classification of Diseases and Related Health Problems, Tenth Revision (ICD–10; World Health Organization, 1992), also summarizes the criteria for disorders that fall under "pervasive developmental disorders"; however, the *DSM–5* criteria are most commonly used by practitioners in the United States.

The current diagnostic criteria for ASD include impairments in the following three areas of social communication and interaction: social-emotional reciprocity; nonverbal communication as it related to social functioning; and developing, maintaining, and understanding interpersonal relationships. These difficulties must be persistent and pervasive and occur across more than one context or situation. Individuals must also exhibit at least two of four RRBs, interests, or activities: stereotyped or repetitive speech, use of objects, or motor movements; ritualized patterns of behavior, inflexibility in regard to routines, and insistence on sameness; extremely restricted interests or fascinations that are unusual in either their intensity or their subject; and unusual sensory interests or responses (i.e., either hyper-reactivity or hyporeactivity) to environmental stimuli. These symptom requirements may be fulfilled either currently or by history, but must have been present early in the child's development and must cause significant impairment or difficulty in the individual's current level of functioning (American Psychiatric Association, 2013).

Although the *DSM–5* includes additional examples of behaviors that would fulfill each criterion, these symptoms can manifest and present in a variety of different ways. Professionals without adequate understanding of the disorder may be likely to either miss ASD symptoms or misinterpret behaviors as characteristic of ASD. For example, certain behaviors, such as a lack of response to name, may be difficult to differentiate as ASD symptoms or as symptoms of medical concerns such as hearing difficulties (Szarkowski, Mood, Shield, Wiley, & Yoshinaga-

Itano, 2014) or seizures (Reilly & Gillberg, 2016). Failure to receive a correct diagnosis is a serious concern across medical and psychological fields, and is particularly deleterious to individuals with ASD as it interferes with access to effective treatment options. Therefore, it is crucial that practitioners be appropriately and extensively trained in the diagnosis of this neurodevelopmental disorder, and that other medical professionals who suspect the presence of ASD refer cases to qualified practitioners in the field.

Although researchers indicate that some children with ASD can be reliably diagnosed by 2 years of age (Chawarska, Klin, Paul, & Volkmar, 2007), there is often a substantial delay in age at diagnosis (Daniels & Mandell, 2013; Mandell, Novak, & Zubritsky, 2005; Shattuck et al., 2009). Increased awareness and sensitive diagnostic assessments have increased the number of children receiving a diagnosis at a young age. Some children with milder symptomology may not exhibit severe difficulties until later in childhood when social demands begin to exceed their abilities (American Psychiatric Association, 2013). However, the importance of early identification and diagnosis of ASD cannot be overemphasized, as researchers have consistently found that the earlier children begin receiving behavioral treatment, the better the potential outcomes (MacDonald, Parry-Cruwys, Dupere, & Ahearn, 2014; Virues-Ortega, Rodríguez, & Yu, 2013).

Many assessment measures have been developed to aid in the diagnosis of ASD. Some include screening measures for young children to facilitate referral for comprehensive evaluation, others are intended to assess a variety of symptoms central to the disorder to determine whether the individual's symptoms meet clinical diagnostic criteria, while still others assess certain domains of symptoms (e.g., RRBs, sensory symptoms, receptive and/or expressive communication). Although it is beyond the scope of this chapter to provide a comprehensive and detailed review of all measures used to assess ASD or related comorbidities, some of the most commonly used assessment measures are mentioned here, and the purpose of different types of instruments is discussed. For a comprehensive list of measures and the publishers, please refer to the Children's

Hospital of Philadelphia Center for Autism Research "Autism Spectrum Disorder Measures" table noted in the tool kit at the end of this chapter.

The high degree of heterogeneity of autism symptoms in the population has been emphasized, and developmental considerations are important in diagnostic practices, as autism symptom presentation can often change with age (Shattuck et al., 2007). Although ASD is a neurodevelopmental disorder and is therefore present early in an individual's development, the *DSM–5* specifies that symptoms may either not become impairing until the social demands of the individual's environment surpass the individual's skills or may become less impairing as the individual learns new skills as they develop (American Psychiatric Association, 2013). Therefore, age and developmental level may influence symptom presentation, and should be taken into account during the diagnostic evaluation.

Screening Tools

There has been a significant increase in research on screening practices in recent years in an attempt to adequately address the need for early identification of ASD in very young children (Barton, Dumont-Mathieu, & Fein, 2012; Robins et al., 2016; Robins & Dumont-Mathieu, 2006; Zwaigenbaum et al., 2015). Screening tools are often utilized for young children by health care providers. If children score in the at-risk range on a screening measure or parents or providers express concerns regarding a child's development, they are often referred for a diagnostic evaluation. The tool kit at the end of this chapter lists a resource from the CDC for "Screening and Diagnosis for Healthcare Providers," which includes screening recommendations as well as a pediatric developmental screening flowchart, which details the process of screening and referral in pediatric and primary care practice.

Screening measures are often based on parent report, which has certain advantages, such as faster and easier administration. However, although parents are able to give information about their child's behavior in multiple settings, a limitation of parent report measures is that some parents may have less knowledge regarding development and therefore be less able to recognize signs of atypical development

(Barton, Dumont-Mathieu, & Fein, 2012). There are many commonly used screening measures; as noted, the tool kit includes a CDC "Screening and Diagnosis for Healthcare Providers" guide. One of the most widely used screeners is the Modified Checklist for Autism in Toddlers, Revised With Follow-Up (M-CHAT-R/F; Robins, Fein, & Barton, 2009); some advantages of this measure are that is quick (5–10 minute administration time) and that positive screens require a follow-up interview, which can be conducted by a staff member other than a medical professional. Other measures include an observation component by a trained professional, which has advantages in terms of recognition of atypical behaviors; however, this is not always feasible, as it sometimes involves the professional observing the child in his or her own home (Barton et al., 2012).

Although there has been some controversy regarding whether universal autism screening is warranted (Al-Qabandi, Gorter, & Rosenbaum, 2011; Siu et al., 2016), most researchers advocate for the widespread use of screening tools in pediatric offices (Robins et al., 2016; Zwaigenbaum et al., 2015), as formal screening combined with surveillance by medical professionals has been shown to be more effective than surveillance alone (Barton et al., 2012). Specifically, the U.S. Preventative Services Task Force found insufficient evidence to support universal screening of all young children 18 to 30 months whose parents or providers have no concerns regarding their development; however, the CDC specified that this is meant to serve as a call for additional future research (CDC, 2016).

Diagnostic Interviews

Comprehensive interviews are also an integral piece of the diagnostic process. One of the most commonly used semistructured interviews is the Autism Diagnostic Interview-Revised (ADI-R; Rutter, Le Couteur, & Lord, 2003), which serves as a complement to the Autism Diagnostic Observation Schedule, Second Edition (ADOS-2; Lord et al., 2012), an observational measure that is discussed later in this chapter. Due to the long administration time of the ADI-R (often 90 minutes or longer), many clinicians utilize their own abbreviated forms of caregiver interviews. The Diagnostic Interview for Social and Communication Disorders (DISCO) is also often utilized in clinical practice for diagnosis as well as to guide recommendations (Wing, Leekam, Libby, Gould, & Larcombe, 2002).

Observation Measures

The use of observational measures in the diagnostic process is particularly useful because it allows the clinician to gain an objective measure of the individual's behavior without potential subjective bias of caregiver perception of behavior. The ADOS-2 is one of the most commonly used observational tools. It includes four standard modules and one toddler module to account for differences in symptom presentation across age and developmental level. The revised algorithm is based on two domains that are consistent with the *DSM–5* diagnostic criteria: social affect and RRBs (Gotham, Risi, Pickles, & Lord, 2007).

Another commonly utilized observation scale is the Childhood Autism Rating Scale, Second Edition (CARS-2; Schopler, Van Bourgondien, Wellman, & Love, 2010). The CARS-2 is based on a combination of parent report and observation of the child's behavior by the clinician. Versions include the standard version as well as a high-functioning version in order to take into account developmental and functioning level, which may impact symptom presentation.

Rating Scales

Parent, teacher, and self-report rating scales are commonly used as supplemental measures of ASD symptomology. A benefit of many of these scales is that they cover a variety of autism symptoms. They also sometimes have multiple versions, so that symptom endorsement can be compared across caregivers, teachers, and in certain cases, self-report. This allows for acquisition of information from multiple informants, which is an important component of diagnostic assessment (Möricke, Buitelaar, & Rommelse, 2016).

There are a large number of rating scales for autism and related symptoms. Some of the most commonly implemented scales include the Social Responsiveness Scale, Second edition (SRS-2; Constantino & Gruber, 2012), the Social Communication Questionnaire

(SCQ; Rutter, Bailey, & Lord, 2003), the Checklist for Autism Spectrum Disorder (CASD; Mayes, 2012), the Gilliam Autism Rating Scale, Third Edition (GARS-3; Gilliam, 2014), the Autism Spectrum Quotient (AQ; Baron-Cohen, Wheelwright, Skinner, Martin, & Clubley, 2001), the Pervasive Developmental Disorder Behavior Inventory (PDDBI; Cohen & Sudhalter, 2005), the Baby and Infant Screen for Children with aUtIsm Traits (BISCUIT; Matson, Boisjoli, & Wilkins, 2007), Autism Spectrum Disorders-Diagnostic for Children (ASD-DC; Matson, González, & Wilkins, 2009; Matson, Gonzalez, Wilkins, & Rivet, 2008), Autism Spectrum Disorders-Diagnosis for Adults with intellectual disability (ASD-DA; Matson, Boisjoli, González, Smith, & Wilkins, 2007), and the Autism Spectrum Rating Scales (ASRS; Goldstein & Naglieri, 2009). Other measures target specific symptom domains, such as sensory symptoms (e.g., the Sensory Profile 2; Dunn, 2014). As noted, the tool kit at the end of this chapter includes a resource from the Children's Hospital of Philadelphia Center for Autism Research on autism spectrum disorder measures, which provides additional information on a variety of measures.

EVIDENCE-BASED PHARMACOLOGICAL TREATMENTS OF AUTISM SPECTRUM DISORDER

There are no U.S. Food and Drug Administration (FDA) approved pharmacological approaches that have been shown to significantly improve the core autism symptoms, such as increasing social-emotional reciprocity and facilitating the development and maintenance of interpersonal relationships, and decreasing unusual reactions to sensory input or overly restricted and intense interests (Baribeau & Anagnostou, 2014; Mohiuddin & Ghaziuddin, 2013; Poling et al., 2017; Siegel, 2012). Therefore, it is important to note that all pharmacological treatments currently target related emotional and behavioral symptoms associated with challenging behavior and comorbid psychopathologies, such as irritability, aggression, anxiety, and hyperactivity, rather than underlying ASD symptoms (Baribeau & Anagnostou, 2014; Mohiuddin & Ghaziuddin, 2013). Common comorbid disorders include anxiety disorders, obsessive-compulsive disorder, attention-deficit/hyperactivity disorder (ADHD), and oppositional defiant disorder (Leyfer et al., 2006; Simonoff et al., 2008).

Ethical and effective treatments in medical and psychological fields must be based on evidence-based practice. Currently, only two psychotropic medications (i.e., risperidone and aripiprazole), both atypical antipsychotics, are approved for treatment of irritability and aggression in individuals with ASD (Baribeau & Anagnostou, 2014; Joshi,

2017; Poling et al., 2017). Therefore, the majority of psychotropic medications prescribed to individuals with ASD are considered off-label (Earle, 2016; McCracken & Gandal, 2016). Information regarding the target behaviors of medications often prescribed for individuals with ASD and the evidence for their effectiveness are presented in Table 17.1. Although studies have yielded different estimates of medication use, reviews of the literature indicate that the majority (i.e., 50%–80%) of individuals with ASD are prescribed psychotropic medications at some

TABLE 17.1

Commonly Used Psychotropic Medications in Individuals With Autism Spectrum Disorder

Class of medication	Common medications in this class (trade names)	Target symptoms	At least one RCT demonstrating effectiveness for target symptoms	FDA approved for individuals with ASD	Broad considerations
Atypical antipsychotic	Risperidone (Risperdal®), Aripiprazole (Abilify®), Olanzapine (Zyprexa®), Clozapine (Clozaril®), Quetiapine (Seroquel®)	Irritability, repetitive behaviors	Risperidone, aripiprazole, olanzapine	Risperidone, aripiprazole	Evidence of effectiveness in treating irritability
Psycho-stimulant	Methylphenidate (Aptensio®, Concerta®, Metadate®, Methylin®, Ritalin®), amphetamine/dextroamphetamine (Adderall®)	Hyperactivity, comorbid ADHD	Methylphenidate	None	Effective for treatment of comorbid ADHD
Alpha-2 agonist	Guanfacine (Intuiv®), Clonidine (Catapres®)	Hyperactivity, comorbid ADHD	Guanfacine, clonidine	None	Effective for treating ADHD in children with ASD; considered second line compared with methylphenidate
Selective serotonin reuptake inhibitor	Fluoxetine (Prozac®), fluvoxamine (Luvox®), sertraline (Zoloft®), citalopram (Celexa®, Cipramil®)	Stereotyped behaviors, depression, anxiety	Fluoxetine, fluvoxamine	None	Some evidence of improvement in repetitive behaviors and mood concerns, but only RCTs demonstrating effectiveness were for adults
Anticonvulsant	Topiramate (Topamax®), divalproex sodium (Depakote®), lamotrigine (Lamictal®), levetiracetam (Keppra®)	Irritability	Divalproex	None	Effective in managing seizures in individuals with ASD, and some evidence that divalproex may improve irritability symptoms

Note. ADHD = attention-deficit/hyperactivity disorder; ASD = autism spectrum disorder; FDA = U.S. Food and Drug Administration; RCT = randomized controlled trial.

point in their lives (Buck et al., 2014; Mandell et al., 2008; Mohiuddin & Ghaziuddin, 2013; Schubart, Camacho, & Leslie, 2014; Taylor, 2016); these rates may be higher in inpatient samples (Wink et al., 2017a). Recent research indicates that rate of psychotropic drug use in this population is increasing, particularly in young children (Schubart et al., 2014).

Mandell and colleagues (2008) found that in an extremely large sample (i.e., 60,641) of children under 21 with ASD who were enrolled in Medicaid, 56% were prescribed at least one psychotropic medication, and 20% were prescribed three or more of these medications. However, other researchers have indicated that psychotropic prescription rates may be higher for young children on Medicaid than those with private insurance (Jackel et al., 2017). Mandell and colleagues (2008) found that the most common drug class was neuroleptics (31%); the second most common was antidepressants (25%), followed by stimulants (22%). Those with at least one additional psychiatric diagnosis were also more likely to have used psychotropic medications.

In a recent systematic review by Jobski and colleagues (2017), the authors also investigated rates of different types of medications. Their findings were somewhat different than Mandell and colleagues (2008). They found that individuals with ASD were most often prescribed antipsychotics, followed by stimulants, and then antidepressants. They noted that the high prevalence of psychotropic medication prescription was likely accounted for by comorbidities and treatment of behaviors other than core ASD symptoms. An earlier study by Rosenberg and colleagues (2010) supported these results, noting that stimulants, neuroleptics, and antidepressants were the most commonly prescribed medications in this population.

Several factors have been found to be related to rates of medication use. Unsurprisingly, presence of externalizing behavior difficulties has been found to be a significant predictor of medication use in individuals with ASD (Coury et al., 2012; Morgan, Roy, & Chance, 2003). Demographic variables such as age and ethnicity have been found to be related to rates of medication use, as older age and White/non-Hispanic ethnicity are associated with increased medication use (Coury et al., 2012;

Mandell et al., 2008). However, researchers have not found a relationship between sex and psychotropic medication (Coury et al., 2012; Houghton et al., 2017; Lake et al., 2017; Wink et al., 2017a).

Medications rates have been found to be higher in inpatient than outpatient samples. Wink and colleagues (2017a) reported that 91.7% of youth with ASD in inpatient psychiatric facilities were prescribed at least one psychotropic medication, and more than 50% were prescribed two or more psychotropic drugs. They noted that the stability of medication use over time indicates that psychotropic medication use is a central aspect of behavior management in inpatient psychiatric care. Children in foster care were also more likely to be prescribed psychotropic medications (Houghton et al., 2017; Mandell et al., 2008). This may be due to the desire to decrease challenging behaviors to facilitate placement stability. Mandell and colleagues (2008) also suggest that children in foster care may be less likely to be enrolled in behavioral interventions, and therefore psychotropic drugs may be the primary method of behavior management.

An important consideration is that many of the large-scale, population-based studies on the prevalence of psychotropic medication use involve samples from the United States. Researchers have indicated that these findings may not be generalizable to the wider population of individuals with ASD. Specifically, Hsia and colleagues (2014) found that psychotropic drug prescription rates for individuals with ASD were highest in North America, followed by Europe and then South America. Wong et al. (2014) also found discrepancies in prescription rates across countries, and suggested that this is likely due at least in part to economic variables.

Antipsychotics

Antipsychotic drugs are one of the most commonly prescribed medications for individuals with ASD (Wink et al., 2017a), and have been shown to decrease challenging behaviors in some children with ASD (Jobski et al., 2017; McQuire, Hassiotis, Harrison, & Pilling, 2015). The historical significance of the use of this drug class is rooted in the belief that autism was an early manifestation of psychosis or schizophrenia; thus, antipsychotics were one of the first classes of psychotropic medication to be investigated in this population (Mohiuddin & Ghaziuddin, 2013). These drugs include risperidone, aripiprazole, and olanzapine, as well as some less commonly used medications such as clomipramine, haloperidol, and quetiapine. As previously stated, risperidone and aripiprazole remain the only two drugs approved by the FDA for treatment of irritability in individuals with ASD (Accordino et al., 2016; Jobski et al., 2017; McQuire et al., 2015). Side effects commonly reported in this population include weight gain, sedation, and elevated levels of prolactin (Jobski et al., 2017; McQuire et al., 2015). Although atypical antipsychotics have the best support for decreasing challenging behaviors in this population, researchers caution that additional research on long-term effectiveness is still needed, particularly since there is evidence that adverse side effects may not occur until several weeks or months into treatment (McQuire et al., 2015).

Risperidone is an atypical antipsychotic designed to treatment schizophrenia, and this second-generation antipsychotic was developed to decrease side effects (Taylor, 2016). It impacts serotonin and dopamine systems, which have been hypothesized to be related to ASD symptoms (Diler, Firat, & Avci, 2002; McDougle et al., 2005). Nonetheless, other researchers have refuted the role of dopamine in ASD (Mohammadi & Akhondzadeh, 2007). Randomized controlled trials (RCTs) of risperidone in individuals with ASD indicate that it is significantly related to decreased scores on the irritability subscales of the Aberrant Behavior Checklist (ABC) and Clinical Global Impression Scale (CGI; Elbe & Lalani, 2012; Mohiuddin & Ghaziuddin, 2013; Pandina, Bossie, Youssef, Zhu, & Dunbar, 2007), as well as improvements on the CARS and Children's Global Assessment Scale (CGAS; Nagaraj, Singhi, & Malhi, 2006). A review by McQuire and colleagues (2015) also indicated that a small number of studies have shown that risperidone may improve adaptive functioning in children with ASD; however, the authors indicate that due to the small number of studies and statistical heterogeneity, these results should be interpreted with caution.

Aripiprazole is a novel antipsychotic typically used for treatment of bipolar disorder (Taylor, 2016).

Aripiprazole has been shown to decrease irritability scores on both the ABC and CGI in individuals with ASD (Mohiuddin & Ghaziuddin, 2013). The review by McQuire and colleagues mentioned in the preceding paragraph also provided some evidence that aripiprazole may improve quality of life, but again, these results were based on relatively few studies.

Olanzapine is another atypical antipsychotic developed for individuals with schizophrenia and other psychoses. It has been shown to be effective in decreasing aggression and agitation in the general population, and although it also has some evidence in adults with ASD, the small samples sizes utilized in these studies call into question the evidence base for this medication (Taylor, 2016). In children, there is some evidence that olanzapine may decrease irritability; it also was associated with more negative side effects than aripiprazole or risperidone (Accordino et al., 2016; Earle, 2016). For example, Hollander and colleagues (2006) found that olanzapine was related to improvements on the CGI in a double-blind placebo-controlled study, but adverse side effects included significant weight gain. Other antipsychotic medications, such as haloperidol, clozapine, paliperidone, and quetiapine, have one or two studies each that indicate that they may decrease problem behaviors in adults; however, these studies tended to have a small number of participants and did not include any placebo-controlled trials, so there is insufficient evidence for their use for adults in this population (Taylor, 2016).

Issues Regarding the Use of Irritability as a Symptom Construct

It should be noted that *irritability* is a commonly used term that essentially serves as a catchall for many types of challenging behaviors exhibited by individuals with ASD and/or intellectual disability (ID); it often encompasses behaviors such as aggression, self-injurious behaviors, and other challenging behaviors (Matson & Konst, 2015). It is often used as a construct to measure medication effectiveness (Fung et al., 2016). However, the prescription of antipsychotics or other classes of medications to treat irritability may obscure the important consideration of the actual etiology of these behaviors. To consider irritability as a separable symptom with a neuro-chemical basis may pose some difficulties in treatment conceptualization, as it may diminish the role of difficulties with social communication that are associated with an ASD diagnosis. The approach to treating irritability as a way to decrease challenging behaviors assumes that these behaviors are symptoms of irritability itself; however, Matson and Neal (2009) note that this conceptualization may underemphasize the role of operant conditioning and the function of these behaviors, which should be a primary consideration in treatment planning. This is further discussed in the subsequent section on the integration of pharmacotherapy with nonpharmacological approaches.

Antidepressants

Antidepressants are utilized in this population not only for depressive symptoms but also for challenging behaviors such as irritability and aggression, as well as the reduction of repetitive behaviors (Mohiuddin & Ghaziuddin, 2013; Taylor, 2016). Commonly studied antidepressants include fluvoxamine, clomipramine, fluoxetine, and citalopram. The evidence for the efficacy of these medications in decreasing repetitive behaviors and challenging behaviors has been mixed, with some studies reporting improvements while others have not found differences from placebo (Mohiuddin & Ghaziuddin, 2013; Taylor, 2016). In Jobski and colleagues' review (2017), antidepressants were found to have little evidence of effectiveness, and so the author cautioned that medical professionals should be judicious in the prescription of these types of medications to patients with ASD.

Selective serotonin reuptake inhibitors (SSRIs) have been studied in this population, as some have suggested that elevated levels of serotonin in the blood stream may serve as a biomarker (Gabriele, Sacco, & Persico, 2014). Therefore, the rationale behind these medications is that they inhibit the reuptake of this additional serotonin and may decrease rates of repetitive behavior and potentially self-injurious and aggressive behaviors as well. According to a review by Taylor (2016), research findings on fluoxetine in the late 1990s were mixed, though more recent studies have

indicated improvements related to anxiety and compulsive behavior in adults with ASD (Buchsbaum et al., 2001), including one double-blind, placebo-controlled trial (Hollander et al., 2012). Similarly, case studies evaluating fluvoxamine have found variability in results, though one controlled trial indicated improvements in aggression, repetitive thoughts, and repetitive behavior in adults (McDougle, Naylor, Cohen, Volkmar, Heninger, & Price, 1996). However, many of the studies reviewed have very small sample sizes, and there were few RCTs. Therefore, Taylor cautions that an evidence base for these medications is not well established, and this is supported by other research reviews (Earle, 2016). A Cochrane review by Williams and colleagues (2013) examined nine RCTs that investigated fluoxetine, fluvoxamine, fenfluramine, and citalopram. They found no evidence that SSRIs were effective for children with ASD, and only limited evidence that they are effective for adults with ASD.

Serotonin and norepinephrine reuptake inhibitors (SNRIs) have been less widely researched. Venlafaxine has been used to treat individuals with obsessive-compulsive disorder, ADHD, and social phobia. However, in the one study identified in Taylor's review (2016), which included two participants, one participant reported improvement in depressive symptoms and obsessive thoughts, while no significant effects were found on autism symptoms. Atomoxetine, a norepinephrine reuptake inhibitor, has been used to treat ADHD symptoms in individuals with ASD. Ghanizadeh (2013) reported that out of six studies on children and adolescents with ASD, only one study, a placebo-controlled trial, noted improvements. Niederhofer and colleagues (2006) reported a reduction in hyperactivity and irritability in one adult with comorbid ID.

Clomipramine, a nonselective 5-HT reuptake inhibitor, has been proposed to potentially improve aggression and obsessive-compulsive behaviors in children with ASD; however, it has been shown to have low tolerability compared with other medications, as the side effects (e.g., seizures, sedation, weight gain, fatigue, insomnia, tremors, nausea, reduced appetite) are often severe and may outweigh any therapeutic gains (Taylor, 2016).

Stimulants

Commonly prescribed stimulants are methyl-phenidate and a combination of amphetamine and dextroamphetamine (Williamson & Martin, 2012). Methylphenidate has been shown to decrease hyperactivity scores on the ABC and CGI (Research Units on Pediatric Psychopharmacology Autism Network, 2005), and there is some evidence that it may also decrease irritability and aggression (Mohiuddin & Ghaziuddin, 2013). Nonetheless, there is evidence that these medications may be less effective in reducing these symptoms in children with ASD than in typically developing children, and children with ASD may also be more susceptible to negative side effects (Williamson & Martin, 2012).

Anticonvulsants

Anticonvulsant medications such as divalproex sodium, lamotrigine, levetiracetam, and topiramate have been investigated as potential treatments for challenging behaviors in individuals with ASD due to potential impact on mood stabilization (Accordino, Kidd, Politte, Henry, & McDougle, 2016; Elbe & Lalani, 2012). The most widely studied is divalproex sodium (Depakote®), which has been shown to improve behaviors such as aggression and mood lability, as well as overall irritability scores on the CGI and ABC (Hollander et al., 2010). One RCT of adjunctive topiramate indicated significant effects on the irritability subscale of the ABC for children prescribed risperidone and topiramate compared with children prescribed risperidone plus placebo (Rezaei et al., 2010). Results of research on lamotrigine did not indicate positive effects, and the results on levetiracetam have been mixed (Accordino et al., 2016; Elbe & Lalani, 2012). Although studies on oxcarbazepine have indicated positive results, these studies do not include controlled trials, and so these results should be interpreted with caution (Accordino et al., 2016). Overall, anticonvulsants do not seem to have as significant positive effects as the antipsychotics previously discussed. A review conducted by Hirota and colleagues (2014) found seven RCTs of anti-epileptic drugs (AEDs) with 171 total participants. Overall, AEDs were not found to significantly improve behavioral symptoms (e.g., irritability, agitation) in participants with ASD.

Although the evidence is not strong for the treatment of behavioral symptoms, anticonvulsants are effective in treating comorbid seizures in individuals with ASD (Tuchman, 2000). Therefore, Accordino and colleagues (2016) note that anti-convulsants may be appropriate for individuals with seizures or those who do not respond well to antipsychotic medications. This is also discussed later in this chapter in the section on comorbidity.

Other Medications

Guanfacine and clonidine, alpha-2 adrenergic agonists thought to have sedative effects as a result of inhibition of norepinephrine, have been used to treat ADHD and irritability symptoms in individuals with ASD. This is thought to be due to the influence of norepinephrine in arousal, so the inhibition of norepinephrine may decrease arousal and thereby ameliorate symptoms of irritability. Researchers indicate that guanfacine may be effective in reducing hyperactivity, impulsivity, and inattention (Scahill et al., 2015). There is also evidence that it may have greater tolerability than stimulants (Earle, 2016). A placebo-controlled, double-blind crossover trial of clonidine indicated improvements on the ABC in regard to irritability and hyperactivity (Jaselskis, Cook, Fletcher, & Leventhal, 1992).

The literature on mood stabilizers in this population is limited, though there is preliminary evidence that lithium may have positive effects on particular subgroups of individuals with ASD, such as those with certain chromosomal abnormalities (Accordino et al., 2016) or with symptoms of mania or elevated mood (Siegel et al., 2014). However, lithium has significant side effects (Handen & Gilchrist, 2006; Siegel et al., 2014). Consequently, substantial future research is warranted before a recommendation for use can be made (see Tool Kit of Resources).

BEST APPROACHES FOR ASSESSING TREATMENT RESPONSE AND MANAGING SIDE EFFECTS

Treatment response is often evaluated by measures such as the CGI, the ABC, the Children's Psychiatric Rating Scale (CPRS), and the Children's Yale-Brown

Obsessive Compulsive Scale (CY-BOCS) modified for pervasive developmental disorder (Kaplan & McCracken, 2012). Although these measures can provide practitioners with valuable information, basing estimates of treatment response on these standardized measures may have certain limitations, as they typically encapsulate more general or broader classes of behavior rather than more specific target behaviors (Matson & Dempsey, 2008; Poling et al., 2017). For example, standardized measures may be restricted in their ability to capture the specific behaviors that are the focus of treatment. Another conceptualization of treatment response is to set goals, conduct implementation, and make decisions based on the specific, operationalized behaviors of interest and the change or lack thereof in these behaviors (Poling et al., 2017).

Side effects of psychotropic drugs are particularly concerning in this population, as there is evidence that individuals with ASD may experience side effects of certain medications more frequently than in the general population (DeFilippis & Wagner, 2016; Earle, 2016). Although atypical antipsychotics are the only types of medications approved by the FDA for use in this population, they also pose serious side effects such as weight gain, sedation, and elevated prolactin levels (Accordino et al., 2016). Adverse effects of SSRIs include hyperactivity and impulsivity, stereotypies, irritability, and aggression (Earle, 2016). Interestingly, these are some of the same symptoms that these medications are supposedly targeting, which may interfere with overall symptom improvement.

As children with ASD are more likely to experience adverse effects of psychotropic medications, physicians tend to follow more cautious prescription practices in this population, such as prescribing lower initial doses and titrating the doses more slowly than they would for typically developing children (Earle, 2016). The integration of behavioral interventions, in addition to ensuring that the individual is receiving comprehensive treatment, can also allow for the reduction of polypharmacy and lower dosages of medications (Earle, 2016).

The increasing prevalence of psychotropic drug prescription in young children carries its own risk. We cite rates of medication use in children younger than 5 later in this chapter, but seek to further emphasize the hazards of this trend. Although some atypical antipsychotics have been approved for use for children aged 5 to 6 or older, there is extremely limited evidence for the safety of psychotropic medications in very young children (Spetie & Arnold, 2007). Spetie and Arnold (2007) caution that little is known regarding the long-term effects and safety of psychotropic medication for very young children who are still in early neurobiological developmental stages. These authors also note concerns regarding potential negative physiological and anatomical effects.

The effectiveness and tolerability of polypharmacy is a topic that has received little attention, considering how many individuals with ASD are prescribed multiple medications. Wink and colleagues (2017b) found that individuals with ASD who received two or more antipsychotic medications showed improvements in target behaviors (e.g., agitation, irritability, aggression, self-injurious behavior). Theses authors did not find significant negative side effects, and their results indicated that the medications were generally well-tolerated. However, researchers such as Jobski and colleagues (2017) caution that psychotropic polypharmacy can be dangerous, as it can increase the risk of interactions between the drugs. They also note that in individuals with ASD, particularly those with comorbid concerns, it may be difficult to differentiate autism or comorbid symptoms from negative side effect such as sleep problems. This issue can impede effective medication monitoring. Poling and colleagues (2017) also warn that there is little research to date on polypharmacy, and therefore little evidence to support this practice.

MEDICATION MANAGEMENT ISSUES

There are many important ethical issues to consider in medication management for individuals in a vulnerable population. One of the most important considerations is that many individuals with ASD, particularly those with comorbid intellectual disability, may not be their own legal guardians and may have a parent or guardian making decisions regarding psychotropic medication prescriptions for them. There are several reasons why parents and guardians may prefer psychopharmacological treatments, particularly when the individual evinces challenging behaviors. These factors include media portrayals by pharmaceutical companies that medications target underlying biological etiologies for behavioral difficulties, as well as a predisposition of guardians to prefer to believe that the cause of these behaviors is neurochemical rather than learned behaviors that have been reinforced by the environment. Medications are also easier and more quickly administered than behavioral interventions, which are time intensive (Matson & Hess, 2011). This point is supported by a finding by Hock and colleagues (2015), who note that parent adherence to treatment was greater for medications than for behavioral or alternative treatments. The influence of insurance companies, which may prefer medications to behavioral treatments due to the high cost of services such as ABA, should not be overlooked. The lack of functional communication in some individuals who are not their own legal guardians also makes them more susceptible to non–evidence-based psychopharmacological treatments, since they may not be able to report on either improvements or side effects as a result of these medications (Poling et al., 2017). Therefore, treatment response is often estimated only based on parent or caregiver report of observable behaviors.

Adherence to medications is also an important consideration. Of a large sample of Medicaid-eligible children with an ASD diagnosis, 44% of those who were prescribed ADHD medications adhered to the medication guidelines, while 43% adhered to antidepressants, and 52% adhered to antipsychotics (Logan et al., 2014). In this study, adherence was defined as the medication being refilled at a rate that indicated that the medication would be available a minimum of 80% of the time from when it was first filled until the end of the study.

The World Health Organization recommends that increased knowledge regarding the condition or medication on the part of the family is related to better adherence (World Health Organization, 2005). Moore and Symons (2009) also stress the importance of investigating why the family is not adhering to the medication regimen in order to develop a plan

to increase adherence. They note that factors such as whether the failure to adhere to the prescription recommendations is accidental or on purpose, caregivers' perceptions of their own adherence (whether they think they are adhering or not), and exactly what the nonadherence consists of (not adhering to the recommended dosage, frequency, etc.) should be considered. Finally, Moore and Symons (2009) also recommend utilizing behavior analytic principles to investigate the antecedents, consequences, and environmental factors associated with medication use to develop a plan in which these components can be altered to increase medication adherence.

EVALUATION OF PHARMACOLOGICAL APPROACHES ACROSS THE LIFESPAN

Individuals' developmental level should be taken into consideration when prescribing medications. Additionally, the longitudinal effects of psychopharmacological agents should also be considered, particularly as little is known about long-term effects of many of the medications reviewed in this chapter.

Although risperidone and aripiprazole are both approved for children with ASD, they are only approved for children at least 5 and 6 years of age, respectively (DeFilippis & Wagner, 2016). However, Mandell and colleagues (2008) found that 18% of children under 3 years of age and 32% of children ages 3 to 5 were prescribed psychotropic medications. A later large-scale study of 5,150 children indicated that 0.52% of 2-year-olds, 1.36% of 3-year-olds, and 2.67% of 4-year-olds were prescribed an atypical antipsychotic (Lake et al., 2017). Although these frequencies are small, and the case could potentially be made that even very young children with significant behavioral difficulties could benefit from atypical antipsychotic use, this finding is concerning due to the lack of research on the effect of these drugs on physical and cognitive development in very young children. Given the lack of evidence that these medications can be safely prescribed to children in this age range, additional research is needed, and physicians should exercise extreme caution in prescribing antipsychotics, or any psychotropic medications, to children this young.

There is substantial evidence that use of psychotropic medication increases with age (Coury et al., 2012; Houghton et al., 2017; Jobski et al., 2017; Lake et al., 2017; Mire, Raff, Brewton, & Goin-Kochel, 2015; Rosenberg et al., 2010). Mire and colleagues found that 16-year-olds were more likely to use psychotropic medication than 11-year-olds, who in turn were more likely to be prescribed medications than 6-year-olds. Lake and colleagues (2017) found rates of psychotropic medication use in 5.41% of children 2 to 11 years old, and 17.71% of children 12 to 17 years old. The frequency of atypical antipsychotic use in young children under 6 years of age was 2.14%. Coury and colleagues (2012) found that 1% of children under age 3, 10% of children aged 3 to 5, 44% of children aged 6 to 11, and 64% of children aged 12 to 17 with ASD were prescribed one or more psychotropic medications.

Rates tend to be even higher in adults with ASD and/or ID. Buck and colleagues found that in a sample of adults with ASD, 59% were prescribed at least one psychotropic medication, 39% were prescribed at least two, 26% were prescribed at least three, and 14% were taking four or more psychotropic medications. Some potential explanations for this upsurge include an increasing willingness of caregivers to use psychotropic interventions for their children, that individuals may develop new behaviors or the severity of challenging behaviors may increase, and behavioral interventions implemented early in development may fail to have positive effects on challenging behaviors or comorbidities (Jobski et al., 2017).

A longitudinal study by Esbensen, Greenberg, Seltzer, and Aman (2009) found that rate of prescription of psychotropic medication increased over a 4.5-year period, and that rates of challenging behaviors decreased. The authors note that additional research is needed to determine whether the improvements in problem behaviors are due to developmental maturation and fewer problem behaviors in older individuals, or due to medication use. An important finding of the study was that once an individual is prescribed psychotropic medication, he or she is 11 times more likely to continue to remain on

some type of medication. Esbensen et al. (2009) suggest that this indicates the importance of psychoeducational programs for family members about recognizing adverse side effects, as the early identification of these effects are crucial for their effective management.

Taylor (2016) reviewed 43 studies on psychopharmacologic intervention for adults with ASD and found that only two medications (i.e., risperidone and fluoxetine) had sufficient evidence to be considered evidence-based approaches to treating symptoms such as irritability and repetitive behaviors. This review suggests that antipsychotic medications are often utilized as a first-line approach for challenging behaviors in adults with ID, and that this treatment approach goes against best-practice guidelines for behavior management.

CONSIDERATION OF POTENTIAL SEX DIFFERENCES

The majority of the research indicates that sex does not increase psychotropic medication rates in individuals with ASD (Coury et al., 2012; Houghton et al., 2017; Lake et al., 2017; Wink et al., 2017a). However, Poling and colleagues (2017) caution that sex differences in drug effects has received inadequate attention in the research literature to date, and future consideration of potential differences in reaction to drugs is warranted.

INTEGRATION OF PHARMACOTHERAPY WITH NONPHARMACOLOGICAL APPROACHES: BENEFITS AND CHALLENGES

As previously mentioned, individualized interventions based on behavioral principles (i.e., ABA) are the gold standard of treatment for individuals with ASD. Many professionals in the field recommend comprehensive behavioral intervention prior to resorting to pharmacotherapy (Canitano & Scandurra, 2011). Earle (2016) recommended ABA to treat RRBs and challenging behaviors and cognitive behavior therapy (CBT) for anxiety concerns.

In the behavior analytic literature, behavioral treatments for challenging or problem behaviors, such as those that typically fall into the irritability categorization, are based on the "function" of the behavior, or, very generally, what is causing and/or maintaining the behavior. Therefore, a functional behavioral assessment (FBA) is typically conducted, and this assessment guides the behavior intervention plan (BIP) for addressing the behavior. The main components of an FBA include identifying the target behavior, the setting events or establishing operations (e.g., hunger, fatigue, illness), the antecedents (or events that occur before the behavior and tend to predict the occurrence of the behavior), and the consequences (or what happens after the behavior that is increasing the likelihood that it will occur again; Cooper, Heron, & Heward, 2007; Newcomer & Lewis, 2004; Sugai, Lewis-Palmer, & Hagan-Burke, 2000). Additional resources for basic information regarding FBAs and BIPs are included in the tool kit at the end of this chapter.

Matson and Neal (2009) point out that for individuals with ID, treating challenging behaviors with psychotropic medications often does not consider the function of the behavior, which should be the variable guiding the treatment for the behavior. By grouping behaviors based on topography—or the form of the behavior (e.g., aggression, self-injury, stereotypy)—and then broadening the definition even more by collapsing all challenging behaviors into one category or attributing these behaviors to "irritability," Matson and Neal caution that specificity of the behavior is lost. This makes determining treatment efficacy and improvements in behavior difficult to measure. As the goal of treatment is to improve behavior, this is clearly a concern. Conducting a functional assessment to determine the functions of the behavior that the clinician seeks to improve, and then using the information gleaned from this assessment to guide treatment planning, is the recommended approach (Matson & Neal, 2009).

Behavioral therapy is a critical aspect of treatment, and researchers have found that behavior therapy in conjunction with pharmacological treatment is more effective than pharmacological treatment alone (Frazier et al., 2010). Best-practice approaches may include psychopharmacological treatment as one component, but should also include behavioral and educational components to ensure a compre-hensive and evidence-based approach (Kaplan & McCracken, 2012). However, a barrier to these services may be that not all communities or schools have trained behavior analysts, making the utilization of integrated approaches difficult.

INTEGRATED APPROACHES FOR ADDRESSING COMMON COMORBID DISORDERS

Although there is significant variability in exact prevalence estimates, the literature indicates that many psychiatric and medical comorbid conditions are extremely common in children and adults with ASD. In a review conducted by Tsai in 2014, prevalence estimates in children with ASD for any comorbid psychiatric disorder were between 27% to 95%. The prevalence estimates for ADHD ranged from 9% to 83%, any anxiety disorder from 26% to 61%, any depressive disorder from 1% to 11%, and any tic disorder between 11% to 26%. Additional consideration of integrated treatment approaches for some of these common comorbidities are discussed briefly below. Table 17.1 indicates some of the behavioral or psychiatric concerns beyond core ASD symptoms that are common targets of psychotropic medication prescription.

As previously discussed, stimulants commonly used to treat ADHD symptoms may be effective for individuals in this population. However, there is evidence that they are less effective than for children without ASD, and have higher rates of adverse side effects in children with ASD (Earle, 2016; Research Units on Pediatric Psychopharmacology Autism Network, 2005). For example, Barnard-Brak and colleagues (2016) found that stimulant medications did not improve either symptoms associated with ASD (i.e., social interaction and communication) or symptoms associated with ADHD (i.e., hyperactivity and task persistence). Conversely, Joshi and colleagues (2017) found that methylphenidate is effective in treatment ADHD symptoms in children with high-functioning ASD. Behavior management plans may also be effective in addressing hyperactivity and impulsivity, either alone or in conjunction with stimulant medications (Pfiffner & Haack, 2014).

CBT is well established as a treatment for mood concerns such as anxiety and depression; however, there is a dearth of literature on the use or adaptation of CBT treatments for individuals with low cognitive abilities, such as those with comorbid ID (Sturmey, 2004). CBT treatments for children with ASD and comorbid anxiety typically employ standard CBT techniques, but with some modifications to address the difficulties associated with ASD symptomology, and these treatment approaches have been shown to be effective in addressing anxiety symptoms in this population (Danial, 2013; Ekman & Hiltunen, 2015; Lang, Regester, Lauderdale, Ashbaugh, & Haring, 2010; Nadeau et al., 2011). There is some evidence that SSRIs may improve anxiety symptoms in individuals with ASD; however, this evidence is limited, and negative side effects have been reported (Nadeau et al., 2011). Therefore, SSRIs may be effective for some individuals with ASD and comorbid anxiety, but clinicians should exercise caution in the prescription of these medications and additional research is needed.

Several medical comorbidities are also more common in individuals with ASD, such as epilepsy and gastrointestinal symptoms (Chandradasa et al., 2017). AEDs may be effective in managing seizures in this population; however, children with developmental disabilities may be at increased risk of negative side effects of these medications. Practitioners should consider factors such as the type of AED, titration to the lowest effective dose, and effects of the use of multiple psychotropic medications (Depositario-Cabacar & Zelleke, 2010).

The prevalence of comorbidities likely also differs across age ranges. For example, a study by Soke and colleagues (2018) found that certain medical and behavioral conditions, such as ADHD, oppositional defiant disorder, anxiety, sleep difficulties, and motor difficulties, among others, were more common in 8-year-olds with ASD than in 4-year-olds. Further, Jones and colleagues (2016) conducted a follow-up study for adults with ASD and found that adults with ASD continued to experience many medical conditions first diagnosed in childhood. Given the high prevalence of comorbid medical, psychological, and behavioral concerns,

attention to potential comorbidities is extremely important in intervention. Notably, treatment of these comorbid concerns often involves additional considerations in comparison to the treatment of these difficulties in typically developing individuals.

EMERGING TRENDS

Research on novel agents has increased in recent years, though no new medications have been clinically recommended for this population. Some such agents include oxytocin, gamma-aminobutyric acid (GABA), glutamatergic agents (Baribeau & Anagnostou, 2014), and insulin-like growth factor 1 (IGF-1; Howes et al., 2017). Although the evidence for the efficacy of these medications for core ASD symptoms is currently too limited to warrant clear recommendation, several large-scale studies are currently underway to investigate oxytocin, vasopressin (NCT1962870), and IGF-1 (NCT01970345; Howes et al., 2017). The results of these studies will be important in furthering the research on their efficacy, feasibility, and tolerability in this population.

There is some evidence that oxytocin, an endogenous neuropeptide, may improve social difficulties in individuals with ASD (Anagnostou et al., 2012; Andari et al., 2010; Parker et al., 2017), and some findings even indicate potential improvements in RRBs (Bernaerts, Dillen, Steyaert, & Alaerts, 2017). A small number of studies utilizing magnetic resonance imaging, RCTs, and case reports have indicated positive effects on social and emotional skills (LeClerc & Easley, 2015). However, some researchers caution that the evidence for beneficial effects of oxytocin is limited, and they stress the need for additional large-scale RCTs (Alvares, Quintana, & Whitehouse, 2017; DeMayo, Song, Hickie, & Guastella, 2017; Howes et al., 2017; Ooi, Weng, Kossowsky, Gerger, & Sung, 2017).

Another newer line of study has emerged that investigates the potential role of an increased rate of excitatory versus inhibitory neurotransmissions in ASD. As such, research on medications that target glutamate and GABA have become more common (Accordino et al., 2016). Overall, the research on glutamatergic agents is sparse, as few studies have investigated their use in individuals with ASD, and the few that have did not indicate significant improvements in behavior (Howes et al., 2017). GABAergic agonists inhibit the release of glutamate, and this is thought to balance neurotransmission for individuals with ASD. However, studies on arbaclofen and pregnenolone have not yielded conclusive enough results to recommend their use in this population (Howes et al., 2017). Piracetam, a GABA derivative that modulates neurotransmission, is prescribed for a wide variety of conditions (Winblad, 2005). One study found that prescription of piracetam plus risperidone was more effective in decreasing challenging behaviors than risperidone alone (McQuire et al., 2015).

Several future research directions have been suggested. Researchers have consistently advocated for additional future research on the long-term effectiveness and safety of psychotropic medication use in this population (Houghton et al., 2017). Joshi (2017) notes that much of the research on psychotropic medication use for individuals with ASD include samples of individuals with comorbid ID, but studies on individuals with average intellectual functioning are scarcer. Because of many of the concerns regarding the prevalence of medication use and limited effectiveness in this population, the authors echo the sentiment of Lake and colleagues (2017) that additional long-term, large-scale studies are necessary to understand best-practice approaches to prescription practices for individuals with ASD.

TOOL KIT OF RESOURCES

Autism Spectrum Disorder

Patient Resources

Autism Speaks Autism Treatment Network: Medication Decision Aid: https://www.autismspeaks.org/science/resources-programs/autism-treatment-network/tools-you-can-use/medication-guide

American Academy of Child & Adolescent Psychiatry: Autism Spectrum Disorder: Parents' Medication Guide: http://www.aacap.org/App_Themes/AACAP/Docs/resource_centers/autism/Autism_Spectrum_Disorder_Parents_Medication_Guide.pdf

Centers for Disease Control and Prevention: Treatment: https://www.cdc.gov/ncbddd/autism/treatment.html

National Institute of Mental Health: A Parents' Guide to Autism Spectrum Disorder: https://www.autism-watch.org/general/nimh.pdf

Schall, C. (2002). A consumer's guide to monitoring psychotropic medication for individuals with autism spectrum disorders. *Focus on Autism and Other Developmental Disabilities, 17*, 229–235. http://dx.doi.org/10.1177/10883576020170040501

Spectrum News: Autism Research News & Opinion: https://spectrumnews.org/

Provider Resources

Children's Hospital of Philadelphia Research Institute: Center for Autism Research: Autism Spectrum Disorder Measures: https://www.carautismroadmap.org/autism-spectrum-disorder-measures/?print=pdf

Children's Hospital of Philadelphia Research Institute: Center for Autism Research: Elements of an Evaluation for Autism Spectrum Disorder: https://www.carautismroadmap.org/elements-of-an-evaluation-for-an-autism-spectrum-disorder/?print=pdf

Centers for Disease Control and Prevention: Screening and Diagnosis for Healthcare Providers: https://www.cdc.gov/ncbddd/autism/hcp-screening.html

Children's Hospital of Philadelphia Research Institute: Center for Autism Research: Functional Behavioral Assessment: What Is It?: https://www.carautismroadmap.org/functional-behavioral-assessment/?print=pdf

Children's Hospital of Philadelphia Research Institute: Center for Autism Research: Behavior Intervention Plan: https://www.carautismroadmap.org/behavior-intervention-plan/?print=pdf

References

Accordino, R. E., Kidd, C., Politte, L. C., Henry, C. A., & McDougle, C. J. (2016). Psychopharmacological interventions in autism spectrum disorder.

*Asterisks indicate assessments or resources.

Expert Opinion on Pharmacotherapy, 17, 937–952. http://dx.doi.org/10.1517/14656566.2016.1154536

Achkova, M., & Manolova, H. (2014). Diagnosis "autism"–From Kanner and Asperger to *DSM–5. Journal of Intellectual Disability–Diagnosis and Treatment, 2,* 112–118.

Al-Qabandi, M., Gorter, J. W., & Rosenbaum, P. (2011). Early autism detection: Are we ready for routine screening? *Pediatrics, 128,* e211–e217. http://dx.doi.org/10.1542/peds.2010-1881

Alvares, G. A., Quintana, D. S., & Whitehouse, A. J. O. (2017). Beyond the hype and hope: Critical considerations for intranasal oxytocin research in autism spectrum disorder. *Autism Research, 10,* 25–41. http://dx.doi.org/10.1002/aur.1692

American Psychiatric Association. (2013). *Diagnostic and statistical manual of mental disorders* (5th ed.). Washington, DC: Author.

Anagnostou, E., Soorya, L., Chaplin, W., Bartz, J., Halpern, D., Wasserman, S., . . . Hollander, E. (2012). Intranasal oxytocin versus placebo in the treatment of adults with autism spectrum disorders: A randomized controlled trial. *Molecular Autism, 3,* 16. http://dx.doi.org/10.1186/2040-2392-3-16

Andari, E., Duhamel, J.-R., Zalla, T., Herbrecht, E., Leboyer, M., & Sirigu, A. (2010). Promoting social behavior with oxytocin in high-functioning autism spectrum disorders. *PNAS Proceedings of the National Academy of Sciences of the United States of America, 107,* 4389–4394. http://dx.doi.org/10.1073/pnas.0910249107

Baio, J., Wiggins, L., Christensen, D. L., Maenner, M. J., Daniels, J., Warren, X., . . . Dowling, N. F. (2018). Prevalence of autism spectrum disorders: Autism and developmental disabilities monitoring network, 11 sites, United States, 2014. *Morbidity and Mortality Weekly Report, 66,* 1–23.

Baribeau, D. A., & Anagnostou, E. (2014). An update on medication management of behavioral disorders in autism. *Current Psychiatry Reports, 16,* 437. http://dx.doi.org/10.1007/s11920-014-0437-0

Barnard-Brak, L., Davis, T. N., Schmidt, M., & Richman, D. M. (2016). Effects associated with on- and off-label stimulant treatment of core autism and ADHD symptoms exhibited by children with autism spectrum disorder. *Developmental Neurorehabilitation, 19,* 46–53. http://dx.doi.org/10.3109/17518423.2014.904949

*Baron-Cohen, S., Wheelwright, S., Skinner, R., Martin, J., & Clubley, E. (2001). The autism-spectrum quotient (AQ): Evidence from Asperger syndrome/high-functioning autism, males and females, scientists and mathematicians. *Journal of Autism and Developmental Disorders, 31,* 5–17. http://dx.doi.org/10.1023/A:1005653411471

Barton, M. L., Dumont-Mathieu, T., & Fein, D. (2012). Screening young children for autism spectrum disorders in primary practice. *Journal of Autism and Developmental Disorders, 42,* 1165–1174. http://dx.doi.org/10.1007/s10803-011-1343-5

Bazzano, A., Zeldin, A., Schuster, E., Barrett, C., & Lehrer, D. (2012). Vaccine-related beliefs and practices of parents of children with autism spectrum disorders. *American Journal on Intellectual and Developmental Disabilities, 117,* 233–242. http://dx.doi.org/10.1352/1944-7558-117.3.233

Bernaerts, S., Dillen, C., Steyaert, J., & Alaerts, K. (2017). 864. The effects of four weeks of intranasal oxytocin on social responsiveness and repetitive and restricted behaviors in autism spectrum disorders: A randomized controlled trial. *Biological Psychiatry, 81*(10, Suppl.), S349–S350. http://dx.doi.org/10.1016/j.biopsych.2017.02.589

Bettelheim, B. (1967). *The empty fortress: Infantile autism and the birth of the self.* New York, NY: Free Press.

Buchsbaum, M. S., Hollander, E., Haznedar, M. M., Tang, C., Spiegel-Cohen, J., Wei, T. C., . . . Mosovich, S. (2001). Effect of fluoxetine on regional cerebral metabolism in autistic spectrum disorders: A pilot study. *International Journal of Neuropsychopharmacology, 4,* 119–125. http://dx.doi.org/10.1017/S1461145701002280

Buck, T. R., Viskochil, J., Farley, M., Coon, H., McMahon, W. M., Morgan, J., & Bilder, D. A. (2014). Psychiatric comorbidity and medication use in adults with autism spectrum disorder. *Journal of Autism and Developmental Disorders, 44,* 3063–3071. http://dx.doi.org/10.1007/s10803-014-2170-2

Canitano, R., & Scandurra, V. (2011). Psychopharmacology in autism: An update. *Progress in Neuro-Psychopharmacology & Biological Psychiatry, 35,* 18–28. http://dx.doi.org/10.1016/j.pnpbp.2010.10.015

Center for Disease Control and Prevention. (2016). *Screening and diagnosis for healthcare providers.* Retrieved from https://www.cdc.gov/ncbddd/autism/hcp-screening.html

Chandradasa, M., Rohanachandra, Y., Dahanayake, D., Hettiarachchi, D., Gunathilake, M., Fernando, R., & Wijetunge, S. (2017). A comparative study on medical comorbidities among children with autism spectrum disorder and controls in a children's hospital. *Sri Lanka Journal of Child Health, 46,* 262–266. http://dx.doi.org/10.4038/sljch.v46i3.8329

Chawarska, K., Klin, A., Paul, R., & Volkmar, F. (2007). Autism spectrum disorder in the second year: Stability and change in syndrome expression. *Journal of Child Psychology and Psychiatry, 48,* 128–138. http://dx.doi.org/10.1111/j.1469-7610.2006.01685.x

Cohen, I. L., & Sudhalter, V. (2005). *Pervasive Developmental Disorder Behavior Inventory (PDDBI)*. Lutz, FL: Psychological Assessment Resources.

*Constantino, J. N., & Gruber, C. P. (2012). *Social Responsiveness Scale* (2nd ed.). Los Angeles, CA: Western Psychological Services.

Cooper, J. O., Heron, T. E., & Heward, W. L. (2007). *Applied behavior analysis.* Upper Saddle River, NJ: Pearson/Merrill-Prentice Hall.

Coury, D. L., Anagnostou, E., Manning-Courtney, P., Reynolds, A., Cole, L., McCoy, R., . . . Perrin, J. M. (2012). Use of psychotropic medication in children and adolescents with autism spectrum disorders. *Pediatrics, 130*(Suppl. 2), S69–S76. http://dx.doi.org/10.1542/peds.2012-0900D

Danial, J. T. (2013). *Cognitive behavior therapy for anxiety: Adapting interventions for children with autism and intellectual disability.* Los Angeles, CA: University of California.

Daniels, A. M., & Mandell, D. S. (2013). Explaining differences in age at autism spectrum disorder diagnosis: A critical review. *Autism: An International Journal of Research and Practice, 18,* 583–597. http://dx.doi.org/10.1177/1362361313480277

DeFilippis, M., & Wagner, K. D. (2016). Treatment of autism spectrum disorder in children and adolescents. *Psychopharmacology Bulletin, 46*(2), 18–41.

DeMayo, M. M., Song, Y. J. C., Hickie, I. B., & Guastella, A. J. (2017). A review of the safety, efficacy and mechanisms of delivery of nasal oxytocin in children: Therapeutic potential for autism and Prader-Willi syndrome, and recommendations for future research. *Paediatric Drugs, 19,* 391–410. http://dx.doi.org/10.1007/s40272-017-0248-y

Depositario-Cabacar, D. F. T., & Zelleke, T. G. (2010). Treatment of epilepsy in children with developmental disabilities. *Developmental Disabilities Research Reviews, 16,* 239–247. http://dx.doi.org/10.1002/ddrr.116

Diler, R. S., Firat, S., & Avci, A. (2002). An open-label trial of risperidone in children with autism. *Current Therapeutic Research, 63,* 91–102. http://dx.doi.org/10.1016/S0011-393X(02)80009-1

*Dunn, W. (2014). *Sensory Profile-2.* San Antonio, TX: Pearson.

Earle, J. F. (2016). An introduction to the psychopharmacology of children and adolescents with autism spectrum disorder. *Journal of Child and Adolescent Psychiatric Nursing, 29,* 62–71. http://dx.doi.org/10.1111/jcap.12144

Ekman, E., & Hiltunen, A. J. (2015). Modified CBT using visualization for autism spectrum disorder (ASD), anxiety and avoidance behavior—a quasi-experimental open pilot study. *Scandinavian Journal of Psychology, 56,* 641–648. http://dx.doi.org/10.1111/sjop.12255

Elbe, D., & Lalani, Z. (2012). Review of the pharmacotherapy of irritability of autism. *Journal of the Canadian Academy of Child and Adolescent Psychiatry, 21*(2), 130–146.

Esbensen, A. J., Greenberg, J. S., Seltzer, M. M., & Aman, M. G. (2009). A longitudinal investigation of psychotropic and non-psychotropic medication use among adolescents and adults with autism spectrum disorders. *Journal of Autism and Developmental Disorders, 39,* 1339–1349. http://dx.doi.org/10.1007/s10803-009-0750-3

Fombonne, E. (2009). Epidemiology of pervasive developmental disorders. *Pediatric Research, 65,* 591–598. http://dx.doi.org/10.1203/PDR.0b013e31819e7203

Frazier, T. W., Youngstrom, E. A., Haycook, T., Sinoff, A., Dimitriou, F., Knapp, J., & Sinclair, L. (2010). Effectiveness of medication combined with intensive behavioral intervention for reducing aggression in youth with autism spectrum disorder. *Journal of Child and Adolescent Psychopharmacology, 20,* 167–177. http://dx.doi.org/10.1089/cap.2009.0048

Fung, L. K., Mahajan, R., Nozzolillo, A., Bernal, P., Krasner, A., Jo, B., . . . Hardan, A. Y. (2016). Pharmacologic treatment of severe irritability and problem behaviors in autism: A systematic review and meta-analysis. *Pediatrics, 137*(Suppl. 2), S124–S135. http://dx.doi.org/10.1542/peds.2015-2851K

Gabriele, S., Sacco, R., & Persico, A. M. (2014). Blood serotonin levels in autism spectrum disorder: A systematic review and meta-analysis. *European Neuropsychopharmacology, 24,* 919–929. http://dx.doi.org/10.1016/j.euroneuro.2014.02.004

Ghanizadeh, A. (2013). Atomoxetine for treating ADHD symptoms in autism: A systematic review. *Journal of Attention Disorders, 17,* 635–640. http://dx.doi.org/10.1177/1087054712443154

*Gilliam, J. E. (2014). *Gilliam Autism Rating Scale* (3rd ed.). Austin, TX: Pro-ed.

*Goldstein, S., & Naglieri, J. A. (2009). *Autism Spectrum Rating Scales (ASRS)*. Toronto, Ontario, Canada: Multi-Health Systems.

Gotham, K., Risi, S., Pickles, A., & Lord, C. (2007). The Autism Diagnostic Observation Schedule: Revised algorithms for improved diagnostic validity. *Journal of Autism and Developmental Disorders, 37,* 613–627. http://dx.doi.org/10.1007/s10803-006-0280-1

Handen, B. L., & Gilchrist, R. (2006). Practitioner review: Psychopharmacology in children and adolescents with mental retardation. *Journal of Child Psychology and Psychiatry, 47,* 871–882. http://dx.doi.org/10.1111/j.1469-7610.2006.01588.x

Hirota, T., Veenstra-Vanderweele, J., Hollander, E., & Kishi, T. (2014). Antiepileptic medications in autism spectrum disorder: A systematic review and meta-analysis. *Journal of Autism and Developmental Disorders, 44*, 948–957. http://dx.doi.org/10.1007/s10803-013-1952-2

Hock, R., Kinsman, A., & Ortaglia, A. (2015). Examining treatment adherence among parents of children with autism spectrum disorder. *Disability and Health Journal, 8*, 407–413. http://dx.doi.org/10.1016/j.dhjo.2014.10.005

Hollander, E., Chaplin, W., Soorya, L., Wasserman, S., Novotny, S., Rusoff, J., . . . Anagnostou, E. (2010). Divalproex sodium vs placebo for the treatment of irritability in children and adolescents with autism spectrum disorders. *Neuropsychopharmacology, 35*, 990–998. http://dx.doi.org/10.1038/npp.2009.202

Hollander, E., Soorya, L., Chaplin, W., Anagnostou, E., Taylor, B. P., Ferretti, C. J., . . . Settipani, C. (2012). A double-blind placebo-controlled trial of fluoxetine for repetitive behaviors and global severity in adult autism spectrum disorders. *The American Journal of Psychiatry, 169*, 292–299. http://dx.doi.org/10.1176/appi.ajp.2011.10050764

Hollander, E., Wasserman, S., Swanson, E. N., Chaplin, W., Schapiro, M. L., Zagursky, K., & Novotny, S. (2006). A double-blind placebo-controlled pilot study of olanzapine in childhood/adolescent pervasive developmental disorder. *Journal of Child and Adolescent Psychopharmacology, 16*, 541–548. http://dx.doi.org/10.1089/cap.2006.16.541

Houghton, R., Ong, R. C., & Bolognani, F. (2017). Psychiatric comorbidities and use of psychotropic medications in people with autism spectrum disorder in the United States. *Autism Research, 10*(12), 2037–2047. http://dx.doi.org/10.1002/aur.1848

Howes, O. D., Rogdaki, M., Findon, J. L., Wichers, R. H., Charman, T., King, B. H., . . . Murphy, D. G. (2017). Autism spectrum disorder: Consensus guidelines on assessment, treatment and research from the British Association for Psychopharmacology. *Journal of Psychopharmacology, 32*, 3–29. http://dx.doi.org/10.1177/0269881117741766

Howlin, P. (2006). Autism spectrum disorders. *Psychiatry, 5*, 320–324. http://dx.doi.org/10.1053/j.mppsy.2006.06.007

Hsia, Y., Wong, A. Y. S., Murphy, D. G. M., Simonoff, E., Buitelaar, J. K., & Wong, I. C. K. (2014). Psychopharmacological prescriptions for people with autism spectrum disorder (ASD): A multinational study. *Psychopharmacology, 231*, 999–1009. http://dx.doi.org/10.1007/s00213-013-3263-x

Huerta, M., & Lord, C. (2012). Diagnostic evaluation of autism spectrum disorders. *Pediatric Clinics of North America, 59*, 103–111, xi. http://dx.doi.org/10.1016/j.pcl.2011.10.018

Hviid, A., Stellfeld, M., Wohlfahrt, J., & Melbye, M. (2003). Association between thimerosal-containing vaccine and autism. *JAMA, 290*, 1763–1766. http://dx.doi.org/10.1001/jama.290.13.1763

Jackel, C., Shults, J., Wiley, S., Meinzen-Derr, J., Augustyn, M., & Blum, N. (2017). Factors associated with developmental behavioral pediatricians prescribing psychotropic medication to children with autism spectrum disorder: A study of three DBPNet sites. *Journal of Developmental and Behavioral Pediatrics, 38*, 584–592. http://dx.doi.org/10.1097/DBP.0000000000000488

Jain, A., Marshall, J., Buikema, A., Bancroft, T., Kelly, J. P., & Newschaffer, C. J. (2015). Autism occurrence by MMR vaccine status among US children with older siblings with and without autism. *JAMA, 313*, 1534–1540. http://dx.doi.org/10.1001/jama.2015.3077

Jaselskis, C. A., Cook, E. H., Jr., Fletcher, K. E., & Leventhal, B. L. (1992). Clonidine treatment of hyperactive and impulsive children with autistic disorder. *Journal of Clinical Psychopharmacology, 12*, 322–327. http://dx.doi.org/10.1097/00004714-199210000-00005

Jobski, K., Höfer, J., Hoffmann, F., & Bachmann, C. (2017). Use of psychotropic drugs in patients with autism spectrum disorders: A systematic review. *Acta Psychiatrica Scandinavica, 135*, 8–28. http://dx.doi.org/10.1111/acps.12644

Jones, K. B., Cottle, K., Bakian, A., Farley, M., Bilder, D., Coon, H., & McMahon, W. M. (2016). A description of medical conditions in adults with autism spectrum disorder: A follow-up of the 1980s Utah/UCLA Autism Epidemiologic Study. *Autism, 20*, 551–561. http://dx.doi.org/10.1177/1362361315594798

Joshi, G. (2017). Are there lessons to be learned from the prevailing patterns of psychotropic drug use in patients with autism spectrum disorder? *Acta Psychiatrica Scandinavica, 135*, 5–7. http://dx.doi.org/10.1111/acps.12683

Joshi, G., Hoskova, B., Fitzgerald, M., Ceranoglu, T. A., Yule, A., Fried, R. S., . . . Biederman, J. (2017). A prospective open-label trial of extended-release liquid methylphenidate for the treatment of attention deficit/hyperactivity disorder (ADHD) in adults with high-functioning autism spectrum disorder: An interim analysis. *Journal of the American Academy of Child & Adolescent Psychiatry, 56*, S259. http://dx.doi.org/10.1016/j.jaac.2017.09.301

Kaplan, G., & McCracken, J. T. (2012). Psychopharmacology of autism spectrum disorders. *Pediatric Clinics of North America, 59*, 175–187, xii. http://dx.doi.org/10.1016/j.pcl.2011.10.005

Kaye, J. A., del Mar Melero-Montes, M., & Jick, H. (2001). Mumps, measles, and rubella vaccine and the incidence of autism recorded by general practitioners: A time trend analysis. *BMJ, 322*, 460–463. http://dx.doi.org/10.1136/bmj.322.7284.460

Lake, J. K., Denton, D., Lunsky, Y., Shui, A. M., Veenstra-VanderWeele, J., & Anagnostou, E. (2017). Medical conditions and demographic, service and clinical factors associated with atypical antipsychotic medication use among children with an autism spectrum disorder. *Journal of Autism and Developmental Disorders, 47*, 1391–1402. http://dx.doi.org/10.1007/s10803-017-3058-8

Lang, R., Regester, A., Lauderdale, S., Ashbaugh, K., & Haring, A. (2010). Treatment of anxiety in autism spectrum disorders using cognitive behaviour therapy: A systematic review. *Developmental Neurorehabilitation, 13*, 53–63. http://dx.doi.org/10.3109/17518420903236288

LeClerc, S., & Easley, D. (2015). Pharmacological therapies for autism spectrum disorder: A review. *P&T, 40*(6), 389–397.

Leyfer, O. T., Folstein, S. E., Bacalman, S., Davis, N. O., Dinh, E., Morgan, J., . . . Lainhart, J. E. (2006). Comorbid psychiatric disorders in children with autism: Interview development and rates of disorders. *Journal of Autism and Developmental Disorders, 36*, 849–861. http://dx.doi.org/10.1007/s10803-006-0123-0

Logan, S. L., Carpenter, L., Leslie, R. S., Hunt, K. S., Garrett-Mayer, E., Charles, J., & Nicholas, J. S. (2014). Rates and predictors of adherence to psychotropic medications in children with autism spectrum disorders. *Journal of Autism and Developmental Disorders, 44*, 2931–2948. http://dx.doi.org/10.1007/s10803-014-2156-0

*Lord, C., Rutter, M., DiLavore, P., Risi, S., Gotham, K., & Bishop, S. (2012). *Autism Diagnostic Observation Schedule* (2nd ed.). Los Angeles, CA: Western Psychological Corporation.

MacDonald, R., Parry-Cruwys, D., Dupere, S., & Ahearn, W. (2014). Assessing progress and outcome of early intensive behavioral intervention for toddlers with autism. *Research in Developmental Disabilities, 35*, 3632–3644. http://dx.doi.org/10.1016/j.ridd.2014.08.036

Magaña, S., Parish, S. L., Rose, R. A., Timberlake, M., & Swaine, J. G. (2012). Racial and ethnic disparities in quality of health care among children with autism and other developmental disabilities. *Intellectual and Developmental Disabilities, 50*, 287–299. http://dx.doi.org/10.1352/1934-9556-50.4.287

Mandell, D. S., Morales, K. H., Marcus, S. C., Stahmer, A. C., Doshi, J., & Polsky, D. E. (2008). Psychotropic medication use among Medicaid-enrolled children with autism spectrum disorders. *Pediatrics, 121*, e441–e448. http://dx.doi.org/10.1542/peds.2007-0984

Mandell, D. S., Novak, M. M., & Zubritsky, C. D. (2005). Factors associated with age of diagnosis among children with autism spectrum disorders. *Pediatrics, 116*, 1480–1486. http://dx.doi.org/10.1542/peds.2005-0185

Mandell, D. S., Wiggins, L. D., Carpenter, L. A., Daniels, J., DiGuiseppi, C., Durkin, M. S., . . . Kirby, R. S. (2009). Racial/ethnic disparities in the identification of children with autism spectrum disorders. *American Journal of Public Health, 99*, 493–498. http://dx.doi.org/10.2105/AJPH.2007.131243

*Matson, J. L., Boisjoli, J. A., González, M. L., Smith, K. R., & Wilkins, J. (2007). Norms and cut off scores for the autism spectrum disorders diagnosis for adults (ASD-DA) with intellectual disability. *Research in Autism Spectrum Disorders, 1*, 330–338. http://dx.doi.org/10.1016/j.rasd.2007.01.001

*Matson, J. L., Boisjoli, J. A., & Wilkins, J. (2007). *The Baby and Infant Screen for Children with aUtIsm Traits (BISCUIT)*. Baton Rouge, LA: Disability Consultants.

Matson, J. L., & Dempsey, T. (2008). Autism spectrum disorders: Pharmacotherapy for challenging behaviors. *Journal of Developmental and Physical Disabilities, 20*, 175–191. http://dx.doi.org/10.1007/s10882-007-9088-y

*Matson, J. L., González, M., & Wilkins, J. (2009). Validity study of the Autism Spectrum Disorders-Diagnostic for Children (ASD-DC). *Research in Autism Spectrum Disorders, 3*, 196–206. http://dx.doi.org/10.1016/j.rasd.2008.05.005

*Matson, J. L., Gonzalez, M. L., Wilkins, J., & Rivet, T. T. (2008). Reliability of the autism spectrum disorder-diagnostic for children (ASD-DC). *Research in Autism Spectrum Disorders, 2*, 533–545. http://dx.doi.org/10.1016/j.rasd.2007.11.001

Matson, J. L., & Hess, J. A. (2011). Psychotropic drug efficacy and side effects for persons with autism spectrum disorders. *Research in Autism Spectrum Disorders, 5*, 230–236. http://dx.doi.org/10.1016/j.rasd.2010.04.004

Matson, J. L., & Konst, M. J. (2015). Why pharmacotherapy is overused among persons with autism spectrum disorders. *Research in Autism Spectrum Disorders, 9*, 34–37. http://dx.doi.org/10.1016/j.rasd.2014.10.006

Matson, J. L., & Kozlowski, A. M. (2011). The increasing prevalence of autism spectrum disorders. *Research in Autism Spectrum Disorders, 5*, 418–425. http://dx.doi.org/10.1016/j.rasd.2010.06.004

Matson, J. L., & Neal, D. (2009). Psychotropic medication use for challenging behaviors in persons with intellectual disabilities: An overview. *Research in Developmental Disabilities, 30*, 572–586. http://dx.doi.org/10.1016/j.ridd.2008.08.007

*Mayes, S. D. (2012). *Checklist for Autism Spectrum Disorder (CASD)*. Los Angeles, CA: Western Psychological Services.

McCracken, J. T., & Gandal, M. (2016). Psychopharmacology of autism spectrum disorder. In C. McDougle (Ed.), *Autism spectrum disorder* (pp. 275–300). New York, NY: Oxford University Press. http://dx.doi.org/10.1093/med/9780199349722.003.0016

McDougle, C. J., Naylor, S. T., Cohen, D. J., Volkmar, F. R., Heninger, G. R., & Price, L. H. (1996). A double-blind, placebo-controlled study of fluvoxamine in adults with autistic disorder. *Archives of General Psychiatry, 53*, 1001–1008. http://dx.doi.org/10.1001/archpsyc.1996.01830110037005

McDougle, C. J., Scahill, L., Aman, M. G., McCracken, J. T., Tierney, E., Davies, M., . . . Vitiello, B. (2005). Risperidone for the core symptom domains of autism: Results from the study by the autism network of the research units on pediatric psychopharmacology. *The American Journal of Psychiatry, 162*, 1142–1148. http://dx.doi.org/10.1176/appi.ajp.162.6.1142

McQuire, C., Hassiotis, A., Harrison, B., & Pilling, S. (2015). Pharmacological interventions for challenging behaviour in children with intellectual disabilities: A systematic review and meta-analysis. *BMC Psychiatry, 15*, 303. http://dx.doi.org/10.1186/s12888-015-0688-2

Miles, J. H. (2011). Autism spectrum disorders—a genetics review. *Genetics in Medicine, 13*, 278–294. http://dx.doi.org/10.1097/GIM.0b013e3181ff67ba

Mire, S. S., Raff, N. S., Brewton, C. M., & Goin-Kochel, R. P. (2015). Age-related trends in treatment use for children with autism spectrum disorder. *Research in Autism Spectrum Disorders, 15–16*, 29–41. http://dx.doi.org/10.1016/j.rasd.2015.03.001

Mohammadi, M. R., & Akhondzadeh, S. (2007). Autism spectrum disorders: Etiology and pharmacotherapy. *Current Drug Therapy, 2*, 97–103. http://dx.doi.org/10.2174/157488507780619095

Mohiuddin, S., & Ghaziuddin, M. (2013). Psychopharmacology of autism spectrum disorders: A selective review. *Autism: An International Journal of Research and Practice, 17*, 645–654. http://dx.doi.org/10.1177/1362361312453776

Moore, T. R., & Symons, F. J. (2009). Adherence to behavioral and medical treatment recommendations by parents of children with autism spectrum disorders. *Journal of Autism and Developmental Disorders, 39*, 1173–1184. http://dx.doi.org/10.1007/s10803-009-0729-0

Morgan, C. N., Roy, M., & Chance, P. (2003). Psychiatric comorbidity and medication use in autism: A community survey. *Psychiatric Bulletin, 27*, 378–381.

Möricke, E., Buitelaar, J. K., & Rommelse, N. N. J. (2016). Do we need multiple informants when assessing autistic traits? The degree of report bias on offspring, self, and spouse ratings. *Journal of Autism and Developmental Disorders, 46*, 164–175. http://dx.doi.org/10.1007/s10803-015-2562-y

Nadeau, J., Sulkowski, M. L., Ung, D., Wood, J. J., Lewin, A. B., Murphy, T. K., . . . Storch, E. A. (2011). Treatment of comorbid anxiety and autism spectrum disorders. *Neuropsychiatry, 1*, 567–578. http://dx.doi.org/10.2217/npy.11.62

Nagaraj, R., Singhi, P., & Malhi, P. (2006). Risperidone in children with autism: Randomized, placebo-controlled, double-blind study. *Journal of Child Neurology, 21*, 450–455. http://dx.doi.org/10.1177/08830738060210060801

Newcomer, L. L., & Lewis, T. J. (2004). Functional behavioral assessment: An investigation of assessment reliability and effectiveness of function-based interventions. *Journal of Emotional and Behavioral Disorders, 12*, 168–181. http://dx.doi.org/10.1177/10634266040120030401

Niederhofer, H., Damodharan, S. K., Joji, R., & Corfield, A. (2006). Atomoxetine treating patients with autistic disorder. *Autism: An International Journal of Research and Practice, 10*, 647–649. http://dx.doi.org/10.1177/1362361306073001

Ooi, Y. P., Weng, S.-J., Kossowsky, J., Gerger, H., & Sung, M. (2017). Oxytocin and autism spectrum disorders: A systematic review and meta-analysis of randomized controlled trials. *Pharmacopsychiatry, 50*(1), 5–13.

Pandina, G. J., Bossie, C. A., Youssef, E., Zhu, Y., & Dunbar, F. (2007). Risperidone improves behavioral symptoms in children with autism in a randomized, double-blind, placebo-controlled trial. *Journal of Autism and Developmental Disorders, 37*, 367–373. http://dx.doi.org/10.1007/s10803-006-0234-7

Parker, K. J., Oztan, O., Libove, R. A., Sumiyoshi, R. D., Jackson, L. P., Karhson, D. S., . . . Hardan, A. Y. (2017). Intranasal oxytocin treatment for social deficits and biomarkers of response in children with autism. *Proceedings of the National Academy of Sciences, 114*, 8119–8124. http://dx.doi.org/10.1073/pnas.1705521114

Pfiffner, L. J., & Haack, L. M. (2014). Behavior management for school-aged children with ADHD. *Child and Adolescent Psychiatric Clinics of North America, 23*, 731–746. http://dx.doi.org/10.1016/j.chc.2014.05.014

Poling, A., Ehrhardt, K., & Li, A. (2017). Psychotropic medications as treatments for people with autism spectrum disorder. In J. L. Matson (Ed.), *Handbook of treatments for autism spectrum disorder* (pp. 459–476). Cham, Switzerland: Springer. http://dx.doi.org/10.1007/978-3-319-61738-1_25

Reilly, C., & Gillberg, C. (2016). Epilepsy. In J. L. Matson (Ed.), *Comorbid conditions in individuals with intellectual disabilities* (pp. 195–286). Switzerland: Springer International Publishing. http://dx.doi.org/10.1007/978-3-319-19183-6_10

Research Units on Pediatric Psychopharmacology Autism Network. (2005). Randomized, controlled, crossover trial of methylphenidate in pervasive developmental disorders with hyperactivity. *Archives of General Psychiatry, 62,* 1266–1274. http://dx.doi.org/10.1001/archpsyc.62.11.1266

Rezaei, V., Mohammadi, M. R., Ghanizadeh, A., Sahraian, A., Tabrizi, M., Rezazadeh, S. A., & Akhondzadeh, S. (2010). Double-blind, placebo-controlled trial of risperidone plus topiramate in children with autistic disorder. *Progress in Neuro-Psychopharmacology & Biological Psychiatry, 34,* 1269–1272. http://dx.doi.org/10.1016/j.pnpbp.2010.07.005

Richdale, A. L., & Schreck, K. A. (2011). Assessment and intervention in autism: An historical perspective. In J. L. Matson (Ed.), *Clinical assessment and intervention for autism spectrum disorders* (pp. 3–24). Oxford, UK: Elsevier.

Robins, D. L., Adamson, L. B., Barton, M., Jr., Connell, J. E., Jr., Dumont-Mathieu, T., Dworkin, P. H., . . . Vivanti, G. (2016). Universal autism screening for toddlers: Recommendations at odds. *Journal of Autism and Developmental Disorders, 46,* 1880–1882. http://dx.doi.org/10.1007/s10803-016-2697-5

Robins, D. L., & Dumont-Mathieu, T. M. (2006). Early screening for autism spectrum disorders: Update on the Modified Checklist for Autism in Toddlers and other measures. *Journal of Developmental and Behavioral Pediatrics, 27*(2, Suppl.), S111–S119. http://dx.doi.org/10.1097/00004703-200604002-00009

*Robins, D. L., Fein, D., & Barton, M. (2009). *Modified Checklist for Autism in Toddlers, revised, with follow-up* (M-CHAT-R/F). Retrieved from http://www2.gsu.edu/~psydlr/M-CHAT/Official_M-CHAT_Website_files/M-CHAT-R_F.pdf

Rosenberg, R. E., Mandell, D. S., Farmer, J. E., Law, J. K., Marvin, A. R., & Law, P. A. (2010). Psychotropic medication use among children with autism spectrum disorders enrolled in a national registry, 2007–2008. *Journal of Autism and Developmental Disorders, 40,* 342–351. http://dx.doi.org/10.1007/s10803-009-0878-1

*Rutter, M., Bailey, A., & Lord, C. (2003). *The Social Communication Questionnaire.* Los Angeles, CA: Western Psychological Services.

*Rutter, M., Le Couteur, A., & Lord, C. (2003). *Autism Diagnostic Interview-Revised (ADI-R).* Los Angeles, CA: Western Psychological Services.

Scahill, L., McCracken, J. T., King, B. H., Rockhill, C., Shah, B., Politte, L., . . . McDougle, C. J. (2015).

Extended-release guanfacine for hyperactivity in children with autism spectrum disorder. *The American Journal of Psychiatry, 172,* 1197–1206. http://dx.doi.org/10.1176/appi.ajp.2015.15010055

*Schopler, E., Van Bourgondien, M. E., Wellman, G. J., & Love, S. R. (2010). *The Childhood Autism Rating Scale* (2nd ed.). Los Angeles, CA: Western Psychological Services.

Schubart, J. R., Camacho, F., & Leslie, D. (2014). Psychotropic medication trends among children and adolescents with autism spectrum disorder in the Medicaid program. *Autism: An International Journal of Research and Practice, 18,* 631–637. http://dx.doi.org/10.1177/1362361313497537

Shattuck, P. T., Durkin, M., Maenner, M., Newschaffer, C., Mandell, D. S., Wiggins, L., . . . Cuniff, C. (2009). Timing of identification among children with an autism spectrum disorder: Findings from a population-based surveillance study. *Journal of the American Academy of Child & Adolescent Psychiatry, 48,* 474–483. http://dx.doi.org/10.1097/CHI.0b013e31819b3848

Shattuck, P. T., Seltzer, M. M., Greenberg, J. S., Orsmond, G. I., Bolt, D., Kring, S., . . . Lord, C. (2007). Change in autism symptoms and maladaptive behaviors in adolescents and adults with an autism spectrum disorder. *Journal of Autism and Developmental Disorders, 37,* 1735–1747. http://dx.doi.org/10.1007/s10803-006-0307-7

Siegel, M. (2012). Psychopharmacology of autism spectrum disorder: Evidence and practice. *Child and Adolescent Psychiatric Clinics of North America, 21,* 957–973. http://dx.doi.org/10.1016/j.chc.2012.07.006

Siegel, M., Beresford, C. A., Bunker, M., Verdi, M., Vishnevetsky, D., Karlsson, C., . . . Smith, K. A. (2014). Preliminary investigation of lithium for mood disorder symptoms in children and adolescents with autism spectrum disorder. *Journal of Child and Adolescent Psychopharmacology, 24,* 399–402. http://dx.doi.org/10.1089/cap.2014.0019

Simonoff, E., Pickles, A., Charman, T., Chandler, S., Loucas, T., & Baird, G. (2008). Psychiatric disorders in children with autism spectrum disorders: Prevalence, comorbidity, and associated factors in a population-derived sample. *Journal of the American Academy of Child & Adolescent Psychiatry, 47,* 921–929. http://dx.doi.org/10.1097/CHI.0b013e318179964f

Siu, A. L., Bibbins-Domingo, K., Grossman, D. C., Baumann, L. C., Davidson, K. W., Ebell, M., . . . Pignone, M. P. (2016). Screening for autism spectrum disorder in young children: U.S. Preventive Services Task Force recommendation statement. *JAMA, 315,* 691–696. http://dx.doi.org/10.1001/jama.2016.0018

Soke, G. N., Maenner, M. J., Christensen, D., Kurzius-Spencer, M., & Schieve, L. A. (2018). Prevalence of co-occurring medical and behavioral conditions/symptoms among 4- and 8-year-old children with autism spectrum disorder in selected areas of the United States in 2010. *Journal of Autism and Developmental Disorders, 48*, 2663–2676. http://dx.doi.org/10.1007/s10803-018-3521-1

Spetie, L., & Arnold, L. E. (2007). Ethical issues in child psychopharmacology research and practice: Emphasis on preschoolers. *Psychopharmacology, 191*, 15–26. http://dx.doi.org/10.1007/s00213-006-0685-8

Sugai, G., Lewis-Palmer, T., & Hagan-Burke, S. (2000). Overview of the functional behavioral assessment process. *Exceptionality, 8*, 149–160. http://dx.doi.org/10.1207/S15327035EX0803_2

Sturmey, P. (2004). Cognitive therapy with people with intellectual disabilities: A selective review and critique. *Clinical Psychology & Psychotherapy, 11*, 222–232. http://dx.doi.org/10.1002/cpp.409

Szarkowski, A., Mood, D., Shield, A., Wiley, S., & Yoshinaga-Itano, C. (2014). A summary of current understanding regarding children with autism spectrum disorder who are deaf or hard of hearing. *Seminars in Speech and Language, 35*, 241–259. http://dx.doi.org/10.1055/s-0034-1389097

Taylor, B., Miller, E., Farrington, C. P., Petropoulos, M.-C., Favot-Mayaud, I., Li, J., & Waight, P. A. (1999). Autism and measles, mumps, and rubella vaccine: No epidemiological evidence for a causal association. *Lancet, 353*, 2026–2029. http://dx.doi.org/10.1016/S0140-6736(99)01239-8

Taylor, L. J. (2016). Psychopharmacologic intervention for adults with autism spectrum disorder: A systematic literature review. *Research in Autism Spectrum Disorders, 25*(Suppl. C), 58–75. http://dx.doi.org/10.1016/j.rasd.2016.01.011

Thomas, P., Zahorodny, W., Peng, B., Kim, S., Jani, N., Halperin, W., & Brimacombe, M. (2012). The association of autism diagnosis with socioeconomic status. *Autism: The International Journal of Research and Practice, 16*, 201–213. http://dx.doi.org/10.1177/1362361311413397

Tidmarsh, L., & Volkmar, F. R. (2003). Diagnosis and epidemiology of autism spectrum disorders. *The Canadian Journal of Psychiatry, 48*, 517–525. http://dx.doi.org/10.1177/070674370304800803

Tsai, L. Y. (2014). Prevalence of comorbid psychiatric disorders in children and adolescents with autism spectrum disorder. *Journal of Experimental and Clinical Medicine, 6*, 179–186. http://dx.doi.org/10.1016/j.jecm.2014.10.005

Tuchman, R. (2000). Treatment of seizure disorders and EEG abnormalities in children with autism spectrum

disorders. *Journal of Autism and Developmental Disorders, 30*, 485–489. http://dx.doi.org/10.1023/A:1005572128200

Virués-Ortega, J. (2010). Applied behavior analytic intervention for autism in early childhood: Meta-analysis, meta-regression and dose-response meta-analysis of multiple outcomes. *Clinical Psychology Review, 30*, 387–399. http://dx.doi.org/10.1016/j.cpr.2010.01.008

Virues-Ortega, J., Rodríguez, V., & Yu, C. T. (2013). Prediction of treatment outcomes and longitudinal analysis in children with autism undergoing intensive behavioral intervention. *International Journal of Clinical and Health Psychology, 13*, 91–100. http://dx.doi.org/10.1016/S1697-2600(13)70012-7

Volkmar, F. R., Lord, C., Bailey, A., Schultz, R. T., & Klin, A. (2004). Autism and pervasive developmental disorders. *Journal of Child Psychology and Psychiatry, 45*, 135–170. http://dx.doi.org/10.1046/j.0021-9630.2003.00317.x

Williams, K., Brignell, A., Randall, M., Silove, N., & Hazell, P. (2013). Selective serotonin reuptake inhibitors (SSRIs) for autism spectrum disorders (ASD). *Cochrane Database of Systematic Reviews, 8*, CD004677. http://dx.doi.org/10.1002/14651858.CD004677.pub3

Williamson, E. D., & Martin, A. (2012). Psychotropic medications in autism: Practical considerations for parents. *Journal of Autism and Developmental Disorders, 42*, 1249–1255. http://dx.doi.org/10.1007/s10803-010-1144-2

Winblad, B. (2005). Piracetam: A review of pharmacological properties and clinical uses. *CNS Drug Reviews, 11*, 169–182. http://dx.doi.org/10.1111/j.1527-3458.2005.tb00268.x

*Wing, L., Leekam, S. R., Libby, S. J., Gould, J., & Larcombe, M. (2002). The Diagnostic Interview for Social and Communication Disorders: Background, inter-rater reliability and clinical use. *Journal of Child Psychology and Psychiatry, 43*, 307–325. http://dx.doi.org/10.1111/1469-7610.00023

Wink, L. K., Pedapati, E. V., Adams, R., Erickson, C. A., Pedersen, K. A., Morrow, E. M., . . . Siegel, M. (2017a). Characterization of medication use in a multicenter sample of pediatric inpatients with autism spectrum disorder. *Journal of Autism and Developmental Disorders, 48*, 3711–3719. http://dx.doi.org/10.1007/s10803-017-3153-x

Wink, L. K., Pedapati, E. V., Horn, P. S., McDougle, C. J., & Erickson, C. A. (2017b). Multiple antipsychotic medication use in autism spectrum disorder. *Journal of Child and Adolescent Psychopharmacology, 27*, 91–94. http://dx.doi.org/10.1089/cap.2015.0123

Wong, A. Y. S., Hsia, Y., Chan, E. W., Murphy, D. G. M., Simonoff, E., Buitelaar, J. K., & Wong, I. C. K. (2014). The variation of psychopharmacological prescription rates for people with autism spectrum disorder (ASD) in 30 countries. *Autism Research, 7,* 543–554. http://dx.doi.org/10.1002/aur.1391

World Health Organization. (1992). *The ICD–10 classification of mental and behavioural disorders: Clinical descriptions and diagnostic guidelines.* Geneva, Switzerland: Author.

World Health Organization. (2005). *Improving access and use of psychotropic medicines. Mental health policy and service guidance package.* Geneva, Switzerland: Author.

Zafeiriou, D. I., Ververi, A., & Vargiami, E. (2007). Childhood autism and associated comorbidities. *Brain & Development, 29,* 257–272. http://dx.doi.org/10.1016/j.braindev.2006.09.003

Zwaigenbaum, L., Bauman, M. L., Fein, D., Pierce, K., Buie, T., Davis, P. A., . . . Wagner, S. (2015). Early screening of autism spectrum disorder: Recommendations for practice and research. *Pediatrics, 136*(Suppl. 1), S41–S59. http://dx.doi.org/10.1542/peds.2014-3667D

CHAPTER 18

PHARMACOLOGICAL TREATMENT OF NEUROCOGNITIVE DISORDERS

Alfredo Carlo Altamura, Matteo Lazzaretti, Andrea Arighi,
Alessandro Pigoni, Elio Scarpini, and Paolo Brambilla

Behavioral or psychiatric symptoms are quite common in several neurological conditions, such as dementias and neurodegenerative disorders (Kales, Gitlin, & Lyketsos, 2015). These symptoms may include depression, apathy, repetitive questioning, agitation, psychosis, aggression, sleep problems, wandering, and a variety of socially inappropriate behaviors, such as personality changes and disinhibition (Lyketsos et al., 2011).

This variegate symptomatology is often referred as *behavioral and psychological symptoms of dementia* (BPSD), and it represents a major concern in health care (Kales et al., 2015). These symptoms are among the most complex, stressful, and costly aspects of care, not only for patients but also for caregivers.

Psychiatric symptoms may be present not only in the last phases of neurodegenerative disorders but also in the early stages or at onset (Grau-Rivera, Gelpi, Carballido-López, Sánchez-Valle, & López-Villegas, 2015). Diagnosis and treatment of psychiatric symptoms in dementia may present many problems, as we review in this chapter, exemplifying the difficulties clinicians confront in dealing with such a fragile population. The treatment of these conditions represents a major issue of concern and should be guided by a multidisciplinary endeavor, including pharmacological and nonpharmacological interventions. In this chapter we review diagnostic and therapeutic issues regarding BPSD in the most common neurodegenerative disorders.

EPIDEMIOLOGY AND PREVALENCE

Alzheimer's Disease

Alzheimer's disease (AD) is the most frequent cause of dementia worldwide, accounting for approximately 70% of diagnoses of dementia, and it is one of the great health care challenges of the century, associated with an estimated health care cost of $172 billion per year in the United States only (Scheltens et al., 2016). The incidence rate for dementia increases exponentially with age, with the most pronounced increase occurring during the 7th and 8th decades of life. Individuals from Western countries (North America and Western Europe) exhibit the highest prevalence and incidence of dementia, followed by Latin America and China (Reitz & Mayeux, 2014). Based on its age of onset, AD is classified into early onset AD (onset < 65 years), accounting for 1% to 5% of all cases, and late-onset AD (onset ≥ 65 years), accounting for greater than 95% of affected individuals (Reitz & Mayeux, 2014).

Frontotemporal Dementia

Frontotemporal dementia (FTD) is an insidious neurodegenerative clinical syndrome observed among the elderly. FTD comprises a heterogeneous group of syndromes caused by progressive and selective degeneration of the frontal lobes and/or temporal lobes, with relative preservation of the posterior regions of the brain. This focal neurodegeneration

P. B. was partially supported by grants funded by the Italian Ministry of Health (RF-2016-02364582).

http://dx.doi.org/10.1037/0000133-018
APA Handbook of Psychopharmacology, S. M. Evans (Editor-in-Chief)

in the anterior areas of the brain leads to disorders of behavior, language, and executive function (Pressman & Miller, 2014). FTD is considered the third most common form of dementia across all age groups, with a prevalence ranging from 3% to 26%, but it is the leading cause of early-onset dementia (Vieira et al., 2013). FTD is commonly clinically divided into three distinct clinical syndromes: behavioral variant frontotemporal degeneration (bvFTD) and two primary progressive aphasias, semantic variant primary progressive aphasia and a nonfluent variant primary progressive aphasia (Bang, Spina, & Miller, 2015). bvFTD is the most common variant and displays the earliest onset, with a mean age at presentation of approximately 58 years (Pressman & Miller, 2014).

Parkinson's Disease

Parkinson's disease (PD) is one of the most common and complex neurological disorders in the elderly population. Classically, it is characterized by evidence for a movement disorder, such as tremor, rigidity, and bradykinesia (i.e., a slowness of movements); however, clinical management requires attention beyond its motor features, given the fact that the vast majority of the patients experience various and polymorph nonmotor symptoms as well (Kalia & Lang, 2015). PD is a neurodegenerative disease characterized by early death of dopaminergic neurons in the substantia nigra pars compacta. PD is recognized as the most common neurodegenerative disorder after AD, with a prevalence higher in Western developed regions, such as Europe, North America, and South America (Dorsey et al., 2007). The incidence ranges from 10 to 18 per 100,000 person-years, and increases nearly exponentially with age, with a peak around 80 years of age (Van Den Eeden et al., 2003). Males are usually more affected than females, with a ratio of approximately 3:2.

Huntington's Disease

Huntington's disease (HD) is an inherited disorder devastating to patients and their families, involving autosomal dominant inheritance (MacDonald & The Huntington's Disease Collaborative Research Group, 1993). This disorder usually shows an onset in the prime of adult life and is characterized by

a progressive course (Bates et al., 2015). HD is a neurodegenerative clinical syndrome that leads to impairment in behavior, emotion, judgment, and cognition (Bates et al., 2015). The worldwide prevalence of this illness is 5 to 10 cases per 100,000 persons, with 30,000 people affected in the United States and Canada (Dayalu & Albin, 2015). There are gross differences in the prevalence of HD by ancestry; the highest rate of the disease is in populations of European descent (Kay, Hayden, & Leavitt, 2017), with an estimated prevalence in the United Kingdom of 12.3 per 100,000 persons in the year 2010.

DIAGNOSING NEUROCOGNITIVE DISORDERS

Alzheimer's Disease

The typical clinical presentation of AD accounts for memory impairment and spatial disorientation interfering with daily life activities. However, atypical presentations are also possible, including language, visual, and executive problems appearing before—and being more pronounced than—memory deficits. For this reason, the presence of memory impairment is no longer a requirement for diagnosis, which is currently based on clinical history and neuropsychological testing, supported by biomarker evidence (Lyketsos et al., 2011). Clinical diagnosis of any dementia syndrome depends on taking a history from the patient and family members, neuropsychological testing, and assessment of symptoms over time. Tests commonly used for AD evaluate global cognition, such as the Mini Mental State Examination (MMSE) or the Montreal Cognitive Assessment (MoCA; Costa et al., 2017). Memory remains one of the most impaired domains that can be assessed through specific tests, such as the Free and Cued Selective Reminding Test (FCSRT). Other memory tests, particularly those based on list learning and delayed recall, can also be effective in identification of the amnestic syndrome of AD. These tests include different versions of the paired-associate learning and the Rey auditory verbal learning tasks. Other promising neuropsychological tests to detect the amnestic impairments that are specific to early pathological involvement of the entorhinal–perirhinal cortex include the Delayed Matching to Sample (DMS), a visual recognition test that is correlated with an AD pattern in patients with mild cognitive impairment (Costa et al., 2017). Atypical variants, however, may need different tests to be fully assessed, such as evaluation of impairment in the visual identification of objects, symbols, words, or faces in the occipito-temporal variant (Costa et al., 2017). One of the most well-known measures is the Visual Object and Space Perception Battery (VOSP; Quental, Brucki, & Bueno, 2013).

The key pathological changes observed in the brain of a person with AD are extracellular deposits of amyloid-β (Aβ) peptide in neuritic plaques, and hyperphosphorylated tau protein, a microtubule assembly protein accumulating inside the neurons as neurofibrillary tangles. The first set of diagnostic criteria previously took into account only clinical symptoms. Currently, with new cerebrospinal fluid (CSF) analysis and the advent of advanced brain imaging techniques, more accurate criteria have been proposed (Dubois et al., 2014). A long predementia stage is now well known and described, when supported by biomarkers suggesting the presence of amyloid and neurodegeneration. These biomarkers are used to attribute the likelihood of an AD diagnosis to the clinical syndrome. Core CSF biomarkers for AD are Aβ42, which shows the amount of amyloid deposition; total tau (t-tau), which reflects the intensity of neurodegeneration; and phosphorylated tau (p-tau), which correlates with neurofibrillary pathological changes (Blennow, Hampel, Weiner, & Zetterberg, 2010). Another clinically available pathophysiological biomarker is positron emission tomography (PET) with ligands for Aβ amyloid. However, brain amyloidosis is a necessary but not sufficient condition for diagnosis of AD; therefore, amyloid PET presents currently a high negative predictive value and just a moderate positive predictive value, given that up to 35% of cognitively healthy elderly people may have positive amyloid PET scans.

Moreover, neuroimaging has a key role in the topographical definition of brain damage in suspected AD. Magnetic resonance imaging (MRI) is the assessment of choice. Hippocampal atrophy represents the most common and more specific finding, often associated with medial temporal atrophy (Kehoe, McNulty, Mullins, & Bokde, 2014). In addition, 18-fluorodeoxyglucose PET (FDG-PET) obtained a great relevance in the diagnostic workout of AD, with a pattern of reduced temporoparietal and posterior cingulate intake (Dukart et al., 2013).

With regard to symptomatology, cognition is not the only domain affected by AD; mood and behavior might also be involved. Most AD patients, indeed, develop BPSD during the course of the illness, often including agitation, apathy, depression, and psychosis (particularly delusions). BPSD are considered to represent a core feature of the disease (Lyketsos et al., 2011). BPSD may occur at any time of the disease but generally become more prominent as dementia severity, along with brain damage, increases. An easy method to assess these symptoms is the Neuropsychiatric Inventory Questionnaire (NPI-Q), which is often used to diagnose and follow up on BPSD. A limited but growing amount of evidence, based on more precise neuroimaging and neurochemistry methods, has led to a better understanding about brain mechanisms underlying BPSD in AD. Although far from conclusive, the results from using these methods might be of great help in understanding brain circuits and consequently tailoring new treatment approaches.

Agitation is one of the most problematic behaviors for patients and caregivers. Even though there is no complete concordance between the results, agitation was consistently associated with loss of grey matter volume in several specific brain regions, including the frontal and anterior cingulate cortices, posterior cingulate cortex (PCC), insula, amygdala, and hippocampus (Hu et al., 2015). Apathy is another common symptom of AD and involves lack of initiative and motivation as well as emotional blunting as core symptoms (Rosenberg et al., 2015). Neuroimaging studies of apathy reported a substantial association with damage to the anterior cingulate cortex, as evidenced by altered perfusion and decrease of gray matter and white matter integrity. Overall, all of these anatomical and functional abnormalities have been found to be associated with increased global amyloid burden and neurofibrillary tangles (Marshall et al., 2013), underlying a more severe course of the disease.

Many genes have been implicated in the pathogenesis of AD. The APOE4 allele is considered the major genetic risk factor for AD and is the most studied (Wood, 2017). APOE is a lipid-binding protein and is expressed in humans as three common isoforms coded for by three alleles. Lifetime risk for AD is more than 50% for APOE4 homozygotes and 20% to 30% for APOE3 and APOE4 heterozygotes. APOE4 contributes to sporadic late onset AD. By contrast, early onset AD has been firmly associated with three genes, namely β-amyloid precursor protein (APP), presenilin 1 (PSEN1), and presenilin 2 (PSEN2). AD-linked mutations in these three genes exhibit high penetrance (>85%), are mostly autosomal dominantly inherited, and lead with certainty to Aβ aggregation and early onset of disease (Reitz & Mayeux, 2014).

Frontotemporal Dementia

Clinical presentation might be widely heterogeneous and may resemble psychiatric disorders, which are often misdiagnosed at the onset of FTD. Behavioral disinhibition is a classic hallmark of bvFTD and often the first symptom presented. Patients can behave contrary to social norms; they may inappropriately touch or behave aggressively toward strangers or even engage in criminal behaviors. Often, this behavioral alteration correlates with atrophy in various brain regions associated with evaluation of potential outcomes from future actions and rewards (Rosen et al., 2005). A common and pervasive initial symptom is apathy, which refers to a general passivity and lack of motivation to pursue previously rewarding activities (Manoochehri & Huey, 2012). This might progress to mutism and immobility in the end stages of the disease and is correlated with dysfunction of brain networks that involve the right anterior cingulate and caudate (Rosen et al., 2005). Early in the disease course, patients can lose the ability to respond to the emotional expressions and needs of others and can be distant, cold, and indifferent. Loss of empathy is correlated with atrophy in the right anterior temporal and medial frontal regions, while an impaired recognition of emotions is associated with gray matter volume

loss in the right lateral inferior temporal and right middle temporal gyri (Rosen et al., 2005). Patients affected by bvFTD often present ritualistic behaviors including counting rituals, hoarding objects, and wandering fixed routes. Moreover, they often change dietary habits, showing hyperorality, developing a strong preference for sweets and carbohydrates, or eating beyond the point of satiety (Manoochehri & Huey, 2012). One of the most widely used neuropsychological exams for FTD is the Frontal Behavioral Inventory, which assesses changes in personality and behavior, such as apathy, judgment, inflexibility, and disinhibition (Ryan et al., 2017). Others useful tools to evaluate neuropsychiatric alterations are the NPI-Q and the Memory Complaint Questionnaire (MAC-Q), which assess age-related memory decline, and the Blessed Dementia Rating Scale, which is a measure of general functioning (Ryan et al., 2017).

In addition, patients affected by bvFTD often present changes within the language domain, including stereotyped speech and echolalia (repetition of words spoken by another person; Pressman & Miller, 2014). These changes represent a disruption of dominant lobar language networks. Neuropsychological assessment in these individuals frequently reveals deficits in executive dysfunction. These domains could be explored using several neuropsychiatric tests, such as the Wisconsin Card Sorting Test (WCST), the total time from the Trail Making Test Part B (TMT-B), or the number of words generated on the Controlled Oral Word Association Test (COWA; Ryan et al., 2017). The assessment of language alterations and impairment requires, therefore, specific measures, and the most widely used are the Peabody Picture Vocabulary Test—Fourth Edition (PPVT-4), the Northwestern Anagram Test (NAT), the Boston Naming Test, the Boston Diagnostic Aphasia Examination, and the Western Aphasia Battery repetition subtest (Mesulam et al., 2009). These tests proved very useful in diagnosing and subtyping aphasias. Although memory can be better preserved in FTD compared with AD, episodic memory may be impaired even in early stages of the disease. By contrast, drawing and other visuospatial functions are often remarkably spared in all of the FTD clinical subtypes. All of these clinical features are included in the criteria for the diagnosis of bvFTD (Rascovsky et al., 2011).

bvFTD presents an MRI pattern of selective atrophy of the anterior regions of the brain, which include the orbitofrontal, anterior cingulate, anterior insular, and anterior temporal cortices, particularly within the right hemisphere. Functional neuroimaging studies such as FDG-PET might be more sensitive than MRI in early stages and show hypometabolism of the frontal, anterior cingulate, and anterior temporal regions in FTD, in contrast to temporoparietal and posterior cingulate hypometabolism in AD (Pressman & Miller, 2014).

Like many neurodegenerative diseases, bvFTD is characterized by the accumulation of abnormal protein deposits (Bang et al., 2015). Tau proteins normally maintain the correct microtubular structure. Mutations in the microtubule-associated protein tau (MAPT) gene have been detected in more than 30% of patients with FTD (Bang et al., 2015).

The two more common genetic mutations associated with another protein (TDP-43) involved in pathology are progranulin and C9orf72. Mutations in the progranulin gene (GRN) accounted for approximately 8% of all familial forms of FTD, while mutations in C9orf72 may account for up to 20% of familial cases (Pressman & Miller, 2014).

Parkinson's Disease

The classical motor symptoms of PD were described more than 200 years ago, and include bradykinesia, muscular rigidity, rest tremor, and postural and gait impairment (Kalia & Lang, 2015). Motor features in patients tend to be heterogeneous and are usually classified into two subgroups: the first with tremor-dominant features and relative absence of other motor symptoms, and the non–tremor-dominant subtype, which includes phenotypes such as akinetic-rigid syndrome and postural instability gait disorder. Moreover, the tremor-dominant subtype is usually characterized by a slower progression and lower impairment.

Additionally, many patients, over the course of the disease, experience nonmotor symptoms such as impaired olfaction; constipation; rapid eye movement sleep behavior disorder; and several neuropsychiatric disturbances, including depression, mood disorders, anxiety, sleep disturbances, psychosis, and behavioral and cognitive alterations. These symptoms are common in the early phases of the disease and are associated with reduced quality of life for patients and for caregivers. Nonmotor features are also frequently present long before the onset of the classical motor symptoms and constitute a premotor or prodromal phase that can last up to 12 to 14 years before the clinical onset of tremors and classical motor features.

Cognitive alterations are also common in the course of PD. Cognitive decline and dementia occur in more than 80% of patients with a 20-year disease duration (Kalia & Lang, 2015). Executive function, memory, and visuospatial abilities seem to be the most involved domains and might also be affected in the early stages of the disease.

Among nonmotor features, depression is one of the most common, even though depressive disturbances are often underrecognized and undertreated (Marsh, 2013). The prevalence of depression in patients affected by PD ranges between 40% and 50%. Subsyndromal depression (i.e., a state of altered and depressed mood that does not fully meet *Diagnostic and Statistical Manual of Mental Disorders* criteria for a depressive episode) is also common and might have a great impact on patients' quality of life. The likelihood of an episode of depression is greater in the immediate premotor years before the clinical diagnosis of PD, providing evidence that the neurodegenerative process contributes to prodromal mood disturbances (Marsh, 2013).

Apart from dopaminergic deficits in the substantia nigra pars compacta, it is well known that in PD, neurological disease involves other brain areas and loss of noradrenergic and serotonergic neurons as well. A prevailing model for the development of depression in PD proposes that degeneration of mesocortical and mesolimbic dopaminergic neurons causes orbitofrontal dysfunction, which leads to serotonergic alterations in the dorsal raphe and consequently to dysfunction of the depression-related orbitofrontal basal ganglia-thalamic network (Hu et al., 2015).

Although the gold standard is neuropathological assessment, the diagnosis of PD is still usually made based on clinical criteria. The most widely used assessment is the Unified Parkinson's Disease Rating Scale, which proved useful for both diagnosis and follow-up. It is composed of six parts, which assess respectively: (a) evaluation of mentation, behavior, and mood; (b) self-evaluation of daily life activities including speech, swallowing, handwriting, dressing, hygiene, falling, salivating, turning in bed, walking, and cutting food; (c) clinician-scored, monitored motor evaluation; (d) complications; (e) staging of severity of PD and prognosis; and (f) disability. Strategies to develop biomarkers for the diagnosis are under investigation, especially to assess the early stages of the disease. Candidate imaging markers include single photon emission computed tomography methods to measure reduction in substantia nigra dopaminergic neurons. These imaging techniques may be very helpful in differentiating PD from other disorders.

As already mentioned, the crucial pathological feature of PD is loss of dopaminergic neurons within the substantia nigra pars compact first and later in other brain regions. Another hallmark of PD is aggregation of abnormally folded proteins, as in many other neurodegenerative disorders. The protein involved in PD pathology is α-synuclein. When misfolded, α-synuclein becomes insoluble and aggregates to form intracellular inclusions within the cell body (Lewy bodies) and processes (Lewy neurites) of neurons (Kalia & Lang, 2015). α-synuclein is coded by the SNCA gene, which is found mutated in a form of monogenic, autosomal dominant parkinsonism. However, the most common causes of genetically inherited parkinsonism are mutations in leucine-rich repeat kinase 2 (LRRK2) and parkin protein, which are responsible for a dominant and a recessive form of PD, respectively. In sporadic PD, the greatest genetic risk factor associated with the illness is mutation in the GBA gene, which provides instructions for making an enzyme involved in lysosomes function. Changes in this gene may contribute to the faulty breakdown of toxic substances in cells, leading to a formation of abnormal protein deposits, which could potentially kill dopamine-producing nerve cells.

Huntington's Disease

Although the first description of an inherited cause for chorea was put forward in 1832, George Huntington provided an accurate and complete description in 1872. HD is caused by a CAG repeat expansion in the huntingtin (HTT) gene on chromosome 4, and the age of HD onset is inversely correlated with the length of the expansion (Ross et al., 2014). The genetic defect causes progressive atrophy of the striatum, the cortex, and extrastriatal structures. Initially, atrophy is selective for the caudate and putamen; in late stages, the atrophy becomes less selective, involving the whole brain, with the exception of the cerebellum.

The clinical course of HD can be divided into premanifest and manifest periods (Ross et al., 2014), although it has been proposed that *prediagnostic HD* may be a more appropriate term, considering that this population includes those that have subtle clinical features and asymptomatic individuals with CAG-expanded HTT (Sturrock & Leavitt, 2010). At clinical examination, common findings in premanifest HD individuals may include subtle oculomotor abnormalities, including a reduction or slowing of normal lateral eye movements (Sturrock & Leavitt, 2010). Classically, the onset of the illness (Huntington Study Group, 1996) is defined as the point when a patient who carries a CAG-expanded HTT allele develops an otherwise unexplained extrapyramidal movement disorder: chorea, a pathology very common in HD, usually involving rapid, rotatory, involuntary, and afinalistic (or dystonic) bradykinesia and rigidity, similarly to that found in individuals with PD (Liu et al., 2015).

The motor disorder of HD can be divided into involuntary and voluntary movement disorders (Bates et al., 2015). Chorea is a type of involuntary movement (from the Greek *choreia*, to dance) involving rapid, irregular, and jerky motion of the limbs, trunk, and face, giving HD its characteristic clinical appearance. Dystonic movements or postures can also occur. The voluntary movement disorders include incoordination, bradykinesia, and rigidity (Bates et al., 2015). This impairment is inexorably progressive, leading to a nonambulatory condition and severe dysarthria and dysphagia (alteration in normal swallowing and speaking due to motor abnormalities of oropharyngeal muscles). In advanced illness, patients are akinetic (they cannot move, or can only perform small, slow movements) and mute.

Patients suffering from HD frequently show cognitive or affective symptoms decades before manifesting motor signs (Paulsen et al., 2008). Cognitive impairment in HD includes slowness of thought and deterioration of complex intellectual functions, with patients often lacking awareness of their disabilities. HD should be considered a subcortical dementia, with principal impairment in executive function, abstract thinking, and working memory; aphasia, agnosia, and apraxia (i.e., difficulty in accomplishing fine movements) are uncommon.

The Unified Huntington's Disease Rating Scale (UHDRS) is a widely used clinical and research tool for the assessment of HD, developed by the Huntington Study Group (Liu et al., 2015). It is divided into six different domains that evaluate motor signs, cognitive symptoms, behavioral alterations, independence from caregivers, functional components, and total functional capacity. Cognitive symptoms could be further assessed with test battery-timed tasks such as the Stroop test, the Trail Making Test, the Symbol Digit Modalities Test, and verbal fluency tests, as well as memory tests such as list learning and tests of emotion recognition such as the Ekman 60 Faces Test (Snowden, 2017).

Psychiatric symptoms are a significant aspect of HD and symptoms also increase with progression of disease severity (Epping et al., 2016). The psychiatric symptoms of HD are the most variable aspect of the HD clinical phenotype (Sturrock & Leavitt, 2010); their behavioral correlates are protean, leading to a sort of organic personality disorder. Depression occurs in 40% of patients, but symptoms like irritability and impulsivity are the most common psychiatric features (Epping et al., 2016) and are associated with white matter changes. Obsessive compulsive and aggressive behaviors can also occur. Psychosis, mania, anxiety, and substance abuse are also seen in some patients (Epping et al., 2016).

EVIDENCE-BASED PHARMACOLOGICAL TREATMENT OF NEUROCOGNITIVE DISORDERS

In this section, we discuss pharmacological treatments for AD, HD, PD, and FTD. Table 18.1 presents a complete review of randomized controlled trials (RCTs) for each of the four neurocognitive disorders.

Alzheimer's Disease

It has been suggested that neuropsychiatric symptoms, rather than cognitive dysfunction, impose the greatest burden on family caregivers and predict caregivers' decisions to institutionalize patients with dementia (Chen et al., 2017). Therefore, efficacious treatment of neuropsychiatric symptoms could have a tremendous impact not only on patients' quality of life but also on caregivers and society. Most of the medications approved for AD by the Food and Drug Administration (FDA), while helping in slowing the progression of the disease, did not prove efficacy in assessing neuropsychiatric and behavioral symptoms. In recent years, both nonpharmacological and pharmacological approaches have been proposed and tested, with often discouraging results.

Memantine, an N-methyl-D-aspartate receptor antagonist, has been approved by the FDA for the treatment of moderate to severe AD (Matsunaga, Kishi, & Iwata, 2015). No significant behavioral benefit was observed in trials assessing the efficacies of such compounds, despite great heterogeneity in the samples assessed (Wang, Yu, Wang, et al., 2015). Memantine has been associated with dizziness, headache, confusion, and constipation, and therefore should be used carefully. Concerning antipsychotics, conventional agents with high potency D2 antagonisms demonstrated low or no efficacy in RCTs (Kales et al., 2015). Haloperidol may have a slight benefit for reducing aggression and agitation, but it is as of yet unclear whether this positive result outweighs its adverse effects (especially extrapyramidal symptoms). Instead, atypical antipsychotics have demonstrated some efficacy in the management of several BPSD in RCTs. The Clinical Antipsychotic Trials of Intervention Effectiveness-Alzheimer's disease trial (CATIE-AD) showed that risperidone and olanzapine proved

TABLE 18.1

Overview of Clinical Trials for the Psychopharmacological Management of Psychiatric Symptoms in Neurodegenerative Disorders

Author	Design	Drug assessed	Sample (M/F)	Results
			Alzheimer's disease	
Ballard et al., 2005	RCT, placebo controlled	quetiapine, rivastigmine	93 (19/74)	Neither quetiapine nor rivastigmine resulted effective in the treatment of agitation measured by CMAI. Compared with placebo, quetiapine was associated with significantly greater cognitive decline.
Brodaty et al., 2005	RCT, placebo controlled	risperidone	93 (14/79)	Risperidone reduced psychosis and improved global functioning in moderate-to-severe AD and MD, assessed by the BEHAVE-AD psychosis subscale.
Carotenuto et al., 2017	RCT, placebo controlled	donepezil plus choline alphoscerate or placebo	113 (43/70)	Significant decrease of distress of the caregiver and mood disorders, as assessed by NPI, in patients treated with donepezil and choline alphoscerate.
De Deyn et al., 2004	RCT, placebo controlled	olanzapine at different doses	652 (163/489)	Olanzapine at 7.5 mg/day significantly decreased psychosis and overall behavioral disturbances in NPI-NH Psychosis Total scores (sum of Delusions and Hallucinations items = primary efficacy measure).
De Deyn et al., 2005	RCT, placebo controlled	risperidone	1155 (381/774)	Improvement in aggression and psychosis, measured by the CMAI and BEHAVE-AD total and subscales.
Finkel et al., 2004	RCT, placebo controlled	sertraline	244 (100/144)	There were no statistically significant differences at endpoint. However, a linear mixed model analysis found modest but statistically significantly greater improvements in the CGI-I score in the sertraline group.
Leonpacher et al., 2016	RCT, placebo controlled	citalopram	186 (not reported)	Participants treated with citalopram were significantly less likely to be reported as showing delusions, anxiety, and irritability/lability, assessed by the NPI.
Lyketsos et al., 2003	RCT, placebo controlled	sertraline	44 (14/30)	Sertraline superior to placebo for the treatment of major depression in AD, measured by The Cornell Scale for Depression in Dementia and the HDRS. Depression reduction was accompanied by less behavior disturbance and improved activities.
Mintzer et al., 2006	RCT, placebo controlled	risperidone	416 (101/315)	Both groups improved; no differences between treatment and placebo. Measures assessed by scores on the BEHAVE-AD Psychosis subscale and CGI-C.
Mintzer et al., 2007	RCT, placebo controlled	aripiprazole	487 (104/383)	Significantly improved psychotic symptoms, agitation, and clinical global impression, measured by NPI-NH version Psychosis Subscale score.
Olin, Fox, Pawluczyk, Taggart, and Schneider, 2001	RCT, placebo controlled	carbamazepine	21 (not reported)	Improvement for the carbamazepine group on the CGI-C and the BPRS Hostility item, with a trend toward worsening on the BPRS Hallucination item.
Porsteinsson et al., 2014	RCT, placebo controlled	citalopram	186 (103/85)	Citalopram compared with placebo significantly reduced agitation and caregiver distress, as assessed by the 18-point Neurobehavioral Rating Scale agitation subscale and the modified Alzheimer's Disease Cooperative Study-Clinical Global Impression of Change.

TABLE 18.1

Overview of Clinical Trials for the Psychopharmacological Management of Psychiatric Symptoms in Neurodegenerative Disorders (*Continued*)

Author	Design	Drug assessed	Sample (M/F)	Results
Schneider et al., 2006	RCT, placebo controlled	risperidone, olanzapine, quetiapine	421 (186/235)	No significant differences were noted among the groups with regard to improvement on the CGI-C scale.
Streim et al., 2008	RCT, placebo controlled	aripiprazole	256 (61/195)	No benefits for the treatment of psychotic symptoms; but improvement in agitation, anxiety, and depression. Measures were obtained from the NPI-NH Psychosis score.
Sultzer et al., 2008	RCT, placebo controlled	olanzapine, quetiapine, risperidone	421(not reported)	Greater improvement with olanzapine or risperidone on the NPI total score, risperidone on the CGI-C, olanzapine and risperidone on the BPRS hostile suspiciousness factor, and risperidone on the BPRS psychosis factor. There was worsening with olanzapine on the BPRS withdrawn depression factor.
Frontotemporal dementia				
Deakin, Rahman, Nestor, Hodges, and Sahakian, 2004	RCT, placebo controlled	paroxetine	10 (7/3)	No significant differences on BPSD, assessed by the NPI and the Cambridge Behavioral Inventory. Paroxetine caused a decrease in accuracy on the paired associates learning task, reversal learning, and a delayed pattern recognition task.
Huey, Garcia, Wassermann, Tierney, and Grafman, 2008	RCT	quetiapine vs dextroamphetamine	8 (not reported)	Treatment with dextroamphetamine improved behavioral symptoms; quetiapine did not. Measures were obtained from the NPI and the Repeatable Battery for the Assessment of Neuropsychological Status.
Jesso et al., 2011	RCT, placebo controlled	oxytocin	20 (not reported)	Improvements in NPI, compared with baseline, via small reductions across multiple items and reduced identification of negative facial expressions, a possible sign of improved cooperative behavior.
Lebert, Stekke, Hasenbroekx, and Pasquier, 2004	RCT	trazodone	31 (15/16)	Significant decrease in the NPI total score compared with baseline.
Parkinson's disease (PD)				
Antonini et al., 2006	RCT	amitriptyline, sertraline	31(not reported)	Both drugs significantly reduced the HDRS score.
Barone et al., 2006	RCT	sertraline, pramipexole	67 (35/32)	The proportion of patients who recovered was significantly higher in the pramipexole group compared with the sertraline group, as defined by the HDRS.
Barone et al., 2010	RCT, placebo controlled	pramipexole	267 (180/97)	Pramipexole improved depressive symptoms compared with placebo in patients with PD, measured with the Beck Depression Inventory.
Devos et al., 2008	RCT, placebo controlled	citalopram, desipramine	48 (21/27)	Desipramine improved depression based on the MADRS score, compared with citalopram and placebo.

(*continues*)

TABLE 18.1

Overview of Clinical Trials for the Psychopharmacological Management of Psychiatric Symptoms in Neurodegenerative Disorders (*Continued*)

Author	Design	Drug assessed	Sample (M/F)	Results
Leentjens, Vreeling, Luijckx, and Verhey, 2003	RCT, placebo controlled	sertraline	12 (8/4)	In spite of a clear treatment effect in both the placebo and the sertraline group, there was no significant difference in response rate or in effect size between the two groups, assessed by means of MADRS.
Pintor et al., 2012	RCT	ziprasidone, clozapine	14 (6/8)	Ziprasidone was at least as effective as clozapine in reducing psychotic symptoms in PD, measured by the BPRS, and the Scale for the Assessment of Positive Symptoms.
Richard et al., 2012	RCT	paroxetine, venlafaxine	115 (not reported)	Both paroxetine and venlafaxine XR significantly improved depression in patients with PD, as measured by the HDRS score.
Weintraub et al., 2010	RCT, placebo controlled	atomoxetine	55 (36/19)	Atomoxetine treatment was not efficacious for the treatment of clinically significant depressive symptoms in PD, but was associated with improvement in global cognitive performance and daytime sleepiness.
Huntington's disease (HD)				
Beglinger et al., 2014	RCT, placebo controlled	citalopram	33 (18/15)	No evidence that short-term treatment with citalopram improved executive functions in HD.

Note. AD = Alzheimer's disease; BEHAVE-AD = Behavioral Pathology of Alzheimer's Disease; BPRS = Brief Psychiatric Rating Scale; CGI-C = Clinical Global Impression of Change; CGI-I = Clinical Global Impression–Improvement scale; CMAI = Cohen-Mansfield Agitation Inventory; HDRS = Hamilton Depression Rating Scale; MADRS = Montgomery-Åsberg Depression Rating Scale; MD = mixed dementia; NPI = Neuropsychiatric Inventory; NPI-NH = Neuropsychiatric Inventory-Nursing Home; PD = Parkinson's disease; RCT = randomized controlled trial; XR = extended release.

overall effective compared with placebo, with the greatest impact on anger, aggression, and paranoid ideation (Sultzer et al., 2008). A meta-analysis reported overall significant improvement in patients treated with atypical antipsychotics compared with placebo (Wang, Yu, Wang, et al., 2015). Specifically, olanzapine, aripiprazole, and risperidone showed the most robust efficacy, while quetiapine presented insufficient efficacy, with mixed positive and negative results (Paleacu, Barak, Mirecky, & Mazeh, 2008; Rocca, Marino, Montemagni, Perrone, & Bogetto, 2007). Olanzapine seems to have a greater impact on aggression and agitation than psychosis (Ballard & Howard, 2006), whereas aripiprazole alleviated predominantly psychotic features and agitation (De Deyn et al., 2013).

However promising, the real impact of antipsychotics on psychosis and behavioral symptoms is modest (Lanctôt et al., 2017) and these compounds are associated with many adverse effects, including somnolence, cognitive decline, movement disorders, infections, edema, weight gain, metabolic syndrome, and hypotension (which leads to an increased risk of falls and stroke; Lanctôt et al., 2017). A greater concern is the increased mortality observed in patients with dementia treated with antipsychotics. A retrospective cohort study (Kales et al., 2012) examined the mortality risk of antipsychotic use in a national sample of more than 33,000 older veterans with dementia treated with haloperidol, risperidone, olanzapine, quetiapine, or valproic acid (as a comparator). Mortality was highest in those receiving haloperidol, followed by risperidone and olanzapine, then valproic acid, and lastly quetiapine. Therefore, the use of antipsychotics in clinical practice in patients with AD, although often necessary, must be considered carefully and done under clinical surveillance.

Cholinesterase inhibitors (ChEIs) are frequently used drugs for cognitive symptoms of dementia and AD. However, these compounds have also been tested in several trials on behavioral disturbances. AD patients significantly benefitted from ChEIs in terms of reduction of behavioral disturbances compared with placebo (Wang, Yu, Wang, et al., 2015). Their effect is low to moderate and they showed higher efficacy in the treatment of agitation than psychosis (Kales et al., 2015). Moreover, open label studies of ChEIs proved efficacious in the treatment of apathy, and the best results on mood symptoms (depression, anxiety, and apathy) were obtained when an acetylcholinesterase inhibitor (donepezil) was combined with a cholinergic precursor (choline alphoscerate; Carotenuto et al., 2017). In terms of side effects, ChEIs are associated with diarrhea, nausea, and vomiting, and less commonly with symptomatic bradycardia and syncope. These drugs should therefore be used with caution in people with low heart rates.

Results regarding using antidepressants to treat neuropsychiatric symptoms are mixed and not always easy to interpret. Earlier meta-analyses suggested a moderate efficacy and good tolerability of tricyclic antidepressants and selective serotonin reuptake inhibitors (SSRIs) for depression in AD (Bains, Birks, & Dening, 2002). Antidepressants have also been used to target agitation and psychosis in AD. A review of such trials found evidence for a reduction in agitation using sertraline and citalopram compared with placebo (Seitz et al., 2011). In a more recent RCT, citalopram demonstrated good efficacy for agitation, which also lowered caregiver distress (Porsteinsson et al., 2014). However, a meta-analysis did not detect any significant differences between antidepressant and placebo, with no clear benefit for depression or agitation in patients with AD (Wang, Yu, Wang, et al., 2015).

Similarly, no clear evidence that mood stabilizers may reduce BPSD in AD has been detected. Studies of valproic acid and derivatives have not shown treatment benefits for patients with AD (Kales et al., 2015), and even meta-analyses suggest a trend that valproate treatment might slightly worsen neuropsychiatric symptoms compared with placebo (Wang, Yu, Wang, et al., 2015). Limited results from small trials of short duration on carbamazepine showed some benefit for agitation and global clinical outcomes in AD (Olin, Fox, Pawluczyk, Taggart, & Schneider, 2001).

In conclusion, ChEIs and atypical antipsychotics have demonstrated the best evidence for treating neuropsychiatric symptoms in AD, but with certain adverse and sometimes severe effects. Although safer, antidepressants and mood stabilizers did not demonstrate sufficient benefits for neuropsychiatric symptoms.

Frontotemporal Dementia

There are currently no FDA-approved medications for treating bvFTD and the proper treatment requires an individually tailored approach. Given the fact that no treatment capable of changing the course of the neurodegenerative disease is currently available, the focus of medical therapy is mainly symptomatic, and the majority of bvFTD patients receive medications that are also used to treat AD, including ChEIs, SSRIs, or atypical antipsychotics (Manoochehri & Huey, 2012).

ChEIs are prescribed for approximately 40% of bvFTD patients (Manoochehri & Huey, 2012). In contrast to AD, however, the cholinergic system in FTD is relatively intact and results from clinical trials have not been particularly positive, especially for galantamine and donezepil (Kertesz et al., 2008; Mendez, Shapira, McMurtray, & Licht, 2007). Rivastigmine showed some improvements in behavioral and depressive symptoms but did not prevent cognitive deterioration (Moretti et al., 2004).

Some clinical trials have been conducted on memantine, with mixed results. The most recent one reported a small improvement only in agitation, with other behavioral domains not affected by the pharmacological treatment (Li et al., 2016).

SSRIs are attractive agents to use for treating bvFTD, since there is evidence of serotonergic neuronal loss in autopsy specimens from FTD patients (Tsai & Boxer, 2014). Fluoxetine, sertraline, paroxetine, fluvoxamine, and citalopram have all been tested to treat the behavioral symptoms of FTD, albeit mainly in small, open-label studies (Tsai & Boxer, 2016). Both citalopram and fluoxetine improved disinhibition, irritability, and depressive symptoms in bvFTD patients (Herrmann et al., 2012). However, the only serotonergic drug that demonstrated clinical efficacy was trazodone, in a small, double-blind, placebo-controlled trial (Lebert, Stekke, Hasenbroekx, & Pasquier, 2004). Subjects treated with trazodone showed significant improvement in agitation, depression, and eating abnormalities. In consideration of these findings, despite the lack of rigorous clinical trials, SSRIs and serotoninergic agents show sufficient benefits for neuropsychiatric symptoms in bvFTD.

Dopaminergic function in bvFTD seems altered not only in association with extrapyramidal symptoms but also directly related to agitation (Engelborghs et al., 2008). Antipsychotic medications can thus help with neurobehavioral symptoms in FTD but should be used with caution, because individuals with bvFTD are predisposed toward parkinsonian symptoms and therefore more vulnerable to extrapyramidal side effects. Aripiprazole, risperidone, and olanzapine also mitigate behavioral disturbances, delusion, and caregiver stress (Fellgiebel, Müller, Hiemke, Bartenstein, & Schreckenberger, 2007; Moretti et al., 2003). In a case series, quetiapine improved agitation in FTD patients (Chow & Mendez, 2002), and it has a good safety profile in terms of side effects, given its relatively small D2 receptor antagonism.

Antiepileptics with mood-stabilizing effects, such as carbamazepine and valproic acid, were reported to improve behavioral symptoms (Poetter & Stewart, 2012). Topiramate, an antimigraine medication commonly used in binge eating disorder, has been shown in several case reports to reduce hyperorality in FTD patients (Nestor, 2012).

In conclusion, SSRIs and atypical antipsychotics seem to be the best choice for treating moderate and severe bvFTD. This remains the case despite some concerns about safety and side effects of second generation antipsychotics.

Parkinson's Disease

A number of different drugs to treat motor symptoms in PD have been approved by the FDA, with levodopa and carbidopa remaining the most widely used. However, these compounds showed a limited efficacy on neuropsychological and behavioral symptoms and

are therefore not the focus of this chapter. Although PD is an incurable illness, pharmacological treatment can help with many of the nonmotor symptoms involved. A variety of treatments are available, and for some patients, these treatments can control psychiatric symptoms like sleep disorders, autonomic dysfunction, depression, and psychosis.

Psychosis in PD is most effectively treated with clozapine (Connolly & Lang, 2014), although quetiapine, which has less efficacy, is more often prescribed first because of the risk of agranulocytosis and the requirement for frequent blood monitoring with clozapine. Other neuroleptics like haloperidol, olanzapine, risperidone, and aripiprazole should not be used for PD, since these medications can induce extrapyramidal symptoms and thus worsen parkinsonism (Goldman, Vaughan, & Goetz, 2011). Moreover, dopamine agonists should be avoided in patients with a history of addiction, obsessive-compulsive disorder, or impulsive personality, because these patients are at high risk for developing impulse control disorders (Kalia & Lang, 2015). Cholinesterase inhibitors, such as donezepil and rivastigmine, might reduce hallucinations—especially visual ones—and delusions in patients with Parkinson-related dementia (Kalia & Lang, 2015).

Depressive symptoms related to PD are usually treated with classical antidepressants. SSRIs (including citalopram, escitalopram, fluoxetine, paroxetine, and sertraline) are the most commonly prescribed treatment despite research supporting the efficacy of tricyclic antidepressants, specifically desipramine and nortriptyline, for the treatment of PD-related depression (Troeung, Egan, & Gasson, 2013). Recent meta-analyses show insufficient evidence to support the use of SSRIs or SNRIs (venlafaxine and duloxetine) in PD, but tricyclic antidepressants were found efficacious (Troeung et al., 2013). The dopamine agonist pramipexole shows some evidence of efficacy in treating depression in PD patients and could be an option, especially when both motor and mood symptoms are being targeted (Connolly & Lang, 2014).

Huntington's Disease

A multidisciplinary treatment for HD is necessary, similarly to other dementias. Nevertheless, an appropriate pharmacotherapy in HD is of unclear benefit for the protean neuropsychiatric symptoms (Wyant et al., 2017). Pharmacological management of HD is actually just symptomatic management. Second generation antipsychotic agents, like quetiapine and olanzapine, can be useful in treating irritability, aggression, and psychotic symptoms (Wyant et al., 2017). The choice to use second generation antipsychotics over traditional anti-psychotics is motivated by their ability to cause weight gain in patients who experienced weight loss, and for the lower risk of inducing tardive dyskinesia and other extrapyramidal side effects (Dayalu & Albin, 2015). Clinical experience also supports the use of these agents to control chorea; however, only the monoamine-depleting agent tetrabenazine has been clearly shown to reduce chorea in an appro-priately double-blind, placebo-controlled study (Huntington Study Group, 2006). Actually, tetra-benazine remains the only treatment for chorea that is approved by FDA, with evidence and indications for HD (Mestre, Ferreira, Coelho, Rosa, & Sampaio, 2009). Depression is the most clinically relevant side effect of tetrabenazine; depletion of dopamine reduces chorea, while depletion of serotonin and norepinephrine may worsen depression and anxiety, leading to an increased risk for suicide. The presence of depression is generally thought of as a relative contraindication to its use. Antipsychotics can be associated with sedation, somnolence, parkinsonism, severe dysphagia. For these reasons, any drug change should be monitored closely, start with a low dose, be tapered slowly, and be switched to a different agent if problems develop.

Benzodiazepines such as clonazepam can also be used to manage chorea and may be particularly useful when taken prophylactically to minimize chorea in individuals who are experiencing exac-erbation of involuntary movements in response to specific circumstances (Sturrock & Leavitt, 2010). SSRIs are commonly used for depressive symptoms because of their additional efficacy in treating obses-sive compulsive symptomatology. The noradrenergic and serotonergic drug mirtazapine and the serotonin antagonist and reuptake inhibitor trazodone could be useful to manage insomnia and sleep disturbance. Cognitive dysfunction in HD disrupts social and

occupational function in the prime of these patients' lives, but good treatment options are lacking at this time (Wyant et al., 2017).

BEST APPROACHES FOR ASSESSING TREATMENT RESPONSE AND MANAGING SIDE EFFECTS

The treatment of neurodegenerative disorders represents a major issue of concern and should be guided by a multidisciplinary approach, including pharmacological and nonpharmacological inter-ventions. The vast majority of drugs are commonly used off-label, since they have not been formally approved by the FDA nor by the European Medicines Agency, due to lack of evidence for their efficacy (Kales et al., 2015). The choice and dosage of pharmacological medications should be guided not only by efficacy but also by potential side effects and unwanted interactions with other medications, following a rigorous risk and benefit assessment. Drug starting doses for elderly patients are usually lower than those recommended for younger adults and should be titrated up or down slowly, according to clinical response and elicitation of side effects. Moreover, given the fact that polytherapies are a typical practice for patients affected by dementia, drugs that do not have clearly demonstrated advantages should be avoided. It should be consid-ered that patients over 80 years of age presented Cumulative Illness Rating Scale (CIRS) scores significantly higher than did patients under age 80, and higher CIRS scores were associated with lower treatment adherence and greater cognitive impair-ment (Sinforiani et al., 2017). Considering that the number of elderly people with cognitive disorders will increase, the approach to neurodegenerative disorders has to change and fit social and epidemio-logical modifications. It is not easy to assess the efficacy of therapeutic interventions in neuro-degenerative disorders, given the fact that we do not have disease-modifying treatments, but only symptomatic drugs. The progression of the diseases is usually assessed by a strict follow-up using the same clinical, neuropsychological, and neuro-psychiatric batteries that are commonly used for diagnosis (refer to the Diagnosing Neurocognitive

Disorders section in this chapter for further information). The Clinical Dementia Rating (CDR) scale is a widely used tool for both research and clinical purposes (Costa et al., 2017). The CDR is a numeric scale used to quantify the severity of symptoms of dementia and its progression during follow-ups. It is a structured interview that assesses cognitive and functional performance in six areas: memory, orientation, judgment and problem-solving, community affairs, home and hobbies, and personal care. Combined scores are used to obtain a composite score ranging from 0 (no impairments) to 3 (severe impairments), which provides a measure of the severity of the disease.

MEDICATION MANAGEMENT ISSUES

BPSD are among the most complex, stressful, and costly aspects of care, not only for patients but also for caregivers. It is important to note that individuals affected by dementia might not be able to take care of themselves, especially in the late phases of the illnesses. Compliance and adherence are often very difficult to assess and are primarily handled by caregivers. Therefore, the role of caregivers in patients' management is of fundamental importance, because they not only have to take care of treatment compliance but also manage the possibility of a relapse or worsening of symptoms. Caregivers, families, and health care professionals are the strongest allies to therapy, and have key roles in outcomes as well. A recent complete review (Kröger et al., 2017) showed that little solid evidence is available regarding how to improve adherence in patients with cognitive disorders. Some promising strategies have been studied, including reducing the number and frequency of prescribed medications, educational strategies, and reminder techniques. A recently developed strategy is named *deprescribing*, an interprofessional process consisting of a detailed medication review (taking the health status and quality of life of the patient into account) and aimed at tapering or discontinuing medications in order to reduce inappropriate polypharmacy and improve health outcomes (Scott et al., 2014).

Regarding specific compounds, dopaminergic therapy for PD can induce neuropsychiatric symptoms.

Hallucinations are both a feature of later stage PD and a consequence of dopaminergic medication, whereas additional psychotic symptoms are generally drug related (Kalia & Lang, 2015). Moreover, dopamine agonists are associated with other neuropsychiatric dopamine-related side effects such as pathological gambling, hypersexuality, binge eating, and compulsive spending (Kalia & Lang, 2015). Moreover, several studies reported the possibility that benzodiazepines produce dependence and motor disability, and therefore must be used with great attention and for limited periods of time (Robles Bayón & Gude Sampedro, 2014).

EVALUATION OF PHARMACOLOGICAL APPROACHES ACROSS THE LIFESPAN

To the best of our knowledge, no study has assessed the differential response to treatment in individuals of different ages across the lifespan. However, several treatments demonstrated the possibility of having a more vigorous effect on mild to moderate symptoms, and therefore in younger subjects who are in early phases of the disease (Salloway et al., 2011).

In general, some considerations can be drawn when treating an elderly and fragile population, which presents a predisposition to adverse events and side effects. In this framework, some drugs should be avoided or handled with care and always in a medical environment.

Benzodiazepines are among the most commonly prescribed drugs for elderly people. However, RCTs comparing benzodiazepines with placebo for BPSD in AD are lacking. Given serious concerns about adverse events, such agents are not recommended except for management of an acute crisis. Indeed, high cumulative doses of benzodiazepines and prolonged duration of treatment have been associated with increased risk of falls as well as dementia and cognitive decline (Islam et al., 2016) and their use in elderly populations should be discouraged.

Some issues have also arisen in the use of antidepressants, and currently tricyclic antidepressants are rarely used with elderly people, especially those in cognitive decline, due to the risk of orthostatic hypotension and falls. Usually, tricyclic antidepressants are used less frequently with older patients who are cognitively impaired because they can often produce adverse events.

CONSIDERATION OF POTENTIAL SEX DIFFERENCES

Dementia has multiple causes and diverse manifestations, and might present with heterogeneity regarding the impact of sex or gender on prevalence, risk factors, and outcomes. Several epidemiologic studies show that neurodegeneration and clinical symptoms in AD occur more rapidly for females; however, males with AD have a shorter survival time (Podcasy & Epperson, 2016). Men usually show greater comorbidity and higher mortality than do women, who instead reported more disability and longer survival. Survival curves showed that women reach partial loss of autonomy faster than men (Sinforiani et al., 2010). These differences may be due to reductions in estradiol levels during the 5th decade of life and beyond, which are possibly responsible for brain metabolic differences across sexes (Podcasy & Epperson, 2016). Inflammation is another risk factor for AD that varies by sex, with inflammatory dysregulation being stronger in females (Podcasy & Epperson, 2016). In contrast, sex differences in symptomatology and progression to dementia among individuals with PD, FTD, and HD are still unclear (Podcasy & Epperson, 2016).

To the best of our knowledge, only a few studies have assessed sex differences in regard to pharmacological treatments in neurodegenerative diseases, most of them in AD. Based on epidemiological data, older women with AD are more likely to use psychotropic medications than older men (Moga et al., 2017), possibly due to different symptomatological course. A recent systematic review of sex differences in treatment response to ChEIs reported no significant differences (Canevelli et al., 2017). A study suggested a sex difference in cognitive response to sertraline (Munro et al., 2004). Indeed, women treated with sertraline demonstrated improved cognition compared with women on placebo; on the other hand, men treated with sertraline worsened significantly in cognition. However, the relatively limited attention to this topic must be taken into account, given the fact that very few RCTs take into consideration sex in post hoc analysis.

INTEGRATION OF PHARMACOTHERAPY WITH NONPHARMACOLOGICAL APPROACHES: BENEFITS AND CHALLENGES

Nonpharmacologic treatments are often suggested as a first-line treatment approach for BPSD in dementia by numerous guidelines, medical organizations, and expert groups. These strategies encompass a vast array of behavioral, environmental, and caregiver-supportive interventions, aimed at assessing potential unmet needs and environmental or interpersonal stressors. These approaches educate caregivers, make changes to the physical environment, increase social engagement, promote exercise and activities, and address sleep problems. Although the evidence of efficacies of these strategies is slim, in an RCT they seemed to produce moderate yet significant positive impacts on neuropsychiatric symptoms (Cohen-Mansfield, Thein, Marx, Dakheel-Ali, & Freedman, 2012). However, these strategies have largely not been translated into real-world clinical management and standard care (Kales et al., 2015), and drugs are often preferred over nonpharmacologic strategies.

INTEGRATED APPROACHES FOR ADDRESSING COMMON COMORBID DISORDERS

Neurodegenerative disorders may present several comorbidities, some regarding a specific disease. For example, there are three neurodegenerative syndromes that frequently overlap both clinically and neuropathologically with FTD: corticobasal syndrome (CBS), progressive supranuclear palsy (PSP), and amyotrophic lateral sclerosis (ALS; Tsai & Boxer, 2014). PSP is defined by early falls and ophthalmoplegia (although other subtypes exist), while ALS is a motor neuron disease with increasingly recognized cognitive dysfunction (Tsai & Boxer, 2014), and CBS is an atypical parkinsonian syndrome, characterized by motor and cognitive disorders.

Regarding PD, depression is one of the most common comorbid diseases and is often under-diagnosed. For diagnosis, the best evidence in PD supports the use of the Geriatric Depression Scale (GDS-15), at a cutoff of 5, along with the Cornell Scale for Depression in Dementia (CSDD) and Hamilton Depression Rating Scale (HDRS; Marsh, 2013). Psychosocial interventions (cognitive behavior therapy, interpersonal therapy, and counseling) proved helpful in treating this condition. However, most patients also need pharmacological therapies (Goodarzi & Ismail, 2017). As explained in more depth in the Evidence-Based Pharmacological Treatment of Neurocognitive Disorders section of this chapter, common antidepressants are widely used, with mixed and inconclusive results in RCTs and meta-analyses (Troeung et al., 2013). The dopamine agonist pramipexole showed some efficacy in treating depression in PD patients.

People affected by neurodegenerative disorders are usually older and display pronounced health frailty, which increases the risk of adverse outcomes, including physical and psychological disabilities. These fragile states account for multiple interrelated physiological systems. There is a gradual decline in physiological reserve with aging that is accelerated by the presence of a neurodegenerative disorder. These complex aging mechanisms are influenced by underlying genetic and environmental factors in combination with epigenetic mechanisms. *Frailty* is considered a common and disabling geriatric syndrome that is characterized by a loss of ability to adapt to environmental stress because of diminished functional reserves. According to this perspective, stressors such as neurodegenerative genetic-based disorders promote chronic inflammatory states, likely contributing to the onset of frailty. These factors directly affect brain structure, inducing loss of hippocampal neurons and causing hippocampal atrophy; these structural effects underlie memory deficits and promote the onset of depression and anxiety (Brambilla et al., 2012).

Analyzing all the possible comorbidities of elderly individuals is not within the scope of this chapter. However, we'd like to raise attention to a common side effect of many drugs and physical states: delirium. *Delirium* is characterized by an acute change in mental status, disturbances of consciousness, and clouded sensorium, which might be accompanied by abnormalities in mood, perception, and behavior. The geriatric population is particularly at risk of developing delirium, which is described to affect up to 50% of the elder hospitalized population and shows a medical and/or multifactorial etiology (Inouye, Westendorp, & Saczynski, 2014). Pre-existing medical conditions, such as uncontrolled diabetes, pulmonary or urinary tract infections, and electrolyte alterations are the most common causes of delirium in the elderly. Additionally, misuse or abuse of prescription drugs (such as benzodiazepines) may lead to delirium. Inappropriate medication use in the elderly is the cause of many hospital admissions and may trigger psychotic symptoms. For all of these reasons, the possible onset of such a condition should be dealt with using great care.

EMERGING TRENDS

Neurocognitive impairments are a core component of both neurodegenerative disorders and psychiatric diseases, and one of the great pharmacological challenges of our time is to identify strategies to correct or at least slow down cognitive decline. A comprehensive assessment of all the possible symptomatic strategies intended to ameliorate and slow cognitive decline is not possible within this chapter; however, we wish to note that several possible treatments have been proposed, from atypical anti-psychotics and mood stabilizers to antioxidant and nutraceutical compounds (Sumiyoshi, Higuchi, & Uehara, 2013). Unfortunately, all of these possible treatments demonstrated only minor efficacy and are still under study.

Alzheimer's Disease

Several RCTs are investigating new compounds for agitation and aggression in dementia and AD. Results are still inconclusive and need further study, but some of them might prove promising. Brexpiprazole is an atypical antipsychotic chemically similar to aripiprazole and is currently being investigated for treating agitation and aggression in AD. Scyllo-inositol, one of the stereoisomers of inositol, has undergone testing in a Phase 2 clinical trial; although it has demonstrated acceptable safety, there was no significant improvement in neuropsychiatric symptoms (Salloway et al., 2011). Some evidence is emerging regarding the possible effectiveness of cannabinoid compounds on aggression and agitation in AD (Ahmed, van der Marck, van den Elsen, & Olde Rikkert, 2015). Moreover, in vitro and in vivo studies have demonstrated that cannabinoids can reduce oxidative stress, neuroinflammation, and the formation of amyloid plaques and neurofibrillary tangles, and therefore might be of great interest in future research. Prazosin, an alpha-1 norepinephrine antagonist used for hypertension and benign prostatic hypertrophy, has demonstrated a good tolerability and improved behavioral symptoms in AD (Wang et al., 2009).

Frontotemporal Dementia

Emerging treatments that have been tested in FTD include dopaminergic therapies and the neuropeptide oxytocin. Dextroamphetamine has been tested along with quetiapine in a small group of bvFTD patients (Rahman et al., 2006). The dextroamphetamine group, but not the quetiapine group, showed improvement, especially in apathy and disinhibition compared with baseline. Another double-blind, placebo-controlled study using a single dose of methylphenidate (a dopamine and norepinephrine reuptake inhibitor) demonstrated improvements in risk-taking behavior (Huey, Garcia, Wassermann, Tierney, & Grafman, 2008). However, larger double-blind studies with long-term follow-up are mandatory to determine the real safety and efficacy of these drugs. Safety, in particular, is a crucial issue for these compounds, in light of their potential behavioral adverse effects such as risk-taking behavior, abuse liability, and hallucinations. Therefore, routine use of stimulants in FTD is not currently recommended.

A randomized, double-blind, placebo-controlled study examined the effects of a single dose of intranasal oxytocin in a small sample of patients affected by bvFTD (Jesso et al., 2011). The study demonstrated small improvements in several behavioral domains, but clear data regarding short- and long-term efficacy are still lacking. All of the presented treatments, however, are merely symptomatic and do not alter the progression of the neurocognitive disease. Apart from relieving symptoms, a disease-modifying therapy is needed. A better understanding of the neurobiology of FTD may lead to protein-specific drugs, involving tau and TDP-43 pathways.

Parkinson's Disease

New trends are emerging from both pharmacologic and nonpharmacologic treatment strategies for PD. For example, one study showed that the selective serotonin 5-HT$_{2A}$ inverse agonist pimavanserin improved psychotic symptoms without worsening motor symptoms (Cummings et al., 2014). Transcranial magnetic stimulation is used for treatment of depression in patients without PD, but there are no RCTs to support its use with PD. The multicenter randomized EARLYSTIM trial showed that deep brain stimulation of the subthalamic nucleus early in the disease course improved several secondary outcome measures, including neuropsychiatric symptoms (see Chapter 32, this volume, for more in-depth discussion of these new techniques).

Huntington's Disease

The dopidines are a novel class of dopamine stabilizers in development for use with patients with HD. Their complex pharmacodynamics result in state-dependent effects on dopamine transmission (Huntington Study Group HART Investigators, 2013). When dopaminergic tone is low, dopidines enhance transmission; when tone is high, they antagonize dopamine receptors, similar to antipsychotics (de Yebenes et al., 2011).

Enhanced peripheral immune activation in patients with HD has to be considered, and the possibility to improve symptoms with nonsteroidal anti-inflammatory drugs like ibuprofen should be explored, as it has been with PD and AD. Because patients with HD can be identified in the premanifest period, this population might provide an ideal test case for interventional trials measuring the neuroprotective effectiveness of anti-inflammatory drugs. A Phase 2 trial of laquinimod, an experimental immune modulatory drug investigated in multiple sclerosis trials (Comi et al., 2008), for use with HD will enable a detailed examination of the relationship between the immune system and disease progression.

Patients with HD show abnormal handling of tryptophan and kynurenine metabolism and increased oxidative stress. Considering the emerging importance of tryptophan, a precursor of several compounds including serotonin and melatonin, an appropriate management of sleep–wake cycles and melatonin-like therapy could improve the quality of therapy in this disease (Kalliolia et al., 2014).

SUMMARY

After this brief review, some conclusions can be drawn. First, There are psychological and behavioral patterns shared by different neurodegenerative diseases. These features could arise early in the course of the disease and could present merely psychiatric symptoms. This factor may delay the diagnosis and make it difficult. Second, no currently known treatment can cure or prevent neurodegenerative diseases or neuropsychological symptoms associated with them. Many different compounds have been assessed, but the number of RCTs is quite limited and they have been conducted on a small cohort of subjects. Third, to the best of our knowledge, no specific drugs have been approved for behavioral and psychological symptoms in neurodegenerative disorders. Most of the compounds used are common psychiatric treatments, which are not specific to symptoms of dementia. Finally, The choice of a drug in patients affected by neurodegenerative processes should follow a risk/benefit assessment, given the fact that these subjects' health is fragile and that they are more prone to adverse events. Please see the Tool Kit of Resources for further suggested reading.

TOOL KIT OF RESOURCES

Alzheimer's Disease

Patient Resources

Symptoms and Diagnosis—The Alzheimer's Association: https://www.alz.org/alzheimers_disease_what_is_alzheimers.asp

Symptoms and Causes—Mayo Clinic: https://www.mayoclinic.org/diseases-conditions/alzheimers-disease/symptoms-causes/syc-20350447

Alzheimer's disease—Diagnosis and treatment—Mayo Clinic: https://www.mayoclinic.org/diseases-conditions/alzheimers-disease/diagnosis-treatment/drc-20350453

Provider Resources

Pharmacotherapies for sleep disturbances in dementia—McCleery—2016—The Cochrane Library—Wiley Online Library: http://onlinelibrary.wiley.com/doi/10.1002/14651858.CD009178.pub3/epdf

Information, support and training for informal caregivers of people with dementia—González-Fraile—2015—The Cochrane Library—Wiley Online Library: http://onlinelibrary.wiley.com/doi/10.1002/14651858.CD006440.pub2/full

Dementia, disability and frailty in later life—midlife approaches to delay or prevent onset | Guidance and guidelines | NICE: https://www.nice.org.uk/guidance/ng16/resources/dementia-disability-and-frailty-in-later-life-midlife-approaches-to-delay-or-prevent-onset-pdf-1837274790085

Dementia: supporting people with dementia and their carers in health and social care | Guidance and guidelines | NICE: https://www.nice.org.uk/guidance/cg42/resources/dementia-supporting-people-with-dementia-and-their-carers-in-health-and-social-care-pdf-975443665093

Withdrawal versus continuation of chronic antipsychotic drugs for behavioural and psychological symptoms in older people with dementia—Declercq—2013—The Cochrane Library—Wiley Online Library: http://onlinelibrary.wiley.com/doi/10.1002/14651858.CD007726.pub2/full

Nonpharmacological interventions for sleep disturbances in people with dementia—Wilfling—2015—The Cochrane Library—Wiley Online Library: http://onlinelibrary.wiley.com/doi/10.1002/14651858.CD011881/full

Bains, J., Birks, J., & Dening, T. (2002). Antidepressants for treating depression in dementia. *Cochrane Database Systematic Reviews, 2002*(4), CD003944. http://dx.doi.org/10.1002/14651858.CD003944

Ballard, C., & Howard, R. (2006). Neuroleptic drugs in dementia: Benefits and harm. *Nature Reviews Neuroscience, 7,* 492–500.

Dietary interventions for maintaining cognitive function in cognitively healthy people in late life—Siervo—2015—The Cochrane Library—Wiley Online Library: http://onlinelibrary.wiley.com/doi/10.1002/14651858.CD011910/full

Vitamin and mineral supplementation for maintaining cognitive function in cognitively healthy people in late life—Al-Assaf—2015—The Cochrane Library—Wiley Online Library: http://onlinelibrary.wiley.com/doi/10.1002/14651858.CD011906/full

Dietary interventions for prevention of dementia in people with mild cognitive impairment—Tang—2015—The Cochrane Library—Wiley Online Library: http://onlinelibrary.wiley.com/doi/10.1002/14651858.CD011909/full

Scheltens, P., Blennow, K., Breteler, M. M., & Van der Flier, W. M. (2016). Alzheimer's disease. *Lancet, 388*(10043), 505–17.

Seitz, D. P., Adunuri, N., Gill, S. S., Gruneir, A., Herrmann, N., & Rochon, P. (2011). Antidepressants for agitation and psychosis in dementia. *Cochrane Database Systematic Reviews, 2011*(2), CD008191. http://dx.doi.org/10.1002/14651858.CD008191.pub2

Low-dose antipsychotics in people with dementia | Guidance and guidelines | NICE: https://www.nice.org.uk/advice/ktt7/resources/lowdose-antipsychotics-in-people-with-dementia-pdf-1632175200709

Huntington's Disease

Patient Resources

The Huntington's Disease | Signs, Symptoms, and Diagnosis: https://www.alz.org/dementia/huntingtons-disease-symptoms.asp

Home—HOPES Huntington's Disease Information: http://web.stanford.edu/group/hopes/cgi-bin/hopes_test/

The Huntington's Disease Society of America: http://hdsa.org/about-hdsa/

Huntington's disease—Symptoms and causes—Mayo Clinic: https://www.mayoclinic.org/diseases-conditions/huntingtons-disease/symptoms-causes/syc-20356117

Huntington's disease—Diagnosis and treatment—Mayo Clinic: https://www.mayoclinic.org/diseases-conditions/huntingtons-disease/diagnosis-treatment/drc-20356122

Provider Resources

Bates, G. P., Dorsey, R., Gusella, J. F., Hayden, M. R., Kay, C., Leavitt, B. R., . . . Tabrizi, S. J. (2015). Huntington disease. *Nature Reviews Disease Primers, 1*, 15005. http://dx.doi.org/10.1038/nrdp.2015.5

Dayalu, P., & Albin, R. L. (2015). Huntington disease: Pathogenesis and treatment. *Neurologic Clinics, 33*(1), 101–14.

Mestre, T., Ferreira, J., Coelho, M. M., Rosa, M., & Sampaio, C. (2009). Therapeutic interventions for symptomatic treatment in Huntington's disease.

Cochrane Database Systematic Reviews, 2009(3), CD006456. http://dx.doi.org/10.1002/14651858.CD006456.pub2

Ross, C. A., Aylward, E. H., Wild, E. J., Langbehn, D. R., Long, J. D., & Tabrizi, S. J. (2014). Huntington disease: Natural history, biomarkers and prospects for therapeutics. *Nature Reviews Neurology, 10*(4), 204–16.

Wyant, K. J., Ridder, A. J., & Dayalu, P. (2017). Huntington's disease: Update on treatments. *Current Neurology and Neuroscience Reports, 17*, 33. http://dx.doi.org/10.1007/s11910-017-0739-9

Frontotemporal Dementia

Patient Resources

Frontotemporal Dementia | Signs, Symptoms, and Diagnosis: https://www.alz.org/dementia/fronto-temporal-dementia-ftd-symptoms.asp

Frontotemporal dementia—Symptoms and causes—Mayo Clinic: https://www.mayoclinic.org/diseases-conditions/frontotemporal-dementia/symptoms-causes/syc-20354737

Frontotemporal dementia—Diagnosis and treatment—Mayo Clinic: https://www.mayoclinic.org/diseases-conditions/frontotemporal-dementia/diagnosis-treatment/drc-20354741

Provider Resources

Bang, J., Spina, S., & Miller, B. L. (2015). Frontotemporal dementia. *Lancet, 386*(10004), 1672–82.

Tsai, R. M., & Boxer, A. L. (2014). Treatment of frontotemporal dementia. *Current Treatment Options in Neurology, 16*(11), 319.

Parkinson's Disease

Patient Resources

Parkinson's Disease | Signs, Symptoms, and Diagnosis/The Alzheimer's Association: https://www.alz.org/dementia/parkinsons-disease-symptoms.asp

Parkinson's disease—Symptoms and causes—Mayo Clinic: https://www.mayoclinic.org/diseases-conditions/parkinsons-disease/symptoms-causes/syc-20376055

Parkinson's disease—Diagnosis and treatment—Mayo Clinic: https://www.mayoclinic.org/diseases-conditions/parkinsons-disease/diagnosis-treatment/drc-20376062

Parkinson's disease in adults | Guidance and guidelines | NICE: https://www.nice.org.uk/guidance/ng71

Provider Resources

Connolly, B. S., & Lang, A. E. (2014). Pharmacological treatment of Parkinson disease: A review. *JAMA, 311*(16), 1670–1683.

Kalia, L. V., & Lang, A. E. (2015). Parkinson's disease. *Lancet, 386*(9996), 896–912.

Anticholinergics (various) for neuroleptic-induced parkinsonism—Dickenson—2014—The Cochrane Library—Wiley Online Library: http://onlinelibrary. wiley.com/doi/10.1002/14651858.CD011113/full

Interventions for improving medication adherence in patients with idiopathic Parkinson's disease— Daley—2014—The Cochrane Library—Wiley Online Library: http://onlinelibrary.wiley.com/ doi/10.1002/14651858.CD011191/full

References

Ahmed, A., van der Marck, M. A., van den Elsen, G., & Olde Rikkert, M. (2015). Cannabinoids in late-onset Alzheimer's disease. *Clinical Pharmacology and Therapeutics, 97*(6), 597–606.

Antonini, A., Tesei, S., Zecchinelli, A., Barone, P., De Gaspari, D., Canesi, M., . . . Pezzoli, G. (2006). Randomized study of sertraline and low-dose amitriptyline in patients with Parkinson's disease and depression: Effect on quality of life. *Movement Disorders, 21*, 1119–1122. http://dx.doi.org/10.1002/ mds.20895

Bains, J., Birks, J., & Dening, T. (2002). Antidepressants for treating depression in dementia. *Cochrane Database of Systematic Reviews, 4*, CD003944.

Ballard, C., & Howard, R. (2006). Neuroleptic drugs in dementia: Benefits and harm. *Nature Reviews Neuroscience, 7*, 492–500. http://dx.doi.org/10.1038/ nrn1926

Ballard, C., Margallo-Lana, M., Juszczak, E., Douglas, S., Swann, A., Thomas, A., . . . Jacoby, R. (2005). Quetiapine and rivastigmine and cognitive decline in Alzheimer's disease: Randomised double blind placebo controlled trial. *BMJ, 330*, 874. http:// dx.doi.org/10.1136/bmj.38369.459988.8F

Bang, J., Spina, S., & Miller, B. L. (2015). Frontotemporal dementia. *Lancet, 386*(10004), 1672–1682.

Barone, P., Poewe, W., Albrecht, S., Debieuvre, C., Massey, D., Rascol, O., . . . Weintraub, D. (2010). Pramipexole for the treatment of depressive symptoms in patients with Parkinson's disease: A randomised, double-blind, placebo-controlled trial. *Lancet Neurology, 9*, 573–580. http://dx.doi.org/ 10.1016/S1474-4422(10)70106-X

Barone, P., Scarzella, L., Marconi, R., Antonini, A., Morgante, L., Bracco, F., . . . Musch, B., & the Depression/Parkinson Italian Study Group. (2006). Pramipexole versus sertraline in the treatment of depression in Parkinson's disease: A national multi-center parallel-group randomized study. *Journal of Neurology, 253*(5), 601–607.

Bates, G. P., Dorsey, R., Gusella, J. F., Hayden, M. R., Kay, C., . . . Tabrizi, S. J. (2015). Huntington disease. *Nature Reviews Disease Primers, Apr 23; 1*, 15005. http://dx.doi.org/10.1038/nrdp.2015.5

Beglinger, L. J., Adams, W. H., Langbehn, D., Fiedorowicz, J. G., Jorge, R., Biglan, K., . . . Paulsen, J. S. (2014). Results of the citalopram to enhance cognition in Huntington disease trial. *Movement Disorders, 29*, 401–405. http://dx.doi.org/10.1002/mds.25750

Blennow, K., Hampel, H., Weiner, M., & Zetterberg, H. (2010). Cerebrospinal fluid and plasma biomarkers in Alzheimer disease. *Neurology, 6*, 131–144. http://dx.doi.org/10.1038/nrneurol.2010.4

Brambilla, P., Como, G., Isola, M., Taboga, F., Zuliani, R., Goljevscek, S., . . . Balestrieri, M. (2012). White-matter abnormalities in the right posterior hemisphere in generalized anxiety disorder: A diffusion imaging study. *Psychological Medicine, 42*, 427–434. http://dx.doi.org/10.1017/S0033291711001255

Brodaty, H., Ames, D., Snowdon, J., Woodward, M., Kirwan, J., Clarnette, R., . . . Greenspan, A. (2005). Risperidone for psychosis of Alzheimer's disease and mixed dementia: Results of a double-blind, placebo-controlled trial. *International Journal of Geriatric Psychiatry, 20*(12), 1153–1157

Canevelli, M., Quarata, F., Remiddi, F., Lucchini, F., Lacorte, E., Vanacore, N., . . . Cesari, M. (2017). Sex and gender differences in the treatment of Alzheimer's disease: A systematic review of random-ized controlled trials. *Pharmacological Research, 115*, 218–223. http://dx.doi.org/10.1016/ j.phrs.2016.11.035

Carotenuto, A., Rea, R., Traini, E., Fasanaro, A. M., Ricci, G., Manzo, V., & Amenta, F. (2017). The effect of the association between donepezil and choline alphoscerate on behavioral disturbances in Alzheimer's disease: Interim results of the ASCOMALVA Trial. *Journal of Alzheimer's Disease, 56*, 805–815. http://dx.doi.org/10.3233/JAD-160675

Chen, C., Chang, C. C., Chang, W. N., Tsai, N. W., Huang, C. C., Chang, Y. T., . . . Lu, C. H. (2017). Neuropsychiatric symptoms in Alzheimer's disease: Associations with caregiver burden and treatment outcomes. *QJM, 110*(9), 565–570.

Chow, T. W., & Mendez, M. F. (2002). Goals in symptom-atic pharmacologic management of frontotemporal

*Asterisks indicate assessments or resources.

lobar degeneration. *American Journal of Alzheimer's Disease and Other Dementias, 17*, 267–272. http://dx.doi.org/10.1177/153331750201700504

Cohen-Mansfield, J., Thein, K., Marx, M. S., Dakheel-Ali, M., & Freedman, L. (2012). Efficacy of non-pharmacologic interventions for agitation in advanced dementia: A randomized, placebo-controlled trial. *The Journal of Clinical Psychiatry, 73*, 1255–1261. http://dx.doi.org/10.4088/JCP.12m07918

Comi, G., Pulizzi, A., Rovaris, M., Abramsky, O., Arbizu, T., Boiko, A., . . . the LAQ/5062 Study Group. (2008). Effect of laquinimod on MRI-monitored disease activity in patients with relapsing-remitting multiple sclerosis: A multicentre, randomised, double-blind, placebo-controlled phase IIb study. *Lancet, 371*(9630), 2085–2092. http://dx.doi.org/10.1016/S0140-6736(08)60918-6.

*Connolly, B. S., & Lang, A. E. (2014). Pharmacological treatment of Parkinson disease: A review. *JAMA, 311*(16), 1670–1683.

Costa, A., Bak, T., Caffarra, P., Caltagirone, C., Ceccaldi, M., Collette, F., . . . Cappa, S. F. (2017). The need for harmonisation and innovation of neuropsychological assessment in neurodegenerative dementias in Europe: Consensus document of the Joint Program for Neurodegenerative Diseases Working Group. *Alzheimer's Research & Therapy, 9*(1), 27.

Cummings, J., Isaacson, S., Mills, R., Williams, H., Chi-Burris, K., Corbett, A., . . . Ballard, C. (2014). Pimavanserin for patients with Parkinson's disease psychosis: A randomised, placebo-controlled phase 3 trial. *The Lancet, 383*, 533–540. http://dx.doi.org/10.1016/S0140-6736(13)62106-6

Dayalu, P., & Albin, R. L. (2015). Huntington disease: Pathogenesis and treatment. *Neurologic Clinics, 3*(1), 101–114.

De Deyn, P. P., Carrasco, M. M., Deberdt, W., Jeandel, C., Hay, D. P., Feldman, P. D., . . . Breier, A. (2004). Olanzapine versus placebo in the treatment of psychosis with or without associated behavioral disturbances in patients with Alzheimer's disease. *International Journal of Geriatric Psychiatry, 19*(2), 115–126.

De Deyn, P. P., Drenth, A. F., Kremer, B. P., Oude Voshaar, R. C., & Van Dam, D. (2013). Aripiprazole in the treatment of Alzheimer's disease. *Expert Opinion on Pharmacotherapy, 14*(4), 459–474.

De Deyn, P. P., Katz, I. R., Brodaty, H., Lyons, B., Greenspan, A., & Burns, A. (2005). Management of agitation, aggression, and psychosis associated with dementia: A pooled analysis including three randomized, placebo-controlled double-blind trials in nursing home residents treated with risperidone. *Clinical Neurology and Neurosurgery, 107*(6), 497–508.

de Yebenes, J. G., Landwehrmeyer, B., Squitieri, F., Reilmann, R., Rosser, A., Barker, R. A., . . . the MermaiHD study investigators. (2011). Pridopidine for the treatment of motor function in patients with Huntington's disease (MermaiHD): A phase 3, randomised, double-blind, placebo-controlled trial. *The Lancet Neurology, 10*, 1049–1057. http://dx.doi.org/10.1016/S1474-4422(11)70233-2

Deakin, J. B., Rahman, S., Nestor, P. J., Hodges, J. R., & Sahakian, B. J. (2004). Paroxetine does not improve symptoms and impairs cognition in frontotemporal dementia: A double-blind randomized controlled trial. *Psychopharmacology, 172*(4), 400–408.

Devos, D., Dujardin, K., Poirot, I., Moreau, C., Cottencin, O., Thomas, P., . . . Defebvre, L. (2008). Comparison of desipramine and citalopram treatments for depression in Parkinson's disease: A double-blind, randomized, placebo-controlled study. *Movement Disorders, 23*(6), 850–857.

Dorsey, E. R., Constantinescu, R., Thompson, J. P., Biglan, K. M., Holloway, R. G., Kieburtz, K., . . . Tanner, C. M. (2007). Projected number of people with Parkinson disease in the most populous nations, 2005 through 2030. *Neurology, 68*, 384–386. http://dx.doi.org/10.1212/01.wnl.0000247740.47667.03

*Dubois, B., Feldman, H. H., Jacova, C., Hampel, H., Molinuevo, J. L., Blennow, K., . . . Cummings, J. L. (2014). Advancing research diagnostic criteria for Alzheimer's disease: The IWG-2 criteria. *Lancet Neurology, 13*(6), 614–629.

Dukart, J., Mueller, K., Barthel, H., Villringer, A., Sabri, O., Schroeter, M. L., & the Alzheimer's Disease Neuroimaging Initiative. (2013). Meta-analysis based SVM classification enables accurate detection of Alzheimer's disease across different clinical centers using FDG-PET and MRI. *Psychiatry Research: Neuroimaging, 212*, 230–236. http://dx.doi.org/10.1016/j.pscychresns.2012.04.007

Engelborghs, S., Vloeberghs, E., Le Bastard, N., Van Buggenhout, M., Mariën, P., Somers, N., . . . De Deyn, P. P. (2008). The dopaminergic neuro-transmitter system is associated with aggression and agitation in frontotemporal dementia. *Neurochemistry International, 52*(6), 1052–1060.

Epping, E. A., Kim, J. I., Craufurd, D., Brashers-Krug, T. M., Anderson, K. E., McCusker, E., . . . Paulsen, J. S., & PREDICT-HD Investigators and Coordinators of the Huntington Study Group. (2016). Longitudinal psychiatric symptoms in prodromal Huntington's disease: A decade of data. *American Journal of Psychiatry, 173*(2), 184–192.

Fellgiebel, A., Müller, M. J., Hiemke, C., Bartenstein, P., & Schreckenberger, M. (2007). Clinical improve-ment in a case of frontotemporal dementia under aripiprazole treatment corresponds to partial recovery of disturbed frontal glucose metabolism. *The World Journal of Biological Psychiatry, 8*, 123–126. http://dx.doi.org/10.1080/15622970601016538

Finkel, S. I., Mintzer, J. E., Dysken, M., Krishnan, K. R., Burt, T., & McRae, T. (2004). A randomized, placebo-controlled study of the efficacy and safety of sertraline in the treatment of the behavioral manifestations of Alzheimer's disease in outpatients treated with donepezil. *International Journal of Geriatric Psychiatry, 19*(1), 9–18.

Goldman, J. G., Vaughan, C. L., & Goetz, C. G. (2011). An update expert opinion on management and research strategies in Parkinson's disease psychosis. *Expert Opinion on Pharmacotherapy, 12,* 2009–2024. http://dx.doi.org/10.1517/14656566.2011.587122

Goodarzi, Z., & Ismail, Z. (2017). A practical approach to detection and treatment of depression in Parkinson disease and dementia. *Neurology Clinical Practice, 7*(2), 128–140.

Grau-Rivera, O., Gelpi, E., Carballido-López, E., Sánchez-Valle, R., López-Villegas, M. D. (2015). Rapidly progressive dementia with psychotic onset in a patient with the C9ORF72 mutation. *Clinical Neuropathology, 34*(5), 294–297.

Herrmann, N., Black, S. E., Chow, T., Cappell, J., Tang-Wai, D. F., & Lanctôt, K. L. (2012). Serotonergic function and treatment of behavioral and psychological symptoms of frontotemporal dementia. *The American Journal of Geriatric Psychiatry, 20,* 789–797. http://dx.doi.org/10.1097/JGP.0b013e31823033f3

Hu, X., Meiberth, D., Newport, B., & Jessen, F. (2015). Anatomical correlates of the neuropsychiatric symptoms in Alzheimer's disease. *Current Alzheimer Research, 12,* 266–277. http://dx.doi.org/10.2174/1567205012666150302154914

Huey, E. D., Garcia, C., Wassermann, E. M., Tierney, M. C., & Grafman, J. (2008). Stimulant treatment of frontotemporal dementia in 8 patients. *The Journal of Clinical Psychiatry, 69,* 1981–1982. http://dx.doi.org/10.4088/JCP.v69n1219a

Huntington Study Group. (1996). Unified Huntington's disease rating scale: Reliability and consistency. *Movement Disorders, 11,* 136–142. http://dx.doi.org/10.1002/mds.870110204

Huntington Study Group. (2006). Tetrabenazine as antichorea therapy in Huntington disease: A randomized controlled trial. *Neurology, 66,* 366–372. http://dx.doi.org/10.1212/01.wnl.0000198586.85250.13

Huntington Study Group HART Investigators. (2013). A randomized, double-blind, placebo-controlled trial of pridopidine in Huntington's disease. *Movement Disorders, 28,* 1407–1415. http://dx.doi.org/10.1002/mds.25362

Inouye, S. K., Westendorp, R. G., & Saczynski, J. S. (2014). Delirium in elderly people. *The Lancet, 383,* 911–922. http://dx.doi.org/10.1016/S0140-6736(13)60688-1

Islam, M. M., Iqbal, U., Walther, B., Atique, S., Dubey, N. K., Nguyen, P. A., . . . Shabbir, S. A. (2016). Benzodiazepine use and risk of dementia in the elderly population: A systematic review and meta-analysis. *Neuroepidemiology, 47,* 181–191. http://dx.doi.org/10.1159/000454881

Jesso, S., Morlog, D., Ross, S., Pell, M. D., Pasternak, S. H., Mitchell, D. G., . . . Finger, E. C. (2011). The effects of oxytocin on social cognition and behaviour in frontotemporal dementia. *Brain: A Journal of Neurology, 134,* 2493–2501. http://dx.doi.org/10.1093/brain/awr171

*Kales, H. C., Gitlin, L. N., & Lyketsos, C. G. (2015). Assessment and management of behavioral and psychological symptoms of dementia. *BMJ, 350,* h369.

Kales, H. C., Kim, H. M., Zivin, K., Valenstein, M., Seyfried, L. S., Chiang, C., . . . Blow, F. C. (2012). Risk of mortality among individual antipsychotics in patients with dementia. *The American Journal of Psychiatry, 169,* 71–79. http://dx.doi.org/10.1176/appi.ajp.2011.11030347

Kalia, L. V., & Lang, A. E. (2015). Parkinson's disease. *Lancet, 386*(9996), 896–912.

Kalliolia, E., Silajdžić, E., Nambron, R., Hill, N. R., Doshi, A., Frost, C., . . . Warner, T. T. (2014). Plasma melatonin is reduced in Huntington's disease. *Movement Disorders, 29*(12), 1511–1515.

Kay, C., Hayden, M. R., & Leavitt, B. R. (2017). Epidemiology of Huntington disease. *Handbook of Clinical Neurology, 144,* 31–46. http://dx.doi.org/10.1016/B978-0-12-801893-4.00003-1

Kehoe, E. G., McNulty, J. P., Mullins, P. G., & Bokde, A. L. (2014). Advances in MRI biomarkers for the diagnosis of Alzheimer's disease. *Biomarkers in Medicine, 8*(9), 1151–1169. http://dx.doi.org/10.2217/bmm.14.42

Kertesz, A., Morlog, D., Light, M., Blair, M., Davidson, W., Jesso, S., & Brashear, R. (2008). Galantamine in frontotemporal dementia and primary progressive aphasia. *Dementia and Geriatric Cognitive Disorders, 25,* 178–185. http://dx.doi.org/10.1159/000113034

*Kröger, E., Tatar, O., Vedel, I., Giguère, A. M. C., Voyer, P., Guillaumie, L., . . . Guénette, L. (2017). Improving medication adherence among community-dwelling seniors with cognitive impairment: A systematic review of interventions. *International Journal of Clinical Pharmacy, 39,* 641–656. http://dx.doi.org/10.1007/s11096-017-0487-6

*Lanctôt, K. L., Amatniek, J., Ancoli-Israel, S., Arnold, S. E., Ballard, C., Cohen-Mansfield, J., . . . Boot, B. (2017). Neuropsychiatric signs and symptoms of Alzheimer's disease: New treatment paradigms. *Alzheimer's & Dementia, 3*(3), 440–449.

Lebert, F., Stekke, W., Hasenbroekx, C., & Pasquier, F. (2004). Frontotemporal dementia: A randomised, controlled trial with trazodone. *Dementia and Geriatric Cognitive Disorders, 17*, 355–359. http://dx.doi.org/10.1159/000077171

Leentjens, A. F., Vreeling, F. W., Luijckx, G. J., & Verhey, F. R. (2003). SSRIs in the treatment of depression in Parkinson's disease. *International Journal of Geriatric Psychiatry, 18*, 552–554. http://dx.doi.org/10.1002/gps.865

Leonpacher, A. K., Peters, M. E., Drye, L. T., Makino, K. M., Newell, J. A., Devanand, D. P., . . . the CitAD Research Group. (2016). Effects of citalopram on neuropsychiatric symptoms in Alzheimer's dementia: Evidence from the CitAD Study. *American Journal of Psychiatry, 173*(5), 473–480.

Li, P., Quan, W., Zhou, Y. Y., Wang, Y., Zhang, H. H., & Liu, S. (2016). Efficacy of memantine on neuropsychiatric symptoms associated with the severity of behavioral variant frontotemporal dementia: A six-month, open-label, self-controlled clinical trial. *Experimental and Therapeutic Medicine, 12*(1), 492–498.

*Liu, D., Long, J. D., Zhang, Y., Raymond, L. A., Marder, K., Rosser, A., . . . the PREDICT-HD Investigators and Coordinators of the Huntington Study Group. (2015). Motor onset and diagnosis in Huntington disease using the diagnostic confidence level. *Journal of Neurology, 262*, 2691–2698. http://dx.doi.org/10.1007/s00415-015-7900-7

Lyketsos, C. G., Carrillo, M. C., Ryan, J. M., Khachaturian, A. S., Trzepacz, P., Amatniek, J., . . . Miller, D. S. (2011). Neuropsychiatric symptoms in Alzheimer's disease. *Alzheimer's & Dementia: The Journal of the Alzheimer's Association, 7*, 532–539. http://dx.doi.org/10.1016/j.jalz.2011.05.2410

Lyketsos, C. G., DelCampo, L., Steinberg, M., Miles, Q., Steele, C. D., Munro, C., . . . Rabins, P. V. (2003). Treating depression in Alzheimer disease: Efficacy and safety of sertraline therapy, and the benefits of depression reduction: The DIADS. *Archives of General Psychiatry, 60*(7), 737–746.

MacDonald, M. E., Ambrose, C. M., Duyao, M. P., Myers, R. H., Lin, C., Srinidhi, L., . . . Harper, P. S. (1993). A novel gene containing a trinucleotide repeat that is expanded and unstable on Huntington's disease chromosomes. *Cell, 72*, 971–983. http://dx.doi.org/10.1016/0092-8674(93)90585-E

*Manoochehri, M., & Huey, E. D. (2012). Diagnosis and management of behavioral issues in frontotemporal dementia. *Current Neurology and Neuroscience Reports, 12*(5), 528–536.

Marsh, L. (2013). Depression and Parkinson's disease: Current knowledge. *Current Neurology and Neuroscience Reports, 13*, 409. http://dx.doi.org/10.1007/s11910-013-0409-5

Marshall, G. A., Donovan, N. J., Lorius, N., Gidicsin, C. M., Maye, J., Pepin, L. C., . . . Johnson, K. A. (2013). Apathy is associated with increased amyloid burden in mild cognitive impairment. *The Journal of Neuropsychiatry and Clinical Neurosciences, 25*, 302–307. http://dx.doi.org/10.1176/appi.neuropsych.12060156

Matsunaga, S., Kishi, T., & Iwata, N. (2015). Memantine monotherapy for Alzheimer's disease: A systematic review and meta-analysis. *PLoS One, 10*, e0123289. http://dx.doi.org/10.1371/journal.pone.0123289

Mendez, M. F., Shapira, J. S., McMurtray, A., & Licht, E. (2007). Preliminary findings: Behavioral worsening on donepezil in patients with frontotemporal dementia. *The American Journal of Geriatric Psychiatry, 15*, 84–87.

Mestre, T., Ferreira, J., Coelho, M. M., Rosa, M., & Sampaio, C. (2009). Therapeutic interventions for symptomatic treatment in Huntington's disease. *Cochrane Database of Systematic Reviews, 2009*(3), CD006456. http://dx.doi.org/10.1002/14651858.CD006456.pub2

Mesulam, M., Wieneke, C., Rogalski, E., Cobia, D., Thompson, C., & Weintraub, S. (2009). Quantitative template for subtyping primary progressive aphasia. *Archives of Neurology, 66*, 1545–1551. http://dx.doi.org/10.1001/archneurol.2009.288

Mintzer, J., Greenspan, A., Caers, I., Van Hove, I., Kushner, S., Weiner, M., . . . Schneider, L. S. (2006). Risperidone in the treatment of psychosis of Alzheimer disease: Results from a prospective clinical trial. *American Journal of Psychiatry, 14*(3), 280–291.

Mintzer, J. E., Tune, L. E., Breder, C. D., Swanink, R., Marcus, R. N., McQuade, R. D., & Forbes, A. (2007). Aripiprazole for the treatment of psychoses in institutionalized patients with Alzheimer dementia: A multicenter, randomized, double-blind, placebo-controlled assessment of three fixed doses. *American Journal of Psychiatry, 15*(11), 918–931.

Moga, D. C., Taipale, H., Tolppanen, A. M., Tanskanen, A., Tiihonen, J., Hartikainen, S., . . . Gnjidic, D. (2017). A comparison of sex differences in psychotropic medication use in older people with Alzheimer's disease in the US and Finland. *Drugs & Aging, 34*(1), 55–65.

Moretti, R., Torre, P., Antonello, R. M., Cattaruzza, T., Cazzato, G., & Bava, A. (2004). Rivastigmine in frontotemporal dementia: An open-label study. *Drugs & Aging, 21*, 931–937. http://dx.doi.org/10.2165/00002512-200421140-00003

Moretti, R., Torre, P., Antonello, R. M., Cazzato, G., Griggio, S., & Bava, A. (2003). Olanzapine as a treatment of neuropsychiatric disorders of Alzheimer's disease and other dementias: A 24-month follow-up of 68 patients. *American Journal of Alzheimer's Disease and Other Dementias, 18*, 205–214. http://dx.doi.org/10.1177/153331750301800410

Munro, C. A., Brandt, J., Sheppard, J. M., Steele, C. D., Samus, Q. M., Steinberg, M., . . . Lyketsos, C. G. (2004). Cognitive response to pharmacological treatment for depression in Alzheimer disease: Secondary outcomes from the depression in

Alzheimer's disease study (DIADS). *The American Journal of Geriatric Psychiatry, 12,* 491–498. http://dx.doi.org/10.1097/00019442-200409000-00007

Nestor, P. J. (2012). Reversal of abnormal eating and drinking behaviour in a frontotemporal lobar degeneration patient using low-dose topiramate. *Journal of Neurology, Neurosurgery, & Psychiatry, 83,* 349–350. http://dx.doi.org/10.1136/jnnp.2010.238899

Olin, J. T., Fox, L. S., Pawluczyk, S., Taggart, N. A., & Schneider, L. S. (2001). A pilot randomized trial of carbamazepine for behavioral symptoms in treatment-resistant outpatients with Alzheimer disease. *The American Journal of Geriatric Psychiatry, 9,* 400–405. http://dx.doi.org/10.1097/00019442-200111000-00008

Paleacu, D., Barak, Y., Mirecky, I., & Mazeh, D. (2008). Quetiapine treatment for behavioural and psychological symptoms of dementia in Alzheimer's disease patients: A 6-week, double-blind, placebo-controlled study. *International Journal of Geriatric Psychiatry, 23*(4), 393–400.

Paulsen, J. S., Langbehn, D. R., Stout, J. C., Aylward, E., Ross, C. A., Nance, M., . . . Hayden, M., & the Predict-HD Investigators and Coordinators of the Huntington Study Group. (2008). Detection of Huntington's disease decades before diagnosis: The Predict-HD study. *Journal of Neurology, Neurosurgery, and Psychiatry, 79*(8), 874–880.

Pintor, L., Valldeoriola, F., Baillés, E., Martí, M. J., Muñiz, A., & Tolosa, E. (2012). Ziprasidone versus clozapine in the treatment of psychotic symptoms in Parkinson disease: A randomized open clinical trial. *Clinical Neuropharmacology, 35*(2), 61–66.

Podcasy, J. L., & Epperson, C. N. (2016). Considering sex and gender in Alzheimer disease and other dementias. *Dialogues in Clinical Neuroscience, 18*(4), 437–446.

Poetter, C. E., & Stewart, J. T. (2012). Treatment of indiscriminate, inappropriate sexual behavior in frontotemporal dementia with carbamazepine. *Journal of Clinical Psychopharmacology, 32,* 137–138. http://dx.doi.org/10.1097/JCP.0b013e31823f91b9

Porsteinsson, A. P., Drye, L. T., Pollock, B. G., Devanand, D. P., Frangakis, C., Ismail, Z., . . . Lyketsos, C. G., & the CitAD Research Group. (2014). Effect of citalopram on agitation in Alzheimer disease: The CitAD randomized clinical trial. *JAMA: Journal of the American Medical Association, 311,* 682–691. http://dx.doi.org/10.1001/jama.2014.93

*Pressman, P. S., & Miller, B. L. (2014). Diagnosis and management of behavioral variant frontotemporal dementia. *Biological Psychiatry, 75*(7), 574–581.

Quental, N. B., Brucki, S. M., & Bueno, O. F. (2013). Visuospatial function in early Alzheimer's disease—the use of the Visual Object and Space Perception (VOSP) battery. *PLoS One, 8*(7), e68398.

Rahman, S., Robbins, T. W., Hodges, J. R., Mehta, M. A., Nestor, P. J., Clark, L., & Sahakian, B. J. (2006). Methylphenidate ("Ritalin") can ameliorate abnormal risk-taking behavior in the frontal variant of frontotemporal dementia. *Neuropsychopharmacology, 31,* 651–658. http://dx.doi.org/10.1038/sj.npp.1300886

Rascovsky, K., Hodges, J. R., Knopman, D., Mendez, M. F., Kramer, J. H., Neuhaus, J., . . . Miller, B. L. (2011). Sensitivity of revised diagnostic criteria for the behavioural variant of frontotemporal dementia. *Brain, 134*(Pt 9), 2456–2477.

Reitz, C., & Mayeux, R. (2014). Alzheimer disease: Epidemiology, diagnostic criteria, risk factors and biomarkers. *Biochemical Pharmacology, 88*(4), 640–651.

Richard, I. H., McDermott, M. P., Kurlan, R., Lyness, J. M., Como, P. G., Pearson, N., . . . McDonald, W., & the SAD-PD Study Group. (2012). A randomized, double-blind, placebo-controlled trial of antidepressants in Parkinson disease. *Neurology, 78*(16), 1229–1236.

Robles Bayón, A., & Gude Sampedro, F. (2014). Inappropriate treatments for patients with cognitive decline. *Neurologia, 29*(9), 523–532.

Rocca, P., Marino, F., Montemagni, C., Perrone, D., & Bogetto, F. (2007). Risperidone, olanzapine and quetiapine in the treatment of behavioral and psychological symptoms in patients with Alzheimer's disease: Preliminary findings from a naturalistic, retrospective study. *Psychiatry and Clinical Neuroscience, 61*(6), 622–629.

Rosen, H. J., Allison, S. C., Schauer, G. F., Gorno-Tempini, M. L., Weiner, M. W., & Miller, B. L. (2005). Neuroanatomical correlates of behavioural disorders in dementia. *Brain, 128*(Pt 11), 2612–2625.

Rosenberg, P. B., Nowrangi, M. A., & Lyketsos, C. G. (2015). Neuropsychiatric symptoms in Alzheimer's disease: What might be associated brain circuits? *Molecular Aspects of Medicine, 43–44,* 25–37. http://dx.doi.org/10.1016.j.mam.2015.05.005

Ross, C. A., Aylward, E. H., Wild, E. J., Langbehn, D. R., Long, J. D., Warner, J. H., . . . Tabrizi, S. J. (2014). Huntington disease: Natural history, biomarkers and prospects for therapeutics. *Nature Reviews Neurology, 10*(4), 204–216.

Ryan, K. A., Hammers, D., DeLeon, A., Bilen, H., Frey, K., Burke, J., . . . Giordani, B. (2017). Agreement among neuropsychological and behavioral data and PiB findings in diagnosing frontotemporal dementia. *Journal of Clinical Neuroscience, 44,* 128–132.

Salloway, S., Sperling, R., Keren, R., Porsteinsson, A. P., van Dyck, C. H., Tariot, P. N., . . . Cedarbaum, J. M., & the ELND005-AD201 Investigators. (2011). A phase 2 randomized trial of ELND005, scyllo-inositol, in mild to moderate Alzheimer disease. *Neurology, 77,* 1253–1262.

Scheltens, P., Blennow, K., Breteler, M. M., de Strooper, B., Frisoni, G. B., Salloway, S., & Van der Flier, W. M. (2016). Alzheimer's disease. *Lancet, 388*(10043), 505–517.

Schneider, L. S., Tariot, P. N., Dagerman, K. S., Davis, S. M., Hsiao, J. K., Ismail, M. S., . . . Lieberman, J. A., & the CATIE-AD Study Group. (2006). Effectiveness of atypical antipsychotic drugs in patients with Alzheimer's disease. *The New England Journal of Medicine, 355,* 1525–1538. http://dx.doi.org/10.1056/NEJMoa061240

Scott, I. A., Anderson, K., Freeman, C. R., & Stowasser, D. A. (2014). First do no harm: A real need to deprescribe in older patients. *The Medical Journal of Australia, 201,* 390–392. http://dx.doi.org/10.5694/mja14.00146

Seitz, D. P., Adunuri, N., Gill, S. S., Gruneir, A., Herrmann, N., & Rochon, P. (2011). Antidepressants for agitation and psychosis in dementia. *Cochrane Database of Systematic Reviews, 2,* CD008191.

Sinforiani, E., Bernini, S., & Picascia, M. (2017). Correlations among age, cognitive impairment, and comorbidities in Alzheimer's disease: Report from a center for cognitive disorders. *Aging Clinical and Experimental Research, 29,* 1299–1300. http://dx.doi.org/10.1007/s40520-017-0807-7

Sinforiani, E., Citterio, A., Zucchella, C., Bono, G., Corbetta, S., Merlo, P., & Mauri, M. (2010). Impact of gender differences on the outcome of Alzheimer's disease. *Dementia and Geriatric Cognitive Disorders, 30,* 147–154. http://dx.doi.org/10.1159/000318842

Snowden, J. S. (2017). The neuropsychology of Huntington's disease. *Archives of Clinical Neuropsychology, Nov; 32*(7), 876–887.

Streim, J. E., Porsteinsson, A. P., Breder, C. D., Swanink, R., Marcus, R., McQuade, R., & Carson, W. H. (2008). A randomized, double-blind, placebo-controlled study of aripiprazole for the treatment of psychosis in nursing home patients with Alzheimer disease. *American Journal of Geriatric Psychiatry, 16*(7), 537–550.

Sturrock, A., & Leavitt, B. R. (2010). The clinical and genetic features of Huntington disease. *Journal of Geriatric Psychiatry and Neurology, 23*(4), 243–259.

Sultzer, D. L., Davis, S. M., Tariot, P. N., Dagerman, K. S., Lebowitz, B. D., Lyketsos, C. G., . . . Schneider, L. S., & the CATIE-AD Study Group. (2008). Clinical symptom responses to atypical antipsychotic medications in Alzheimer's disease: Phase 1 outcomes from the CATIE-AD effectiveness trial. *The American Journal of Psychiatry, 165,* 844–854. http://dx.doi.org/10.1176/appi.ajp.2008.07111779

Sumiyoshi, T., Higuchi, Y., & Uehara, T. (2013). Neural basis for the ability of atypical antipsychotic drugs to improve cognition in schizophrenia. *Frontiers in Behavioral Neuroscience, 7,* 140.

Troeung, L., Egan, S. J., & Gasson, N. (2013). A meta-analysis of randomised placebo-controlled treatment trials for depression and anxiety in Parkinson's disease. *PLoS One, 8,* e79510. http://dx.doi.org/10.1371/journal.pone.0079510

Tsai, R. M., & Boxer, A. L. (2014). Treatment of frontotemporal dementia. *Current Treatment Options in Neurology, 16,* 319. http://dx.doi.org/10.1007/s11940-014-0319-0

*Tsai, R. M., & Boxer, A. L. (2016). Therapy and clinical trials in frontotemporal dementia: Past, present, and future. *Journal of Neurochemistry, 138*(Suppl. 1), 211–221.

Van Den Eeden, S. K., Tanner, C. M., Bernstein, A. L., Fross, R. D., Leimpeter, A., Bloch, D. A., & Nelson, L. M. (2003). Incidence of Parkinson's disease: Variation by age, gender, and race/ethnicity. *American Journal of Epidemiology, 157*(11), 1015–1022.

Vieira, R. T., Caixeta, L., Machado, S., Silva, A. C., Nardi, A. E., Arias-Carrión, O., & Carta, M. G. (2013). Epidemiology of early-onset dementia: A review of the literature. *Clinical Practice and Epidemiology in Mental Health, 9,* 88–95. http://dx.doi.org/10.2174/1745017901309010088

Wang, J., Yu, J. T., & Tan, L. (2015). PLD3 in Alzheimer's disease. *Molecular Neurobiology, 51*(2), 480–486.

*Wang, J., Yu, J. T., Wang, H. F., Meng, X. F., Wang, C., Tan, C. C., & Tan, L. (2015). Pharmacological treatment of neuropsychiatric symptoms in Alzheimer's disease: A systematic review and meta-analysis. *Journal of Neurology, Neurosurgery, and Psychiatry, 86,* 101–109. http://dx.doi.org/10.1136/jnnp-2014-308112

Wang, L. Y., Shofer, J. B., Rohde, K., Hart, K. L., Hoff, D. J., McFall, Y. H., . . . Peskind, E. R. (2009). Prazosin for the treatment of behavioral symptoms in patients with Alzheimer disease with agitation and aggression. *American Journal of Geriatric Psychiatry, 17*(9), 744–751.

Weintraub, D., Mavandadi, S., Mamikonyan, E., Siderowf, A. D., Duda, J. E., Hurtig, H. I., . . . Stern, M. B. (2010). Atomoxetine for depression and other neuropsychiatric symptoms in Parkinson disease. *Neurology, 75*(5), 448–455.

Wood, H. (2017). Alzheimer disease: ApoE4 implicated in tau-mediated neurodegeneration. *Nature Reviews. Neurology, 13*(12), 706–707.

*Wyant, K. J., Ridder, A. J., & Dayalu, P. (2017). Huntington's disease—update on treatments. *Current Neurology and Neuroscience Reports, 17*(4), 33.

Chapter 19

PHARMACOLOGICAL TREATMENT OF PAIN AND PAIN-RELATED DISORDERS

Julie R. Price, Micah J. Price, and Amie Hall

Pain dates back to the beginning of humankind. Physiological interventions for pain management, such as trepanning or drilling holes in the skull, have been found as far back as 6500 B.C., as evidenced in prehistoric skulls from France (Restak, 2000). Acupuncture—inserting needles into the body for pain relief or as a form of physical therapy—dates back to ancient China, with estimates ranging to around 4000 years ago, and is still in use today. Pharmacological treatments derived from plants have long been documented for pain management. Hippocrates used salicylic acid, the active ingredient in aspirin harvested from the willow tree, for women in childbirth for its pain-relieving benefits. After the discovery of the opium poppy in Mesopotamia in 3400 B.C., the opium trade began to sweep the world. This movement halted in Europe in 1300 A.D. during the Holy Inquisition, as opium was viewed as demonic. In 1527, Paracelsus reintroduced opium as laudanum in the European literature and it was prescribed as a painkiller. It was not until 1803 that morphine was synthesized as "God's own medicine" for its reliability, long-lasting effects, and safety (Booth, 1998, p. 81). In 1874 heroin was synthesized and introduced commercially. After only 5 years on the market, heroin addiction rose to alarming rates and in 1905 the U.S. Congress banned opium. In 2009, the World Health Organization reported that around 80% of the world's population did not have adequate access to pain relief, with the U.S. Food and Drug Administration (FDA) further planning to restrict access to opioid-based pain relievers (A Brief History of Opium, 2015). As a result, guidelines were established in 2016 by the Centers for Disease Control and Prevention (CDC) that recommends the use of nonpharmacological and nonopioid pharmacological treatments for pain, shorter durations for opioid prescriptions, and keeping opioid doses lower than the equivalent of 90 milligrams of morphine.

The perception of pain (nociception) has been a point of discussion since ancient times. Pain (nociception) occurs as a result of a perceived noxious stimulus activating receptors called nociceptors in the peripheral nervous system (PNS). This information is then transmitted to the central nervous system (CNS), where the perception of pain is generated (National Research Council, 2009). The experience of pain is a result of higher cognitive processing, whereas nociception can occur in either the presence or absence of pain. Suffering is the affective or emotional responses to pain and to the adverse events associated with the pain. Pain, a normal physiological process, is connected to, but is not mutually exclusive with suffering. Rakel and Weil (2012) indicate that suffering influences how the body perceives pain. Targeted interventions for

http://dx.doi.org/10.1037/0000133-019
APA Handbook of Psychopharmacology, S. M. Evans (Editor-in-Chief)

suffering will impact pain severity and overall quality of life, thereby decreasing the patient's overall pain presentation and experience. Thus, suffering is an option and can be viewed as an opportunity for growth (Rakel & Weil, 2012).

Mind–body medicine is not a new concept. However, it was not until around the mid-20th century that medical science shifted from the dualistic view to the understanding that pain is a subjective experience with both physiological and psychological components. In 1994, the International Association for the Study of Pain (IASP) defined pain as an "unpleasant sensory and emotional experience associated with actual or potential tissue damage" (Merskey & Spear, 1967, p. 59).

EPIDEMIOLOGY AND PREVALENCE

The treatment of nonmalignant/noncancer-related pain and pain-related conditions have varied greatly over time, with mixed success. However, over the past century the knowledge, theories, and understanding of pain has increased dramatically. Pain receptors have been identified and mechanisms of drug interactions have become better understood, all leading to the development of more advanced theories. Treatments have also improved, with the development of research-driven medications, technologically advanced devices to block pain signaling, and less invasive surgical techniques. Despite this, pain is the most common reason Americans access the health care system. It is a leading cause of disability and a major contributor to health care costs. An Institute of Medicine (IOM) report (2011) indicated that chronic pain impacts more than 100 million U.S. adults—more than heart disease, diabetes, and cancer combined, with a cost of $560 to $635 billion annually. This figure includes the estimated cost of associated pain-related health care and disability and lost wages and productivity, though it does not take into account the emotional or personal costs to individuals and their families. The CDC (2016) collected data over a 3-month period on adults age 18 and older who experience headache/migraine, low back, and neck pain. The data indicated that

15.4% reported severe headache or migraine pain, 29.1% reported low back pain, and 15.7% reported neck pain.

Pediatric populations also experience significant distress associated with chronic pain. King et al. (2011) found that headaches were the most commonly studied, with an estimated median prevalence rate of 23%. Other types of pain (back, abdominal, musculoskeletal) are highly prevalent in children and adolescents with median prevalence rates ranging from 11% to 38%, with an increase over the last several decades (King et al., 2011). Huguet and Miró (2008) discussed results that found 37.3% of school-aged children reported experiencing chronic pain within the past 3 months, with 5.1% of the children reporting moderate or severe chronic pain-related concerns. The American Pain Society (2012) suggests that chronic pain affects between 20% and 35% of children and adolescents worldwide. These effects may predispose children to the development of pain conditions later in life (Young & Kemper, 2013) similar to their older counterparts, and have been shown to interfere significantly with daily functioning. Decreased quality of life, missed work/school days, changes in academic/job performance, mood- and sleep-related changes, impacts on social development and relationships, missed income and time at work by parents and family, and increased medical and medication utilization are all common secondary pain-associated experiences that affect more than just the patient (King et al., 2011).

Patients with chronic pain often present primarily for and with physical pain-related complaints, despite the reciprocal nature and relationship with emotional suffering. Therefore, both mental and physical pain-related disorders will be discussed.

Somatic Symptom Disorder

High rates of medically unexplained somatic pain complaints are consistently found in the literature (Joergen Grabe et al., 2003; Schumacher & Brahler, 1999). In 2006, a study by Hiller et al. was conducted with 2,552 people, of which 81.6% (4 out of 5 people) reported at least one somatic symptom causing at least mild impairment in the last 7 days. Of these individuals 22.1% also endorsed at least one frequent, chronic somatic symptom causing severe disabling impairment. There was overwhelming endorsement of back pain in every second person, with 40% experiencing headaches. Given the widespread somatic complaints coupled with the previous conceptualization of the disorder, the specific prevalence of somatic symptom disorder is unknown. However, estimates suggest it occurs in 5% to 7% of the general adult population, with an estimated female to male ratio of 10:1 (American Psychiatric Association [APA], 2013; Kurlansik & Maffei, 2016).

Genito-Pelvic Pain/Penetration Disorder

The exact prevalence of this disorder is unknown, though it is estimated that 15% of North American women seek help for pain during intercourse (American Psychiatric Association, 2013). Sungur (2013) noted that in some group-oriented cultures, referrals to sexual dysfunction treatment centers were between 52% and 73% of those seeking treatment.

Other Nonmental/Medical Pain-Related Disorders

Chronic low back pain (CLBP) is the most common type of pain in the United States, with a prevalence rate between 60% and 80% (Stevens & Saper, 2012). Given these percentages, it is safe to say that most adults will experience LBP at some point in their lifetime. Peripheral neuropathy is nerve damage caused by high blood sugar leading to numbness, loss of sensation, and pain in feet, legs, or hands. Sixty percent to 70% of all individuals with diabetes will develop peripheral neuropathy (Bril et al., 2011). Headaches are a common complaint, with prevalence rates between 8% and 18%, whereas 16% of women and 6% of men suffer with migraine headaches (Jackson, Kuriyama, & Hayashino, 2012). Migraines include throbbing head pain (unilateral or bilateral), and usually present with nausea, vomiting, photophobia, or sonophobia. Fibromyalgia is a cluster of symptoms that include chronic widespread pain, cognitive disturbance, fatigue, joint pain, and sleep difficulties. The American College of Rheumatology indicates that

2% to 4% of people have fibromyalgia, with it occurring more often in women than men (Bhana, 2017). Complex regional pain syndrome (CRPS) is a syndrome that usually develops after a traumatic/harmful event, and is identified by severe pain, hypersensitivity, swelling, and temperature and color changes in the skin. Neuropathic pain is the primary feature and presentation usually begins in one limb, but can spread. CRPS can by divided into type I (previously reflex sympathetic dystrophy) and type II, when nerve injury is apparent (previously causalgia). CRPS can affect anyone at any time, though more often seen in women (Perez et al., 2010).

DIAGNOSING PAIN AND PAIN-RELATED DISORDERS

Medical disorders can present as psychological disorders and psychological disorders can present as medical disorders. Thus, the integration of a comprehensive clinical interview with screening instruments (as indicated), an extensive chart review, laboratory and radiological imaging, collateral information where available (spouse, family, school, etc.), and collaboration with attending providers is necessary to achieve diagnostic clarification. It is also important to keep in mind that available medical information can change, either as a result of a new or different diagnostic test or via the scientific literature. In addition, the reciprocal nature of mind and body is still not fully understood, thus it is crucial to revisit a diagnosis as new information becomes available. See the Tool Kit of Resources at the end of the chapter for additional patient and provider resources.

Somatic Symptom Disorder

Somatic symptom disorder with predominant pain (previously pain disorder) in the *Diagnostic and Statistical Manual of Mental Disorders* (5th ed.; *DSM–5*; American Psychiatric Association, 2013) was reconceptualized and now "emphasizes diagnosis made on the basis of positive symptoms and signs (distressing somatic symptoms plus abnormal thoughts, feelings, and behaviors in response to these symptoms) rather than the absence of a medical explanation for somatic symptoms" (p. 309). This reconceptualization was aimed at providing greater clarification for individuals working in medical settings including primary care and pain management clinics. It was also made to reinforce the mind–body connection (vs. mind–body dualism), as the patient's suffering is real and genuine. Furthermore, this reconceptualized diagnosis allows for a more inclusive frame, shifting from the biomedical model and taking into account the biopsychosocial–spiritual model of conceptualization. In the past somatization disorders have been viewed as not real and labeled as psychogenic pain when no medical explanations were present. This view often left patients hearing the infamous words, "It's all is your head . . . There is nothing more I can do." It also added to their feelings of demoralization, at which point they were referred to mental health professionals for psychotropic medication evaluation and management.

Somatic symptom disorder is most effectively diagnosed via a comprehensive clinical interview to assess for specific diagnostic criteria. Patients meet somatic symptom disorder diagnostic criteria when they experience somatic (bodily) symptoms that cause significant distress in their ability to function on a daily basis (Criteria A). They also experience excessive thoughts, feelings, or behaviors related to the somatic symptoms (Criteria B), which might include illness anxiety, identity fusion with health concerns, avoidance behaviors, and high levels of medical utilization. Finally, their symptomatology lasts longer than 6 months in duration (Criteria C; American Psychiatric Association, 2013). See the *DSM–5* for diagnostic specifiers. In addition, screening instruments can provide useful diagnostic information. The most widely utilized is the Patient Health Questionnaire somatic symptoms scale (PHQ-15) used to evaluate potential somatic symptomatology (Spitzer, Kroenke, & Williams, 2002). Other useful assessment instruments and measures include but are not limited to the Pain Catastrophizing Scale (PCS; Sullivan, 2009), Millon Behavioral Medicine Diagnostic (Millon, Antoni, Millon, Minor, & Grossman, 2001), and the Minnesota Multiphasic Personality Inventory—2—Restructured Form (Ben-Porath & Tellegen, 2008). However, caution should be used, as these measures often poorly diagnostically differentiate between

somatic and psychological manifestation of symptomatology. Frances and Chapman (2013) described this caution with

> the golden rule: an underlying medical illness or medication side effect has to be ruled out before ever deciding that someone's symptoms are caused by mental disorder. . . . There are serious risks attached to over-psychologizing somatic symptoms and mislabeling the normal reactions to being sick—especially when the judgments are based on vague wording that can't possibly lead to reliable diagnosis. (p. 484)

Genito-Pelvic Pain/Penetration Disorder

Genito-pelvic pain/penetration disorder (previously vaginismus) is characterized by persistent or recurrent symptoms including difficulties with penetration, genito-pelvic pain, fear of pain or penetration, and/or pelvic floor muscle tension. The symptomatology lasts at least 6 months in duration and the symptoms cause significant distress. Additionally, the dysfunction is not better accounted for by another disorder or condition (e.g., nonsexual mental disorder, relationship distress, medication effects; American Psychiatric Association, 2013). See the *DSM–5* for diagnostic specifiers.

Other Nonmental/Medical Pain-Related Disorders

The following pain disorders are medical in nature, and therefore the diagnosis is established by a medical provider, not a mental health provider: CLBP, diabetic peripheral neuropathic pain, migraine, fibromyalgia, and complex regional pain syndrome. The diagnosis of such medical disorders is outside of a psychologists' scope of practice and thus will not be discussed in this chapter. However, given the controversy surrounding the diagnosis of fibromyalgia, it is important to at least dispel the myth that fibromyalgia is the result of solely a psychiatric disorder and/or a trauma history. Understanding current research and imaging studies has challenged stereotypical provider beliefs by providing direct evidence of alterations in the hypothalamic–pituitary–adrenal axis (HPA axis), which results in central pain sensitivities (central sensitization/hyperreactivity). The HPA axis regulates responses to trauma, stress, and injury and is associated with functional impairment in the fascia in fibromyalgia patients. Similar pathophysiological responses have been found in patients suffering from posttraumatic stress disorder (PTSD) and thus may lead to the increased likelihood of comorbidity of these diagnoses.

EVIDENCE-BASED PHARMACOLOGICAL TREATMENTS OF PAIN AND PAIN-RELATED DISORDERS

The treatment of pain and pain-related disorders relies heavily on the incorporation of the underlying physiological pain diagnosis (headache, fibromyalgia, low back pain, etc.). This diagnostic information gets coupled with mental health comorbidities and/or symptomatology (anxiety, depression, insomnia, etc.), and potential side effect profiles when differentially developing the psychopharmacological treatment plan. Thus, psychopharmacological interventions for pain and pain-related disorders do not necessarily lend themselves to starting with a particular class of medications. For example, if a patient presented with a diagnosis of depression and fibromyalgia, a starting point for medication management might be duloxetine, a serotonin and norepinephrine reuptake inhibitor (SNRI). However, if the patient presented with a diagnosis of depression and migraine headaches, a starting point for medication management might be amitriptyline, a tricyclic antidepressant (TCA).

Pharmacologic analgesics for the treatment of nonmalignant pain and pain-related disorders are still the most widely utilized interventions for chronic pain management. Table 19.1 provides examples of medications with usual dosing ranges for selected pain syndromes, common/adverse drug reactions, and clinical pearls. Psychopharmacological treatment of pain, while not a novel concept, remains underutilized. This underutilization occurs despite significant research demonstrating the effectiveness of antidepressants and anticonvulsants in treatment of patients with

chronic pain. Overall, the disinhibition and imbalance of serotonin and norepinephrine in endogenous pain inhibitory pathways are thought to contribute to persistent pain (Marks et al., 2009). Thus, antidepressants such as TCAs, selective serotonin reuptake inhibitors (SSRIs), and SNRIs are the mainstay treatments of pain and pain-related disorders, due to their pain-modulating effects via increasing levels of serotonin and norepinephrine. Antidepressants also have the potential to improve other symptomatology including mood, fatigue, and sleep via these same mechanisms. Much like antidepressants, anticonvulsants are used for the treatment of pain and pain-related disorders because of their pain-modulating properties. However, the mechanism of action is less clear for pain modulation with anticonvulsants. Researchers have found that neurochemical mechanisms for neuropathic pain and epilepsy are similar, making the use of anticonvulsants for the treatment of neuropathic pain a reasonable choice (Ryder & Stannard, 2005). Listed in the next sections are some of the more common nonmalignant pain-related syndromes, two of which are included in the *DSM–5*.

Somatic Symptom Disorder

Psychopharmacological treatment for somatic symptom disorder includes off label use of TCAs, SSRIs, SNRIs, and St. John's wort (a dietary supplement). A meta-analysis by O'Malley et al. (1999), indicated that amitriptyline, the most studied TCA, was more likely to be effective than SSRIs. Amitriptyline is metabolized to nortriptyline, which inhibits the reuptake of norepinephrine and serotonin. It not only improves pain but also has benefits for fatigue, functional symptoms, sleep, and other symptomatology. Fluoxetine (an SSRI) has been shown to decrease pain and other symptoms, as well as improve functional status and sleep (Kurlansik & Maffei, 2016; O'Malley et al., 1999). SNRIs may also help to improve physical symptoms, anxiety, and depression for patients with somatic symptom disorder (Kleinstäuber et al., 2014). Research indicates that some medications, specifically opioids, are not effective for somatic symptom disorder and should be avoided (Croicu, Chwastiak, & Katon, 2014). However, it is important to consider new

TABLE 19.1

Examples of Medications Used for Treating Pain and Pain-Related Disorders

Select drugs	Usual adult dose range	Pain syndromes for which evidence of efficacy exists	Common/adverse drug reactions	Clinical pearls
I. Antidepressants				
SSRIs				
Citalopram Fluoxetine Paroxetine	20–40 mg/d 20–80 mg/d 20–60 mg/d	Somatic symptom disorder Fibromyalgia	Citalopram: QTc-prolongation > 40 mg/d Class effects: nausea, sedation, insomnia, nervousness, agitation, restlessness, diarrhea, decreased libido, dry mouth, diaphoresis, anorgasmia, erectile dysfunction, weight gain (to varying degrees)	▪ Take with food to help with nausea ▪ Use lower doses in elderly and patients with hepatic or renal impairment ▪ Start low and titrate up slowly to lowest effective dose; improves tolerability ▪ Taper slowly when discontinuing to prevent withdrawal symptoms
SNRIs				
Duloxetine	60–120 mg/d (target dose 60 mg/d; doses > 60 mg/d have not been shown to be more efficacious)	Somatic symptom disorder Chronic back pain Fibromyalgia Migraine prophylaxis Neuropathic pain	Venlafaxine: blood pressure changes at high doses, HTN risk Class effects: nausea, dry mouth, headache, excessive sweating, nervousness, dizziness, anorexia, dry mouth, diaphoresis, constipation, weakness, sedation, insomnia	▪ Take with food to help with nausea ▪ Monitor blood pressure ▪ Start low and go slow ▪ Taper down
Venlafaxine	37.5–225 mg/d (target dose for migraine prevention 75–150 mg/d)			
Milnacipran	50–100 mg bid			
TCAs				
Amitriptyline Nortriptyline	25–150 mg/d 25–150 mg/d	Somatic symptom disorder Fibromyalgia Migraine prophylaxis Neuropathic pain, Postherpetic neuralgia	Class effects: anticholinergic effects (dry mouth, constipation, blurred vision, confusion), sedation, weight gain, sexual dysfunction, low seizure threshold, rash, blood disorders, behavioral disturbances, orthostatic hypotension, QTc prolongation	▪ Avoid or use lower doses in elderly ▪ Give at bedtime ▪ Start low and go slow ▪ Taper down
Tetracyclic Antidepressant				
Trazodone	50–150 mg/d; max 200 mg	Insomnia	Sedation, dry mouth, constipation, orthostatic hypotension, dizziness; rare, but serious side effect: priapism	▪ Avoid or use lower doses in elderly ▪ Give at bedtime ▪ Start low and go slow ▪ Taper down

II. Anticonvulsants

Drug	Dose	Indications	Side effects	Monitoring
Carbamazepine	100–400 mg bid; max dose 1,200 mg/d	Trigeminal neuralgia	Side effects are usually dose dependent; dizziness, drowsiness, ataxia nausea, anorexia, nystagmus, diplopia. Rare, but serious side effects: Stevens–Johnson syndrome/toxic epidermal necrolysis; idiosyncratic blood dyscrasias—aplastic anemia and agranulocytosis; hyponatremia	▪ Monitor CBC, liver, renal, and thyroid function tests ▪ Conduct ophthalmic exam ▪ Is an enzyme inducer, therefore has many drug interactions
Oxcarbazepine	300–900 mg bid	Trigeminal neuralgia	Side effects are usually less frequent and severe than carbamazepine; nausea, vomiting, dizziness, fatigue, tremors, hyponatremia	▪ Monitor CBC, liver, renal, and thyroid function tests ▪ Conduct ophthalmic exam ▪ Is an enzyme inducer, therefore has many drug interactions
Gabapentin	900–3,600 mg tid (doses > 1,800 mg/d have not been shown to be more efficacious)	CRPS Fibromyalgia Migraine prophylaxis Neuropathic pain Postherpetic neuralgia	Dizziness, drowsiness, peripheral edema, weight gain, poor concentration	▪ Monitor renal function; dosage adjustments necessary for renal impairment
Pregabalin	150–600 mg bid/tid	Fibromyalgia Migraine prophylaxis Neuropathic pain Postherpetic neuralgia	Dizziness, drowsiness, peripheral edema, weight gain, poor concentration	▪ Monitor renal function; dosage adjustments necessary for renal impairment
Topiramate	50 mg bid	Migraine prophylaxis	Cognitive dysfunction, sedation, kidney stones, weight loss, metabolic acidosis	▪ Monitor liver and kidney function, electrolytes ▪ Dosage adjustments necessary for renal impairment

Note. SSRIs = selective serotonin reuptake inhibitors; d = day; QTc = measure of time between start of the Q wave and the T wave in the heart's electrical cycle; SNRIs = serotonin and norepinephrine reuptake inhibitors; HTN = hypertension; bid = twice a day; TCAs = tricyclic antidepressants; CBC = complete blood count; tid = three times a day; CRPS = complex regional pain syndrome.

symptomatology in patients who carry this diagnosis, as patients may develop new or additional pain-related conditions that might require short-term opioid analgesics.

Genito-Pelvic Pain/Penetration Disorder

Unfortunately, few psychopharmacological agents have been studied in genito-pelvic pain/penetration disorder. However, research and case reports have shown that topical anesthetics (lidocaine), muscle relaxants (nitroglycerin ointment), and botulinum toxin injections may be beneficial (Lahaie, Boyer, Amsel, Khalifé, & Binik, 2010). Anxiolytics such as diazepam have also been shown to help when used in conjunction with psychotherapy.

Chronic Low Back Pain

The first line treatments for CLBP include analgesics such as acetaminophen (APAP), nonsteroidal anti-inflammatory drugs (NSAIDs), and opioids. While APAP is reasonably safe, evidence supporting its efficacy is lacking (Davies, Maher, & Hancock, 2008). However, when combined with opioids, it has been shown to have an opioid-sparing effect such that the opioid dose can be lowered without jeopardizing pain relief (Last & Hulbert, 2009). Research indicates moderate to strong evidence for NSAIDs for CLBP (Stevens & Saper, 2012), with empirical support indicating that use decreases both pain intensity and patient disability (Enthoven, Roelofs, Deyo, van Tulder, & Koes, 2016). Opioids including tramadol should be reserved for patients with disabling pain that is not controlled or likely to be controlled with NSAIDs or APAP (Chou et al., 2007). Even though these medications have been shown to decrease pain, the reduction may not be clinically significant for or improve function in patients with CLBP (Abdel Shaheed, Maher, Williams, Day, & McLachlan, 2016; Chaparro et al., 2013). Tapentadol, a novel opioid that also inhibits the reuptake of norepinephrine, decreases pain in patients with moderate to severe CLBP (Santos et al., 2015).

Duloxetine, an SNRI, is the only antidepressant that is FDA approved for the treatment of CLBP and has been shown to decrease pain (Skljarevski et al., 2009, 2010). Research on TCAs for CLBP is conflicting. Low dose TCAs (amitriptyline, 10–25 mg nightly) may be effective, particularity as an adjunct for pain relief (Stevens & Saper, 2012). However, in other studies TCAs were not found to be beneficial (Urquhart, Hoving, Assendelft, Roland, & van Tulder, 2008). SSRIs have not been shown to be effective and are not recommended in the treatment of CLBP (Last & Hulbert, 2009; Urquhart et al., 2008). Muscle relaxants including both benzodiazepines (BZDs) and non-BZDs are used off-label for acute CLBP flares, though they do have significant potential for abuse/dependence and should only be used on a short-term basis.

Diabetic Peripheral Neuropathic Pain

Evidenced-based guidelines developed by the IASP Neuropathic Pain Special Interest Group indicate the first-line pharmacological treatments are second-generation anticonvulsants (gabapentin, pregabalin), SNRIs (duloxetine, venlafaxine), and TCAs (amitriptyline; Bril et al., 2011; Finnerup et al., 2015). If these treatments fail, then first-generation anticonvulsants (sodium valproate) and opioid analgesics including tramadol should be considered, even though there is limited evidence to support the use of valproic acid or sodium valproate for neuropathic pain (Wiffen, Derry, Moore, & Kalso, 2014). Topical agents such as a lidocaine patch or capsaicin can be added as adjunctive treatments (Bril et al., 2011).

Migraine Headache

NSAIDs and triptans (frovatriptan) have both been shown effective for acute/abortive migraine treatment. However, NSAIDs alone or in combination with caffeine should be considered as first-line treatment for mild to moderate migraines or severe migraines that have been previously responsive to NSAID treatment (Silberstein, 2000). Analgesics that contain butalbital have also been shown effective, but their use should be limited/monitored due to risk of overuse leading to rebound headaches (Silberstein, 2000).

Preventive migraine treatments include beta blockers (propranolol, metoprolol), TCAs (amitriptyline, nortriptyline), and the second-generation anticonvulsant topiramate. Other treatment options may include anticonvulsants (divalproex, gabapentin),

SNRIs (venlafaxine), beta blockers (atenolol, nadolol), and antihypertensives (lisinopril, candesartan; Silberstein et al., 2012), with beta blockers demonstrating more tolerability (Shamliyan et al., 2013). In patients who have 15 or more headache days a month, botulinum toxin injections may decrease headache frequency (Jackson et al., 2012). For women who have menstrual migraines, premenstrual treatment with triptans may be prophylactic (Pringsheim, Davenport, & Dodick, 2008).

Fibromyalgia

Treatment guidelines for fibromyalgia recommend using antidepressants (TCAs, SNRIs, SSRIs) and second-generation anticonvulsants (gabapentin, pregabalin) for their pain-modulating properties (Fitzcharles et al., 2013). However, low-dose TCAs are the gold standard for treatment, given sleep-related benefits. Medications approved by the FDA include pregabalin, duloxetine, and milnacipran. Antidepressants in general for fibromyalgia have been widely studied and have demonstrated mixed results, but appear useful when depressive symptomatology is present (Fitzcharles et al., 2013), specifically paroxetine, fluoxetine, citalopram, and trazodone, given its sedating properties (Walitt, Urrútia, Nishishinya, Cantrell, & Häuser, 2015). Amitriptyline, a TCA, has been shown to decrease pain as well as improve sleep and fatigue (Moore, Derry, Aldington, Cole, & Wiffen, 2015), though SNRIs (duloxetine and milnacipran) appear to be favored over amitriptyline. Duloxetine has been studied extensively and has demonstrated to benefit not only pain, but quality of life and sleep, while milnacipran has been shown to improve pain, fatigue, and quality of life (Lunn, Hughes, & Wiffen, 2014). Second-generation anticonvulsants (gabapentin and pregabalin) have been used given their pain-relieving properties and do appear to improve sleep and quality of life (Häuser, Bernardy, Uçeyler, & Sommer, 2009). In addition, pregabalin also has been shown to help with anxiety and fatigue (Derry et al., 2016).

Due to the mechanism of action of traditional opioids, which predicts their lack of efficacy, there is no evidence from clinical trials that opioids are effective for fibromyalgia. Therefore, guidelines recommend against the use of opioid analgesics in this patient population (Goldenberg, Clauw, Palmer, & Clair, 2016). Cyclobenzaprine, a skeletal muscle relaxant that may help with myofacial pain associated with fibromyalgia, and analgesics such as APAP and NSAIDs may also be considered as adjuncts for pain control. Patients with fibromyalgia may require combination therapy for optimal control of their pain and other symptoms (Fitzcharles et al., 2013).

Complex Regional Pain Syndrome

CRPS treatment may consist of the following: bisphosphonates, calcitonin, gabapentin, ketamine, and steroids (Perez et al., 2010). Bisphosphonates, which are generally used to treat osteoporosis and improve bone strength, have been shown to decrease pain and signs of inflammation; however, dose, frequency, and duration remains unclear (Borchers & Gershwin, 2014; Perez et al., 2010). Research is conflicting, but calcitonin, another medication generally used to treat osteoporosis, may also be effective for treating pain (O'Connell, Wand, McAuley, Marston, & Moseley, 2013). Oral corticosteroids may decrease pain and improve symptoms and quality of life (Atalay, Ercidogan, Akkaya, & Sahin, 2014). Gabapentin has documented benefit with neuropathic pain syndromes and was found to provide mild pain relief with significantly reduced sensory deficits (hyperesthesia and allodynia) in the affected limb (van de Vusse et al., 2004). In addition, intermittent ketamine infusions at subanesthetic doses may decrease pain, though this effect may not be sustained over time and may not provide functional improvements (Sigtermans et al., 2009). Daily intravenous ketamine, however, may provide repeated pain relief (O'Connell et al., 2013). Oral corticosteroids may also decrease pain and improve symptoms and quality of life (Atalay, Ercidogan, Akkaya, & Sahin, 2014).

BEST APPROACHES FOR ASSESSING TREATMENT RESPONSE AND MANAGING SIDE EFFECTS

When utilizing psychopharmacological interventions it is imperative for the provider to monitor safety and efficacy. While the primary goal of the patient may be pain reduction, it is important to communicate realistic expectations, establish realistic goals (increased function, quality of life), and discuss the treatment of comorbidities, as patients may not understand that pain reduction might be a byproduct versus a primary outcome of pharmacological interventions. Establishing appropriate expectations initially provides a foundation for accurately assessing and monitoring psychopharmacologic interventions. For example, functionality, quality of life, sleep, and/or either increases or decreases to mood symptomatology might be the primary target, thereby reducing the patient's overall pain presentation. Passik and Weinreb (2000) proposed the use of the "Four As" to assess pain treatment response in patients on opioids; however, it is also useful for nonopioid analgesics:

1. Analgesia—monitor a patient's pain relief (e.g., using 0 to 10 scale).
2. Activities of daily living (ADLs)—monitor physical and psychosocial functioning, specifically quality of life and functionality.
3. Adverse effects—the goal is the highest analgesia with the lowest possible side effect profile.
4. Aberrant behaviors—be aware of behaviors suggestive of drug use, abuse, or diversion.

Periodic readministration of initial pain assessment measures can be beneficial for evaluating treatment responses. Additionally, one should also utilize appropriate measures to assess for the development of potential comorbidities (e.g., anxiety, depression, sleep problems).

Patients should also be monitored for side effects, adverse drug events, and drug toxicity to ensure tolerability and safety. Side effects (e.g., nausea, sedation, weight gain, decreased libido, suicidal ideation, Stevens-Johnson syndrome), should be assessed by utilizing both open- and closed-ended questions as necessary to evaluate any potential changes since beginning or changing dosages. This approach is important because patients might not realize or remember, even if they were informed, that a particular symptom is associated with a medication or modification in dosing. Ongoing monitoring is also important as side effects can lead

to anxious and depressive symptomatology, low self-image, lower quality of life, and even life-threatening difficulties. Physical and neurological examination; laboratory and electrocardiography testing; and routine monitoring of vital signs including weight, heart rate, pulse, and blood pressure can all aid in this process and should be tracked continually. Thus, knowledge of drug-to-drug interactions, toxic dose ranges, black box warnings, physiological and behavioral indications for toxicity, therapeutic index, and methods of monitoring are necessary (Burns, Walker, & Rey, 2012).

MEDICATION MANAGEMENT ISSUES

When considering medication management issues, several key concepts are important and should be assessed when working with pain and pain-related disorders. First, is the patient adherent to medication recommendations and regimens? If adherence appears to be an issue, assess underlying reasons for nonadherence, as it could be related to side effect profile, financial or insurance issues, insurance formulary restrictions, cognitive difficulties or forgetting, misunderstanding, or lack of perceived efficacy. Second, is tolerance the issue? Tolerance is the body's adaptation to repeated exposure of a drug after continued use, thus requiring increasing dosages (Price, Hawkins, & Passik, 2015). Third, is the patient physiologically dependent and/or experiencing withdrawal symptomatology? Physiological dependence is the body's adaptation for potentially developing a withdrawal syndrome that can be produced by rapid and abrupt dose reduction or cessation, decreased bioavailability, and/or administration of an antagonist (Price, Hawkins, & Passik, 2015). This third concept is important to understand to avoid stigmatization, the use of the label of addict, and inappropriate management. Fourth, does the patient have an opioid or other substance use disorder? Fifth, is the patient chemically coping? Chemical coping is a term used to describe the behavior of patients who utilize their medications to cope with psychosocial issues (e.g., underlying anxious and depressive symptomatology, sleep problems, interpersonal relationships, trauma history). These patients are usually rigid and not willing or interested in nonpharmacological interventions, spending most of their time obtaining medications for pain management; thus, they do not adhere to an integrative pain management treatment plan, including recommendations for pain psychology or physical therapy. Some aberrant behaviors are usually present, but many patients are adherent enough to avoid being discharged from treatment (Feinberg, Feinberg, Pohl, Bokarius, & Darnall, 2017). Finally, are aberrant drug-related behaviors (misuse, diversion) suspected? If aberrancy appears to be an issue, this is usually indicative of a larger substance use disorder (dependency syndrome) for which a differential diagnosis should be constructed to fully address and manage those issues (Price, Hawkins, & Passik, 2015). However, addiction should be differentiated from pseudo-addiction, which is an intense desire for adequate pain control, causing a patient to request escalating dosage as a result of inadequate pain control. Failure to differentiate could lead to medication mismanagement, misdiagnosis, and/or a missed opportunity for psychological interventions targeted at suffering.

Antidepressants and Anticonvulsants in Pain and Pain-Related Disorders

In general, antidepressants have been shown to be effective in the treatment of neuropathic pain, fibromyalgia, CLBP, migraines and tension headaches, and musculoskeletal and malignant pain. Anticonvulsants have been shown to decrease pain in patients with neuropathy, trigeminal neuralgia, CRPS, and fibromyalgia, and they are used for migraine prophylaxis. Medications should be started at low dosages and titrated up slowly until the lowest effective dose is obtained, as slow titration improves tolerability. SSRIs and SNRIs may initially cause stomach upset or nausea, though these effects are often manageable if dosages "start low and go slow." Common side effects include sedation, insomnia, diarrhea, weight gain, dizziness, dry mouth, and sexual dysfunction, all to varying degrees and based on the particular agent. Dawood, Schlaich, Brown, and Lambert (2009) found that SNRIs and TCAs, increase blood pressure, but not SSRIs. SSRIs and SNRIs are also generally better tolerated than TCAs.

TCAs increase the risk of CNS depression; use caution when combining with opioid or BZDs. Common TCA side effects include anticholinergic effects: blurred vision, dry mouth, constipation, urine retention, and orthostatic hypotension.

Often patients require combination therapy or polypharmacy, which may include the use of TCAs combined with SSRIs or SNRIs. This combination, while sometimes necessary, does increase the risk of drug interactions for patients, including serotonin syndrome, which is the overaccumulation of serotonin in the body leading to a triad (cognitive, autonomic, somatic) of side effects. Antidepressants combined with triptans, tramadol and other opioid analgesics (meperidine, tapentadol), and/or cyclobenzaprine—a skeletal muscle relaxant structurally similar to TCAs—can increase the risk of serotonin syndrome in patients with chronic pain. Carbamazepine is a potent CYP3A4 enzyme inducer, which increases risk of drug interactions as it may decrease serum concentrations and therefore reduce efficacy of medications that are CYP3A4 substrates. These include medications that may be used for the treatment of pain-related disorders, such as APAP, codeine, diazepam, and SSRIs (e.g., citalopram). Gabapentin and pregabalin are renally eliminated; therefore, to decrease risk of adverse drug events, renal function laboratory tests should be monitored and adjusted according to creatinine clearance.

When the decision has been made to discontinue a psychotropic medication, a slow, tapered approach should be utilized to decrease risk of withdrawal symptoms. Tapering off of antidepressants is especially important with many SSRIs or SNRIs in an effort to avoid antidepressant discontinuation syndrome, which may involve, for example, flu-like symptoms, insomnia, nausea, hyperarousal, sensory disturbance, and imbalance (Schatzberg et al., 2006). When discontinuing anticonvulsants, tapering reduces the risk of rebound or worsening of the underlying condition being treated (Hixson, 2010). In addition, patients may experience withdrawal symptoms if anticonvulsants—especially gabapentin and pregabalin—are discontinued without tapering.

EVALUATION OF PHARMACOLOGICAL APPROACHES ACROSS THE LIFESPAN

While there may be some variation in subjective experiences of pain, there is no age group that is immune to its effects. Given that much of the information elsewhere in this chapter relates heavily to adulthood, this section will focus on psychotropic pain management considerations in children and adolescents, during pregnancy, and with the elderly.

Pediatrics

Is it estimated that chronic pain affects 20% to 40% of children worldwide, with musculoskeletal, headache, and abdominal pain being the most common (Feinberg et al., 2017). Treating chronic pain in children and adolescents can be challenging given underlying developmental changes; children may even have difficulties relaying and describing their pain adequately and effectively. Despite these challenges, it is imperative to address these issues, as exposure to physical pain and/or reoccurring medical procedures early in life is strongly associated with the development of fear and anxiety disorders later in life (Pao & Bosk, 2011). These experiences have also been shown to affect pain processing by modifying neural pathways. This sensitization then leads to changes in a child's experience of pain later in life (Harvey & Morton, 2007). These neural pathways/sensitization changes, when combined with anxiety or phobias, can lead to challenges in avoidance and nonadherence in regard to future medical treatments.

The selection of psychotropic medication for the management of pediatric pain often involves understanding variations in metabolism and physiology that can occur in children, such as the dynamic response to a given plasma concentration or increase in protein binding (Burns, Walker, & Rey, 2012). Given these variations, it is imperative not to make the assumption that children are just smaller versions of adults.

Selecting appropriate psychotropic medications and corresponding dosages that are safe for the pediatric population also pose challenges. These challenges are in part due to the highly controlled nature of pediatric research. In general, FDA approval is limited in regard to psychotropic medications for use in children and adolescents (Hieber, 2013), but approval is almost nonexistent for psychotropic use in pediatric pain management. In April 2017, as a result of opioid-related deaths, the FDA made an announcement restricting the use of codeine (to treat pain and cough) and tramadol (to treat pain) in children under 12 years, and tramadol (to treat pain after surgery) in children younger than 18 years of age. Recent findings also suggest that NSAIDs may actually be equally or more effective than morphine for outpatient postoperative pain (Poonai et al., 2017).

When prescribing psychotropic medications for pediatric pain, one should closely evaluate black box warnings, approved age ranges, therapeutic dosages, and potentially confounding medical comorbidities. Some medications also require pretreatment laboratory tests with ongoing monitoring to guard against hepatic or renal issues. Prior to prescribing, close collaboration with the treating pediatric providers is recommended, as underlying chronic pain conditions typically suggest a complex medical history. One should also consider the possibility of pregnancy, substance use, and/or illicit medication use/abuse. Even with all of the cautions, research suggests that psychotropic medications have been found helpful in the treatment of pediatric peripheral neuropathies, chronic abdominal pain, and migraines (Pao, 2004).

The following medical conditions and corresponding psychotropic medications have multiple studies suggesting potential efficacy. The subsequent medications, unless otherwise specified, have been FDA approved for children at varying ages for mental health disorders only. This list is not exhaustive, but is meant to provide a starting point in the development of an individualized pain management treatment plan.

For migraine prophylaxis, both amitriptyline and divalproex have been repeatedly discussed as an effective treatment for pediatric patients. Amitriptyline is commonly used in pain management as a prophylactic agent for migraines. Studied dosages varied from 0.1 to 0.4 mg/kg/d with possible increases if needed every 2 weeks, and a maximum dosage ranging from 100 to 200 mg/d with 84% to 89% of children reporting decreases in headache severity and frequency (Pao, 2004). Drowsiness was the primary side effect reported, but other mild as well as more adverse effects are possible. Divalproex, an anticonvulsant, is FDA approved for migraine prophylaxis in children. It is converted to valproic acid in the stomach and increases the concentration of gamma-aminobutyric acid (GABA) in the brain. The studied dosages varied, but typically ranged from 3.1 to 45 mg/kg/d, with starting dose at 250 mg bid and gradual increase up to 1,000 mg/d if needed, with 79% to 91% of children reporting decreases in headache severity and frequency (Eiland, Jenkins, & Durham, 2007; Pao, 2004). Typical side effects include gastrointestinal upset, weight gain, somnolence, dizziness, and tremor, but other mild and more severe side effects are possible, so standard therapeutic drug monitoring is suggested (Pao, 2004).

For neuropathic and other pain-related issues, gabapentin has been repeatedly described to be effective for pediatric patients (Butkovic, Toljan, & Mihovilovic-Novak, 2006; Eiland et al., 2007; Pao, 2004). Gabapentin is commonly used to treat neuropathic, migraine (occasionally), cancer, and other pain-related complaints. The specific mechanism of action (MOA) involved in pain control is unknown, but it appears to inhibit excitatory neuron activity. Dosages varied from 2 to 40 mg/kg/d, with a starting dose of 300 mg/d, slow titration up, and a maximum dosage of 2,400 to 3,600 mg/d suggested (Eiland et al., 2007; Pao, 2004). Side effects during evaluated dosages included sedation, confusion, dizziness, and ataxia, but other mild and more adverse effects are possible. Dosage should be tapered off over a week or longer (Butkovic, Toljan, & Mihovilovic-Novak, 2006). Fluoxetine has also been discussed for use in pediatric pain management; however, multiple studies appeared to demonstrate mixed to poor results (Moulin et al., 2014).

Pregnant Women

Management of psychotropic medications during pregnancy can be a significant challenge. Medications have a potential for teratogenic effect on the undeveloped fetus, as medications by the mother are carried through the blood supply to the fetal brain. In regard to psychotropic pain management, it should be noted that no medication has been determined by the FDA to be completely safe for use during pregnancy (Ahmed et al., 2016). While some have not been found to cause increased risk of fetal malformation, others have well-established teratogenic effects (Ahmed et al., 2016). These factors do not suggest that women who are pregnant cannot benefit from psychotropic medication, but extra caution is warranted. The FDA developed pregnancy risk categories (A, B, C, D, and X) to help identify systemic drug absorption causing birth defects. Significant risks and complexities are involved with psychopharmacologic management in pregnant women with preexisting comorbid health issues. Therefore, nonpharmacological interventions (e.g., psychotherapy) are strongly recommended, as well as a consultation with a provider specializing in pregnancy and pain management.

Elderly

Pain is common and increases with age. Musculoskeletal conditions, neuropathies, and cancer pain are the primary reasons elderly patients seek out medical care. Cavalieri (2007) reported that between 25% and 50% of community-dwelling elderly endorsed chronic pain-related complaints, compared to 45% and 80% of nursing home residents. Burns, Walker, and Rey (2012), reported that more than 80% of elderly patients suffer from at least one chronic illness. Elderly patients experience reductions in gastrointestinal, liver, and other systemic functioning, which can lead to issues with altered distribution and excretion. The elderly are more likely to attribute pain to the process of aging, which can lead to underreporting and thus poor pain management either in the form of undertreatment or improper treatment (Zacharoff, Pujol, & Corsini, 2010). This can be the result of poor communication, provider biases, or even underlying concerns regarding overprescribing and/or addiction. Furthermore, reduced awareness and sensitivity to certain medications can result in unnecessarily high dosages and/or require reductions in medication dosages to prevent adverse effects (Burns, Walker, & Rey, 2012). Feinberg et al. (2017) suggested that one third of all prescribed pain medications are prescribed for those over age 65, with adverse drug-related events or effects occurring from the combination of opioids and sedatives in 30% of elderly hospital admissions. Combine these challenges with polypharmacy issues and it is easy to understand why pain management in the elderly can pose tremendous challenges.

In an attempt to address these challenges, the American Geriatrics Society (American Geriatrics Society Panel on Pharmacological Management of Persistent Pain in Older Persons, 2009) developed extensive guidelines in regard to pharmacological pain management in the geriatric population. The AGS provides a strong recommendation against prescribing tertiary TCAs (amitriptyline, imipramine, doxepin), due to elevated risk for adverse effects (delirium, syncope, sedation, ataxia, arrhythmias, QTc prolongation). Thus, appropriate medication selection and management is critical. The AGS guidelines also strongly recommend that treatment should begin with the lowest possible dose and be titrated up slowly, while monitoring both the desired response and effectiveness and possible adverse effects (Cavalieri, 2007). Given the variations in health and polypharmacy challenges among the elderly, consultation with geriatric providers (e.g., palliative care, rheumatology, cardiology, oncology) can provide additional useful information regarding complex comorbid medical histories.

CONSIDERATION OF POTENTIAL SEX DIFFERENCES

Research has consistently demonstrated significant differences in prevalence rates of chronic pain and pain perception between males and females (IOM, 2011), though underlying mechanisms are not fully understood. Biological, psychological, and social factors, as well as inaccurate stereotypes and individual biases, all play a varying role in these differences. Male and female sex differences in regard to pain have been found in hormonal, genetic, and positron emission tomography brain studies (Paulson, Minoshima, Morrow, & Casey, 1998). Therefore, understanding pain-related gender and sex differences is an objective physiological necessity if a patient's experience of pain is to be adequately addressed.

Before addressing male/female pain-related differences, it is importance to briefly discuss the definitions of the terms sex and gender. The term sex refers to the physical or biological traits that distinguish males and females (American Psychological Association, 2015). Richardson and Holdcroft (2009) refer to sex differences as classification of living things via their reproductive organs or chromosomes. The term gender refers to the psychological, behavioral, social, and cultural components of being male or female (American Psychological Association, 2015). Some published pain-related materials address the issues of sex and gender differences (e.g., IOM, 2011; Richardson & Holdcroft, 2009), while others make no mention of these characterizations. Unless noted otherwise, this chapter will consider the terms male and female to be associated with corresponding norms for sex and gender characteristics.

The *DSM–5* (American Psychiatric Association, 2013) indicates that females endorse a greater number of somatic symptoms than males. The increased report of somatic symptoms in females is also consistent with an increased experience of pain in females, which has been documented to change across the lifespan, often in response to sex hormone alterations (Cairns, 2007). Women are not only at a greater risk for experiencing many pain conditions (Fillingim, King, Ribeiro-Dasilva, Rahim-Williams, & Riley, 2009), but also report more types of pain and are twice as likely to experience head-related pain compared with men (CDC, 2009). The diagnosis of genito-pelvic pain/penetration disorder is exclusive to women, though the *DSM–5* does suggest that men experiencing similar painful issues concerning urological pelvic pain could be classified in the other specific or unspecified sexual dysfunction categories.

Women dominate a majority of the statistics in pain research. Women are more likely to report pain, use greater overall amounts of pain medication, and experience greater amounts of pain in response to laboratory stimuli (Olson, 2016; Richardson & Holdcroft, 2009). Paulson et al. (1998) reported that females perceive a noxious heat stimulus more intensely and experience greater activation in the contralateral thalamus and anterior insula parts of the brain. Additionally, Portenoy, Ugarte, Fuller, and Haas (2004) suggested that among other factors, being female itself is even a risk factor for experiencing a statistically significant higher likelihood of disabling pain. Interestingly, and unique to females, is a hormone-sensitive analgesic phenomenon called pregnancy-induced analgesia. Several studies have demonstrated hormonal changes during gestation with peak analgesia immediately before childbirth (Fillingim & Ness, 2000; Jarvis et al., 1997). However, there is a growing body of evidence that indicates higher resting blood pressure is associated with lower pain sensitivity. Fillingim and Maixner (1996) confirmed that systolic, diastolic, and mean arterial pressures were significantly correlated with pain response in males but not females, demonstrating an inverse relationship between blood pressure and pain sensitivity. Research also found that men experience greater amounts of shoulder pain and are more likely to die from opioid overdose than women (CDC, 2016; IOM, 2011).

Not all sex differences in pain management involve just the physiological experience of pain. There are also psychological, emotional, and sociocultural experiences that are sculpted through gender role expectations that influence pain experiences, including beliefs about controllability and anxiety, for example (Olson, 2016; Richardson & Holdcroft, 2009). In relation to sex differences and reaction to pain, research has found that anxiety was associated with increased pain sensitivity in men but not women (Riley, Robinson, Wise, Myers, & Fillingim, 1998). These biopsychosocial experiences play an important role in acceptance or acknowledgment of pain, as well as in adherence issues involving recommended psychotropic pain management plans. However, Chin and Rosenquist (2009) do suggest that some bias may exist in pain research. They found male patients were less prone to report pain to female interviewers and female patients were more willing to report pain to male interviewers (Chin & Rosenquist, 2009).

No discussion on sex differences and pain would be complete without reference to pain among transgender patients. Research in this area is limited; however, some interesting findings have been reported. Aloisi et al. (2007) indicate that one third of the male-to-female patients reported the development of chronic pain during their treatment with estrogen and androgens, yet more than half of the female-to-male patients reported a decrease in prior chronic pain once starting testosterone treatment. Male-to-female patients also endorsed decreased pain tolerance, increased sensitivity to thermal stimuli, increased musculoskeletal pain and headaches, and breast pain, which could be at least somewhat attributed to tissue growth (Aloisi et al., 2007). The Aloisi et al. study was limited in size ($n = 73$) and duration (1 year postinitiation of hormonal treatment), and psychological effects cannot be discounted. However, the results do appear to support some influence of hormones on pain experience.

Given the above research, the stereotype that females have a higher tolerance for pain than males is inaccurate at best. At worst, these biases can result in suboptimal pain management, which is already common among both men and women (Richardson & Holdcroft, 2009). Given the biopsychosocial challenges and subjectivity in pain experiences, it is extremely important that sex/gender biases and assumptions be set aside when engaging in pain evaluation and management.

INTEGRATION OF PHARMACOTHERAPY WITH NONPHARMACOLOGICAL APPROACHES: BENEFITS AND CHALLENGES

Within the last 15 to 20 years, meta-analyses have emerged regarding the effectiveness of psychotherapy, psychopharmacology, or combined integrative treatments. Stahl (2012) proposed that both successful psychotherapy and psychopharmacotherapy may act on similar neurocircuit mechanisms to improve psychiatric symptomatology, creating a synergistic effect. Schwartz and Sachdeva (2014) discussed several studies that integrated psychotherapeutic and psychopharmacologic interventions and demonstrated increased effectiveness as well as neurobiologic changes across many psychiatric disorders. For example, combining psychotherapy and psychopharmacological interventions for the treatment of both adolescent depression and children with attention-deficit/hyperactivity disorder provide superior results, with medication providing early benefit and psychotherapy providing long-term benefit (Hollon et al., 2005; LeVine & Foster, 2010). Despite the research on the efficacy of combined treatment, psychopharmacology—specifically, antidepressant medication—remains the most commonly prescribed intervention with individuals less likely to utilize psychotherapy (Olfson & Marcus, 2009).

Unfortunately, the integration of psychological and pharmacological interventions for chronic pain has proceeded along independent tracks, with psychological interventions being primarily cognitive behavioral in nature. However, that has begun to change with more recent studies. Landa, Peterson, and Fallon (2012) concluded that psychotherapeutic and/or pharmacological interventions, which lead to the development of affect regulation can alter brain circuits, and thus is beneficial in somatoform-related pain. Muse and Moore (2012) also describe the opportunity to integrate behavioral therapy and modification with pharmacotherapy within the operant conditioning paradigm for motivating adherence and rehabilitation in chronic pain syndromes.

Psychobiosocial–Spiritual Approach

As discussed, pain and pain-related disorders are multimodal in nature and are perpetuated by a number of factors. Thus, pain treatment requires the integration of biochemical, psychological, social, and cultural factors (Bial & Cope, 2011). This approach has been recognized in the CDC's guidelines for prescribing opioids for chronic pain. Their first recommendation states,

> Nonpharmacologic therapy and non-opioid pharmacologic therapy are preferred for chronic pain. Clinicians should consider opioid therapy only if expected benefits for both pain and function are anticipated to outweigh risks to the patient. If opioids are used,

they should be combined with non-pharmacologic therapy and nonopioid pharmacologic therapy, as appropriate. (Dowell, Haegerich, & Chou, 2016, p. 12)

Medical psychology is the integration of both psychotherapeutic and somatic modalities for the treatment of mental illness. Medical psychologists may, where allowed by law, consult, prescribe and monitor medications, as well as order and interpret laboratory tests and other medical diagnostic studies (Quillin, 2007). For prescribing medical psychologists, given their extended training, this becomes encapsulated in the "psychobiosocial model of care" (LeVine & Foster, 2010, p. 106). See Chapter 29, this volume, for a more in-depth discussion. Sundblom, Haikonen, Niemi-Pynttäri, and Tigerstedt (1994) also identified the existence of a spiritual domain in chronic pain and demonstrated that some patients (50%) found benefit from subjective spiritual healing, even when there were no changes to physical pain or psychological distress. They also found there was a tendency to reduce analgesic intake and endorse fewer sleep difficulties, with slight increases in social, recreational, and sexual activities (Sundblom et al., 1994).

Evidenced-Based Psychotherapeutic Modalities for Pain

Cognitive behavior therapy (CBT) is the most commonly accepted psychological modality utilized for chronic pain (Morley, Eccleston, & Williams, 1999). This acceptance is due to the wealth of research indicating its efficacy in improving pain and pain-related problems across a wide range of chronic pain syndromes (Ehde, Dillworth, & Turner, 2014), as it focuses on the relationships between cognitions (or thoughts), emotions (or feelings), and behaviors. In CBT for chronic pain, the primary tenant focuses on cognitive factors over behavioral (operant conditioning) factors, specifically cognitive restructuring (distorted thinking, ruminative thoughts, catastrophizing, anticipation, fear, negative expectations regarding ability to control pain/pain efficacy), self-concept, avoidance, coping skills training (active versus passive), psychophysiologic techniques (relaxation, imagery, pacing, etc.), stress management, communication, and self-monitoring techniques (Price, Hawkins, Adams, Breitbart, & Passik, 2015; Turk, 2014; Zacharoff et al., 2010).

Acceptance and commitment therapy (ACT) is a third-wave approach that further enhances previous cognitive and behavioral models and based on relational frame theory. ACT for chronic pain emphasizes pain acceptance with the primary goal of developing psychological flexibility in order to improve function (Veehof, Trompetter, Bohlmeijer, & Schreurs, 2016). Hayes, Luoma, Bond, Masuda, and Lillis (2006) described psychological flexibility as the process of being fully present in the moment while either maintaining or changing behaviors in order to move in the direction of chosen goals and value systems. Attention is shifted to the here and now (mindful present moment awareness) rather than ruminating (on the past) or catastrophizing (about the future). Thoughts, feelings, and sensations that arise as a part of the pain experience are no longer rejected, avoided, or suppressed, leading to acceptance. Behaviors shift from pain control to value-based actions (McCracken & Vowles, 2014). Psychological flexibility is an inherently integrative process, and when applied to chronic pain this allows for flexibility in pain responses. ACT is an empirically supported treatment with strong research support for general chronic pain (Society of Clinical Psychology, American Psychological Association, Division 12, 2011), with consistent positive outcomes including increased physical and social functioning and decreased pain-related medical visits; changes were still demonstrated 3 years after treatment (McCracken & Vowles, 2014).

Other mindfulness-based therapies, including mindfulness-based stress reduction (MBSR) and mindfulness-based cognitive therapy (MBCT), have been shown to be effective for chronic pain. Jon Kabat-Zinn and colleagues have published numerous studies on the effectiveness of mindfulness meditation/MBSR in patients with chronic pain, low back pain, and pain coping responses (Kabat-Zinn, Lipworth, & Burney, 1985). The Gotink et al. (2015) systematic review of randomized controlled trials for patients with chronic pain identified significant improvements in pain burden,

depressive symptomatology, and overall physical health as well as decreased pain intensity and disability.

Other Nonpharmacology Modalities

Other nonpharmacological interventions for chronic pain management include interventional pain management (epidural steroid and trigger point injections, nerve and facet blocks, radio frequency ablations, spinal cord stimulator), surgical interventions (rhizotomy, discectomy, laminectomy), pain and health psychology (CBT, ACT, biofeedback, mindfulness, meditation, relaxation), chiropractic and osteopathic manipulation, graded motor imagery/mirror-box therapy, electrical stimulation devices (transcutaneous electrical nerve stimulation; TENS), acupuncture, yoga, tai chi, qigong, physical therapy, aquatic therapy, nutrition, herbal medicine, essential oils, and hyperbaric oxygen.

In addition, chronic pain functional restoration programs have demonstrated successful outcomes. Evidence suggests 3-week programs are most effective and supports the utilization of the biopsychosocial–spiritual model of health care with the goal of functional restoration. This is done via mind–body skills acquisition and behavioral change, empowering the patient to regain or maximize independence and ADLs, with the goal of returning to activities through active modalities. Treatment plans consist of medication management with opioid discontinuation, physical conditioning/exercise, psychological interventions, functional goal setting, adherence, reevaluation, and family education.

Benefits and Challenges

Psychotherapy has taken a back seat to pharmacotherapy due to many factors, including but not limited to theories regarding mechanisms of action/neurobiology, insurance coverage and reimbursement rates, visit times/the primary care model, expected work load, and potential influence from pharmaceutical companies, with both recognized benefits and challenges to such integration. The challenge is to incorporate the biomedical concepts without neglecting the psychosocial ones. Medical history taking must include a review of major organ systems, genetic history, a neurocognitive/mental status examination, activities of daily living, use of alcohol/drugs/illicit substances, physical and neurological examinations, an understanding of medical equipment, psychopharmacology, an understanding of how and when to order laboratory testing, considerations for special populations, therapeutic drug monitoring, patient's ability to provide informed consent, and knowledge of differential diagnosis—particularly when to refer to other biomedical health care professionals (Burns, Walker, & Rey, 2012). In addition, Rief and Martin (2014), found that patients, with or without medically explained somatic symptoms, initially present with a biomedical concept about their pain, and that psychoeducation is required to help facilitate the understanding of the mind–body connection. This becomes challenging if somatic symptomatology derives from a serious medical condition such as cancer pain or chest/cardiac pain. Thus, it is imperative to accurately identify the role of the specific treatments and techniques, understanding that processes are likely to vary considerably between pain-related disorders (Rief & Martin, 2014). Other challenges involve the current opioid epidemic, with some if not the majority of pain patients seeking passive (vs. active) and immediate interventions in an effort "fix" or "cure" their pain. Based on the current reimbursement system, it is often more expensive up front to utilize integrative approaches. This leads to the continued use of passive interventions, including prescription medications, despite frequent failed medication trials and poor pain management outcomes. Additionally, stigma regarding psychotropic medications, especially in military settings and with older generations, is still prevalent.

Hollon et al. (2005) described three benefits of utilizing combined psychotherapeutic and pharmacological treatments—specifically, the enhancement in the magnitude, probability, and breath of treatment response. Combined treatment has been associated with higher response rates, reduced dropout rates with the addition of psychotherapy, increased adherence, and more willingness to maintain pharmacotherapy and tolerate the side effect profile when accompanied by psychotherapy (Hollon et al., 2005; Pampallona, Bollini, Tibaldi, Kupelnick, & Munizza, 2004).

INTEGRATED APPROACHES FOR ADDRESSING COMMON COMORBID DISORDERS

As discussed, pain is pervasive across individuals and settings and can result in emotional distress and exacerbate existing underlying mental health disorders. Among various mental health disorders, pain is more common in individuals with depression, anxiety and PTSD, sleep disorders, and substance-related disorders (Outcalt et al., 2015).

Depression

Pain is the most common somatic symptom and depression is the most common mental health symptom endorsed by patients in primary care settings (Otis & Hughes, 2010), with 60% to 65% of depressed patients reporting symptoms of pain (Bair, Robinson, Katon, & Kroenke, 2003; Clark, Holbelmann, & Levenson, 2017). A study by Kroenke, Shen, Oxman, Williams, and Dietrich (2008) found that pain improved over time with the remission of depressive symptomology. They also found increased pain severity lead to decreased treatment outcomes for depression. Given the complex reciprocal relationship between pain and depression, a combination of psychotherapy and psychopharmacotherapy is recommended for the treatment of comorbid pain and depression. Research indicated that a combination of CBT and antidepressants was effective at reducing the symptoms and relapse of major depressive disorder (Bair et al., 2003; Guidi, Tomba, & Fava, 2015). For comorbid neuropathic pain and depressive symptomatology, SNRIs and TCAs each demonstrate faster rates of improvement and less relapse in regard to both pain and depression as compared with SSRIs alone (Clark, Holbelmann, & Levenson, 2017).

Anxiety/Posttraumatic Stress Disorder

Anxiety elevates the sympathetic nervous system response, a psychophysiological reaction. Elevated levels of anxiety then increase the perception of pain, which has been found to be independent of the intensity of the painful stimulus (Tang & Gibson, 2005). The experience of pain can lead to kinesophobia (fear of movement), panic attacks, phobias, and even the development of PTSD. Kroenke et al. (2013) reported that 45% of patients with chronic pain reported significant anxious symptomatology in the primary care setting. Prevalence rates for PTSD range from 10% to 50% among chronic pain patients (Sharp, 2004).

Treatment for comorbid pain and anxiety/PTSD primarily involves the use of psychotherapy and psychotropic medications. Widely utilized trauma-based therapies include prolonged exposure therapy, cognitive processing therapy, and eye-movement desensitization and reprocessing. Price, Hawkins, Adams, et al. (2015) recommend a multimodal approach including psychological, rehabilitative, interventional, and psychopharmacologic treatments, specifically antidepressants (SNRIs, SSRIs) and short-term use of anxiolytics, such as clonazepam or buspirone, as needed. Interventional procedures are utilized for both pain and PTSD symptomatology to include stellate ganglion blocks, which block the activation of the sympathetic ganglion, the body's danger alert system. Jeffreys (2017), in the "Clinician's Guide to Medications for PTSD," recommends the use of trauma-focused psychotherapy over pharmacotherapy as first-line treatment. However, SSRIs are also recommended, and both sertraline and paroxetine have been FDA approved for PTSD. Otis, Keane, and Kerns (2003) focus on cognitive behavioral techniques as potentially most beneficial for comorbid pain and PTSD treatment. A study by Guina, Rossetter, DeRhodes, Nahhas, and Welton (2015) found that BZDs are ineffective, worsened symptom outcomes for patients with PTSD, and interfered with the efficacy of psychotherapeutic interventions; therefore it is strongly recommended against the use of BZDs for comorbid pain and PTSD.

Sleep
Insomnia is a tremendous challenge in the chronic pain population. Research has demonstrated that pain and poor sleep are directly associated (Fielding & Wong, 2012). Koffel et al. (2016) found a reciprocal relationship; poor sleep predicted increased pain, and, to a lesser extent, increased pain predicted less sleep. Prevalence rates comparing sleep difficulties and pain often vary by medical condition, but in a study of chronic pain by Karaman et al. (2014),

it was found that 40.7% of patients with chronic pain experience sleep-related difficulties. Integrating psychotherapy and psychopharmacology for sleep disturbances can be beneficial both in the short and long term. Both cognitive behavior therapy for insomnia (CBT-I) and acceptance and commitment therapy for insomnia (ACT-I) have been shown to be beneficial in the management of sleep and warrant strong consideration. The most effective strategy for psychotropic medication management of these comorbidities is to first evaluate the currently prescribed medication regimen for efficacy and counterproductivity. A corresponding medication change might be sufficient. If not, the addition of a psychotropic medication that has sleep or drowsiness side effects could be appropriate. In general, medications that have been found beneficial for patients with both pain and sleep difficulties include amitriptyline or trazodone (Morin, 2001).

Substance-Related Disorders
Pain, insomnia, depression, and anxiety are all risk factors for substance abuse, though substance abuse is also a risk factor for any of these conditions. These conditions are also common features associated with substance withdrawal, which has been shown to lead to the use of, or dependence on, other analgesic medications or substances to reduce withdrawal symptoms or cravings (American Psychiatric Association, 2013). However, it should be noted that it is not uncommon for individuals with chronic pain to demonstrate pseudoaddiction: concern about opioid availability or drug-seeking behaviors that resolve when the pain is relieved (Price, Hawkins, & Passik, 2015). These individuals are open to other integrative modalities, tend to utilize active interventions, are adherent to medication regimens, and fears may be legitimate as opposed to true substance use disorder (Clark, Holbelmann, & Levenson, 2017; Price, Hawkins, & Passik, 2015).

Opioid use and other analgesic-based substance-related disorders are often associated with or mentioned in relation to escalating prescribing practices in an effort to maximize control of pain symptomatology (Kolodny et al., 2015). Therefore, treating the underlying substance use disorder must also involve pain-related interventions in order to maximize treatment success (Ilgen et al., 2016). Nonmedication pain treatment for comorbid substance use disorders (e.g., psychotherapy) is desirable (Ilgen et al., 2016), and due to the propensity for abuse, psychopharmacological medication options are limited. If psychopharmacological medications are considered, those with the lowest possibility of abuse should be selected. Ultimately, this area of pain management is best addressed in consultation with the addictionologist and/or as part of substance abuse treatment, with a plan involving both individual and group psychotherapy in an environment designed to monitor outcomes effectively (e.g., urine drug screens, pill counts), as significant comorbidities make effective pain management treatment for this population highly challenging and specialized.

EMERGING TRENDS

Advances in technology have been the driver for a number of recent trends gaining traction in the world of pain management. The use of video conferencing for medical and mental health treatment, technology miniaturization that provides a more exact blockade of specific neural pain pathways, ketamine for pain and depression, chronic pain functional restoration programs, and genomics testing for medication management have all made journal news. In regard to psychopharmacological advances, perhaps the most interesting of these advances involves the use of pharmacogenetic biomarker testing, which offers a way to assess a patient's metabolism profile, risk of adverse events, and the likelihood of efficacy for certain medications (Agarwal, Udoji, & Trescot, 2017). This information can then be used to guide both the selection of a particular psychotropic medication and help with dosages. Psychotropic medications for which testing might be beneficial include antipsychotics, stimulants, and antidepressants (Tennant & Hocum, 2015). It should be noted that pharmacogenetic testing for wide-scale use is still in its infancy. Thus, it can be expensive and may or may not be covered by insurance. Testing is also not instantaneous, and results can take a day for in-house labs or longer if sent out for results. Finally, the research on effectiveness of pharmacogenetics testing is still limited,

and efficacy for the general population has yet to be established (Agarwal, Udoji, & Trescot, 2017).

CONCLUSION

Most physicians, psychologists, and other clinicians working in comprehensive pain management programs already offer a limited combined psychopharmacological approach (Keefe, Gil, & Rose, 1986). While research has increased knowledge, understanding, and available treatment interventions, many questions still remain. The societal cost of pain and pain-related disorders is just beginning to be grasped. Given individualistic vulnerabilities and variabilities, we are also still unable to objectively measure a person's experience of pain. The goal of integrative pain management should be healing through the lens of functional rehabilitation and quality of life; a "fix" or "cure" is unrealistic and likely not possible with chronic pain syndromes. Optimal pain management requires an integrative treatment plan consisting of pharmacological, psychological, interventional, rehabilitative, complementary and alternative medicine, nutrition, and spiritual interventions via a transdisciplinary approach to pain management in order to influence the health and disease of the patient.

TOOL KIT OF RESOURCES

Pharmacological Treatment of Pain and Pain-Related Disorders

Patient Resources

American Academy of Pain Medicine, Patient Center: http://www.painmed.org/patientcenter/

American Chronic Pain Association (ACPA), Pain Management Tools: https://www.theacpa.org/pain-management-tools/

Stanford Medicine, Division of Pain Medicine, Patient Resources: http://med.stanford.edu/pain/patient-resources.html

Provider Resources

American Chronic Pain Association (ACPA). ACPA Resource Guide To Chronic Pain Management: An Integrated Guide to Medical, Interventional, Behavioral, Pharmacologic and Rehabilitation

Therapies: https://www.theacpa.org/wp-content/uploads/2018/05/ACPA_Resource_Guide_2018-Final_Feb.pdf

American Geriatric Society. Pharmacological Management of Persistent Pain in Older Persons: https://www.americangeriatrics.org/publications-tools

American Pain Society, Clinical Practice Guidelines: http://www.americanpainsociety.org/education/guidelines/overview

Centers for Disease Control and Prevention. Health, United States: Annual Report on Trends in Health Statistics: https://www.cdc.gov/nchs/hus/index.htm

PainEDU, Articles and Clinical Tools: https://www.painedu.org

Millon Behavioral Medicine Diagnostic: https://www.pearsonclinical.com/psychology/products/100000231/millon-behavioral-medicine-diagnostic-mbmd.html

Minnesota Multiphasic Personality Inventory-2 Restructured Form: https://www.upress.umn.edu/test-division/MMPI-2-RF

Screener: The Pain Catastrophizing Scale: http://sullivan-painresearch.mcgill.ca/pdf/pcs/PCSManual_English.pdf

Screener: Patient Health Questionnaire 15: http://www.phqscreeners.com/

U.S. Department of Veterans Affairs, National Center for PTSD, Clinician's Guide to Medications for PTSD: https://www.ptsd.va.gov/professional/treat/txessentials/clinician_guide_meds.asp

References

A Brief History of Opium. (2015). Retrieved from https://www.opioids.com/timeline/

Abdel Shaheed, C., Maher, C. G., Williams, K. A., Day, R., & McLachlan, A. J. (2016). Efficacy, tolerability, and dose-dependent effects of opioid analgesics for low back pain: A systematic review and meta-analysis. *JAMA Internal Medicine, 176,* 958–968. http://dx.doi.org/10.1001/jamainternmed.2016.1251

Agarwal, D., Udoji, M. A., & Trescot, A. (2017). Genetic testing for opioid pain management: A primer. *Pain and Therapy, 6,* 93–105. http://dx.doi.org/10.1007/s40122-017-0069-2

Ahmed, S., Moukaddam, N., Worley, A. V., Patel, K. R., Shah, A., & Tucci, V. (2016). Teratogenic potential of commonly prescribed psychotropic drugs. *Medical Journal of Obstetrics and Gynecology, 4*(4), 1091.

Aloisi, A. M., Bachiocco, V., Costantino, A., Stefani, R., Ceccarelli, I., Bertaccini, A., & Meriggiola, M. C. (2007). Cross-sex hormone administration changes pain in transsexual women and men. *Pain, 132* (1, Suppl. 1), S60–S67. http://dx.doi.org/10.1016/j.pain.2007.02.006

American Geriatrics Society Panel on Pharmacological Management of Persistent Pain in Older Persons. (2009). Pharmacological management of persistent pain in older persons. *Journal of the American Geriatrics Society, 57,* 1331–1346. http://dx.doi.org/10.1111/j.1532-5415.2009.02376.x

American Pain Society. (2012). *Assessment and management of children with chronic pain: A position statement from the American Pain Society.* Chicago, IL: Author.

American Psychiatric Association. (2013). *Diagnostic and statistical manual of mental disorders* (5th ed.). Washington, DC: Author.

American Psychological Association. (2015). *APA dictionary of psychology* (2nd ed.). Washington, DC: Author.

Atalay, N. S., Ercidogan, O., Akkaya, N., & Sahin, F. (2014). Prednisolone in complex regional pain syndrome. *Pain Physician, 17*(2), 179–185.

Bair, M. J., Robinson, R. L., Katon, W., & Kroenke, K. (2003). Depression and pain comorbidity: A literature review. *Archives of Internal Medicine, 163,* 2433–2445. http://dx.doi.org/10.1001/archinte.163.20.2433

Ben-Porath, Y. S., & Tellegen, A. (2008). *Minnesota Multiphasic Personality Inventory-2-Restructured Form* (MMPI-2 RF) [Measurement Instrument]. Minneapolis, MN: University of Minnesota Press.

Bhana, S. (2017). *Patient Fact Sheet: Fibromyalgia.* Atlanta, GA: American College of Rheumatology.

*Bial, E., & Cope, D. K. (2011). Introduction to pain management, historical perspectives, and careers in pain management. In N. Vadivelu, R. D. Urman, & R. L. Hines (Eds.), *Essentials of pain management* (pp. 3–16). New York, NY: Springer Science Business Media.

Booth, M. (1998). *Opium: A History.* New York, NY: St. Martin.

Borchers, A. T., & Gershwin, M. E. (2014). Complex regional pain syndrome: A comprehensive and critical review. *Autoimmunity Reviews, 13,* 242–265. http://dx.doi.org/10.1016/j.autrev.2013.10.006

*Bril, V., England, J., Franklin, G. M., Backonja, M., Cohen, J., Del Toro, D., . . . Zochodne, D., the American Academy of Neurology, the American Association of Neuromuscular and Electrodiagnostic

*Asterisks indicate assessments or resources.

Medicine, & the American Academy of Physical Medicine and Rehabilitation. (2011). Evidence-based guideline: Treatment of painful diabetic neuropathy: Report of the American Academy of Neurology, the American Association of Neuromuscular and Electrodiagnostic Medicine, and the American Academy of Physical Medicine and Rehabilitation. *Neurology, 76,* 1758–1765. http://dx.doi.org/10.1212/WNL.0b013e3182166ebe

*Burns, W., Walker, L., & Rey, J. (2012). The practice of clinical psychopharmacology. In M. Muse & B. Moore (Eds.), *Handbook of Clinical Psychopharmacology for Psychologists* (pp. 353–430). Hoboken, NJ: Wiley.

Butkovic, D., Toljan, S., & Mihovilovic-Novak, B. (2006). Experience with gabapentin for neuropathic pain in adolescents: Report of five cases. *Paediatric Anaesthesia, 16,* 325–329. http://dx.doi.org/10.1111/j.1460-9592.2005.01687.x

Cairns, B. E. (2007). The influence of gender and sex steroids on craniofacial nociception. *Headache, 47,* 319–324. http://dx.doi.org/10.1111/j.1526-4610.2006.00708.x

Cavalieri, T. A. (2007). Managing pain in geriatric patients. *The Journal of the American Osteopathic Association, 107*(4), ES10–ES16.

Centers for Disease Control and Prevention. (2009). Summary Health Statistics for U.S. Adults: National Health Interview Survey, 2009. Retrieved from http://www.cdc.gov/nchs/data/series/sr_10/sr10_249.pdf

Centers for Disease Control and Prevention. (2016). Health, United States, 2016: With chartbook on long-term trends in health. Retrieved from https://www.cdc.gov/nchs/data/hus/hus16.pdf

Chaparro, L. E., Furlan, A. D., Deshpande, A., Mailis-Gagnon, A., Atlas, S., & Turk, D. C. (2013). Opioids compared to placebo or other treatments for chronic low-back pain. *Cochrane Database of Systematic Reviews, 8,* CD004959. http://dx.doi.org/10.1002/14651858.cd004959.pub4

Chin, M., & Rosenquist, R. (2009). Sex, gender, and pain: Men are from Mars, women are from Venus. . . . *Obstetric Anesthesia Digest, 29,* 57. http://dx.doi.org/10.1097/01.aoa.0000350590.05970.1e

Chou, R., Qaseem, A., Snow, V., Casey, D., Cross, J. T., Jr., Shekelle, P., Owens, D. K., the Clinical Efficacy Assessment Subcommittee of the American College of Physicians, the American College of Physicians, & the American Pain Society Low Back Pain Guidelines Panel. (2007). Diagnosis and treatment of low back pain: A joint clinical practice guideline from the American College of Physicians and the American Pain Society. *Annals of Internal Medicine, 147,* 478–491. http://dx.doi.org/10.7326/0003-4819-147-7-200710020-00006

Clark, M., Holbelmann, J. G., & Levenson, J. (2017). Pain management. In J. L. Levenson & S. Ferrando (Eds.), *Clinical manual of psychopharmacology in the medically ill* (2nd ed., pp. 633–674). Arlington, VA: American Psychiatric Association Publishing.

Croicu, C., Chwastiak, L., & Katon, W. (2014). Approach to the patient with multiple somatic symptoms. *The Medical Clinics of North America, 98,* 1079–1095. http://dx.doi.org/10.1016/j.mcna.2014.06.007

Davies, R. A., Maher, C. G., & Hancock, M. J. (2008). A systematic review of paracetamol for non-specific low back pain. *European Spine Journal, 17,* 1423–1430. http://dx.doi.org/10.1007/s00586-008-0783-x

Dawood, T., Schlaich, M., Brown, A., & Lambert, G. (2009). Depression and blood pressure control: All antidepressants are not the same. *Hypertension, 54,* e1. http://dx.doi.org/10.1161/HYPERTENSIONAHA.109.133272

Derry, S., Cording, M., Wiffen, P. J., Law, S., Phillips, T., & Moore, R. A. (2016). Pregabalin for pain in fibromyalgia in adults. *Cochrane Database of Systematic Reviews, 9,* CD011790. http://dx.doi.org/10.1002/14651858.CD011790.pub2

*Dowell, D., Haegerich, T. M., & Chou, R. (2016). CDC guideline for prescribing opioids for chronic pain: United States, 2016. *MMWR Recommendations and Reports, 65,* 1–49. http://dx.doi.org/10.15585/mmwr.rr6501e1

Ehde, D. M., Dillworth, T. M., & Turner, J. A. (2014). Cognitive-behavioral therapy for individuals with chronic pain: Efficacy, innovations, and directions for research. *American Psychologist, 69,* 153–166. http://dx.doi.org/10.1037/a0035747

Eiland, L. S., Jenkins, L. S., & Durham, S. H. (2007). Pediatric migraine: Pharmacologic agents for prophylaxis. *The Annals of Pharmacotherapy, 41,* 1181–1190. http://dx.doi.org/10.1345/aph.1K049

Enthoven, W. T., Roelofs, P. D., Deyo, R. A., van Tulder, M. W., & Koes, B. W. (2016). Non-steroidal anti-inflammatory drugs for chronic low back pain. *Cochrane Database of Systematic Reviews, 2,* CD012087. http://dx.doi.org/10.1002/14651858.cd012087

*Feinberg, S., Feinberg, R., Pohl, M., Bokarius, V., & Darnall, B. (2017). *ACPA resource guide to chronic pain management: An integrated guide to medical, interventional, behavioral, pharmacologic and rehabilitation therapies.* Rocklin, CA: American Chronic Pain Association.

Fielding, R., & Wong, W. S. (2012). Prevalence of chronic pain, insomnia, and fatigue in Hong Kong. *Hong Kong Medical Journal, 18*(3, Suppl. 3), 9–12.

Fillingim, R. B., King, C. D., Ribeiro-Dasilva, M. C., Rahim-Williams, B., & Riley, J. L., III. (2009). Sex, gender, and pain: A review of recent clinical and experimental findings. *The Journal of Pain, 10*, 447–485. http://dx.doi.org/10.1016/j.jpain.2008.12.001

Fillingim, R. B., & Maixner, W. (1996). The influence of resting blood pressure and gender on pain responses. *Psychosomatic Medicine, 58*, 326–332. http://dx.doi.org/10.1097/00006842-199607000-00005

Fillingim, R. B., & Ness, T. J. (2000). Sex-related hormonal influences on pain and analgesic responses. *Neuroscience and Biobehavioral Reviews, 24*, 485–501. http://dx.doi.org/10.1016/S0149-7634(00)00017-8

Finnerup, N. B., Attal, N., Haroutounian, S., McNicol, E., Baron, R., Dworkin, R. H., . . . Wallace, M. (2015). Pharmacotherapy for neuropathic pain in adults: A systematic review and meta-analysis. *The Lancet Neurology, 14*, 162–173. http://dx.doi.org/10.1016/S1474-4422(14)70251-0

*Fitzcharles, M. A., Ste-Marie, P. A., Goldenberg, D. L., Pereira, J. X., Abbey, S., Choinière, M., . . . Shir, Y., & the National Fibromyalgia Guideline Advisory Panel. (2013). 2012 Canadian Guidelines for the diagnosis and management of fibromyalgia syndrome: Executive summary. *Pain Research & Management, 18*, 119–126. http://dx.doi.org/10.1155/2013/918216

Frances, A., & Chapman, S. (2013). DSM–5 somatic symptom disorder mislabels medical illness as mental disorder. *Australian and New Zealand Journal of Psychiatry, 47*, 483–484. http://dx.doi.org/10.1177/0004867413484525

Goldenberg, D. L., Clauw, D. J., Palmer, R. E., & Clair, A. G. (2016). Opioid use in fibromyalgia. *Mayo Clinic Proceedings, 91*, 640–648. http://dx.doi.org/10.1016/j.mayocp.2016.02.002

Gotink, R. A., Chu, P., Busschbach, J. J. V., Benson, H., Fricchione, G. L., & Hunink, M. G. M. (2015). Standardised mindfulness-based interventions in healthcare: An overview of systematic reviews and meta-analyses of RCTs. *PLoS ONE, 10*, e0124344. http://dx.doi.org/10.1371/journal.pone.0124344

Guidi, J., Tomba, E., & Fava, G. A. (2015). The sequential integration of pharmacotherapy and psychotherapy in the treatment of major depressive disorder: A meta-analysis of the sequential model and a critical review of the literature. *The American Journal of Psychiatry, 173*, 128–137. http://dx.doi.org/10.1176/appi.ajp.2015.15040476

Guina, J., Rossetter, S. R., DeRhodes, B. J., Nahhas, R. W., & Welton, R. S. (2015). Benzodiazepines for PTSD: A systematic review and meta-analysis. *Journal of Psychiatric Practice, 21*, 281–303. http://dx.doi.org/10.1097/PRA.0000000000000091

Harvey, A. J., & Morton, N. S. (2007). Management of procedural pain in children. *Archives of Disease in Childhood. Education and Practice, 92*, ep20–ep26. http://dx.doi.org/10.1136/adc.2005.085936

Häuser, W., Bernardy, K., Uçeyler, N., & Sommer, C. (2009). Treatment of fibromyalgia syndrome with gabapentin and pregabalin—a meta-analysis of randomized controlled trials. *Pain, 145*, 69–81. http://dx.doi.org/10.1016/j.pain.2009.05.014

Hayes, S. C., Luoma, J. B., Bond, F. W., Masuda, A., & Lillis, J. (2006). Acceptance and commitment therapy: Model, processes and outcomes. *Behaviour Research and Therapy, 44*, 1–25. http://dx.doi.org/10.1016/j.brat.2005.06.006

Hieber, R. (2013, May). Toolbox: Psychotropic medications approved in children and adolescents. *Mental Health Clinician, 2*, 344–346. http://dx.doi.org/10.9740/mhc.n145473

Hiller, W., Rief, W., & Brähler, E. (2006). Somatization in the population: From mild bodily misperceptions to disabling symptoms. *Social Psychiatry and Psychiatric Epidemiology, 41*, 704–712. http://dx.doi.org/10.1007/s00127-006-0082-y

Hixson, J. D. (2010). Stopping antiepileptic drugs: When and why? *Current Treatment Options in Neurology, 12*, 434–442. http://dx.doi.org/10.1007/s11940-010-0083-8

Hollon, S. D., Jarrett, R. B., Nierenberg, A. A., Thase, M. E., Trivedi, M., & Rush, A. J. (2005). Psychotherapy and medication in the treatment of adult and geriatric depression: Which monotherapy or combined treatment? *The Journal of Clinical Psychiatry, 66*, 455–468. http://dx.doi.org/10.4088/JCP.v66n0408

Huguet, A., & Miró, J. (2008). The severity of chronic pediatric pain: An epidemiological study. *The Journal of Pain, 9*, 226–236. http://dx.doi.org/10.1016/j.jpain.2007.10.015

Ilgen, M. A., Bohnert, A. S. B., Chermack, S., Conran, C., Jannausch, M., Trafton, J., & Blow, F. C. (2016). A randomized trial of a pain management intervention for adults receiving substance use disorder treatment. *Addiction, 111*, 1385–1393. http://dx.doi.org/10.1111/add.13349

Institute of Medicine. (2011). *Relieving pain in America: A blueprint for transforming prevention, care, education, and research.* Washington, DC: The National Academies Press.

Jackson, J. L., Kuriyama, A., & Hayashino, Y. (2012). Botulinum toxin A for prophylactic treatment of migraine and tension headaches in adults: A meta-analysis. *JAMA, 307*, 1736–1745. http://dx.doi.org/10.1001/jama.2012.505

Jarvis, S., McLean, K. A., Chirnside, J., Deans, L. A., Calvert, S. K., Molony, V., & Lawrence, A. B. (1997). Opioid-mediated changes in nociceptive threshold during pregnancy and parturition in the sow. *Pain, 72*, 153–159. http://dx.doi.org/10.1016/S0304-3959(97)00027-4

Jeffreys, M. (2017). Clinician's guide to medications for PTSD. Washington, DC: National Center for PTSD. Retrieved from https://www.ptsd.va.gov/professional/treat/txessentials/clinician_guide_meds.asp

Joergen Grabe, H. J., Meyer, C., Hapke, U., Rumpf, H. J., Freyberger, H. J., Dilling, H., & John, U. (2003). Specific somatoform disorder in the general population. *Psychosomatics: Journal of Consultation and Liaison Psychiatry, 44*, 304–311. http://dx.doi.org/10.1176/appi.psy.44.4.304

Kabat-Zinn, J., Lipworth, L., & Burney, R. (1985). The clinical use of mindfulness meditation for the self-regulation of chronic pain. *Journal of Behavioral Medicine, 8*, 163–190. http://dx.doi.org/10.1007/BF00845519

Karaman, S., Karaman, T., Dogru, S., Onder, Y., Citil, R., Bulut, Y. E., . . . Suren, M. (2014). Prevalence of sleep disturbance in chronic pain. *European Review for Medical and Pharmacological Sciences, 18*, 2475–2481.

Keefe, E. J., Gil, K. M., & Rose, S. C. (1986). Behavioral approaches in the multidisciplinary management of chronic pain: Programs and issues. *Clinical Psychology Review, 6*, 87–113. http://dx.doi.org/10.1016/0272-7358(86)90007-3

King, S., Chambers, C. T., Huguet, A., MacNevin, R. C., McGrath, P. J., Parker, L., & MacDonald, A. J. (2011). The epidemiology of chronic pain in children and adolescents revisited: A systematic review. *Pain, 152*, 2729–2738. http://dx.doi.org/10.1016/j.pain.2011.07.016

Kleinstäuber, M., Witthöft, M., Steffanowski, A., van Marwijk, H., Hiller, W., & Lambert, M. J. (2014). Pharmacological interventions for somatoform disorders in adults. *Cochrane Database of Systematic Reviews*, CD010628. http://dx.doi.org/10.1002/14651858.cd010628.pub2

Koffel, E., Kroenke, K., Bair, M. J., Leverty, D., Polusny, M. A., & Krebs, E. E. (2016). The bidirectional relationship between sleep complaints and pain: Analysis of data from a randomized trial. *Health Psychology, 35*, 41–49. http://dx.doi.org/10.1037/hea0000245

Kolodny, A., Courtwright, D. T., Hwang, C. S., Kreiner, P., Eadie, J. L., Clark, T. W., & Alexander, G. C. (2015). The prescription opioid and heroin crisis: A public health approach to an epidemic of addiction. *Annual Review of Public Health, 36*, 559–574. http://dx.doi.org/10.1146/annurev-publhealth-031914-122957

Kroenke, K., Outcalt, S., Krebs, E., Bair, M. J., Wu, J., Chumbler, N., & Yu, Z. (2013). Association between anxiety, health-related quality of life and functional impairment in primary care patients with chronic pain. *General Hospital Psychiatry, 35*, 359–365. http://dx.doi.org/10.1016/j.genhosppsych.2013.03.020

Kroenke, K., Shen, J., Oxman, T. E., Williams, J. W., Jr., & Dietrich, A. J. (2008). Impact of pain on the outcomes of depression treatment: Results from the RESPECT trial. *Pain, 134*, 209–215. http://dx.doi.org/10.1016/j.pain.2007.09.021

Kurlansik, S. L., & Maffei, M. S. (2016). Somatic symptom disorder. *American Family Physician, 93*(1), 49–54.

Lahaie, M. A., Boyer, S. C., Amsel, R., Khalifé, S., & Binik, Y. M. (2010). Vaginismus: A review of the literature on the classification/diagnosis, etiology and treatment. *Women's Health, 6*, 705–719. http://dx.doi.org/10.2217/WHE.10.46

Landa, A., Peterson, B. S., & Fallon, B. A. (2012). Somatoform pain: A developmental theory and translational research review. *Psychosomatic Medicine, 74*, 717–727. http://dx.doi.org/10.1097/PSY.0b013e3182688e8b

Last, A. R., & Hulbert, K. (2009). Chronic low back pain: Evaluation and management. *American Family Physician, 79*(12), 1067–1074.

LeVine, E. S., & Foster, E. O. (2010). Integration of psychotherapy and pharmacotherapy by prescribing–medical psychologists: A psychobiosocial model of care. In R. E. McGrath & B. A. Moore (Eds.), *Pharmacotherapy for psychologists: Prescribing and collaborative roles* (pp. 105–131). Washington, DC: American Psychological Association. http://dx.doi.org/10.1037/12167-006

Lunn, M. P., Hughes, R. A., & Wiffen, P. J. (2014). Duloxetine for treating painful neuropathy, chronic pain or fibromyalgia. *Cochrane Database of Systematic Reviews*, CD007115. http://dx.doi.org/10.1002/14651858.cd007115.pub3

Marks, D. M., Shah, M. J., Patkar, A. A., Masand, P. S., Park, G.-Y., & Pae, C.-U. (2009). Serotonin-norepinephrine reuptake inhibitors for pain control: Premise and promise. *Current Neuropharmacology, 7*, 331–336. http://dx.doi.org/10.2174/157015909790031201

McCracken, L. M., & Vowles, K. E. (2014). Acceptance and commitment therapy and mindfulness for chronic pain: Model, process, and progress. *American Psychologist, 69*, 178–187. http://dx.doi.org/10.1037/a0035623

Merskey, H., & Spear, F. G. (1967). The concept of pain. *Journal of Psychosomatic Research, 11*, 59–67. http://dx.doi.org/10.1016/0022-3999(67)90057-8

*Millon, T., Antoni, M., Millon, C., Minor, S., & Grossman, S. (2001). Millon Behavioral Medicine Diagnostic (MBMD) [Measurement instrument]. Bloomington, MN: Pearson Clinical Assessment Group.

Moore, R. A., Derry, S., Aldington, D., Cole, P., & Wiffen, P. J. (2015). Amitriptyline for neuropathic pain in adults. *Cochrane Database of Systematic Reviews, 2015*(7), CD008242. http://dx.doi.org/10.1002/14651858.cd008242.pub3

Morin, C. M. (2001). Combined treatments of insomnia. In M. T. Sammons & N. B. Schmidt (Eds.), *Combined treatments for mental disorders: A guide to psychological and pharmacological interventions* (pp. 111–129). Washington, DC: American Psychological Association. http://dx.doi.org/10.1037/10415-005

Morley, S., Eccleston, C., & Williams, A. (1999). Systematic review and meta-analysis of randomized controlled trials of cognitive behaviour therapy and behaviour therapy for chronic pain in adults, excluding headache. *Pain, 80*(1,2), 1–13

*Moulin, D., Boulanger, A., Clark, A. J., Clarke, H., Dao, T., Finley, G. A., . . . Williamson, O. D., & the Canadian Pain Society. (2014). Pharmacological management of chronic neuropathic pain: Revised consensus statement from the Canadian Pain Society. *Pain Research & Management, 19*, 328–335. http://dx.doi.org/10.1155/2014/754693

Muse, M., & Moore, B. (2012). Integrating clinical psychopharmacology within the practice of medical psychology. In M. Muse & B. Moore (Eds.), *Handbook of Clinical Psychopharmacology for Psychologists* (pp. 17–43). Hoboken, NJ: John Wiley & Sons.

National Research Council. (2009). *Recognition and alleviation of pain in laboratory animals.* Washington, DC: National Academies Press. Retrieved from https://www.ncbi.nlm.nih.gov/books/NBK32659/

O'Connell, N. E., Wand, B. M., McAuley, J., Marston, L., & Moseley, G. L. (2013). Interventions for treating pain and disability in adults with complex regional pain syndrome: An overview of systematic reviews. *Cochrane Database of Systematic Reviews, 2013*(4), CD009416. http://dx.doi.org/10.1002/14651858.cd009416.pub2

Olfson, M., & Marcus, S. C. (2009). National patterns in antidepressant medication treatment. *Archives of General Psychiatry, 66*, 848–856. http://dx.doi.org/10.1001/archgenpsychiatry.2009.81

Olson, K. (2016). Gender and the pain experience. *Practical Pain Management, 16*(2), 1–3. Retrieved from https://www.practicalpainmanagement.com/pain/gender-pain-experience

O'Malley, P. G., Jackson, J. L., Santoro, J., Tomkins, G., Balden, E., & Kroenke, K. (1999). Antidepressant therapy for unexplained symptoms and symptom syndromes. *The Journal of Family Practice, 48*(12), 980–990.

Otis, J. D., & Hughes, D. H. (2010). Psychiatry and chronic pain. *The Psychiatric Times, 27*(12). Retrieved from http://www.psychiatrictimes.com/special-reports/psychiatry-and-chronic-pain

Otis, J. D., Keane, T. M., & Kerns, R. D. (2003). An examination of the relationship between chronic pain and post-traumatic stress disorder. *Journal of Rehabilitation Research and Development, 40*, 397–405. http://dx.doi.org/10.1682/JRRD.2003.09.0397

Outcalt, S. D., Kroenke, K., Krebs, E. E., Chumbler, N. R., Wu, J., Yu, Z., & Bair, M. J. (2015). Chronic pain and comorbid mental health conditions: Independent associations of posttraumatic stress disorder and depression with pain, disability, and quality of life. *Journal of Behavioral Medicine, 38*, 535–543. http://dx.doi.org/10.1007/s10865-015-9628-3

Pampallona, S., Bollini, P., Tibaldi, G., Kupelnick, B., & Munizza, C. (2004). Combined pharmacotherapy and psychological treatment for depression: A systematic review. *Archives of General Psychiatry, 61*, 714–719. http://dx.doi.org/10.1001/archpsyc.61.7.714

Pao, M. (2004). An exploration of psychotropic medications for pain. *Patient Care, 38*(9), 59–80.

Pao, M., & Bosk, A. (2011). Anxiety in medically ill children/adolescents. *Depression and Anxiety, 28*, 40–49. http://dx.doi.org/10.1002/da.20727

Passik, S. D., & Weinreb, H. J. (2000). Managing chronic nonmalignant pain: Overcoming obstacles to the use of opioids. *Advances in Therapy, 17*, 70–83. http://dx.doi.org/10.1007/BF02854840

Paulson, P. E., Minoshima, S., Morrow, T. J., & Casey, K. L. (1998). Gender differences in pain perception and patterns of cerebral activation during noxious heat stimulation in humans. *Pain, 76*, 223–229. http://dx.doi.org/10.1016/S0304-3959(98)00048-7

Perez, R. S., Zollinger, P. E., Dijkstra, P. U., Thomassen-Hilgersom, I. L., Zuurmond, W. W., Rosenbrand, K. C., . . . the CRPS I task force. (2010). Evidence based guidelines for complex regional pain syndrome type 1. *BMC Neurology, 10*, 20. http://dx.doi.org/10.1186/1471-2377-10-20

Poonai, N., Datoo, N., Ali, S., Cashin, M., Drendel, A. L., Zhu, R., . . . Bartley, D. (2017). Oral morphine versus ibuprofen administered at home for post-operative orthopedic pain in children: A randomized controlled trial. *Canadian Medical Association Journal, 189*, E1252–E1258. http://dx.doi.org/10.1503/cmaj.170017

Portenoy, R. K., Ugarte, C., Fuller, I., & Haas, G. (2004). Population-based survey of pain in the United States: Differences among White, African American, and Hispanic subjects. *The Journal of Pain, 5*, 317–328. http://dx.doi.org/10.1016/j.jpain.2004.05.005

Price, J. R., Hawkins, A. D., Adams, M. L., Breitbart, W. S., & Passik, S. D. (2015). Psychological and psychiatric interventions in pain control. In N. I. Cherny,

M. T. Fallon, S. Kaasa, R. K. Portenoy, & D. C. Currow (Eds.), *Oxford textbook of palliative medicine* (pp. 612–627). Oxford, United Kingdom: Oxford University Press.

Price, J. R., Hawkins, A. D., & Passik, S. D. (2015). Opioid therapy: Managing risk of abuse, addiction, and diversion. In N. I. Cherny, M. T. Fallon, S. Kaasa, R. K. Portenoy, & D. C. Currow (Eds.), *Oxford textbook of palliative medicine* (pp. 560–566). Oxford, United Kingdom: Oxford University Press.

Pringsheim, T., Davenport, W. J., & Dodick, D. (2008). Acute treatment and prevention of menstrually related migraine headache: Evidence-based review. *Neurology, 70,* 1555–1563. http://dx.doi.org/10.1212/01.wnl.0000310638.54698.36

Quillin, J. W. (2007). Medical psychology defined. *ASAP Tablet, 8.* Retrieved from http://www.apadivisions.org/division-55/publications/tablet/2007/12-issue.pdf

Rakel, D., & Weil, A. (2012). Philosophy of integrative medicine. In D. Rakel (Ed.), *Integrative medicine* (3rd ed., pp. 588–598). Philadelphia, PA: Elsevier Saunders.

Restak, R. M. (2000). *Mysteries of the Mind.* Washington, DC: National Geographic Society.

Richardson, J., & Holdcroft, A. (2009). Gender differences and pain medication. *Women's Health, 5,* 79–88. http://dx.doi.org/10.2217/17455057.5.1.79

Rief, W., & Martin, A. (2014). How to use the new *DSM–5* somatic symptom disorder diagnosis in research and practice: A critical evaluation and a proposal for modifications. *Annual Review of Clinical Psychology, 10,* 339–367. http://dx.doi.org/10.1146/annurev-clinpsy-032813-153745

Riley, J. L., III, Robinson, M. E., Wise, E. A., Myers, C. D., & Fillingim, R. B. (1998). Sex differences in the perception of noxious experimental stimuli: A meta-analysis. *Pain, 74,* 181–187. http://dx.doi.org/10.1016/S0304-3959(97)00199-1

Ryder, S., & Stannard, C. F. (2005). Treatment of chronic pain: Antidepressant, antiepileptic and antiarrhythmic drugs. *Continuing Education in Anaesthesia, Critical Care & Pain, 5,* 18–21. http://dx.doi.org/10.1093/bjaceaccp/mki003

Santos, J., Alarcão, J., Fareleira, F., Vaz-Carneiro, A., & Costa, J. (2015). Tapentadol for chronic musculo-skeletal pain in adults. *Cochrane Database of Systematic Reviews, 5,* CD009923. http://dx.doi.org/10.1002/14651858.cd009923.pub2

Schatzberg, A. F., Blier, P., Delgado, P. L., Fava, M., Haddad, P. M., & Shelton, R. C. (2006). Antidepressant discontinuation syndrome: Consensus panel recommendations for clinical management and additional research. *The Journal of Clinical Psychiatry, 67*(Suppl. 4), 27–30.

Schumacher, J., & Brahler, E. (1999). The prevalence of pain in the elderly German population: Results of population-based studies with the Giessen Subjective Complaints List. *Schmerz, 16,* 249–254.

Schwartz, T. L., & Sachdeva, S. (2014). Integrating psychotherapy and psychopharmacology: Outcomes, endophenotypes, and theoretical underpinnings regarding effectiveness. In I. Reis de Oliveira, T. Schwartz, & S. Stahl (Eds.), *Integrating psychotherapy and psychopharmacology: A handbook for clinicians* (pp. 1–23). New York, NY: Routledge.

Shamliyan, T. A., Choi, J. Y., Ramakrishnan, R., Miller, J. B., Wang, S. Y., Taylor, F. R., & Kane, R. L. (2013). Preventive pharmacologic treatments for episodic migraine in adults. *Journal of General Internal Medicine, 28,* 1225–1237. http://dx.doi.org/10.1007/s11606-013-2433-1

Sharp, T. J. (2004). The prevalence of post-traumatic stress disorder in chronic pain patients. *Current Pain and Headache Reports, 8,* 111–115. http://dx.doi.org/10.1007/s11916-004-0024-x

Sigtermans, M. J., van Hilten, J. J., Bauer, M. C., Arbous, M. S., Marinus, J., Sarton, E. Y., & Dahan, A. (2009). Ketamine produces effective and long-term pain relief in patients with complex regional pain syndrome type 1. *Pain, 145,* 304–311. http://dx.doi.org/10.1016/j.pain.2009.06.023

Silberstein, S., Holland, S., Freitag, F., Dodick, D., Argoff, C., & Ashman, E. (2012). Evidence-based guideline update: Pharmacologic treatment for episodic migraine prevention in adults: Report of the quality standards subcommittee of the American academy of neurology and the American headache society: Table 1. *Neurology, 78,* 1337–1345. http://dx.doi.org/10.1212/WNL.0b013e3182535d20

Silberstein, S. D. (2000). Practice parameter: Evidence-based guidelines for migraine headache (an evidence-based review): Report of the Quality Standards Subcommittee of the American Academy of Neurology. *Neurology, 55,* 754–762. http://dx.doi.org/10.1212/WNL.55.6.754

Skljarevski, V., Desaiah, D., Liu-Seifert, H., Zhang, Q., Chappell, A. S., Detke, M. J., . . . Backonja, M. (2010). Efficacy and safety of duloxetine in patients with chronic low back pain. *Spine, 35,* E578–E585. http://dx.doi.org/10.1097/BRS.0b013e3181d3cef6

Skljarevski, V., Ossanna, M., Liu-Seifert, H., Zhang, Q., Chappell, A., Iyengar, S., . . . Backonja, M. (2009). A double-blind, randomized trial of duloxetine versus placebo in the management of chronic low back pain. *European Journal of Neurology, 16,* 1041–1048. http://dx.doi.org/10.1111/j.1468-1331.2009.02648.x

Society of Clinical Psychology, American Psychological Association, Division 12. (2011). *Acceptance and commitment therapy for chronic pain.* Retrieved from http://www.div12.org/PsychologicalTreatments/treatments/chronicpain_act.html

Spitzer, R. L., Kroenke, K., & Williams, J. (2002). Patient Health Questionnaire-15 (PHQ-15) [Measurement Instrument]. Retrieved from http://www.phqscreeners.com

Stahl, S. M. (2012). Psychotherapy as an epigenetic "drug": Psychiatric therapeutics target symptoms linked to malfunctioning brain circuits with psychotherapy as well as with drugs. *Journal of Clinical Pharmacy and Therapeutics, 37*, 249–253.

Stevens, J. M., & Saper, R. B. (2012). Chronic low back pain. In D. Rakel (Ed.), *Integrative medicine* (3rd ed., pp. 588–598). Philadelphia, PA: Elsevier Saunders.

Sullivan, M. A. (2009). *The Pain Catastrophizing Scale (PCS)* [Measurement Instrument]. Retrieved from http://sullivan-painresearch.mcgill.ca/pdf/pcs/PCSManual_English.pdf

Sundblom, D. M., Haikonen, S., Niemi-Pynttäri, J., & Tigerstedt, I. (1994). Effect of spiritual healing on chronic idiopathic pain: A medical and psychological study. *The Clinical Journal of Pain, 10*, 296–302. http://dx.doi.org/10.1097/00002508-199412000-00009

Sungur, M. (2013). The role of cultural factors in the course and treatment of sexual problems. In K. S. Hall & C. A. Graham (Eds.), *The cultural context of sexual pleasure and problems* (1st ed., pp. 308–332). New York, NY: Routledge.

Tang, J., & Gibson, S. J. (2005). A psychophysical evaluation of the relationship between trait anxiety, pain perception, and induced state anxiety. *The Journal of Pain, 6*, 612–619. http://dx.doi.org/10.1016/j.jpain.2005.03.009

Tennant, F., & Hocum, B. (2015). Pharmacogenetics and pain management: Clinical use and interpretation of the common pharmacogenetic tests. *Practical Pain Management, 15*, 1–3. Retrieved from http://www.practicalpainmanagement.com/resources/diagnostic-tests/pharmacogenetics-pain-management

Turk, D. C. (2014). Psychological interventions. In H. T. Benzon, J. P. Rathmell, C. L. Wu, D. C. Turk, C. E. Argoff, & R. W. Hurley (Eds.), *Practical management of pain* (5th ed., pp. 615–628). Philadelphia, PA:

Elsevier. http://dx.doi.org/10.1016/B978-0-323-08340-9.00045-1

Urquhart, D. M., Hoving, J. L., Assendelft, W. W., Roland, M., & van Tulder, M. W. (2008). Antidepressants for non-specific low back pain. *Cochrane Database of Systematic Reviews, 1*, CD001703. http://dx.doi.org/10.1002/14651858.cd001703.pub3

U.S. Food and Drug Administration. (2017). *FDA restricts use of prescription codeine pain and cough medicines and tramadol pain medicines in children; recommends against use in breastfeeding women.* Retrieved from https://www.fda.gov/downloads/Drugs/DrugSafety/UCM553814.pdf

van de Vusse, A. C., Stomp-van den Berg, S. G., Kessels, A. H., & Weber, W. E. (2004). Randomised controlled trial of gabapentin in complex regional pain syndrome type 1 [ISRCTN84121379]. *BMC Neurology, 4*, 13. http://dx.doi.org/10.1186/1471-2377-4-13

Veehof, M. M., Trompetter, H. R., Bohlmeijer, E. T., & Schreurs, K. M. G. (2016). Acceptance- and mindfulness-based interventions for the treatment of chronic pain: A meta-analytic review. *Cognitive Behaviour Therapy, 45*, 5–31. http://dx.doi.org/10.1080/16506073.2015.1098724

Walitt, B., Urrútia, G., Nishishinya, M. B., Cantrell, S. E., & Häuser, W. (2015). Selective serotonin reuptake inhibitors for fibromyalgia syndrome. *Cochrane Database of Systematic Reviews, 6*, CD011735. http://dx.doi.org/10.1002/14651858.CD011735

Wiffen, P. J., Derry, S., Moore, R. A., & Kalso, E. A. (2014). Carbamazepine for chronic neuropathic pain and fibromyalgia in adults. *Cochrane Database of Systematic Reviews, 4*, CD005451. http://dx.doi.org/10.1002/14651858.cd005451.pub3

Young, L., & Kemper, K. J. (2013). Integrative care for pediatric patients with pain. *The Journal of Alternative and Complementary Medicine 19*, 627–632. http://dx.doi.org/10.1089/acm.2012.0368

*Zacharoff, K. L., Pujol, L. M., & Corsini, E. (2010). *The PainEDU.org Manual: A Pocket Guide to Pain Management* (4th ed.). Waltham, MA: Inflexxion, Inc.

CHAPTER 20

PHARMACOLOGICAL TREATMENT OF BORDERLINE PERSONALITY DISORDER

Amit Bhaduri, Katherine Thompson, and Andrew Chanen

Borderline personality disorder (BPD) is a severe mental disorder characterized by pervasive and persistent instability of sense of self, extreme sensitivity to perceived interpersonal slights, intense and unstable emotionality, and impulsive behaviors that are often self-destructive. In this chapter, BPD refers to the *Diagnostic and Statistical Manual of Mental Disorders* (fifth edition; *DSM–5*) definition of the disorder, which comprises nine diagnostic criteria (American Psychiatric Association, 2013).

BPD is associated with severe adverse personal, social, and economic consequences. These include persistent functional disability (Gunderson et al., 2011), high levels of burden for family and carers (Bailey & Grenyer, 2013), lower educational attainment and high unemployment (Chanen, 2015), poor physical health (Quirk et al., 2015), a greater number of co-occurring mental disorders (Thompson et al., 2018; Zimmerman, Chelminski, Young, Dalrymple, & Martinez, 2013), recurrent self-harm, and a suicide rate of around 8% (Leichsenring, Leibing, Kruse, New, & Leweke, 2011).

Despite the clinical needs of people with BPD, the nature of their disorder (especially interpersonal dysfunction) often leads them to have adverse interactions with both clinicians and the health care system, consequently resulting in inappropriate or poor treatment. This is most evident in the prescribing of medication, as clinicians frequently overprescribe or do not follow the treatment guidelines (Zanarini, Frankenburg, Bradford Reich, Harned, & Fitzmaurice, 2015).

In this chapter, we briefly outline BPD, give a practical review of the pharmacotherapy literature, and present clinical recommendations for prescribing for individuals with BPD.

EPIDEMIOLOGY AND PREVALENCE

The point prevalence of BPD is estimated to be between 0.5% and 3.9% according to cross-sectional community-based surveys across North America and Europe (Coid, Yang, Tyrer, Roberts, & Ullrich, 2006; Lenzenweger, 2008; Torgersen, Kringlen, & Cramer, 2001; Trull, Jahng, Tomko, Wood, & Sher, 2010). Lifetime prevalence among adults in the United States has been estimated to be as high as 5.9% (Grant et al., 2008). The only prospective, multiwave study assessing BPD from adolescence through to adulthood found that by the mean age of 33 years, 5.5% had met diagnostic criteria for BPD (Johnson, Cohen, Kasen, Skodol, & Oldham, 2008). In primary care settings, the prevalence of BPD is 4 times that of the general population (Gross et al., 2002). BPD affects around one in five psychiatric outpatients (Chanen et al., 2008; Korzekwa, Dell, Links, Thabane, & Webb, 2008; Zimmerman, Chelminski, & Young, 2008). In community samples, there is an equal prevalence of BPD among males and females (Lenzenweger, 2008) but in mental health service

http://dx.doi.org/10.1037/0000133-020
APA Handbook of Psychopharmacology, S. M. Evans (Editor-in-Chief)

settings, 75% to 80% of BPD patients are female (Chanen & Thompson, 2016a).

DIAGNOSING BORDERLINE PERSONALITY DISORDER

A diagnosis of BPD is made when any five out of the nine *DSM–5* BPD criteria are present (American Psychiatric Association, 2013). These diagnostic features need to occur in an inflexible and pervasive pattern across a variety of different contexts, usually beginning in adolescence or early adulthood.

Although BPD usually has its onset in the period between puberty and emerging adulthood, assessment and diagnosis of BPD are often delayed in clinical service settings. This is often due to a fear of stigmatizing clients, a misplaced belief that the diagnosis cannot be made in people under the age of 18 years, or a lack of appropriate specialized early intervention treatment services for BPD (Chanen & McCutcheon, 2013). However, there is now a solid evidence base confirming that BPD is as reliable and valid a diagnosis in adolescence as it is in adulthood (Chanen, Sharp, Hoffman, & the Global Alliance for Prevention and Early Intervention for Borderline Personality Disorder, 2017). Moreover, although the *DSM–5* has continued the tradition of syndrome-based categorical diagnosis of personality disorder, it is widely acknowledged that the threshold for distinguishing patients with and without a personality disorder is arbitrary (Clark, 2007). Both adult and adolescent patients with levels of borderline pathology below the diagnostic threshold (i.e., one–four *DSM–5* BPD criteria) still experience substantial increases in psychosocial impairment, even if they meet only one or two of the BPD criteria (Thompson et al., 2018; Zimmerman, Chelminski, Young, Dalrymple, & Martinez, 2012; Zimmerman et al., 2013).

Individuals with BPD commonly present for care following a suicide attempt or nonsuicidal self-injury, during a psychosocial crisis (e.g., breakdown of a relationship), or when experiencing an acute mental state disorder (e.g., depressive, anxiety, posttraumatic, eating, or substance use disorder). In fact, co-occurring (*comorbid*) mental state disorders are the norm in BPD. Therefore, a key task of clinical assessment is to distinguish *state phenomena* (transient aberrations in mental state; e.g., depressive episodes) from *trait phenomena* (long-standing patterns of thinking, feeling, behaving, perceiving, and relating; Chanen & Thompson, 2016b). What distinguishes BPD (and personality disorder in general) from other mental disorders is that the features are present most of the time and comprise part of the patient's usual self. Such patients will report that this is how they "usually are" on a day-to-day basis. Reliability and validity of assessment can be enhanced by interviewing informants, such as family members, a partner, or close friends.

In most settings, assessment for BPD is via clinical interview and application of *DSM–5* BPD criteria. There is evidence that clinicians tend not to adhere to the *DSM* criteria during an unstructured clinical interview (Morey & Benson, 2016), and that there is often poor agreement among clinicians when they rely on a "gut feeling" (Chanen & Thompson, 2016b; Mellsop, Varghese, Joshua, & Hicks, 1982). The reliability and validity of clinical assessment can be enhanced by the use of diagnostic instruments. Most semistructured diagnostic instruments are arranged according to the *DSM–IV* or *DSM–5* diagnostic criteria (which are identical) or according to functional domains (work, self, interpersonal relationships, etc.), and they are used mainly for research purposes, as they can be time-consuming to administer. For example, the Structured Clinical Interview for DSM–5 Personality Disorders (SCID-5-PD; First, Spitzer, Benjamin, & Williams, 2015) comprehensively assesses for each of the *DSM–5* personality disorders. A diagnosis of personality disorder is given when the patient reaches the threshold for the number of criteria outlined in the *DSM* for each particular personality disorder. Using instruments such as this, it is usual for patients to meet criteria for more than one personality disorder, as there is a high rate of co-occurrence (Kaess et al., 2013; Zanarini, Frankenburg, Vujanovic, et al., 2004). For more information, see the Tool Kit of Resources at the end of this chapter, which outlines helpful resources for clinicians. These include treatment guidelines and assessment tools, along with information sheets and online resources, that can assist with psychoeducation of patients, family members, and friends of people with BPD.

There are two instruments that solely assess for BPD: the Diagnostic Interview for BPD–Revised (DIB-R; Zanarini, Gunderson, Frankenburg, & Chauncey, 1989) for adults and the Childhood Interview for DSM–IV BPD (Sharp, Ha, Michonski, Venta, & Carbone, 2012). In addition, the Structured Clinical Interview for the DSM–5 Alternative Model for Personality Disorders Module III (SCID-5-AMPD; First, Skodol, Bender, & Oldham, 2017) assesses personality disorders (including BPD) within an alternative diagnostic framework developed for the *DSM–5*.

In routine clinical practice, both screening and self-report diagnostic instruments can provide a convenient adjunct to clinical assessment. These are not intended to be used as the only source of clinical diagnosis, but they can guide further information gathering. Instruments that have been used for screening adults and adolescents include the 15 BPD items from the Structured Clinical Interview for DSM–IV Personality Disorders Personality Questionnaire (SCID-II-PQ BPD; First, Gibbon, Benjamin, Spitzer, & Williams, 1997), the McLean Screening Instrument for BPD (MSI-BPD; Zanarini et al., 2003a), and the Borderline Personality Questionnaire (BPQ; Poreh et al., 2006). The 11-item Borderline Personality Features Scale for Children (Sharp, Steinberg, Temple, & Newlin, 2014) is designed solely for use in children and adolescents. It has both child and parent versions.

EVIDENCE-BASED PHARMACOLOGICAL TREATMENTS FOR BORDERLINE PERSONALITY DISORDER

There is a general lack of evidence to support the use of pharmacological treatments for BPD. Studies that have been conducted are limited by methodological problems (see Table 20.1 for a summary). In comparison, there is a much stronger research base for the use of BPD-specific psychosocial interventions.

Treatment Guidelines

National BPD treatment guidelines have been developed in the United States (American Psychiatric Association, 2001), United Kingdom (National Collaborating Centre for Mental Health, 2011), Australia (National Health and Medical Research Council, 2012), the Netherlands (Richtlijnontwikkeling, 2008), and Germany (DGPPN, 2009). Although each set of guidelines is based on similar research evidence, each differs in the interpretation of this evidence and subsequent recommendations (Martín-Blanco et al., 2017). Nonetheless, one consistent recommendation is that the primary treatment for BPD should be structured psychosocial interventions. Although the various guidelines differ in their emphasis on the role and utility of pharmacotherapy for BPD, all agree that pharmacotherapy should not be the primary treatment modality.

It is noteworthy that real-world clinician prescribing practices differ markedly from research evidence (Zanarini, Frankenburg, Hennen, & Silk, 2004) and from the recommendations of the various national guidelines, regardless of country. It remains unclear why this might be the case (Martín-Blanco et al., 2017) but it is possible that this deviation reflects clinical factors such as poor access to evidence-based psychosocial treatments, day-to-day pressures faced by frontline clinicians with limited core professional training in evidence-based BPD treatment, and the absence of high-quality evidence for many medicines used for BPD (Chanen & Thompson, 2016b).

The American Psychiatric Association guidelines, published in 2001, proposed a prescribing algorithm, based on Soloff's (1998, 2000) heuristic model of target symptoms within three clinical domains of psychopathology. The first domain, cognitive-perceptual symptoms, includes suspiciousness, paranoid ideation, ideas of reference, dissociation, illusions, odd or eccentric thinking, and transitory (stress-related) hallucinations. The second domain, affective dysregulation, includes lability of mood, rejection sensitivity, "mood crashes," inappropriate intense anger, and temper outbursts. The third domain, impulsive-behavioral dyscontrol, comprises recurrent suicidal threats and behaviors, impulsive aggression, violence against people or property, binge behaviors (drugs, alcohol, sex, or food), and cognitive impulsivity with low frustration tolerance.

TABLE 20.1

Summary of Medication Evidence

Medication	Target symptoms	Amount of evidence
Antidepressants		
amitriptyline (e.g., Elavil®) fluoxetine (e.g., Prozac®) fluvoxamine (e.g., Luvox®) mianserin (e.g., Tolvon®) phenelzine (e.g., Nardil®)	depressive symptoms, anger, irritability, aggression	Some evidence for fluoxetine and amitriptyline in depression. Some evidence for fluoxetine in reducing anger, irritability, and aggression. No evidence for the rest.
Mood stabilizers		
carbamazepine (e.g., Tegretol®) lamotrigine (e.g., Lamictal®) topiramate (e.g., Topamax®) valproate (e.g., Depakote®)	interpersonal problems, depression, anger, anxiety, hostility	Some evidence for valproate in reducing interpersonal problems, depression, and anger. Some evidence for lamotrigine in reducing anger. Some evidence for topiramate in reducing anger, anxiety, depression, and hostility No evidence for the rest.
Antipsychotics		
aripiprazole (e.g., Abilify™) haloperidol (e.g., Haldol®) olanzapine (e.g., Zyprexa®) quetiapine (e.g., Seroquel®) ziprasidone (e.g., Geodon®)	depressive symptoms, hostility, impulsivity, anger, anxiety, interpersonal problems, paranoia, psychotic symptoms, affective instability	Some evidence for haloperidol in reducing depressive symptoms, hostility, impulsivity, and anger. Some evidence for olanzapine in interpersonal sensitivity, anxiety, anger, hostility, paranoia, psychoticism, and global functioning. Some evidence for aripiprazole in anger, anxiety, depression, hostility, impulsivity, interpersonal problems, and psychotic symptoms. Some evidence for quetiapine in affective instability, anger, interpersonal difficulties, and cognitive-perceptual difficulties. No evidence for the rest.

The American Psychiatric Association algorithm was subsequently updated with new clinical trial data by the Dutch (Richtlijnontwikkeling, 2008) and German (DGPPN, 2009) guideline groups. The most recent update of the algorithm was made by the Cochrane systematic review of randomized controlled trials for pharmacotherapy of BPD (Lieb, Völlm, Rücker, Timmer, & Stoffers, 2010). Their updated guideline recommends haloperidol, aripiprazole, olanzapine, lamotrigine, sodium valproate, and topiramate for affective dysregulation; aripiprazole, topiramate, and lamotrigine for impulsive/behavioral symptoms; and aripiprazole and olanzapine for cognitive-perceptual symptoms. This symptom-domain model has been criticized because it is speculative, has not been tested in hypothesis-driven studies (Kendall, Burbeck, & Bateman, 2010), and relies too heavily on low-quality evidence (e.g., uncontrolled trials or underpowered randomized controlled trials) or clinical trials of questionable scientific integrity (Stoffers & Lieb, 2015).

The National Institute for Clinical Excellence (NICE) guidelines were first published in the United Kingdom in 2009 and then revised in 2015 (National Collaborating Centre for Mental Health, 2009; National Institute for Health and Care Excellence, 2015). The NICE review of pharmaceutical trials for BPD called into question the trustworthiness of findings relating to topiramate (Loew et al., 2006; Nickel et al., 2004, 2005), lamotrigine (Tritt et al., 2005), and aripiprazole (Nickel et al., 2006) due to alleged misconduct from the research group that conducted the trials. These trials played a substantial role in informing the Cochrane review's recommendations. The NICE guideline recommended against the use of any medication as a primary treatment for BPD but were in favor of antipsychotic or sedative medication only for short-term (up to 1 week) crisis management. Curiously, this recommendation is unsupported by any clinical trial (Chanen, 2010).

In Australia, the National Health and Medical Research Council (NHMRC) guidelines were published in 2012, recommending a more permissive version of the NICE guideline recommendations. The NHMRC committee recognized that there was an absence of evidence, rather than definitive evidence, for ineffectiveness of medications for BPD. They concluded that medication has modest and inconsistent effects but does not change the nature or course of BPD. The NHMRC guidelines suggest that time-limited use of medication can be an adjunct to psychological therapy to manage specific symptoms. In agreement with the NICE guidelines (National Institute for Health and Care Excellence, 2015), the NHMRC guidelines recommend that medicines can be considered for acute crises, if psychological intervention is insufficient.

Pharmacological Studies

No medication has been approved for treating BPD by the U.S. Food and Drug Administration, the U.K.'s Medicines and Healthcare Products Regulatory Agency (Bozzatello, Ghirardini, Uscinska, Rocca, & Bellino, 2017), or Australia's Therapeutic Goods Administration. Controlled clinical trials of pharmacological intervention for BPD have focused on specific symptoms of the disorder, with some evidence of positive outcomes. The quality of evidence for pharmacological treatments for BPD has been limited by small research sample sizes, co-occurring psychopathology, short follow-up periods, lack of consensus regarding core outcome measures, and nonrepresentative samples of BPD patients (e.g., less severe BPD, absence of male patients, exclusion of patients with co-occurring mental disorders; Bozzatello et al., 2017; Hancock-Johnson, Griffiths, & Picchioni, 2017; Herpertz et al., 2007), which thereby affects the generalizability of findings.

Antidepressant medications. In keeping with both the NICE (National Institute for Health and Care Excellence, 2015) and NHMRC (National Health and Medical Research Council, 2012) guidelines for the treatment of BPD, antidepressant medication should only be used to treat co-occurring depressive or anxiety disorders (Bozzatello et al., 2017; Lieb et al., 2010), especially as there is little support for the effectiveness of selective serotonin reuptake inhibitors (SSRIs) in reducing the core BPD features of unstable mood, unstable relationships and/or self-image, or impulsivity (Chanen & Thompson, 2016b). The tetracyclic antidepressant mianserin (Montgomery, Montgomery, & Roy, 1983), the SSRIs fluoxetine and fluvoxamine (Rinne, van den Brink, Wouters, & van Dyck, 2002; Salzman et al., 1995; Simpson et al., 2004), the monoamine oxidase inhibitor phenelzine (Soloff et al., 1993), and the tricyclic antidepressant amitriptyline (Soloff et al., 1989) have all been tested for BPD in randomized controlled trials. Both amitriptyline and fluoxetine have been associated with a significant reduction in depressive symptoms (Bozzatello et al., 2017; Markovitz, 1995; Soloff et al., 1989), and fluoxetine with a reduction in anger and irritability and aggression (Salzman et al., 1995). However, given the potentially life-threatening effects of overdose, tricyclic antidepressants and monoamine oxidase inhibitors should be prescribed with extreme caution in people with BPD (Bozzatello et al., 2017).

Mood stabilizer medications. There have been trials of varying quality and reliability examining valproate, lamotrigine, topiramate, and carbamazepine in patients with BPD. These agents are commonly prescribed for the management of bipolar disorder (see Chapter 8, this handbook) or epilepsy.

Valproate is available as sodium valproate, valproic acid, and semisodium valproate. Its mechanism of action is believed to be potentiation of gamma-aminobutyric acid pathways. Two small randomized controlled trials of valproate for BPD reported a significant reduction in interpersonal problems and depression (Frankenburg & Zanarini, 2002; Hollander et al., 2001) and a significant decrease in anger (Hollander et al., 2001). However, valproate is not recommended for use in women with BPD because it is both a significant teratogen and it is also associated with an increased prevalence of polycystic ovary syndrome (Bilo & Meo, 2008; Okanović & Zivanović, 2016), a condition that appears to be overrepresented among women with BPD (Roepke et al., 2010).

Lamotrigine works by blocking sodium channels and reducing glutamatergic neurotransmission. A small study reported that doses of up to 200 mg were associated with a significant reduction in anger (Tritt et al., 2005). However, this is one of the clinical trials of dubious scientific integrity, as noted earlier (Stoffers & Lieb, 2015).

Topiramate blocks sodium channels, potentiates gamma-aminobutyric acid activity, and weakly antagonizes specific glutamate receptor subtypes. At mean doses of 200 mg to 250 mg, topiramate has been associated with a significant reduction in symptoms of anger, anxiety, depression, and hostility in people with BPD when compared with placebo but it also has been associated with weight loss (Loew et al., 2006; Nickel et al., 2004, 2005). Again, doubt has been expressed about the integrity of these clinical trials (Stoffers & Lieb, 2015).

Carbamazepine blocks sodium channels, decreasing glutamate release and reducing the turnover of noradrenaline and dopamine. Carbamazepine has not shown any significant benefit over placebo in the treatment of depression, hostility, or overall psychopathology in people with BPD (De La Fuente & Lotstra, 1994).

Antipsychotic medications. Antipsychotic medications are primarily dopamine antagonists, except for aripiprazole, which is a partial agonist at the dopamine D2 receptor. Some antipsychotics also affect serotonin pathways. First-generation antipsychotics, which have a higher affinity for and occupancy of D2 receptors, are more likely to cause extrapyramidal symptoms. Second-generation antipsychotic medications have a lower occupancy of D2 receptors but cause greater blockade of the serotonin $5HT_{2A}$ receptor (Abi-Dargham & Laruelle, 2005), and they show a higher propensity toward weight gain and metabolic side effects.

The first-generation antipsychotic haloperidol has been investigated in BPD and has shown some evidence of effectiveness in reducing depressive symptoms, hostility, impulsivity, and anger (Soloff et al., 1989, 1993), but it also has been associated with a high attrition rate due to extrapyramidal side effects. It should be noted that haloperidol can also prolong the cardiac QT interval (the period of time between the electrical depolarization and repolarization of the heart's ventricles), with potentially fatal consequences.

Olanzapine is the most commonly studied second-generation antipsychotic in people with BPD. Olanzapine has been associated with a significant improvement in interpersonal sensitivity, anxiety, anger, hostility, paranoia, psychoticism, and global functioning (Bogenschutz & Nurnberg, 2004; Zanarini et al., 2011; Zanarini & Frankenburg, 2001). However, one large randomized controlled trial did not demonstrate any significant improvement following treatment (Schulz et al., 2008), and it should be noted that olanzapine is also associated with significant increase in appetite, weight gain, and the metabolic syndrome.

In one 8-week placebo-controlled trial in 52 patients with BPD, aripiprazole was found to significantly reduce anger, anxiety, depression and hostility, psychotic symptoms, impulsivity, and interpersonal problems (Nickel et al., 2006). Again, this is one of the clinical trials whose scientific integrity was called into question by the NICE guideline group (Stoffers & Lieb, 2015).

Ziprasidone was found to have no significant effect when compared with placebo on a range of measures in a study of 60 adults with BPD taking a mean dose of 84 mg daily, over 12 weeks (Pascual et al., 2008).

A placebo-controlled randomized controlled trial of extended-release quetiapine reported a significant improvement in the BPD symptoms of affective instability, anger, interpersonal difficulties, and cognitive-perceptual problems (Black et al., 2014). Adverse events reported by study participants included sedation, changes in appetite, and dry mouth.

Omega-3 fatty acids. The long-chain omega-3 polyunsaturated fatty acids (omega-3 PUFAs) eicosapentaenoic acid and docosahexaenoic acid are a component of cell membranes and are essential in maintaining normal neuronal activity. Their levels have been found to be reduced in the red blood cell membranes of people with a range of psychiatric disorders, leading to trials of omega-3 fatty acid supplements for a range of conditions (Freeman et al., 2006; Sinn, Milte, & Howe, 2010). In BPD, omega-3 fatty acids have been reported to reduce depressive symptoms (Hallahan, Hibbeln, Davis, & Garland, 2007; Zanarini & Frankenburg, 2003) and suicidality (Hallahan et al., 2007) and to improve global functioning scores (Amminger et al., 2013).

Opioid antagonists. There is some evidence pointing toward the role of endogenous opiates in contributing to the development of dissociative symptoms. Two small trials investigated the use of the opioid antagonists naloxone and naltrexone in the treatment of dissociative symptoms in patients with BPD, but no significant improvement was shown (Philipsen, Schmahl, & Lieb, 2004; Schmahl et al., 2012).

Oxytocin. A small randomized controlled trial of 14 patients with BPD found that 40 IU of intranasal oxytocin reduced stress-induced dysphoria (Simeon et al., 2011).

Summary. These pharmacological studies do not support any role for SSRIs in the treatment of BPD, other than for the treatment of co-occurring depression and anxiety. Other psychotropic medications require further investigation. There is limited evidence that mood stabilizers such as topiramate, sodium valproate, and lamotrigine might reduce affective dysregulation and impulsive aggression. Antipsychotics such as aripiprazole, olanzapine, and quetiapine might reduce cognitive-perceptual symptoms and affective dysregulation, and omega-3 fatty acids might reduce the overall severity of BPD. However, the overall quality of the evidence for pharmacological treatments for BPD is poor. Studies have been limited by small sample sizes, co-occurring psychopathology, short follow-up periods, lack of consensus regarding core outcome measures, and nonrepresentative patient samples. Importantly, this stands in marked contrast to the much stronger and more consistent evidence for the effectiveness of psychosocial interventions for BPD (Cristea et al., 2017), albeit with small to medium effect sizes.

As the Australian NHMRC guidelines committee (National Health and Medical Research Council,

2012) recognized, there is an absence of evidence, rather than definitive evidence, for ineffectiveness of medications for BPD. This "evidence vacuum" leads to wide variability in the actual prescribing habits of clinicians treating people with BPD.

BEST APPROACHES FOR ASSESSING TREATMENT RESPONSE AND MANAGING SIDE EFFECTS

Collaboration on realistic and specific goals for treatment, arrangements for monitoring progress toward these goals, and anticipating the duration of treatment provides a strong platform for successful prescribing (Chanen & Thompson, 2016b). The goals for pharmacological intervention will vary for each patient. For example, the goal of treatment with an antipsychotic medication might be to reduce the experience of paranoid ideas or auditory verbal hallucinations, while treatment with a mood stabilizer might be to reduce the frequency or severity of dysphoric states. Ideally, there should be a priori agreement not only on the target symptom but also on the maximum dose to be trialed, the criteria for discontinuation of the medication, and whether subsequent medications or augmentation strategies will be trialed, if goals are not met within the agreed trial period.

Treatment response is best determined by clinical assessment, including collateral history, and can be supported by encouraging patients to keep diaries monitoring their targeted symptoms. Goal-based outcome measures are a useful tool to demonstrate progress toward individually tailored goals (Law & Jacob, 2013).

The management of side effects is specific to each medication, not to each disorder. Guidance on managing side effects arising from specific medications is covered in other chapters of this handbook, such as those on depressive, psychotic, and bipolar disorders (see Chapters 7, 10, & 8, respectively). As with any prescribing, an open, honest, and realistic discussion about the side-effect burden and other risks, including long-term risks of taking medication (e.g., the metabolic syndrome or movement disorders), should precede any prescription. Treatment-emergent side effects, such as increased agitation or suicidal ideation for young people (< 25 years old) taking SSRI medication, should be discussed explicitly and planned for at the outset.

MEDICATION MANAGEMENT ISSUES

The principles of responsible prescribing for BPD are outlined in Exhibit 20.1. The highly interpersonal nature of the difficulties associated with BPD means that patients can elicit strong emotional, cognitive, and behavioral responses from clinicians. Clinicians might feel pulled or pushed into inappropriately prescribing medication, which is often heralded by clinician feelings of anger, dismissiveness, or helplessness, or by the belief that the patient needs rescuing. Alternatively, clinicians might feel cheated or manipulated, leading to an excessively rigid and inflexible response to a request for a trial of medication. Medication must never be used in a punitive manner or as a substitute for other more appropriate forms of care and treatment.

In severe and complex presentations of BPD, where the absence of evidence for prescribing is most pronounced, time-limited use of medication might be indicated for the management of specific symptoms, ideally as an adjunct to structured psychological therapy. Under these circumstances, the risks of prescribing medication might outweigh

---

EXHIBIT 20.1

Key Considerations in the Pharmacological Treatment of Borderline Personality Disorder

---

Medication only has modest and inconsistent effects and therefore should not be used as a primary treatment in place of structured psychological therapies.

Time-limited use of medication can be a helpful adjunct to psychological therapy in more complex and severe cases to manage specific symptoms.

Collaboration, with open and honest discussion, with patients and other team members is needed in agreeing about the rationale for prescribing, the duration of the trial medication period, and the monitoring of progress toward treatment goals.

Medication should be withdrawn if it is not having the intended effect after a reasonable trial period.

Polypharmacy should be avoided.

Safeguards against overdose and dependence need to be considered.

---

the risks of not prescribing, bearing in mind the high suicide rate (Pompili, Girardi, Ruberto, & Tatarelli, 2005) and other adverse outcomes in BPD. In these situations, open and honest discussions with the patient about the rationale for prescribing are essential. It is recommended that prescribing take the form of serial trials of monotherapy (i.e., sequential use of single agents). There also needs to be a consensus between prescribers and other professionals involved in the patient's care, and a primary prescriber should be designated to mitigate the risk of multiple prescriptions and concurrent or overlapping medication strategies. Polypharmacy should be avoided, given the absence of evidence for its effectiveness and the potential for increased side effects and long-term harms.

Safeguards are also needed to minimize the risk of overdose, due to the high risk of suicide (Pompili et al., 2005) in patients with BPD. Measures include using medications that are relatively safe in overdose as well as prescribing fewer tablets, with more frequent administrations, during times of heightened acute risk. The potential for interaction of prescribed medication with alcohol and other substances needs to established and openly discussed with the patient.

In acute crisis situations, short-term prescribing of sedative medication for a duration of no longer than 1 week can be considered, if psychological strategies are clinically insufficient (National Institute for Health and Care Excellence, 2015). Caution should be exercised if prescribing medication that is associated with dependence, such as benzodiazepines, and this medication should be withdrawn as soon as a crisis has resolved.

Despite the limited evidence base for the use of medication and the recommendations of national guidelines for minimizing or avoiding medications, medication usage is paradoxically high in patients with BPD. The McLean Study of Adult Development found that medications were prescribed for 78% of patients with BPD, for more than 75% of the 6-year follow-up period posthospitalization (Zanarini, Frankenburg, Hennen, & Silk, 2004). Over this same period, polypharmacy was common, with 37% of patients taking three or more, 20% taking four or more, and 12% taking five or more concurrent standing medications. (A standing medication is a prewritten medication order with specific instructions from a medical practitioner to administer the medication in person [e.g., a nurse] in defined circumstances.) At 16-year follow-up, the rates were 36%, 19%, and 7%, respectively (Zanarini, Frankenburg, Reich, Conkey, & Fitzmaurice, 2015). Patients with BPD were more likely to receive every type of psychotropic medication, except for tricyclic antidepressants and monoamine oxidase inhibitors (Zanarini, Frankenburg, Bradford Reich, et al., 2015). These prescription rates suggest that prescribing practice strays from evidence-based recommendations, despite the publication of systematic reviews (Martín-Blanco et al., 2017). The main improvement identified in prescribing practice over time has been greater adherence in prescribing atypical antipsychotics more frequently and limiting the use of SSRIs, tricyclic antidepressants, and benzodiazepines (Martín-Blanco et al., 2017). The reasons for this shift in practice are unclear, as are the long-term effects of prescribing second-generation antipsychotics to patients with BPD (e.g., the metabolic syndrome; Balon, 2017).

EVALUATION OF PHARMACOLOGICAL APPROACHES ACROSS THE LIFESPAN

There has been significant growth in knowledge about BPD in adolescents and emerging adults over the past 2 decades (e.g., Kaess, Brunner, & Chanen, 2014; Sharp & Fonagy, 2015). BPD has been shown to be as valid and reliable a diagnosis in adolescence as it is in adulthood, based on the following: evidence for its genetic basis; similarity in prevalence, phenomenology, stability, and risk factors; evidence for marked separation of course and outcome of adolescent BPD and other disorders; and efficacy of disorder-specific treatment (Chanen et al., 2017). The weight of empirical evidence has led the *DSM–5*, and the U.K. and Australian national treatment guidelines, to legitimize the diagnosis of BPD prior to age 18, and the "first wave" of evidence-based treatments has demonstrated that structured psychological treatments for BPD in young people are effective (Chanen, 2015). This has provided a firm basis for establishing early diagnosis and treatment (i.e., early

intervention) for BPD and for subthreshold borderline personality pathology (Chanen & McCutcheon, 2013). Consequent upon this, young people are increasingly likely to be exposed to the same pressures to prescribe and prescribing hazards that accompany adults with BPD. These hazards are compounded by the absence of high-quality controlled clinical trials of pharmacotherapy for BPD in young people. Although the general principles of prescribing, described earlier in this chapter, can be applied to young people, caution should prevail and medications should only be used in extreme circumstances and in specialized psychiatric settings.

The implications of BPD in the elderly population (> 65 years old) is limited by a scarcity of research (Cruitt & Oltmanns, 2018). BPD features have been linked to suicidal ideation, poorer physical health, and cognitive decline in later life. As is the case for young people, there are no high-quality controlled clinical trials of pharmacotherapy for BPD in the elderly.

CONSIDERATION OF POTENTIAL SEX DIFFERENCES

Although the *DSM–5* states that BPD is predominantly diagnosed in women (75%) in clinical settings (American Psychiatric Association, 2013), high-quality epidemiological studies have reported that there is no significant sex difference in the rate of this disorder in adults (Coid et al., 2006; Grant et al., 2008; Lenzenweger, Lane, Loranger, & Kessler, 2007; Torgersen, Kringlen, & Cramer, 2001) or adolescents (Zanarini et al., 2011) in the community. It has been suggested that the discrepancy between the prevalence in clinical versus community settings might be due to sex differences in help-seeking behavior, with men being more likely to present to alcohol and drug treatment services rather than to access pharmacological or psychological treatment (Sansone & Sansone, 2011). This assumption has been supported in part by a large community study that reported men with BPD were more likely to present with co-occurring substance disorders as well as schizotypal, narcissistic, and antisocial personality disorders (Johnson et al., 2003). Sociocultural factors are another possible explanation for the overrepresentation of women in clinical services, as the same behaviors displayed in men and women are often judged differently (Chanen & Thompson, 2016a). Evidence does not support sex differences in clinical presentation being attributable to biased application of the diagnostic criteria (Anderson, Sankis, & Widiger, 2001; Widiger, 1998) or any systematic sex bias in the *DSM* criteria (Aggen et al., 2009). For a review of the topic, see Chanen and Thompson (2016a).

INTEGRATION OF PHARMACOTHERAPY WITH NONPHARMACOLOGICAL APPROACHES: BENEFITS AND CHALLENGES

The development of evidence-based psychotherapies for BPD challenges the myth that BPD is an untreatable condition (Bateman, Gunderson, & Mulder, 2015), with more than 13 manualized psychotherapies having been tested in controlled clinical trials (Choi-Kain, Finch, Masland, Jenkins, & Unruh, 2017). Among the more common treatments are dialectical behavior therapy (Linehan et al., 2006), mentalization-based treatment (Bateman & Fonagy, 2016), schema-focused therapy (van Asselt et al., 2008), transference-focused psychotherapy (van Asselt et al., 2008), cognitive analytic therapy (Ryle, 1997), systems training for emotional predictability and problem-solving (Blum et al., 2008), dynamic deconstructive psychotherapy (Gregory, DeLucia-Deranja, & Mogle, 2010), and good psychiatric management (Links, Ross, & Gunderson, 2015). These approaches have several common characteristics: Their approach to BPD problems is structured (manualized); patients are encouraged to have a sense of agency; therapists assist patients to connect feelings to events and actions; and therapists are active, validating, and supervised in their practice (Bateman et al., 2015).

Both the NICE and NHMRC guidelines for the treatment of BPD recognize that these psychological treatments are the most effective form of intervention for the core features of this disorder. The NICE guidelines (National Institute for Health and Care Excellence, 2015) recommend that people with BPD should be offered psychological therapies that help

them manage their condition, so they can choose the type and length of session and treatment frequency. Likewise the mental health professionals providing the treatment and support need to have their supervision tailored to their role and needs, due to the stress associated with supporting patients with BPD (National Institute for Health and Care Excellence, 2015). The NHMRC guidelines (National Health and Medical Research Council, 2012) recommend that people with BPD should be provided with specialized psychological therapy that has been developed for the treatment of BPD and that this treatment should be delivered by adequately trained health professionals who receive regular clinical supervision.

Some clinical trials have studied the combination of medication and psychotherapy in BPD but they are universally low-quality randomized controlled trials. In a 12-week randomized controlled trial, 20 females with BPD who were receiving dialectical behavioral therapy received either 40 mg of fluoxetine or placebo. No between-group differences were found on self-report measures of depression, anxiety, anger, dissociation, or global functioning (Simpson et al., 2004). In a 32-week randomized controlled trial, 55 outpatients with BPD were randomized to fluoxetine 20 mg to 40 mg per day plus clinical management or to fluoxetine 20 mg to 40 mg per day plus interpersonal psychotherapy adapted to BPD (Bellino, Rinaldi, & Bogetto, 2010). Completer analysis found that the interpersonal psychotherapy plus fluoxetine treatment group had a greater reduction on measures of core symptoms of the disorder (interpersonal relationships, affective instability, and impulsivity), anxiety, and quality of life, a reduction that was maintained after 2 years of research follow-up (Bozzatello & Bellino, 2016). Finally, in a trial of sequential psychotherapy and pharmacotherapy, 15 BPD patients who had received 4 weeks of condensed dialectical behavior therapy were randomized to either divalproex extended release or placebo for 12 weeks. No significant between-group differences were found at the trial endpoint (Moen et al., 2012). These studies provide inconclusive evidence for the effectiveness of combined or sequential pharmacotherapy and psychotherapy for the core features of BPD.

INTEGRATED APPROACHES FOR ADDRESSING COMMON COMORBID DISORDERS

Typical rates of comorbidity among clinical samples of adults with BPD are 87% major depression, 62% substance disorder, 89% anxiety, 58% posttraumatic stress disorder, and 54% eating disorder (Zanarini, Frankenburg, Hennen, Reich, & Silk, 2004). Typical rates among adolescents are 41% to 71% mood disorder, 32% to 37% substance disorder, 16% to 35% anxiety, 6% to 52% eating disorder, and 13% to 17% disruptive behavior disorder (Chanen, Jovev, & Jackson, 2007; Kaess et al., 2013).

The treatment of co-occurring disorders should be the most common reason for prescribing medication to patients with BPD. Lifetime prevalence for at least one co-occurring mental disorder is almost 100% in BPD (Bender et al., 2001). Recommendations for pharmacological treatment of comorbid disorders should follow evidence-based guidelines for the relevant comorbidity. Once again, caution needs to be exercised when prescribing these medications in BPD due to the high risk of overdose or misuse of medication, and to high-risk sexual behavior among this patient group with regard to potentially teratogenic effects on an unborn fetus. This can be particularly challenging when patients with BPD have a co-occurring psychotic illness, such as schizophrenia or schizoaffective disorder. This is not uncommon, with 28% of patients with psychotic disorder screening positive for a co-occurring personality disorder in a multicenter U.K. study (Moran et al., 2003).

EMERGING TRENDS

The controlled clinical trial literature in BPD is notable for its unsystematic approach. Many classes of agent have been studied across diverse primary outcomes and with an inconsistent approach to measurement of these outcomes. Many trials have failed to progress beyond pilot studies, despite promising findings. For example, pilot studies (Zanarini & Frankenburg, 2003) and post hoc analyses (Amminger et al., 2013) suggest that a randomized controlled trial of omega-3 fish oils in BPD is warranted. Several trials involving oxytocin are underway targeting social trust and emotion recognition. Ongoing trials examining

drugs that affect N-methyl-D-aspartate signaling, including ketamine, are underway, as glutamatergic pathways have effects on disinhibition, social cognition, and dissociative symptoms (Ripoll, 2012). Clinical trial registries include treatments as diverse as the glucocorticoid receptor antagonist mifepristone (which affects the hypothalamic–pituitary–adrenal axis) and various second-generation antipsychotics. Neurostimulatory treatments, such as repetitive transcranial magnetic stimulation, magnetic seizure therapy, and transcranial direct current stimulation, are also being tested in BPD.

Further research is needed on the causes of BPD and the neurobiological mechanisms involved. Particular emphasis in terms of treatment needs to be placed on improving social and vocational outcomes associated with the disorder.

SUMMARY

BPD is a leading cause of disability and mortality and is commonly encountered in clinical practice. Once considered untreatable, the outlook for patients is much improved, with a range of effective psychosocial treatments available for the disorder. In comparison, the quality of evidence for pharmacological treatments for BPD is poor. Controlled clinical trials are generally low quality and have yielded inconsistent evidence of positive outcomes for specific features of the disorder. There is general agreement among international clinical guidelines that medications should not be used as primary therapy for BPD because of these modest and inconsistent effects, because they do not change the nature or course of the disorder, and because the risk of adverse short- and long-term effects is high. However, several factors mean that pharmacotherapy for BPD is common in real-world clinical practice. These include the absence of evidence of effectiveness, rather than definitive evidence for ineffectiveness, of medications for BPD; the low external validity of clinical trials (due to unrepresentative patient samples); and the limited availability of and high dropout rates from psychosocial treatments. Pharmacotherapy for BPD should be approached with a high degree of caution and be intended for management of specific symptoms, using time-limited trials of single agents, with collaborative and clearly defined treatment goals, and preferably as an adjunct to psychological therapy. Medication should be withdrawn if it is not having the intended effect after a reasonable trial period. Polypharmacy should be avoided at all times and safeguards should be considered to minimize the risk of overdose or dependence. In order to advance the field, there is an urgent need to conduct high-quality randomized controlled trials, with relevant and BPD-specific outcome measures.

TOOL KIT OF RESOURCES

Borderline Personality Disorder (BPD)

Patient Resources

Information sheet for young people (aged 15–25 years) with BPD: https://goo.gl/XvL8w5

Online information for carers of young people (aged 15–25 years) with BPD: https://goo.gl/erzkpc; https://goo.gl/V6EUsg

Online information for adults and adolescents with BPD: https://www.borderlinepersonalitydisorder.com

Online information for family and friends of people with BPD: https://goo.gl/yoCacK

Provider Resources

Information sheet for clinicians working with young people (aged 15–25 years) with BPD: https://goo.gl/Q4MeJA

Treatment Guidelines for BPD:

Australia: https://www.nhmrc.gov.au/guidelines-publications/mh25

United Kingdom: https://www.nice.org.uk/guidance/cg78; www.nice.org.uk/guidance/qs88

United States: American Psychiatric Association, 2001

Selected Semistructured Interview Measures for Assessing Borderline Personality Disorder

Measures for adults that assess all *DSM–IV* personality disorders: Diagnostic Interview for DSM–IV Personality Disorders (DIPD-IV; Zanarini, Frankenburg, Chauncey, & Gunderson, 1987)

International Personality Disorders Examination (IPDE; Loranger, Janca, & Sartorius, 1997)–DSM–IV Version

Structured Clinical Interview for DSM–IV Axis II Disorders (SCID-II; First et al., 1997 [has been used with adolescent patients in published studies])

Structured Interview for DSM–IV Personality Disorders (SIDP-IV; Pfohl, Blum, & Zimmerman, 1997)

Measure for adults that assesses all six *DSM–5* alternative model personality disorders: Structured Clinical Interview for the DSM–5 Alternative Model for Personality Disorders Module III (SCID-5-AMPD; First et al., 2017)

Measure for adults that assesses BPD alone: Revised Diagnostic Interview for Borderlines (DIB-R; Zanarini et al., 1989)

Measure for adolescents that assesses BPD alone: Childhood Interview for DSM–IV Borderline Personality Disorder (CI-BPD; Sharp et al., 2012)

Measures for assessing change in BPD severity over time in adults: Zanarini Rating Scale for Borderline Personality Disorder (ZAN-BPD; Zanarini et al., 2003b)

Measures for assessing change in BPD severity over time in adults or adolescents: Borderline Personality Disorder Severity Index–IV (BPDSI-IV; Arntz et al., 2003)

References

Abi-Dargham, A., & Laruelle, M. (2005). Mechanisms of action of second generation antipsychotic drugs in schizophrenia: Insights from brain imaging studies. *European Psychiatry, 20,* 15–27. http://dx.doi.org/10.1016/j.eurpsy.2004.11.003

Aggen, S. H., Neale, M. C., Røysamb, E., Reichborn-Kjennerud, T., & Kendler, K. S. (2009). A psychometric evaluation of the *DSM–IV* borderline personality disorder criteria: Age and sex moderation of criterion functioning. *Psychological Medicine, 39,* 1967–1978. http://dx.doi.org/10.1017/S0033291709005807

American Psychiatric Association. (2001). *Practice guideline for the treatment of patients with borderline personality disorder.* Washington, DC: American Psychiatric Publishing.

American Psychiatric Association. (2013). *Diagnostic and statistical manual of mental disorders* (5th ed.). Washington, DC: Author.

Amminger, G. P., Chanen, A. M., Ohmann, S., Klier, C. M., Mossaheb, N., Bechdolf, A., . . . Schäfer, M. R. (2013). Omega-3 fatty acid supplementation in adolescents with borderline personality disorder and ultra-high risk criteria for psychosis: A post hoc subgroup analysis of a double-blind, randomized controlled trial. *The Canadian Journal of Psychiatry, 58,* 402–408. http://dx.doi.org/10.1177/070674371305800705

Anderson, K. G., Sankis, L. M., & Widiger, T. A. (2001). Pathology versus statistical infrequency: Potential

*Asterisks indicate assessments or resources.

sources of gender bias in personality disorder criteria. *Journal of Nervous and Mental Disease, 189*, 661–668.

Arntz, A., van den Hoorn, M., Cornelis, J., Verheul, R., van den Bosch, W. M. C., & de Bie, A. J. H. T. (2003). Reliability and validity of the borderline personality disorder severity index. *Journal of Personality Disorders, 17*, 45–59. http://dx.doi.org/10.1521/pedi.17.1.45.24053

Bailey, R. C., & Grenyer, B. F. S. (2013). Burden and support needs of carers of persons with borderline personality disorder: A systematic review. *Harvard Review of Psychiatry, 21*(5), 248–258.

Balon, R. (2017). Changes in psychopharmacological management of persons with borderline personality disorder. *Acta Psychiatrica Scandinavica, 136*, 332. http://dx.doi.org/10.1111/acps.12779

Bateman, A., & Fonagy, P. (2016). *Mentalization-based treatment for personality disorders: A practical guide.* Oxford, United Kingdom: Oxford University Press.

Bateman, A. W., Gunderson, J., & Mulder, R. (2015). Treatment of personality disorder. *The Lancet, 385*(9969), 735–743. http://dx.doi.org/10.1016/S0140-6736(14)61394-5

Bellino, S., Rinaldi, C., & Bogetto, F. (2010). Adaptation of interpersonal psychotherapy to borderline personality disorder: A comparison of combined therapy and single pharmacotherapy. *The Canadian Journal of Psychiatry, 55*, 74–81. http://dx.doi.org/10.1177/070674371005500203

Bender, D. S., Dolan, R. T., Skodol, A. E., Sanislow, C. A., Dyck, I. R., McGlashan, T. H., . . . Gunderson, J. G. (2001). Treatment utilization by patients with personality disorders. *The American Journal of Psychiatry, 158*, 295–302. http://dx.doi.org/10.1176/appi.ajp.158.2.295

Bilo, L., & Meo, R. (2008). Polycystic ovary syndrome in women using valproate: A review. *Gynecological Endocrinology, 24*, 562–570. http://dx.doi.org/10.1080/09513590802288259

Black, D. W., Zanarini, M. C., Romine, A., Shaw, M., Allen, J., & Schulz, S. C. (2014). Comparison of low and moderate dosages of extended-release quetiapine in borderline personality disorder: A randomized, double-blind, placebo-controlled trial. *The American Journal of Psychiatry, 171*, 1174–1182. http://dx.doi.org/10.1176/appi.ajp.2014.13101348

Blum, N., St John, D., Pfohl, B., Stuart, S., McCormick, B., Allen, J., . . . Black, D. W. (2008). Systems Training for Emotional Predictability and Problem Solving (STEPPS) for outpatients with borderline personality disorder: A randomized controlled trial and 1-year follow-up. *American Journal of Psychiatry, 165*, 468–478. http://dx.doi.org/10.1176/appi.ajp.2007.07071079

Bogenschutz, M. P., & Nurnberg, G. H. (2004). Olanzapine versus placebo in the treatment of borderline person-

ality disorder. *The Journal of Clinical Psychiatry, 65*, 104–109. http://dx.doi.org/10.4088/JCP.v65n0118

Bozzatello, P., & Bellino, S. (2016). Combined therapy with interpersonal psychotherapy adapted for borderline personality disorder: A two-years follow-up. *Psychiatry Research, 240*, 151–156. http://dx.doi.org/10.1016/j.psychres.2016.04.014

Bozzatello, P., Ghirardini, C., Uscinska, M., Rocca, P., & Bellino, S. (2017). Pharmacotherapy of personality disorders: What we know and what we have to search for. *Future Neurology, 12*, 199–222. http://dx.doi.org/10.2217/fnl-2017-0010

Chanen, A., Sharp, C., Hoffman, P., & the Global Alliance for Prevention and Early Intervention for Borderline Personality Disorder. (2017). Prevention and early intervention for borderline personality disorder: A novel public health priority. *World Psychiatry, 16*, 215–216. http://dx.doi.org/10.1002/wps.20429

Chanen, A. M. (2010). The National Institute for Health and Clinical Excellence guideline for borderline personality disorder: More realistic than nihilistic. *Personality and Mental Health, 4*, 41–44. http://dx.doi.org/10.1002/pmh.116

Chanen, A. M. (2015). Borderline personality disorder in young people: Are we there yet? *Journal of Clinical Psychology, 71*, 778–791. http://dx.doi.org/10.1002/jclp.22205

Chanen, A. M., Jovev, M., Djaja, D., McDougall, E., Yuen, H. P., Rawlings, D., & Jackson, H. J. (2008). Screening for borderline personality disorder in outpatient youth. *Journal of Personality Disorders, 22*, 353–364. http://dx.doi.org/10.1521/pedi.2008.22.4.353

Chanen, A. M., Jovev, M., & Jackson, H. J. (2007). Adaptive functioning and psychiatric symptoms in adolescents with borderline personality disorder. *The Journal of Clinical Psychiatry, 68*, 297–306. http://dx.doi.org/10.4088/JCP.v68n0217

Chanen, A. M., & McCutcheon, L. (2013). Prevention and early intervention for borderline personality disorder: Current status and recent evidence. *The British Journal of Psychiatry. Supplement, 202*, s24–s29. http://dx.doi.org/10.1192/bjp.bp.112.119180

Chanen, A. M., & Thompson, K. (2016a). Borderline personality disorder: Sex differences. In D. J. Castle & K. M. Abel (Eds.), *Comprehensive Women's Mental Health* (pp. 137–147). Cambridge, UK: Cambridge University Press. http://dx.doi.org/10.1017/CBO9781107045132.013

Chanen, A. M., & Thompson, K. N. (2016b). Prescribing and borderline personality disorder. *Australian Prescriber, 39*, 49–53. http://dx.doi.org/10.18773/austprescr.2016.019

Choi-Kain, L. W., Finch, E. F., Masland, S. R., Jenkins, J. A., & Unruh, B. T. (2017). What works in the treatment of borderline personality disorder. *Current Behavioral Neuroscience Reports, 4,* 21–30. http://dx.doi.org/10.1007/s40473-017-0103-z

Clark, L. A. (2007). Assessment and diagnosis of personality disorder: Perennial issues and an emerging reconceptualization. *Annual Review of Psychology, 58,* 227–257. http://dx.doi.org/10.1146/annurev.psych.57.102904.190200

Coid, J., Yang, M., Tyrer, P., Roberts, A., & Ullrich, S. (2006). Prevalence and correlates of personality disorder in Great Britain. *The British Journal of Psychiatry, 188,* 423–431. http://dx.doi.org/10.1192/bjp.188.5.423

Cristea, I. A., Gentili, C., Cotet, C. D., Palomba, D., Barbui, C., & Cuijpers, P. (2017). Efficacy of psychotherapies for borderline personality disorder: A systematic review and meta-analysis. *JAMA Psychiatry, 74,* 319–328. http://dx.doi.org/10.1001/jamapsychiatry.2016.4287

Cruitt, P. J., & Oltmanns, T. F. (2018). Age-related outcomes associated with personality pathology in later life. *Current Opinion in Psychology, 21,* 89–93. http://dx.doi.org/10.1016/j.copsyc.2017.09.013

De La Fuente, J. M., & Lotstra, F. (1994). A trial of carbamazepine in borderline personality disorder. *European Neuropsychopharmacology, 4,* 479–486. http://dx.doi.org/10.1016/0924-977X(94)90296-8

DGPPN. (2009). *Behandlungsleitlinie persönlichkeitsstörungen* [Personality disorders. Practice guidelines]. Heidelberg, Germany: Steinkopff Verlag.

First, M. B., Gibbon, M., Benjamin, L. S., Spitzer, R. L., & Williams, J. B. (1997). *Structured Clinical Interview for DSM–IV Axis II Personality Disorders (SCID-II): Set of user's guide, interview and questionnaire.* Washington, DC: American Psychiatric Publishing.

First, M. B., Skodol, A. E., Bender, D. S., & Oldham, J. M. (2017). *User's guide for the Structured Clinical Interview for the DSM–5® Alternative Model for Personality Disorders (SCID-5-AMPD).* Washington, DC: American Psychiatric Publishing.

First, M. B., Spitzer, R. L., Benjamin, L. S., & Williams, J. B. W. (2015). *User's guide for the Structured Clinical Interview for DSM–5 Personality Disorders (SCID-5-PD).* Washington, DC: American Psychiatric Publishing.

Frankenburg, F. R., & Zanarini, M. C. (2002). Divalproex sodium treatment of women with borderline personality disorder and bipolar II disorder: A double-blind placebo-controlled pilot study. *The Journal of Clinical Psychiatry, 63,* 442–446. http://dx.doi.org/10.4088/JCP.v63n0511

Freeman, M. P., Hibbeln, J. R., Wisner, K. L., Davis, J. M., Mischoulon, D., Peet, M., . . . Stoll, A. L. (2006). Omega-3 fatty acids: Evidence basis for treatment and future research in psychiatry. *The Journal of Clinical Psychiatry, 67,* 1954–1967. http://dx.doi.org/10.4088/JCP.v67n1217

Grant, B. F., Chou, S. P., Goldstein, R. B., Huang, B., Stinson, F. S., Saha, T. D., . . . Ruan, W. J. (2008). Prevalence, correlates, disability, and comorbidity of *DSM–IV* borderline personality disorder: Results from the Wave 2 National Epidemiologic Survey on Alcohol and Related Conditions. *The Journal of Clinical Psychiatry, 69,* 533–545. http://dx.doi.org/10.4088/JCP.v69n0404

Gregory, R. J., DeLucia-Deranja, E., & Mogle, J. A. (2010). Dynamic deconstructive psychotherapy for borderline personality disorder comorbid with alcohol use disorders: 30-month follow-up. *Journal of the American Psychoanalytic Association, 58,* 560–566. http://dx.doi.org/10.1177/0003065110376303

Gross, R., Olfson, M., Gameroff, M., Shea, S., Feder, A., Fuentes, M., . . . Weissman, M. M. (2002). Borderline personality disorder in primary care. *Archives of Internal Medicine, 162,* 53–60. http://dx.doi.org/10.1001/archinte.162.1.53

Gunderson, J. G., Stout, R. L., McGlashan, T. H., Shea, M. T., Morey, L. C., Grilo, C. M., . . . Skodol, A. E. (2011). Ten-year course of borderline personality disorder: Psychopathology and function from the Collaborative Longitudinal Personality Disorders Study. *Archives of General Psychiatry, 68,* 827–837. http://dx.doi.org/10.1001/archgenpsychiatry.2011.37

Hallahan, B., Hibbeln, J. R., Davis, J. M., & Garland, M. R. (2007). Omega-3 fatty acid supplementation in patients with recurrent self-harm. Single-centre double-blind randomised controlled trial. *The British Journal of Psychiatry, 190,* 118–122. http://dx.doi.org/10.1192/bjp.bp.106.022707

Hancock-Johnson, E., Griffiths, C., & Picchioni, M. (2017). A focused systematic review of pharmacological treatment for borderline personality disorder. *CNS Drugs, 31,* 345–356. http://dx.doi.org/10.1007/s40263-017-0425-0

Herpertz, S. C., Zanarini, M., Schulz, C. S., Siever, L., Lieb, K., Möller, H.-J., . . . Möller, H.-J., & the WFSBP Task Force on Personality Disorders. (2007). World Federation of Societies of Biological Psychiatry (WFSBP) guidelines for biological treatment of personality disorders. *The World Journal of Biological Psychiatry, 8,* 212–244. http://dx.doi.org/10.1080/15622970701685224

Hollander, E., Allen, A., Lopez, R. P., Bienstock, C. A., Grossman, R., Siever, L. J., . . . Stein, D. J. (2001). A preliminary double-blind, placebo-controlled trial of divalproex sodium in borderline personality disorder. *The Journal of Clinical Psychiatry, 62,* 199–203. http://dx.doi.org/10.4088/JCP.v62n0311

Johnson, D., Shea, M. T., Yen, S., Battle, C. L., Zlotnick, C., Sanislow, C. A., . . . Zanarini, M. C. (2003). Gender differences in borderline personality disorder: Findings from the collaborative longitudinal personality disorders study. *Comprehensive Psychiatry, 44,* 284–292. http://dx.doi.org/10.1016/S0010-440X(03)00090-7

Johnson, J. G., Cohen, P., Kasen, S., Skodol, A. E., & Oldham, J. M. (2008). Cumulative prevalence of personality disorders between adolescence and adulthood. *Acta Psychiatrica Scandinavica, 118,* 410–413. http://dx.doi.org/10.1111/j.1600-0447.2008.01231.x

Kaess, M., Brunner, R., & Chanen, A. (2014). Borderline personality disorder in adolescence. *Pediatrics, 134,* 782–793. http://dx.doi.org/10.1542/peds.2013-3677

Kaess, M., von Ceumern-Lindenstjerna, I.-A., Parzer, P., Chanen, A., Mundt, C., Resch, F., & Brunner, R. (2013). Axis I and II comorbidity and psychosocial functioning in female adolescents with borderline personality disorder. *Psychopathology, 46,* 55–62. http://dx.doi.org/10.1159/000338715

Kendall, T., Burbeck, R., & Bateman, A. (2010). Pharmacotherapy for borderline personality disorder: NICE guideline. *The British Journal of Psychiatry, 196,* 158–159. http://dx.doi.org/10.1192/bjp.196.2.158

Korzekwa, M. I., Dell, P. F., Links, P. S., Thabane, L., & Webb, S. P. (2008). Estimating the prevalence of borderline personality disorder in psychiatric outpatients using a two-phase procedure. *Comprehensive Psychiatry, 49,* 380–386. http://dx.doi.org/10.1016/j.comppsych.2008.01.007

Law, D., & Jacob, J. (2013). *Goals and goal based outcomes (GBOs): Some useful information* (3rd ed.). London, UK: CAMHS Press.

Leichsenring, F., Leibing, E., Kruse, J., New, A. S., & Leweke, F. (2011). Borderline personality disorder. *The Lancet, 377,* 74–84. http://dx.doi.org/10.1016/S0140-6736(10)61422-5

Lenzenweger, M. F. (2008). Epidemiology of personality disorders. *Psychiatric Clinics of North America, 31*(3), 395–403, vi. http://dx.doi.org/10.1016/j.psc.2008.03.003

Lenzenweger, M. F., Lane, M. C., Loranger, A. W., & Kessler, R. C. (2007). *DSM–IV* personality disorders in the National Comorbidity Survey Replication. *Biological Psychiatry, 62,* 553–564. http://dx.doi.org/10.1016/j.biopsych.2006.09.019

Lieb, K., Völlm, B., Rücker, G., Timmer, A., & Stoffers, J. M. (2010). Pharmacotherapy for borderline personality disorder: Cochrane systematic review of randomised trials. *The British Journal of Psychiatry, 196,* 4–12. http://dx.doi.org/10.1192/bjp.bp.108.062984

Linehan, M. M., Comtols, K. A., Murray, A. M., Brown, M. Z., Gallop, R. J., Heard, H. L., . . . Lindenboim, N. (2006). Two-year randomized controlled trial and follow-up of dialectical behavior therapy vs

therapy by experts for suicidal behaviors and borderline personality disorder. *Archives of General Psychiatry, 63,* 757–766. http://dx.doi.org/10.1001/archpsyc.63.7.757

Links, P. S., Ross, J., & Gunderson, J. G. (2015). Promoting good psychiatric management for patients with borderline personality disorder. *Journal of Clinical Psychology, 71,* 753–763. http://dx.doi.org/10.1002/jclp.22203

Loew, T. H., Nickel, M. K., Muehlbacher, M., Kaplan, P., Nickel, C., Kettler, C., . . . Egger, C. (2006). Topiramate treatment for women with borderline personality disorder: A double-blind, placebo-controlled study. *Journal of Clinical Psychopharmacology, 26,* 61–66. http://dx.doi.org/10.1097/01.jcp.0000195113.61291.48

Loranger, A. W., Janca, A., & Sartorius, N. (Eds.). (1997). *Assessment and diagnosis of personality disorders: The ICD–10 International Personality Disorder Examination (IPDE).* Cambridge, UK: Cambridge University Press. http://dx.doi.org/10.1017/CBO9780511663215

Markovitz, P. J. (1995). Pharmacotherapy of impulsivity, aggression, and related disorders. In E. Hollander & D. Stein (Eds.), *Impulsivity and aggression* (pp. 263–287). New York, NY: Wiley.

Martín-Blanco, A., Ancochea, A., Soler, J., Elices, M., Carmona, C., & Pascual, J. C. (2017). Changes over the last 15 years in the psychopharmacological management of persons with borderline personality disorder. *Acta Psychiatrica Scandinavica, 136,* 323–331. http://dx.doi.org/10.1111/acps.12767

Mellsop, G., Varghese, F., Joshua, S., & Hicks, A. (1982). The reliability of Axis II of *DSM–III. The American Journal of Psychiatry, 139,* 1360–1361. http://dx.doi.org/10.1176/ajp.139.10.1360

Moen, R., Freitag, M., Miller, M., Lee, S., Romine, A., Song, S., . . . Schulz, S. C. (2012). Efficacy of extended-release divalproex combined with "condensed" dialectical behavior therapy for individuals with borderline personality disorder. *Annals of Clinical Psychiatry, 24*(4), 255–260.

Montgomery, D., Montgomery, S., & Roy, D. (1983). Mianserin in the prophylaxis of suicidal behaviour: A double blind placebo controlled trial. In J. P. Soubrier & J. Vedrinne (Eds.), *Depression and suicide* (pp. 786–790). Paris, France: Pergamon Press.

Moran, P., Walsh, E., Tyrer, P., Burns, T., Creed, F., & Fahy, T. (2003). Does co-morbid personality disorder increase the risk of suicidal behaviour in psychosis? *Acta Psychiatrica Scandinavica, 107,* 441–448. http://dx.doi.org/10.1034/j.1600-0447.2003.00125.x

Morey, L. C., & Benson, K. T. (2016). An investigation of adherence to diagnostic criteria, revisited: Clinical diagnosis of the *DSM–IV/DSM–5* Section II personality disorders. *Journal of Personality Disorders, 30*, 130–144. http://dx.doi.org/10.1521/pedi_2015_29_188

National Collaborating Centre for Mental Health. (2009). *Borderline personality disorder: Treatment and management.* London, UK: Royal College of Psychiatrists.

National Collaborating Centre for Mental Health. (2011). *Borderline personality disorder: Treatment and management.* Leicester, UK: British Psychological Society.

National Health and Medical Research Council. (2012). *Clinical practice guideline for the management of borderline personality disorder.* Melbourne, Australia. Author.

National Institute for Health and Care Excellence. (2015). *Personality disorders: Borderline and antisocial* (Quality Standard No. 88). Retrieved from http://nice.org.uk/guidance/qs88

Nickel, M. K., Muehlbacher, M., Nickel, C., Kettler, C., Gil, F. P., Bachler, E., . . . Kaplan, P. (2006). Aripiprazole in the treatment of patients with borderline personality disorder: A double-blind, placebo-controlled study. *The American Journal of Psychiatry, 163*, 833–838. http://dx.doi.org/10.1176/ajp.2006.163.5.833

Nickel, M. K., Nickel, C., Kaplan, P., Lahmann, C., Mühlbacher, M., Tritt, K., . . . Loew, T. H. (2005). Treatment of aggression with topiramate in male borderline patients: A double-blind, placebo-controlled study. *Biological Psychiatry, 57*, 495–499. http://dx.doi.org/10.1016/j.biopsych.2004.11.044

Nickel, M. K., Nickel, C., Mitterlehner, F. O., Tritt, K., Lahmann, C., Leiberich, P. K., . . . Loew, T. H. (2004). Topiramate treatment of aggression in female borderline personality disorder patients: A double-blind, placebo-controlled study. *The Journal of Clinical Psychiatry, 65*, 1515–1519. http://dx.doi.org/10.4088/JCP.v65n1112

Okanović, M., & Zivanović, O. (2016). Valproate, bipolar disorder and polycystic ovarian syndrome. *Medicinski Pregled, 69*(3–4), 121–126. http://dx.doi.org/10.2298/MPNS1604121O

Pascual, J. C., Soler, J., Puigdemont, D., Pérez-Egea, R., Tiana, T., Alvarez, E., & Pérez, V. (2008). Ziprasidone in the treatment of borderline personality disorder: A double-blind, placebo-controlled, randomized study. *The Journal of Clinical Psychiatry, 69*, 603–608. http://dx.doi.org/10.4088/JCP.v69n0412

Pfohl, B., Blum, N., & Zimmerman, M. (1997). *Structured Interview for DSM–IV Personality: SIDP-IV.* Washington, DC: American Psychiatric Publishing.

Philipsen, A., Schmahl, C., & Lieb, K. (2004). Naloxone in the treatment of acute dissociative states in female patients with borderline personality disorder. *Pharmacopsychiatry, 37*, 196–199. http://dx.doi.org/10.1055/s-2004-827243

Pompili, M., Girardi, P., Ruberto, A., & Tatarelli, R. (2005). Suicide in borderline personality disorder: A meta-analysis. *Nordic Journal of Psychiatry, 59*, 319–324. http://dx.doi.org/10.1080/08039480500320025

*Poreh, A. M., Rawlings, D., Claridge, G., Freeman, J. L., Faulkner, C., & Shelton, C. (2006). The BPQ: A scale for the assessment of borderline personality based on *DSM–IV* criteria. *Journal of Personality Disorders, 20*, 247–260. http://dx.doi.org/10.1521/pedi.2006.20.3.247

Quirk, S. E., Berk, M., Chanen, A. M., Koivumaa-Honkanen, H., Brennan-Olsen, S. L., Pasco, J. A., & Williams, L. J. (2015). Population prevalence of personality disorder and associations with physical health comorbidities and health care service utilization: A review. *Personality Disorders: Theory, Research, and Treatment, 7*, 136–146. http://dx.doi.org/10.1037/per0000148

Richtlijnontwikkeling, L. S. M. (2008). *Richtlijn voor de diagnostiek en behandeling van volwassen patiënten met een persoonlijkheidsstoornis. [Guideline for the diagnosis and treatment of adult patients with a personality disorder.]* Utrecht: Trimbos-Instituut.

Rinne, T., van den Brink, W., Wouters, L., & van Dyck, R. (2002). SSRI treatment of borderline personality disorder: A randomized, placebo-controlled clinical trial for female patients with borderline personality disorder. *The American Journal of Psychiatry, 159*, 2048–2054. http://dx.doi.org/10.1176/appi.ajp.159.12.2048

Ripoll, L. H. (2012). Clinical psychopharmacology of borderline personality disorder: An update on the available evidence in light of the *Diagnostic and Statistical Manual of Mental Disorders–5. Current Opinion in Psychiatry, 25*, 52–58. http://dx.doi.org/10.1097/YCO.0b013e32834c3f19

Roepke, S., Ziegenhorn, A., Kronsbein, J., Merkl, A., Bahri, S., Lange, J., . . . Lammers, C.-H. (2010). Incidence of polycystic ovaries and androgen serum levels in women with borderline personality disorder. *Journal of Psychiatric Research, 44*, 847–852. http://dx.doi.org/10.1016/j.jpsychires.2010.01.007

Ryle, A. (1997). *Cognitive analytic therapy of borderline personality disorder: The model and the method.* New York, NY, John Wiley & Sons.

Salzman, C., Wolfson, A. N., Schatzberg, A., Looper, J., Henke, R., Albanese, M., . . . Miyawaki, E. (1995). Effect of fluoxetine on anger in symptomatic volunteers with borderline personality disorder. *Journal of Clinical Psychopharmacology, 15*, 23–29. http://dx.doi.org/10.1097/00004714-199502000-00005

Sansone, R. A., & Sansone, L. A. (2011). Gender patterns in borderline personality disorder. *Innovations in Clinical Neuroscience, 8*(5), 16–20.

Schmahl, C., Kleindienst, N., Limberger, M., Ludäscher, P., Mauchnik, J., Deibler, P., . . . Bohus, M. (2012). Evaluation of naltrexone for dissociative symptoms in borderline personality disorder. *International Clinical Psychopharmacology, 27,* 61–68. http://dx.doi.org/10.1097/YIC.0b013e32834d0e50

Schulz, S. C., Zanarini, M. C., Bateman, A., Bohus, M., Detke, H. C., Trzaskoma, Q., . . . Corya, S. (2008). Olanzapine for the treatment of borderline personality disorder: Variable dose 12-week randomised double-blind placebo-controlled study. *The British Journal of Psychiatry, 193,* 485–492. http://dx.doi.org/10.1192/bjp.bp.107.037903

Sharp, C., & Fonagy, P. (2015). Practitioner review: Borderline personality disorder in adolescence—recent conceptualization, intervention, and implications for clinical practice. *Journal of Child Psychology and Psychiatry, 56,* 1266–1288. http://dx.doi.org/10.1111/jcpp.12449

*Sharp, C., Ha, C., Michonski, J., Venta, A., & Carbone, C. (2012). Borderline personality disorder in adolescents: Evidence in support of the Childhood Interview for DSM–IV Borderline Personality Disorder in a sample of adolescent inpatients. *Comprehensive Psychiatry, 53,* 765–774. http://dx.doi.org/10.1016/j.comppsych.2011.12.003

Sharp, C., Steinberg, L., Temple, J., & Newlin, E. (2014). An 11-item measure to assess borderline traits in adolescents: Refinement of the BPFSC using IRT. *Personality Disorders: Theory, Research, and Treatment, 5,* 70–78. http://dx.doi.org/10.1037/per0000057

Simeon, D., Bartz, J., Hamilton, H., Crystal, S., Braun, A., Ketay, S., & Hollander, E. (2011). Oxytocin administration attenuates stress reactivity in borderline personality disorder: A pilot study. *Psychoneuroendocrinology, 36,* 1418–1421. http://dx.doi.org/10.1016/j.psyneuen.2011.03.013

Simpson, E. B., Yen, S., Costello, E., Rosen, K., Begin, A., Pistorello, J., & Pearlstein, T. (2004). Combined dialectical behavior therapy and fluoxetine in the treatment of borderline personality disorder. *The Journal of Clinical Psychiatry, 65,* 379–385. http://dx.doi.org/10.4088/JCP.v65n0314

Sinn, N., Milte, C., & Howe, P. R. C. (2010). Oiling the brain: A review of randomized controlled trials of omega-3 fatty acids in psychopathology across the lifespan. *Nutrients, 2,* 128–170. http://dx.doi.org/10.3390/nu2020128

Soloff, P. H. (1998). Algorithms for pharmacological treatment of personality dimensions: Symptom-specific treatments for cognitive-perceptual, affective, and impulsive-behavioral dysregulation. *Bulletin of the Menninger Clinic, 62*(2), 195–214.

Soloff, P. H. (2000). Psychopharmacology of borderline personality disorder. [ix.]. *Psychiatric Clinics of North America, 23,* 169–192. http://dx.doi.org/10.1016/S0193-953X(05)70150-7

Soloff, P. H., Cornelius, J., George, A., Nathan, S., Perel, J. M., & Ulrich, R. F. (1993). Efficacy of phenelzine and haloperidol in borderline personality disorder. *Archives of General Psychiatry, 50,* 377–385. http://dx.doi.org/10.1001/archpsyc.1993.01820170055007

Soloff, P. H., George, A., Nathan, S., Schulz, P. M., Cornelius, J. R., Herring, J., & Perel, J. M. (1989). Amitriptyline versus haloperidol in borderlines: Final outcomes and predictors of response. *Journal of Clinical Psychopharmacology, 9,* 238–246. http://dx.doi.org/10.1097/00004714-198908000-00002

Stoffers, J. M., & Lieb, K. (2015). Pharmacotherapy for borderline personality disorder—current evidence and recent trends. *Current Psychiatry Reports, 17,* 534. http://dx.doi.org/10.1007/s11920-014-0534-0

Thompson, K. N., Jackson, H., Cavelti, M., Betts, J., McCutcheon, L., Jovev, M., & Chanen, A. M. (2018). The clinical significance of subthreshold borderline personality disorder features in outpatient youth. *Journal of Personality Disorders, 32,* 1–11. http://dx.doi.org/10.1521/pedi_2018_32_330

Torgersen, S., Kringlen, E., & Cramer, V. (2001). The prevalence of personality disorders in a community sample. *Archives of General Psychiatry, 58,* 590–596. http://dx.doi.org/10.1001/archpsyc.58.6.590

Tritt, K., Nickel, C., Lahmann, C., Leiberich, P. K., Rother, W. K., Loew, T. H., & Nickel, M. K. (2005). Lamotrigine treatment of aggression in female borderline-patients: A randomized, double-blind, placebo-controlled study. *Journal of Psychopharmacology, 19,* 287–291. http://dx.doi.org/10.1177/0269881105051540

Trull, T. J., Jahng, S., Tomko, R. L., Wood, P. K., & Sher, K. J. (2010). Revised NESARC personality disorder diagnoses: Gender, prevalence, and comorbidity with substance dependence disorders. *Journal of Personality Disorders, 24,* 412–426. http://dx.doi.org/10.1521/pedi.2010.24.4.412

van Asselt, A. D., Dirksen, C. D., Arntz, A., Giesen-Bloo, J. H., van Dyck, R., Spinhoven, P., . . . Severens, J. L. (2008). Out-patient psychotherapy for borderline personality disorder: Cost-effectiveness of schema-focused therapy v. transference-focused psychotherapy. *British Journal of Psychiatry, 192,* 450–457. http://dx.doi.org/10.1192/bjp.bp.106.033597

Widiger, T. A. (1998). Four out of five ain't bad. *Archives of General Psychiatry, 55,* 865–866. http://dx.doi.org/10.1001/archpsyc.55.10.865

Zanarini, M. C., & Frankenburg, F. R. (2001). Olanzapine treatment of female borderline personality disorder patients: A double-blind, placebo-controlled pilot study. *The Journal of Clinical Psychiatry, 62,* 849–854. http://dx.doi.org/10.4088/JCP.v62n1103

Zanarini, M. C., & Frankenburg, F. R. (2003). Omega-3 fatty acid treatment of women with borderline personality disorder: A double-blind, placebo-controlled pilot study. *The American Journal of Psychiatry, 160,* 167–169. http://dx.doi.org/10.1176/appi.ajp.160.1.167

Zanarini, M. C., Frankenburg, F. R., Bradford Reich, D., Harned, A. L., & Fitzmaurice, G. M. (2015). Rates of psychotropic medication use reported by borderline patients and axis II comparison subjects over 16 years of prospective follow-up. *Journal of Clinical Psychopharmacology, 35,* 63–67. http://dx.doi.org/10.1097/JCP.0000000000000232

Zanarini, M. C., Frankenburg, F. R., Chauncey, D. L., & Gunderson, J. G. (1987). The diagnostic Interview for Personality Disorders: Interrater and test-retest reliability. *Comprehensive Psychiatry, 28,* 467–480. http://dx.doi.org/10.1016/0010-440X(87)90012-5

Zanarini, M. C., Frankenburg, F. R., Hennen, J., Reich, D. B., & Silk, K. R. (2004). Axis I comorbidity in patients with borderline personality disorder: 6-year follow-up and prediction of time to remission. *The American Journal of Psychiatry, 161,* 2108–2114. http://dx.doi.org/10.1176/appi.ajp.161.11.2108

Zanarini, M. C., Frankenburg, F. R., Hennen, J., & Silk, K. R. (2004). Mental health service utilization by borderline personality disorder patients and Axis II comparison subjects followed prospectively for 6 years. *The Journal of Clinical Psychiatry, 65,* 28–36. http://dx.doi.org/10.4088/JCP.v65n0105

Zanarini, M. C., Frankenburg, F. R., Reich, D. B., Conkey, L. C., & Fitzmaurice, G. M. (2015). Treatment rates for patients with borderline personality disorder and other personality disorders: A 16-year study. *Psychiatric Services, 66,* 15–20. http://dx.doi.org/10.1176/appi.ps.201400055

Zanarini, M. C., Frankenburg, F. R., Vujanovic, A. A., Hennen, J., Reich, D. B., & Silk, K. R. (2004). Axis II comorbidity of borderline personality disorder: Description of 6-year course and prediction to time-to-remission. *Acta Psychiatrica Scandinavica, 110,* 416–420. http://dx.doi.org/10.1111/j.1600-0447.2004.00362.x

*Zanarini, M. C., Gunderson, J. G., Frankenburg, F. R., & Chauncey, D. L. (1989). The Revised Diagnostic Interview for Borderlines: Discriminating BPD from other Axis II disorders. *Journal of Personality Disorders, 3,* 10–18. http://dx.doi.org/10.1521/pedi.1989.3.1.10

Zanarini, M. C., Schulz, S. C., Detke, H. C., Tanaka, Y., Zhao, F., Lin, D., . . . Corya, S. (2011). A dose comparison of olanzapine for the treatment of borderline personality disorder: A 12-week randomized, double-blind, placebo-controlled study. *The Journal of Clinical Psychiatry, 72,* 1353–1362. http://dx.doi.org/10.4088/JCP.08m04138yel

*Zanarini, M. C., Vujanovic, A. A., Parachini, E. A., Boulanger, J. L., Frankenburg, F. R., & Hennen, J. (2003a). A screening measure for BPD: The McLean Screening Instrument for Borderline Personality Disorder (MSI-BPD). *Journal of Personality Disorders, 17,* 568–573. http://dx.doi.org/10.1521/pedi.17.6.568.25355

*Zanarini, M. C., Vujanovic, A. A., Parachini, E. A., Boulanger, J. L., Frankenburg, F. R., & Hennen, J. (2003b). Zanarini Rating Scale for Borderline Personality Disorder (ZAN-BPD): A continuous measure of *DSM–IV* borderline psychopathology. *Journal of Personality Disorders, 17,* 233–242. http://dx.doi.org/10.1521/pedi.17.3.233.22147

Zimmerman, M., Chelminski, I., & Young, D. (2008). The frequency of personality disorders in psychiatric patients. *Psychiatric Clinics of North America, 31,* 405–420. http://dx.doi.org/10.1016/j.psc.2008.03.015

Zimmerman, M., Chelminski, I., Young, D., Dalrymple, K., & Martinez, J. (2012). Does the presence of one feature of borderline personality disorder have clinical significance? Implications for dimensional ratings of personality disorders. *The Journal of Clinical Psychiatry, 73,* 8–12. http://dx.doi.org/10.4088/JCP.10m06784

Zimmerman, M., Chelminski, I., Young, D., Dalrymple, K., & Martinez, J. (2013). Is dimensional scoring of borderline personality disorder important only for subthreshold levels of severity? *Journal of Personality Disorders, 27,* 244–251. http://dx.doi.org/10.1521/pedi.2013.27.2.244

PHARMACOLOGICAL TREATMENT OF SUBSTANCE USE DISORDERS AND ADDICTION

CHAPTER 21

GENERAL INTRODUCTION: ISSUES AND PERSPECTIVE ON MEDICATION ASSISTED TREATMENT

Kyle K. Kampman

Medication assisted treatment (MAT) is an important part of the management of addictive disorders. In this section of the *APA Handbook of Psychopharmacology* (Pharmacological Treatment of Substance Use Disorders and Addiction), the use of MAT for the treatment of specific addictive disorders will be discussed including: alcohol, cannabis, stimulants, opioids, sedatives, nicotine, and gambling. Prior to discussing the specific addictions, it is important to understand the origins of MAT, including many of the barriers that slowed its progression and still impede full utilization today. This introduction will provide an overview of the development of MAT and the rationale behind its adoption. Barriers to use, including conceptual barriers as well as practical barriers, are also reviewed. In understanding the usefulness of MAT, it is also important to understand the goals of treatment. What should an efficacious medication be expected to do, and what are the best strategies to employ to extract the best effect from a medication? Finally, how to best integrate medications into existing psychosocial treatment has been a topic of great controversy that needs to be understood in order to maximize the effect of MAT.

ORIGINS OF ADDICTION TREATMENT AND MEDICATION ASSISTED TREATMENT

Addiction treatment in the United States has been heavily influenced by the Minnesota Model (MM) of treatment, which was first developed at a state mental hospital in Minnesota in the 1950s and included the blending of professional staff and trained nonprofessional staff (who themselves were in recovery; Anderson, McGovern, & DuPont, 1999). The MM included the use of the principles and practices of Alcoholics Anonymous. In the MM, addiction is conceived of as an involuntary disability, or a true disease, as opposed to a moral failing. This model relies heavily on the use of inpatient treatment with the goal of complete abstinence from all drugs that can be abused. Although the MM espouses the disease concept of addiction, an implicit assumption in the design of treatment and measured outcomes was that the disease of addiction could be cured. Long-term treatments, especially the long-term use of medications, were not thought to be indicated. The use of medications, particularly agonist medications such as methadone, were highly discouraged in this model.

For many years, the influence of the MM was an impediment to the use of MAT. However, over time, a number of factors have combined to overcome some of the misconceptions about the disease of addiction and have opened the door for the use of MAT, even among very traditional MM programs (Galanter, Seppala, & Klein, 2016). Among the factors that have altered our conception of the disease of addiction and its appropriate treatment are a remarkable increase in our understanding of the neurobiology of addiction and the failure of

http://dx.doi.org/10.1037/0000133-021
APA Handbook of Psychopharmacology, S. M. Evans (Editor-in-Chief)

traditional drug treatment programs to effectively prevent relapse in a number of addictive disorders, most prominently alcohol use disorder and opioid use disorder (Campbell, Lawrence, & Perry, 2018; Davison et al., 2006; Ling et al., 2009).

ADDICTION AS A BRAIN DISEASE

Over the past several decades, much has been learned about the neurobiology of addiction. This new knowledge has stimulated research into pharmacotherapy as a strategy for treatment. Processes involved in addictive disorders can be divided into those that mediate reward and craving for reward, and those that mediate withdrawal and negative reinforcement. The rewarding aspects of drug use include the euphoria associated with drug use and the desire to experience the pleasurable aspects of drug use again. These aspects of drug use are often more compelling early in the process of addiction. After continued use, however, other processes such as drug withdrawal also become important motivators of continued drug use. Once a drug user becomes physically dependent on a drug, he or she will experience unpleasant effects, including physical symptoms, when the drug is abruptly discontinued. These unpleasant effects of discontinuation punish the drug user for discontinuing the use of a drug. This process, called *negative reinforcement*, is often a more prominent cause for continued drug use after repetitive drug use for a prolonged period of time. Both drug reward and negative reinforcement involve changes in the neurobiology of the brain that promote continued drug use and provide targets for pharmacotherapy.

Most drug users start to use drugs in order to feel good. The pleasurable effects of all addictive drugs are mediated by activation of the reward center in the brain caused by increases in the release of dopamine (Wise, 2008). Along with the drug itself, environmental cues that are consistently present before the drug user experiences the effects of the drug may become associated with drug use and trigger drug-like responses in a process called *conditioning* (O'Brien, Childress, McLellan, & Ehrman, 1992). These conditioned reminders of the rewarding experiences themselves can trigger a rapid release of

dopamine in anticipation of the reward. These fast surges of dopamine release a trigger craving for the drug (Volkow et al., 2006). The response to conditioned cues of drug use involves the same molecular mechanisms associated with learning and memory formation called long-term potentiation. Long-term potentiation is a brain process in which the transmission of signals between neurons increases. Signal strength is increased by the insertion of receptors at the synapses that are stimulated by the excitatory neurotransmitter glutamate. Glutamate acts through α-amino-3-hydroxy-5-methyl-4-isoxazolepropionic acid (AMPA) and N-methyl-D-aspartate (NMDA) receptors. The insertion of AMPA receptors into the synapse enhances the efficiency of transmission and has been shown to contribute to long-term potentiation in animal studies of addiction (Volkow, Koob, & McLellan, 2016; Wolf & Ferrario, 2010). Medications acting on glutamatergic receptors such as topiramate and acamprosate have been shown to be efficacious for the treatment of alcohol use disorder and possibly also cocaine use disorder (Kampman et al., 2004, 2013; Kranzler et al., 2014; Mason, Goodman, Chabac, & Lehert, 2006).

Medications can be used to intervene in this reward process by blocking the trigger of dopamine release. Naltrexone, a mu opiate receptor antagonist, can prevent the rewarding effects of opiates directly by preventing activation of the opiate receptor. Naltrexone may also block the rewarding effects of alcohol in some patients by preventing activation of the opiate receptor caused by the stimulated release of beta endorphins produced by alcohol (Volpicelli, Watson, King, Sherman, & O'Brien, 1995). Varenicline, which is an effective medication for tobacco use disorder, blocks nicotine receptors and can prevent their activation, thus preventing the initiation of the reward process caused by smoking. Buprenorphine also reduces the rewarding effects of opiates by blocking the mu opiate receptor. Methadone, which is a long-acting mu opiate agonist, can block the euphoric effects of opiates by conferring tolerance to abused opiates. Other medications may influence craving by altering glutamatergic activity. Acamprosate may reduce conditioned cue-induced alcohol craving by reducing glutamatergic activity at NMDA receptors (Mason & Ownby,

2000). Topiramate may also reduce cue-induced alcohol and cocaine craving by blocking AMPA receptors (Kranzler et al., 2014).

Negative reinforcement of continued drug use involves neurobiological changes that support addiction and may offer different pharmacological targets (Koob & Mason, 2016). Many substances including opiates, alcohol, stimulants, and cannabis produce dysphoria, craving, and other adverse withdrawal symptoms when the substance is abruptly stopped or taken at much lower doses. Treating withdrawal symptoms and preventing acute withdrawal is an important part of the treatment of opiate, nicotine, and alcohol withdrawal. Methadone, as a full opiate agonist, and buprenorphine, as a partial opiate agonist, are effective in reducing acute withdrawal symptoms in patients with opioid use disorder. Likewise, nicotine replacement and the partial nicotine agonist varenicline may alleviate nicotine withdrawal symptoms in tobacco users. In alcohol-dependent patients, the use of benzodiazepines or gabapentin can alleviate acute alcohol withdrawal symptoms and help patients achieve initial abstinence. Protracted withdrawal symptoms thought to be associated with increases in glutamatergic activity that are linked with chronic alcohol use may be alleviated with medications such as acamprosate (Mason et al., 2006).

THE NEED FOR MEDICATION ASSISTED TREATMENT

A common theme in the development of all the medications for the treatment of substance use disorders (SUDs) is a tremendous need for a better treatment. For example, patients with opioid use disorder treated with withdrawal management and psychosocial treatment will relapse more often than not (Davison et al., 2006). In addition, withdrawal management followed by psychosocial treatment alone significantly increases the risk of overdose and death (Ravndal & Amundsen, 2010). Rates of relapse among patients with alcohol use disorder is also high (Moos & Moos, 2006). Quit rates among smokers without pharmacotherapy are close to 5%. Even with nicotine, replacement rates only increase to 20%, which is what stimulated the search for more

efficacious nonnicotine medications (Prochaska & Benowitz, 2016). Psychosocial treatment alone is often ineffective for the treatment of SUDs, and thus medications that improve efficacy are a welcome addition to the antiaddiction armamentarium.

TARGETS FOR PHARMACOTHERAPY AND THE DEVELOPMENT OF MEDICATION ASSISTED TREATMENT

As discussed in the previous section, advances in our understanding of the neurobiology of addictions have provided targets for potential pharmacological intervention. These targets may need to be engaged by medications to promote a useful outcome. The question becomes: What do we want a medication to do for the treatment of addiction? There are a limited number of potentially useful effects of medications. Medications can (a) alleviate withdrawal symptoms, in a process called *withdrawal management*; (b) reduce craving; or (c) block the euphoric effects of drugs of abuse or punish drug use by promoting toxic effects of drug use.

Withdrawal Management

Managing withdrawal can be an important first step for the treatment of most addictions. Alcohol withdrawal is a potentially life-threatening illness associated with seizures and delirium tremens. Opiate withdrawal, though not generally considered life-threatening, is associated with a number of uncomfortable symptoms including nausea, vomiting, diarrhea, abdominal cramping, tremor anxiety, tachycardia, and muscle pain. Patients with opioid use disorder often have an intense fear of withdrawal symptoms and withdrawal avoidance is a large part of the motivation to use drugs.

Stimulant withdrawal produces less dramatic physical symptoms compared with opiate and alcohol withdrawal, but withdrawal symptom severity is associated with poor outcome in the treatment of cocaine and amphetamine use disorder (Kampman et al., 2001; McGregor et al., 2005). Likewise, marijuana withdrawal is generally not medically significant but is associated with increased rates of relapse (Budney, Hughes, Moore, & Vandrey, 2004; Moore & Budney, 2003).

Effective medications have been available for the treatment of alcohol and opioid withdrawal for many years. For alcohol, sedatives of all types, including alcohol itself, have been effectively used to manage alcohol withdrawal symptoms. Benzodiazepines are most commonly used for alcohol withdrawal because of their relative safety (Mayo-Smith, 1997). For opioid withdrawal, simply replacing short-acting opiates of abuse, such as heroin, with longer acting opiates, such as methadone, has been an effective treatment. More recently, the development of the partial opiate agonist buprenorphine has provided an effective withdrawal management drug that increases treatment flexibility by allowing for outpatient withdrawal management outside of the context of an opiate treatment program. For marijuana and stimulant withdrawal, there are no medications approved by the Food and Drug Administration (FDA) for withdrawal management.

As important as withdrawal management can be for initiating abstinence, it is a mistake to believe that simply alleviating withdrawal symptoms is all that is necessary to provide effective treatment. Relapse prevention is just as important. For example, for the treatment of opioid use disorder, it has been shown that simply treating withdrawal symptoms and referring a patient to psychosocial treatment will result in relapse in the vast majority of cases (Davison et al., 2006). It has also been shown that simply managing withdrawal symptoms can put patients at risk for subsequent overdose and death (Ravndal & Amundsen, 2010). High rates of relapse after withdrawal symptoms have been alleviated have also been shown for other SUDs, including alcohol, cannabis, cocaine, and amphetamine.

Craving

Managing craving is another important medication target. A medication that does not address the overwhelming drive to use drugs is unlikely to be effective, especially if it is short acting. Craving can be extremely uncomfortable for patients, whether it is promoted by withdrawal symptoms or by conditioned reminders of prior drug use. Medication adherence can be a problem for a medication that does not address craving effectively. Oral naltrexone for the treatment of opioid use disorder is a good

example. Except in patients with a strong motivation to maintain abstinence, oral naltrexone has not been shown to be very effective (Sullivan et al., 2007). On the other hand, longer acting forms of naltrexone that do not depend on daily adherence, such as extended release injectable naltrexone and implantable naltrexone, have been shown to be effective for the treatment of opioid use disorder (Krupitsky et al., 2011).

Reinforcement

The ability to block the euphoric effects of a drug of abuse is another aspect of the effect of antiaddiction medications. If a medication is able to prevent a patient from getting high, should he or she slip and use a drug, it will greatly improve the chances that the patient will remain in treatment. An example is methadone for the treatment of opioid use disorder.

Methadone maintenance began in 1965. The first clinic was established as part of Rockefeller University (Salsitz & Wiegand, 2016). Methadone maintenance treatment was developed in response to a dramatic increase in heroin-related overdose deaths in New York City. Prior to the introduction of methadone, treatment was nonpharmacological. The most effective treatment was thought to be the Federal Narcotic Farms, which were an early form of therapeutic community. Patients were detoxified from opiates and then worked on the farms for 6 months. Unfortunately, most patients relapsed when they left the farms and returned home (Salsitz & Wiegand, 2016). Methadone was chosen as the maintenance drug because it could be taken orally, caused little euphoria or sedation, and did not promote tolerance. Patients treated with methadone had little drug craving and could function normally. In addition, methadone given at sufficient doses provided a pharmacological blockade to the euphoric effects of heroin. Dole and Nyswander (1965) combined methadone with a comprehensive treatment program, with the goal of returning patients to full functioning in their community.

It has been shown that higher doses of methadone are more effective than lower doses, and finding "the blocking dose" of methadone is often a target in methadone maintenance treatment (Strain, Stitzer, Liebson, & Bigelow, 1993). Another example is the effectiveness of long-acting injectable naltrexone for the treatment of opioid use disorder. Its primary mechanism of action is preventing the euphoric effects of opiates, although it has been shown to have anti-craving effects as well (Krupitsky et al., 2011).

The ability to punish drug use is also the mechanism of action of disulfiram. Disulfiram was the first medication approved for the treatment of a SUD. Like many psychiatric medications, its discovery was serendipitous. Disulfiram is used in the production of rubber. Disulfiram was first considered as a possible treatment for alcohol use disorder in 1937. E. E. Williams, an American chemical plant physician, observed that a group of disulfiram-exposed workers became sick after drinking alcohol. These individuals abstained from alcohol. Williams thought that disulfiram's aversive properties to alcohol could be useful as a treatment for alcohol use disorder (Williams, 1937). Two Danish researchers, Hald and Jacobsen, independently discovered the disulfiram–ethanol reaction during their investigation on disulfiram as a vermicide (Suh, Pettinati, Kampman, & O'Brien, 2006). They collaborated with a clinician, Martensen-Larsen. In subsequent clinical trials, Hald and Jacobsen (1948) and Martensen-Larsen (1948) found disulfiram to be therapeutic for its deterrent effects on drinking. Disulfiram was approved by the FDA for the treatment of alcohol use disorder in 1951.

In patients taking disulfiram, the use of alcohol provokes an uncomfortable syndrome that may include flushing, tachycardia, nausea, and vomiting. This provides a deterrent to drinking alcohol. The problem with this mechanism of action is, again, adherence. Disulfiram is most effective when adherence is observed (Brewer, Streel, & Skinner, 2017). In trials in which dosing was not observed, adherence has been noted to be a problem (Fuller et al., 1986).

BARRIERS TO THE USE OF MEDICATIONS

Despite evidence of efficacy, pharmacotherapy for the treatment of addictions is underutilized. Knudsen, Abraham, and Roman (2011) published a study showing that less than 30% of contemporary addiction treatment programs offer medications, and less than half of eligible patients in programs that offer medications actually receive medications. Although the recent opioid use epidemic has stimulated more use of MAT for opioids, the use of medications for the treatment of alcohol use disorder is still lagging.

There are a number of potential causes for the underutilization of medications for the treatment of SUDs. Some of the causes are related to perceived cultural barriers in treatment programs. Many treatment programs, especially in the United States, utilize a 12-step facilitation model. Some participants in 12-step programs do not support the use of medications for the treatment of addictions and will discourage their use. This sometimes occurs despite the fact that Alcoholics Anonymous recommends that medication use be a private issue between patient and physician (Chappel & DuPont, 1999). Stigma can also play a role in discouraging the use of medications (Woods & Joseph, 2015). Methadone use is limited to opiate treatment programs wherein medications are dispensed daily. The need to go to an opiate treatment program daily may discourage some individuals from seeking treatment due to stigma. Education may also be a barrier. Simply not being aware of the availability of effective medications for the treatment of SUDs may prevent full utilization of effective treatments.

Knudsen and colleagues (Knudsen, Roman, & Oser, 2010; Knudsen et al., 2011), in their study of barriers to the use of medications for the treatment of SUDs, found that stigma and other cultural barriers were not the biggest barriers to treatment. Instead, they found that access to medical personnel was the greatest barrier. Many, if not most, of the treatment programs they studied did not have medical personnel on staff, and this lack of medical staff was identified as the greatest barrier to the provision of MAT. For many years, SUD treatment has been conducted in programs separate from general medical treatment. This is especially true for publicly funded programs, in which most SUD treatment is provided.

Ensuring that patients have access to MAT is important. As more effective medications are identified and as more providers become available, some of the cultural and educational barriers will be overcome. The most important barrier to overcome is simply making effective forms of MAT available in all treatment programs, especially publicly funded programs.

INTEGRATION OF MEDICATIONS AND PSYCHOSOCIAL TREATMENT

Evidence suggests that MAT is more effective with the inclusion of some type of psychosocial treatment. Psychosocial treatments have included a range of therapies such as 12-step facilitation, cognitive behavior therapy (CBT), contingency management, and motivational interviewing, to name a few. There is no consistent evidence supporting one particular type of psychosocial treatment as being more effective (Dugosh et al., 2016). Forms of psychosocial treatment that support medication adherence may be particularly useful.

The overall goal of psychosocial treatment is to modify the underlying processes that serve to maintain addictive behavior, encourage engagement with pharmacotherapy, and treat underlying comorbid psychiatric illness (Dugosh et al., 2016). What particular type of psychosocial treatment is chosen and where it is provided do not seem to be critical variables. There is little evidence supporting any type of matching of therapy to a particular type of medication or illness severity measure. This was shown to be true for alcohol use disorder in a large multicenter trial comparing CBT, motivational enhancement therapy, and 12-step facilitation therapy. In this trial, all the therapies provided benefit and there were no significant differences between the three in efficacy. Out of a number of baseline variables, the only variable that predicted better outcome in any of the treatments was psychiatric severity. Patients with lower psychiatric severity had more abstinent days when treated with 12-step facilitation therapy (Project Match Research Group, 1997). Patients have been shown to experience improved outcomes after receiving psychosocial treatment, in both individual and group formats, using a variety of approaches. Many types of psychosocial treatment have been found to be efficacious when combined with pharmacotherapy. Some examples include: social skills training, couples counseling, CBT, contingency management, 12-step facilitation therapy, motiva-

tional interviewing, and family therapy (Carroll & Onken, 2005). Participation in mutual help programs is generally considered beneficial.

Although many types of psychosocial treatment may be successfully combined with MAT, brief interventions—especially interventions that support adherence to the MAT—may be particularly useful. Starosta, Leeman, and Volpicelli (2006) found that a type of brief counseling they labeled BRENDA was particularly useful when coupled with naltrexone for the treatment of alcohol use disorder (Starosta et al., 2006). The brief nature of treatment that could be provided by the prescribing physician and the inclusion of interventions aimed at promoting medication adherence were identified as particular strengths of the treatment. Fiellin et al. (2006) also found that brief counseling combined with buprenorphine was effective for the treatment of opioid use disorder.

Psychosocial treatment generally improves outcome in MAT, although the provision of MAT with limited psychosocial treatment has also been shown to be effective (Dunlop et al., 2017; Schwartz et al., 2006). There is no single type of psychosocial treatment that has been proven to be more effective than another. The use of brief psychosocial treatments, especially treatments provided by the prescribing practitioner, are convenient and may provide the additional benefit of supporting medication adherence. For a good review of the integration of medications and psychosocial treatment, see Treatment Improvement Protocol 63 (Substance Abuse and Mental Health Services Administration, 2018).

MAT is becoming an increasingly more important aspect of therapy for all addictions. The specific medications shown to be effective for each addiction and how they are used will be covered in more detail in the chapters that follow. In using MAT, it is important to understand the role that medications play in the treatment of addictions. Although the research to date has demonstrated that changes occur in the brain as a result of addiction and medications can address some of these changes, it is important to remember that MAT by itself is rarely sufficient to address all aspects of the addictive process. No medications that have been developed so far can completely achieve the three-part goal of eliminating withdrawal symptoms, alleviating craving, and blocking the high of abused drugs. Integrating MAT with effective psychosocial treatment is still the best treatment for addictive disorders.

References

Anderson, D. J., McGovern, J. P., & DuPont, R. L. (1999). The origins of the Minnesota model of addiction treatment—A first person account. *Journal of Addictive Diseases, 18*, 107–14. http://dx.doi.org/10.1300/J069v18n01_10

Brewer, C., Streel, E., & Skinner, M. (2017). Supervised disulfiram's superior effectiveness in alcoholism treatment: Ethical, methodological, and psychological aspects. *Alcohol and Alcoholism, 52*(2), 213–219.

Budney, A. J., Hughes, J. R., Moore, B. A., & Vandrey, R. (2004). Review of the validity and significance of cannabis withdrawal syndrome. *The American Journal of Psychiatry, 161*, 1967–1977. http://dx.doi.org/10.1176/appi.ajp.161.11.1967

Campbell, E. J., Lawrence, A. J., & Perry, C. J. (2018). New steps for treating alcohol use disorder. *Psychopharmacology, 235*, 1759–1773. http://dx.doi.org/10.1007/s00213-018-4887-7

Carroll, K. M., & Onken, L. S. (2005). Behavioral therapies for drug abuse. *The American Journal of Psychiatry, 162*, 1452–1460. http://dx.doi.org/10.1176/appi.ajp.162.8.1452

Chappel, J. N., & DuPont, R. L. (1999). Twelve-step and mutual-help programs for addictive disorders. *Psychiatric Clinics of North America, 22*, 425–446. http://dx.doi.org/10.1016/S0193-953X(05)70085-X

Davison, J. W., Sweeney, M. L., Bush, K. R., Davis Correale, T. M., Calsyn, D. A., Reoux, J. P., . . . Kivlahan, D. R. (2006). Outpatient treatment engagement and abstinence rates following inpatient opioid detoxification. *Journal of Addictive Diseases, 25*(4), 27–35. http://dx.doi.org/10.1300/J069v25n04_03

Dole, V. P., & Nyswander, M. (1965). A medical treatment for diacetylmorphine (heroin) addiction. A clinical trial with methadone hydrochloride. *Journal of the American Medical Association, 193*, 646–650. http://dx.doi.org/10.1001/jama.1965.03090080008002

*Dugosh, K., Abraham, A., Seymour, B., McLoyd, K., Chalk, M., & Festinger, D. (2016). A systematic review on the use of psychosocial interventions in conjunction with medications for the treatment of opioid addiction. *Journal of Addiction Medicine, 10*, 93–103. http://dx.doi.org/10.1097/ADM.0000000000000193

Dunlop, A. J., Brown, A. L., Oldmeadow, C., Harris, A., Gill, A., Sadler, C., . . . Lintzeris, N. (2017). Effectiveness and cost-effectiveness of unsupervised buprenorphine-naloxone for the treatment of heroin dependence in a randomized waitlist controlled trial. *Drug and Alcohol Dependence, 174*, 181–191. http://dx.doi.org/10.1016/j.drugalcdep.2017.01.016

Fiellin, D. A., Pantalon, M. V., Chawarski, M. C., Moore, B. A., Sullivan, L. E., O'Connor, P. G., & Schottenfeld, R. S. (2006). Counseling plus buprenorphine–naloxone maintenance therapy for opioid dependence. *The New England Journal of Medicine, 355*, 365–374. http://dx.doi.org/10.1056/NEJMoa055255

Fuller, R. K., Branchey, L., Brightwell, D. R., Derman, R. M., Emrick, C. D., Iber, F. L., . . . Shaw, S. (1986). Disulfiram treatment of alcoholism: A Veterans Administration cooperative study. *Journal of the American Medical Association, 256*, 1449–1455. http://dx.doi.org/10.1001/jama.1986.03380110055026

Galanter, M., Seppala, M., & Klein, A. (2016). Medication-assisted treatment for opioid dependence in Twelve Step–oriented residential rehabilitation settings. *Substance Abuse, 37*, 381–383. http://dx.doi.org/10.1080/08897077.2016.1187241

Hald, J., & Jacobsen, E. (1948). A drug sensitising the organism to ethyl alcohol. *Lancet, 252*, 1001–1004. http://dx.doi.org/10.1016/S0140-6736(48)91514-1

Kampman, K. M., Alterman, A. I., Volpicelli, J. R., Maany, I., Muller, E. S., Luce, D. D., . . . O'Brien, C. P. (2001). Cocaine withdrawal symptoms and initial urine toxicology results predict treatment attrition in outpatient cocaine dependence treatment. *Psychology of Addictive Behaviors, 15*, 52–59. http://dx.doi.org/10.1037/0893-164X.15.1.52

Kampman, K. M., Pettinati, H., Lynch, K. G., Dackis, C., Sparkman, T., Weigley, C., & O'Brien, C. P. (2004). A pilot trial of topiramate for the treatment of cocaine dependence. *Drug and Alcohol Dependence, 75*, 233–240. http://dx.doi.org/10.1016/j.drugalcdep.2004.03.008

Kampman, K. M., Pettinati, H. M., Lynch, K. G., Spratt, K., Wierzbicki, M. R., & O'Brien, C. P. (2013). A double-blind, placebo-controlled trial of topiramate for the treatment of comorbid cocaine and alcohol dependence. *Drug and Alcohol Dependence, 133*, 94–99. http://dx.doi.org/10.1016/j.drugalcdep.2013.05.026

Koob, G. F., & Mason, B. J. (2016). Existing and Future Drugs for the Treatment of the Dark Side of Addiction. *Annual Review of Pharmacology and Toxicology, 56*, 299–322. http://dx.doi.org/10.1146/annurev-pharmtox-010715-103143

Knudsen, H. K., Abraham, A. J., & Roman, P. M. (2011). Adoption and implementation of medications in addiction treatment programs. *Journal of Addiction*

*Asterisks indicate assessments or resources.

Medicine, 5, 21–27. http://dx.doi.org/10.1097/ADM.0b013e3181d41ddb

*Knudsen, H. K., Roman, P. M., & Oser, C. B. (2010). Facilitating factors and barriers to the use of medications in publicly funded addiction treatment organizations. *Journal of Addiction Medicine, 4*, 99–107. http://dx.doi.org/10.1097/ADM.0b013e3181b41a32

Kranzler, H. R., Covault, J., Feinn, R., Armeli, S., Tennen, H., Arias, A. J., . . . Kampman, K. M. (2014). Topiramate treatment for heavy drinkers: Moderation by a GRIK1 polymorphism. *The American Journal of Psychiatry, 171*, 445–452. http://dx.doi.org/10.1176/appi.ajp.2013.13081014

Krupitsky, E., Nunes, E. V., Ling, W., Illeperuma, A., Gastfriend, D. R., & Silverman, B. L. (2011). Injectable extended-release naltrexone for opioid dependence: A double-blind, placebo-controlled, multicentre randomised trial. *Lancet, 377*, 1506–1513. http://dx.doi.org/10.1016/S0140-6736(11)60358-9

Ling, W., Hillhouse, M., Domier, C., Doraimani, G., Hunter, J., Thomas, C., . . . Bilangi, R. (2009). Buprenorphine tapering schedule and illicit opioid use. *Addiction, 104*, 256–265. http://dx.doi.org/10.1111/j.1360-0443.2008.02455.x

Martensen-Larsen, O. (1948). Treatment of alcoholism with a sensitising drug. *Lancet, 252*, 1004–1005. http://dx.doi.org/10.1016/S0140-6736(48)91515-3

Mason, B. J., Goodman, A. M., Chabac, S., & Lehert, P. (2006). Effect of oral acamprosate on abstinence in patients with alcohol dependence in a double-blind, placebo-controlled trial: The role of patient motivation. *Journal of Psychiatric Research, 40*, 383–393. http://dx.doi.org/10.1016/j.jpsychires.2006.02.002

Mason, B. J., & Ownby, R. L. (2000). Acamprosate for the treatment of alcohol dependence: A review of double-blind, placebo-controlled trials. *CNS Spectrums, 5*, 58–69. http://dx.doi.org/10.1017/S1092852900012827

Mayo-Smith, M. F. (1997). Pharmacological management of alcohol withdrawal. A meta-analysis and evidence-based practice guideline. *Journal of the American Medical Association, 278*, 144–151. http://dx.doi.org/10.1001/jama.1997.03550020076042

McGregor, C., Srisurapanont, M., Jittiwutikarn, J., Laobhripatr, S., Wongtan, T., & White, J. M. (2005). The nature, time course and severity of methamphetamine withdrawal. *Addiction, 100*, 1320–1329. http://dx.doi.org/10.1111/j.1360-0443.2005.01160.x

Moore, B. A., & Budney, A. J. (2003). Relapse in outpatient treatment for marijuana dependence. *Journal of Substance Abuse Treatment, 25*, 85–89. http://dx.doi.org/10.1016/S0740-5472(03)00083-7

Moos, R. H., & Moos, B. S. (2006). Rates and predictors of relapse after natural and treated remission from alcohol use disorders. *Addiction, 101*, 212–222. http://dx.doi.org/10.1111/j.1360-0443.2006.01310.x

O'Brien, C. P., Childress, A. R., McLellan, A. T., & Ehrman, R. (1992). Classical conditioning in drug-dependent humans. *Annals of the New York Academy of Sciences, 654*, 400–415. http://dx.doi.org/10.1111/j.1749-6632.1992.tb25984.x

Prochaska, J. J., & Benowitz, N. L. (2016). The past, present, and future of nicotine addiction therapy. *Annual Review of Medicine, 67*, 467–486. http://dx.doi.org/10.1146/annurev-med-111314-033712

Project Match Research Group. (1997). Matching alcoholism treatments to client heterogeneity: Project MATCH posttreatment drinking outcomes. *Journal of Studies on Alcohol, 58*, 7–29. http://dx.doi.org/10.15288/jsa.1997.58.7

Ravndal, E., & Amundsen, E. J. (2010). Mortality among drug users after discharge from inpatient treatment: An 8-year prospective study. *Drug and Alcohol Dependence, 108*, 65–69. http://dx.doi.org/10.1016/j.drugalcdep.2009.11.008

Salsitz, E., & Wiegand, T. (2016). Pharmacotherapy of opioid addiction: "Putting a real face on a false demon." *Journal of Medical Toxicology; Official Journal of the American College of Medical Toxicology, 12*, 58–63. http://dx.doi.org/10.1007/s13181-015-0517-5

Schwartz, R. P., Highfield, D. A., Jaffe, J. H., Brady, J. V., Butler, C. B., Rouse, C. O., . . . Battjes, R. J. (2006). A randomized controlled trial of interim methadone maintenance. *Archives of General Psychiatry, 63*, 102–109. http://dx.doi.org/10.1001/archpsyc.63.1.102

Starosta, A. N., Leeman, R. F., & Volpicelli, J. R. (2006). The BRENDA model: Integrating psychosocial treatment and pharmacotherapy for the treatment of alcohol use disorders. *Journal of Psychiatric Practice, 12*, 80–89. http://dx.doi.org/10.1097/00131746-200603000-00003

Strain, E. C., Stitzer, M. L., Liebson, I. A., & Bigelow, G. E. (1993). Dose-response effects of methadone in the treatment of opioid dependence. *Annals of Internal Medicine, 119*, 23–27. http://dx.doi.org/10.7326/0003-4819-119-1-199307010-00004

*Substance Abuse and Mental Health Services Administration. (2018). *Medications to treat opioid use disorder. Treatment Improvement Protocol (TIP) Series 63, full document. HHS Publication No. (SMA) 18-5063FULLDOC.* Rockville, MD: Substance Abuse and Mental Health Services Administration.

Suh, J. J., Pettinati, H. M., Kampman, K. M., & O'Brien, C. P. (2006). The status of disulfiram: A half of a century later. *Journal of Clinical Psychopharmacology, 26*, 290–302. http://dx.doi.org/10.1097/01.jcp.0000222512.25649.08

Sullivan, M. A., Garawi, F., Bisaga, A., Comer, S. D., Carpenter, K., Raby, W. N., . . . Nunes, E. V. (2007). Management of relapse in naltrexone maintenance for heroin dependence. *Drug and Alcohol Dependence*, *91*, 289–292. http://dx.doi.org/10.1016/j.drugalcdep.2007.06.013

Volkow, N. D., Koob, G. F., & McLellan, A. T. (2016). Neurobiologic advances from the brain disease model of addiction. *The New England Journal of Medicine*, *374*, 363–371. http://dx.doi.org/10.1056/NEJMra1511480

Volkow, N. D., Wang, G. J., Telang, F., Fowler, J. S., Logan, J., Childress, A. R., . . . Wong, C. (2006). Cocaine cues and dopamine in dorsal striatum: Mechanism of craving in cocaine addiction. *The Journal of Neuroscience*, *26*, 6583–6588. http://dx.doi.org/10.1523/JNEUROSCI.1544-06.2006

Volpicelli, J. R., Watson, N. T., King, A. C., Sherman, C. E., & O'Brien, C. P. (1995). Effect of naltrexone on alcohol "high" in alcoholics. *The American Journal of Psychiatry*, *152*, 613–615. http://dx.doi.org/10.1176/ajp.152.4.613

Williams, E. E. (1937). Effects of alcohol on workers with carbon disulfide. *Journal of the American Medical Association*, *109*, 1472–1473.

Wise, R. A. (2008). Dopamine and reward: The anhedonia hypothesis 30 years on. *Neurotoxicity Research*, *14*, 169–183. http://dx.doi.org/10.1007/BF03033808

Wolf, M. E., & Ferrario, C. R. (2010). AMPA receptor plasticity in the nucleus accumbens after repeated exposure to cocaine. *Neuroscience and Biobehavioral Reviews*, *35*, 185–211. http://dx.doi.org/10.1016/j.neubiorev.2010.01.013

Woods, J. S., & Joseph, H. (2015). Stigma from the viewpoint of the patient. *Journal of Addictive Diseases*, *34*, 238–247. http://dx.doi.org/10.1080/10550887.2015.1059714

CHAPTER 22

PHARMACOLOGICAL TREATMENT OF ALCOHOL USE DISORDER

Barbara J. Mason

Alcohol misuse costs the United States economy about $249 billion annually, based on factors such as lost productivity, health care expenses, and law enforcement costs (U.S. Department of Health and Human Services (HHS), Office of the Surgeon General, 2016). Alcohol is responsible for the deaths of about 88,000 Americans per year, and accounts for half of all liver disease in the United States (National Center for Health Statistics, 2016). Individuals with *untreated* alcohol use disorder (AUD) utilize twice as much health care and cost twice as much as those with *treated* AUD (Holder, 1998); accordingly, total health care costs were found to decrease following AUD treatment initiation. Furthermore, combining medication approved by the U.S. Food and Drug Administration (FDA) for treating AUD with evidence-based behavioral therapy has been found to be associated with fewer inpatient admissions and 30% lower total health care costs than for those individuals not receiving medication-assisted treatment (Baser, Chalk, Rawson, & Gastfriend, 2011). These statistics make a compelling case for considering FDA-approved medication in conjunction with evidence-based behavioral therapy for all patients with AUD. In this chapter, we provide a brief review of the epidemiology and diagnosis of AUD, with a focus on FDA-approved medications and management issues associated with these

medications. We conclude with a section on emerging pharmacotherapies for AUD.

EPIDEMIOLOGY AND PREVALENCE

Approximately 6% (14.6 million) of American adults (Substance Abuse and Mental Health Services Administration [SAMHSA], 2017) meet the *Diagnostic and Statistical Manual of Mental Disorders, 5th edition* (*DSM–5*; American Psychiatric Association, 2013) criteria for AUD. *DSM–5* criteria for AUD include symptoms of compulsive drinking despite harmful consequences, craving, and a loss of control over alcohol intake; symptoms of physiological dependence, tolerance and withdrawal, may also be present. The presence of two to three out of 11 possible symptoms indicates AUD of mild severity; four to five symptoms indicate AUD of moderate severity, and six or more symptoms is severe AUD.

Binge drinking is the most common, costly, and deadly pattern of excessive alcohol use. Binge drinking is defined by the National Institute on Alcohol Abuse and Alcoholism (NIAAA) as drinking that brings blood alcohol concentration (BAC) levels to 0.08 g/dL. This BAC level typically occurs after four drinks for women and five drinks for men within about 2 hours. Binge drinking accounts for about three quarters of alcohol-related costs to our society,

Appreciation is expressed to Michael Skinner, MD, PharmD, for his review of this chapter, and to Sam Reed for his editorial assistance in the preparation of this chapter. Support for this work was provided by the Pearson Center for Alcoholism and Addiction Research and Grants R01AA023152, U01AA025476, and P60AA006420 from the National Institute on Alcohol Abuse and Alcoholism.

http://dx.doi.org/10.1037/0000133-022
APA Handbook of Psychopharmacology, S. M. Evans (Editor-in-Chief)

such as motor vehicle crashes, violence, child abuse, suicide, alcohol overdose, and fetal alcohol spectrum disorders. About 26.2% of Americans (64.1 million) had one or more binge drinking days in the past month (SAMHSA, 2017).

Chronic heavy drinking is defined by the NIAAA in women as routinely drinking more than 3 drinks per day or more than 7 drinks per week, and in men as routinely drinking more than 4 drinks per day or more than 14 drinks per week. Chronic heavy drinking is the third leading cause of preventable death in the United States, and is causally associated with various cancers, heart disease, and liver disease (NIAAA, 2010). About 6.6% of Americans (16.1 million) are heavy drinkers (SAMHSA, 2017).

DIAGNOSING ALCOHOL USE DISORDER

A common reason individuals with AUD do not seek treatment is that they are unaware that they need it (HHS, 2016). Individuals may never have been told they have AUD or may not consider themselves to have a drinking problem. Underestimating the severity of one's drinking problem and overestimating one's ability to control it are associated with alcohol-induced changes in brain circuits that control incentive salience, negative affect, and executive function (Koob & Le Moal, 1997; HHS, 2016). These factors underscore the importance of adequate screening and accurate diagnosis as a first step in treating AUD.

There are brief screening instruments that can be routinely incorporated into an initial evaluation to probe for pathological alcohol use (see *Assessing Alcohol Problems: A Guide for Clinicians and Researchers*, listed in the Tool Kit of Resources at the end of this chapter). Examples include the 3-item Alcohol Use Disorders Identification Test-Concise (AUDIT-C), which assesses drinking quantity and frequency (Bush, Kivlahan, McDonell, Fihn, & Bradley, 1998), or the NIAAA single-question screen "How many times in the past year have you had 'X' or more drinks in a day?", with X being 5 for men and 4 for women, and responses greater than 1 indicating a positive screen (Smith, Schmidt, Allensworth-Davies, & Saitz, 2009; HHS, 2016). These quick drinking quantity/frequency questions do not provide a diagnosis of AUD that is based on *DSM–5*

criteria. However, a positive screen can serve as a signal that further evaluation is warranted, because chronic heavy alcohol use may lead to the development of AUD.

The International Classification of Diseases, 10th Revision (ICD–10; World Health Organization [WHO], 1992), draft of the ICD–11(WHO, 2016), and the *Diagnostic and Statistical Manual of Mental Disorders, 4th edition* (*DSM–4*; American Psychiatric Association, 2000) use the term *alcohol dependence*. *DSM–5* combines earlier diagnostic criteria for alcohol abuse and dependence under the term *alcohol use disorder*, with severity modifiers of mild, moderate, or severe, based on the number of criteria met. *DSM–5* criteria for AUD of moderate or greater severity is essentially equivalent to *DSM–4* and *ICD–10* criteria for alcohol dependence (Compton, Dawson, Goldstein, & Grant, 2013). Given that *DSM–5* was first published in 2013, the admission criteria for the studies mentioned in this chapter are based on alcohol dependence, unless otherwise noted.

EVIDENCE-BASED PHARMACOLOGICAL APPROACHES TO ALCOHOL USE DISORDER

There are three medications that are approved by the FDA for the treatment of AUD: disulfiram (Antabuse® and generic, oral), naltrexone (Revia® and generic, oral; Vivitrol®, long-acting injectable) and acamprosate (Campral® and generic, oral). A fourth drug, nalmefene (Selincro®, oral), is approved throughout the European Union, and is to be taken on an as needed basis prior to anticipated drinking occasions. All are obtainable by prescription and share the following key characteristics:

- Not a cure for AUD, but rather a tool in the toolkit for treatment of AUD
- Not a treatment for alcohol withdrawal
- Should be initiated following detoxification and/or an abstinent baseline (see Table 22.1)
- Not alcohol substitution drugs
- Not addictive or habit forming
  - Increasing doses are not needed to achieve the desired effect (no tolerance)
  - Drug discontinuation does not precipitate rebound craving or drinking

TABLE 22.1

Summary of Disulfiram, Naltrexone (Oral and Injectable), and Acamprosate Treatment Parameters*

	Disulfiram (oral)	Naltrexone (oral)	Naltrexone (injectable)	Acamprosate (oral)
Primary evidence-based outcome	No drinking Double-blind trials, n.s.[a] Open label trials, moderate effect size[a] Supervised administration trials, large effect size[a]	No heavy drinking NNT = 12[b]	Heavy drinking days WMD = −4.6%[b]	No drinking NNT = 12[b]
Median trial duration	6.5 months[a]	3 months[b]	6 months[c]	6 months[b]
Dosing	500 mg daily weeks 1 and 2; 250 mg daily thereafter	One 50-mg tablet, daily	One 380-mg injection, monthly	Two 333-mg tablets, 3 times daily
Cost per month[c]	$48	$33	$1,308	$142
Abstinent baseline	≥12 hours (mandatory)	≈4 days[d]	7 days[c,e]	≈6 days[d]
Treatment goal	Abstinence[e]	Nonabstinence[d]	n.s.[c]	Abstinence[d]
Medical contraindications[e]	Use of metronidazole, paraldehyde, alcohol-containing preparations Severe myocardial disease or coronary occlusion Psychosis	Opioid dependence, withdrawal, or use Acute hepatitis or liver failure *Not studied in moderate or severe renal impairment*	Opioid dependence, withdrawal, or use within 7–10 days Acute hepatitis or liver failure *Caution in moderate or severe renal impairment*	Severe renal impairment (creatinine clearance ≤30 mL/min) *Dose adjustment in creatinine clearance 30 mL/min to 50 mL/min*
Dropout due to adverse events	Unknown	NNH = 48[b]	14.1% (placebo 6.7%)[c]	n.s.[b]
Adverse events	Neuritis, neuropathy[e] Hepatitis, hepatic failure[e] Psychosis[e] Drowsiness, fatigue[e] Impotence[e] Headache[e] Acne, allergic dermatitis[e] Metallic, garlic aftertaste[e]	Dizziness NNH = 16[b] Nausea NNH = 9[b] Vomiting NNH = 24[b]	≥5% and 2 times placebo[e] Vomiting, nausea Injection site reactions Muscle cramps Dizziness, syncope Somnolence, sedation Decreased appetite	Diarrhea 17% (placebo 10%)[e]

Note. Monthly cost estimates provided by local discount pharmacy (Costco), and are based on generic formulations when available. NNH = number needed to harm; NNT = number needed to treat; n.s. = not significant; WMD = weighted mean difference.
*Review each drug's package insert for full prescribing information. [a]Skinner, Lahmek, Pham, and Aubin, 2014. [b]Jonas et al., 2014. [c]Garbutt et al., 2005. [d]Maisel, Blodgett, Wilbourne, Humphreys, and Finney, 2013. [e]Information derived from package inserts (Alkermes Inc., 2010; Duramed Pharmaceuticals, Inc., 2013; Merck Santé, 2005; Physicians Total Care, Inc., 2010).

- Drug administration does not induce euphoria or other subjective effects associated with abuse potential
- No "street value" as illicit drugs
- Should be prescribed as part of a comprehensive treatment plan that considers medical contraindications, treatment goals, and concurrent disorders in selecting a pharmacological treatment, and which monitors medication adherence, adverse events, and treatment response after treatment initiation.
- Associated with better drinking outcomes (with counseling) than placebo (with counseling) in meta-analyses of clinical trials

A comparative summary of treatment parameters for the FDA-approved medications is presented in Table 22.1. Each variable depicted in Table 22.1 is derived from the most comprehensive database available, including meta-analyses, package inserts and multicenter trials.

Pharmacological treatment is typically considered for AUD of moderate or greater severity. This stage of the disorder usually follows a chronic, relapsing course characterized by compulsive heavy alcohol drinking despite harmful consequences (American Psychiatric Association, 2013). The emergence of an acute (up to 5 days duration) withdrawal syndrome upon marked reduction in or abrupt cessation of drinking is typically followed by a protracted withdrawal phase of indeterminate duration, with a high risk of relapse to pathological drinking; the cyclical nature of the disorder is illustrated in the outer ring of Figure 22.1.

Practice guidelines developed by the American Psychiatric Association for the pharmacological treatment of patients with AUD recommend the use of acamprosate or naltrexone in patients with moderate to severe AUD who wish to cut down or quit drinking, who prefer medication or who have not responded to nonpharmacological treatments, and who have no contraindications to the use of these medications (American Psychiatric Association, 2017). These guidelines suggest that disulfiram generally not be chosen as an initial treatment for AUD, given the potential risk of severe reactions and physiological consequences of drinking in combination with disulfiram, and given

the evidence for the efficacy of acamprosate and naltrexone.

Recent large-scale meta-analyses found that either acamprosate or naltrexone combined with counseling have superior efficacy for increasing rates of abstinence (acamprosate, NNT = 12) or no heavy drinking (naltrexone, NNT = 12) relative to counseling administered in conjunction with placebo (Jonas et al., 2014). A NNT = 12 indicates that about 12 people would need to be treated to achieve a case of no drinking or no heavy drinking. No significant difference was found between acamprosate and naltrexone for return to any drinking or heavy drinking in meta-analyses of trials that compared acamprosate and naltrexone (Jonas et al., 2014). Despite these evidence-based findings for efficacy, results from a nationwide pharmacy survey indicate that fewer than 9% of 8.4 million afflicted Americans fill a prescription for one of the FDA-approved medications for alcohol dependence (Mark, Kassed, Vandivort-Warren, Levit, & Kranzler, 2009).

Early FDA-approved medications for AUD targeted the binge/intoxication stage, either by serving as a psychological deterrent (disulfiram) or antagonist of the reinforcing effects of alcohol (naltrexone). However, such drugs can also produce side effects that limit medication adherence (Mitchell, Bergren, Chen, Rowbotham, & Fields, 2009). Acamprosate supports abstinence through modulation of activity in the glutamatergic system that is associated with craving and the preoccupation/anticipation stage of protracted withdrawal. Acamprosate tends to have a more benign side effect profile and to be better tolerated, with better rates of adherence than earlier medications (Mason & Lehert, 2012). To date, there are no FDA-approved drugs associated with the withdrawal/negative affect phase of AUD, but drug targets specific to this phase are under investigation (see Figure 22.1). The negative affect stage of protracted withdrawal includes symptoms of anxiety, dysphoria, and irritability (Geller, 1991), and is associated with activation of brain stress systems, particularly overexpression of corticotropin releasing factor (CRF) in the extended amygdala (Koob, 2008). Such neuroadaptations extend into the preoccupation/anticipation stage of protracted withdrawal (inner ring of Figure 22.1).

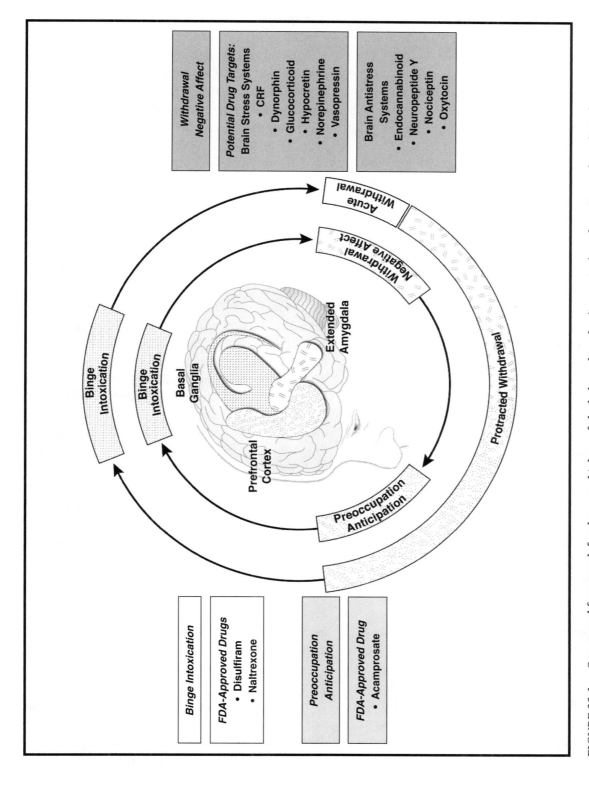

FIGURE 22.1.   Conceptual framework for the neurobiology of alcohol use disorder (inner ring), with corresponding clinical states (outer ring). From "Neurocircuitry of Addiction," by G. F. Koob and N. D. Volkow, 2010, *Neuropsychopharmacology, 35,* p. 228. Copyright 2010 by Nature Publishing Group, and "Reward, Motivation, and Addiction," by G. F. Koob, B. J. Everitt, and T. W. Robbins, in *Fundamental Neuroscience, Third Edition* (pp. 987–1016), by L. R. Squire, F. E. Bloom, N. C. Spitzer, S. du Lac, A. Ghosh, and D. Berg (Eds.), 2008, Amsterdam, the Netherlands: Academic Press. Copyright 2008 by Elsevier. Adapted with permission.

Dysregulation of the prefrontal cortex during the preoccupation/anticipation stage drives symptoms of craving, and perpetuates residual negative emotional states and sleep disturbances. All of the above symptoms of protracted withdrawal have been identified as risk factors for drinking relapse (Brower, Aldrich, & Hall, 1998; Clark et al., 1998; Foster & Peters, 1999; Gillin et al., 1994; Lowman, Allen, Stout, & The Relapse Research Group, 1996), and the underlying neurobiology offers a multitude of potential drug targets, as shown in Figure 22.1.

Disulfiram (Antabuse and generic formulations) was the first drug approved for the treatment of alcoholism (in 1951) by the FDA. It is an inhibitor of the enzyme aldehyde dehydrogenase; if even small amounts of alcohol are consumed, acetaldehyde quickly accumulates, with rapid onset of a disulfiram–alcohol interaction that includes flushing, nausea, vomiting, and multiple cardiac and respiratory symptoms that could result in death in severe reactions. Disulfiram is used as a deterrent to alcohol use and should never be given to a patient when in a state of alcohol intoxication, or without their full knowledge. The psychological threat of the disulfiram–alcohol interaction may be the primary mechanism of disulfiram's deterrent effect, as opposed to the drug's pharmacodynamic properties (Skinner, Lahmek, Pham, & Aubin, 2014). The fear of a disulfiram–alcohol interaction is equivalent across treatment groups in placebo-controlled double-blind trials, which mitigates against detecting disulfiram treatment effects relative to placebo. A meta-analysis of randomized, open label trials found a moderate effect of disulfiram relative to various comparison groups; the effect of disulfiram was found to be large under conditions of supervised administration (Skinner et al., 2014). This meta-analysis also found more serious adverse events with disulfiram than with comparison treatments (Skinner et al., 2014). Disulfiram may be considered for patients with a clear goal of complete abstinence, who are capable of understanding the risks of an alcohol–disulfiram interaction, who prefer disulfiram or have not responded to acamprosate and naltrexone, and have no medical contraindications (American Psychiatric Association, 2017). Medication compliance is a demonstrated problem

with disulfiram (Fuller et al., 1986) and outcomes are optimized with supervised administration (e.g., by a spouse or roommate, in compliant patients who wish to remain abstinent; Jørgensen, Pedersen, & Tønnesen, 2011). Disulfiram tablets are taken orally each morning, starting with 500 mg for the first 1 to 2 weeks, and then 250 mg each morning thereafter.

Disulfiram is medically contraindicated in patients who have had a recent myocardial infarction or coronary artery disease, or have a history of a seizure disorder, or who are psychotic. Metronidazole, paraldehyde, and alcohol-containing preparations like sertraline oral concentrate and cough syrups are contraindicated, as are alcohol-containing mouthwash, hand sanitizers, aftershaves, sauces, and desserts, to avoid precipitating an alcohol–disulfiram interaction. The intensity of the interaction varies across individuals, but is generally proportional to the amounts of disulfiram and alcohol ingested. The duration of the reaction varies from 30 to 60 minutes to several hours, or as long as there is alcohol in the blood. Patients should be instructed to abstain from alcohol for at least 12 hours before taking disulfiram, and be advised that reactions with alcohol can occur up to 14 days after taking disulfiram. This prolonged duration of action has the potential benefit of discouraging impulsive drinking.

Prior to initiating treatment with disulfiram, patients should receive a physical exam with electrocardiogram and liver function tests (LFTs; alanine aminotransferase [ALT], aspartate aminotransferase [AST], gamma-glutamyl transferase [GGT]). Repeat LFTs should be obtained periodically, as elevations in hepatic enzymes commonly occur—and more rarely, potentially fatal acute hepatotoxicity, even after months of treatment and in patients with normal baseline liver function. Patients should be instructed to seek immediate medical attention if signs and symptoms of liver toxicity occur (fatigue, weakness, persistent abdominal pain, nausea, vomiting, jaundice, or dark urine). It is suggested that patients carry a wallet card noting that they are taking disulfiram, in case of an alcohol–disulfiram interaction or other drug-related medical emergency.

The alcohol–disulfiram interaction has inherent risks, which some patients prefer to strengthen their motivation to abstain from alcohol. Disulfiram is typically well tolerated when taken as prescribed (Chick, 1999). The potential benefits of disulfiram for appropriately selected patients who prefer this treatment has been found to outweigh the harms, particularly given the risks of continued alcohol use (American Psychiatric Association, 2017).

Naltrexone is a pure opioid receptor antagonist that was approved by the FDA first for opioid dependence (in 1984), and later for alcohol dependence (as an oral medication in 1994; as a long-acting injectable in 2006). Opioid receptor antagonism as a treatment strategy for alcohol dependence was based on the hypothesis that if alcohol consumption was less rewarding, drinking would decrease. A systematic review and meta-analysis was conducted that included 53 randomized controlled trials of oral naltrexone (50 mg) for the treatment of AUD (Jonas et al., 2014). The included studies involved 9,140 patients and treatment durations of 12 weeks or longer. Naltrexone was found to significantly decrease the likelihood of a return to heavy drinking (NNT = 12, 95% confidence interval [CI], 8 to 26) and, to a lesser extent, a return to any drinking (NNT = 20, 95% CI, 11 to 500). This finding replicates results from an earlier meta-analysis that found an NNT = 8.6 for reduction in heavy drinking associated with naltrexone (Maisel, Blodgett, Wilbourne, Humphreys, & Finney, 2013).

This earlier meta-analysis also assessed moderators of naltrexone treatment response and found that about 4 days of abstinence prior to beginning treatment significantly improved naltrexone treatment response. Additionally, treatment goals other than abstinence were associated with a larger effect size on reducing heavy drinking than the goal of complete abstinence. Two early 3-month studies followed up with patients and found treatment effects were no longer significant relative to placebo at 1 to 3 months posttreatment (Anton et al., 2001; O'Malley et al., 1996). These data pose a conundrum in that the meta-analysis of predictors of treatment response found naltrexone efficacy to be optimized in patients who do not have abstinence as their treatment goal, but who are abstinent at baseline (Maisel et al., 2013), and the antagonist effect of the drug does not persist long beyond drug elimination. Hence,

pairing naltrexone with a relapse prevention form of cognitive behavior therapy focused on coping skills may offer an optimal treatment strategy (O'Malley et al., 1992), wherein heavy drinking is blocked pharmaceutically and behavioral therapy facilitates the alcohol-free lifestyle characteristic of long-term recovery.

Another strategy to understand variability in naltrexone response has focused on μ opioid receptor gene polymorphism status. Initial enthusiasm for this pharmacogenetic approach was based on secondary analyses from completed clinical trials that found that patients might be more responsive if they had at least one G allele of A118G polymorphism of OPRM1 (Anton, Oroszi, et al., 2008; Kranzler, Armeli, Covault, & Tennen, 2013; Oslin et al., 2003) However, subsequent studies have not found an association between genotype and naltrexone response, including a negative clinical trial that prospectively stratified patients on the basis of their OPRM1 genotype (Oslin et al., 2015). These conflicting results do not support a role for OPRM1 genotype determination in current clinical practice.

There have been no head-to-head comparisons of the efficacy of oral versus injectable naltrexone to date. A meta-analysis of drinking outcomes from 1,926 participants in two trials of different formulations of injectable naltrexone found no significant effects of treatment on return to any drinking or heavy drinking, but did find a reduction in the number of heavy drinking days (weighted mean difference −4.6%; 95 CI, −8.5% to −0.56%). The trial conducted in support of FDA approval found a similar effect of Vivitrol 380 mg, but only in men and in individuals with 7 days of abstinence prior to randomization (Garbutt et al., 2005).

Any form of naltrexone treatment for AUD is contraindicated in patients who have physiologic dependence on opioids, are in opioid withdrawal, who have used prescribed or illicit forms of opioids within the past 7 to 10 days, or who have a urine drug screen positive for opioids. The reason for these prohibitions is to avoid unintended precipitation of opioid withdrawal through administration of an opioid antagonist. Naltrexone also has the capacity to cause hepatocellular injury when used in higher than recommended doses, and is contraindicated in patients with acute hepatitis or liver failure. Naltrexone has not been evaluated in patients with severe hepatic impairment, and clinical trials of naltrexone tend to exclude patients with LFTs greater than 3 times the upper limit of normal. Caution is also advised in patients with moderate to severe renal impairment, because naltrexone and its primary metabolite are excreted primarily in the urine, and it has not been studied in patients with ≥ moderate renal impairment. To manage risk, baseline medical screening for naltrexone treatment may include tests of renal and hepatic function and a urine drug screen. Repeat LFTs (ALT, AST, GGT) may verify the absence of naltrexone-related hepatic enzyme abnormalities, as well as reflect beneficial effects of cutting down or quitting drinking (GGT). A recent meta-analysis found a higher risk for discontinuation due to adverse events with naltrexone relative to placebo (Jonas et al., 2014). Common side effects of naltrexone include nausea, vomiting, and dizziness (Duramed Pharmaceuticals, Inc., 2013; Jonas et al., 2014). Patients receiving Vivitrol may also experience a range of injection site reactions. Patients should be advised not to drive or operate heavy machinery until they feel confident that the drug does not affect their ability to perform such functions. Patients should be advised to seek medical attention if they experience symptoms of acute hepatitis (e.g., persistent stomach pain, dark urine, tiredness, yellowing of the whites of the eyes).

Patients may be advised to carry a wallet card indicating that they are receiving naltrexone. In the case of an emergency situation requiring pain management, nonopioid analgesics or regional analgesia can be used. Naltrexone will also antagonize the effects of opioid-based remedies (e.g., for coughs or diarrhea), and nonopioid-based treatments should be selected.

Acamprosate is a synthetic compound with a chemical structure similar to that of the endogenous amino acid homotaurine, which is a structural analogue of the amino acid neurotransmitter γ-aminobutyric acid and the amino acid neuromodulator taurine. Acamprosate was developed in France in the 1980s and approved by the FDA for the maintenance of abstinence in detoxified patients with alcohol dependence in 2004. Repeated cycles of heavy drinking and withdrawal dysregulate the balance between neuronal excitation (e.g., glutamatergic) and inhibition (e.g., GABAergic). Much of the preclinical literature suggests that acamprosate treats alcohol dependence by restoring homeostasis in N-methyl-D-aspartate (NMDA) mediated glutamatergic neurotransmission (Littleton, 2007; Mason & Heyser, 2010). Glutamatergic hyperactivity is associated with alcohol craving and the preoccupation/anticipation phase of protracted withdrawal (Figure 22.1).

In contrast to disulfiram, which causes aversive behavior through negative physical effects, or naltrexone, which tempers the pleasurable effects of alcohol, acamprosate acts to normalize dysregulation in neurochemical systems that have been implicated in the biological mechanisms of alcohol dependence. For example, a randomized, double-blind, placebo-controlled, crossover study using dynamic magnetic resonance spectroscopy found decreases in the brain regions for which N-acetylaspartate and glutamate are the main signal contributors (Bolo et al., 1998), suggesting a central glutamatergic effect of acamprosate. Acamprosate appears to have a sustained effect on the withdrawal-related hyperexcitatory state which allows alcohol-dependent patients to return to a normal level of neural activity more rapidly than with placebo (Boeijinga et al., 2004). Acamprosate requires around a week to reach steady-state levels in the nervous system, and its effects on drinking behavior typically persist after the treatment is completed, consistent with its role in restoring homeostasis in brain glutamate activity (Mason & Heyser, 2010).

The majority of acamprosate clinical trials are 6 to 12 months in duration. Meta-analyses of 27 acamprosate randomized controlled trials found that the NNT to prevent a return to any drinking with acamprosate was 12 (95% CI, 8 to 26; Jonas et al., 2014). This finding replicates the results from an earlier meta-analysis that found an NNT = 7.5 for complete abstinence associated with acamprosate (Maisel et al., 2013); detoxification and required abstinence (mean = 6.21 ± 5.49 days) prior to acamprosate administration was associated with increased efficacy (Maisel et al., 2013). A meta-analysis that obtained individual records from over 6,000 individuals who participated in 22 acamprosate studies found an incremental gain of 10.4% (95% CI 7.1 to 13.7, $p < 0.001$) in percentage of abstinent days, an incremental gain of 11.0% (7.4 to 14.6, $p < 0.001$) in percentage of no heavy drinking days, an odds ratio of 1.9 (1.6 to 2.2, $p < 0.001$) for rate of complete abstinence, and an odds ratio of 1.9 (1.6 to 2.3, $p < 0.001$) for rate of no heavy drinking over the study duration (Mason & Lehert, 2012), with no differences in the rate of discontinuation due to adverse events or severity or type of adverse event. Acamprosate was also associated with significantly higher rates of treatment completion ($p = 0.004$) and medication compliance ($p < 0.001$) than placebo. A limited number of posttreatment follow-up studies have shown the effects of acamprosate to be sustained for periods up to 1 year after the last dose (Mason & Heyser, 2010). Additionally, sleep lab (Staner et al., 2006) and clinical data (Perney, Lehert, & Mason, 2012; Perney, Rigole, Mason, Dematteis, & Lehert, 2015) indicate that acamprosate reverses alcohol-related changes in sleep architecture, which may yield added value when treating patients with comorbid psychiatric disorders characterized by sleep disturbance, such as posttraumatic stress disorder and anxiety and depressive disorders.

Acamprosate has low bioavailability, requiring divided dosing (two 333 mg tablets) taken three times per day. It is suggested that patients place a 1-week supply of acamprosate in an over-the-counter pill tray with day and time of dose indicated to avoid missed doses. Identification of phenotypes and genotypes associated with acamprosate response may further optimize treatment effect size; for example, an association has recently been reported between acamprosate treatment response and polymorphisms in candidate genes in glycine and glutamate neurotransmission pathways (Karpyak et al., 2014). Another pharmacogenomics analysis found the efficacy of acamprosate to be enhanced depending on the C-allele frequency of the GABARA6 gene and the T-allele homozygotes for the C+1412T polymorphism of the GABARB2 gene (Ooteman et al., 2009). A pharmacometabolomic study identified elevated baseline serum glutamate as a biomarker of acamprosate response in 120 alcohol-dependent patients; baseline serum glutamate levels were found to be significantly higher in responders compared with nonresponders, and serum glutamate levels of responders were normalized after acamprosate treatment, whereas there was no significant glutamate change in nonresponders (Nam et al., 2015). These results suggest that elevated baseline serum glutamate levels are a potential biomarker associated with positive acamprosate response. By developing such predictors, it may be possible to improve patient treatment matching and the overall success rate of acamprosate—and to that end, any pharmacotherapy used in the treatment of AUD.

Acamprosate is excreted primarily by the kidney. Due to the risk of accumulation of acamprosate with prolonged administration of therapeutic doses in renally impaired patients (Wilde & Wagstaff, 1997), the use of acamprosate is contraindicated in patients with severe renal impairment (creatinine clearance <30 mL/min); a dosage adjustment to one 333-mg tablet administered three times daily is recommended in patients with moderate renal impairment (creatinine clearance 30–50 mL/min; Saivin et al., 1998; Wilde & Wagstaff, 1997). No dose adjustment is required for patients with mild renal impairment (creatinine clearance >50 mL/min). Acamprosate is not metabolized by the liver, and is not associated with drug–drug interactions. It does not interact with alcohol (as does disulfiram), nor precipitate opioid withdrawal in patients using opioids (as does naltrexone). Acamprosate has also been found to not interact with medications commonly prescribed for patients with AUD, including disulfiram, antidepressants, anxiolytics, or hypnotics. Pharmacokinetic studies found that coadministration with naltrexone increased the rate and extent of acamprosate absorption without compromising its tolerability (Johnson et al., 2003; Mason et al., 2002). These results suggest that such combination therapy may improve acamprosate's bioavailability. Diarrhea, typically mild to moderate at the start of treatment, is the side effect most commonly associated with acamprosate (17%) relative to placebo (10%; Merck Santé, 2005). Meta-analyses found acamprosate to have no significant difference in risk of withdrawal from treatment due to adverse events compared with placebo (Jonas et al., 2014).

In summary, acamprosate, naltrexone, and disulfiram are evidence-based pharmacotherapies for AUD that have been used safely and effectively for decades. The potential benefits for appropriately selected patients have been found to outweigh the harms, particularly given the risks of continued alcohol misuse (American Psychiatric Association, 2017).

BEST APPROACHES FOR ASSESSING TREATMENT RESPONSE AND MANAGING SIDE EFFECTS

Recovery is historically characterized as a voluntarily maintained lifestyle of abstinence from alcohol and all other nonprescribed drugs in dependent individuals (Betty Ford Institute Consensus Panel, 2007). Although abstinence is considered to be an optimal treatment outcome, the FDA may also consider no heavy drinking as a clinically meaningful outcome for assessing medication efficacy, given the association between alcohol-related harms and heavy drinking (see the Epidemiology and Prevalence section in this chapter). Responder analyses, such as the rate of abstinence or no heavy drinking, predict clinical benefit. As such, they are preferable to analyses of mean differences, which are difficult to interpret with regard to clinical relevance. AUD clinical trials tend to follow patients for 3 to 6 months. Such treatment durations may be too brief to measure change in alcohol-related harms such as driving under the influence or impaired quality of life. Therefore, rates of abstinence and no heavy drinking are the outcomes most commonly assessed. A standardized self-report and a biochemical measure of alcohol intake are thus important metrics for assessing AUD pharmacotherapy response.

Urine dipstick measures of alcohol glucuronide (EtG) and handheld analyzers of alcohol in expired breath can provide an immediate direct indication of drinking at the time of a clinic visit. However, alcohol use cannot be detected in breath, urine, or plasma over an extended interval between study visits. For example, a breathalyzer reports the concentration of alcohol currently present in a patient's blood. Alcohol is metabolized at a rate of .015 of BAC per hour, and so a patient who had

a .08 BAC at noon and then did not drink would likely have a .00 BAC at a 6 pm clinic visit. Urinary EtG and plasma phosphatidylethanol are measures of alcohol metabolites that have high sensitivity and specificity like BAC, but with a slightly longer window of detection, depending on the amount of alcohol consumed. For example, EtG will detect one to two drinks consumed the previous day or 10 drinks consumed 4 to 5 days earlier (Litten, Bradley, & Moss, 2010). Indirect biomarkers of alcohol use between clinic visits (e.g., GGT, and carbohydrate-deficient transferrin [CDT]) have limitations with regard to sensitivity and/or specificity. GGT has moderate sensitivity to chronic heavy drinking. GGT levels in the blood may initially exceed the upper limit of normal and remain elevated for 2 to 3 weeks after heavy drinking cessation. Most clinical laboratories routinely measure GGT. False positives may occur due to smoking, non–alcohol-related diseases, and various medications. The relative amount of CDT to total transferrin in serum (% CDT) becomes abnormal after 7 to 10 days of heavy drinking. After cessation of drinking, 2 to 3 weeks are required for % CDT values to return to normal. Analysis of % CDT requires relatively expensive specialized testing. Improvements in methods to measure CDT have resulted in incremental gains in specificity related to effects of smoking, body weight, gender, and liver diseases on CDT values (Litten et al., 2010).

A standardized interview using a calendar format, typically a variation of the Timeline Followback (Sobell & Sobell, 1992), employs prompts such as weekend versus weekdays, paydays, or holidays to assess quantity and frequency of alcohol used between clinic visits, using a "standard" drink metric (see the link to *Assessing Alcohol Problems: A Guide for Clinicians and Researchers* in the Tool Kit of Resources at the end of this chapter). One standard drink is defined as containing about 14 grams of pure alcohol, which is found in 12 ounces of regular beer, 5 ounces of wine, and 1.5 ounces of distilled spirits. Computerized administration is also available to encourage accurate reporting by patients. Keeping a daily diary of dose(s) taken, abstinence, or drinking, and the circumstances associated with a drinking episode for review at patient visits may facilitate treatment outcome as well as accurate reporting. Periodic interviews with close friends or relatives of the patient may be used in conjunction with biological measures to validate the patient's Timeline Followback interview self-report measures of alcohol use. If discrepancies between sources cannot be resolved, the most negative outcome is typically assumed to be accurate.

Projects to develop noninvasive, transdermal alcohol biosensors that can be worn on the wrist to measure alcohol consumption in real time are under development. Additionally, smartphone apps have been developed for ecological momentary assessment of various behaviors and experiences in real time in the natural environment (Shiffman, Stone, & Hufford, 2008). Such technology may be applied to measure drinking and identify triggers for relapse or medication nonadherence in real time and in the patient's own environment, in order to develop personalized strategies to enhance treatment outcome.

Approaches that use neurostimulation are in early stages of investigation as novel treatments for AUD. For example, repetitive transcranial magnetic stimulation (rTMS) devices are FDA approved for the treatment of depression that has not responded to antidepressant medication. Small short-term studies of rTMS effects on craving in response to alcohol cues in AUD have used varying treatment parameters with mixed results; drinking outcomes in clinical trials have yet to be investigated (Gorelick, Zangen, & George, 2014).

If a relapse to heavy drinking occurs in patients taking acamprosate or naltrexone, they should be instructed to continue taking the medication as prescribed. Relapses may be briefer in duration and of less severity if medication is continued, and neither medication interacts with alcohol.

Patient safety is optimized by adhering to the recommended dose and to the medical contraindications and cautions on the product label. A physical exam and laboratory testing is recommended before treatment is initiated and may help with subsequent monitoring of treatment response and adverse events. Useful baseline laboratory tests include alcohol breath, blood concentration, or alcohol glucuronide testing; urine drug screen; liver function tests (GGT, ALT,

AST); compete blood count; testing for vitamin deficiencies; renal function tests (standard panel for urea [blood urea nitrogen], electrolytes, and serum creatinine); and a pregnancy test for women of childbearing potential. Obtaining a baseline urine drug screen and measures of hepatic function and creatinine clearance may guide medication selection. A urine drug screen may provide information about otherwise undisclosed drug use, including opioid use, which is exclusionary for naltrexone treatment of AUD. Baseline liver function tests may detect hepatic impairment that would mitigate against treatment with disulfiram and naltrexone. Similarly, a baseline test of creatinine clearance may identify severe impairment (<30 mL/min) in creatinine clearance that would contraindicate the choice of acamprosate and necessitate caution if using naltrexone. In addition to obtaining medical clearance for a patient to receive a pharmacotherapy for AUD, the pros and cons of these treatments should be reviewed with the patient and their preference identified, taking into consideration their treatment goals, the medication's cost, dosing schedule, and potential risks and side effects. If a treatment provider is unfamiliar with these medications, suggestions are to read the package insert and the SAMHSA link in the Tool Kit of Resources, and to ask a respected colleague to discuss their clinical experience with these medications.

Other than the relatively unobtrusive blood and urine tests and discussions specific to the medications described previously, the intake for AUD should proceed as usual. A baseline of alcohol misuse should be established, preferably using quantitative self-report and biochemical measures, against which treatment effects can be tracked, as discussed further later in this chapter. Likewise, harmful effects of alcohol on the patient's health, functioning, and legal status should be documented, and comorbid disorders ruled out, including nicotine dependence, that may influence AUD outcome if left untreated. Risk of suicide may be elevated in patients with AUD and, although rare, suicide has occurred in patients taking these pharmacotherapies for AUD. Therefore, screening for suicidality at baseline and periodically thereafter may identify increased suicide risk that requires further intervention. An integrated treatment plan specific to the patient should be developed to address both AUD and clinically significant concurrent conditions.

A patient should be informed about what to expect from taking a medication, how it may help with AUD, and potential risks and side effects. A patient information sheet providing this information in writing can be taken home by the patient for future reference. A phone call to the patient a few days after a prescription has been provided, to address any concerns and assess medication adherence and side effects, may facilitate successful medication initiation. Common side effects (e.g., dizziness, nausea, diarrhea) are usually mild, associated with treatment initiation, and resolve quickly. Advise patients to avoid driving a car or operating heavy machinery until they are reasonably certain that the drug does not affect their ability to engage in such activities. Over-the-counter remedies (e.g., Pepto-Bismol) may be suggested for diarrhea and nausea. Patients should be given a phone number to call and instructed to inform their treatment provider immediately if suicide ideation or depression develops, or if symptoms of acute hepatitis or liver failure emerge (in the case of naltrexone and disulfiram). It is recommended that patients taking disulfiram have repeat bilirubin and LFTs at 2 weeks, then monthly for 6 months and every 3 months thereafter. Carrying a wallet card is advisable to notify emergency personnel that the patient is taking naltrexone, should anesthesia or pain management be required, or disulfiram, in case an alcohol—disulfiram interaction is precipitated.

Medication nonadherence may negatively impact pharmacotherapy outcome in AUD. Determine if adverse events are undermining medication adherence and intervene accordingly. As noted above, disulfiram adherence and effect size increased with observed administration. Long-acting injectable naltrexone was developed to offset the adherence problems noted with daily oral dosing. Acamprosate has a 3 times daily dosing schedule; to ensure adherence, patients may package their medication in over-the-counter weekly pill trays with day and time of day indicated for each dose. Identify frequently missed doses by asking the patient to bring their pill tray and unused medication at every visit, and link commonly missed doses with an activity of daily living such as eating meals or brushing teeth as a reminder for the patient to take their medication at that time.

There is little scientific evidence to guide the optimal duration of pharmacological treatments of AUD. A patient's history of relapses and the potential consequences of a relapse, the severity of AUD at baseline, and the patient's clinical response and side effects may be determining factors. These factors should be explored with the patient if a wish to discontinue treatment is expressed before a stable recovery has been achieved.

An option for treatment nonresponse may be to consider switching to an alternative medication, barring any medical contraindications. Partial response to an adequate trial at the recommended dose of a medication is a treatment challenge. For example, a patient may have reduced their drinking by half from baseline, but continue to have episodes of heavy drinking. One may consider the use of combined treatments on a case-by-case basis. There are data that lend support to the safety of acamprosate combined with naltrexone or disulfiram (Besson, Aeby, Kasas, Lehert, & Potgieter, 1998; Johnson et al., 2003; Jonas et al., 2014; Mason et al., 2002), but efficacy data are insufficient to support a general recommendation for combined use as a first-line treatment approach to AUD (American Psychiatric Association, 2017). Given a potentially increased risk of hepatotoxicity when naltrexone and disulfiram are used in combination, this combination is rarely considered.

EVALUATION OF PHARMACOLOGICAL APPROACHES ACROSS THE LIFESPAN

Drinking is illegal under the age of 21 years throughout the United States, and alcohol misuse, rather than dependence, is more characteristic of this age group. Nevertheless, it is never too early (or too late) to treat AUD. Small ($N = 26$), double-blind, placebo-controlled studies in adolescents report good tolerability and higher rates of abstinence with acamprosate and disulfiram relative to placebo (Niederhofer & Staffen, 2003a; Niederhofer & Staffen, 2003b). Patients over the age of 65 years have been included in some clinical trials of disulfiram (De Sousa & Jagtap, 2009), naltrexone (Garbutt et al., 2005), and acamprosate (Mason, Goodman, Chabac, & Lehert, 2006), but not in sufficient numbers to analyze differences in safety and efficacy from younger patients. Older patients may be at increased risk for hepatic, renal, or cardiac problems; other disorders; or use of concomitant medications that may influence the choice of pharmacotherapy for AUD and indicate a need for closer monitoring.

CONSIDERATION OF POTENTIAL SEX DIFFERENCES

A recent national survey (Center for Behavioral Health Statistics and Quality [CBHSQ], 2015) found that 5.6 million American women (4.1%) met criteria for AUD in the past year. Prevalence is highest among women in the childbearing ages of 18 to 29 years, with associated risk of fetal alcohol symptoms in their children (Grant et al., 2004). Alcohol use by pregnant women can have profound effects on the developing fetus. These effects can lead to a wide range of disabilities, including fetal alcohol spectrum disorder, which is characterized by intellectual disabilities, speech and language delays, poor social skills, and sometimes facial deformities. In addition, women generally experience liver damage and other health problems after consuming less alcohol than men, in part because of sex differences in total body water and alcohol metabolism (Bradley, Badrinath, Bush, Boyd-Wickizer, & Anawalt, 1998; Greenfield, 2002). Among women, chronic consumption of more than two drinks per day is associated with increased risk of mortality, breast cancer, hypertension, stroke, and reproductive problems (Bradley et al., 1998). Binge drinking among women (e.g., consuming four or more drinks in a row) may incur increased risk of accident, rape, assault, and unprotected sex (Wechsler, Dowdall, Davenport, & Rimm, 1995). Comorbid depression and anxiety disorders comorbid with AUD are also more prevalent among women than men, with associated risk of suicidality (Conway, Compton, Stinson, & Grant, 2006). Given the significant disease burden of alcohol dependence in women, early intervention and effective treatment options are clearly needed.

Women with childbearing potential who do not use a reliable method of birth control or who are lactating must be excluded from medication trials to avoid risk of exposing the fetus or newborn to medication. However, women need to be represented in clinical trials of AUD, because sex may be associated with differential drug efficacy. For example, although sex does not influence the pharmacokinetics of Vivitrol, it showed efficacy in men but not in women in the pivotal multicenter trial for AUD (Garbutt et al., 2005), and oral naltrexone did not differ from placebo in the only trial exclusively studying women (O'Malley et al., 2007). Potential differences in drug metabolism due to ethnicity or sex hormones, and consequent effects on drug efficacy or safety, require adequate representation of minorities and women in clinical trials. The majority of clinical trials of disulfiram were conducted primarily in men; women comprised less than 10% of all patients included in a recent meta-analysis (Skinner et al., 2014).

A sex-specific meta-analysis of individual records obtained from 1,317 women and 4,794 men who participated in 22 acamprosate clinical trials found a significant effect of acamprosate relative to placebo on rates of abstinence and no heavy drinking, and effect sizes did not differ between men and women (Mason & Lehert, 2012). Despite a history of significantly more anxiety, depression, suicide attempts, drug abuse, interpersonal loss, and greater liver impairment at baseline than men, women responded comparably well to alcoholism treatment. The side effect and tolerability profile of acamprosate was comparable to that of placebo in number as well as type and severity of adverse events, and did not differ between women and men. Importantly, acamprosate was associated with significantly higher rates of treatment completion and medication compliance than placebo among both women and men.

There are no adequate and well-controlled studies of pharmacotherapies for AUD in pregnant women. It is recommended that these medications should not be used during pregnancy unless treating acute alcohol withdrawal with benzodiazepines (American Psychiatric Association, 2017).

It is not known whether acamprosate, disulfiram, or naltrexone are excreted in human milk. Because so many drugs are excreted in human milk, caution should be used when administering acamprosate or naltrexone to a nursing woman, and disulfiram should be avoided (Alkermes Inc., 2010; Duramed Pharmaceuticals, Inc., 2013; Merck Santé, 2005; Physicians Total Care, Inc., 2010).

INTEGRATION OF PHARMACOTHERAPY WITH NONPHARMACOLOGICAL APPROACHES: BENEFITS AND CHALLENGES

Nonpharmacological approaches to AUD have long been the standard of the field, whether in a clinical setting or by participating in a self-help group. Essentially all of the clinical trials covered in this chapter studied a medication in addition to either the routine AUD treatment patients would ordinarily receive in that setting, or used a manual-guided form of behavioral therapy. See the Tool Kit of Resources at the end of this chapter for links to four such behavioral treatment manuals: *AlcoholFree Therapist's Manual*, *Motivation Enhancement Therapy Manual*, *Cognitive Behavioral Coping Skills Therapy Manual*, and *Medical Management Treatment Manual*.

The goal of most pharmacotherapy trials was to demonstrate that behavioral therapy combined with medication had a higher rate of treatment response than behavioral therapy alone (i.e., combined with placebo). Meta-analyses show that, on average, pharmacotherapies for AUD have a small but significant treatment effect size relative to placebo in patients provided with concomitant behavioral therapy (Jonas et al., 2014). Efforts to identify phenotypes, genotypes, and biomarkers of response (described previously) are aimed at guiding the selection of a pharmacotherapy to optimize the likelihood of response for a given patient. However, it is human nature to expect that "pill = cure," and medication should be presented as one tool in a tool kit of evidence-based treatments for AUD. On the other hand, some members of self-help groups have criticized members who take AUD medication as not having a "true, drug-free" recovery. None of the pharmacotherapies for AUD are an alcohol-substitution drug like methadone is for heroin, and this criticism reflects a lack of understanding of drug mechanism. Physician members of Alcoholics

Anonymous (AA) drafted a pamphlet that patients can be given (link in the Tool Kit of Resources), advising that AA members should not "play doctor," and the authors offer useful guidelines to discriminate appropriate from risky use of medications in patients with AUD and other drug use disorders (Alcoholics Anonymous, 2011).

Medications can help restore normal brain functioning, reduce relapse risk, and decrease symptoms of protracted withdrawal (e.g., craving), thereby facilitating better engagement in behavioral treatment. Behavioral therapies, in turn, enhance pharmacotherapy response by modifying attitudes and behaviors related to alcohol, increasing healthy life skills, and helping people to stay in treatment. The NIAAA Navigator (see the Tool Kit of Resources for link) is a new website designed to assist in locating clinicians who provide evidence-based behavioral and/or pharmacological treatments for AUD. Integrating pharmacological and behavioral treatments for AUD increases the likelihood of a patient meeting their goals for treatment.

PHARMACOTHERAPY FOR ADDRESSING COMORBID DISORDERS

A recent nationwide survey found that among people ages 12 and older who had AUD or another substance use disorder (SUD), 13% had both AUD and SUD, and 41% also had a psychiatric disorder (CBHSQ, 2015). Ninety percent of completed suicides involve a mental disorder (primarily depression) and/or SUD (primarily AUD; Center for Substance Abuse Treatment, 2008). Depression may promote increased alcohol intake; alcohol may promote dysphoria, hopelessness, impaired problem-solving, and aggression. Twenty-five percent of completed suicides showed alcohol intoxication at time of death, and AUD is associated with 6.2 times greater suicide risk (SAMHSA, 2012). Co-occurring disorders should be considered the expectation rather than the exception, and be treated concurrently to help reduce the risk of suicide when one disorder is left untreated.

An accurate psychiatric diagnosis cannot be made when a patient is drinking or withdrawing from alcohol; alcohol may reduce some psychiatric symptoms, and conversely, symptoms of anxiety and depression may be mistaken as withdrawal instead of an underlying disorder that requires independent treatment. Symptoms of alcohol withdrawal should be managed before trying to treat comorbid disorders; then, symptoms of psychiatric disorders should lead to further integrated assessment and treatment planning, with both AUD and comorbid disorders considered primary disorders. Patients with AUD and comorbid disorders may benefit from a chronic care management approach that includes evidence-based behavioral and pharmacological treatments; social support services; and clinical monitoring of adverse events, medication adherence, and symptoms of relapse. It is important to work collaboratively with the patient and involved significant others, communicating the risks and benefits of each treatment option relative to the patient's recovery goals, and ensuring that the patient comprehends this information. The selection of psychiatric medications in patients with AUD requires consideration of abuse potential and potential interactions with other medications, tobacco, illicit drugs, and alcohol, which may affect drug metabolism and safety and warrant enhanced monitoring.

Naltrexone (oral and injectable) is approved by the FDA both for treatment of AUD and for the prevention of relapse to opioid use following opioid detoxification. Patients with AUD and comorbid opioid use disorder (OUD) who wish to remain opioid-free and to cut down or quit drinking can receive this single treatment for both disorders, in conjunction with a comprehensive management program that includes psychosocial support. Naltrexone is an opioid antagonist and will induce withdrawal in opioid-using patients. Patients receiving Vivitrol must be opioid-free for 7 to 10 days before treatment. It is vital for patients to comprehend that an attempt to overcome the blockade produced by naltrexone by taking opioids is very dangerous and may lead to fatal overdose. Similarly, use of lower doses of opioids after Vivitrol is discontinued (at the end of a Vivitrol dosing interval, or after missing a Vivitrol dose) could result in life-threatening opioid intoxication (e.g., respiratory arrest and circulatory collapse).

Acamprosate may be used safely in patients with AUD and comorbid OUD who choose opioid substitution therapy with methadone or buprenorphine. Acamprosate is not metabolized in the liver, and thus drug–drug interactions via cytochrome P450 inhibition are unlikely. The pharmacokinetics of acamprosate were not altered by coadministration with an anxiolytic, an antidepressant medication, or alcohol (Rosenthal, Gage, Perhach, & Goodman, 2008), suggesting that it can be used safely in patients with AUD who are receiving concomitant medications for comorbid psychiatric disorders. Several studies suggest that acamprosate may help to normalize the underlying neurobiological mechanisms of alcohol-related disturbances in sleep. Sleep disturbances are a challenge often faced by recently detoxified patients. A sleep laboratory study showed that acamprosate improved alcohol-related changes in sleep continuity, Stage 3 sleep, and rapid eye movement sleep latency (Staner et al., 2006), all of which are classically described as important determinants of relapse (Brower, Aldrich, Robinson, Zucker, & Greden, 2001). Subjective sleep data obtained from randomized controlled trials of acamprosate in AUD lent clinical validation to the sleep laboratory findings (Perney et al., 2012; Perney et al., 2015). A beneficial effect of acamprosate on alcohol-related sleep disturbance may be particularly germane to comorbid disorders in which sleep disruption is a factor (e.g., depression, anxiety, posttraumatic stress disorder).

Practice guidelines recommend that antidepressant medication and benzodiazepines not be used for the treatment of AUD, unless there is a concurrent disorder for which these are indicated treatments, or unless benzodiazepines are used to treat acute alcohol withdrawal (American Psychiatric Association, 2017). Patients with AUD and concurrent major depressive disorder have been found to respond to antidepressant medications (Mason, Kocsis, Ritvo, & Cutler, 1996; McGrath et al., 1996; Pettinati et al., 2010; Roy-Byrne et al., 2000). Conversely, use of antidepressant medication to reduce drinking relapse is generally not supported in patients with AUD who are not depressed (American Psychiatric Association, 2017). Similarly, the use of antipsychotics to reduce risk of drinking relapse is not supported as a first-line treatment for AUD, but may be particularly useful in patients with AUD who have a concurrent disorder for which the drug is indicated (Anton, Kranzler, et al., 2008; Bender et al., 2007). Bipolar disorder concurrent with AUD is effectively treated with bipolar medications, with concomitant benefit for drinking outcomes (Brown, Garza, & Carmody, 2008; Salloum et al., 2005). The use of bipolar medications to reduce risk of drinking relapse is not effective in patients with AUD who are not bipolar (Brown et al., 2008; Brown et al., 2014; Fawcett et al., 2000; Litten et al., 2012). Anxiety disorders concurrent with AUD respond to some antianxiety medications such as sertraline (Brady, Sonne, & Roberts, 1995) and paroxetine (Book, Thomas, Randall, & Randall, 2008; Thomas, Randall, Book, & Randall, 2008), but not to others such as venlafaxine (Ciraulo et al., 2013). The use of an antianxiety medication to reduce risk of drinking relapse in patients with AUD who do not have anxiety disorders has not been found to be effective in a double-blind, placebo-controlled trial of buspirone (Fawcett et al., 2000).

EMERGING TRENDS

Medications development for AUD can benefit from use of a framework for stages of the AUD cycle that is linked to neurocircuitry. Dysregulation in the brain reward and stress systems that results in the symptoms of acute and protracted withdrawal during the withdrawal/negative affect and preoccupation/anticipation stages of the AUD cycle is a neglected focus for drug development for AUD. Much previous work on medications for AUD focused on blocking the rewarding effects of drugs in the binge/intoxication stage of the AUD cycle, but identification of a clear role for the motivational signs of withdrawal as reflected by negative emotional states in the withdrawal/negative affect stage represent a compelling rationale for focusing on neurobiological targets in this domain. The dramatic surge in our understanding of the neurocircuitry and neuropharmacological mechanisms that are involved in the development and maintenance of the withdrawal/negative affect stage have provided numerous unique and viable targets for future drug development, as shown in Figure 22.1.

Some of these potential targets have advanced to clinical testing. For example, a mixed glucocorticoid/progesterone receptor antagonist, mifepristone, was found to decrease craving and drinking in recently abstinent participants with AUD in a human laboratory model of protracted withdrawal (Vendruscolo et al., 2015), and is now under study in a randomized controlled trial. Glucocorticoid receptor signaling in the hypothalamic–pituitary–adrenal axis and extrahypothalamic system may be a potential target for drug development because of a putative dual role (i.e., to normalize reward function and desensitize stress systems).

Vasopressin is a prostress, prodysphoria-inducing brain neurotransmitter system that converges on the extended amygdala and contributes to negative emotional states associated with alcohol withdrawal (Koob, 2008). A vasopressin V1b receptor antagonist, ABT-436, was found to increase the rate of abstinence in a multicenter trial of AUD (Ryan et al., 2017). Furthermore, participants who reported high levels of stress responded better, as evidenced by decreases in both the frequency of drinking and the number of heavy drinking days (Ryan et al., 2017). These trials lend support to desensitization of brain systems mediating negative emotional states in protracted withdrawal as a valid pharmacological target for AUD. A complementary pharmacological approach is to activate antistress buffering systems in the brain as a strategy for restoring homeostasis in protracted withdrawal (Koob, 2008). Oxytocin is a neuropeptide that is an emerging candidate as a stress buffer, and is currently under clinical investigation for the treatment of AUD and withdrawal. Preliminary work has shown that intranasal oxytocin was superior to placebo in reducing symptoms of relatively mild alcohol withdrawal (Pedersen et al., 2013) and had a dual effect on alcohol craving in a human lab study; more socially anxious subjects with alcohol abuse showed decreased craving, and less socially anxious individuals showed increased craving with oxytocin relative to placebo (Mitchell, Arcuni, Weinstein, & Woolley, 2016).

Another pharmacological strategy to address desensitization of brain systems mediating negative emotional states involves partial agonists. Partial agonists can be defined as drugs that bind to a receptor and have low efficacy, often with high affinity. As such, partial agonists will show antagonism when there is high agonist tone but agonism when there is low agonist tone. In terms of the AUD cycle, partial agonists could theoretically block the reinforcing effects of alcohol during the binge/intoxication stage, but in addition block or blunt the negative motivational effects that characterize the withdrawal/negative affect stage. Varenicline, an FDA-approved treatment for smoking cessation (Jorenby et al., 2006), has shown positive effects for the treatment of AUD in a multicenter, double-blind, placebo-controlled clinical trial, in which varenicline lowered weekly percent of heavy drinking days, drinks per drinking day, and alcohol craving, compared with the placebo group (Litten et al., 2013).

The underutilization of existing pharmacotherapies and their modest effect sizes point to a need for new medications to safely and effectively treat AUD. The repurposing of existing medications approved for other indications may help to expeditiously meet this need. Topiramate and gabapentin are two drugs that were originally developed as antiepileptic medications and have recently shown therapeutic potential for AUD. Practice guidelines recommend that topiramate or gabapentin be offered to patients who have a goal of decreasing or quitting drinking; who prefer topiramate or gabapentin, or are intolerant to or have not responded to acamprosate and naltrexone; and have no contraindications to the use of these medications (American Psychiatric Association, 2017). Co-occurring disorders, concomitant medications, and side effect profile are additional factors that may guide the selection of topiramate or gabapentin.

Topiramate (Topamax® and generics) is approved by the FDA for the treatment of epilepsy and for the prophylaxis of migraine. A meta-analysis of randomized controlled trials of 3 months duration and dose titration to a target dose of 200 to 300 mg/d in outpatients with AUD found topiramate to be associated with fewer drinking days (WMD, −6.5%; 95% CI, −12.0% to −1%), fewer heavy drinking days (WMD, −9%; 95% CI, −15.3% to −2.7%), and fewer drinks per drinking day (WMD, −1.0; 95% CI, −1.6 to −0.48) than placebo (Jonas et al., 2014).

While topiramate has no contraindications, it has a number of warnings and precautions. Recommended lab tests include baseline and periodic measures of serum bicarbonate to detect treatment-emergent metabolic acidosis; baseline tests of renal function, as creatinine clearance less than 70 mL/min requires a dose adjustment to half the starting and maintenance dose; and baseline tests of hepatic function, as topiramate plasma concentration is increased in hepatic impairment. Meta-analyses found patients with AUD who were treated with topiramate had a higher risk of cognitive dysfunction (NNH, 12; 95% CI, 7 to 84), paresthesias (NNH, 4; 95% CI, 3 to 7), and taste abnormalities (NNH 7; 95% CI, 5 to 15) than did patients treated with placebo. The cognitive dysfunction is an adverse event commonly associated with treatment discontinuation, symptoms of which may include confusion, psychomotor slowing, attention, concentration and memory impairment, and speech or language problems (particularly word-finding difficulties; Salinsky et al., 2005). Other central nervous system adverse events include dizziness, somnolence, fatigue, depression, or mood problems. Warnings include risk of acute myopia and secondary angle closure glaucoma, decreased sweating and increased body temperature, suicidal behavior and ideation, kidney stones, hyperammonemia and encephalopathy. Patients with or without a seizure history should be gradually withdrawn from topiramate to minimize the potential for seizures. Topiramate interacts pharmacokinetically with some antiepileptic drugs, central nervous system depressants, oral contraceptives, metformin, lithium, and carbonic anhydrase inhibitors, with significant changes in drug plasma concentrations; refer to the package insert for guidance. Infants exposed to topiramate in utero have an increased risk of cleft lip and/or palate, particularly if exposure occurs in the first trimester (when many women do not know they are pregnant). Topiramate passes into breast milk.

Gabapentin (Neurontin® and generics) is FDA approved for the treatment of epilepsy and postherpetic neuralgia. A systematic review found the efficacy of gabapentin for treatment of AUD supported by five of six single-site treatment studies reporting drinking outcomes (Mason, Quello, & Shadan, 2018). Studies evaluating two doses of gabapentin found greater efficacy associated with the higher dose relative to the lower dose. For instance, a 12-week trial ($N = 150$) of 0, 900, and 1800 mg/d of gabapentin found significant linear dose effects on rates of abstinence and no heavy drinking; number of drinks per week; number of drinking days per week; GGT; and on standardized measures of craving, negative affect, and insomnia (Mason et al., 2014). The 1800 mg/d dose was associated with a NNT = 5 (95% CI, 3 to 75) for no heavy drinking and a NNT = 8 (95% CI, 6 to ∞) for rate of complete abstinence. All gabapentin treatment studies were conducted with patients who concomitantly received behavioral treatment. The preponderance of evidence suggests that combining gabapentin with behavioral support provides an incremental advantage in drinking outcomes relative to behavioral support with placebo.

Six of eight AUD studies with sleep measures reported a significant beneficial effect of gabapentin on alcohol-related sleep disturbance, a key precipitant of relapse in protracted withdrawal; beneficial effects on sleep were not associated with daytime drowsiness or dysfunction (Mason et al., 2018). Gabapentin-related decreases in negative affect were shown in alcohol withdrawal measures and in weekly Beck Depression Inventory scores over a 12-week randomized clinical trial of AUD treatment (Mason et al., 2018).

There are no contraindications to gabapentin, other than known hypersensitivity to the medication. Gabapentin is not metabolized in the liver. It is eliminated from systemic circulation by renal excretion as unchanged drug. A baseline test of creatinine clearance is indicated. Dose should be adjusted in patients with reduced renal function (creatinine clearance <60 mL/min). Gabapentin (≤1800 mg/d) has shown no safety concerns among the 655 outpatients with AUD who participated in the 11 studies included in a systematic review (Mason et al., 2018). Adverse events tended to be mild to moderate, and to not differ from placebo. Common adverse events included headache, insomnia, fatigue, muscle aches, and various gastrointestinal complaints in both gabapentin- and placebo-treated patients with AUD.

Alcohol was not found to interact meaningfully with gabapentin in a pharmacokinetic/pharmacodynamic (PK/PD) alcohol-gabapentin drug interaction study; gabapentin was not found to increase blood alcohol concentrations nor intoxicating, stimulating, or sedating effects of alcohol (Bisaga & Evans, 2006). The lack of appreciable hepatic metabolism is a PK advantage of gabapentin, as chronic heavy drinking is often associated with liver injury. Importantly, gabapentin treatment outcomes and adverse effects do not appear to differ between men and women with AUD.

Based on significant clinical and postmarketing experience for approved pain and epilepsy indications, gabapentin is considered to have a good safety and tolerability profile. The most commonly reported adverse events with gabapentin in comparison with placebo-treated patients in non-AUD pivotal trials include dizziness, somnolence, peripheral edema, ataxia, fatigue, and nystagmus. As with any centrally active drug, patients should be advised not to drive motor vehicles or operate heavy machinery until they have ascertained that the drug does not affect their performance.

Antiepileptic drugs, including gabapentin and topiramate, increase the risk of suicidal thoughts or behavior in about one in 500 patients taking these drugs for any indication. Abrupt withdrawal from gabapentin and topiramate has precipitated seizures and status epilepticus; on and off titration is indicated. Reports of abuse of gabapentinoids, such as gabapentin and pregabalin, are increasingly being documented in high-risk populations, notably opioid and prescription drug abusers. Gabapentin is not a controlled or scheduled substance. There was no evidence of tolerance to gabapentin dose or rebound with titration off drug, nor evidence of abuse potential in studies of alcohol dependence. However, patients undergoing opioid withdrawal, those who misuse prescriptions recreationally, and prison populations may be at increased risk to misuse gabapentin, with self-administered doses often far exceeding the therapeutic range (Chiappini & Schifano, 2016; Smith, Havens, & Walsh, 2016). Hence, patients with risk histories should be monitored for potential gabapentinoid misuse or diversion (e.g., self-dose escalation, a "need" for unusually high doses, repeated requests to replace "lost" medication, and other drug-seeking behaviors).

The recent surge in our understanding of the neurocircuitry and neuropharmacological mechanisms that are involved in protracted withdrawal/negative affect and relapse in AUD have provided abundant targets for future medication development for treating AUD. Both repurposed drugs like gabapentin, topiramate, and the glucocorticoid receptor antagonist, and new molecular entities such as the vasopressin V1b receptor antagonist, are all selective for these targets and are showing promise as emerging new treatments for AUD.

TOOL KIT OF RESOURCES

Behavioral Therapies Used in Pharmacotherapy Trials

- AlcoholFree.today: http://alcoholfree.today
  Patient and therapist materials from the U.S. multisite acamprosate study
- COMBINE Monograph Series: Volume 2: Medical Management Treatment Manual: https://pubs.niaaa.nih.gov/publications/combine/Combine%202.pdf
  Treatment issues specific to pharmacotherapy trials in AUD
- Project MATCH Monograph Series: https://pubs.niaaa.nih.gov/publications/projectmatch/matchintro.htm
  Motivational Enhancement Therapy Manual
  Cognitive-Behavioral Coping Skills Therapy Manual

Pharmacotherapy Guidance

- The A.A. Member—Medications & Other Drugs: https://www.aa.org/assets/en_US/p-11_aamembersMedDrug.pdf
  Developed by physician members of Alcoholics Anonymous to guide prescription use in AUD
- American Psychiatric Association Practice Guideline for the Pharmacological Treatment of Patients With Alcohol Use Disorder: https://psychiatryonline.org/doi/book/10.1176/appi.books.9781615371969
- Incorporating Alcohol Pharmacotherapies Into Medical Practice: https://store.samhsa.gov/shin/content//SMA13-4380/SMA13-4380.pdf

Diagnosis and Treatment Information

- Assessing Alcohol Problems: A Guide for Clinicians and Researchers: https://pubs.niaaa.nih.gov/publications/AssessingAlcohol/index.htm
- NIAAA Navigator: https://alcoholtreatment.niaaa.nih.gov
  To identify local evidence-based AUD treatment options.
- The Surgeon General's Report on Alcohol, Drugs, and Health: https://addiction.surgeongeneral.gov/surgeon-generals-report.pdf

References

*Alcoholics Anonymous. (2011). *The A.A. member—medications & other drugs*. New York, NY: Author. Retrieved from https://www.aa.org/assets/en_US/p-11_aamembersMedDrug.pdf

Alkermes Inc. (2010). Vivitrol highlights of prescribing information. Waltham, MA: Author. Retrieved from https://www.accessdata.fda.gov/drugsatfda_docs/label/2010/021897s015lbl.pdf

American Psychiatric Association. (2000). *Diagnostic and statistical manual of mental disorders* (4th ed., text rev). Washington, DC: Author.

American Psychiatric Association. (2013). *Diagnostic and statistical manual of mental disorders* (5th ed.). Washington, DC: Author.

*American Psychiatric Association. (2017). *Practice guideline for the pharmacological treatment of patients with alcohol use disorder*. Washington, DC: American Psychiatric Association. Retrieved from https://psychiatryonline.org/doi/pdf/10.1176/appi.books.9781615371969

Anton, R. F., Kranzler, H., Breder, C., Marcus, R. N., Carson, W. H., & Han, J. (2008). A randomized, multicenter, double-blind, placebo-controlled study of the efficacy and safety of aripiprazole for the treatment of alcohol dependence. *Journal of Clinical Psychopharmacology, 28*, 5–12. http://dx.doi.org/10.1097/jcp.0b013e3181602fd4

Anton, R. F., Moak, D. H., Latham, P. K., Waid, L. R., Malcolm, R. J., Dias, J. K., & Roberts, J. S. (2001). Posttreatment results of combining naltrexone with cognitive-behavior therapy for the treatment of alcoholism. *Journal of Clinical Psychopharmacology, 21*, 72–77. http://dx.doi.org/10.1097/00004714-200102000-00013

Anton, R. F., Oroszi, G., O'Malley, S., Couper, D., Swift, R., Pettinati, H., & Goldman, D. (2008). An evaluation of mu-opioid receptor (OPRM1) as a predictor of

*Asterisks indicate assessments or resources.

naltrexone response in the treatment of alcohol dependence: Results from the Combined Pharmacotherapies and Behavioral Interventions for Alcohol Dependence (COMBINE) study. *Archives of General Psychiatry, 65,* 135–144. http://dx.doi.org/10.1001/archpsyc.65.2.135

Baser, O., Chalk, M., Rawson, R., & Gastfriend, D. R. (2011). Alcohol dependence treatments: Comprehensive healthcare costs, utilization outcomes, and pharmacotherapy persistence. *The American Journal of Managed Care, 17*(8, Suppl. 8), S222–S234.

Bender, S., Scherbaum, N., Soyka, M., Rüther, E., Mann, K., & Gastpar, M. (2007). The efficacy of the dopamine D2/D3 antagonist tiapride in maintaining abstinence: A randomized, double-blind, placebo-controlled trial in 299 alcohol-dependent patients. *International Journal of Neuropsychopharmacology, 10,* 653–660. http://dx.doi.org/10.1017/S1461145706007164

Besson, J., Aeby, F., Kasas, A., Lehert, P., & Potgieter, A. (1998). Combined efficacy of acamprosate and disulfiram in the treatment of alcoholism: A controlled study. *Alcoholism: Clinical and Experimental Research, 22,* 573–579. http://dx.doi.org/10.1111/j.1530-0277.1998.tb04295.x

Betty Ford Institute Consensus Panel. (2007). What is recovery? A working definition from the Betty Ford Institute. *Journal of Substance Abuse Treatment, 33,* 221–228. http://dx.doi.org/10.1016/j.jsat.2007.06.001

Bisaga, A., & Evans, S. M. (2006). The acute effects of gabapentin in combination with alcohol in heavy drinkers. *Drug and Alcohol Dependence, 83,* 25–32. http://dx.doi.org/10.1016/j.drugalcdep.2005.10.008

Boeijinga, P. H., Parot, P., Soufflet, L., Landron, F., Danel, T., Gendre, I., . . . Luthringer, R. (2004). Pharmacodynamic effects of acamprosate on markers of cerebral function in alcohol-dependent subjects administered as pretreatment and during alcohol abstinence. *Neuropsychobiology, 50,* 71–77. http://dx.doi.org/10.1159/000077944

Bolo, N., Nédélec, J. F., Muzet, M., De Witte, P., Dahchour, A., Durbin, P., & Macher, J. P. (1998). Central effects of acamprosate: Part 2. Acamprosate modifies the brain in-vivo proton magnetic resonance spectrum in healthy young male volunteers. *Psychiatry Research: Neuroimaging, 82,* 115–127. http://dx.doi.org/10.1016/S0925-4927(98)00017-1

Book, S. W., Thomas, S. E., Randall, P. K., & Randall, C. L. (2008). Paroxetine reduces social anxiety in individuals with a co-occurring alcohol use disorder. *Journal of Anxiety Disorders, 22,* 310–318. http://dx.doi.org/10.1016/j.janxdis.2007.03.001

Bradley, K. A., Badrinath, S., Bush, K., Boyd-Wickizer, J., & Anawalt, B. (1998). Medical risks for women who drink alcohol. *Journal of General Internal Medicine,*

13, 627–639. http://dx.doi.org/10.1046/j.1525-1497.1998.cr187.x

Brady, K. T., Sonne, S. C., & Roberts, J. M. (1995). Sertraline treatment of comorbid posttraumatic stress disorder and alcohol dependence. *The Journal of Clinical Psychiatry, 56*(11), 502–505.

Brower, K. J., Aldrich, M. S., & Hall, J. M. (1998). Polysomnographic and subjective sleep predictors of alcoholic relapse. *Alcoholism, Clinical and Experimental Research, 22,* 1864–1871. http://dx.doi.org/10.1111/j.1530-0277.1998.tb03995.x

Brower, K. J., Aldrich, M. S., Robinson, E. A., Zucker, R. A., & Greden, J. F. (2001). Insomnia, self-medication, and relapse to alcoholism. *The American Journal of Psychiatry, 158,* 399–404. http://dx.doi.org/10.1176/appi.ajp.158.3.399

Brown, E. S., Davila, D., Nakamura, A., Carmody, T. J., Rush, A. J., Lo, A., . . . Bret, M. E. (2014). A randomized, double-blind, placebo-controlled trial of quetiapine in patients with bipolar disorder, mixed or depressed phase, and alcohol dependence. *Alcoholism: Clinical and Experimental Research, 38,* 2113–2118. http://dx.doi.org/10.1111/acer.12445

Brown, E. S., Garza, M., & Carmody, T. J. (2008). A randomized, double-blind, placebo-controlled add-on trial of quetiapine in outpatients with bipolar disorder and alcohol use disorders. *The Journal of Clinical Psychiatry, 69,* 701–705. http://dx.doi.org/10.4088/JCP.v69n0502

*Bush, K., Kivlahan, D. R., McDonell, M. B., Fihn, S. D., & Bradley, K. A. (1998). The AUDIT alcohol consumption questions (AUDIT-C): An effective brief screening test for problem drinking. Ambulatory Care Quality Improvement Project (ACQUIP). Alcohol Use Disorders Identification Test. *Archives of Internal Medicine, 158,* 1789–1795. http://dx.doi.org/10.1001/archinte.158.16.1789

Center for Behavioral Health Statistics and Quality. (2015). Behavioral health trends in the United States: Results from the 2014 National Survey on Drug Use and Health (HHS Publication No. SMA 15-4927, NSDUH Series H-50). Rockville, MD: Center for Behavioral Health Statistics and Quality, Substance Abuse and Mental Health Services. Retrieved from https://www.samhsa.gov/data/sites/default/files/NSDUH-FRR1-2014/NSDUH-FRR1-2014.pdf

Center for Substance Abuse Treatment. (2008). *Substance Abuse and Suicide Prevention: Evidence and Implications—A White Paper.* DHHS Pub. No. SMA-08-4352. Rockville, MD: Substance Abuse and Mental Health Services Administration.

Chiappini, S., & Schifano, F. (2016). A decade of gabapentinoid misuse: An analysis of the European Medicines Agency's "suspected adverse drug reactions" database. *CNS Drugs, 30,* 647–654. http://dx.doi.org/10.1007/s40263-016-0359-y

Chick, J. (1999). Safety issues concerning the use of disulfiram in treating alcohol dependence. *Drug Safety, 20*, 427–435. http://dx.doi.org/10.2165/00002018-199920050-00003

Ciraulo, D. A., Barlow, D. H., Gulliver, S. B., Farchione, T., Morissette, S. B., Kamholz, B. W., . . . Knapp, C. M. (2013). The effects of venlafaxine and cognitive behavioral therapy alone and combined in the treatment of co-morbid alcohol use-anxiety disorders. *Behaviour Research and Therapy, 51*, 729–735. http://dx.doi.org/10.1016/j.brat.2013.08.003

Clark, C. P., Gillin, J. C., Golshan, S., Demodena, A., Smith, T. L., Danowski, S., . . . Schuckit, M. (1998). Increased REM sleep density at admission predicts relapse by three months in primary alcoholics with a lifetime diagnosis of secondary depression. *Biological Psychiatry, 43*, 601–607. http://dx.doi.org/10.1016/S0006-3223(97)00457-5

Compton, W. M., Dawson, D. A., Goldstein, R. B., & Grant, B. F. (2013). Crosswalk between *DSM–IV* dependence and *DSM–5* substance use disorders for opioids, cannabis, cocaine and alcohol. *Drug and Alcohol Dependence, 132*, 387–390. http://dx.doi.org/10.1016/j.drugalcdep.2013.02.036

Conway, K. P., Compton, W., Stinson, F. S., & Grant, B. F. (2006). Lifetime comorbidity of *DSM–IV* mood and anxiety disorders and specific drug use disorders: Results from the National Epidemiologic Survey on Alcohol and Related Conditions. *The Journal of Clinical Psychiatry, 67*, 247–258. http://dx.doi.org/10.4088/JCP.v67n0211

De Sousa, A., & Jagtap, J. (2009). An open label trial of naltrexone versus disulfiram in elderly patients with alcohol dependence. *Journal of Pakistan Psychiatric Society, 6*(2), 85–89.

Duramed Pharmaceuticals, Inc. (2013). *REVIA (naltrexone hydrochloride tablets USP)*. Pomona, NY: Author; Retrieved from https://www.accessdata.fda.gov/drugsatfda_docs/label/2013/018932s017lbl.pdf

Fawcett, J., Kravitz, H. M., McGuire, M., Easton, M., Ross, J., Pisani, V., . . . Teas, G. (2000). Pharmacological treatments for alcoholism: Revisiting lithium and considering buspirone. *Alcoholism: Clinical and Experimental Research, 24*, 666–674. http://dx.doi.org/10.1111/j.1530-0277.2000.tb02038.x

Foster, J. H., & Peters, T. J. (1999). Impaired sleep in alcohol misusers and dependent alcoholics and the impact upon outcome. *Alcoholism: Clinical and Experimental Research, 23*, 1044–1051. http://dx.doi.org/10.1111/j.1530-0277.1999.tb04223.x

Fuller, R. K., Branchey, L., Brightwell, D. R., Derman, R. M., Emrick, C. D., Iber, F. L., . . . Shaw, S. (1986). Disulfiram treatment of alcoholism. A Veterans Administration cooperative study. *Journal of the American Medical Association, 256*, 1449–1455. http://dx.doi.org/10.1001/jama.1986.03380110055026

Garbutt, J. C., Kranzler, H. R., O'Malley, S. S., Gastfriend, D. R., Pettinati, H. M., Silverman, B. L., . . . the Vivitrex Study Group. (2005). Efficacy and tolerability of long-acting injectable naltrexone for alcohol dependence: A randomized controlled trial. *JAMA: Journal of the American Medical Association, 293*(13), 1617–1625. http://dx.doi.org/10.1001/jama.293.13.1617

Geller, A. (1991). Protracted abstinence. In N. S. Miller (Ed.), *Comprehensive handbook of drugs and alcohol addiction* (pp. 905–913). New York, NY: Marcel Dekker.

Gillin, J. C., Smith, T. L., Irwin, M., Butters, N., Demodena, A., & Schuckit, M. (1994). Increased pressure for rapid eye movement sleep at time of hospital admission predicts relapse in nondepressed patients with primary alcoholism at 3-month follow-up. *Archives of General Psychiatry, 51*, 189–197. http://dx.doi.org/10.1001/archpsyc.1994.03950030025003

Gorelick, D. A., Zangen, A., & George, M. S. (2014). Transcranial magnetic stimulation in the treatment of substance addiction. *Annals of the New York Academy of Sciences, 1327*, 79–93.

Grant, B. F., Stinson, F. S., Dawson, D. A., Chou, S. P., Dufour, M. C., Compton, W., . . . Kaplan, K. (2004). Prevalence and co-occurrence of substance use disorders and independent mood and anxiety disorders: Results from the National Epidemiologic Survey on Alcohol and Related Conditions. *Archives of General Psychiatry, 61*, 807–816. http://dx.doi.org/10.1001/archpsyc.61.8.807

Greenfield, S. F. (2002). Women and alcohol use disorders. *Harvard Review of Psychiatry, 10*, 76–85. http://dx.doi.org/10.1080/10673220216212

Holder, H. D. (1998). Cost benefits of substance abuse treatment: An overview of results from alcohol and drug abuse. *The Journal of Mental Health Policy and Economics, 1*, 23–29. http://dx.doi.org/10.1002/(SICI)1099-176X(199803)1:1<23::AID-MHP3>3.0.CO;2-Q

Johnson, B. A., O'Malley, S. S., Ciraulo, D. A., Roache, J. D., Chambers, R. A., Sarid-Segal, O., & Couper, D. (2003). Dose-ranging kinetics and behavioral pharmacology of naltrexone and acamprosate, both alone and combined, in alcohol-dependent subjects. *Journal of Clinical Psychopharmacology, 23*, 281–293. http://dx.doi.org/10.1097/01.jcp.0000084029.22282.bb

*Jonas, D. E., Amick, H. R., Feltner, C., Bobashev, G., Thomas, K., Wines, R., . . . Garbutt, J. C. (2014). Pharmacotherapy for adults with alcohol use disorders in outpatient settings: A systematic review and meta-analysis. *JAMA: Journal of the American Medical Association, 311*, 1889–1900. http://dx.doi.org/10.1001/jama.2014.3628

Jorenby, D. E., Hays, J. T., Rigotti, N. A., Azoulay, S., Watsky, E. J., Williams, K. E., . . . Reeves, K. R.

(2006). Efficacy of varenicline, an α4β2 nicotinic acetylcholine receptor partial agonist, vs placebo or sustained-release bupropion for smoking cessation: A randomized controlled trial. *JAMA: The Journal of the American Medical Association, 296*, 56–63.

Jørgensen, C. H., Pedersen, B., & Tønnesen, H. (2011). The efficacy of disulfiram for the treatment of alcohol use disorder. *Alcoholism: Clinical and Experimental Research, 35*, 1749–1758. http://dx.doi.org/10.1111/j.1530-0277.2011.01523.x

Karpyak, V. M., Biernacka, J. M., Geske, J. R., Jenkins, G. D., Cunningham, J. M., Rüegg, J., . . . Choi, D. S. (2014). Genetic markers associated with abstinence length in alcohol-dependent subjects treated with acamprosate. *Translational Psychiatry, 4*, e453. http://dx.doi.org/10.1038/tp.2014.103

Koob, G. F. (2008). A role for brain stress systems in addiction. *Neuron, 59*, 11–34. http://dx.doi.org/10.1016/j.neuron.2008.06.012

Koob, G. F., & Le Moal, M. (1997). Drug abuse: Hedonic homeostatic dysregulation. *Science, 278*, 52–58. http://dx.doi.org/10.1126/science.278.5335.52

Koob, G. F., & Volkow, N. D. (2010). Neurocircuitry of addiction. *Neuropsychopharmacology, 35*, 217–238. http://dx.doi.org/10.1038/npp.2009.110

Kranzler, H. R., Armeli, S., Covault, J., & Tennen, H. (2013). Variation in OPRM1 moderates the effect of desire to drink on subsequent drinking and its attenuation by naltrexone treatment. *Addiction Biology, 18*, 193–201. http://dx.doi.org/10.1111/j.1369-1600.2012.00471.x

Litten, R. Z., Bradley, A. M., & Moss, H. B. (2010). Alcohol biomarkers in applied settings: Recent advances and future research opportunities. *Alcoholism, Clinical and Experimental Research, 34*, 955–967. http://dx.doi.org/10.1111/j.1530-0277.2010.01170.x

Litten, R. Z., Fertig, J. B., Falk, D. E., Ryan, M. L., Mattson, M. E., Collins, J. F., . . . Stout, R., & the NCIG 001 Study Group. (2012). A double-blind, placebo-controlled trial to assess the efficacy of quetiapine fumarate XR in very heavy-drinking alcohol-dependent patients. *Alcoholism: Clinical and Experimental Research, 36*, 406–416. http://dx.doi.org/10.1111/j.1530-0277.2011.01649.x

Litten, R. Z., Ryan, M. L., Fertig, J. B., Falk, D. E., Johnson, B., Dunn, K. E., . . . Stout, R., & the NCIG (National Institute on Alcohol Abuse and Alcoholism Clinical Investigations Group) Study Group. (2013). A double-blind, placebo-controlled trial assessing the efficacy of varenicline tartrate for alcohol dependence. *Journal of Addiction Medicine, 7*, 277–286. http://dx.doi.org/10.1097/ADM.0b013e31829623f4

Littleton, J. M. (2007). Acamprosate in alcohol dependence: Implications of a unique mechanism of action. *Journal of Addiction Medicine, 1*, 115–125. http://dx.doi.org/10.1097/ADM.0b013e318156c26f

Lowman, C., Allen, J., Stout, R. L., & The Relapse Research Group. (1996). Replication and extension of Marlatt's taxonomy of relapse precipitants: Overview of procedures and results. The research group. *Addiction, 91*(Suppl.), S51–S71. http://dx.doi.org/10.1046/j.1360-0443.91.12s1.16.x

Maisel, N. C., Blodgett, J. C., Wilbourne, P. L., Humphreys, K., & Finney, J. W. (2013). Meta-analysis of naltrexone and acamprosate for treating alcohol use disorders: When are these medications most helpful? *Addiction, 108*, 275–293. http://dx.doi.org/10.1111/j.1360-0443.2012.04054.x

Mark, T. L., Kassed, C. A., Vandivort-Warren, R., Levit, K. R., & Kranzler, H. R. (2009). Alcohol and opioid dependence medications: Prescription trends, overall and by physician specialty. *Drug and Alcohol Dependence, 99*, 345–349. http://dx.doi.org/10.1016/j.drugalcdep.2008.07.018

Mason, B. J., Goodman, A. M., Chabac, S., & Lehert, P. (2006). Effect of oral acamprosate on abstinence in patients with alcohol dependence in a double-blind, placebo-controlled trial: The role of patient motivation. *Journal of Psychiatric Research, 40*, 383–393. http://dx.doi.org/10.1016/j.jpsychires.2006.02.002

Mason, B. J., Goodman, A. M., Dixon, R. M., Hameed, M. H., Hulot, T., Wesnes, K., . . . Boyeson, M. G. (2002). A pharmacokinetic and pharmacodynamic drug interaction study of acamprosate and naltrexone. *Neuropsychopharmacology, 27*, 596–606. http://dx.doi.org/10.1016/S0893-133X(02)00368-8

Mason, B. J., & Heyser, C. J. (2010). Acamprosate: A prototypic neuromodulator in the treatment of alcohol dependence. *CNS & Neurological Disorders - Drug Targets, 9*, 23–32. http://dx.doi.org/10.2174/187152710790966641

Mason, B. J., Kocsis, J. H., Ritvo, E. C., & Cutler, R. B. (1996). A double-blind, placebo-controlled trial of desipramine for primary alcohol dependence stratified on the presence or absence of major depression. *JAMA: Journal of the American Medical Association, 275*, 761–767. http://dx.doi.org/10.1001/jama.1996.03530340025025

Mason, B. J., & Lehert, P. (2012). Acamprosate for alcohol dependence: A sex-specific meta-analysis based on individual patient data. *Alcoholism: Clinical and Experimental Research, 36*, 497–508. http://dx.doi.org/10.1111/j.1530-0277.2011.01616.x

Mason, B. J., Quello, S., Goodell, V., Shadan, F., Kyle, M., & Begovic, A. (2014). Gabapentin treatment for alcohol dependence: A randomized clinical trial. *JAMA*

Internal Medicine, 174, 70–77. http://dx.doi.org/10.1001/jamainternmed.2013.11950

Mason, B. J., Quello, S., & Shadan, F. (2018). Gabapentin for the treatment of alcohol use disorder. *Expert Opinion on Investigational Drugs, 27,* 113–124. http://dx.doi.org/10.1080/13543784.2018.1417383

McGrath, P. J., Nunes, E. V., Stewart, J. W., Goldman, D., Agosti, V., Ocepek-Welikson, K., & Quitkin, F. M. (1996). Imipramine treatment of alcoholics with primary depression: A placebo-controlled clinical trial. *Archives of General Psychiatry, 53,* 232–240. http://dx.doi.org/10.1001/archpsyc.1996.01830030054009

Merck Santé. (2005). *CAMPRAL (acamprosate calcium) delayed-release tablets.* Lyon, France: Author. Retrieved from https://www.accessdata.fda.gov/drugsatfda_docs/label/2010/021431s013lbl.pdf

Mitchell, J. M., Arcuni, P. A., Weinstein, D., & Woolley, J. D. (2016). Intranasal oxytocin selectively modulates social perception, craving, and approach behavior in subjects with alcohol use disorder. *Journal of Addiction Medicine, 10,* 182–189. http://dx.doi.org/10.1097/ADM.0000000000000213

Mitchell, J. M., Bergren, L. J., Chen, K. S., Rowbotham, M. C., & Fields, H. L. (2009). Naltrexone aversion and treatment efficacy are greatest in humans and rats that actively consume high levels of alcohol. *Neurobiology of Disease, 33,* 72–80. http://dx.doi.org/10.1016/j.nbd.2008.09.018

Nam, H. W., Karpyak, V. M., Hinton, D. J., Geske, J. R., Ho, A. M., Prieto, M. L., . . . Choi, D. S. (2015). Elevated baseline serum glutamate as a pharmaco-metabolomic biomarker for acamprosate treatment outcome in alcohol-dependent subjects. *Translational Psychiatry, 5,* e621. http://dx.doi.org/10.1038/tp.2015.120

National Center for Health Statistics. (2016, revised 2017). *Health, United States, 2015: With special feature on racial and ethnic health disparities* (DHHS Publication No. 2016–1232). Hyattsville, MD: U.S. Department of Health and Human Services.

*National Institute on Alcohol Abuse and Alcoholism. (2010, revised May 2016). Rethinking drinking: Alcohol and your health (NIH Publication No. 15-3770). Washington, DC: U.S. Government Printing Office. Retrieved from https://pubs.niaaa.nih.gov/publications/RethinkingDrinking/Rethinking_Drinking.pdf

Niederhofer, H., & Staffen, W. (2003a). RETRACTED ARTICLE: Acamprosate and its efficacy in treating alcohol dependent adolescents. *European Child & Adolescent Psychiatry, 12,* 144–148. http://dx.doi.org/10.1007/s00787-003-0327-1

Niederhofer, H., & Staffen, W. (2003b). Comparison of disulfiram and placebo in treatment of alcohol dependence of adolescents. *Drug and Alcohol Review, 22,* 295–297. http://dx.doi.org/10.1080/0959523031000154436

O'Malley, S. S., Jaffe, A. J., Chang, G., Rode, S., Schottenfeld, R., Meyer, R. E., & Rounsaville, B. (1996). Six-month follow-up of naltrexone and psychotherapy for alcohol dependence. *Archives of General Psychiatry, 53,* 217–224. http://dx.doi.org/10.1001/archpsyc.1996.01830030039007

O'Malley, S. S., Jaffe, A. J., Chang, G., Schottenfeld, R. S., Meyer, R. E., & Rounsaville, B. (1992). Naltrexone and coping skills therapy for alcohol dependence. A controlled study. *Archives of General Psychiatry, 49,* 881–887. http://dx.doi.org/10.1001/archpsyc.1992.01820110045007

O'Malley, S. S., Sinha, R., Grilo, C. M., Capone, C., Farren, C. K., McKee, S. A., . . . Wu, R. (2007). Naltrexone and cognitive behavioral coping skills therapy for the treatment of alcohol drinking and eating disorder features in alcohol-dependent women: A randomized controlled trial. *Alcoholism: Clinical and Experimental Research, 31*(4), 625–634.

Ooteman, W., Naassila, M., Koeter, M. W., Verheul, R., Schippers, G. M., Houchi, H., . . . van den Brink, W. (2009). Predicting the effect of naltrexone and acamprosate in alcohol-dependent patients using genetic indicators. *Addiction Biology, 14,* 328–337. http://dx.doi.org/10.1111/j.1369-1600.2009.00159.x

Oslin, D. W., Berrettini, W., Kranzler, H. R., Pettinati, H., Gelernter, J., Volpicelli, J. R., & O'Brien, C. P. (2003). A functional polymorphism of the mu-opioid receptor gene is associated with naltrexone response in alcohol-dependent patients. *Neuropsychopharmacology, 28,* 1546–1552. http://dx.doi.org/10.1038/sj.npp.1300219

Oslin, D. W., Leong, S. H., Lynch, K. G., Berrettini, W., O'Brien, C. P., Gordon, A. J., & Rukstalis, M. (2015). Naltrexone vs placebo for the treatment of alcohol dependence: A randomized clinical trial. *JAMA Psychiatry, 72,* 430–437. http://dx.doi.org/10.1001/jamapsychiatry.2014.3053

Pedersen, C. A., Smedley, K. L., Leserman, J., Jarskog, L. F., Rau, S. W., Kampov-Polevoi, A., . . . Garbutt, J. C. (2013). Intranasal oxytocin blocks alcohol withdrawal in human subjects. *Alcoholism: Clinical and Experimental Research, 37,* 484–489. http://dx.doi.org/10.1111/j.1530-0277.2012.01958.x

Perney, P., Lehert, P., & Mason, B. J. (2012). Sleep disturbance in alcoholism: Proposal of a simple measurement, and results from a 24-week randomized controlled study of alcohol-dependent patients assessing acamprosate efficacy. *Alcohol and*

Alcoholism, 47, 133–139. http://dx.doi.org/10.1093/alcalc/agr160

Perney, P., Rigole, H., Mason, B., Dematteis, M., & Lehert, P. (2015). Measuring sleep disturbances in patients with alcohol use disorders: A short questionnaire suitable for routine practice. *Journal of Addiction Medicine, 9*, 25–30. http://dx.doi.org/10.1097/ADM.0000000000000063

Pettinati, H. M., Oslin, D. W., Kampman, K. M., Dundon, W. D., Xie, H., Gallis, T. L., . . . O'Brien, C. P. (2010). A double-blind, placebo-controlled trial combining sertraline and naltrexone for treating co-occurring depression and alcohol dependence. *The American Journal of Psychiatry, 167*, 668–675. http://dx.doi.org/10.1176/appi.ajp.2009.08060852

Physicians Total Care, Inc. (2010). Antabuse® (disulfiram tablets USP) in alcoholism. Tulsa, OK: Author. Retrieved from https://dailymed.nlm.nih.gov/dailymed/getFile.cfm?setid=12850de3-c97c-42c1-b8d3-55dc6fd05750&usg=AOvVaw2YOGPqBcurzytr2C6wsM2R

Rosenthal, R. N., Gage, A., Perhach, J. L., & Goodman, A. M. (2008). Acamprosate: Safety and tolerability in the treatment of alcohol dependence. *Journal of Addiction Medicine, 2*, 40–50. http://dx.doi.org/10.1097/ADM.0b013e31816319fd

Roy-Byrne, P. P., Pages, K. P., Russo, J. E., Jaffe, C., Blume, A. W., Kingsley, E., . . . Ries, R. K. (2000). Nefazodone treatment of major depression in alcohol-dependent patients: A double-blind, placebo-controlled trial. *Journal of Clinical Psychopharmacology, 20*, 129–136. http://dx.doi.org/10.1097/00004714-200004000-00003

Ryan, M. L., Falk, D. E., Fertig, J. B., Rendenbach-Mueller, B., Katz, D. A., Tracy, K. A., . . . Litten, R. Z. (2017). A phase 2, double-blind, placebo-controlled randomized trial assessing the efficacy of ABT-436, a novel V1b receptor antagonist, for alcohol dependence. *Neuropsychopharmacology, 42*, 1012–1023. http://dx.doi.org/10.1038/npp.2016.214

Saivin, S., Hulot, T., Chabac, S., Potgieter, A., Durbin, P., & Houin, G. (1998). Clinical pharmacokinetics of acamprosate. *Clinical Pharmacokinetics, 35*, 331–345. http://dx.doi.org/10.2165/00003088-199835050-00001

Salinsky, M. C., Storzbach, D., Spencer, D. C., Oken, B. S., Landry, T., & Dodrill, C. B. (2005). Effects of topiramate and gabapentin on cognitive abilities in healthy volunteers. *Neurology, 64*, 792–798. http://dx.doi.org/10.1212/01.WNL.0000152877.08088.87

Salloum, I. M., Cornelius, J. R., Daley, D. C., Kirisci, L., Himmelhoch, J. M., & Thase, M. E. (2005). Efficacy of valproate maintenance in patients with bipolar disorder and alcoholism: A double-blind placebo-controlled study. *Archives of General Psychiatry, 62*, 37–45. http://dx.doi.org/10.1001/archpsyc.62.1.37

Shiffman, S., Stone, A. A., & Hufford, M. R. (2008). Ecological momentary assessment. *Annual Review of Clinical Psychology, 4*, 1–32. http://dx.doi.org/10.1146/annurev.clinpsy.3.022806.091415

Skinner, M. D., Lahmek, P., Pham, H., & Aubin, H. J. (2014). Disulfiram efficacy in the treatment of alcohol dependence: A meta-analysis. *PLoS One, 9*, e87366. http://dx.doi.org/10.1371/journal.pone.0087366

Smith, P. C., Schmidt, S. M., Allensworth-Davies, D., & Saitz, R. (2009). Primary care validation of a single-question alcohol screening test. *Journal of General Internal Medicine, 24*, 783–788. http://dx.doi.org/10.1007/s11606-009-0928-6

Smith, R. V., Havens, J. R., & Walsh, S. L. (2016). Gabapentin misuse, abuse and diversion: A systematic review. *Addiction, 111*, 1160–1174. http://dx.doi.org/10.1111/add.13324

Sobell, L. C., & Sobell, M. B. (1992). Timeline Follow-back: A technique for assessing self-reported ethanol consumption. In J. Allen & R. Z. Litten (Eds.), *Measuring Alcohol Consumption: Psychosocial and Biological Methods* (pp. 41–72). Totowa, NJ: Humana Press. http://dx.doi.org/10.1007/978-1-4612-0357-5_3

Staner, L., Boeijinga, P., Danel, T., Gendre, I., Muzet, M., Landron, F., & Luthringer, R. (2006). Effects of acamprosate on sleep during alcohol withdrawal: A double-blind placebo-controlled polysomnographic study in alcohol-dependent subjects. *Alcoholism: Clinical and Experimental Research, 30*, 1492–1499. http://dx.doi.org/10.1111/j.1530-0277.2006.00180.x

Substance Abuse and Mental Health Services Administration (SAMHSA). (2008). Results from the 2007 National Survey on Drug Use and Health: National Findings (Office of Applied Studies, NSDUH Series H-34, DHHS Publication No. SMA 08-4343). Rockville, MD: Author. Retrieved from http://www.dpft.org/resources/NSDUHresults2007.pdf

Substance Abuse and Mental Health Services Administration (SAMHSA). (2012). General principles for the use of pharmacological agents to treat individuals with co-occurring mental and substance use disorders. HHS Publication No. SMA12-4689, Rockville, MD: Author. Retrieved from https://store.samhsa.gov/shin/content//SMA12-4689/SMA12-4689.pdf

Substance Abuse and Mental Health Services Administration (SAMHSA). (2017). Key substance use and mental health indicators in the United States: Results from the 2016 National Survey on Drug Use and Health (HHS Publication No. SMA 17-5044, NSDUH Series H-52). Rockville, MD: Center for Behavioral Health Statistics and Quality, Substance Abuse and Mental Health Services Administration. Retrieved from https://store.samhsa.gov/shin/content//SMA17-5044/SMA17-5044.pdf

Thomas, S. E., Randall, P. K., Book, S. W., & Randall, C. L. (2008). A complex relationship between co-occurring social anxiety and alcohol use disorders: What effect does treating social anxiety have on drinking? *Alcoholism: Clinical and Experimental Research, 32,* 77–84. http://dx.doi.org/10.1111/j.1530-0277.2007.00546.x

U.S. Department of Health and Human Services (HHS), Office of the Surgeon General. (2016). Facing addiction in America: The Surgeon General's report on alcohol, drugs, and health. Washington, DC: Author. Retrieved from https://addiction.surgeongeneral.gov/surgeon-generals-report.pdf

Vendruscolo, L. F., Estey, D., Goodell, V., Macshane, L. G., Logrip, M. L., Schlosburg, J. E., . . . Mason, B. J. (2015). Glucocorticoid receptor antagonism decreases alcohol seeking in alcohol-dependent individuals. *The Journal of Clinical Investigation, 125,* 3193–3197. http://dx.doi.org/10.1172/JCI79828

Wechsler, H., Dowdall, G. W., Davenport, A., & Rimm, E. B. (1995). A gender-specific measure of binge drinking among college students. *American Journal of Public Health, 85,* 982–985. http://dx.doi.org/10.2105/AJPH.85.7.982

Wilde, M. I., & Wagstaff, A. J. (1997). Acamprosate. A review of its pharmacology and clinical potential in the management of alcohol dependence after detoxification. *Drugs, 53,* 1038–1053. http://dx.doi.org/10.2165/00003495-199753060-00008

World Health Organization. (1992). *The ICD–10 classification of mental and behavioural disorders: Clinical descriptions and diagnostic guidelines.* Geneva, Switzerland: Author.

World Health Organization. (2016). ICD–11 beta draft. Geneva, Switzerland: Author. Retrieved from https://icd.who.int/dev11/l-m/en

CHAPTER 23

PHARMACOLOGICAL TREATMENT OF CANNABIS USE DISORDER

Jan Copeland

Cannabis is the most widely used and variably regulated drug in the world, with increasing trends of use being reported in the United States, Australia, Asia, and Africa (Copeland & Pokorski, 2016). With the relatively recent promotion and commercialization of the use of cannabis for medical and nonmedical purposes, particularly in the United States, there has been a rapid rise in use, particularly in daily use (Davenport & Caulkins, 2016). The term cannabis is used to describe the various products (e.g., marijuana, hashish, wax) and chemical compounds (e.g., nabiximols) of what are typically the most common species, *Cannabis sativa* and *Cannabis indica* (Copeland, Rook, & Matalon, 2015). Despite rising use and rapidly changing legislative approaches, conclusive evidence of its effects and safety in the short and long term have not been well established (National Academies of Sciences, Engineering and Medicine, 2017). Evidence has shown a decrease in the age of commencement of cannabis use in some developed countries, and a prolongation of risk of initiation to cannabis use beyond adolescence amongst more recent users. This chapter will provide an overview of the best evidence available on the epidemiology of cannabis use disorder (CUD), assessment, research, and promising pharmacotherapies for cannabis withdrawal and dependence. While there are currently no approved pharmacotherapies for CUD, 20 years of committed and high-quality research in the human laboratory and clinical settings have been based on the recent understanding that endocannabinoid signaling is involved in reward and addiction (Sloan et al., 2017). This work has led to medications with promise of efficacy in the treatment of cannabis withdrawal, improved retention in treatment, reduced cannabis use, and results that point to promising future work. This chapter outlines the range of medications that have been assessed, including cannabinoids, and discusses the need to consider particular characteristics of clients, such as sex, impulsivity, and severity of cannabis use, when selecting a medication in the off-label treatment of CUD or cannabis withdrawal.

EPIDEMIOLOGY AND PREVALENCE

Cannabis is the most commonly used illicit drug across Western countries, including Europe (6.6% reporting recent past year use; European Monitoring Centre for Drugs and Drug Addiction, 2015), North America (13.9% reporting recent use; Center for Behavioral Health Statistics, 2014), and Australia (10.2% reporting recent use; Australian Institute of Health and Welfare, 2017). It has a history of use for thousands of years as a crop, and has held commercial, medicinal, and spiritual value across a number of cultures. Cannabis plants are believed to have evolved in Central Asia in the regions of Mongolia and southern Siberia from around 4,000 B.C. Prior to the development of modern science, cannabis

http://dx.doi.org/10.1037/0000133-023
APA Handbook of Psychopharmacology, S. M. Evans (Editor-in-Chief)

was used as a medicine. It enjoyed a brief period of popularity as a medicinal herb in Europe and the United States in the 1800s, being prescribed for various conditions including menstrual cramps, asthma, cough, insomnia, birth labor, migraine, throat infection, and withdrawal from opiate use (Zuardi, 2006). Because of problems with titrating the dose, there were issues with patients being given too little or too much, resulting in anything from no effect to adverse effects. Cannabis was removed from the register of medicines in the early 20th century in the United States and made illegal at around the same time. There was no recognition of CUD historically, so there is no record of other substances being used to manage the disorder in Western medicine beyond symptomatic relief with agents available at the time, such as morphine and alcohol.

Most cannabis users do not smoke frequently and report either unproblematic experimental or irregular use, or abstinence following the experience of a negative consequence from use (Swift, Coffey, Carlin, Degenhardt, & Patton, 2008; von Sydow et al., 2001). However, a developing evidence base suggests that health-related consequences are likely if the drug is used frequently or from an early age (Silins et al., 2014). This evidence base shows greatest consistency for four particular health concerns that are often experienced by heavy cannabis users. First, there are concerns for the mental health of users, with associations between cannabis use and some affective disorders (Agrawal et al., 2017) and the onset of psychosis (Murray et al., 2017). Second, heavy users can experience cognitive impairments which can make it harder to learn and commit information to memory (Lisdahl et al., 2014) and are thought to be associated with school dropout (Silins et al., 2014) and unsafe driving (Asbridge, Hayden, & Cartwright, 2012). Third, smoking cannabis impairs respiratory health, particularly by increasing the risk of developing a wheeze, cough, and problems with bronchial dynamics (Gates, Jaffe, & Copeland, 2014). Finally, an estimated one in 10 of all cannabis users, and one in two daily users, will develop a CUD (Hall & Pacula, 2003). Those with CUD are characterized by clinically significant psychological distress (often presenting with clinical diagnoses), social problems,

and an inability to stop use despite such problems (Budney et al., 2003; Copeland, Swift, & Rees, 2001).

Given the prevalence of CUD in the general population, many individuals seek treatment for cannabis use. Data taken from the Australian National Minimum Data Set of Alcohol and Other Drug Treatment Services shows that, between 2013 and 2014, cannabis was the primary drug of concern in 24% of presentations to government-funded alcohol and drug treatment services, second only to alcohol (41%; Australian Institute of Health and Welfare, 2013). Comparable data on treatment seeking in the United States is reported in the Treatment Episode Data Set by the Substance Abuse and Mental Health Services Administration (SAMHSA). Using the same timeline, admissions to state-funded treatment services primarily for cannabis use were reported as 16% in 2003, increasing to 23.1% in 2009, and then decreasing again to 17% in 2013 (SAMHSA, 2015). In Europe, the number of first-time presentations to treatment facilities for cannabis rose from 45,000 in 2006 to 69,000 in 2014, with an 8% increase in reported daily use (European Monitoring Centre for Drugs and Drug Addiction, 2015).

Although cannabis is the second most commonly reported drug of concern in substance use disorder (SUD) treatment services, this still leaves a larger proportion of individuals in need of treatment who do not access it (Copeland & Swift, 2009). Reports suggest that only between one in 10 to just over one in three individuals with CUD will go on to access treatment in the United States and Australia (Agosti & Levin, 2004; Dennis, Babor, Roebuck, & Donaldson, 2002; Stinson, Ruan, Pickering, & Grant, 2006). More recent estimates are available from the United States, where in 2013, 2.9% of the population of persons at least 12 years old needed treatment for an illicit drug use problem (7.6 million people), and only one in five of this group (19.5%) received treatment at a specialist facility in the previous year (Center for Behavioral Health Statistics, 2014).

Compared with alcohol treatment, a larger proportion of cannabis treatment episodes come from mandated treatment through the criminal justice system (Australian Institute of Health and Welfare,

2013). Also, the majority of cannabis treatment seekers are self-referred, and in Australia diversion from criminal justice is the most common source of referral (32%; Australian Institute of Health and Welfare, 2013). The road to cannabis treatment can often be a particularly long and arduous journey. One of the reasons has been the historical view that cannabis use did not cause neuroadaptation and physical symptoms of tolerance and withdrawal over time (Budney & Hughes, 2006). As the evidence base has developed with animal and human studies and a valid and reliable measure of cannabis withdrawal became available (Allsop et al., 2012), cannabis withdrawal is now a discrete diagnosis in the *Diagnostic and Statistical Manual of Mental Disorders* (5th ed.; *DSM–5*; American Psychiatric Association, 2013). This diagnostic category has assisted in the recognition of the need for specialized CUD interventions. A survey of those who have accessed treatment found that, prior to seeking treatment, the average cannabis user will have attempted to quit an average of more than six times (Dennis et al., 2002), reported near daily use over 10 years, or a CUD diagnosis for 3 years (Stephens, Roffman, & Simpson, 1993). Finally, previous studies of cannabis treatment seekers in the United States and Australia have identified some important differences between those who do and do not seek this kind of treatment: Treatment seekers are more likely to be single, male, younger than 30 years old, have dropped out from schooling, and report comorbid problems with alcohol use (Gates, Copeland, Swift, & Martin, 2012), compared with similar cannabis users not seeking treatment.

DIAGNOSING CANNABIS USE DISORDER

Increasing prevalence, particularly daily cannabis use, among those reporting they use for medical conditions (Lin, Ilgen, Jannausch, & Bohnert, 2016) means that screening and intervention for CUD is of growing importance in a range of treatment settings.

Additional venues for screening and intervention are mental health and related settings. Comorbidity of CUD with other SUDs (e.g., alcohol use disorder) and with other mental health disorders (e.g., anxiety, depression, schizophrenia) is a clinical concern and

occurs relatively frequently. Cannabis use among those vulnerable to psychotic disorders precipitates the disorder on average 3 years earlier, increases rates of noncompliance with medication, and increases hospitalizations (Myles, Myles, & Large, 2016).

Despite the harms associated with CUD, only a minority will identify their cannabis use as problematic (von Sydow et al., 2001). Cannabis users may seek assistance for problems such as poor sleep, anger, depression, anxiety, psychosis, relationship issues, or respiratory problems (Copeland et al., 2001), but not mention their use of cannabis to the clinician. Various barriers can inhibit treatment seeking, such as not being aware of treatment options, thinking treatment is unnecessary, wanting to avoid the stigma associated with accessing treatment, concerns about confidentiality, lack of accessibility, and costs of treatment (Gates, Copeland et al., 2012). When adults do present for cannabis treatment, they typically have used cannabis for 10 or more years, with multiple failed attempts to quit (Copeland et al., 2001). Adolescent cannabis users who present for treatment are typically coerced, with families, schools, or the legal system often initiating efforts to access assistance for the adolescent (Copeland, 2016).

Having identified high-risk groups for CUD and how they may present to various workplace and health care settings, it is important to screen and assess them for the disorder. There are three major cannabis-related disorders in the two classification schemes of the *DSM–5* (American Psychiatric Association, 2013) and the *International Statistical Classification of Diseases and Related Health Problems 10th Revision* (ICD–10; World Health Organization, 1992). Acute cannabis intoxication (characterized by difficulty with coordination, lethargy, decreased concentration, slowed reaction time, slurred speech, and red eyes, with high doses of tetrahydrocannabinol [THC] producing confusion, amnesia, delusions, hallucinations, anxiety, and agitation) is a recognized diagnosis in both systems, but is not relevant to the discussion of pharmacological treatment of CUD and related conditions. Cannabis withdrawal is now recognized as a discrete disorder in *DSM–5*, while CUD is covered by codes such as cannabis abuse, uncomplicated, and cannabis dependence, uncomplicated (use disorder moderate and severe) for medical billing purposes in ICD–10. Assessing the nature and extent of cannabis use is fundamental regarding decisions about the need for treatment and preparing a treatment plan. While there are no agreed upon cutoffs for the level of cannabis use that constitutes a threat to an individual's health and well-being, it is well understood that early initiation to cannabis use (before the age of 16 years in particular), more than weekly use, and using in risky situations increases the risk of negative consequences. In formal psychiatric/psychological or medical settings, the diagnosis of CUD is made in the same way as other SUDs. The most comprehensive assessment is via a structured interview, more typically used in research settings to generate a *DSM–5* diagnosis of CUD—for example, using the Structured Clinical Interview for DSM–5 (SCID-5) with various versions for clinical and research purposes (First, Williams, Karg, & Spitzer, 2015).

In day-to-day clinical practice, a briefer measure, while still evidence-based, is preferred and logistically more likely to be systematically implemented. There are several valid and reliable screening tools for the detection of current and 12-month cannabis use-related problems. There are a number of cannabis-specific issues that affect meaningful assessment of quantity and frequency of cannabis use in the absence of an agreed upon standard cannabis unit (Norberg, Mackenzie, & Copeland, 2012). The relevant issues are discussed in detail by Bashford (Bashford, 2009) and López-Pelayo and colleagues (López-Pelayo, Batalla, Balcells, Colom, & Gual, 2015), and issues specific to primary care by Winstock and colleagues (Winstock, Ford, & Witton, 2010). The latter reference also contains a helpful flowchart for clinical assessment of CUD and appropriate responses, as does the online resource https://cannabissupport.com.au/media/4481/gp-factsheets-for-patients-and-gps-2016-combined-version.pdf. The flowchart contained in that kit sets out the steps in the assessment and brief management of cannabis-related problems. It is focused around the Severity of Dependence Scale (SDS), which will help determine if a patient is dependent on cannabis, along with scoring and suggested feedback. This scale has also been validated for use with adolescents (Martin, Copeland, Gilmour, Gates, &

Swift, 2006). There are other brief instruments to assess CUD (Bashford, 2009), and the Cannabis Use Problems Identification Test to assess high-risk adolescents for the short-term development of CUD (Bashford, Flett, & Copeland, 2010). For further information on these and other measures go to https://cannabissupport.com.au/media/1594/management-of-cannabis-use-disorder-and-related-issues-a-clinicians-guide.pdf, and see the Tool Kit of Resources at the end of this chapter.

In many nonspecialized addiction settings, clients rarely present thinking about changing their cannabis use, so they may require some time to take in the information and make a commitment to change. It is important to be supportive of this process and encourage clients whose cannabis use is of concern to return when they are ready to discuss making changes in their patterns of use. They may only be ready to cut down at first, but any change is positive and supports further reduction. The flowcharts referred to previously outline the series of questions and circumstances and responses that should ensue. Within more specialist services, the assessment of cannabis-related problems is also appropriate and may include measures such as the Cannabis Problems Questionnaire for adults (Copeland et al., 2005) and adolescents (Martin et al., 2006), among other measures available (López-Pelayo et al., 2015).

EVIDENCE-BASED PHARMACOLOGICAL TREATMENTS OF CANNABIS USE DISORDER

As prevalence of CUD increases, so does demand for treatment (Hasin et al., 2015). To date, psychosocial treatment remains the primary approach utilized, despite high nonresponse and relapse rates (70%; Balter, Cooper, & Haney, 2014). These approaches are discussed in a later section. There is a clear need to improve current treatment options and medications may be a useful adjunct to aid in successful treatment outcomes; however, there are currently no approved medications for the treatment of CUD (Gorelick, 2016). This chapter aims to present information on the pharmacotherapies that have been trialed as a treatment for CUD. The strategies that have been explored include agonist substitution, antagonists, or modulators of noncannabinoid neurotransmitter systems, assessing the effects on different aspects of cannabis use (e.g., intoxication, withdrawal, self-administration). Research to date is limited to human laboratory studies and small open-label or placebo-controlled clinical trials. All the studies conducted have provided useful information regarding safety and tolerability of medications combined with cannabis, as well as clinically relevant outcomes to guide the selection of medications to test in expensive and time-consuming clinical trials.

Unlike other psychoactive drugs, cannabis is a very complex drug class, and in order to understand potential pharmacotherapies a brief overview is required. While cannabis has been used and cultivated for at least 6,000 years, our nascent understanding of its pharmacology is little more than a century old (Atakan, 2012). It was wrongly assumed that cannabinol, the first compound isolated from the plant, was responsible for its psychoactive effects (Mechoulam & Hanuš, 2000). The second compound found was cannabidiol (CBD), which is receiving much research attention for its antiepileptic effects in particular (Mechoulam & Hanuš, 2002). The following year the principal psychoactive compound, delta-9-THC, was isolated by the same group, led by Mechoulam (Gaoni & Mechoulam, 1964). The next important development in this research was the identification of the endogenous (i.e., within the body) cannabinoid receptor system (ECS) that recognized the specific binding sites of cannabinoids as partial agonists of the CB1 and CB2 receptor systems (Atakan, 2012). While knowledge of the role of the ECS is still evolving, the available evidence indicates that it has multiple regulatory roles in neuronal, vascular, metabolic, immune, and reproduction systems, along with its on-demand regulatory role on other neurotransmitter systems that affects functions such as cognition, memory, motor movement, and pain perception (Gaoni & Mechoulam, 1964). An exciting new development in the field of cannabinoid pharmacology is the ability of allosteric modulators (i.e., a substance that alters effects) to selectively engage specific transduction pathways, which can potentially be used to produce tailored therapeutic strategies for a range of condi-

tions including CUD and withdrawal management (Cheer & Hurd, 2017). Another frontier in the development of responses to CUD is an improved understanding of the role of prenatal cannabis exposure and epigenetic inheritance (which refers to external modifications to DNA that turn genes "on" or "off" while not changing the DNA sequence; instead, they affect how cells "read" genes), which increase susceptibility to all SUDs including CUD, and will be the area in which preventative approaches will be further supported (Melis et al., 2017). Similar to the acute action of other rewarding psychoactive drugs such as alcohol, stimulants, opioids, and nicotine, activation of the CB1 receptor by THC releases presynaptic dopamine in the reward circuit (Gaoni & Mechoulam, 1964). In principle, CUD could be pharmacologically treated using the following approaches: (a) use of agents to suppress withdrawal and craving, analogous to nicotine replacement therapy for tobacco; and (b) chronic blockade of the drug's site of action—the CB1 receptor—or other modulation of the neurotransmitter systems directly engaged by the drug—the ECS—or indirect modulation of its actions on the brain's mesolimbic dopaminergic reward circuit (Gorelick, 2016). The ECS has bidirectional interactions with several other neurotransmitter systems in the brain, which may offer a range of potential targets for CUD treatment (Curran et al., 2016). Such potential targets include dopamine, noradrenaline, serotonin, glutamate, gamma-aminobutyric acid (GABA), and acetylcholine. To follow is a narrative review of the literature on pharmacotherapies that have been assessed in some way for the management of cannabis withdrawal and/or CUD. The studies mentioned, along with some additional ones, are set out in Table 23.1.

Cannabinoid Medications

During chronic cannabis use, a series of brain changes occur, which continue to be poorly understood. These changes however, are thought to lead to the development of dependence. Downregulation (a decrease in the number of receptors to a molecule, such as a hormone or neurotransmitter), which reduces the cell's sensitivity, and desensitization (the equivalent of drug tolerance of the CB1 receptors)

TABLE 23.1

Pharmacological Trials for Cannabis Use Disorder—Including Withdrawal Only*

Drug	N =	Sex M/F	Dose	Design	Results	Authors
Cannabinoid agonists						
Oral THC	7	7 M/0 F	10 mg	Nonclinical, experimental laboratory	Reduced withdrawal symptoms.	Haney et al., 2004
Oral THC	8	6 M/2 F	30, 90 mg	Randomized double-blind placebo-controlled cross-over	Reduced withdrawal symptoms.	Budney, Vandrey, Hughes, Moore, and Bahrenburg, 2007
Nabilone	11	8 M/3 F	6, 8 mg	Nonclinical, experimental laboratory	Reduced withdrawal symptoms and cannabis use.	Haney et al., 2013
Dronabinol	2	2 M/0 F	10–50 mg	Case studies	Mixed results.	Levin and Kleber, 2008
Dronabinol	156	128 M/28 F	20 mg BD	Randomized double-blind placebo-controlled trial	No difference between groups.	Levin et al., 2011
Dronabinol and Lofexidine	122	84 M/38 F	20 mg Dronabinol TDS and 0.6 mg Lofexidine TDS	Randomized double-blind placebo-controlled trial	No difference between groups.	Levin et al., 2016
Cannabidiol	1	0 M/1 F	300–600 mg	Case study	Reduced withdrawal symptoms and cannabis use.	Crippa et al., 2013
Cannabidiol	8	7 M/1 F	600 mg/day times 5 and 600 mg/day times 3	Open-label trial	5/8 completed full treatment and abstinence was maintained by 4/8 at day 28 follow-up. All those receiving the higher dose completed treatment and achieved abstinence at follow-up.	Pokorski et al., 2017
Nabiximols	51	40 M/11 F	166.4 mg	Randomized double-blind placebo-controlled cross-over	Reduced withdrawal (Cannabis Withdrawal Scale) and increased retention.	Allsop et al., 2015
Nabiximols	40	29 M/11 F	Max 113.4 mg THC/105 mg CBD	Randomized double-blind clinical trial	No effect on retention, abstinence, or cannabis withdrawal, but reduced cannabis use.	Trigo et al., 2018
Rimonabant	63	63 M/0 F	1, 3, 10, 30, 90 mg	Randomized double-blind placebo-controlled cross-over	Attenuated effects of cannabis, potentially serious side effects.	Huestis et al., 2001
Rimonabant	42	42 M/0 F	40 mg	Double-blind parallel groups	Attenuated cardiovascular effects of cannabis, removed from the market.	Huestis et al., 2007

Other agents

Opioid antagonists

Drug	N	M/F	Dose	Study design	Results	Reference
Naltrexone	14	8 M/6 F	50 mg	Double-blind placebo-controlled cross-over	Failed to attenuate dronabinol.	Wachtel and de Wit, 2000
Naltrexone	22	10 M/12 F	12 mg	Nonclinical, experimental laboratory	Mixed results by dose and effect type, no sex differences.	Haney, 2007
Naltrexone	29	15 M/14 F	12, 25, 50, or 100 mg	Nonclinical, experimental laboratory	Enhanced subjective effects of cannabis.	Cooper and Haney, 2010
Naltrexone	5	9 M/4 F	50 or 200 mg	Double-blind placebo-controlled cross-over	No difference between groups.	Greenwald and Stitzer, 2000

Antidepressants

Drug	N	M/F	Dose	Study design	Results	Reference
Bupropion	10	8 M/2 F	300 mg	Nonclinical, experimental laboratory	Worsened withdrawal.	Haney et al., 2001
Nefazodone	7	6 M/1 F	450 mg	Nonclinical, experimental laboratory	Improved anxiety but not withdrawal overall.	Haney, Hart, Ward, and Foltin, 2003
Fluoxetine	10 Adolescent major depression and substance use disorder	8 M/2 F	20–40 mg	Randomized double-blind placebo-controlled cross-over	Reduced cannabis use at 5-year follow-up.	Cornelius et al., 2005
Lofexidine + THC	8	8 M/0 F	2.4 mg; 60 mg	Nonclinical, experimental laboratory	Reduced withdrawal.	Haney et al., 2008
Nefazodone Bupropion	106	81 M/25 F	300 mg; 150 mg	Randomized double-blind placebo	No difference between groups.	Carpenter, McDowell, Brooks, Cheng, and Levin, 2009
Baclofen or Mirtazapine	10	10 M/0 F	30, 60, 90 mg; 30 mg	Nonclinical, experimental laboratory	No difference between groups.	Haney et al., 2010
Fluoxetine	70 Adolescent major depression and CUD	43 M/27 F	20 mg	Randomized double-blind placebo-controlled cross-over	No difference between groups.	Cornelius et al., 2010
Venlafaxine-extended release (Ven-XR)	103	76 M/27 F	375 mg CUD and comorbid depression	Randomized double-blind placebo-controlled	No difference between groups on mood, abstinence rates low and poorer for those receiving Ven-XR.	Levin et al., 2013
Escitalopram	52	39 M/13 F	10 mg/day	Double-blind, placebo-controlled	No difference between groups, high attrition rate (50%).	Weinstein et al., 2014
Vilazodone	76	60 M/17 F	40 mg/day	Randomized, controlled pilot	No difference between groups, but women did more poorly than men.	McRae-Clark et al., 2016

(continues)

513

TABLE 23.1

Pharmacological Trials for Cannabis Use Disorder—Including Withdrawal Only* (*Continued*)

Drug	N =	Sex M/F	Dose	Design	Results	Authors
Glutamate						
N-acetylcysteine	24	18 M/6 F	1,200 mg	Open-label	Reduced self-reported use, but not urine cannabinoid levels.	Gray, Watson, Carpenter, and Larowe, 2010
N-acetylcysteine	116	84 M/32 F	1,200 mg	Randomized double-blind placebo-controlled	Increased negative urine cannabi-noid tests during treatment.	Gray et al., 2012
N-acetylcysteine	309	216 M/93 F	120 mg	Randomized, placebo-controlled	No difference between groups.	Gray et al., 2017
Anxiolytic						
Buspirone	11	10 M/1 F	up to 60 mg	Open-label	Reduced craving and irritability.	McRae, Brady, and Carter, 2006
Buspirone	50	27 M/23 F	up to 60 mg	Double blind, placebo controlled	Reduced cannabis use.	McRae-Clark et al., 2009
Antiepileptics						
Divalproex	7	7 M/0 F	1500 mg	Nonclinical, experimental laboratory	Worsened withdrawal.	Haney et al., 2004
Divalproex	25	23 M/2 F	1,500–2,000 mg	Randomized double-blind placebo-controlled cross-over	No difference between groups.	Levin et al., 2004
Topiramate	66 15–24 years	32 M/34 F	200 mg/day	Randomized, placebo-controlled	Superior to placebo for quantity smoked but not frequency or abstinence. Poorly tolerated with 52% attrition.	Miranda et al., 2017

Other

Drug	N	M/F	Dose	Study design	Outcome	Reference
Gabapentin	50	44 M/6 F	1,200 mg	Randomized double-blind placebo-controlled cross-over	Decreased withdrawal severity, high attrition.	Mason et al., 2012
Oxytocin	16	12 M/4 F	40 international units (IU)	Randomized double-blind placebo-controlled cross-over	Decreased craving and anxiety.	McRae-Clark, Baker, Maria, and Brady, 2013
Oxytocin	16	10 M/6 F	40 IU pretreatment to MET	Randomized, placebo-controlled pilot study	Oxytocin led to reduced amount of cannabis use.	Sherman, Baker, and McRae-Clark, 2017
Quetiapine	14	12 M/2F	200 mg	Nonclinical, experimental laboratory double-blind, counter-balanced, within-subject study	Decreased withdrawal, increased cannabis use.	Cooper, Foltin, et al., 2013
Varenicline	5	3 M/2 F	0.5–1 mg	Case series	Reduced use, zero completion of study due to side effects.	Newcombe, Walker, Sheridan, and Galea, 2015
Zolpidem	20	17 M/3 F	12.5 mg extended release (ER)	Within-subject, placebo crossover study	Zolpidem improved sleep during withdrawal. Zolpidem was not associated with any significant side effects or next-day cognitive performance impairments.	Vandrey, Smith, McCann, Budney, and Curran, 2011
Zolpidem vs Zolpidem and nabilone	11	11 M/0 F	12.5 mg ER 3 mg	Nonclinical, experimental laboratory	Both decreased sleep withdrawal symptoms; only combination reduced mood and food intake; cf. placebo.	Hermann et al., 2016
Ziprasidone Clozapine	30 CUD and schizophrenia	26 M/4 F	NS	Randomized clinical study	Both groups reduced cannabis use, clozapine associated with fewer positive symptoms of schizophrenia, more side effects, and poorer compliance.	Schnell et al., 2014

Note. M = male; F = female; THC = tetrahydrocannabinol; BD = twice a day; TDS = three times a day; CBD = cannabidiol; CUD = cannabis use disorder; MET = motivational enhancement therapy; NS = no significant difference.
*This table is intended to be a brief overview and includes additional studies; please see text for further details where relevant.

are also thought to occur. This suggests that withdrawal is driven by compensatory downregulation of the endocannabinoid system (Breivogel et al., 2003). These withdrawal symptoms promote relapse into drug use, implying that pharmacological strategies aimed at alleviating cannabis withdrawal might prevent relapse and reduce dependence. Cannabinoid replacement therapy and CB1 receptor antagonism are two potential treatments for cannabis dependence that are currently under investigation (Breivogel et al., 2003; Ramesh & Haney, 2015).

CB1 receptor antagonists. Rimonabant is a CB1-selective cannabinoid receptor antagonist that was found to block the effects of THC in animals. This strategy targets the addiction to cannabis by blocking the positive subjective and reinforcing effects of the drug (Ramesh & Haney, 2015). In a placebo-controlled experimental study by Huestis and colleagues (2001) of nontreatment seekers; rimonabant was tested in 63 individuals with a history of cannabis use. All participants were given a cannabis joint 2 hours after taking the medication. The medication was found to decrease feelings of intoxication and decrease heart rate. This study was among the first to show that blocking the cannabis receptor was effective in decreasing the subjective cannabis effects (Huestis et al., 2001). However, rimonabant, which was initially approved in Europe as a drug to treat obesity, was withdrawn from that market in 2009 due to potentially serious side effects, such as severe depression and suicidal thoughts (Christensen, Kristensen, Bartels, Bliddal, & Astrup, 2007). Novel cannabinoid receptor antagonists are believed to be in development (Sloan et al., 2017).

CB1 receptor agonists. Agonist substitution involves replacing the drug of concern with the same or a similar drug in a safer form and route of administration. It is hypothesized that CB1 receptor agonists should decrease cannabis use by activating the same key binding sites as cannabis, reducing withdrawal and cravings (Benyamina, Lecacheux, Blecha, Reynaud, & Lukasiewcz, 2008). Agonist therapy is also thought to attenuate the acute effects of cannabis through competition at the receptor sites, facilitating abstinence. The agonist is then generally tapered off once acute withdrawal symptoms

have passed (Benyamina et al., 2008). The cannabis agonist therapies have shown greatest promise in recent trials. Due to the experimental nature of the following studies, there are no known standard dosages for testing not only whether the drug worked, but also whether there was an overall benefit after accounting for side effects (Sloan et al., 2017).

Dronabinol is an oral synthetic form of THC that acts as a cannabinoid receptor agonist at the CB1 receptor. It is approved for use in the United States for AIDS-related anorexia and for nausea as a result of chemotherapy (Haney et al., 2004). It has shown some benefit in doses of 10 mg to 50 mg in reducing cannabis withdrawal symptoms with minimal side effects in several laboratory and open-label studies (Budney, Vandrey, Hughes, Moore, & Bahrenburg, 2007; Haney, 2005). Early studies testing dronabinol on cannabis withdrawal found significant reductions in craving, anxiety, chills, depression, trouble sleeping and decreased appetite (Haney et al., 2004; Haney, 2005; Levin et al., 2011). A follow-up trial was conducted wherein dronabinol decreased symptoms of withdrawal but produced mild intoxication and did not decrease relapse to cannabis (Levin et al., 2011; Bedi et al., 2013). There are two case reports testing dronabinol in combination with other medications. One patient was medicated for 6 months with dronabinol (40 mg/day) and divalproex (250 mg/day), a mood stabilizer that reduces irritability and mood swings in bipolar disorder and during alcohol withdrawal (Levin & Kleber, 2008). A second patient was maintained on dronabinol (10–15 mg/day) while also receiving venlafaxine (25 mg/day) for depression and modafinil (100 mg pro re nata [PRN]) to counter the energy decreases experienced with dronabinol. In both cases, patients achieved and maintained abstinence (Levin & Kleber, 2008).

In a randomized, double-blind, placebo-controlled study by Levin et al. (2011), dronabinol was provided in twice daily 20 mg doses during a 12-week trial with 156 cannabis-dependent adults. Both groups received weekly motivational enhancement therapy (MET) and cognitive behavior therapy (CBT). Dronabinol appeared to lower withdrawal symptoms and promote treatment retention (77% vs. 61%, respectively), but did not affect abstinence at weeks 7 and 8 (17.7% and 15.6% for dronabinol and placebo, respectively). Four serious adverse events were reported, but none were deemed to be study related. Although there is evidence that dronabinol decreases withdrawal, it does not appear to significantly alter levels of cannabis use.

Nabilone is a cannabinoid agonist with superior bioavailability compared with dronabinol, a more predictable dose–response, and less individual variability in drug response (Haney et al., 2013). Promisingly, nabilone has been found to improve both cannabis withdrawal symptoms and prevent relapse in a nonclinical, experimental laboratory-based study (Haney et al., 2013). Nabilone was tested in three 8-day inpatient phases, with each phase assessing a different nabilone dose (0, 6, and 8 mg/day). Both nabilone doses were shown to reverse withdrawal-induced irritability, sleep disturbance, and appetite reduction. Nabilone in either dose also decreased laboratory measures of cannabis relapse, with patients choosing to smoke fewer doses of cannabis while on nabilone compared to placebo (Haney et al., 2013). These positive results support further testing of nabilone in clinical populations.

The most innovative and promising agonist pharmacotherapy currently being explored is nabiximols (Sativex®), which has a 1:1 ratio of delta-9-THC to CBD in an oromucosal, botanically-derived, cannabinoid-based spray. Nabiximols is available in 15 countries for symptomatic relief of spasticity in multiple sclerosis and is being assessed for cancer-related pain (Vermersch, 2011). In a relatively small ($n = 51$) inpatient randomized controlled trial in Australia, nabiximols was efficacious in the reduction of both the severity and time course of cannabis withdrawal, and in retaining participants in withdrawal treatment (Allsop et al., 2014). A later, small Canadian randomized controlled trial of 40 cannabis treatment seekers in the community found no effect on rates of abstinence or levels of cannabis use (Trigo et al., 2018) across the 12-week trial. This does not appear to be dose-related, as participants in the nabiximols arm could dose as required and averaged 113.4 mg THC/ 105 mg CBD daily for the 12 weeks. There was also no difference in levels of symptoms of cannabis withdrawal, although this was not measured using a validated measure (the Marijuana Withdrawal Checklist; Trigo et al., 2018). Similarly, compared with the study in which abstinence was validated (Allsop et al., 2014), there was no improvement in retention in treatment for nabiximols compared with placebo groups in the later study.

The THC component of nabiximols provides the agonist substitution; the CBD content of nabiximols is potentially a major innovation over other CB1 receptor agonists, such as dronabinol and nabilone, because CBD has psychoactive but not intoxicating effects (Pertwee, 2008). CBD is present in varying degrees across different cannabis strains, although it appears largely bred out of modern illicit strains (Swift, Wong, Li, Arnold, & McGregor, 2013). CBD has notable anxiolytic, antidepressant, and anti-psychotic properties, and can attenuate paranoia and other adverse psychological effects of THC in humans (Bergamaschi, Queiroz, Zuardi, & Crippa, 2011; Hayakawa et al., 2007; Iffland & Grotenhermen, 2017; Mechoulam, Peters, Murillo-Rodriguez, & Hanuš, 2007).

CBD appears to operate at both CB1 and CB2 receptors, indirectly stimulating endogenous cannabinoid signaling by suppressing the fatty acid amide hydrolase (FAAH), the enzyme that breaks down anandamide, the endogenous cannabinoid produced by the human body (Mechoulam et al., 2007). This enables more anandamide to remain at the receptors, reducing the sudden withdrawal produced by abrupt cessation of cannabis use. It has also been shown to be an inverse agonist of CB2 receptors (Bergamaschi et al., 2011). It has been tested extensively on animals and humans and is just entering the clinical trials phase for cannabis use. It has shown some promise in a single case study in which it was effective in reducing withdrawal symptoms and sustaining the withdrawal attempt of a cannabis-dependent patient with multiple failed quit attempts. Following maintenance on CBD (300–600 mg/day) for 11 days, the patient demonstrated no self-reported abstinence symptoms (Morgan, Freeman, Schafer, & Curran, 2010). A small open-label trial with 8 participants assessed the feasibility of CBD for the management of cannabis withdrawal (Pokorski et al., 2017). Eight participants were admitted to an inpatient detoxification facility for a 7-day open-label trial of CBD. Five participants received 600 mg of CBD and three participants received 1,200 mg of CBD, returning for a 28-day follow-up interview. CBD was well tolerated by all participants. Five completed the full treatment period, and abstinence was maintained by four participants at day 28 follow-up. All those receiving the higher dose completed treatment and achieved abstinence at follow-up. This pilot study provides support for the further exploration of CBD as a pharmacological adjunctive therapy for cannabis withdrawal and dependence (Pokorski et al., 2017). All of these potential treatments need, and are undergoing, much further testing and replication in order to enter the first line of treatment recommendations.

Other Medications

Various noncannabinoid medications already used to treat other SUDs have been evaluated in controlled inpatient studies for the treatment of cannabis withdrawal, largely with negative results.

Opioid agonists and antagonists. Naltrexone is an opioid μ antagonist approved for treatment of alcohol and opioid dependence, and has also been assessed for the treatment of CUD (Cooper & Haney, 2010; Greenwald & Stitzer, 2000; Haney, 2007; Wachtel & de Wit, 2000).

An outpatient within-subject, randomized, double-blind, placebo-controlled study examining the interaction of naltrexone with smoked cannabis (0% or 3.27% THC) found that an acute dose of naltrexone alone or in combination with 3.27% THC increased ratings of "liking," "take again," "stimulated," "high," "good," and "strength," suggesting that naltrexone may actually increase the abuse liability of cannabinoids (Cooper & Haney, 2010). In a subsequent laboratory study, however, chronic administration of naltrexone decreased the positive subjective effects of cannabis, as well as cannabis self-administration (Haney et al., 2015).

Antidepressants. Nefazodone and mirtazapine are both antidepressants with sedative properties that enhance noradrenergic and serotonergic activity (Carpenter, McDowell, Brooks, Cheng, & Levin, 2009; Haney et al., 2010). Increased sedation reduces

subjective feelings of agitation and irritability and reduces sleep disturbances during cannabis withdrawal. Nefazodone is a serotonin and norepinephrine reuptake inhibitor and a serotonin 5-HT_{2A} receptor antagonist, approved for the treatment of depression (Carpenter et al., 2009). During cannabis withdrawal, nefazodone at 450 mg/day for 26 days decreased symptoms such as anxiety and muscle pain, but did not alleviate irritability, misery, or troubled sleep (Haney et al., 2003). Conversely, in an experimental study, mirtazapine (30 mg/day for 14 days) reversed sleep disruption and appetite loss during cannabis withdrawal, but did not improve participants' mood and did not decrease relapse (Haney et al., 2010). Consistent with the laboratory data, clinical trials with bupropion and nefazodone were also negative. A randomized study of cannabis-dependent participants taking bupropion (300 mg/day divided into two oral doses) and nefazodone (600 mg/day divided into two oral doses) were compared to placebo in a 13-week trial. The study included 1 week of placebo lead in and a 2-week placebo wash-out period. All patients were given weekly sessions with a psychosocial intervention. There was no difference in cannabis use or withdrawal symptoms among those receiving bupropion, nefazodone, or placebo, and only half of the patients completed the 10-week medication phase (Carpenter et al., 2009).

Mood disorders, especially depression, are a common comorbidity associated with cannabis use, hence the use of antidepressant medication in this population has been explored to promote abstinence (Cornelius et al., 2005; Levin et al., 2013). In a 12-week study, no advantage was discovered for the antidepressant fluoxetine (10–20 mg/day for 12 weeks) over placebo on either depression or cannabis use outcomes in depressed cannabis-dependent adolescents (Cornelius et al., 2010). A trial with 103 adult patients found that extended-release venlafaxine (375 mg/day for 12 weeks) was also not effective relative to placebo in reducing depression, and found fewer abstinent participants in the venlafaxine group (11.8% and 36.5%, respectively; Levin et al., 2013). Overall, neither laboratory nor clinical studies provide compelling evidence for the utility of antidepressants to treat CUDs.

Anxiolytics and mood stabilizers. Given that anxiety can be a symptom of cannabis withdrawal, it was hypothesized that anxiety symptoms may be a useful treatment target. The nonbenzodiazepine anxiolytic buspirone was tested in a randomized, controlled clinical trial for CUD (McRae-Clark et al., 2009). Cannabis-dependent patients were randomized to buspirone (60 mg/day) or placebo for 12 weeks in conjunction with a psychological intervention (two or three sessions of motivational interviewing during the first 4 weeks). The study reported a high dropout rate (50%) and no direct effect of buspirone on self-reported anxiety, withdrawal symptoms, or craving. However, exploratory analyses suggested that a reduction in anxiety, regardless of treatment condition, predicted cannabis abstinence (McRae-Clark et al., 2009).

Divalproex has also been investigated for its mood stabilizing properties arising from its effects on GABA transmission. Divalproex is an anticonvulsant approved for the treatment of seizures and bipolar disorder as well as for migraine prophylaxis. Administered at 1,500 mg/day for 29 days, divalproex decreased cannabis cravings, but increased anxiety, irritability, and fatigue, and decreased cognitive performance compared with placebo (Haney et al., 2004). In a randomized, placebo-controlled pilot study with 25 cannabis-dependent adults, the dose of divalproex was adjusted to individual patient response (ranging from 250 to 2,000 mg/day) in conjunction with CBT for a period of 8 weeks. Patients who completed the 8 weeks reported decreased irritability, cannabis craving, and cannabis use. However, there was an increased incidence of adverse reactions related to the medication, such as fatigue, headaches, drowsiness, and nausea (Levin et al., 2004). The adverse events related to the medication as well as poor patient compliance do not support the clinical utility of divalproex.

Another mood stabilizer tested for the treatment of cannabis withdrawal is lithium carbonate. Two small preliminary open-label inpatient laboratory studies with participants receiving 600 mg to 900 mg/day for 6 days and 1,000 mg/day for 7 days reported moderate reductions in withdrawal symptoms (Bowen et al., 2005; Winstock, Lea, & Copeland, 2009). A recent small randomized controlled study of lithium carbonate, however, found a reduction in some specific withdrawal symptoms such as stomachaches and nightmares, but no significant difference in overall cannabis withdrawal scale scores or levels of cannabis use compared with placebo (Johnston et al., 2014). In this same underpowered study, the authors found that nitrazepam improved participant's sleep during withdrawal regardless of medication condition (Allsop et al., 2015).

There are potential concerns regarding the safety of outpatient administration of lithium due to its toxicity at high doses. As the mechanism of action of lithium carbonate is thought to be on oxytocin release, direct research on the impact of oxytocin on aspects of cannabis interventions was warranted. A small laboratory study evaluated the impact of oxytocin pretreatment on craving, stress, and anxiety responses following a psychosocial stress task with cannabis-dependent participants (McRae-Clark, Baker, Maria, & Brady, 2013). While preliminary, the findings suggested that oxytocin may play a role in the amelioration of stress-induced reactivity and craving in cannabis-dependent individuals. A small randomized clinical study of oxytocin as an adjunct to MET among cannabis-dependent adults found that participants receiving oxytocin showed reductions in the amount of cannabis used daily and number of sessions per day compared with placebo (Sherman, Baker, & McRae-Clark, 2017). These studies suggest that further research exploring the efficacy of oxytocin in cannabis withdrawal management and relapse prevention is warranted.

Additional medications. Quetiapine, an atypical antipsychotic that is a $5\text{-}HT_{2A}$ and dopamine D2 antagonist and a partial agonist at the $5\text{-}HT_{1A}$ receptor, inhibits the norepinephrine transporter. Quetiapine was given to cannabis users with schizophrenia or bipolar disorder and was reported to reduce cannabis use over the course of treatment (Potvin, Stip, & Roy, 2004). An inpatient laboratory study comparing quetiapine at 200 mg/day for 15 days to placebo found improved sleep quality and decreased anorexia during cannabis withdrawal (Cooper, Foltin, et al., 2013). There was, however, increased craving for, and self-administration of, cannabis, indicating that this drug is not an appropriate potential treatment for CUDs.

A small ($n = 38$) randomized controlled study has evaluated the effects of atomoxetine on the symptoms of attention-deficit/hyperactivity disorder (ADHD) and cannabis use among cannabis-dependent adults. In conjunction with motivational interviewing, atomoxetine had no effect on self-rated ADHD symptoms nor cannabis use outcomes (McRae-Clark et al., 2010). An earlier open-label pilot study among a similar study population also did not find any significant influence on cannabis use, but reported high levels of adverse gastrointestinal effects of atomoxetine (Tirado et al., 2008).

An α_2-adrenergic receptor agonist, lofexidine, currently used to treat opioid withdrawal, has been assessed in clinical studies for CUD in combination with cannabinoid agonists, but not tested as a single medication. Combining lofexidine and dronabinol produced the most significant improvements in sleep, withdrawal, craving, and relapse compared to placebo (Haney et al., 2008). A recent laboratory study of another adrenergic receptor agonist, guanfacine, for cannabis withdrawal with an outpatient phase reported that a single daily administration at varying doses at bedtime improved sleep and mood relative to placebo and warranted further clinical research (Haney et al., 2018).

Alternative pharmacotherapy approaches continue to be explored as the understanding of the neuropharmacology of CUDs improves. These alternative medications have been found to treat other drugs of dependence or target similar pathways as cannabis. Animal studies showed that N-acetylcysteine (NAC), an antioxidant, reversed alterations to the glutamine system associated with self-administration of a range of addictive drugs. In an open-label study, adolescents received 2,400 mg of NAC daily over a 4-week period with no other intervention. The medication decreased self-reported cannabis use as well as cannabis craving. It was generally well tolerated but did produce some mild-to-moderate side effects such as heartburn, insomnia, vivid dreams, and irritability (Gray, Watson, Carpenter, & Larowe, 2010). In a follow-up 8-week double-blind, randomized, placebo-controlled trial, 116 treatment-seeking cannabis-dependent adolescents aged 15 to 21 years received NAC (1,200 mg) or placebo twice daily, as well as contingency management and brief cessation counseling weekly (Gray et al., 2012). There was no significant influence on cannabis use at 1-month follow-up. Similarly, a more recent randomized, placebo-controlled trial of NAC with 302 adults with CUD across six sites over 12 weeks with contingency management also found no difference in THC-free urine toxicology at follow-up (Gray et al., 2017). This series of studies suggests NAC is not of value for the management of CUD for adults or adolescents.

A medication primarily used as a muscle relaxant, baclofen, similarly did not reduce cannabis relapse, had negative effects on mood and behavior, and reduced cognitive performance across conditions in a laboratory model of cannabis withdrawal (Haney et al., 2010). These results fail to support the use of baclofen for cannabis withdrawal.

Gabapentin is an alkylated analogue of GABA, approved in the United States for the treatment of seizures and postherpetic neuralgia. In a 12-week randomized double-blind placebo-controlled trial with 50 adults with cannabis dependence, 1,200 mg of gabapentin was divided into three daily doses. Participants also received individualized weekly manualized abstinence-oriented counseling. Although there was a high dropout rate, the authors found statistically significant reductions in amount of cannabis used and days of use, along with reductions in cannabis withdrawal symptoms, marijuana cravings, sleep problems, and depression scores. Improvements in measures of executive functioning were also seen and there were no serious adverse events (Mason et al., 2012). There have, however, been reports regarding the misuse potential of gabapentin, which may be an important consideration in future studies (Schifano et al., 2011; Smith, Higgins, Baldacchino, Kidd, & Bannister, 2012).

Varenicline is a tobacco cessation aid with demonstrated efficacy. It is a partial agonist at the $\alpha 4\beta 2$ subtype of the nicotinic acetylcholine receptor (nAChR) and a full agonist at the $\alpha 7$nAChR, which has also been shown to bind with THC. In light of this binding similarity and the common concurrent use of cannabis with tobacco, varenicline was tested on five cannabis and tobacco users in a small case series. Four of the participants reported a reduction in the enjoyment obtained from cannabis and the amount they used (Newcombe, Walker, Sheridan,

& Galea, 2015). Nevertheless, all patients failed to complete the 12-week course of medication due to a variety of reported side effects such as headache, vomiting, and anger. The reasons reported by participants for ceasing varenicline included feeling flat, experiencing nausea and vomiting, feeling angry, and being short tempered. A further small ($n = 7$) pilot study that evaluated the feasibility and preliminary effectiveness of varenicline for co-occurring cannabis and tobacco use recruited from an urban, outpatient opioid treatment program. Due to the setting of opioid replacement therapy, retention at 8 weeks was 100%, but in this study no adverse effects prompted varenicline discontinuation and it was associated with reduced cannabis craving, cannabis use, and tobacco use compared with placebo (Adams, Arnsten, Ning, & Nahvi, 2018). A larger study would be required to assess the utility of varenicline in the treatment of cannabis dependence, as well as close monitoring of adverse events.

One of the more recent drugs to be tested, vilazodone, a selective serotonin reuptake inhibitor and partial $5\text{-}HT_{1A}$ agonist, was tested against placebo on a randomized group of 76 cannabis-dependent adults. Participants received 40 mg of vilazodone a day for 8 weeks, with brief motivational enhancement therapy intervention and contingency management to encourage study retention. Vilazodone was found to provide no advantage over placebo in reducing cannabis use (McRae-Clark et al., 2016).

Summary

Increasing cannabis prevalence results in an increase in harms associated with cannabis use, including CUD. With a growing number of users seeking treatment for CUDs, there is a demand for targeted treatments and a wider range of evidence-based options. Comorbid SUDs and mental health conditions are common and should be assessed and treated concurrently. Although there is currently no evidence-based pharmacotherapy for the treatment of CUD, Table 23.1 provides a summation of many of the trials that have been conducted, and highlights the therapies that were least successful, such as the antagonist rimonabant. The most promising are the newer agonist therapies, such as nabiximols and nabilone, which have been found to reduce

measures of withdrawal and relapse without serious adverse effects, warranting further exploration in the management of aspects of CUD.

It is anticipated that as the evidence base for full and partial CB1 receptor agonists is developed, these medications will become cost effective and accessible. Pilot data and theoretical support for CBD makes it an important cannabinoid to evaluate for the treatment of CUDs with comorbid psychoactive and anxiety disorders. Different approaches yet to be explored include the inhibition of endocannabinoid catabolic enzymes, FAAH, and monoacylglycerol lipase, which reduces cannabinoid withdrawal in animal models with cannabinoid dependence. FAAH inhibitors appear to lack the abuse liability associated with cannabinoid agonists (Panlilio, Justinova, & Goldberg, 2013). A study examining the efficacy of FAAH inhibitors in reducing cannabis withdrawal in cannabis-dependent participants is currently underway at Yale University. However, the catastrophic preclinical trial of the FAAH inhibitor BIA 10-2474-101, which led to the death of one participant and serious injury to a further five, sounds a new note of caution for future studies of compounds impacting the ECS for a range of indications.

BEST APPROACHES FOR ASSESSING TREATMENT RESPONSE AND MANAGING SIDE EFFECTS

Given there are no pharmacological treatments for the management of cannabis withdrawal or CUD that have been approved, there is no agreed upon approach to assessing treatment responses outside the research environment. The efficacy of medications other than cannabinoids is poor and only typically show promise when combined with a cannabinoid in clinical trials, hence they will be the focus.

As with all clinical trials, the use of valid and reliable measures should be standardized practice in order to generate comparable data for meta-analytical approaches and development of the evidence-base for the management of CUD. The key outcome for trials assessing a pharmacotherapy for cannabis withdrawal is appropriate measure of the syndrome. The only validated measure is the Cannabis Withdrawal Scale (Allsop et al., 2012; Allsop,

Norberg, Copeland, Fu, & Budney, 2011). Similarly, retention in treatment, quantity/frequency of cannabis use (preferably using a standardized calendar prompt method such as Timeline Followback; Norberg et al., 2012; Tomko et al., 2018), and presence/severity of CUD should be primary study outcomes. It might also be advantageous to enable prospective observational studies through creation of registries, protocols, and mandatory reporting of adverse events (Deshpande, Mailis-Gagnon, Zoheiry, & Lakha, 2015).

The adverse effects of THC are not yet well understood, especially in the long term, and nothing is known of the effects of pediatric use of cannabinoids over the life course. Given the paucity of research on the use of cannabinoids for the management of CUD, the wider literature on their use for other conditions may be helpful. The review by Whiting and colleagues (2015) assessed adverse events associated with trials to date and showed that cannabinoid trials were associated with a significant adverse event burden. Common adverse effects included asthenia, balance problems, confusion, dizziness, disorientation, diarrhea, euphoria, drowsiness, dry mouth, fatigue, hallucinations, nausea, somnolence, and vomiting, with no differences with mode or type of cannabinoid studied (Whiting et al., 2015). This study reported typically narrow confidence intervals indicating high precision of estimates and the heterogeneity across trials was mostly low to moderate, indicating findings were similar across studies (Andrade, 2016). Clinical trials in the management of CUD are typically short term (12 weeks, and often fewer of dosing), with small sample sizes and short follow-up periods (4–12 weeks) at the end of dosing only, little objective monitoring of medication compliance, and no biological validation of self-reported cannabis use. More complete toxicological evaluations of compounds, such as genotoxicity and assessment of the effects of cannabinoids on hormones and immune function, are scarce, as are data on drug–cannabinoid interactions (Iffland & Grotenhermen, 2017).

MEDICATION MANAGEMENT ISSUES

As there are no approved medications for CUD, there is no postmarket testing of medication management in a community setting. Treatment

retention is poor in many trials of medications that modulate neurotransmitter systems other than the ECS (Gorelick, 2016). The extant trials typically have tight inclusion criteria that exclude the majority of those with CUD, as they frequently use alcohol and other drugs and have comorbid mental health disorders/psychological distress (Okuda et al., 2010), and this will affect guidelines for medication management into the future as pharmacotherapies are approved for CUD. The sex ratios of participants typically reflect those of the population of people with CUD, around 60% to 70% male, and no studies have examined differences in adverse events and their management at this early stage of the evidence base development.

EVALUATION OF PHARMACOLOGICAL APPROACHES ACROSS THE LIFESPAN

There has been no evaluation of these pharmacological approaches across the lifespan (childhood, adolescence, emerging adulthood, adulthood, elderly). An overarching consideration when contemplating prescribing a cannabinoid preparation is the general risk-to-benefit ratio. When the condition being treated is not severe and life limiting, such as with CUD, and where there is no evidence of the efficacy—let alone the effectiveness—of the compound for that condition, the risks potentially associated with the prescribing of a potent THC product for the young and the elderly should be prioritized. For those aged younger than 16 years, THC may disrupt brain development (Kolb, Li, Robinson, & Parker, 2017; Renard et al., 2016) and increase the risk of developing CUD and mental health conditions such as a psychotic illness (Silins et al., 2014; Whitfield-Gabrieli et al., 2018). Trials of relatively low-dose THC exposure in the evaluation of nabiximols for multiple sclerosis in an aging population found that the most common relevant adverse events likely to increase the risk of slips and falls were dizziness, fatigue, somnolence, and vertigo, at typically mild to moderate intensity and resolving within a few days, even with continued THC/CBD treatment (Keating, 2017). A further concern is the interaction of THC with alcohol, affecting coordination, concentration, and the ability to respond quickly (Keating, 2017).

CONSIDERATION OF POTENTIAL SEX DIFFERENCES

There is considerable intersubject variation in response to the psychotogenic effects of cannabinoids (Atakan, 2012) and there are sex differences in the analgesic effects of THC (Cooper, Comer, & Haney, 2013). Recent research has demonstrated that among cannabis smokers, men exhibit greater cannabis-induced analgesia relative to women that is independent of cannabis-elicited subjective effects associated with abuse liability, which were consistent between men and women. As such, sex-dependent differences in cannabis's analgesic effects warrant further investigation when considering the potential therapeutic effects of cannabinoids for pain relief (Cooper & Haney, 2016). A recent review of the potential mechanisms of sex differences in cannabis use reported variations in the endocannabinoid system by sex, along with differences in cannabis exposure effects on brain structure and function and in the co-occurrence of cannabis use with symptoms of anxiety, depression, and schizophrenia (Calakos, Bhatt, Foster, & Cosgrove, 2017). Further, female cannabis users are reported to be especially vulnerable to earlier onset of schizophrenia, and mixed trends emerge in the correlation of depressive symptoms with cannabis exposure in females and males (Calakos et al., 2017).

INTEGRATION OF PHARMACOTHERAPY WITH NONPHARMACOLOGICAL APPROACHES: BENEFITS AND CHALLENGES

The intervention approaches for adults and adolescents with the strongest evidence base to date are based on the combination of MET and CBT, particularly in assisting with reduction of cannabis use frequency at early follow-up—although no intervention was consistently effective at 9-month follow-up or later. MET is a counseling approach that helps individuals resolve their ambivalence about engaging in treatment and changing/stopping their drug use. This approach aims to evoke rapid and internally motivated change, rather than guide the patient stepwise through the recovery process (Copeland, 2017). CBT is a relatively short-term,

focused approach to treatment of many types of behavioral and psychiatric conditions. It is a collaborative and individualized intervention that helps the individual identify unhelpful thoughts and behaviors and learn and relearn healthier skills and habits. Techniques include managing craving, high-risk situation management, and relapse prevention (González-Ortega, Echeburúa, García-Alocén, Vega, & González-Pinto, 2016).

In addition, some studies support the utility of adding voucher-based incentives for cannabis-negative urine screens, known as contingency management, to enhance treatment effect on cannabis use frequency (Schuster et al., 2016). In line with treatments for other substance use, abstinence rates were relatively low overall, with approximately one quarter of participants abstinent at final follow-up (Gates, Sabioni, Copeland, Le Foll, & Gowing, 2016).

Given that psychosocial approaches to CUD typically yield low and unstable abstinence rates, which are nonetheless comparable with treatments for other SUD (Gates et al., 2016), the addition of a pharmacological agent will be an important development in the management of CUD. As the development of an approved medication for CUD has not yet been achieved, all clinical trials of medications should include key elements of CBT and MET to improve recruitment to studies and enhance medication compliance, retention in treatment, and relapse prevention. The major challenge to incorporation of psychosocial interventions is the additional staff time and training. As a result it is reasonable to suggest that such elements included in clinical trials may not always be implemented in general clinical practice. This may be offset by the use of a telephone helpline (Gates, Norberg, Copeland, & Digiusto, 2012), web-based delivery (Rooke, Thorsteinsson, Karpin, Copeland, & Allsop, 2010), or the use of smartphone applications (Bakker, Kazantzis, Rickwood, & Rickard, 2016). Unfortunately there is no evidence-based intervention for those with comorbid CUD and other mental health conditions; hence no recommendation for either pharmacotherapy or psychosocial intervention can be made at this stage (Krawczyk et al., 2017).

INTEGRATED APPROACHES FOR ADDRESSING COMMON COMORBID DISORDERS

CUD is frequently associated with concurrent substance use and/or comorbid SUDs. A recent U.S. epidemiological study of adults aged 18 and older from Wave 3 of the National Epidemiologic Survey on Alcohol and Related Conditions (NESARC-III) found that a current *DSM–5* CUD was associated with greater lifetime use of all examined drug classes and previous 12-month use of several newer-class illicit and prescription stimulant-based substances, and with sedative, cocaine, stimulant, club drugs, opioids, and alcohol use disorders but not heroin use disorder (Hasin et al., 2016). In addition to other substance use disorders, the most common psychiatric conditions comorbid with current CUD in the same data set, were mood disorders (odds ratio [OR] = 2.7–5.0), anxiety disorders (OR = 1.7–3.7), posttraumatic stress disorder (PTSD; OR = 3.8), and personality disorders (OR = 3.8–5.0). Lifetime CUD was also associated with mood disorders (OR = 2.6–3.8), anxiety disorders (OR = 2.1–3.2), PTSD (OR = 5.0), and personality disorders (OR = 4.0–4.7). Across severity levels, 12-month and lifetime CUDs were associated with other disorders. Further, with few exceptions (12-month bipolar II disorder, agoraphobia, and specific phobia), associations became stronger (i.e., progressively higher odds ratios) as the severity of CUD increased (Hasin et al., 2016). Given the prevalence of the comorbidity of CUD with a range of other mental health conditions, most commonly other SUDs, it is concerning that there is no evidence-based psychosocial or pharmacological intervention for their management. General clinical guidelines are the only sources of assessment and management at this time (Copeland, 2016).

EMERGING TRENDS

The nascent stage of development of the field of pharmacological interventions for CUD makes all studies emerging trends. Perusal of the www.ClinicalTrials.gov website for the registration of current research reveals studies of some of the medications for CUD described in Table 23.1 and discussed in the 2014 Cochrane review (Marshall, Gowing, Ali, & Le Foll, 2014), and

also some novel medications. These include the anti-obesity drug lorcaserin, the glutamatergic modulator CI-581a, the anticonvulsant pregabalin, the monoamine oxidase B inhibitor selegiline, and the substance P antagonist aprepitant. There are also novel cannabinoids such as tetrahydrocannabivarin (Englund et al., 2016). The most promising of the cannabinoids that has been subject to even Phase II trials is CBD, as set out earlier in the chapter. Studies of the use of CBD as an adjunctive therapy for those with schizophrenia (McGuire et al., 2018) lend further support to the importance of trials of its efficacy among young people with developing mood or psychotic disorders who also use cannabis or have CUD. It may be hypothesized that it may positively impact cannabis craving and levels of use, in addition to improvement in psychiatric functioning.

CUD commonly occurs and carries a notable economic and functional burden at both the individual and societal levels. While there are no clearly efficacious medication treatments for CUD, 20 years of committed and high-quality research in the human laboratory and in clinical settings has resulted in medications with demonstrated effectiveness in the treatment of cannabis withdrawal, the ability to reduce cannabis use, and results that point to promising future work. The current state of pharmacology research for CUD highlights the need to consider particular characteristics of patients, such as sex, impulsivity, and severity of cannabis use, when selecting a medication in the off-label treatment of CUD or cannabis withdrawal. As a field, the body of work also exposes some areas in need of improvement in study design, selection of outcome measures, interpretation of results, and the overall process of evaluating candidate medications. Coming to a consensus as a field and addressing these gaps in future research will likely lend itself to further advances in improving the lives of patients with CUD.

TOOL KIT OF RESOURCES

Cannabis Use Disorder

Patient Resources

Cannabis Information and Support: A website containing evidence-based information and cannabis, CUD and a range of interventions: https://cannabissupport.com.au/

Includes a free web-based intervention with six sessions of CBT: https://cannabissupport.com.au/treatment/tools-to-quit/reduce-your-use/

Also includes a harm reduction intervention for young people: https://cannabissupport.com.au/treatment/tools-to-quit/clear-your-vision/

Government Websites: Websites such as the ones below should be monitored for new developments and guidelines: https://www.drugabuse.gov/drugs-abuse/marijuana/nida-research-marijuana-cannabinoids; https://clinicaltrials.gov/

Provider Resources

Cannabis Information and Support: A tool kit for primary health care practitioners: https://cannabissupport.com.au/media/4481/gp-factsheets-for-patients-and-gps-2016-combined-version.pdf

Cannabis Information and Support: Screening and assessment of cannabis use disorder: https://cannabissupport.com.au/media/1604/screening-and-assessment-for-cannabis-use-disorders.pdf

Marijuana Brief Intervention: Clinical guidelines on the delivery of a range of CUD interventions known as Marijuana Brief Intervention: https://www.hazelden.org/OA_HTML/ibeCCtpItmDspRte.jsp?item=442137&sitex=10020:22372:US

References

Adams, T. R., Arnsten, J. H., Ning, Y., & Nahvi, S. (2018). Feasibility and preliminary effectiveness of varenicline for treating co-occurring cannabis and tobacco use. *Journal of Psychoactive Drugs, 50,* 12–18. http://dx.doi.org/10.1080/02791072.2017.1370746

Agosti, V., & Levin, F. R. (2004). Predictors of treatment contact among individuals with cannabis dependence. *The American Journal of Drug and Alcohol Abuse, 30,* 121–127. http://dx.doi.org/10.1081/ADA-120029869

Agrawal, A., Nelson, E. C., Bucholz, K. K., Tillman, R., Grucza, R. A., Statham, D. J., . . . Lynskey, M. T. (2017). Major depressive disorder, suicidal thoughts and behaviours, and cannabis involvement in discordant twins: A retrospective cohort study. *The Lancet Psychiatry, 4,* 706–714. http://dx.doi.org/10.1016/S2215-0366(17)30280-8

Allsop, D. J., Bartlett, D. J., Johnston, J., Helliwell, D., Winstock, A., McGregor, I. S., & Lintzeris, N. (2015). The effects of lithium carbonate supple-

mented with nitrazepam on sleep disturbance during cannabis abstinence. *Journal of Clinical Sleep Medicine, 11,* 1153–1162. http://dx.doi.org/10.5664/jcsm.5090

Allsop, D. J., Copeland, J., Lintzeris, N., Dunlop, A. J., Montebello, M., Sadler, C., . . . McGregor, I. S. (2014). Nabiximols as an agonist replacement therapy during cannabis withdrawal: A randomized clinical trial. *JAMA Psychiatry, 71,* 281–291. http://dx.doi.org/10.1001/jamapsychiatry.2013.3947

Allsop, D. J., Copeland, J., Norberg, M. M., Fu, S., Molnar, A., Lewis, J., & Budney, A. J. (2012). Quantifying the clinical significance of cannabis withdrawal. *PLoS ONE, 7,* e44864. http://dx.doi.org/10.1371/journal.pone.0044864

Allsop, D. J., Norberg, M. M., Copeland, J., Fu, S., & Budney, A. J. (2011). The Cannabis Withdrawal Scale development: Patterns and predictors of cannabis withdrawal and distress. *Drug and Alcohol Dependence, 119,* 123–129. http://dx.doi.org/10.1016/j.drugalcdep.2011.06.003

American Psychiatric Association. (2013). *Diagnostic and statistical manual of mental disorders* (5th ed.). Washington, DC: Author.

Andrade, C. (2016). Cannabis and neuropsychiatry, 1: Benefits and risks. *The Journal of Clinical Psychiatry, 77,* e551–e554. http://dx.doi.org/10.4088/JCP.16f10841

Asbridge, M., Hayden, J. A., & Cartwright, J. L. (2012). Acute cannabis consumption and motor vehicle collision risk: Systematic review of observational studies and meta-analysis. *BMJ: British Medical Journal, 344,* e536. http://dx.doi.org/10.1136/bmj.e536

Atakan, Z. (2012). Cannabis, a complex plant: Different compounds and different effects on individuals. *Therapeutic Advances in Psychopharmacology, 2,* 241–254. http://dx.doi.org/10.1177/2045125312457586

Australian Institute of Health and Welfare. (2013). *Alcohol and other drug treatment services in Australia 2013–14.* Canberra, Australia: Author.

Australian Institute of Health and Welfare. (2017). *National Drug Strategy Household Survey 2016: Detailed findings.* Retrieved from https://www.aihw.gov.au/reports/illicit-use-of-drugs/ndshs-2016-detailed/contents/table-of-contents

*Bakker, D., Kazantzis, N., Rickwood, D., & Rickard, N. (2016). Mental health smartphone apps: Review and evidence-based recommendations for future developments. *JMIR Mental Health, 3,* e7. http://dx.doi.org/10.2196/mental.4984

Balter, R. E., Cooper, Z. D., & Haney, M. (2014). Novel pharmacologic approaches to treating Cannabis Use

*Asterisks indicate assessments or resources.

Disorder. *Current Addiction Reports, 1*, 137–143. http://dx.doi.org/10.1007/s40429-014-0011-1

Bashford, J. (2009). *Screening and assessment for cannabis use disorders*. Retrieved from https://cannabissupport.com.au/media/1604/screening-and-assessment-for-cannabis-use-disorders.pdf

*Bashford, J., Flett, R., & Copeland, J. (2010). The Cannabis Use Problems Identification Test (CUPIT): Development, reliability, concurrent and predictive validity among adolescents and adults. *Addiction, 105*, 615–625. http://dx.doi.org/10.1111/j.1360-0443.2009.02859.x

Bedi, G., Cooper, Z. D., & Haney, M. (2013). Subjective, cognitive and cardiovascular dose-effect profile of nabilone and dronabinol in marijuana smokers. *Addiction Biology, 18*, 872–881. http://dx.doi.org/10.1111/j.1369-1600.2011.00427.x

Benyamina, A., Lecacheux, M., Blecha, L., Reynaud, M., & Lukasiewcz, M. (2008). Pharmacotherapy and psychotherapy in cannabis withdrawal and dependence. *Expert Review of Neurotherapeutics, 8*, 479–491. http://dx.doi.org/10.1586/14737175.8.3.479

Bergamaschi, M. M., Queiroz, R. H. C., Zuardi, A. W., & Crippa, J. A. (2011). Safety and side effects of cannabidiol, a Cannabis sativa constituent. *Current Drug Safety, 6*, 237–249. http://dx.doi.org/10.2174/157488611798280924

Bowen, R., McIlwrick, J., Baetz, M., & Zhang, X. (2005). Lithium and marijuana withdrawal. *The Canadian Journal of Psychiatry, 50*, 240–241. http://dx.doi.org/10.1177/070674370505000410

Breivogel, C. S., Scates, S. M., Beletskaya, I. O., Lowery, O. B., Aceto, M. D., & Martin, B. R. (2003). The effects of Δ⁹-tetrahydrocannabinol physical dependence on brain cannabinoid receptors. *European Journal of Pharmacology, 459*, 139–150. http://dx.doi.org/10.1016/S0014-2999(02)02854-6

Budney, A. J., & Hughes, J. R. (2006). The cannabis withdrawal syndrome. *Current Opinion in Psychiatry, 19*(3), 233–238. http://dx.doi.org/10.1097/01.yco.0000218592.00689.e5

Budney, A. J., Moore, B. A., Vandrey, R. G., & Hughes, J. R. (2003). The time course and significance of cannabis withdrawal. *Journal of Abnormal Psychology, 112*, 393–402. http://dx.doi.org/10.1037/0021-843X.112.3.393

Budney, A. J., Vandrey, R. G., Hughes, J. R., Moore, B. A., & Bahrenburg, B. (2007). Oral delta-9-tetrahydrocannabinol suppresses cannabis withdrawal symptoms. *Drug and Alcohol Dependence, 86*, 22–29. http://dx.doi.org/10.1016/j.drugalcdep.2006.04.014

Calakos, K. C., Bhatt, S., Foster, D. W., & Cosgrove, K. P. (2017). Mechanisms underlying sex differences in cannabis use. *Current Addiction Reports, 4*, 439–453. http://dx.doi.org/10.1007/s40429-017-0174-7

Carpenter, K. M., McDowell, D., Brooks, D. J., Cheng, W. Y., & Levin, F. R. (2009). A preliminary trial: Double-blind comparison of nefazodone, bupropion-SR, and placebo in the treatment of cannabis dependence. *The American Journal on Addictions, 18*, 53–64. http://dx.doi.org/10.1080/10550490802408936

Center for Behavioral Health Statistics. (2014). Results from the 2013 National Survey on Drug Use and Health: Summary of National Findings. Retrieved from https://www.samhsa.gov/data/sites/default/files/NSDUHresultsPDFWHTML2013/Web/NSDUHresults2013.pdf

Cheer, J. F., & Hurd, Y. L. (2017). A new dawn in cannabinoid neurobiology: The road from molecules to therapeutic discoveries. *Neuropharmacology, 124*, 1–2. http://dx.doi.org/10.1016/j.neuropharm.2017.07.004

Christensen, R., Kristensen, P. K., Bartels, E. M., Bliddal, H., & Astrup, A. (2007). Efficacy and safety of the weight-loss drug rimonabant: A meta-analysis of randomised trials. *The Lancet, 370*, 1706–1713. http://dx.doi.org/10.1016/S0140-6736(07)61721-8

Cooper, Z. D., Comer, S. D., & Haney, M. (2013). Comparison of the analgesic effects of dronabinol and smoked marijuana in daily marijuana smokers. *Neuropsychopharmacology, 38*, 1984–1992. http://dx.doi.org/10.1038/npp.2013.97

Cooper, Z. D., Foltin, R. W., Hart, C. L., Vosburg, S. K., Comer, S. D., & Haney, M. (2013). A human laboratory study investigating the effects of quetiapine on marijuana withdrawal and relapse in daily marijuana smokers. *Addiction Biology, 18*, 993–1002. http://dx.doi.org/10.1111/j.1369-1600.2012.00461.x

Cooper, Z. D., & Haney, M. (2010). Opioid antagonism enhances marijuana's effects in heavy marijuana smokers. *Psychopharmacology, 211*, 141–148. http://dx.doi.org/10.1007/s00213-010-1875-y

Cooper, Z. D., & Haney, M. (2016). Sex-dependent effects of cannabis-induced analgesia. *Drug and Alcohol Dependence, 167*, 112–120. http://dx.doi.org/10.1016/j.drugalcdep.2016.08.001

Copeland, J. (2016). Cannabis use and its associated disorders: Clinical care. *Australian Family Physician, 45*, 874–877. http://www.ncbi.nlm.nih.gov/pubmed/27903036

*Copeland, J. (2017). *Marijuana Brief intervention: An SBIRT Approach*. Center City, Minnesota: Hazelden Publishing.

*Copeland, J., Gilmour, S., Gates, P., & Swift, W. (2005). The Cannabis Problems Questionnaire: Factor structure, reliability, and validity. *Drug and Alcohol Dependence, 80*, 313–319. http://dx.doi.org/10.1016/j.drugalcdep.2005.04.009

*Copeland, J., & Pokorski, I. (2016). Progress toward pharmacotherapies for cannabis-use disorder: An evidence-based review. *Substance Abuse and

Rehabilitation, 7, 41–53. http://dx.doi.org/10.2147/SAR.S89857

Copeland, J., Rook, S., & Matalon, E. (2015). *Quit cannabis*. Sydney, Australia: Allen & Unwin.

Copeland, J., & Swift, W. (2009). Cannabis use disorder: Epidemiology and management. *International Review of Psychiatry, 21*, 96–103. http://dx.doi.org/10.1080/09540260902782745

Copeland, J., Swift, W., & Rees, V. (2001). Clinical profile of participants in a brief intervention program for cannabis use disorder. *Journal of Substance Abuse Treatment, 20*, 45–52. http://dx.doi.org/10.1016/S0740-5472(00)00148-3

Cornelius, J. R., Bukstein, O. G., Douaihy, A. B., Clark, D. B., Chung, T. A., Daley, D. C., . . . Brown, S. J. (2010). Double-blind fluoxetine trial in comorbid MDD-CUD youth and young adults. *Drug and Alcohol Dependence, 112*, 39–45. http://dx.doi.org/10.1016/j.drugalcdep.2010.05.010

Cornelius, J. R., Clark, D. B., Bukstein, O. G., Birmaher, B., Salloum, I. M., & Brown, S. A. (2005). Acute phase and five-year follow-up study of fluoxetine in adolescents with major depression and a comorbid substance use disorder: A review. *Addictive Behaviors, 30*, 1824–1833. http://dx.doi.org/10.1016/j.addbeh.2005.07.007

Crippa, J. A. S., Hallak, J. E. C., Machado-de-Sousa, J. P., Queiroz, R. H. C., Bergamaschi, M., Chagas, M. H. N., & Zuardi, A. W. (2013). Cannabidiol for the treatment of *cannabis* withdrawal syndrome: A case report. *Journal of Clinical Pharmacy and Therapeutics, 38*, 162–164. http://dx.doi.org/10.1111/jcpt.12018

Curran, H. V., Freeman, T. P., Mokrysz, C., Lewis, D. A., Morgan, C. J. A., & Parsons, L. H. (2016). Keep off the grass? Cannabis, cognition and addiction. *Nature Reviews Neuroscience, 17*, 293–306. http://dx.doi.org/10.1038/nrn.2016.28

Davenport, S. S., & Caulkins, J. P. (2016). Evolution of the United States marijuana market in the decade of liberalization before full legalization. *Journal of Drug Issues, 46*, 411–427. http://dx.doi.org/10.1177/0022042616659759

Dennis, M., Babor, T. F., Roebuck, M. C., & Donaldson, J. (2002). Changing the focus: The case for recognizing and treating cannabis use disorders. *Addiction, 97*(Suppl. 1), 4–15. http://dx.doi.org/10.1046/j.1360-0443.97.s01.10.x

Deshpande, A., Mailis-Gagnon, A., Zoheiry, N., & Lakha, S. F. (2015). Efficacy and adverse effects of medical marijuana for chronic noncancer pain: Systematic review of randomized controlled trials. *Canadian Family Physician: Medecin de Famille Canadien, 61*, e372–e381. http://www.ncbi.nlm.nih.gov/pubmed/26505059

Englund, A., Atakan, Z., Kralj, A., Tunstall, N., Murray, R., & Morrison, P. (2016). The effect of five day dosing with THCV on THC-induced cognitive, psychological and physiological effects in healthy male human volunteers: A placebo-controlled, double-blind, crossover pilot trial. *Journal of Psychopharmacology, 30*, 140–151. http://dx.doi.org/10.1177/0269881115615104

European Monitoring Centre for Drugs and Drug Addiction. (2015). *European Drug Report 2015: Trends and Developments*. Lisbon, Portugal: Author.

First, M. B., Williams, J. B. W., Karg, R. S., & Spitzer, R. L. (2015). *Structured Clinical Interview for DSM–5—Research Version (SCID-5 for DSM–5, Research Version; SCID-5-RV)*. Arlington, VA: American Psychiatric Association. http://www.scid5.org/

Gaoni, Y., & Mechoulam, R. (1964). Isolation, structure, and partial synthesis of an active constituent of hashish. *Journal of the American Chemical Society, 86*, 1646–1647. http://dx.doi.org/10.1021/ja01062a046

Gates, P., Copeland, J., Swift, W., & Martin, G. (2012). Barriers and facilitators to cannabis treatment. *Drug and Alcohol Review, 31*, 311–319. http://dx.doi.org/10.1111/j.1465-3362.2011.00313.x

Gates, P., Jaffe, A., & Copeland, J. (2014). Cannabis smoking and respiratory health: Consideration of the literature. *Respirology, 19*, 655–662. http://dx.doi.org/10.1111/resp.12298

Gates, P. J., Norberg, M. M., Copeland, J., & Digiusto, E. (2012). Randomized controlled trial of a novel cannabis use intervention delivered by telephone. *Addiction, 107*, 2149–2158. http://dx.doi.org/10.1111/j.1360-0443.2012.03953.x

Gates, P. J., Sabioni, P., Copeland, J., Le Foll, B., & Gowing, L. (2016). Psychosocial interventions for cannabis use disorder. *Cochrane Database of Systematic Reviews*, (5): CD005336.

González-Ortega, I., Echeburúa, E., García-Alocén, A., Vega, P., & González-Pinto, A. (2016). Cognitive behavioral therapy program for cannabis use cessation in first-episode psychosis patients: Study protocol for a randomized controlled trial. *Trials, 17*, 372. http://dx.doi.org/10.1186/s13063-016-1507-x

Gorelick, D. A. (2016). Pharmacological treatment of cannabis-related disorders: A narrative review. *Current Pharmaceutical Design, 22*, 6409–6419. http://dx.doi.org/10.2174/1381612822666160822150822

Gray, K. M., Carpenter, M. J., Baker, N. L., DeSantis, S. M., Kryway, E., Hartwell, K. J., . . . Brady, K. T. (2012). A double-blind randomized controlled trial of N-acetylcysteine in cannabis-dependent adolescents. *The American Journal of Psychiatry, 169*, 805–812. http://dx.doi.org/10.1176/appi.ajp.2012.12010055

Gray, K. M., Sonne, S. C., McClure, E. A., Ghitza, U. E., Matthews, A. G., McRae-Clark, A. L., . . . Levin, F. R.

(2017). A randomized placebo-controlled trial of N-acetylcysteine for cannabis use disorder in adults. *Drug and Alcohol Dependence, 177*, 249–257. http://dx.doi.org/10.1016/j.drugalcdep.2017.04.020

Gray, K. M., Watson, N. L., Carpenter, M. J., & Larowe, S. D. (2010). N-acetylcysteine (NAC) in young marijuana users: An open-label pilot study. *The American Journal on Addictions, 19*, 187–189. http://dx.doi.org/10.1111/j.1521-0391.2009.00027.x

Greenwald, M. K., & Stitzer, M. L. (2000). Antinociceptive, subjective and behavioral effects of smoked marijuana in humans. *Drug and Alcohol Dependence, 59*, 261–275. http://dx.doi.org/10.1016/S0376-8716(99)00128-3

Hall, W. D., & Pacula, R. L. (2003). *Cannabis use and dependence: Public health and public policy.* Cambridge, United Kingdom: Cambridge University Press. http://dx.doi.org/10.1017/CBO9780511470219

Haney, M. (2005). The marijuana withdrawal syndrome: Diagnosis and treatment. *Current Psychiatry Reports, 7*, 360–366. http://dx.doi.org/10.1007/s11920-005-0036-1

Haney, M. (2007). Opioid antagonism of cannabinoid effects: Differences between marijuana smokers and nonmarijuana smokers. *Neuropsychopharmacology, 32*, 1391–1403. http://dx.doi.org/10.1038/sj.npp.1301243

Haney, M., Cooper, Z. D., Bedi, G., Herrmann, E., Comer, S. D., Collins Reed, S., . . . Levin, F. R. (2018). Guanfacine decreases symptoms of cannabis withdrawal in daily cannabis smokers. *Addiction Biology.* Advance online publication. http://dx.doi.org/10.1111/adb.12621

Haney, M., Cooper, Z. D., Bedi, G., Vosburg, S. K., Comer, S. D., & Foltin, R. W. (2013). Nabilone decreases marijuana withdrawal and a laboratory measure of marijuana relapse. *Neuropsychopharmacology, 38*, 1557–1565. http://dx.doi.org/10.1038/npp.2013.54

Haney, M., Hart, C. L., Vosburg, S. K., Comer, S. D., Reed, S. C., Cooper, Z. D., & Foltin, R. W. (2010). Effects of baclofen and mirtazapine on a laboratory model of marijuana withdrawal and relapse. *Psychopharmacology, 211*, 233–244. http://dx.doi.org/10.1007/s00213-010-1888-6

Haney, M., Hart, C. L., Vosburg, S. K., Comer, S. D., Reed, S. C., & Foltin, R. W. (2008). Effects of THC and lofexidine in a human laboratory model of marijuana withdrawal and relapse. *Psychopharmacology, 197*, 157–168. http://dx.doi.org/10.1007/s00213-007-1020-8

Haney, M., Hart, C. L., Vosburg, S. K., Nasser, J., Bennett, A., Zubaran, C., & Foltin, R. W. (2004). Marijuana withdrawal in humans: Effects of oral THC or divalproex. *Neuropsychopharmacology, 29*, 158–170. http://dx.doi.org/10.1038/sj.npp.1300310

Haney, M., Hart, C. L., Ward, A. S., & Foltin, R. W. (2003). Nefazodone decreases anxiety during marijuana withdrawal in humans. *Psychopharmacology, 165*, 157–165. http://dx.doi.org/10.1007/s00213-002-1210-3

Haney, M., Ramesh, D., Glass, A., Pavlicova, M., Bedi, G., & Cooper, Z. D. (2015). Naltrexone maintenance decreases cannabis self-administration and subjective effects in daily cannabis smokers. *Neuropsychopharmacology, 40*, 2489–2498. http://dx.doi.org/10.1038/npp.2015.108

Haney, M., Ward, A. S., Comer, S. D., Hart, C. L., Foltin, R. W., & Fischman, M. W. (2001). Bupropion SR worsens mood during marijuana withdrawal in humans. *Psychopharmacology, 155*, 171–179. http://dx.doi.org/10.1007/s002130000657

Hasin, D. S., Kerridge, B. T., Saha, T. D., Huang, B., Pickering, R., Smith, S. M., . . . Grant, B. F. (2016). Prevalence and correlates of DSM–5 cannabis use disorder, 2012–2013: Findings from the National Epidemiologic Survey on Alcohol and Related Conditions-III. *The American Journal of Psychiatry, 173*, 588–599. http://dx.doi.org/10.1176/appi.ajp.2015.15070907

Hasin, D. S., Saha, T. D., Kerridge, B. T., Goldstein, R. B., Chou, S. P., Zhang, H., . . . Grant, B. F. (2015). Prevalence of marijuana use disorders in the United States between 2001–2002 and 2012–2013. *JAMA Psychiatry, 72*, 1235–1242. http://dx.doi.org/10.1001/jamapsychiatry.2015.1858

Hayakawa, K., Mishima, K., Nozako, M., Ogata, A., Hazekawa, M., Liu, A.-X., . . . Fujiwara, M. (2007). Repeated treatment with cannabidiol but not Δ^9-tetrahydrocannabinol has a neuroprotective effect without the development of tolerance. *Neuropharmacology, 52*, 1079–1087. http://dx.doi.org/10.1016/j.neuropharm.2006.11.005

Hermann, E. S., Cooper, Z. D., Bedi, G., Ramesh, D., Reed, S. C., Comer, S. D., . . . Haney, M. (2016). Effects of zolpidem alone and in combination with nabilone on cannabis withdrawal and a laboratory model of relapse in cannabis users. *Psychopharmacology, 233*, 2469–2478. http://dx.doi.org/10.1007/s00213-016-4298-6

Huestis, M. A., Boyd, S. J., Heishman, S. J., Preston, K. L., Bonnet, D., Le Fur, G., & Gorelick, D. A. (2007). Single and multiple doses of rimonabant antagonize acute effects of smoked cannabis in male cannabis users. *Psychopharmacology, 194*, 505–515. http://dx.doi.org/10.1007/s00213-007-0861-5

Huestis, M. A., Gorelick, D. A., Heishman, S. J., Preston, K. L., Nelson, R. A., Moolchan, E. T., & Frank, R. A. (2001). Blockade of effects of smoked marijuana by the CB1-selective cannabinoid receptor antagonist SR141716. *Archives of General*

Psychiatry, 58, 322–328. http://dx.doi.org/10.1001/archpsyc.58.4.322

Iffland, K., & Grotenhermen, F. (2017). An update on safety and side effects of cannabidiol: A review of clinical data and relevant animal studies. *Cannabis and Cannabinoid Research, 2*, 139–154. http://dx.doi.org/10.1089/can.2016.0034

Johnston, J., Lintzeris, N., Allsop, D. J., Suraev, A., Booth, J., Carson, D. S., . . . McGregor, I. S. (2014). Lithium carbonate in the management of cannabis withdrawal: A randomized placebo-controlled trial in an inpatient setting. *Psychopharmacology, 231*, 4623–4636. http://dx.doi.org/10.1007/s00213-014-3611-5

Keating, G. M. (2017). Delta-9-Tetrahydrocannabinol/Cannabidiol oromucosal spray (Sativex®): A review in multiple sclerosis-related spasticity. *Drugs, 77*, 563–574. http://dx.doi.org/10.1007/s40265-017-0720-6

Kolb, B., Li, Y., Robinson, T., & Parker, L. A. (2017). THC alters morphology of neurons in medial prefrontal cortex, orbital prefrontal cortex, and nucleus accumbens and alters the ability of later experience to promote structural plasticity. *Synapse, 72*, e22020. http://dx.doi.org/10.1002/syn.22020

Krawczyk, N., Feder, K. A., Saloner, B., Crum, R. M., Kealhofer, M., & Mojtabai, R. (2017). The association of psychiatric comorbidity with treatment completion among clients admitted to substance use treatment programs in a U.S. national sample. *Drug and Alcohol Dependence, 175*, 157–163. http://dx.doi.org/10.1016/j.drugalcdep.2017.02.006

Levin, F. R., & Kleber, H. D. (2008). Use of dronabinol for cannabis dependence: Two case reports and review. *The American Journal on Addictions, 17*, 161–164. http://dx.doi.org/10.1080/10550490701861177

Levin, F. R., Mariani, J., Brooks, D. J., Pavlicova, M., Nunes, E. V., Agosti, V., . . . Carpenter, K. M. (2013). A randomized double-blind, placebo-controlled trial of venlafaxine-extended release for co-occurring cannabis dependence and depressive disorders. *Addiction, 108*, 1084–1094. http://dx.doi.org/10.1111/add.12108

Levin, F. R., Mariani, J. J., Brooks, D. J., Pavlicova, M., Cheng, W., & Nunes, E. V. (2011). Dronabinol for the treatment of cannabis dependence: A randomized, double-blind, placebo-controlled trial. *Drug and Alcohol Dependence, 116*(1–3), 142–150. http://dx.doi.org/10.1016/j.drugalcdep.2010.12.010

Levin, F. R., Mariani, J. J., Pavlicova, M., Brooks, D., Glass, A., Mahony, A., . . . Choi, J. C. (2016). Dronabinol and lofexidine for cannabis use disorder: A randomized, double-blind, placebo-controlled trial. *Drug and Alcohol Dependence, 159*, 53–60. http://dx.doi.org/10.1016/j.drugalcdep.2015.11.025

Levin, F. R., McDowell, D., Evans, S. M., Nunes, E., Akerele, E., Donovan, S., & Vosburg, S. K. (2004).

Pharmacotherapy for marijuana dependence: A double-blind, placebo-controlled pilot study of divalproex sodium. *The American Journal on Addictions, 13*, 21–32. http://dx.doi.org/10.1080/10550490490265280

Lin, L. A., Ilgen, M. A., Jannausch, M., & Bohnert, K. M. (2016). Comparing adults who use cannabis medically with those who use recreationally: Results from a national sample. *Addictive Behaviors, 61*, 99–103. http://dx.doi.org/10.1016/j.addbeh.2016.05.015

Lisdahl, K. M., Wright, N. E., Medina-Kirchner, C., Maple, K. E., & Shollenbarger, S. (2014). Considering cannabis: The effects of regular cannabis use on neurocognition in adolescents and young adults. *Current Addiction Reports, 1*, 144–156. http://dx.doi.org/10.1007/s40429-014-0019-6

*López-Pelayo, H., Batalla, A., Balcells, M. M., Colom, J., & Gual, A. (2015). Assessment of cannabis use disorders: A systematic review of screening and diagnostic instruments. *Psychological Medicine, 45*, 1121–1133. http://dx.doi.org/10.1017/S0033291714002463

Marshall, K., Gowing, L., Ali, R., & Le Foll, B. (2014). Pharmacotherapies for cannabis dependence. In L. Gowing (Ed.), *Cochrane database of systematic reviews* (p. CD008940). Chichester, UK: Wiley.

Martin, G., Copeland, J., Gilmour, S., Gates, P., & Swift, W. (2006). The Adolescent Cannabis Problems Questionnaire (CPQ-A): Psychometric properties. *Addictive Behaviors, 31*, 2238–2248. http://dx.doi.org/10.1016/j.addbeh.2006.03.001

Mason, B. J., Crean, R., Goodell, V., Light, J. M., Quello, S., Shadan, F., . . . Rao, S. (2012). A proof-of-concept randomized controlled study of gabapentin: Effects on cannabis use, withdrawal and executive function deficits in cannabis-dependent adults. *Neuropsychopharmacology, 37*, 1689–1698. http://dx.doi.org/10.1038/npp.2012.14

McGuire, P., Robson, P., Cubala, W. J., Vasile, D., Morrison, P. D., Barron, R., . . . Wright, S. (2018). Cannabidiol (CBD) as an adjunctive therapy in schizophrenia: A multicenter randomized controlled trial. *American Journal of Psychiatry, 175*, 225–231. http://dx.doi.org/10.1176/appi.ajp.2017.17030325

McRae, A. L., Brady, K. T., & Carter, R. E. (2006). Buspirone for treatment of marijuana dependence: A pilot study. *The American Journal on Addictions, 15*, 404. http://dx.doi.org/10.1080/10550490600860635

McRae-Clark, A. L., Baker, N. L., Gray, K. M., Killeen, T., Hartwell, K. J., & Simonian, S. J. (2016). Vilazodone for cannabis dependence: A randomized, controlled pilot trial. *The American Journal on Addictions, 25*, 69–75. http://dx.doi.org/10.1111/ajad.12324

McRae-Clark, A. L., Baker, N. L., Maria, M. M.-S., & Brady, K. T. (2013). Effect of oxytocin on craving and stress response in marijuana-dependent individuals:

A pilot study. *Psychopharmacology, 228,* 623–631. http://dx.doi.org/10.1007/s00213-013-3062-4

McRae-Clark, A. L., Carter, R. E., Killeen, T. K., Carpenter, M. J., Wahlquist, A. E., Simpson, S. A., & Brady, K. T. (2009). A placebo-controlled trial of buspirone for the treatment of marijuana dependence. *Drug and Alcohol Dependence, 105,* 132–138. http://dx.doi.org/10.1016/j.drugalcdep.2009.06.022

McRae-Clark, A. L., Carter, R. E., Killeen, T. K., Carpenter, M. J., White, K. G., & Brady, K. T. (2010). A placebo-controlled trial of atomoxetine in marijuana-dependent individuals with attention deficit hyperactivity disorder. *The American Journal on Addictions, 19,* 481–489. http://dx.doi.org/10.1111/j.1521-0391.2010.00076.x

Mechoulam, R., & Hanuš, L. (2000). A historical overview of chemical research on cannabinoids. *Chemistry and Physics of Lipids, 108,* 1–13. http://dx.doi.org/10.1016/S0009-3084(00)00184-5

Mechoulam, R., & Hanuš, L. (2002). Cannabidiol: An overview of some chemical and pharmacological aspects. Part I: Chemical aspects. *Chemistry and Physics of Lipids, 121,* 35–43. http://dx.doi.org/10.1016/S0009-3084(02)00144-5

Mechoulam, R., Peters, M., Murillo-Rodriguez, E., & Hanuš, L. O. (2007). Cannabidiol—recent advances. *Chemistry & Biodiversity, 4,* 1678–1692. http://dx.doi.org/10.1002/cbdv.200790147

Melis, M., Frau, R., Kalivas, P. W., Spencer, S., Chioma, V., Zamberletti, E., . . . Parolaro, D. (2017). New vistas on cannabis use disorder. *Neuropharmacology, 124,* 62–72. http://dx.doi.org/10.1016/j.neuropharm.2017.03.033

Miranda, R., Treloar, H., Blanchard, A., Justus, A., Monti, P. M., Chun, T., . . . Gwaltney, C. J. (2017). Topiramate and motivational enhancement therapy for cannabis use among youth: A randomized placebo-controlled pilot study. *Addiction Biology, 22,* 779–790. http://dx.doi.org/10.1111/adb.12350

Morgan, C. J. A., Freeman, T. P., Schafer, G. L., & Curran, H. V. (2010). Cannabidiol attenuates the appetitive effects of Δ^9-tetrahydrocannabinol in humans smoking their chosen cannabis. *Neuropsychopharmacology, 35,* 1879–1885. http://dx.doi.org/10.1038/npp.2010.58

Murray, R. M., Englund, A., Abi-Dargham, A., Lewis, D. A., Di Forti, M., Davies, C., . . . D'Souza, D. C. (2017). Cannabis-associated psychosis: Neural substrate and clinical impact. *Neuropharmacology, 124,* 89–104. http://dx.doi.org/10.1016/j.neuropharm.2017.06.018

Myles, H., Myles, N., & Large, M. (2016). Cannabis use in first episode psychosis: Meta-analysis of prevalence, and the time course of initiation and continued use. *Australian and New Zealand Journal of Psychiatry, 50,* 208–219. http://dx.doi.org/10.1177/0004867415599846

National Academies of Sciences, Engineering and Medicine. (2017). *The health effects of cannabis and cannabinoids: The current state of evidence and recommendations for research.* Washington, DC: The National Academies Press. http://dx.doi.org/10.17226/24625

Newcombe, D. A. L., Walker, N., Sheridan, J., & Galea, S. (2015). The effect of varenicline administration on cannabis and tobacco use in cannabis and nicotine dependent individuals—A case-series. *Journal of Addiction Research & Therapy, 6,* 1–5. http://dx.doi.org/10.4172/2155-6105.1000222

Norberg, M. M., Mackenzie, J., & Copeland, J. (2012). Quantifying cannabis use with the timeline followback approach: A psychometric evaluation. *Drug and Alcohol Dependence, 121,* 247–252. http://dx.doi.org/10.1016/j.drugalcdep.2011.09.007

Okuda, M., Hasin, D. S., Olfson, M., Khan, S. S., Nunes, E. V., Montoya, I., . . . Blanco, C. (2010). Generalizability of clinical trials for cannabis dependence to community samples. *Drug and Alcohol Dependence, 111,* 177–181. http://dx.doi.org/10.1016/j.drugalcdep.2010.04.009

Panlilio, L. V., Justinova, Z., & Goldberg, S. R. (2013). Inhibition of FAAH and activation of PPAR: New approaches to the treatment of cognitive dysfunction and drug addiction. *Pharmacology & Therapeutics, 138,* 84–102. http://dx.doi.org/10.1016/j.pharmthera.2013.01.003

Pertwee, R. G. (2008). The diverse CB_1 and CB_2 receptor pharmacology of three plant cannabinoids: Δ^9-tetrahydrocannabinol, cannabidiol and Δ^9-tetrahydrocannabivarin. *British Journal of Pharmacology, 153,* 199–215. http://dx.doi.org/10.1038/sj.bjp.0707442

Pokorski, I., Clement, N., Phung, N., Weltman, M., Fu, S., & Copeland, J. (2017). Cannabidiol in the management of in-patient cannabis withdrawal: Clinical case series. *Future Neurology, 12,* 133–140. http://dx.doi.org/10.2217/fnl-2016-0035

Potvin, S., Stip, E., & Roy, J.-Y. (2004). The effect of quetiapine on cannabis use in 8 psychosis patients with drug dependency. *The Canadian Journal of Psychiatry, 49,* 711–711. http://dx.doi.org/10.1177/070674370404901020

Ramesh, D., & Haney, M. (2015). Treatment of cannabis use disorders. In N. el-Guebaly, G. Carrà, & M. Galanter (Eds.), *Textbook of addiction treatment: International perspectives* (pp. 367–380). New York, NY: Springer. http://dx.doi.org/10.1007/978-88-470-5322-9_14

Renard, J., Rosen, L. G., Loureiro, M., De Oliveira, C., Schmid, S., Rushlow, W. J., & Laviolette, S. R.

(2016). Adolescent cannabinoid exposure induces a persistent sub-cortical hyper-dopaminergic state and associated molecular adaptations in the prefrontal cortex. *Cerebral Cortex, 27,* 1297–1310. http://dx.doi.org/10.1093/cercor/bhv335

Rooke, S., Thorsteinsson, E., Karpin, A., Copeland, J., & Allsop, D. (2010). Computer-delivered interventions for alcohol and tobacco use: A meta-analysis. *Addiction, 105*(8), 1381–1390. http://dx.doi.org/10.1111/j.1360-0443.2010.02975.x

SAMHSA. (2015). *Treatment Episode Data Set (TEDS) 2003-2013 state admissions to substance abuse treatment services.* Rockville, MD: Author. Retrieved from https://www.samhsa.gov/data/sites/default/files/2013_TED_State_Final/2013_Treatement_Episode_Data_Set_State_final.pdf

Schifano, F., D'Offizi, S., Piccione, M., Corazza, O., Deluca, P., Davey, Z., . . . Scherbaum, N. (2011). Is there a recreational misuse potential for pregabalin? Analysis of anecdotal online reports in comparison with related gabapentin and clonazepam data. *Psychotherapy and Psychosomatics, 80,* 118–122. http://dx.doi.org/10.1159/000321079

Schnell, T., Koethe, D., Krasnianski, A., Gairing, S., Schnell, K., Daumann, J., & Gouzoulis-Mayfrank, E. (2014). Ziprasidone versus clozapine in the treatment of dually diagnosed (DD) patients with schizophrenia and cannabis use disorders: A randomized study. *The American Journal on Addictions, 23,* 308–312. http://dx.doi.org/10.1111/j.1521-0391.2014.12126.x

Schuster, R. M., Hanly, A., Gilman, J., Budney, A., Vandrey, R., & Evins, A. E. (2016). A contingency management method for 30-days abstinence in non-treatment seeking young adult cannabis users. *Drug and Alcohol Dependence, 167,* 199–206. http://dx.doi.org/10.1016/j.drugalcdep.2016.08.622

Sherman, B. J., Baker, N. L., & McRae-Clark, A. L. (2017). Effect of oxytocin pretreatment on cannabis outcomes in a brief motivational intervention. *Psychiatry Research, 249,* 318–320. http://dx.doi.org/10.1016/j.psychres.2017.01.027

Silins, E., Horwood, L. J., Patton, G. C., Fergusson, D. M., Olsson, C. A., Hutchinson, D. M., . . . Mattick, R. P., & the Cannabis Cohorts Research Consortium. (2014). Young adult sequelae of adolescent cannabis use: An integrative analysis. *The Lancet Psychiatry, 1,* 286–293. http://dx.doi.org/10.1016/S2215-0366(14)70307-4

Sloan, M. E., Gowin, J. L., Ramchandani, V. A., Hurd, Y. L., & Le Foll, B. (2017). The endocannabinoid system as a target for addiction treatment: Trials and tribulations. *Neuropharmacology, 124,* 73–83. http://dx.doi.org/10.1016/j.neuropharm.2017.05.031

Smith, B. H., Higgins, C., Baldacchino, A., Kidd, B., & Bannister, J. (2012). Substance misuse of gabapentin. *The British Journal of General Practice, 62,* 406–407. http://dx.doi.org/10.3399/bjgp12X653516

Stephens, R. S., Roffman, R. A., & Simpson, E. E. (1993). Adult marijuana users seeking treatment. *Journal of Consulting and Clinical Psychology, 61,* 1100–1104. http://dx.doi.org/10.1037/0022-006X.61.6.1100

Stinson, F. S., Ruan, W. J., Pickering, R., & Grant, B. F. (2006). Cannabis use disorders in the USA: Prevalence, correlates and co-morbidity. *Psychological Medicine, 36,* 1447–1460. http://dx.doi.org/10.1017/S0033291706008361

Swift, W., Coffey, C., Carlin, J. B., Degenhardt, L., & Patton, G. C. (2008). Adolescent cannabis users at 24 years: Trajectories to regular weekly use and dependence in young adulthood. *Addiction, 103,* 1361–1370. http://dx.doi.org/10.1111/j.1360-0443.2008.02246.x

Swift, W., Wong, A., Li, K. M., Arnold, J. C., & McGregor, I. S. (2013). Analysis of cannabis seizures in NSW, Australia: Cannabis potency and cannabinoid profile. *PLoS ONE, 8,* e70052. http://dx.doi.org/10.1371/journal.pone.0070052

Tirado, C. F., Goldman, M., Lynch, K., Kampman, K. M., & Obrien, C. P. (2008). Atomoxetine for treatment of marijuana dependence: A report on the efficacy and high incidence of gastrointestinal adverse events in a pilot study. *Drug and Alcohol Dependence, 94,* 254–257. http://dx.doi.org/10.1016/j.drugalcdep.2007.10.020

Tomko, R. L., Baker, N. L., McClure, E. A., Sonne, S. C., McRae-Clark, A. L., Sherman, B. J., & Gray, K. M. (2018). Incremental validity of estimated cannabis grams as a predictor of problems and cannabinoid biomarkers: Evidence from a clinical trial. *Drug and Alcohol Dependence, 182,* 1–7. http://dx.doi.org/10.1016/j.drugalcdep.2017.09.035

Trigo, J. M., Soliman, A., Quilty, L. C., Fischer, B., Rehm, J., Selby, P., . . . Le Foll, B. (2018). Nabiximols combined with motivational enhancement/cognitive behavioral therapy for the treatment of cannabis dependence: A pilot randomized clinical trial. *PLoS One, 13,* e0190768. http://dx.doi.org/10.1371/journal.pone.0190768

Vandrey, R., Smith, M. T., McCann, U. D., Budney, A. J., & Curran, E. M. (2011). Sleep disturbance and the effects of extended-release zolpidem during cannabis withdrawal. *Drug and Alcohol Dependence, 117,* 38–44. http://dx.doi.org/10.1016/j.drugalcdep.2011.01.003

Vermersch, P. (2011). Sativex® (tetrahydrocannabinol + cannabidiol), an endocannabinoid system modulator: Basic features and main clinical data. *Expert Review of Neurotherapeutics, 11,* 15–19. http://dx.doi.org/10.1586/ern.11.27

von Sydow, K., Lieb, R., Pfister, H., Höfler, M., Sonntag, H., & Wittchen, H.-U. (2001). The natural course of cannabis use, abuse and dependence over four years: A longitudinal community study of adolescents and young adults. *Drug and Alcohol Dependence, 64,* 347–361. http://dx.doi.org/10.1016/S0376-8716(01)00137-5

Wachtel, S. R., & de Wit, H. (2000). Naltrexone does not block the subjective effects of oral Δ⁹-tetrahydrocannabinol in humans. *Drug and Alcohol Dependence, 59,* 251–260. http://dx.doi.org/10.1016/S0376-8716(99)00127-1

Weinstein, A. M., Miller, H., Bluvstein, I., Rapoport, E., Schreiber, S., Bar-Hamburger, R., & Bloch, M. (2014). Treatment of cannabis dependence using escitalopram in combination with cognitive-behavior therapy: A double-blind placebo-controlled study. *The American Journal of Drug and Alcohol Abuse, 40,* 16–22. http://dx.doi.org/10.3109/00952990.2013.819362

Whitfield-Gabrieli, S., Fischer, A. S., Henricks, A. M., Khokhar, J. Y., Roth, R. M., Brunette, M. F., & Green, A. I. (2018). Understanding marijuana's effects on functional connectivity of the default mode network in patients with schizophrenia and co-occurring cannabis use disorder: A pilot investigation. *Schizophrenia Research, 194,* 70–77. http://dx.doi.org/10.1016/j.schres.2017.07.029

Whiting, P. F., Wolff, R. F., Deshpande, S., Di Nisio, M., Duffy, S., Hernandez, A. V., . . . Kleijnen, J. (2015). Cannabinoids for medical use: A systematic review and meta-analysis. *JAMA, 313,* 2456–2473. http://dx.doi.org/10.1001/jama.2015.6358

*Winstock, A. R., Ford, C., & Witton, J. (2010). Assessment and management of cannabis use disorders in primary care. *BMJ (Clinical Research Ed.), 340,* c1571. http://dx.doi.org/10.1136/bmj.c1571

Winstock, A. R., Lea, T., & Copeland, J. (2009). Lithium carbonate in the management of cannabis withdrawal in humans: An open-label study. *Journal of Psychopharmacology, 23,* 84–93. http://dx.doi.org/10.1177/0269881108089584

World Health Organization. (1992). *The ICD–10 classification of mental and behavioural disorders: Clinical descriptions and diagnostic guidelines.* Geneva, Switzerland: Author. Retrieved from https://www.who.int/classifications/icd/en/bluebook.pdf

Zuardi, A. W. (2006). History of *cannabis* as medicine: A review. *Revista Brasileira de Psiquiatria, 28,* 153–157. http://www.scielo.br/pdf/rbp/v28n2/29785.pdf

CHAPTER 24

PHARMACOLOGICAL TREATMENT OF PSYCHOSTIMULANT USE DISORDERS

Joy M. Schmitz, Margaret C. Wardle, Michael F. Weaver,
Angela M. Heads, Jin H. Yoon, and Scott D. Lane

This chapter focuses on cocaine and methamphetamine, the two most commonly abused psychostimulants, which were initially popularized in the United States for medical purposes (Center for Substance Abuse Treatment, 1999). Cocaine was an ingredient in a variety of patent medicines in the early 1900s, until increasing concerns about abuse led to sharp restrictions as part of the Harrison Narcotic Act of 1914. Amphetamine-like stimulants followed in the 1930s, being used as prescription medications for sleep disorders and performance enhancement in military pilots, until concerns about black market usage led to restrictions in the Controlled Substances Act of 1970. However, easing of social taboos about illicit drug use during the 1960s and 1970s, combined with the industrialization of cocaine production in the hands of cartels, led to exponential increases in cocaine importing to the United States by the 1980s (Center for Substance Abuse Treatment, 1999). New "freebase" manufacturing methods, which produced a readily smokable form of cocaine commonly known as "crack," contributed to a cocaine epidemic in the 1980s and 1990s. During these years, crack cocaine use was identified as the primary substance use problem in the United States (SAMHSA, 1988). During the 1980s, illicit methamphetamine use also continued, but the drug was primarily produced by small-scale distributors in rural areas and on the West Coast, and showed similarly restricted patterns of usage (Maxwell & Brecht, 2011). However, after key precursors of methamphetamine were scheduled in the United States in 1980, manufacturing began to shift to large cartel-supplied "super labs," and an increase in illicit production and use of methamphetamine was seen during the 1990s and early 2000s, up until passage of the Combat Methamphetamine Epidemic Act of 2005 (Courtney & Ray, 2014; Maxwell & Brecht, 2011). Since these peaks of use for cocaine and methamphetamine in the 1980s to 1990s and 1990s to early 2000s respectively, rates of stimulant use disorders in the United States have been in gradual decline (Center for Substance Abuse Treatment, 1999; Courtney & Ray, 2014).

EPIDEMIOLOGY AND PREVALENCE

Currently, stimulant use ranks third in drug use prevalence behind marijuana and misuse of prescription opioids, with approximately 2.8 million Americans reporting past month use and 1.8 million reporting a past-year stimulant use disorder (Center for Behavioral Health Statistics and Quality, 2016). Globally, long-term trends show declines in use, although stimulant use disorder remains the second most common use disorder. Early indicators, including coca bush cultivation and seizure numbers, indicate that stimulant use may be poised for resurgence (United Nations Office on Drugs and Crime, 2017). Stimulants continue to represent a significant health burden, often via cardiovascular side effects and

http://dx.doi.org/10.1037/0000133-024
APA Handbook of Psychopharmacology, S. M. Evans (Editor-in-Chief)

overdose deaths (Degenhardt et al., 2014; Martins, Sampson, Cerdá, & Galea, 2015). Furthermore, there is significant unmet treatment need. Globally, only one in six individuals with any kind of substance use disorder receives treatment, and stimulant users are underrepresented in treatment relative to their numbers in the population (United Nations Office on Drugs and Crime, 2017). This may be due in part to the lack of approved medication treatments for stimulant use disorders, further discussed in the rest of this chapter.

Historically, pharmacological treatment for stimulant use disorders was confined to management of acute symptoms of overdose via beta-blockers, sedatives, or antipsychotics for psychotic episodes (Smith, 1984). Initial approaches to pharmacological treatment of stimulant use disorders per se focused on use of tricyclic antidepressants, either to treat depression when it was perceived as an underlying causal factor for stimulant use (Smith, 1984), or to treat withdrawal symptoms that can resemble depression (Resnick & Resnick, 1984). With growing recognition of the centrality of dopamine (DA) in rewarding effects of stimulants, the focus shifted to both agonist and antagonist strategies involving DA, as reviewed in the following sections. The failure of these approaches to produce an FDA-approved medication have more recently led to consideration of nonneurotransmitter options, including antidrug vaccines and anti-inflammatory medications, as will be detailed in the Emerging Trends section.

DIAGNOSING STIMULANT USE DISORDERS

Diagnosis of a stimulant use disorder relies on *Diagnostic and Statistical Manual of Mental Disorders, 5th edition* (*DSM–5*; American Psychiatric Association, 2013) criteria, with simple reports of frequency of use or physical dependence (e.g., withdrawal, tolerance) being insufficient for diagnosis. Thus, diagnosis is best accomplished via validated semistructured clinical interviews, such as the Structured Clinical Interview for DSM–5 (First, Williams, Karg, & Spitzer, 2015). However, in nonspecialty or primary care settings, brief screening instruments may be useful to determine which patients need additional

diagnostic follow-up or referral. There are no screening instruments specific to stimulant use, but one recommended broad screening approach is the self-report Substance Use Brief Screen (SUBS), which simply establishes past year use of illicit drugs (McNeely et al., 2015), with positive endorsements followed by the World Health Organization Alcohol, Smoking and Substance Involvement Screening Test, Version 3.0 (ASSIST), a brief clinician-administered interview. For all substances used in the past 3 months, the ASSIST probes for problematic use with brief questions (e.g., "During the past 3 months, how often has your use of cocaine led to health, social, legal, or financial problems?" with response options ranging from "0 = never" to "7 = daily or almost daily"). Although this instrument is not diagnostic, and the questions do not exactly parallel *DSM–5* criteria, they do capture aspects relevant to diagnosis, including frequency of use and drug-related urges and problems (Humeniuk et al., 2008). There are also measures of severity of addiction that provide historical information and qualitative information relevant to treatment, such as the Addiction Severity Index, a semistructured interview that provides information on duration and patterns of use and quantifies functional impacts of drug use across life domains for drugs including cocaine and methamphetamine (McLellan, Luborsky, Woody, & O'Brien, 1980).

EVIDENCE-BASED PHARMACOLOGICAL TREATMENT OF STIMULANT USE DISORDERS

Currently, there are no approved medications for the treatment of cocaine or methamphetamine use disorders. Various pharmacological approaches have been investigated and fall into four broad categories. Tables 24.1 through 24.4 provide a focused review of randomized controlled trials (RCTs) assessing candidate medications within each pharmacological approach. An exhaustive review of this literature is beyond the scope of this chapter and the reader is referred elsewhere (Bhatt et al., 2016; Minozzi et al., 2015).

The first category of pharmacological approaches involves using stimulants to treat cocaine and methamphetamine use disorders (see Table 24.1), largely

TABLE 24.1

Randomized Placebo-Controlled Trials of Agonist-Like Medications for Treatment of Primary Stimulant Use Disorder

Agent (trade name)	Stimulant disorder/ sample size (% male)	Doses	Summary of primary outcomes
bupropion (Wellbutrin®)			
(Margolin et al., 1995)	cocaine *n* = 150 (70%)	bupropion: 300 mg/d	No group differences in cocaine-positive urines; subgroup effect in depressed patients receiving bupropion
(Elkashef et al., 2008)	methamphetamine *n* = 151 (67%)	bupropion SR: 150 mg/b.i.d.	No group differences in methamphetamine-positive urines
(Shoptaw, Heinzerling, Rotheram-Fuller, Steward, et al., 2008)	methamphetamine *n* = 73 (64.4%)	bupropion SR: 150 mg/b.i.d.	No group differences in methamphetamine-positive urines
(Shoptaw, Heinzerling, Rotheram-Fuller, Kao, et al., 2008)	cocaine *n* = 70 (84%)	bupropion: 300 mg/d	No group differences in cocaine-positive urines
(Das et al., 2010)	methamphetamine *n* = 30 (100%)	bupropion SR: 150 mg/b.i.d.	No group differences in methamphetamine-positive urines
(Heinzerling et al., 2013)	methamphetamine *n* = 19 (47.4%)	bupropion SR: 150 mg/b.i.d.	No group differences in methamphetamine-positive urines
(Heinzerling et al., 2014)	methamphetamine *n* = 84 (80.9%)	bupropion SR: 150 mg/b.i.d.	No group differences in methamphetamine-positive urines
(Anderson et al., 2015)	methamphetamine *n* = 204 (65%)	bupropion SR: 150 mg/b.i.d.	No group differences in methamphetamine-positive urines
disulfiram (Antabuse®)			
(Carroll et al., 2004)	cocaine *n* = 121 (74%)	disulfiram: 250 mg/d	Reduced cocaine-positive urines in disulfiram group
(Carroll et al., 2016)	cocaine *n* = 99 (72.7%)	disulfiram: 250 mg/d	No effect of disulfiram on cocaine use
modafinil (Provigil®)			
(Dackis, Kampman, Lynch, Pettinati, & O'Brien, 2005)	cocaine *n* = 62 (71%)	modafinil: 400 mg/d	Reduced cocaine-positive urines in modafinil treatment group
(Anderson et al., 2009)	cocaine *n* = 210 (71.9%)	modafinil: 200 mg/d; 400 mg/d	Improved percentage of cocaine nonuse days in 200 mg/d group; post hoc effect favored subgroup without a history of alcohol dependence
(Shearer et al., 2009)	methamphetamine *n* = 80 (62.4%)	modafinil: 200 mg/d	No group differences in methamphetamine-positive urines
(Heinzerling et al., 2010)	methamphetamine *n* = 71 (70.4%)	modafinil: 400 mg/d	No group differences in methamphetamine-positive urines
(Anderson et al., 2012)	methamphetamine *n* = 210 (59.1%)	modafinil: 200 mg/d; 400 mg/d	No group differences in methamphetamine-positive urines
(Dackis et al., 2012)	cocaine *n* = 210 (73.7%)	modafinil: 200 mg/d; 400 mg/d	No group differences in cocaine-positive urines
(Kampman et al., 2015)	cocaine *n* = 94 (81%)	modafinil: 300 mg/d	Higher abstinence rates in modafinil group

(continues)

TABLE 24.1

Randomized Placebo-Controlled Trials of Agonist-Like Medications for Treatment of Primary Stimulant Use Disorder (*Continued*)

Agent (trade name)	Stimulant disorder/ sample size (% male)	Doses	Summary of primary outcomes
d-amphetamine (Dexedrine®)			
(Grabowski et al., 2001)	cocaine *n* = 128 (79%)	d-amphetamine: 15–30 mg/d; 30–60 mg/d	Improved retention in 15–30 mg/d group; Reduced cocaine-positive urines in 30–60 mg/d group
(Shearer, Wodak, van Beek, Mattick, & Lewis, 2003)	cocaine *n* = 30 (not reported)	d-amphetamine: 60 mg/d	No group differences on retention or cocaine-positive urines; within-group analysis showed improvements favoring d-amphetamine group for self-reported cocaine use
(Grabowski et al., 2004)	cocaine *n* = 94 (67%)	d-amphetamine: 15–30 mg/d; 30–60 mg/d	Reduced cocaine-positive urines in 30–60 mg/d group
(Longo et al., 2010)	methamphetamine *n* = 49 (61.2%)	d-amphetamine: 110 mg/d	No group differences in methamphetamine-positive hair samples
(Galloway et al., 2011)	methamphetamine *n* = 60 (56.7%)	d-amphetamine: 60 mg/d	No group differences in methamphetamine-positive urines
methylphenidate (Ritalin®)			
(Grabowski et al., 1997)	cocaine *n* = 24 (78%)	methylphenidate, immediate and extended release: 45 mg/d	No group differences in retention or cocaine-positive urines
(Tiihonen et al., 2007)	methamphetamine *n* = 34 (70.6%)	methylphenidate, extended release: 54 mg/d	Fewer methamphetamine-positive urines in methylphenidate group
(Miles et al., 2013)	methamphetamine *n* = 78 (62.8%)	methylphenidate, extended release: 54 mg/d	No group differences in methamphetamine-positive urines
(Ling et al., 2014)	methamphetamine *n* = 110 (81.8%)	methylphenidate, extended release: 54 mg/d	Reduced self-reported methamphetamine use days during treatment in methylphenidate group
(Rezaei et al., 2015)	methamphetamine *n* = 56 (73.2%)	methylphenidate, extended release: 54 mg/d	Reduced methamphetamine-positive urines in methylphenidate group
lisdexamfetamine (Vyvanse®)			
(Mooney et al., 2015)	cocaine *n* = 43 (81.3%)	lisdexamfetamine: 70 mg/d	No group differences in cocaine-positive urines
methamphetamine (Desoxyn®)			
(Mooney et al., 2009)	cocaine *n* = 82 (65.8%)	Immediate release methamphetamine: 5 mg/ 6 times a day; sustained release methamphetamine 30 mg/d	Reduced cocaine-positive urines in the sustained release methamphetamine group

Note. SR = sustained release; b.i.d. = two times a day.

based on the agonist or replacement therapy model that has shown efficacy for treating nicotine and opiate dependence. Because stimulants do not bind to a single receptor, this pharmacological approach has been aimed at directly or indirectly increasing brain monoamines in the same way that cocaine and methamphetamine act acutely, but with lower addictive potential. For cocaine use disorder (CUD), two agents, modafinil and amphetamine, appear promising. Modafinil, an FDA-approved medication for the treatment of narcolepsy, binds to the DA transporter, resulting in increased synaptic DA levels. Promising initial results (Dackis, Kampman, Lynch, Pettinati, & O'Brien, 2005) have been followed by larger trials reporting negative findings or effects only in select patient subgroups, such as cocaine-dependent patients without a history of alcohol dependence (Anderson et al., 2009). However, in the most recent RCT, Kampman et al. (2015) found modafinil, at a dose of 300 mg daily, was superior to placebo at promoting abstinence during the last 3 weeks of the trial (Kampman et al., 2015).

Sustained-release amphetamine as an agonist treatment has shown evidence of therapeutic efficacy. Dextroamphetamine (Dexedrine Spansule®) in escalating dose regimens up to 60 mg daily was superior to lower doses (up to 30 mg) and placebo in reducing drug use in patients with CUD (Grabowski et al., 2001; Shearer et al., 2003). Along similar lines, the use of sustained-release methamphetamine (Desoxyn®) for cocaine dependence reduced cocaine-positive urines in a single-site trial (Mooney et al., 2009). The efficacy of these agents is offset by controversy over the idea of treating an addiction with a controlled substance that has the potential for misuse and diversion (Kollins, 2007; Negus & Henningfield, 2015). In response, novel formulations with lower abuse potential have been considered. Lisdexamfetamine (Vyvanse®) is a prodrug of dextroamphetamine and has the advantage of being inactive until it is converted to active dextroamphetamine in the blood by red blood cells, resulting in slower onset and longer duration of action compared to immediate release dextroamphetamine (Banks, Hutsell, Blough, Poklis, & Negus, 2015). Mooney et al. (2015) showed that lisdexamfetamine was safe and well tolerated

in patients with CUD. This pilot study was underpowered to detect efficacy, however, reduction in craving was reported.

For methamphetamine use disorder, available evidence from RCTs does not support the use of modafinil or dextroamphetamine. Most recently, Rezaei et al. (2015) reported that once-daily, sustained-release methylphenidate treatment for 10 weeks was safe, well tolerated, and associated with reduced methamphetamine use, warranting further investigation. These results are in accordance with some (Ling et al., 2014; Tiihonen et al., 2007) but not all (Miles et al., 2013) previous studies.

The second category of pharmacological approaches involves the use of medications intended to antagonize the reinforcing effects of stimulants, with the most commonly studied agents being antipsychotics (Table 24.2). Conceptually, by blocking DA receptors, these medications may be able to reduce craving and use of stimulants. Practically, a main disadvantage in antagonist treatment has been low patient acceptability and compliance. Unlike agonist medications, antagonists do not produce cross-tolerance to the effects of the abused drug and therefore have a low probability of functioning as effective reinforcers in patients. Moreover, antipsychotics are not risk free, and nontrivial neuroleptic-induced side effects have been reported (Gawin, Khalsa-Denison, & Jatlow, 1996; Kumor, Sherer, & Jaffe, 1986). Results of several systematic reviews and meta-analyses (Álvarez, Pérez-Mañá, Torrens, & Farré, 2013; Amato, Minozzi, Pani, & Davoli, 2007; Kishi, Matsuda, Iwata, & Correll, 2013) fail to support this approach as an effective treatment for cocaine or methamphetamine use disorder.

The third category of pharmacological approaches involves use of antidepressants (Table 24.3), based in part on the central and overlapping role of the DA system in depression and stimulant use disorders. Conceptually, by targeting areas of the brain involved in regulation of mood, antidepressants may alleviate dysphoria and craving associated with downregulation of monoamine systems characterized by chronic stimulant use. This is another category in which empirical evidence from the RCT literature for cocaine treatment is not uniformly supportive

TABLE 24.2

Randomized Placebo-Controlled Trials of Antagonist-Like Medications for Treatment of Primary Stimulant Use Disorder

Agent (trade name)	Stimulant disorder/ sample size (% male)	Doses	Summary of primary outcomes
ritanserin (Risperdal®)			
(Johnson et al., 1997)	cocaine $n = 65$ (80.8%)	ritanserin: 10 mg/d	No group differences in cocaine-positive urines
risperidone			
(Levin et al., 1999)	cocaine $n = 14$ (71%)	tisperidone: 2.1 mg/d	No group differences in cocaine-positive urines
(Grabowski et al., 2000)	cocaine $n = 193$ (74%)	risperidone: 2 mg/d; 4 mg/d	No group differences in cocaine-positive urines
(Loebl et al., 2008)	cocaine $n = 31$ (100%)	risperidone: long-acting (IM) 25 mg	No group differences in cocaine-positive urines
reserpine (Raudixin®)			
(Winhusen, Somoza, Sarid-Segal, et al., 2007)	cocaine $n = 119$ (70%)	reserpine: 0.50 mg/d	No group differences in cocaine-positive urines
olanzapine (Zyprexa®)			
(Kampman, Pettinati, Lynch, Sparkman, & O'Brien, 2003)	cocaine $n = 30$ (73.3%)	olanzapine: 10 mg/d	Reduced cocaine-positive urines in the placebo group
(Reid, Casadonte, et al., 2005)	cocaine $n = 63$ (79.3%)	olanzapine: 10 mg/d	No group differences in cocaine-positive urines
(Hamilton, Nguyen, Gerber, & Rubio, 2009)	cocaine $n = 48$ (100%)	lanzapine: 20 mg/d	No group differences in cocaine-positive urines
quetiapine (Seroquel®)			
(Tapp et al., 2015)	cocaine $n = 60$ (86.6%)	quetiapine: 400 mg/d	No group differences in cocaine-positive urines
ondansetron (Zofran®)			
(Johnson et al., 2006)	cocaine $n = 63$ (87%)	ondansetron: 0.25 mg/b.i.d.; 1.0 mg/b.i.d.; 4.0 mg/b.i.d.	Reduced cocaine-positive urines in the ondansetron 4.0 mg/b.i.d. group
(Johnson et al., 2008)	methamphetamine $n = 150$ (96%)	ondansetron: 0.25 mg/b.i.d.; 1.0 mg/b.i.d.; 4 mg/b.i.d.	No group differences in methamphetamine-positive urines
mirtazapine (Remeron®)			
(Colfax et al., 2011)	methamphetamine $n = 60$ (100%)	mirtazapine: 30 mg/d	Reduced methamphetamine use in mirtazapine group

Note. IM = intramuscular; b.i.d. = two times a day.

TABLE 24.3

Randomized Placebo-Controlled Trials of Antidepressant Medications for Treatment of Primary Stimulant Use Disorder

Agent (trade name)	Stimulant disorder/ sample size (% male)	Doses	Summary of primary outcomes
fluoxetine (Prozac®)			
(Covi, Hess, Kreiter, & Haertzen, 1995)	cocaine $n = 59$ (80%)	fluoxetine: 20 mg/d; 40 mg/d; 60 mg/d	No group differences in cocaine-positive urines
(Grabowski et al., 1995)	cocaine $n = 155$ (72%)	fluoxetine: 20 mg/d; 40 mg/d	No group differences in cocaine-positive urines
(Batki, Washburn, Delucchi, & Jones, 1996)	cocaine $n = 32$ (66%)	fluoxetine: 40 mg/d	No group differences in cocaine-positive urines
(Schmitz et al., 2001)	cocaine $n = 68$ (57.3%)	fluoxetine: 40 mg/d	No group differences in cocaine-positive urines
citalopram (Celexa®)			
(Moeller et al., 2007)	cocaine $n = 76$ (86.8%)	citalopram: 20 mg/d	Reduced cocaine-positive urines in the citalopram group
sertraline (Zoloft®)			
(Winhusen et al., 2005)	cocaine $n = 67$ (73%)	sertraline: 100 mg/d Donepezil: 10 mg/d Tiagabine: 20 mg/d	No group differences in cocaine-positive urines
(Shoptaw et al., 2006)	methamphetamine $n = 229$ (61.6 %)	sertraline: 50 mg/d	No group differences in methamphetamine-positive urines
(Oliveto et al., 2012)	cocaine $n = 86$ (61.6%)	sertraline: 50 mg/d	Sertraline delayed relapse in recently abstinent cocaine dependent patients with depressive symptoms
(Mancino et al., 2014)	cocaine $n = 99$ (77%)	sertraline: 200 mg/d gabapentin augmentation: 1,200 mg/d	Reduced cocaine-positive urines in the sertraline group
imipramine (Tofranil®)			
(Nunes et al., 1995)	cocaine $n = 113$ (73%)	imipramine: 150–300 mg/d	Higher abstinence rates in subgroup with comorbid depression or nasal users
desipramine (Norpramin®)			
(Gawin et al., 1989)	cocaine $n = 72$ (76%)	desipramine: 2.5 mg/kg/d lithium carbonate: 600 mg/d	Higher rates of abstinence in desipramine group
(Weddington et al., 1991)	cocaine $n = 54$ (76%)	desipramine: 200 mg/d Amantadine: 400 mg/d	No group differences in cocaine-positive urines
(Carroll et al., 1994)	cocaine $n = 110$ (72%)	desipramine: 300 mg/d	Higher rates of abstinence in subgroup with lower baseline severity of cocaine use
(Hall et al., 1994)	cocaine $n = 94$ (100%)	desipramine: 200 mg/d	No group differences in cocaine-positive urines

(continues)

TABLE 24.3

Randomized Placebo-Controlled Trials of Antidepressant Medications for Treatment of Primary Stimulant Use Disorder (*Continued*)

Agent (trade name)	Stimulant disorder/ sample size (% male)	Doses	Summary of primary outcomes
(Campbell et al., 2003)	cocaine *n* = 146 (74.5%)	desipramine: 200 mg/d carbamazepine: 800 mg/d	No group differences in cocaine-positive urines
(McDowell et al., 2005)	cocaine *n* = 111 (75%)	desipramine: 300 mg/d	No group differences in cocaine-positive urines
bupropion (Wellbutrin®)			
(Elkashef et al., 2008)	methamphetamine *n* = 151 (67%)	bupropion: 150 mg/b.i.d.	Reduced methamphetamine-positive urines in subgroup with lower baseline use of methamphetamine
(Shoptaw, Heinzerling, Rotheram-Fuller, Kao, et al., 2008)	cocaine *n* = 70 (86%)	bupropion: 300 mg/d	No group differences in cocaine-positive urines
(Shoptaw, Heinzerling, Rotheram-Fuller, Steward, et al., 2008)	methamphetamine *n* = 73 (64.3%)	bupropion: 150 mg/b.i.d.	Reduced methamphetamine-positive urines in bupropion in subgroup with lower baseline use of methamphetamine
nefazodone (Serzone®)			
(Ciraulo et al., 2005)	cocaine *n* = 69 (71%)	nefazodone: 400 mg/d	Reduced level of benzoylecgonine in nefazodone group
(Passos, Camacho, Lopes, & Borges dos Santos, 2005)	cocaine *n* = 210 (92.4%)	nefazodone: 300 mg/d	No group differences in cocaine-positive urines
selegiline (Emsam®)			
(Elkashef et al., 2006)	cocaine *n* = 300 (78%)	selegiline trans-dermal system: 6 mg per 24 h	No group differences in cocaine-positive urines

Note. b.i.d. = two times a day.

(Lima, Reisser, Soares, & Farrell, 2003; Pani, Trogu, Vecchi, & Amato, 2011), though efficacy has been suggested in individual studies of citalopram (Moeller et al., 2007) and sertraline (Mancino et al., 2014; Oliveto et al., 2012). That these two selective serotonin reuptake inhibitors have greater affinity for the serotonin transporter has been suggested as an explanation for their positive effects as compared with fluoxetine, a more potent inhibitor of 5-HT_{2C} receptors. Notably, the two trials demonstrating the clinical efficacy of sertraline used a relapse paradigm, in which participants abstained from cocaine while residing at a residential facility during medication

induction (Mancino et al., 2014; Oliveto et al., 2012). Additionally, both studies enrolled cocaine-dependent patients with depressive symptoms, another condition that may define the bounds of efficacy with this medication. For methamphetamine addiction, there is some evidence to suggest that bupropion may be effective in a certain subgroup of patients. Post hoc analysis of data from two separate trials indicated reduced methamphetamine use in patients who had low to moderate baseline use (less than 18 days a month) compared with heavier users (Elkashef et al., 2008; Shoptaw, Heinzerling, Rotheram-Fuller, Steward, et al., 2008). As of yet, no prospective clinical trials have been conducted to confirm this patient–treatment interaction.

The fourth category of pharmacological approaches involves use of anticonvulsants, based on the goal of increasing GABAergic function or regulating glutamate to produce decreased DA activity (Table 24.4). Systematic reviews of current evidence fail to support the clinical use of anticonvulsants as a group in the treatment of cocaine (Minozzi et al., 2008; Minozzi et al., 2015) or methamphetamine dependence (Elkashef et al., 2012). A relatively recent systematic review and meta-analysis of five RCTs evaluated topiramate for CUD (Singh, Keer, Klimas, Wood, & Werb, 2016). Three of the trials showed that topiramate improved rates of continuous abstinence compared with placebo (Johnson et al., 2013; Kampman et al., 2004; Kampman et al., 2013), suggesting limited evidence of efficacy. These positive effects were reported in trials that included ongoing psychosocial therapy (e.g., cognitive behavior therapy [CBT]) and slow titration over several weeks to a month to mitigate adverse events. Two trials of topiramate for methamphetamine use disorder have been conducted; both reported benefit in reducing methamphetamine use (Elkashef et al., 2012; Rezaei, Ghaderi, Mardani, Hamidi, & Hassanzadeh, 2016).

In summary, there is currently no medication with FDA approval for the management of psychostimulant use disorders (cocaine or methamphetamine). The partial success or lack of success with single agents has prompted consideration of combination pharmacotherapy to address the complexity of these disorders using agents with distinct mechanisms of action. For cocaine, an initial trial of amphetamine in combination with topiramate demonstrated significantly higher rates of abstinence compared with placebo (Mariani et al., 2012), warranting further evaluation in a larger multicenter study. For methamphetamine, the combination of injectable, extended-release naltrexone (Vivitrol®) plus once-daily bupropion extended-release tablets is currently being evaluated in a multisite RCT within the National Institute on Drug Abuse (NIDA) Clinical Trials Network (CTN: NCT03078075). Thus, novel medication combinations for stimulant use disorders appear warranted as a means to enhance the therapeutic effects of monotherapies.

BEST APPROACHES FOR ASSESSING TREATMENT RESPONSE AND MANAGING SIDE EFFECTS

There is no single definitive method to assess response to treatment of stimulant use disorders. It is important for clinicians to conduct ongoing reassessment of benefit from a trial of pharmacotherapy for stimulant use, including complete documentation of the initial evaluation and any positive or negative changes with each reassessment. The goal for long-term treatment of stimulant use disorders is overall improvement in function, not just reduction of stimulant use quantity or frequency. Improvement in function includes improvement in physical and mental health, employment, relationships, or criminal activity. Patients should be asked regularly about these areas of function to help determine treatment response.

The gold standard to assess treatment response is self-reported drug use. Asking about stimulant use at every follow-up visit is essential, including amount, frequency, route of administration, context, and triggers for use. The Timeline Followback (TLFB) is a method that can be used as a clinical tool to obtain a variety of quantitative estimates of stimulant use (Robinson, Sobell, Sobell, & Leo, 2014). It can be self-administered or administered by an interviewer or by computer, and it involves asking clients to retrospectively estimate their stimulant use ranging from 7 days to 2 years prior to the interview date. Quantitative estimates can be used to measure change in stimulant use levels in outcome monitoring. The TLFB can also be used as a motivational feedback tool to analyze clients' stimulant use and to increase motivation to change.

Drug testing for stimulant metabolites provides objective confirmation of the patient's self-report of recent use or abstinence. Urine testing is inexpensive, noninvasive and widely available through approved laboratories or point-of-care collection (done in the practitioner's office), and results are ready in minutes. Screening assays are available for a variety of stimulant compounds (amphetamine, methamphetamine, cocaine, etc.). While screening assays for cocaine have high reliability and few false positives, screening for amphetamine may be

TABLE 24.4

Randomized Placebo-Controlled Trials of GABAergic Agents for Treatment of Primary Stimulant Use Disorder

Agent (trade name)	Stimulant disorder/ sample size (% male)	Doses	Summary of primary outcomes
carbamazepine (Tegretol®)			
(Cornish et al., 1995)	cocaine *n* = 95 (98%)	carbamazepine: 200 mg/d increased to reach serum level of 4 to 12 µg/mL	No group differences in cocaine-positive urines
(Kranzler, Bauer, Hersh, & Klinghoffer, 1995)	cocaine *n* = 40 (100%)	carbamazepine: Up to 600 mg/d	No group differences in cocaine-use
(Montoya, Levin, Fudala, & Gorelick, 1995)	cocaine *n* = 72 (79%)	carbamazepine: Up to 800 mg/d	No group differences in cocaine-positive urines
(Halikas, Crosby, Pearson, & Graves, 1997)	cocaine *n* = 183 (71%)	carbamazepine: 400 mg/d; 800 mg/d	Reduction in cocaine-positive urines in the 400 mg/d group
(Campbell et al., 2003)	cocaine *n* = 146 (69.6%)	carbamazepine: Up to 800 mg/d	No group differences in cocaine-positive urines
tiagabine (Gabitril®)			
(Winhusen et al., 2005)	cocaine *n* = 34 (82%)	tiagabine: 20 mg/d; Sertraline: 100 mg/d; Donepezil: 10 mg/d	No group differences in cocaine-positive urines
(González et al., 2007)	cocaine *n* = 76 (76%)	tiagabine: 24 mg/d; gabapentin: 2,400 mg/d	Reduction in cocaine-positive urines in the tiagabine group
(Winhusen, Somoza, Ciraulo, et al., 2007)	cocaine *n* = 141 (67%)	tiagabine: 20 mg/d	No group differences in cocaine-positive urines
baclofen (Lioresal®)			
(Heinzerling et al., 2006)	methamphetamine *n* = 88 (69.3%)	baclofen: 30 mg/t.i.d.	No group differences in methamphetamine-positive urines
gabapentin (Neurontin®)			
(Berger et al., 2005)	cocaine *n* = 60 (70%)	gabapentin: 1,800 mg/d; reserpine: 0.5 mg/d; lamotrigine: 150 mg/d	Reduction in cocaine-positive urines for the reserpine group
(Bisaga et al., 2006)	cocaine *n* = 99 (88%)	gabapentin: 1,600 mg/b.i.d.	No group differences in cocaine-positive urines
(Heinzerling et al., 2006)	methamphetamine *n* = 88 (69.3%)	gabapentin: 800 mg/t.i.d.	No group differences in methamphetamine-positive urines
topiramate (Topamax®)			
(Kampman et al., 2004)	cocaine *n* = 40 (97.5%)	topiramate: 200 mg/d	Higher 3-week continuous abstinence in topiramate group
(Elkashef et al., 2012)	methamphetamine *n* = 890 (63.6%)	topiramate: 200 mg/d	No group differences in methamphetamine-positive urines. Reduction in weekly median urine methamphetamine levels in topiramate group.
(Johnson et al., 2013)	cocaine *n* = 142 (72.5%)	topiramate: 300 mg/d	Reduction in cocaine-positive urines for the topiramate group

TABLE 24.4

Randomized Placebo-Controlled Trials of GABAergic Agents for Treatment of Primary Stimulant Use Disorder (*Continued*)

Agent (trade name)	Stimulant disorder/ sample size (% male)	Doses	Summary of primary outcomes
(Kampman et al., 2013)	cocaine $n = 170$ (79%)	topiramate: 300 mg/d	Reduction in cocaine-positive urines for topiramate group with comorbid alcohol dependence and more severe cocaine withdrawal symptoms
(Nuijten, Blanken, van den Brink, & Hendriks, 2014)	cocaine $n = 82$ (81.6%)	topiramate: 200 mg/d	No group differences in cocaine-positive urines
(Umbricht et al., 2014)	cocaine $n = 171$ (52%)	topiramate: 300 mg/d	No group differences in cocaine-positive urines
(Rezaei et al., 2016)	Methamphetamine $n = 62$ (not reported)	topiramate: 200 mg/d	Reduction in methamphetamine-positive urines for the topiramate group
baclofen (Lioresal)			
(Shoptaw et al., 2003)	cocaine $n = 70$ (68.5%)	baclofen: 20 mg/t.i.d.	Reduced cocaine-positive urines in baclofen treatment group

Note. t.i.d. = three times a day; b.i.d. = two times a day.

confounded by several legitimate medications that patients may take for attention-deficit/hyperactivity disorder (e.g., dextroamphetamine salts [Adderall®], methylphenidate [Ritalin®], or lisdexamfetamine [Vyvanse]). This can, however, be verified by requesting information from the patient's prescriber or pharmacy. A false positive result may occur with common over-the-counter medications such as pseudoephedrine (Sudafed®), although this usually requires large doses. Confirmatory testing can identify not only the specific stimulant present in the patient's urine, but also the relative quantity (which can indicate high dose or recent use). Patients in early recovery may have drug testing at nearly every visit. This is not to "catch them in the act," but to deter undesirable behavior and assist patients in achieving abstinence for better treatment outcomes. As patients demonstrate appropriate ability to maintain abstinence and engage in recovery activities, the frequency of monitoring can be gradually reduced.

There are validated measures of specific symptoms of stimulant use disorders that may be useful for assessing treatment response. These include measures of craving (Lievaart et al., 2015; Northrup, Green, Walker, Greer, & Trivedi, 2015; Sussner

et al., 2006) and withdrawal (Kampman et al., 1998; Zorick et al., 2010), such as the Stimulant Craving Questionnaire (Northrup et al., 2015). The Cocaine Selective Severity Assessment (CSSA) is a validated instrument used for assessing cocaine withdrawal. The 18-item CSSA combines objective indicators (bradycardia) with self-reported symptoms, such as anxiety, craving for sweets, and anhedonia, rated on a scale of 0 to 7 (Kampman et al., 1998). For methamphetamine, the Methamphetamine Withdrawal Questionnaire is a 30-item, rater-scored instrument that uses a 4-point Likert scale to assess functional, emotional, physical, and additional symptoms of methamphetamine withdrawal, along with a review of vital signs (Zorick et al., 2010).

Each category of pharmacological approaches for treatment of psychostimulant disorders has its own set of side effects to consider. Most studies have shown the various pharmacotherapies that have been tried to be relatively well tolerated and, certainly, not more severe than the effects of ongoing stimulant use. No significant adverse events have been reported in studies of modafinil or sustained-release dextroamphetamine, suggesting that stimulant substitution treatment may be safe in patients using cocaine

(Gorelick, 2014). Common side effects of modafinil include anxiety, nausea, and headache; common side effects of dextroamphetamine include reduced appetite, insomnia, anxiety, and irritability.

Disulfiram is a functional DA agonist, which acts by blocking conversion of DA to norepinephrine (Gaval-Cruz & Weinshenker, 2009). Several human laboratory studies have given conflicting results about the safety of cocaine–disulfiram interactions (Baker, Jatlow, & McCance-Katz, 2007; Roache et al., 2011). Common side effects of disulfiram are drowsiness, headache, and a metallic taste in the mouth. Antipsychotic medications should be used with caution, especially in patients who use psychostimulants, because of the risk of developing antipsychotic-induced movement disorders (van Harten, van Trier, Horwitz, Matroos, & Hoek, 1998) or neuroleptic malignant syndrome (Akpaffiong & Ruiz, 1991). Other common side effects of typical antipsychotics include constipation, dry mouth, blurred vision, and weight gain. Antidepressant medications have been widely used for decades with no unexpected or medically serious side effects reported in published clinical trials in populations that include users of psychostimulants (Gorelick, 2014). However, there is an increased risk of cardiovascular side effects, especially arrhythmias, if a patient suffers a relapse to stimulant use while taking an antidepressant. One study demonstrated that concurrent administration of desipramine with cocaine in human volunteers caused additive elevations of heart rate and blood pressure (Fischman, Foltin, Nestadt, & Pearlson, 1990). Typical side effects of antidepressants experienced by patients include dizziness, headache, dry mouth, constipation, nausea, and tremor. Overall, pharmacotherapy for stimulant use disorders is well tolerated by patients and most dangerous side effects occur in the context of relapse to psychostimulant use. Patients should be cautioned about potential adverse effects that can happen if relapse occurs.

MEDICATION MANAGEMENT ISSUES

Medication management interventions to optimize treatment adherence play a critical role in evaluating pharmacotherapy for stimulant use disorders.

Broadly speaking, a number of factors contribute to not taking medications, including dosing frequency, cost, side effects, general illness factors, cognitive deficits, and comorbid psychiatric conditions (Swift, Oslin, Alexander, & Forman, 2011). Some of these issues can be mitigated by properly educating the patient about the rationale and potential benefit of the medication, as well as possible side effects and how to deal with them. It is important to assess perceived difficulty of the medication regimen as soon as possible, either at the initial visit or by scheduling a follow-up visit soon after the first appointment. If possible, doctors should discuss alternative medications that might be less costly, be taken less often, or have less aversive side effects. Finally, doctors may want to be proactive in promoting practical compliance aids (e.g., reminder text services, a calendar, pillboxes, incorporating assistance of friends and family members), particularly for individuals with cognitive and psychiatric conditions. For individuals with stimulant use disorders, the lack of an established effective medication may lower positive treatment expectations, resulting in poor compliance. Few of the medications evaluated to date have shown rapid onset of clinical benefit, another issue in medication management. As discussed later in this chapter, supportive behavioral interventions can be used to offset the relative weaknesses of pharmacotherapies for stimulant use disorders.

Indirect measures of medication compliance include self-report, pill counts, and electronic pill bottles. Self-report measures are the simplest and easiest to administer but are susceptible to memory lapses as well as deceptive reporting, generally resulting in overestimation of actual medication compliance (Stirratt et al., 2015). While electronic pill bottles can keep track of when the medication bottle is opened, and presumably consumed, this approach may be cost prohibitive or impractical in a community or private practice clinic setting, and patients can circumvent it by taking multiple pills when the bottle is opened or simply not taking the medication after removing it from the pill bottle.

As a more direct measure of pill consumption, compounds can be added to medications that are later detectable in urine. While a number of tracer assays have been employed (e.g., sodium bromide, methylene blue, phenol red, fluorescein, bromide, phenazopyridine), riboflavin (vitamin B_2) is most commonly utilized. Riboflavin is excreted in urine and can be detected under ultraviolet lighting using visual inspection as well as more rigorous quantitative assessments, but visual inspection has substantial interrater variability and a high rate of false positive readings (Herron et al., 2013; Mooney, Sayre, Green, Rhoades, & Schmitz, 2004). From a practical standpoint, these methods require a research pharmacy and are likely beyond the scope of a clinical setting.

Relapse is another medication management issue in the treatment of stimulant use disorders. As with other chronic medical illnesses, relapse is not only possible but likely (McLellan, Lewis, O'Brien, & Kleber, 2000). For individuals recovering from a stimulant use disorder, relapse may be perceived as a sign that their treatment has failed. Managing this issue typically involves patient education and counseling on understanding lapses and relapses as indications that medication needs to be reinstated or adjusted. It has been hypothesized that certain medications may be more effective for initiating abstinence in active stimulant users versus relapse prevention in abstinent users (Oliveto et al., 2012; Schmitz et al., 2014; Schmitz et al., 2018); however, this distinction has not been empirically established.

Another issue is the diversion of medications, including amphetamine analogs, in patients with stimulant use disorders. In the aforementioned RCTs of dextroamphetamine, methamphetamine, methylphenidate, and mazindol there were no reports of misuse, diversion, or addiction. Careful evaluation of risk in patients, along with repeated assessment at each visit for signs of misuse (e.g., discordant pill count, repeated lost prescription, symptoms of intoxication or withdrawal), should be conducted. Sustained release preparations are lower risk than immediate release preparations. As the field moves forward with development of prescribed controlled medications for stimulant use disorders, medication management strategies that reduce risk and resistance from the field will become increasingly important (Mariani & Levin, 2012).

EVALUATION OF PHARMACOLOGICAL APPROACHES ACROSS THE LIFESPAN

There has been scant research on pharmacotherapy for stimulant use disorders in adolescents. All of the medication RCTs reviewed previously (see Tables 24.1–24.4) targeted adults older than 18 years of age. Consequently, the safety and efficacy of potential medications for adolescent cocaine or methamphetamine users cannot be inferred from adult data. From a neurodevelopmental perspective, brain differences between adults and adolescents have implications in terms of how medications engage putative mechanisms of action. We found one pilot RCT of bupropion for adolescent (ages 14 to 21 years) methamphetamine abuse/dependence (Heinzerling et al., 2013). Twelve adolescents receiving bupropion sustained release 150 twice daily for 8 weeks were more likely to submit methamphetamine-positive urines compared with 7 participants receiving placebo, contrary to the positive effects of bupropion in reducing methamphetamine use in adults (Elkashef et al., 2008; Shoptaw, Heinzerling, Rotheram-Fuller, Steward, et al., 2008). Key questions remain regarding if and how medication could benefit youth. Medication development research is critically needed to curb substance-related problems during later development and adulthood.

Pharmacological treatment of stimulant use disorders among the elderly has been an understudied area as well. Traditionally, RCTs of medication treatments have excluded patients over the age of 65. The general belief is that the older population represents those with a lifetime history of drug use and not newly diagnosed cases. The extent to which medications tested for younger adults can be applied with equal success to older adults is unknown. Treatment approaches need to take into account unique vulnerabilities for older adults, including medical and mental health comorbidities (Kuerbis, Sacco, Blazer, & Moore, 2014).

CONSIDERATION OF POTENTIAL SEX DIFFERENCES

There are important sex differences in prevalence, course, treatment, and consequences of stimulant use disorders. According to SAMHSA (2016), approximately 34% of individuals in the United States who reported cocaine use in 2014 were women. There is some evidence that women use methamphetamines and other stimulants at equal or greater rates than men (SAMHSA, 2016). It is estimated that among adult users, about 60% are male, while in adolescent populations, more than half of methamphetamine users are female (Chen et al., 2014).

Across all substances, women tend to advance from first use to problematic use of substances earlier, relapse sooner, and suffer more health and social consequences than men (Becker, McClellan, & Reed, 2016; Najavits & Lester, 2008). Women typically seek specialized substance use disorders treatment at lower rates than men (Brady & Ashley, 2005), most likely because men have greater access to treatment through referral sources such as the criminal justice system (Cotto et al., 2010), while women more often seek help through primary care and mental health treatment services (Greenfield et al., 2007).

Despite the importance of considering sex differences in clinical research, a relatively small number of published results from RCTs report outcomes specific to sex. Most do not have sufficient power to detect sex differences or are more representative of men's treatment response. In a study that pooled results from five RCTs of disulfiram treatment for CUD, sex by medication effects were found, with disulfiram-treated women less likely to achieve 3 or more weeks of abstinence when compared with men receiving disulfiram (DeVito, Babuscio, Nich, Ball, & Carroll, 2014). Differential treatment outcomes were not explained by baseline sex differences or differences in medication dose, compliance, or days in treatment. Given that pharmacological treatments for addiction work through different mechanisms of action, it is important to understand how biological sex differences may affect response to treatments.

Modafinil is another DA agonist explored for possible differential sex effects. An RCT testing the effectiveness of modafinil along with CBT in 210 treatment-seeking cocaine users (male $n = 157$, female $n = 53$) found no overall significant effect on the primary outcome of cocaine-positive urines (see Table 24.1), but reported a greater tendency (though not significant) for males to be cocaine-abstinent than females (Dackis et al., 2012). Although the mechanisms for these sex differences with disulfiram and modafinil are not clear, these drugs may alter the reinforcing effects of cocaine, which may be different in men and women.

A study of high-dose (150 mg/day) naltrexone found sex differences in treatment of patients with co-occurring alcohol and cocaine dependence. Compared with placebo, men treated with naltrexone showed greater reduction in cocaine use and drug use severity, whereas women treated with naltrexone showed an increase in cocaine use (Pettinati, Kampman, Lynch, Xie, et al., 2008). The most likely reason for these differential responses is that women experienced more side effects with naltrexone. Men taking naltrexone had a slightly higher rate of medication adherence than women taking naltrexone, while women assigned to naltrexone tended to have higher attrition rates than men. Women's attrition rates were associated with more reported nausea in those receiving naltrexone (Pettinati, Kampman, Lynch, Suh, et al., 2008; Suh, Pettinati, Kampman, & O'Brien, 2008).

Studies examining sex differences in response to medication treatments for other stimulant use disorders (amphetamine and methamphetamine) have been equally scarce. One study noted that bupropion (vs. placebo) significantly reduced methamphetamine use in male participants with low to moderate use at baseline. This result did not hold for female participants in the study. Researchers suggested that the greater percentage of women in this sample with high baseline methamphetamine use might explain these sex differences (Elkashef et al., 2008). These results were not replicated in a similar trial examining bupropion in the treatment of nondaily methamphetamine users (Anderson et al., 2015).

INTEGRATION OF PHARMACOTHERAPY WITH NONPHARMACOLOGICAL APPROACHES: BENEFITS AND CHALLENGES

There are several rationales for using integrated approaches to treat stimulant use disorders. First, the neurobiological and behavioral complexity of these disorders calls for a multicomponent approach that "attends to the multiple needs of the individual, not just his or her drug abuse" (NIDA, 2012, p. 5). A medication, even when found to be effective, cannot by itself address associated social, vocational, or legal problems resulting from chronic drug abuse. Second, in the absence of approved pharmacotherapy, effective nonpharmacological behavioral and psychosocial approaches, including motivational interviewing, CBT, individual drug counseling, and contingency management, have been the mainstays of treatment for cocaine and methamphetamine use disorders (Dutra et al., 2008; Jhanjee, 2014; Roll et al., 2006). Third, combining pharmacological and behavioral interventions that target shared or complementary processes of addiction has the potential to yield additive or synergistic treatment effects. A few examples of such combinations are discussed in this section.

One well-studied pharmacologic approach has been to target the DA neurotransmitter system in the brain with agonist-like medications that may improve reward function. In corresponding fashion, contingency management is a behavioral intervention aimed at increasing access to nondrug rewards contingent on achievement of therapeutic goals, such as abstinence (Petry, Alessi, Olmstead, Rash, & Zajac, 2017). When paired with a DA agent, the combined effects would be expected to enhance response to contingency management treatment. This integrated model of using medications to facilitate contingency management responding has been tested with agonist-like medications (Mooney et al., 2009; Schmitz, Lindsay, Stotts, Green, & Moeller, 2010) as well as antidepressants, including desipramine, bupropion, and citalopram (Kosten et al., 2003; Moeller et al., 2007; Poling et al., 2006), showing some evidence of clinical efficacy.

Another integrated model has been to use pharmacotherapies to facilitate the effects of behavioral interventions on so-called "top down" executive control processes. CBT, for example, attempts to change cognitions and behaviors by heightening awareness of drug-related cues and developing new coping skills. Medications that have cognitive-enhancing effects may optimize response to CBT by addressing impairments that predict poor treatment

engagement and outcome (Sofuoglu, DeVito, Waters, & Carroll, 2013). Galantamine (Sofuoglu, Waters, Poling, & Carroll, 2011) and rivastigmine (Mahoney et al., 2014) have been evaluated for cognitive-enhancing effects in chronic cocaine users; both drugs improved measures of cognitive performance. The potential efficacy of these medications for treatment of stimulant use disorders is being evaluated in current RCTs (e.g., NCT01030692, NCT00809835). It remains to be determined whether the integration of cognitive-enhancing pharmacological and behavioral treatments improves drug use outcomes.

Adherence has been another target for integrated treatment. Elkashef et al. (2012), in their multi-center placebo-controlled trial of topiramate for the treatment of methamphetamine addiction, delivered concurrent brief behavioral compliance enhancement treatment (BBCET) to offset the lengthy 6-week upward dose titration of topiramate. BBCET is a manual-driven, low-intensity psychosocial procedure that emphasizes the importance of medication adherence in changing addictive behavior (Johnson, DiClemente, & Ait-Daoud, 2003). In an ongoing multicenter RCT sponsored by the National Drug Abuse Treatment Clinical Trials Network, the combination of extended-release bupropion and long-acting injectable naltrexone is being evaluated in methamphetamine users (NCT03078075), utilizing nonpharmacological interventions, such as a smartphone video adherence procedure, to maximize compliance with these medications.

INTEGRATED APPROACHES FOR ADDRESSING COMMON COMORBID DISORDERS

Stimulant use disorders commonly co-occur with other substance use (e.g., tobacco cigarettes, alcohol, marijuana, opioids) and psychiatric disorders. The high prevalence of multiple drug use and its clinical impact has prompted efforts toward developing integrated approaches for addressing this comorbidity, with nicotine dependence being a case in point. SAMHSA issued an advisory to promote tobacco smoking cessation among individuals receiving treatment for substance use disorders (SAMHSA, 2011). The advisory cites a seminal

11-year retrospective cohort study among 845 individuals receiving addiction treatment, showing that 51% of deaths in that population resulted from tobacco smoking-related causes. This rate is twice that found in the general population and nearly 1.5 times greater than any other addiction-related causes. Overall, there appears to be no reason not to provide nicotine replacement therapy to individuals with stimulant use disorders that smoke tobacco cigarettes. A recent review of smoking cessation interventions for adults in treatment for substance use disorders, including stimulant use disorders, found no evidence of negative effects on treatment outcomes (Thurgood, McNeill, Clark-Carter, & Brose, 2016).

Alcohol use disorder also commonly co-occurs with stimulant use disorders and is associated with greater negative drug-related health consequences, greater psychosocial problems, poorer treatment adherence, and higher rates of treatment recidivism (Flannery, Morgenstern, McKay, Wechsberg, & Litten, 2004). Early studies assessing the effects of the opioid antagonist naltrexone for the treatment of alcohol dependence, failed to see any effects on alcohol or cocaine use in dual-dependent patients (Hersh, Van Kirk, & Kranzler, 1998; Schmitz, Stotts, Sayre, DeLaune, & Grabowski, 2004). Later studies testing higher doses of naltrexone (150 mg/day), however, reported positive effects in reducing both cocaine and alcohol use (Oslin et al., 1999; Pettinati, Kampman, Lynch, Suh, et al., 2008). Pettinati, Kampman, Lynch, Xie, et al. (2008) assessed the effects of disulfiram (250 mg/day) and naltrexone (100 mg/day) alone and in combination among individuals (*n* = 208) with comorbid CUD and AUD. Individuals receiving disulfiram alone or in combination with naltrexone were the most likely to achieve combined abstinence from cocaine and alcohol.

Common comorbid psychiatric disorders in stimulant use disorders include schizophrenia, depression, and anxiety (including PTSD). With no approved medications for stimulant use disorders, one treatment strategy has been to reduce substance use indirectly by targeting psychiatric symptoms with psychotropic drugs. The atypical antipsychotic medication olanzapine has been evaluated for treatment of schizophrenia and comorbid substance

use disorders in two trials, demonstrating benefit in terms of reducing both psychotic symptoms and drug use (Littrell, Petty, Hilligoss, Peabody, & Johnson, 2001; Smelson et al., 2006). Some evidence supports the efficacy of antidepressants in treating co-occurring CUD and depression (Moeller et al., 2007; Oliveto et al., 2012; Rounsaville, 2004). In a RCT examining the efficacy of imipramine in the treatment of individuals with CUD, compared with the placebo group, individuals treated with imipramine and CBT had greater reductions in depression, cocaine craving, and consecutive abstinence. This favorable response occurred more frequently among the subgroup of cocaine users that had a primary or secondary depressive disorder according to *DSM–III–R* criteria. The researchers suggested that efficacy of imipramine may be limited to clinically defined subgroups of depressed cocaine users; however, these findings have not undergone replication. (Nunes et al., 1995).

Oliveto et al. (2012) enrolled 86 cocaine-dependent patients with depressive symptoms (Hamilton score > 15) in a double-blind RCT consisting of a 2-week residential treatment program followed by a 10-week outpatient treatment program with random assignment to sertraline or placebo. Compared with placebo, the sertraline group showed a trend toward longer time before their first cocaine-positive urine during treatment (lapse) and had significantly more days until relapse (consecutive cocaine-positive urines). Depression scores for both groups decreased over time, with the sharpest decline occurring during the first week of treatment, suggesting that depression at the start of treatment for this sample was indicative of an acute state (Oliveto et al., 2012). A follow-up study evaluating sertraline plus gabapentin in depressed cocaine-dependent patients failed to find the combination to be superior to sertraline alone in delaying relapse (Mancino et al., 2014).

EMERGING TRENDS

Pharmacotherapies for psychostimulant use disorders have predominantly focused on the modulation of monoamines, the details of which are summarized in preceding sections of this chapter. Unfortunately, despite considerable effort and expense, in absentia to date are controlled clinical trials that demonstrate a safety and efficacy profile sufficient to warrant evidence for an indication in the treatment of psychostimulant drug of abuse. This has led investigators to consider novel alternative pharmacological intervention strategies for psychostimulant use disorders. Three emerging trends will be described in this section: vaccines, anti-inflammatories, and the anesthetic agent ketamine.

Vaccines portend to reduce or eliminate the penetration of the abused drug into the central nervous system through a unique pharmacokinetic mechanism (Brimijoin, Shen, Orson, & Kosten, 2013). Clinical trials using active vaccine approaches to treat cocaine abuse have provided mixed results. Early phase trials demonstrated safety, proof of concept in the generation of cocaine antibodies, and reduction in cocaine's subjective rewarding effects (Haney, Gunderson, Jiang, Collins, & Foltin, 2010; Kosten & Domingo, 2013; Kosten, Domingo, Orson, & Kinsey, 2014; Orson et al., 2014; Pravetoni, 2016) and in reducing cocaine-positive urines (Martell et al., 2009). However, in a subsequent multisite clinical trial, the vaccine was not statistically different than placebo (Kosten, Domingo, Shorter, et al., 2014). Importantly, this trial revealed considerable individual variation in the production of cocaine antibodies. Participants who produced a high antibody response had the most cocaine-free urines at the end of treatment (Kosten, Domingo, Shorter, et al., 2014). Clinical trials are underway for CUD using a novel gene transfer method to promote higher antibody levels (Weill Medical College of Cornell University, 2015) and human studies of enzyme biologics (cholinesterases) for CUD are currently in Phase 1 and 2 testing (Indivior, 2013; Teva Pharmaceutical Industries, 2013).

The first vaccines for methamphetamine use disorder are presently being examined in humans. One vaccine developed by InterveXion Therapeutics (Little Rock, Arkansas) provided evidence of safety and efficacy in Phase 1 studies (InterveXion Therapeutics LLC, 2012; Stevens, Henry, Owens, Schutz, & Gentry, 2014) and has now been funded to initiate an initial Phase 2 clinical trial (Stevens & Owens, 2017). A second vaccine for methamphetamine (Kadvax Technologies, Houston, TX) will use

a new method to generate substantially higher antibody levels than first generation vaccines. This project is currently funded to test human Phase 1 and 2 studies (Kogan & Kosten, 2017).

Preclinical and human studies provide evidence that psychostimulant abuse is associated with both acute and chronic inflammation (Sajja, Rahman, & Cucullo, 2016); however, only a small number of clinical trials have explicitly examined medications based on their anti-inflammatory properties. An earlier clinical trial of the COX-2 nonsteroidal anti-inflammatory medication celecoxib in cocaine users found no differences from placebo in primary cocaine use outcomes (Reid, Angrist, et al., 2005). Preliminary evidence suggests that ibudilast, a compound with strong anti-inflammatory properties and neuroprotective effects, may improve aspects of cognition during early methamphetamine abstinence (Birath et al., 2017). A clinical trial for treatment of methamphetamine use disorder with ibudilast is currently in progress (University of California Los Angeles, 2013). Pioglitazone is a peroxisome proliferator-activated receptor gamma (PPAR-γ) agonist that exerts a range of anti-inflammatory and antioxidative effects that promote neuroprotection (Feinstein, 2003; Neher, Weckbach, Huber-Lang, & Stahel, 2012). A preliminary clinical trial of pioglitazone provided evidence for improved white matter integrity and reduced craving intensity in patients with primary CUD (Schmitz et al., 2017).

The anesthetic ketamine has made a distinct impact in psychiatry for the treatment of refractory depression (Murrough, Abdallah, & Mathew, 2017; Sanacora et al., 2017). It is believed that ketamine's rapid-onset efficacy in depression is facilitated via modulation of glutamate in the prefrontal cortex. These glutamate-mediated effects have led investigators to speculate that ketamine administration might stabilize dysphoric mood and enhance motivation and behavior change in substance abusers, particularly when combined with psychotherapy (Dakwar, Anerella, et al., 2014). Initial laboratory-based studies for CUD demonstrated efficacy in reducing cocaine-cue induced craving and motivation to stop cocaine use (Dakwar, Levin, Foltin, Nunes, & Hart, 2014), and robust attenuation of cocaine self-administration (Dakwar, Hart, Levin, Nunes, &

Foltin, 2017). The results prompted a recently completed outpatient clinical trial in participants with CUD, the results of which are completed but not yet in the public domain (New York State Psychiatric Institute, 2012).

SUMMARY

Implementation of psychopharmacology for the treatment of stimulant use disorders remains a challenge, with no medications specifically approved to treat cocaine or methamphetamine addiction. In the absence of an approved medication, behavioral interventions are the mainstay of treatment. The Tool Kit of Resources provides clinicians with comprehensive reviews of available evidence on pharmacologic treatment strategies. For patients, there are several websites that provide reliable information on understanding and overcoming addiction.

TOOL KIT OF RESOURCES

Patient Resources

National Institute on Drug Abuse (NIDA) Drug Use Screening Tool Support Materials: https://www.drugabuse.gov/sites/default/files/files/QuickScreen_Updated_2013%281%29.pdf

National Institute on Drug Abuse (NIDA), Advancing Addiction Science: Methamphetamine: https://www.drugabuse.gov/drugs-abuse/methamphetamine

National Institute on Drug Abuse (NIDA), Advancing Addiction Science: Cocaine: https://www.drugabuse.gov/drugs-abuse/cocaine

SMART Recovery® Self-Management and Recovery Training: http://www.smartrecovery.org/resources/toolchest.htm

Weaver, M. F. (2017). *Addiction treatment.* Newburyport, MA: Carlat Publishing.

Provider Resources

Ballester, J., Valentine, G., & Sofuoglu, M. (2017). Pharmacological treatments for methamphetamine addiction: Current status and future directions. *Expert Review of Clinical Pharmacology, 10,* 305–314. http://dx.doi.org/10.1080/17512433.2017.1268916

*Asterisks indicate assessments or resources.

Brensilver, M., Heinzerling, K. G., & Shoptaw, S. (2013). Pharmacotherapy of amphetamine-type stimulant dependence: An update. *Drug and Alcohol Review, 32,* 449–460. http://dx.doi.org/10.1111/dar.12048

Center for Substance Abuse Treatment. (1999). *Treatment for stimulant use disorders (Treatment Improvement Protocol [TIP] Series, No. 33).* Rockville, MD: Substance Abuse and Mental Health Services Administration.

Negus, S. S., & Henningfield J. (2015). Agonist medications for the treatment of cocaine use disorder. *Neuropsychopharmacology, 40,* 1815–1825. http://dx.doi.org/10.1038/npp.2014.322

Shorter, D., Domingo, C. B., & Kosten, T. R. (2014). Emerging drugs for the treatment of cocaine use disorder: A review of neurobiological targets and pharmacotherapy. *Expert Opinion on Emerging Drugs, 20,* 15–29. http://dx.doi.org/10.1517/14728214.2015.985203

Weaver, M. F. (2017). *Addiction treatment.* Newburyport, MA: Carlat Publishing.

References

Akpaffiong, M. J., & Ruiz, P. (1991). Neuroleptic malignant syndrome: A complication of neuroleptics and cocaine abuse. *Psychiatric Quarterly, 62,* 299–309. http://dx.doi.org/10.1007/BF01958798

Álvarez, Y., Pérez-Mañá, C., Torrens, M., & Farré, M. (2013). Antipsychotic drugs in cocaine dependence: A systematic review and meta-analysis. *Journal of Substance Abuse Treatment, 45,* 1–10. http://dx.doi.org/10.1016/j.jsat.2012.12.013

Amato, L., Minozzi, S., Pani, P. P., & Davoli, M. (2007). Antipsychotic medications for cocaine dependence. *Cochrane Database of Systematic Reviews, 2007*(3): CD006306. http://dx.doi.org/10.1002/14651858.CD006306.pub2

American Psychiatric Association. (2013). *Diagnostic and statistical manual of mental disorders* (5th ed.). Washington, DC: Author.

Anderson, A. L., Li, S. H., Biswas, K., McSherry, F., Holmes, T., Iturriaga, E., . . . Elkashef, A. M. (2012). Modafinil for the treatment of methamphetamine dependence. *Drug and Alcohol Dependence, 120,* 135–141. http://dx.doi.org/10.1016/j.drugalcdep.2011.07.007

Anderson, A. L., Li, S. H., Markova, D., Holmes, T. H., Chiang, N., Kahn, R., . . . Elkashef, A. M. (2015). Bupropion for the treatment of methamphetamine dependence in non-daily users: A randomized, double-blind, placebo-controlled trial. *Drug and Alcohol Dependence, 150,* 170–174. http://dx.doi.org/10.1016/j.drugalcdep.2015.01.036

Anderson, A. L., Reid, M. S., Li, S. H., Holmes, T., Shemanski, L., Slee, A., . . . Elkashef, A. M. (2009). Modafinil for the treatment of cocaine dependence. *Drug and Alcohol Dependence, 104,* 133–139. http://dx.doi.org/10.1016/j.drugalcdep.2009.04.015

Baker, J. R., Jatlow, P., & McCance-Katz, E. F. (2007). Disulfiram effects on responses to intravenous cocaine administration. *Drug and Alcohol Dependence, 87,* 202–209. http://dx.doi.org/10.1016/j.drugalcdep.2006.08.016

Banks, M. L., Hutsell, B. A., Blough, B. E., Poklis, J. L., & Negus, S. S. (2015). Preclinical assessment of lisdexamfetamine as an agonist medication candidate for cocaine addiction: Effects in rhesus monkeys trained to discriminate cocaine or to self-administer cocaine in a cocaine versus food choice procedure. *International Journal of Neuropsychopharmacology, 18,* 1–10. http://dx.doi.org/10.1093/ijnp/pyv009

Batki, S. L., Washburn, A. M., Delucchi, K., & Jones, R. T. (1996). A controlled trial of fluoxetine in crack cocaine dependence. *Drug and Alcohol Dependence, 41,* 137–142. http://dx.doi.org/10.1016/0376-8716(96)01233-1

Becker, J. B., McClellan, M., & Reed, B. G. (2016). Sociocultural context for sex differences in addiction. *Addiction Biology, 21,* 1052–1059. http://dx.doi.org/10.1111/adb.12383

Berger, S. P., Winhusen, T. M., Somoza, E. C., Harrer, J. M., Mezinskis, J. P., Leiderman, D. B., . . . Elkashef, A. (2005). A medication screening trial evaluation of reserpine, gabapentin and lamotrigine pharmacotherapy of cocaine dependence. *Addiction, 100*(Suppl. 1), 58–67. http://dx.doi.org/10.1111/j.1360-0443.2005.00983.x

Bhatt, M., Zielinski, L., Baker-Beal, L., Bhatnagar, N., Mouravska, N., Laplante, P., . . . Samaan, Z. (2016). Efficacy and safety of psychostimulants for amphetamine and methamphetamine use disorders: A systematic review and meta-analysis. *Systematic Reviews, 5,* 189. http://dx.doi.org/10.1186/s13643-016-0370-x

Birath, J. B., Briones, M., Amaya, S., Shoptaw, S., Swanson, A. N., Tsuang, J., . . . Wright, M. J. (2017). Ibudilast may improve attention during early abstinence from methamphetamine. *Drug and Alcohol Dependence, 178,* 386–390. http://dx.doi.org/10.1016/j.drugalcdep.2017.05.016

Bisaga, A., Aharonovich, E., Garawi, F., Levin, F. R., Rubin, E., Raby, W. N., & Nunes, E. V. (2006). A randomized placebo-controlled trial of gabapentin for cocaine dependence. *Drug and Alcohol Depen-*dence, 81, 267–274. http://dx.doi.org/10.1016/j.drugalcdep.2005.07.009

Brady, T. M., & Ashley, O. S. (2005). *Women in substance abuse treatment: Results from the Alcohol and Drug Services Study (ADSS).* Rockville, MD: Substance Abuse and Mental Health Services Administration.

Brimijoin, S., Shen, X., Orson, F., & Kosten, T. (2013). Prospects, promise and problems on the road to effective vaccines and related therapies for substance abuse. *Expert Review of Vaccines, 12,* 323–332. http://dx.doi.org/10.1586/erv.13.1

Campbell, J., Nickel, E. J., Penick, E. C., Wallace, D., Gabrielli, W. F., Rowe, C., . . . Thomas, H. M. (2003). Comparison of desipramine or carbamazepine to placebo for crack cocaine-dependent patients. *The American Journal on Addictions, 12,* 122–136. http://dx.doi.org/10.1111/j.1521-0391.2003.tb00610.x

Carroll, K. M., Fenton, L. R., Ball, S. A., Nich, C., Frankforter, T. L., Shi, J., & Rounsaville, B. J. (2004). Efficacy of disulfiram and cognitive behavior therapy in cocaine-dependent outpatients: A randomized placebo-controlled trial. *Archives of General Psychiatry, 61,* 264–272. http://dx.doi.org/10.1001/archpsyc.61.3.264

Carroll, K. M., Nich, C., Petry, N. M., Eagan, D. A., Shi, J. M., & Ball, S. A. (2016). A randomized factorial trial of disulfiram and contingency management to enhance cognitive behavioral therapy for cocaine dependence. *Drug and Alcohol Dependence, 160,* 135–142. http://dx.doi.org/10.1016/j.drugalcdep.2015.12.036

Carroll, K. M., Rounsaville, B. J., Gordon, L. T., Nich, C., Jatlow, P., Bisighini, R. M., & Gawin, F. H. (1994). Psychotherapy and pharmacotherapy for ambulatory cocaine abusers. *Archives of General Psychiatry, 51,* 177–187. http://dx.doi.org/10.1001/archpsyc.1994.03950030013002

Center for Behavioral Health Statistics and Quality. (2016). Key substance use and mental health indicators in the United States: Results from the 2015 National Survey on Drug Use and Health (HHS Publication No. SMA 16-4984, NSDUH Series H-51). http://www.samhsa.gov/data

Center for Substance Abuse Treatment. (1999). Introduction. In Center for Substance Abuse Treatment, *Treatment for Stimulant Use Disorders* (pp. 1–9). Rockville, MD: Substance Abuse and Mental Health Services Administration.

Chen, L.-Y., Strain, E. C., Alexandre, P. K., Alexander, G. C., Mojtabai, R., & Martins, S. S. (2014). Correlates of nonmedical use of stimulants and methamphetamine use in a national sample. *Addictive Behaviors, 39,* 829–836. http://dx.doi.org/10.1016/j.addbeh.2014.01.018

Ciraulo, D. A., Knapp, C., Rotrosen, J., Sarid-Segal, O., Ciraulo, A. M., LoCastro, J., . . . Leiderman, D.

(2005). Nefazodone treatment of cocaine dependence with comorbid depressive symptoms. *Addiction, 100*(Suppl. 1), 23–31. http://dx.doi.org/10.1111/j.1360-0443.2005.00984.x

Colfax, G. N., Santos, G. M., Das, M., Santos, D. M., Matheson, T., Gasper, J., . . . Vittinghoff, E. (2011). Mirtazapine to reduce methamphetamine use: A randomized controlled trial. *Archives of General Psychiatry, 68*, 1168–1175. http://dx.doi.org/10.1001/archgenpsychiatry.2011.124

Cornish, J. W., Maany, I., Fudala, P. J., Neal, S., Poole, S. A., Volpicelli, P., & O'Brien, C. P. (1995). Carbamazepine treatment for cocaine dependence. *Drug and Alcohol Dependence, 38*, 221–227. http://dx.doi.org/10.1016/0376-8716(95)01102-5

Cotto, J. H., Davis, E., Dowling, G. J., Elcano, J. C., Staton, A. B., & Weiss, S. R. (2010). Gender effects on drug use, abuse, and dependence: A special analysis of results from the National Survey on Drug Use and Health. *Gender Medicine, 7*, 402–413. http://dx.doi.org/10.1016/j.genm.2010.09.004

Courtney, K. E., & Ray, L. A. (2014). Methamphetamine: An update on epidemiology, pharmacology, clinical phenomenology, and treatment literature. *Drug and Alcohol Dependence, 143*(Suppl. C), 11–21. http://dx.doi.org/10.1016/j.drugalcdep.2014.08.003

Covi, L., Hess, J. M., Kreiter, N. A., & Haertzen, C. A. (1995). Effects of combined fluoxetine and counseling in the outpatient treatment of cocaine abusers. *The American Journal of Drug and Alcohol Abuse, 21*, 327–344. http://dx.doi.org/10.3109/00952999509002701

Dackis, C. A., Kampman, K. M., Lynch, K. G., Pettinati, H. M., & O'Brien, C. P. (2005). A double-blind, placebo-controlled trial of modafinil for cocaine dependence. *Neuropsychopharmacology, 30*, 205–211. http://dx.doi.org/10.1038/sj.npp.1300600

Dackis, C. A., Kampman, K. M., Lynch, K. G., Plebani, J. G., Pettinati, H. M., Sparkman, T., & O'Brien, C. P. (2012). A double-blind, placebo-controlled trial of modafinil for cocaine dependence. *Journal of Substance Abuse Treatment, 43*, 303–312. http://dx.doi.org/10.1016/j.jsat.2011.12.014

Dakwar, E., Anerella, C., Hart, C. L., Levin, F. R., Mathew, S. J., & Nunes, E. V. (2014). Therapeutic infusions of ketamine: Do the psychoactive effects matter? *Drug and Alcohol Dependence, 136*, 153–157. http://dx.doi.org/10.1016/j.drugalcdep.2013.12.019

Dakwar, E., Hart, C. L., Levin, F. R., Nunes, E. V., & Foltin, R. W. (2017). Cocaine self-administration disrupted by the N-methyl-D-aspartate receptor antagonist ketamine: A randomized, crossover trial. *Molecular Psychiatry, 22*, 76–81. http://dx.doi.org/10.1038/mp.2016.39

Dakwar, E., Levin, F., Foltin, R. W., Nunes, E. V., & Hart, C. L. (2014). The effects of subanesthetic ketamine infusions on motivation to quit and cue-induced craving in cocaine-dependent research volunteers. *Biological Psychiatry, 76*, 40–46. http://dx.doi.org/10.1016/j.biopsych.2013.08.009

Das, M., Santos, D., Matheson, T., Santos, G. M., Chu, P., Vittinghoff, E., . . . Colfax, G. N. (2010). Feasibility and acceptability of a phase II randomized pharmacologic intervention for methamphetamine dependence in high-risk men who have sex with men. *AIDS, 24*, 991–1000. http://dx.doi.org/10.1097/QAD.0b013e328336e98b

Degenhardt, L., Baxter, A. J., Lee, Y. Y., Hall, W., Sara, G. E., Johns, N., . . . Vos, T. (2014). The global epidemiology and burden of psychostimulant dependence: Findings from the Global Burden of Disease Study 2010. *Drug and Alcohol Dependence, 137*, 36–47. http://dx.doi.org/10.1016/j.drugalcdep.2013.12.025

DeVito, E. E., Babuscio, T. A., Nich, C., Ball, S. A., & Carroll, K. M. (2014). Gender differences in clinical outcomes for cocaine dependence: Randomized clinical trials of behavioral therapy and disulfiram. *Drug and Alcohol Dependence, 145*, 156–167. http://dx.doi.org/10.1016/j.drugalcdep.2014.10.007

Dutra, L., Stathopoulou, G., Basden, S. L., Leyro, T. M., Powers, M. B., & Otto, M. W. (2008). A meta-analytic review of psychosocial interventions for substance use disorders. *The American Journal of Psychiatry, 165*, 179–187. http://dx.doi.org/10.1176/appi.ajp.2007.06111851

Elkashef, A., Fudala, P. J., Gorgon, L., Li, S. H., Kahn, R., Chiang, N., . . . Sather, M. (2006). Double-blind, placebo-controlled trial of selegiline transdermal system (STS) for the treatment of cocaine dependence. *Drug and Alcohol Dependence, 85*, 191–197. http://dx.doi.org/10.1016/j.drugalcdep.2006.04.010

Elkashef, A., Kahn, R., Yu, E., Iturriaga, E., Li, S. H., Anderson, A., . . . Johnson, B. A. (2012). Topiramate for the treatment of methamphetamine addiction: A multi-center placebo-controlled trial. *Addiction, 107*, 1297–1306. http://dx.doi.org/10.1111/j.1360-0443.2011.03771.x

Elkashef, A. M., Rawson, R. A., Anderson, A. L., Li, S. H., Holmes, T., Smith, E. V., . . . Weis, D. (2008). Bupropion for the treatment of methamphetamine dependence. *Neuropsychopharmacology, 33*, 1162–1170. http://dx.doi.org/10.1038/sj.npp.1301481

Feinstein, D. L. (2003). Therapeutic potential of peroxisome proliferator-activated receptor agonists for neurological disease. *Diabetes Technology & Therapeutics, 5*, 67–73. http://dx.doi.org/10.1089/152091503763816481

First, M. B., Williams, J. B., Karg, R. S., & Spitzer, R. L. (2015). *Structured clinical interview for DSM–5:*

Research Version. Arlington, VA: American Psychiatric Association.

Fischman, M. W., Foltin, R. W., Nestadt, G., & Pearlson, G. D. (1990). Effects of desipramine maintenance on cocaine self-administration by humans. *The Journal of Pharmacology and Experimental Therapeutics, 253*, 760–770.

Flannery, B. A., Morgenstern, J., McKay, J., Wechsberg, W. M., & Litten, R. Z. (2004). Co-occurring alcohol and cocaine dependence: Recent findings from clinical and field studies. *Alcoholism: Clinical and Experimental Research, 28*, 976–981. http://dx.doi.org/10.1097/01.ALC.0000128232.30331.65

Galloway, G. P., Buscemi, R., Coyle, J. R., Flower, K., Siegrist, J. D., Fiske, L. A., . . . Mendelson, J. (2011). A randomized, placebo-controlled trial of sustained-release dextroamphetamine for treatment of methamphetamine addiction. *Clinical Pharmacology and Therapeutics, 89*, 276–282. http://dx.doi.org/10.1038/clpt.2010.307

Gaval-Cruz, M., & Weinshenker, D. (2009). Mechanisms of disulfiram-induced cocaine abstinence: Antabuse and cocaine relapse. *Molecular Interventions, 9*, 175–187. http://dx.doi.org/10.1124/mi.9.4.6

Gawin, F. H., Khalsa-Denison, M. E., & Jatlow, P. (1996). Flupentixol-induced aversion to crack cocaine. *The New England Journal of Medicine, 334*, 1340–1341. http://dx.doi.org/10.1056/NEJM199605163342018

Gawin, F. H., Kleber, H. D., Byck, R., Rounsaville, B. J., Kosten, T. R., Jatlow, P. I., & Morgan, C. (1989). Desipramine facilitation of initial cocaine abstinence. *Archives of General Psychiatry, 46*, 117–121. http://dx.doi.org/10.1001/archpsyc.1989.01810020019004

González, G., Desai, R., Sofuoglu, M., Poling, J., Oliveto, A., Gonsai, K., & Kosten, T. R. (2007). Clinical efficacy of gabapentin versus tiagabine for reducing cocaine use among cocaine dependent methadone-treated patients. *Drug and Alcohol Dependence, 87*, 1–9. http://dx.doi.org/10.1016/j.drugalcdep.2006.07.003

Gorelick, D. A. (2014). Pharmacologic interventions for cocaine, methamphetamine, and other stimulant addiction. In R. K. Ries, D. A. Fiellin, S. C. Miller, & R. Saitz (Eds.), *The ASAM principles of addiction medicine, 5th edition*. Philadelphia, PA: Lippincott Williams & Wilkins.

Grabowski, J., Rhoades, H., Elk, R., Schmitz, J., Davis, C., Creson, D., & Kirby, K. (1995). Fluoxetine is ineffective for treatment of cocaine dependence or concurrent opiate and cocaine dependence: Two placebo-controlled, double-blind trials. *Journal of Clinical Psychopharmacology, 15*, 163–174. http://dx.doi.org/10.1097/00004714-199506000-00004

Grabowski, J., Rhoades, H., Schmitz, J., Stotts, A., Daruszka, L. A., Creson, D., & Moeller, F. G. (2001). Dextroamphetamine for cocaine-dependence treatment:

A double-blind randomized clinical trial. *Journal of Clinical Psychopharmacology, 21*, 522–526. http://dx.doi.org/10.1097/00004714-200110000-00010

Grabowski, J., Rhoades, H., Silverman, P., Schmitz, J. M., Stotts, A., Creson, D., & Bailey, R. (2000). Risperidone for the treatment of cocaine dependence: Randomized, double-blind trial. *Journal of Clinical Psychopharmacology, 20*, 305–310. http://dx.doi.org/10.1097/00004714-200006000-00003

Grabowski, J., Rhoades, H., Stotts, A., Cowan, K., Kopecky, C., Dougherty, A., . . . Schmitz, J. (2004). Agonist-like or antagonist-like treatment for cocaine dependence with methadone for heroin dependence: Two double-blind randomized clinical trials. *Neuropsychopharmacology, 29*, 969–981. http://dx.doi.org/10.1038/sj.npp.1300392

Grabowski, J., Roache, J. D., Schmitz, J. M., Rhoades, H., Creson, D., & Korszun, A. (1997). Replacement medication for cocaine dependence: Methylphenidate. *Journal of Clinical Psychopharmacology, 17*, 485–488. http://dx.doi.org/10.1097/00004714-199712000-00008

Greenfield, S. F., Brooks, A. J., Gordon, S. M., Green, C. A., Kropp, F., McHugh, R. K., . . . Miele, G. M. (2007). Substance abuse treatment entry, retention, and outcome in women: A review of the literature. *Drug and Alcohol Dependence, 86*, 1–21. http://dx.doi.org/10.1016/j.drugalcdep.2006.05.012

Halikas, J. A., Crosby, R. D., Pearson, V. L., & Graves, N. M. (1997). A randomized double-blind study of carbamazepine in the treatment of cocaine abuse. *Clinical Pharmacology and Therapeutics, 62*, 89–105. http://dx.doi.org/10.1016/S0009-9236(97)90155-7

Hall, S. M., Tunis, S., Triffleman, E., Banys, P., Clark, H. W., Tusel, D., . . . Presti, D. (1994). Continuity of care and desipramine in primary cocaine abusers. *Journal of Nervous and Mental Disease, 182*, 556–575. http://dx.doi.org/10.1097/00005053-199410000-00007

Hamilton, J. D., Nguyen, Q. X., Gerber, R. M., & Rubio, N. B. (2009). Olanzapine in cocaine dependence: A double-blind, placebo-controlled trial. *The American Journal on Addictions, 18*, 48–52. http://dx.doi.org/10.1080/10550490802544318

Haney, M., Gunderson, E. W., Jiang, H., Collins, E. D., & Foltin, R. W. (2010). Cocaine-specific antibodies blunt the subjective effects of smoked cocaine in humans. *Biological Psychiatry, 67*, 59–65. http://dx.doi.org/10.1016/j.biopsych.2009.08.031

Heinzerling, K. G., Gadzhyan, J., van Oudheusden, H., Rodriguez, F., McCracken, J., & Shoptaw, S. (2013). Pilot randomized trial of bupropion for adolescent methamphetamine abuse/dependence. *Journal of Adolescent Health, 52*, 502–505. http://dx.doi.org/10.1016/j.jadohealth.2012.10.275

Heinzerling, K. G., Shoptaw, S., Peck, J. A., Yang, X., Liu, J., Roll, J., & Ling, W. (2006). Randomized, placebo-controlled trial of baclofen and gabapentin for the treatment of methamphetamine dependence. *Drug and Alcohol Dependence, 85,* 177–184. http://dx.doi.org/10.1016/j.drugalcdep.2006.03.019

Heinzerling, K. G., Swanson, A. N., Hall, T. M., Yi, Y., Wu, Y., & Shoptaw, S. J. (2014). Randomized, placebo-controlled trial of bupropion in methamphetamine-dependent participants with less than daily methamphetamine use. *Addiction, 109,* 1878–1886. http://dx.doi.org/10.1111/add.12636

Heinzerling, K. G., Swanson, A. N., Kim, S., Cederblom, L., Moe, A., Ling, W., & Shoptaw, S. (2010). Randomized, double-blind, placebo-controlled trial of modafinil for the treatment of methamphetamine dependence. *Drug and Alcohol Dependence, 109,* 20–29. http://dx.doi.org/10.1016/j.drugalcdep.2009.11.023

Herron, A. J., Mariani, J. J., Pavlicova, M., Parrinello, C. M., Bold, K. W., Levin, F. R., . . . Bisaga, A. (2013). Assessment of riboflavin as a tracer substance: Comparison of a qualitative to a quantitative method of riboflavin measurement. *Drug and Alcohol Dependence, 128,* 77–82. http://dx.doi.org/10.1016/j.drugalcdep.2012.08.007

Hersh, D., Van Kirk, J. R., & Kranzler, H. R. (1998). Naltrexone treatment of comorbid alcohol and cocaine use disorders. *Psychopharmacology, 139,* 44–52. http://dx.doi.org/10.1007/s002130050688

Humeniuk, R., Ali, R., Babor, T. F., Farrell, M., Formigoni, M. L., Jittiwutikarn, J., . . . Simon, S. (2008). Validation of the alcohol, smoking and substance involvement screening test (ASSIST). *Addiction, 103,* 1039–1047. http://dx.doi.org/10.1111/j.1360-0443.2007.02114.x

Indivior. (2013). *A randomized, 4-sequence, 2-period, double-blind, placebo controlled study with a DSM–IV–TR diagnosis of cocaine abuse (RBP-8000).* Retrieved from https://ClinicalTrials.gov/show/NCT01846481

InterveXion Therapeutics LLC. (2012). *Safety study of Ch-mAb7F9 for methamphetamine abuse.* Retrieved from https://ClinicalTrials.gov/show/NCT01603147

Jhanjee, S. (2014). Evidence based psychosocial interventions in substance use. *Indian Journal of Psychological Medicine, 36,* 112–118. http://dx.doi.org/10.4103/0253-7176.130960

Johnson, B. A., Ait-Daoud, N., Elkashef, A. M., Smith, E. V., Kahn, R., Vocci, F., . . . Bloch, D. A., & the Methamphetamine Study Group. (2008). A preliminary randomized, double-blind, placebo-controlled study of the safety and efficacy of ondansetron in the treatment of methamphetamine dependence. *International Journal of Neuropsychopharmacology, 11,* 1–14. http://dx.doi.org/10.1017/S1461145707007778

Johnson, B. A., Ait-Daoud, N., Wang, X. Q., Penberthy, J. K., Javors, M. A., Seneviratne, C., & Liu, L. (2013). Topiramate for the treatment of cocaine addiction:

A randomized clinical trial. *JAMA Psychiatry, 70,* 1338–1346. http://dx.doi.org/10.1001/jamapsychiatry.2013.2295

Johnson, B. A., Chen, Y. R., Swann, A. C., Schmitz, J., Lesser, J., Ruiz, P., . . . Clyde, C. (1997). Ritanserin in the treatment of cocaine dependence. *Biological Psychiatry, 42,* 932–940. http://dx.doi.org/10.1016/S0006-3223(96)00490-8

*Johnson, B. A., DiClemente, C. C., & Ait-Daoud, N. (2003). Brief Behavioral Compliance Enhancement Treatment (BBCET) manual. In B. A. Johnson, P. Ruiz, & M. Galanter (Eds.), *Handbook of clinical alcoholism treatment* (pp. 282–301). Baltimore, MD: Lippincott Williams & Wilkins.

Johnson, B. A., Roache, J. D., Ait-Daoud, N., Javors, M. A., Harrison, J. M., Elkashef, A., . . . Bloch, D. A. (2006). A preliminary randomized, double-blind, placebo-controlled study of the safety and efficacy of ondansetron in the treatment of cocaine dependence. *Drug and Alcohol Dependence, 84,* 256–263. http://dx.doi.org/10.1016/j.drugalcdep.2006.02.011

Kampman, K. M., Lynch, K. G., Pettinati, H. M., Spratt, K., Wierzbicki, M. R., Dackis, C., & O'Brien, C. P. (2015). A double blind, placebo controlled trial of modafinil for the treatment of cocaine dependence without co-morbid alcohol dependence. *Drug and Alcohol Dependence, 155,* 105–110. http://dx.doi.org/10.1016/j.drugalcdep.2015.08.005

Kampman, K. M., Pettinati, H., Lynch, K. G., Dackis, C., Sparkman, T., Weigley, C., & O'Brien, C. P. (2004). A pilot trial of topiramate for the treatment of cocaine dependence. *Drug and Alcohol Dependence, 75,* 233–240. http://dx.doi.org/10.1016/j.drugalcdep.2004.03.008

Kampman, K. M., Pettinati, H., Lynch, K. G., Sparkman, T., & O'Brien, C. P. (2003). A pilot trial of olanzapine for the treatment of cocaine dependence. *Drug and Alcohol Dependence, 70,* 265–273. http://dx.doi.org/10.1016/S0376-8716(03)00009-7

Kampman, K. M., Pettinati, H. M., Lynch, K. G., Spratt, K., Wierzbicki, M. R., & O'Brien, C. P. (2013). A double-blind, placebo-controlled trial of topiramate for the treatment of comorbid cocaine and alcohol dependence. *Drug and Alcohol Dependence, 133,* 94–99. http://dx.doi.org/10.1016/j.drugalcdep.2013.05.026

*Kampman, K. M., Volpicelli, J. R., McGinnis, D. E., Alterman, A. I., Weinrieb, R. M., D'Angelo, L., & Epperson, L. E. (1998). Reliability and validity of the cocaine selective severity assessment. *Addictive Behaviors, 23,* 449–461. http://dx.doi.org/10.1016/S0306-4603(98)00011-2

Kishi, T., Matsuda, Y., Iwata, N., & Correll, C. U. (2013). Antipsychotics for cocaine or psychostimulant dependence: Systematic review and meta-analysis of randomized, placebo-controlled trials. *The Journal of*

Clinical Psychiatry, 74, e1169–e1180. http://dx.doi.org/10.4088/JCP.13r08525

Kogan, Y., & Kosten, T. R. (2017). Methamphetamine vaccine for humans. NIH NIDA: R42DA043311.

Kollins, S. H. (2007). Abuse liability of medications used to treat attention-deficit/hyperactivity disorder (ADHD). *American Journal on Addictions, 16*(Suppl. 1), 35–42; quiz 43–34. http://dx.doi.org/10.1080/10550490601082775

Kosten, T., Domingo, C., Orson, F., & Kinsey, B. (2014). Vaccines against stimulants: Cocaine and MA. *British Journal of Clinical Pharmacology, 77*, 368–374. http://dx.doi.org/10.1111/bcp.12115

Kosten, T., Oliveto, A., Feingold, A., Poling, J., Sevarino, K., McCance-Katz, E., . . . Gonsai, K. (2003). Desipramine and contingency management for cocaine and opiate dependence in buprenorphine maintained patients. *Drug and Alcohol Dependence, 70*, 315–325. http://dx.doi.org/10.1016/S0376-8716(03)00032-2

Kosten, T. R., & Domingo, C. B. (2013). Can you vaccinate against substance abuse? *Expert Opinion on Biological Therapy, 13*, 1093–1097. http://dx.doi.org/10.1517/14712598.2013.791278

Kosten, T. R., Domingo, C. B., Shorter, D., Orson, F., Green, C., Somoza, E., . . . Kampman, K. (2014). Vaccine for cocaine dependence: A randomized double-blind placebo-controlled efficacy trial. *Drug and Alcohol Dependence, 140*, 42–47. http://dx.doi.org/10.1016/j.drugalcdep.2014.04.003

Kranzler, H. R., Bauer, L. O., Hersh, D., & Klinghoffer, V. (1995). Carbamazepine treatment of cocaine dependence: A placebo-controlled trial. *Drug and Alcohol Dependence, 38*, 203–211. http://dx.doi.org/10.1016/0376-8716(95)01100-D

Kuerbis, A., Sacco, P., Blazer, D. G., & Moore, A. A. (2014). Substance abuse among older adults. *Clinics in Geriatric Medicine, 30*, 629–654. http://dx.doi.org/10.1016/j.cger.2014.04.008

Kumor, K., Sherer, M., & Jaffe, J. (1986). Haloperidol-induced dystonia in cocaine addicts. *Lancet, 328*, 1341–1342. http://dx.doi.org/10.1016/S0140-6736(86)91478-9

Levin, F. R., McDowell, D., Evans, S. M., Brooks, D., Spano, C., & Nunes, E. V. (1999). Pergolide mesylate for cocaine abuse: A controlled preliminary trial. *The American Journal on Addictions, 8*, 120–127. http://dx.doi.org/10.1080/105504999305929

Lievaart, M., Erciyes, F., van der Veen, F. M., van de Wetering, B. J., Muris, P., & Franken, I. H. (2015). Validation of the cocaine versions of the Obsessive Compulsive Drug Use Scale and the Desires for Drug Questionnaire. *The American Journal of Drug and Alcohol Abuse, 41*, 358–365. http://dx.doi.org/10.3109/00952990.2015.1043210

Lima, M. S., Reisser, A. A., Soares, B. G., & Farrell, M. (2003). Antidepressants for cocaine dependence. *Cochrane Database of Systematic Reviews, 2003*(2): CD002950. http://dx.doi.org/10.1002/14651858.CD002950

Ling, W., Chang, L., Hillhouse, M., Ang, A., Striebel, J., Jenkins, J., . . . Esagoff, A. (2014). Sustained-release methylphenidate in a randomized trial of treatment of methamphetamine use disorder. *Addiction, 109*, 1489–1500. http://dx.doi.org/10.1111/add.12608

Littrell, K. H., Petty, R. G., Hilligoss, N. M., Peabody, C. D., & Johnson, C. G. (2001). Olanzapine treatment for patients with schizophrenia and substance abuse. *Journal of Substance Abuse Treatment, 21*, 217–221. http://dx.doi.org/10.1016/S0740-5472(01)00205-7

Loebl, T., Angarita, G. A., Pachas, G. N., Huang, K. L., Lee, S. H., Nino, J., . . . Evins, A. E. (2008). A randomized, double-blind, placebo-controlled trial of long-acting risperidone in cocaine-dependent men. *The Journal of Clinical Psychiatry, 69*, 480–486. http://dx.doi.org/10.4088/JCP.v69n0321

Longo, M., Wickes, W., Smout, M., Harrison, S., Cahill, S., & White, J. M. (2010). Randomized controlled trial of dexamphetamine maintenance for the treatment of methamphetamine dependence. *Addiction, 105*, 146–154. http://dx.doi.org/10.1111/j.1360-0443.2009.02717.x

Mahoney, J. J., III, Kalechstein, A. D., Verrico, C. D., Arnoudse, N. M., Shapiro, B. A., & De La Garza, R., II. (2014). Preliminary findings of the effects of rivastigmine, an acetylcholinesterase inhibitor, on working memory in cocaine-dependent volunteers. *Progress in Neuro-Psychopharmacology & Biological Psychiatry, 50*, 137–142. http://dx.doi.org/10.1016/j.pnpbp.2013.11.001

Mancino, M. J., McGaugh, J., Chopra, M. P., Guise, J. B., Cargile, C., Williams, D. K., . . . Oliveto, A. (2014). Clinical efficacy of sertraline alone and augmented with gabapentin in recently abstinent cocaine-dependent patients with depressive symptoms. *Journal of Clinical Psychopharmacology, 34*, 234–239. http://dx.doi.org/10.1097/JCP.0000000000000062

Margolin, A., Kosten, T. R., Avants, S. K., Wilkins, J., Ling, W., Beckson, M., . . . Bridge, P. (1995). A multicenter trial of bupropion for cocaine dependence in methadone-maintained patients. *Drug and Alcohol Dependence, 40*, 125–131. http://dx.doi.org/10.1016/0376-8716(95)01198-6

Mariani, J. J., & Levin, F. R. (2012). Psychostimulant treatment of cocaine dependence. *Psychiatric Clinics of North America, 35*, 425–439. http://dx.doi.org/10.1016/j.psc.2012.03.012

Mariani, J. J., Pavlicova, M., Bisaga, A., Nunes, E. V., Brooks, D. J., & Levin, F. R. (2012). Extended-release mixed amphetamine salts and topiramate for cocaine dependence: A randomized controlled trial. *Biological Psychiatry, 72*, 950–956.

Martell, B. A., Orson, F. M., Poling, J., Mitchell, E., Rossen, R. D., Gardner, T., & Kosten, T. R. (2009). Cocaine vaccine for the treatment of cocaine dependence in methadone-maintained patients: A randomized, double-blind, placebo-controlled efficacy trial. *Archives of General Psychiatry, 66*, 1116–1123. http://dx.doi.org/10.1001/archgenpsychiatry.2009.128

Martins, S. S., Sampson, L., Cerdá, M., & Galea, S. (2015). Worldwide prevalence and trends in unintentional drug overdose: A systematic review of the literature. *American Journal of Public Health, 105*, e29–e49. http://dx.doi.org/10.2105/AJPH.2015.302843

Maxwell, J. C., & Brecht, M. L. (2011). Methamphetamine: Here we go again? *Addictive Behaviors, 36*, 1168–1173. http://dx.doi.org/10.1016/j.addbeh.2011.07.017

McDowell, D., Nunes, E. V., Seracini, A. M., Rothenberg, J., Vosburg, S. K., Ma, G. J., & Petkova, E. (2005). Desipramine treatment of cocaine-dependent patients with depression: A placebo-controlled trial. *Drug and Alcohol Dependence, 80*, 209–221. http://dx.doi.org/10.1016/j.drugalcdep.2005.03.026

McLellan, A. T., Lewis, D. C., O'Brien, C. P., & Kleber, H. D. (2000). Drug dependence, a chronic medical illness: Implications for treatment, insurance, and outcomes evaluation. *Journal of the American Medical Association, 284*, 1689–1695. http://dx.doi.org/10.1001/jama.284.13.1689

McLellan, A. T., Luborsky, L., Woody, G. E., & O'Brien, C. P. (1980). An improved diagnostic evaluation instrument for substance abuse patients: The Addiction Severity Index. *Journal of Nervous and Mental Disease, 168*, 26–33. http://dx.doi.org/10.1097/00005053-198001000-00006

*McNeely, J., Strauss, S. M., Saitz, R., Cleland, C. M., Palamar, J. J., Rotrosen, J., & Gourevitch, M. N. (2015). A brief patient self-administered substance use screening tool for primary care: Two-site validation study of the Substance Use Brief Screen (SUBS). *The American Journal of Medicine, 128*, 784.e9–784.e19. http://dx.doi.org/10.1016/j.amjmed.2015.02.007

Miles, S. W., Sheridan, J., Russell, B., Kydd, R., Wheeler, A., Walters, C., . . . Tiihonen, J. (2013). Extended-release methylphenidate for treatment of amphetamine/methamphetamine dependence: A randomized, double-blind, placebo-controlled trial. *Addiction, 108*, 1279–1286. http://dx.doi.org/10.1111/add.12109

Minozzi, S., Amato, L., Davoli, M., Farrell, M., Lima Reisser, A. A., Pani, P. P., . . . Vecchi, S. (2008). Anticonvulsants for cocaine dependence. *Cochrane Database of Systematic Reviews, 2008*(2): CD006754. http://dx.doi.org/10.1002/14651858.CD006754.pub2

Minozzi, S., Cinquini, M., Amato, L., Davoli, M., Farrell, M. F., Pani, P. P., & Vecchi, S. (2015). Anticonvulsants for cocaine dependence. *Cochrane Database of Systematic Reviews, 2015*(4): CD006754. http://dx.doi.org/10.1002/14651858.CD006754.pub4

Moeller, F. G., Schmitz, J. M., Steinberg, J. L., Green, C. M., Reist, C., Lai, L. Y., . . . Grabowski, J. (2007). Citalopram combined with behavioral therapy reduces cocaine use: A double-blind, placebo-controlled trial. *The American Journal of Drug and Alcohol Abuse, 33*, 367–378. http://dx.doi.org/10.1080/00952990701313686

Montoya, I. D., Levin, F. R., Fudala, P. J., & Gorelick, D. A. (1995). Double-blind comparison of carbamazepine and placebo for treatment of cocaine dependence. *Drug and Alcohol Dependence, 38*, 213–219. http://dx.doi.org/10.1016/0376-8716(95)01101-4

Mooney, M., Sayre, S., Green, C., Rhoades, H., & Schmitz, J. (2004). Comparing measures of medication taking in a pharmacotherapy trial for cocaine dependence. *Addictive Disorders & Their Treatment, 3*, 165–173. http://dx.doi.org/10.1097/01.adt.0000132509.65041.bf

Mooney, M. E., Herin, D. V., Schmitz, J. M., Moukaddam, N., Green, C. E., & Grabowski, J. (2009). Effects of oral methamphetamine on cocaine use: A randomized, double-blind, placebo-controlled trial. *Drug and Alcohol Dependence, 101*, 34–41. http://dx.doi.org/10.1016/j.drugalcdep.2008.10.016

Mooney, M. E., Herin, D. V., Specker, S., Babb, D., Levin, F. R., & Grabowski, J. (2015). Pilot study of the effects of lisdexamfetamine on cocaine use: A randomized, double-blind, placebo-controlled trial. *Drug and Alcohol Dependence, 153*, 94–103. http://dx.doi.org/10.1016/j.drugalcdep.2015.05.042

Murrough, J. W., Abdallah, C. G., & Mathew, S. J. (2017). Targeting glutamate signalling in depression: Progress and prospects. *Nature Reviews: Drug Discovery, 16*, 472–486. http://dx.doi.org/10.1038/nrd.2017.16

Najavits, L. M., & Lester, K. M. (2008). Gender differences in cocaine dependence. *Drug and Alcohol Dependence, 97*, 190–194. http://dx.doi.org/10.1016/j.drugalcdep.2008.04.012

Negus, S. S., & Henningfield, J. (2015). Agonist Medications for the Treatment of Cocaine Use Disorder. *Neuropsychopharmacology, 40*, 1815–1825. http://dx.doi.org/10.1038/npp.2014.322

Neher, M. D., Weckbach, S., Huber-Lang, M. S., & Stahel, P. F. (2012). New insights into the role of peroxisome proliferator-activated receptors in regulating the inflammatory response after tissue injury. *PPAR Research, 2012*, article ID 728461, 1–13. http://dx.doi.org/10.1155/2012/728461

New York State Psychiatric Institute. (2012). *The effect of brief potent glutamatergic modulation on cocaine dependence.* Retrieved from https://ClinicalTrials.gov/show/NCT01535937

NIDA. (2012). *Principles of drug addiction treatment: A research-based guide* (3rd ed.). North Bethesda, MD: National Institute of Drug Abuse.

Northrup, T. F., Green, C., Walker, R., Greer, T. L., & Trivedi, M. H. (2015). On the invariance of the Stimulant Craving Questionnaire (STCQ) across cocaine and methamphetamine users. *Addictive Behaviors*, *42*(Suppl. C), 144–147. http://dx.doi.org/10.1016/j.addbeh.2014.11.020

Nuijten, M., Blanken, P., van den Brink, W., & Hendriks, V. (2014). Treatment of crack-cocaine dependence with topiramate: A randomized controlled feasibility trial in The Netherlands. *Drug and Alcohol Dependence*, *138*, 177–184. http://dx.doi.org/10.1016/j.drugalcdep.2014.02.024

Nunes, E. V., McGrath, P. J., Quitkin, F. M., Ocepek-Welikson, K., Stewart, J. W., Koenig, T., . . . Klein, D. F. (1995). Imipramine treatment of cocaine abuse: Possible boundaries of efficacy. *Drug and Alcohol Dependence*, *39*, 185–195. http://dx.doi.org/10.1016/0376-8716(95)01161-6

Oliveto, A., Poling, J., Mancino, M. J., Williams, D. K., Thostenson, J., Pruzinsky, R., . . . Kosten, T. R. (2012). Sertraline delays relapse in recently abstinent cocaine-dependent patients with depressive symptoms. *Addiction*, *107*, 131–141. http://dx.doi.org/10.1111/j.1360-0443.2011.03552.x

Orson, F. M., Wang, R., Brimijoin, S., Kinsey, B. M., Singh, R. A., Ramakrishnan, M., . . . Kosten, T. R. (2014). The future potential for cocaine vaccines. *Expert Opinion on Biological Therapy*, *14*, 1271–1283. http://dx.doi.org/10.1517/14712598.2014.920319

Oslin, D. W., Pettinati, H. M., Volpicelli, J. R., Wolf, A. L., Kampman, K. M., & O'Brien, C. P. (1999). The effects of naltrexone on alcohol and cocaine use in dually addicted patients. *Journal of Substance Abuse Treatment*, *16*, 163–167. http://dx.doi.org/10.1016/S0740-5472(98)00039-7

Pani, P. P., Trogu, E., Vecchi, S., & Amato, L. (2011). Antidepressants for cocaine dependence and problematic cocaine use. *Cochrane Database of Systematic Reviews*, *2011*(12): CD002950. http://dx.doi.org/10.1002/14651858.CD002950.pub3

Passos, S. R., Camacho, L. A., Lopes, C. S., & Borges dos Santos, M. A. (2005). Nefazodone in out-patient treatment of inhaled cocaine dependence: A randomized double-blind placebo-controlled trial. *Addiction*, *100*, 489–494. http://dx.doi.org/10.1111/j.1360-0443.2005.01041.x

Petry, N. M., Alessi, S. M., Olmstead, T. A., Rash, C. J., & Zajac, K. (2017). Contingency management treatment for substance use disorders: How far has it come, and where does it need to go? *Psychology of Addictive Behaviors*, *31*, 897–906. http://dx.doi.org/10.1037/adb0000287

Pettinati, H. M., Kampman, K. M., Lynch, K. G., Suh, J. J., Dackis, C. A., Oslin, D. W., & O'Brien, C. P. (2008). Gender differences with high-dose naltrexone in patients with co-occurring cocaine and alcohol dependence. *Journal of Substance Abuse Treatment*, *34*, 378–390. http://dx.doi.org/10.1016/j.jsat.2007.05.011

Pettinati, H. M., Kampman, K. M., Lynch, K. G., Xie, H., Dackis, C., Rabinowitz, A. R., & O'Brien, C. P. (2008). A double blind, placebo-controlled trial that combines disulfiram and naltrexone for treating co-occurring cocaine and alcohol dependence. *Addictive Behaviors*, *33*, 651–667. http://dx.doi.org/10.1016/j.addbeh.2007.11.011

Poling, J., Oliveto, A., Petry, N., Sofuoglu, M., Gonsai, K., Gonzalez, G., . . . Kosten, T. R. (2006). Six-month trial of bupropion with contingency management for cocaine dependence in a methadone-maintained population. *Archives of General Psychiatry*, *63*, 219–228. http://dx.doi.org/10.1001/archpsyc.63.2.219

Pravetoni, M. (2016). Biologics to treat substance use disorders: Current status and new directions. *Human Vaccines & Immunotherapeutics*, *12*, 3005–3019. http://dx.doi.org/10.1080/21645515.2016.1212785

Reid, M. S., Angrist, B., Baker, S., Woo, C., Schwartz, M., Montgomery, A., . . . Rotrosen, J. (2005). A placebo-controlled screening trial of celecoxib for the treatment of cocaine dependence. *Addiction*, *100*(Suppl. 1), 32–42. http://dx.doi.org/10.1111/j.1360-0443.2005.00989.x

Reid, M. S., Casadonte, P., Baker, S., Sanfilipo, M., Braunstein, D., Hitzemann, R., . . . Rotrosen, J. (2005). A placebo-controlled screening trial of olanzapine, valproate, and coenzyme Q10/L-carnitine for the treatment of cocaine dependence. *Addiction*, *100*(Suppl. 1), 43–57. http://dx.doi.org/10.1111/j.1360-0443.2005.00990.x

Resnick, R. B., & Resnick, E. B. (1984). Cocaine abuse and its treatment. *Psychiatric Clinics of North America*, *7*, 713–728. http://dx.doi.org/10.1016/S0193-953X(18)30725-1

Rezaei, F., Emami, M., Zahed, S., Morabbi, M. J., Farahzadi, M., & Akhondzadeh, S. (2015). Sustained-release methylphenidate in methamphetamine dependence treatment: A double-blind and placebo-controlled trial. *DARU Journal of Pharmaceutical Sciences*, *23*, 2. http://dx.doi.org/10.1186/s40199-015-0092-y

Rezaei, F., Ghaderi, E., Mardani, R., Hamidi, S., & Hassanzadeh, K. (2016). Topiramate for the management of methamphetamine dependence: A pilot randomized, double-blind, placebo-controlled trial. *Fundamental & Clinical Pharmacology*, *30*, 282–289. http://dx.doi.org/10.1111/fcp.12178

Roache, J. D., Kahn, R., Newton, T. F., Wallace, C. L., Murff, W. L., De La Garza, R., II, . . . Elkashef, A.

(2011). A double-blind, placebo-controlled assessment of the safety of potential interactions between intravenous cocaine, ethanol, and oral disulfiram. *Drug and Alcohol Dependence, 119*(1–2), 37–45. http://dx.doi.org/10.1016/j.drugalcdep.2011.05.015

Robinson, S. M., Sobell, L. C., Sobell, M. B., & Leo, G. I. (2014). Reliability of the Timeline Followback for cocaine, cannabis, and cigarette use. *Psychology of Addictive Behaviors, 28*, 154–162. http://dx.doi.org/10.1037/a0030992

Roll, J. M., Petry, N. M., Stitzer, M. L., Brecht, M. L., Peirce, J. M., McCann, M. J., . . . Kellogg, S. (2006). Contingency management for the treatment of methamphetamine use disorders. *The American Journal of Psychiatry, 163*, 1993–1999. http://dx.doi.org/10.1176/ajp.2006.163.11.1993

Rounsaville, B. J. (2004). Treatment of cocaine dependence and depression. *Biological Psychiatry, 56*(10), 803–809. http://dx.doi.org/10.1016/j.biopsych.2004.05.009

Sajja, R. K., Rahman, S., & Cucullo, L. (2016). Drugs of abuse and blood-brain barrier endothelial dysfunction: A focus on the role of oxidative stress. *Journal of Cerebral Blood Flow and Metabolism, 36*, 539–554. http://dx.doi.org/10.1177/0271678X15616978

SAMHSA. (1988). *National Household Survey on Drug Abuse*. Rockville, MD: Substance Abuse and Mental Health Services Administration.

SAMHSA. (2011). *Tobacco use cessation during substance abuse treatment counseling*. (Report No. (SMA) 11–4636). Rockville, MD: Substance Abuse and Mental Health Services Administration.

SAMHSA. (2016). *Substance Abuse and Mental Health Services Administration, Behind the Term: Serious Mental Illness* (Vol. DHHS 2832 0120 0037 ref no. 283-12-3702).

Sanacora, G., Frye, M. A., McDonald, W., Mathew, S. J., Turner, M. S., Schatzberg, A. F., . . . Nemeroff, C. B., & the American Psychiatric Association (APA) Council of Research Task Force on Novel Biomarkers and Treatments. (2017). A consensus statement on the use of ketamine in the treatment of mood disorders. *JAMA Psychiatry, 74*, 399–405. http://dx.doi.org/10.1001/jamapsychiatry.2017.0080

Schmitz, J. M., Averill, P., Stotts, A. L., Moeller, F. G., Rhoades, H. M., & Grabowski, J. (2001). Fluoxetine treatment of cocaine-dependent patients with major depressive disorder. *Drug and Alcohol Dependence, 63*, 207–214. http://dx.doi.org/10.1016/S0376-8716(00)00208-8

Schmitz, J. M., Green, C. E., Hasan, K. M., Vincent, J., Suchting, R., Weaver, M. F., . . . Lane, S. D. (2017). PPAR-gamma agonist pioglitazone modifies craving intensity and brain white matter integrity in patients with primary cocaine use disorder: A double-blind

randomized controlled pilot trial. *Addiction, 112*, 1861–1868. http://dx.doi.org/10.1111/add.13868

Schmitz, J. M., Green, C. E., Stotts, A. L., Lindsay, J. A., Rathnayaka, N. S., Grabowski, J., & Moeller, F. G. (2014). A two-phased screening paradigm for evaluating candidate medications for cocaine cessation or relapse prevention: Modafinil, levodopa-carbidopa, naltrexone. *Drug and Alcohol Dependence, 136*, 100–107. http://dx.doi.org/10.1016/j.drugalcdep.2013.12.015

Schmitz, J. M., Lindsay, J. A., Stotts, A. L., Green, C. E., & Moeller, F. G. (2010). Contingency management and levodopa-carbidopa for cocaine treatment: A comparison of three behavioral targets. *Experimental and Clinical Psychopharmacology, 18*, 238–244. http://dx.doi.org/10.1037/a0019195

Schmitz, J. M., Stotts, A. L., Sayre, S. L., DeLaune, K. A., & Grabowski, J. (2004). Treatment of cocaine-alcohol dependence with naltrexone and relapse prevention therapy. *The American Journal on Addictions, 13*, 333–341. http://dx.doi.org/10.1080/10550490490480982

Schmitz, J. M., Stotts, A. L., Vujanovic, A. A., Weaver, M. F., Yoon, J. H., Vincent, J., & Green, C. E. (2018). A sequential multiple assignment randomized trial for cocaine cessation and relapse prevention: Tailoring treatment to the individual. *Contemporary Clinical Trials, 65*, 109–115. http://dx.doi.org/10.1016/j.cct.2017.12.015

Shearer, J., Darke, S., Rodgers, C., Slade, T., van Beek, I., Lewis, J., . . . Wodak, A. (2009). A double-blind, placebo-controlled trial of modafinil (200 mg/day) for methamphetamine dependence. *Addiction, 104*, 224–233. http://dx.doi.org/10.1111/j.1360-0443.2008.02437.x

Shearer, J., Wodak, A., van Beek, I., Mattick, R. P., & Lewis, J. (2003). Pilot randomized double blind placebo-controlled study of dexamphetamine for cocaine dependence. *Addiction, 98*, 1137–1141. http://dx.doi.org/10.1046/j.1360-0443.2003.00447.x

Shoptaw, S., Heinzerling, K. G., Rotheram-Fuller, E., Kao, U. H., Wang, P. C., Bholat, M. A., & Ling, W. (2008). Bupropion hydrochloride versus placebo, in combination with cognitive behavioral therapy, for the treatment of cocaine abuse/dependence. *Journal of Addictive Diseases, 27*, 13–23. http://dx.doi.org/10.1300/J069v27n01_02

Shoptaw, S., Heinzerling, K. G., Rotheram-Fuller, E., Steward, T., Wang, J., Swanson, A. N., . . . Ling, W. (2008). Randomized, placebo-controlled trial of bupropion for the treatment of methamphetamine dependence. *Drug and Alcohol Dependence, 96*, 222–232. http://dx.doi.org/10.1016/j.drugalcdep.2008.03.010

Shoptaw, S., Huber, A., Peck, J., Yang, X., Liu, J., Dang, J., . . . Ling, W. (2006). Randomized, placebo-controlled trial of sertraline and contingency management for the treatment of methamphetamine dependence. *Drug and Alcohol Dependence, 85,* 12–18. http://dx.doi.org/10.1016/j.drugalcdep.2006.03.005

Shoptaw, S., Yang, X., Rotheram-Fuller, E. J., Hsieh, Y. C., Kintaudi, P. C., Charuvastra, V. C., & Ling, W. (2003). Randomized placebo-controlled trial of baclofen for cocaine dependence: Preliminary effects for individuals with chronic patterns of cocaine use. *The Journal of Clinical Psychiatry, 64,* 1440–1448. http://dx.doi.org/10.4088/JCP.v64n1207

Singh, M., Keer, D., Klimas, J., Wood, E., & Werb, D. (2016). Topiramate for cocaine dependence: A systematic review and meta-analysis of randomized controlled trials. *Addiction, 111,* 1337–1346. http://dx.doi.org/10.1111/add.13328

Smelson, D. A., Ziedonis, D., Williams, J., Losonczy, M. F., Williams, J., Steinberg, M. L., & Kaune, M. (2006). The efficacy of olanzapine for decreasing cue-elicited craving in individuals with schizophrenia and cocaine dependence: A preliminary report. *Journal of Clinical Psychopharmacology, 26,* 9–12. http://dx.doi.org/10.1097/01.jcp.0000194624.07611.5e

Smith, D. E. (1984). Diagnostic, treatment and aftercare approaches to cocaine abuse. *Journal of Substance Abuse Treatment, 1,* 5–9. http://dx.doi.org/10.1016/0740-5472(84)90047-3

Sofuoglu, M., DeVito, E. E., Waters, A. J., & Carroll, K. M. (2013). Cognitive enhancement as a treatment for drug addictions. *Neuropharmacology, 64,* 452–463. http://dx.doi.org/10.1016/j.neuropharm.2012.06.021

Sofuoglu, M., Waters, A. J., Poling, J., & Carroll, K. M. (2011). Galantamine improves sustained attention in chronic cocaine users. *Experimental and Clinical Psychopharmacology, 19,* 11–19. http://dx.doi.org/10.1037/a0022213

Stevens, M. W., Henry, R. L., Owens, S. M., Schutz, R., & Gentry, W. B. (2014). First human study of a chimeric anti-methamphetamine monoclonal antibody in healthy volunteers. *mAbs, 6,* 1649–1656. http://dx.doi.org/10.4161/19420862.2014.976431

Stevens, M. W., & Owens, S. M. (2017). A methamphetamine conjugate vaccine: From manufacturing to ind. NIH NIDA: U01DA035511.

*Stirratt, M. J., Dunbar-Jacob, J., Crane, H. M., Simoni, J. M., Czajkowski, S., Hilliard, M. E., . . . Nilsen, W. J. (2015). Self-report measures of medication adherence behavior: Recommendations on optimal use. *Translational Behavioral Medicine, 5,* 470–482. http://dx.doi.org/10.1007/s13142-015-0315-2

Suh, J. J., Pettinati, H. M., Kampman, K. M., & O'Brien, C. P. (2008). Gender differences in predictors of

treatment attrition with high dose naltrexone in cocaine and alcohol dependence. *The American Journal on Addictions, 17,* 463–468. http://dx.doi.org/10.1080/10550490802409074

Sussner, B. D., Smelson, D. A., Rodrigues, S., Kline, A., Losonczy, M., & Ziedonis, D. (2006). The validity and reliability of a brief measure of cocaine craving. *Drug and Alcohol Dependence, 83,* 233–237. http://dx.doi.org/10.1016/j.drugalcdep.2005.11.022

Swift, R., Oslin, D. W., Alexander, M., & Forman, R. (2011). Adherence monitoring in naltrexone pharmacotherapy trials: A systematic review. *Journal of Studies on Alcohol and Drugs, 72,* 1012–1018. http://dx.doi.org/10.15288/jsad.2011.72.1012

Tapp, A., Wood, A. E., Kennedy, A., Sylvers, P., Kilzieh, N., & Saxon, A. J. (2015). Quetiapine for the treatment of cocaine use disorder. *Drug and Alcohol Dependence, 149,* 18–24. http://dx.doi.org/10.1016/j.drugalcdep.2014.12.037

Teva Pharmaceutical Industries. (2013). *Efficacy and safety of TV-1380 as treatment for facilitation of abstinence in cocaine-dependent subjects.* Retrieved from https://ClinicalTrials.gov/show/NCT01887366

Thurgood, S. L., McNeill, A., Clark-Carter, D., & Brose, L. S. (2016). A Systematic Review of Smoking Cessation Interventions for Adults in Substance Abuse Treatment or Recovery. *Nicotine & Tobacco Research, 18,* 993–1001. http://dx.doi.org/10.1093/ntr/ntv127

Tiihonen, J., Kuoppasalmi, K., Föhr, J., Tuomola, P., Kuikanmäki, O., Vorma, H., . . . Meririnne, E. (2007). A comparison of aripiprazole, methylphenidate, and placebo for amphetamine dependence. *The American Journal of Psychiatry, 164,* 160–162. http://dx.doi.org/10.1176/ajp.2007.164.1.160

Umbricht, A., DeFulio, A., Winstanley, E. L., Tompkins, D. A., Peirce, J., Mintzer, M. Z., . . . Bigelow, G. E. (2014). Topiramate for cocaine dependence during methadone maintenance treatment: A randomized controlled trial. *Drug and Alcohol Dependence, 140,* 92–100. http://dx.doi.org/10.1016/j.drugalcdep.2014.03.033

United Nations Office on Drugs and Crime. (2017). *World Drug Report 2017.* Retrieved from www.unodc.org/wdr2017

University of California Los Angeles. (2013). *Trial of ibudilast for methamphetamine dependence (IBUD ph II).* Retrieved from https://ClinicalTrials.gov/show/NCT01860807

van Harten, P. N., van Trier, J. C., Horwitz, E. H., Matroos, G. E., & Hoek, H. W. (1998). Cocaine as a risk factor for neuroleptic-induced acute dystonia. *The Journal of Clinical Psychiatry, 59,* 128–130. http://dx.doi.org/10.4088/JCP.v59n0307

Weddington, W. W., Jr., Brown, B. S., Haertzen, C. A., Hess, J. M., Mahaffey, J. R., Kolar, A. F., & Jaffe, J. H. (1991). Comparison of amantadine and desipramine combined with psychotherapy for treatment of cocaine dependence. *The American Journal of Drug and Alcohol Abuse, 17*, 137–152. http://dx.doi.org/10.3109/00952999108992817

Weill Medical College of Cornell University. (2015). *Safety study of a disrupted adenovirus (Ad) serotype cocaine vaccine for cocaine-dependent individuals.* Retrieved from https://ClinicalTrials.gov/show/NCT02455479

Winhusen, T., Somoza, E., Ciraulo, D. A., Harrer, J. M., Goldsmith, R. J., Grabowski, J., . . . Elkashef, A. (2007). A double-blind, placebo-controlled trial of tiagabine for the treatment of cocaine dependence. *Drug and Alcohol Dependence, 91*, 141–148. http://dx.doi.org/10.1016/j.drugalcdep.2007.05.028

Winhusen, T., Somoza, E., Sarid-Segal, O., Goldsmith, R. J., Harrer, J. M., Coleman, F. S., . . . Elkashef, A. (2007). A double-blind, placebo-controlled trial of reserpine for the treatment of cocaine dependence. *Drug and Alcohol Dependence, 91*, 205–212. http://dx.doi.org/10.1016/j.drugalcdep.2007.05.021

Winhusen, T. M., Somoza, E. C., Harrer, J. M., Mezinskis, J. P., Montgomery, M. A., Goldsmith, R. J., . . . Elkashef, A. (2005). A placebo-controlled screening trial of tiagabine, sertraline and donepezil as cocaine dependence treatments. *Addiction, 100*(Suppl. 1), 68–77. http://dx.doi.org/10.1111/j.1360-0443.2005.00992.x

Zorick, T., Nestor, L., Miotto, K., Sugar, C., Hellemann, G., Scanlon, G., . . . London, E. D. (2010). Withdrawal symptoms in abstinent methamphetamine-dependent subjects. *Addiction, 105*, 1809–1818. http://dx.doi.org/10.1111/j.1360-0443.2010.03066.x

CHAPTER 25

PHARMACOLOGICAL TREATMENT OF OPIOID USE DISORDERS

Hilary S. Connery and R. Kathryn McHugh

The term *opioid use disorder* (OUD) refers to the problematic use of heroin and/or licit or illicit opioid analgesics (prescription opioids) resulting in negative health, social, financial and occupational consequences, despite which an individual persists in problematic use (American Psychiatric Association, 2013). OUD severity ranges from mild to severe and may or may not include physiological dependence (i.e., tolerance to the effects of the drug and an aversive withdrawal syndrome during abstinence states). OUD is associated with substantial morbidity and mortality, including risk for overdose and suicide. In 2015, over 33,000 people died of opioid overdose (Rudd, Seth, David, & Scholl, 2016), a more than 400% increase since the late 1990s. Several pharmacological treatments are effective for the treatment of OUD, and drastically reduce opioid use and overdose risk (see Connery, 2015). Nonetheless, approximately half of individuals treated for OUD fail to adequately respond to treatment, highlighting the importance of further treatment development for this disabling disorder. In this chapter, we review the epidemiology, diagnosis, and treatment of OUD, with a particular focus on pharmacological treatment.

EPIDEMIOLOGY AND PREVALENCE

Prevalence of OUD in the United States has increased dramatically. Beginning in the late 1990s, a rapid increase in nonmedical use and diversion of prescription opioids resulted in increases in negative opioid-related outcomes, such as initiation of heroin use, incidence of OUD, and opioid overdose (Compton & Volkow, 2006). Approximately 2.6 million people in the United States currently have OUD (Center for Behavioral Health Statistics and Quality, 2016).

Furthermore, in 2015 approximately 12.5 million people of ages 12 and older misused prescription opioids (i.e., used without a prescription or at a dose or frequency higher than prescribed) and over 800,000 used heroin (Center for Behavioral Health Statistics and Quality, 2016). Most heroin users reported opioid initiation with prescription opioids (>80%), suggesting that opioid analgesic access creates a primary entry point for problematic opioid use (C. M. Jones, 2013). Indeed, the population of heroin users has changed substantially in recent years, and is now older, more rural, more likely to identify as non-Hispanic White, and more likely to have initiated via prescription opioids relative to previous cohorts (Cicero, Ellis, Surratt, & Kurtz, 2014). Of concern, access to highly potent synthetic opioids—particularly fentanyl analogues—has rapidly increased, with a corresponding increase in overdose fatalities (Rudd et al., 2016).

Young adults (i.e., ages 18–25) comprise the highest risk age group for use of heroin (Center for Behavioral Health Statistics and Quality, 2016) and prescription opioid misuse (Hughes et al., 2016).

Funding support was provided by the National Institute on Drug Abuse DA035297 (R. K. M.).

http://dx.doi.org/10.1037/0000133-025
APA Handbook of Psychopharmacology, S. M. Evans (Editor-in-Chief)

However, opioid misuse and OUD impact all age groups, and are underrecognized and undertreated in adolescents and older adults (Beaudoin, Merchant, & Clark, 2016; Hadland et al., 2017). Although prescription opioid misuse and heroin use are more common among men overall (Centers for Disease Control and Prevention, 2015; Hughes et al., 2016), there are several concerning trends indicating an increasing impact of OUD in women (see the Consideration of Potential Sex Differences section in this chapter). OUD historically impacted racial groups relatively equally, yet the largest increases in both prescription opioid use and heroin use in recent years have been among those identifying as non-Hispanic White (Cicero et al., 2014; Martins et al., 2017). Regionally, OUD and opioid overdose is concentrated in socioeconomically strained communities (especially rural ones), where access to treatment is limited by low availability of mental health and substance use services, inadequate provider knowledge and training in evidence-based treatments, and workforce shortages. Patient barriers to treatment include inadequate health insurance and transportation and childcare barriers (Cicero et al., 2014; E. B. Jones, 2017).

Psychiatric and medical comorbidities are highly prevalent with OUD and complicate treatment. More than one in 10 people with mental illness reported prescription opioid misuse in 2015 (Hughes et al., 2016), and those with OUD report high rates of anxiety, depressive, and traumatic stress disorders (Conway, Compton, Stinson, & Grant, 2006; Grella, Karno, Warda, Niv, & Moore, 2009). Risk for suicide attempt is elevated among those with OUD, even relative to other substance use disorders (Bohnert, Ilgen, Louzon, McCarthy, & Katz, 2017); an estimated 30% to 45% of those with OUD report a history of suicide attempt (Darke et al., 2015; Maloney, Degenhardt, Darke, Mattick, & Nelson, 2007).

Nonmedical use of prescription opioids is common among people with chronic pain, with the majority self-reporting that their misuse began to relieve pain (Han et al., 2017). Moreover, pain is associated with risk for developing OUD and negative outcomes among those diagnosed with OUD (Blanco et al., 2016; Griffin et al., 2016). Among injection users, infectious diseases of blood-borne transmission (e.g., hepatitis C virus [HCV], human immunodeficiency virus [HIV]) and dermal trauma are common.

DIAGNOSING OPIOID USE DISORDER

Given the high national prevalence of prescription opioid misuse/OUD and lethal overdose, universal screening and detection is recommended, especially for subpopulations known to be at elevated risk (e.g., youth, individuals with mental health and/or substance use disorders or chronic pain, individuals experiencing severe distress). Evidence-based screening tools exist to detect opioid misuse; however, no single assessment is yet validated across all populations at risk for opioid misuse/OUD (reviewed in Kaye et al., 2017).

Pragmatically, universal drug screening is feasible using a patient self-administered single question ("How many times in the past year have you used an illegal drug or used a prescription medication for non-medical reasons [for example, because of the experience or feeling it caused]?"; McNeely et al., 2015), to which any response other than zero is considered positive and warrants more careful assessment with a structured and validated questionnaire, such as long or brief versions of the Drug Abuse Screen Test (Yudko, Lozhkina, & Fouts, 2007), or computerized versions of the more comprehensive Alcohol, Smoking, and Substance Involvement Screening Tool (ASSIST; Kumar et al., 2016). Validated assessments are available in the public domain through the Substance Abuse and Mental Health Services Agency online screening tools (https://www.integration.samhsa.gov/clinical-practice/screening-tools#drugs; see the Tool Kit of Resources at the end of this chapter).

Among patients with pain, several screening assessments are recommended to assess risk of future prescription opioid misuse, with the gold standard being the 24-item Screener and Opioid Assessment for Patients with Pain-Revised (SOAPP-R; Butler, Fernandez, Benoit, Budman, & Jamison, 2008), and briefer versions being validated for greater feasibility within busy office practices (Finkelman et al., 2017). In studies of both drug-using populations and prescription OUD populations, self-reported opioid use is concordant with toxicological data in the majority

(74% and 77%, respectively; Gryczynski, Schwartz, Mitchell, O'Grady, & Ondersma, 2014; Hilario et al., 2015), although denial of opioid misuse may be observed more commonly in patients with pain (Hilario et al., 2015; Saroyan et al., 2016).

Detection of any opioid misuse warrants further assessment for OUD as defined by the *Diagnostic and Statistical Manual of Mental Disorders, 5th edition* (*DSM–5*; American Psychiatric Association, 2013). OUD is defined by meeting two or more of 11 impairment criteria during a consecutive 12-month episode and is scaled from mild to severe based on number of criteria met. Criteria reflect abnormal allotment of time and energy spent using opioids with negative consequences. Cardinal criteria include failed attempts to stop opioid use, craving opioids, and persistent use despite serious consequences.

Physical examination may provide signs of active OUD. Signs of opioid intoxication include pupillary constriction ("pinpoint pupils"), sedation, and cognitive slowing; signs of opioid withdrawal include pupillary dilatation, heightened blood pressure and heart rate, yawning, runny nose, tearing, restlessness, piloerection ("gooseflesh"), and anxiety. The latter, in combination with subjective complaints of nausea, vomiting, diarrhea, insomnia, and opioid craving, can be assessed quickly in an office setting using the Clinical Opiate Withdrawal Scale (COWS; Wesson & Ling, 2003). Signs of injection drug use such as scarring or infection along superficial blood vessels ("track marks") may be visible on hands, arms, legs, or neck.

When opioid misuse is suspected, toxicology is the gold standard for confirmation. Office-based urine screening is most commonly used, although blood, saliva, hair, or fingernail analyses may be used. Adulteration of urine samples is a common problem among those not wishing to disclose substance misuse (Jaffee, Trucco, Levy, & Weiss, 2007) and may be avoided by supervising sample collection or having chemical standards by which to normalize an unadulterated urine sample (e.g., temperature checks, creatinine, or other indicators of an intentionally diluted sample). Routine "5-drug" screening for substances of abuse (opiates, cocaine, amphetamines, cannabis, and benzodiazepines) will capture the metabolites of heroin use, codeine, and morphine, but will not detect many frequently prescribed opioids of abuse, including oxycodone, oxymorphone, hydrocodone, hydromorphone, tramadol, fentanyl, methadone, and buprenorphine. Therefore, opioid panels should be tailored to individual patient concern and regional trends.

We emphasize that clinicians should be sensitive to the shame and denial associated with opioid misuse/OUD. Toxicological results are used as objective data to help engage a patient in treatment and improve their understanding of the risks of opioid misuse, and not to coerce patients into care or to restrict their access to care.

EVIDENCE-BASED PHARMACOLOGICAL TREATMENTS OF OPIOID USE DISORDER

Pharmacological treatments have been available for OUD with physiological dependence for over 40 years. Initial development focused on targeting the physiological symptoms of OUD, such as drug withdrawal and craving, both of which are potent drivers of ongoing use and relapse (Kreek & Vocci, 2002; Vocci, Acri, & Elkashef, 2005). Early research focused on identifying potential maintenance medications: opioid agonists (i.e., medications that bind to and activate opioid receptors and block the effects of other opioids) that could be administered safely on an ongoing basis and reduce the risk of illicit opioid use (e.g., tolerance, potent reward or "high," overdose). A series of studies in the 1960s and 1970s examined the efficacy of methadone, a long-acting synthetic opioid initially manufactured for the management of pain. Due to its long-acting nature and slow onset, daily-dosed methadone was not associated with a significant high in opioid-tolerant individuals. Clinical trials demonstrated the efficacy of methadone (Dole & Nyswander, 1965; Dole et al., 1969), and later the related opioid agonist levomethadyl acetate (LAAM; Ling, Charuvastra, Kaim, & Klett, 1976) for the treatment of OUD. Methadone was approved by the FDA in 1972, followed by the approval of the opioid antagonist naltrexone in 1984, and LAAM in 1993. Methadone maintenance was the predominant treatment for OUD for many years because of its efficacy (Mattick, Breen, Kimber,

& Davoli, 2009) and the limitations of alternative approaches (e.g., poor adherence to oral naltrexone, risk for adverse cardiac events with LAAM that later resulted in the FDA removing it from market). Nonetheless, there were, and continue to be, several limitations to methadone treatment, such as the need for daily dosing at a specialty clinic and tolerability/safety challenges.

Buprenorphine and buprenorphine-naloxone were approved by the FDA in 2002, which first allowed for office-based agonist therapy for OUD in the United States. The approval of buprenorphine, as well as recent advances in delivery methods for OUD medications (e.g., extended-release injectable naltrexone and buprenorphine), have expanded the options available and have reduced the time burden for OUD treatment. Nonetheless, access to care remains problematic; most OUD patients do not receive any medication treatment (Feder, Krawczyk, & Saloner, 2017; E. B. Jones, 2017; Wu, Zhu, & Swartz, 2016).

Dysregulation of Central Opioid Neurocircuitry in the Pathogenesis of Opioid Use Disorder: Rationale for Mu-Opioid Targeted Pharmacotherapies

Opioid use disorder has known heritability (Jensen, 2016) but requires repeated environmental exposure to illicit/prescribed opioids for expression of the illness. As such, primary prevention of opioid exposure is highly effective in mitigating risk for developing OUD. For those who develop OUD, stabilization of central mu-opioid receptor (MOR) signaling is the main pharmacological strategy in current practice, as this opioid receptor subtype is to date most implicated in neurocircuitry that becomes highly sensitized and dysregulated in OUD (Koob & Volkow, 2016; Kreek et al., 2012).

Opioids also activate other subtypes of central opioid receptors, including kappa and delta opioid receptors, which appear important in moderating affect, pain, reward, and learning and memory associated with the development of drug use disorder in animal studies (reviewed in Bodnar, 2017), but whose roles in the development and treatment of OUD in humans remain unclear. The nociceptin opioid receptor (NOP) is structurally related to

the kappa opioid receptor yet has low affinity for naturally occurring brain opioid receptor ligands (enkephalin, endorphin, and dynorphin) and the opioid-selective antagonist naloxone. Instead, NOP receptors are activated by a NOP-selective, naturally occurring peptide ligand (nociceptin/orphanin FQ), and functionally, NOP activation in animal models appears to modulate opioid analgesic response and the development of opioid tolerance (reviewed by Witkin et al., 2014). Its role in human development of OUD is not yet known.

Acute MOR activation is associated with euphoria, relaxation, and relief from anxiety and pain, all of which are pleasurable and reinforce opioid taking. Yet, chronic misuse of opioids alters MOR functional response and the neural pathways affected. This biological process is called *allostasis*, and refers to a stress-reactive baseline state which may be transiently relieved by opioid use to feel "normal" (George, Le Moal, & Koob, 2012). Both the pleasurable acute MOR activation phase that reinforces repeated opioid use and the later aversive state that develops with chronic MOR activation appear to be integral in the human development of OUD; a distinct transition point from opioid misuse to OUD is unknown (see also Wise & Koob, 2014). In real-world settings, OUD is largely detected at advanced stages of illness when opioid withdrawal presents and/or negative consequences occur, due to low rates of treatment-seeking in earlier stages.

Pharmacotherapy of Opioid Use Disorder: Basic Principles of Agonist Versus Antagonist Therapy

Three FDA-approved medications for OUD with physiological dependence exist (methadone, buprenorphine, and naltrexone), with varying formulations for administration (see Tables 25.1, 25.2, and 25.3). These are pharmacologically *agonist therapies* (methadone and buprenorphine), which stabilize MOR signaling by activating receptors in a predictable, steady-state manner and preventing (through competitive binding to MOR) irregular activation of MOR by opioids of abuse, or *antagonist therapy* (naltrexone), which stabilizes MOR signaling by competitively blocking opioid binding and thus preventing response to opioid misuse, without

TABLE 25.1

TABLE 25.1

Methadone Maintenance in Clinical Treatment of Opioid Use Disorder (OUD): Full Agonist at Mu-Opioid Receptor

Schedule II medication	Requires federally regulated opioid treatment program dispensation with diversion control policy and limited take-home medication privileges
Formulary in United States	Brand, generic, and sugar-free oral concentrate available in 5 and 10 mg/ml
Induction dosing	5–10 mg every 4 hours up to 40 mg during the first 24 hours Titrate to 60–120 mg over 2 weeks with close medical supervision
Maintenance dosing	60–120 mg each morning; rapid metabolizers may have higher dosing requirements; peak and trough monitoring advisable
Half-life	8–59 hours with long terminal half-life up to 120 hours
Metabolism	Hepatic; significantly affected by cytochrome P450 isoenzymes and drug–drug interactions which may reduce trough levels precipitating opioid withdrawal, or increase peak levels posing risk of oversedation and opioid toxicity, including overdose
Adverse effects	Significant; opioid class effects (gastrointestinal hypomotility, sweating, sedation/"nodding," urinary retention, neurocognitive effects, sexual side effects, hypogonadal syndrome, weight gain, apathy, acute dosing euphoria, sleep-disordered breathing) and risk for cardiac arrhythmia and sudden death
Contraindications	Baseline cardiac arrhythmia or significant pulmonary compromise
Pregnancy	Gold standard for OUD in pregnant women, safe for breastfeeding
Diversion potential	High; supervised dosing mitigates this risk
Overdose risk	High; greatest when not retained in treatment; coprescribing intranasal naloxone rescue kit advised

itself introducing opioid activation. In brief, agonist therapies provide a combined effect of stable opioid substitution plus competitive prevention of opioid misuse effects, whereas antagonist therapy provides only competitive prevention of opioid misuse effects. Randomized controlled clinical trials demonstrate that for all three medications, adding medication to evidence-based psychosocial treatment (such as psychoeducation/medical management, contingency management, and cognitive behavior therapy [CBT] for relapse prevention) will at least double the probability of achieving early opioid abstinence compared with placebo or psychosocial treatment alone (reviewed in Connery, 2015; Mattick et al., 2009; Nunes et al., 2018; see also Fudala et al., 2003; Krupitsky et al., 2011; Weiss et al., 2011; Woody et al., 2008). The difference is more stark when comparing ongoing medication to detoxification alone, with a large, multisite randomized controlled trial (RCT) indicating an approximately 50% treatment response to agonist therapy relative to a 7% treatment

response to detoxification alone (Weiss et al., 2011). It is important to note that no medication has any demonstrated efficacy when prescribed in the absence of psychosocial treatment for OUD (see Carroll & Weiss, 2017).

There are several clinical implications of selecting agonist versus antagonist therapy (see Table 25.4). With agonist therapy, side effects general to opioid class effects will persist, albeit in a more tolerable range (e.g., constipation, sedation, potential neurocognitive effects such as cognitive slowing and slowing of motor reaction responses, sweating, lowered blood pressure, urinary retention, sleep-disordered breathing, hypogonadal syndrome, sexual side effects such as decreased libido and erectile dysfunction). Antagonist therapy maintains no opioid class symptoms. During early stabilization, agonist therapies rapidly and directly reduce opioid craving and withdrawal symptoms due to substitution effects, whereas antagonist therapy may not immediately reduce opioid craving and may worsen withdrawal symptoms if

TABLE 25.2

Buprenorphine Maintenance in Clinical Treatment of Opioid Use Disorder (OUD): Partial Agonist at Mu-Opioid Receptor

Schedule III medication	Currently requires 8-hour certification training to obtain DEA waiver to prescribe, patient caseload capped to 275 per prescriber in second year of practice. These policies are highly debated during the present epidemic need for increased access to care.
Formulary in United States	Generic buprenorphine mono tablet, 2 mg, 8 mg Brand (Probuphine®) buprenorphine mono subdermal rod slow-release implant, 296.8 mg lasting 6 months duration Brand (Sublocade®) buprenorphine mono monthly injection depot, 100 mg, 300 mg *Buprenorphine/naloxone combination to prevent diversion:* Brand (Zubsolv®) sublingual tablet, 1.4/0.36 mg, 5.7/1.4 mg Generic sublingual tablet, 2/0.5 mg, 8/2 mg Brand (Suboxone®) sublingual film, 2/0.5 mg, 4/1 mg, 8/2 mg, 12/3 mg Brand (Bunavail®) buccal film, 2.1/0.3 mg, 4.2/0.7 mg, 6.3/1 mg
Induction dosing	*Transmucosal dosing*: Flexible depending on current opioid use (12–16 mg in first 24 hours in divided doses for active users) versus low-dose induction in those with recent opioid abstinence (2–4 mg initial dose). Those with active OUD should have mild-moderate opioid withdrawal (COWS > 8) prior to initial dosing to avoid precipitated withdrawal. *Injectable dosing*: 300 mg administered to those stabilized on a fixed transmucosal dose for a minimum of 7 days; 300 mg for second injection 4 weeks later, then 100 mg every 4 weeks
Maintenance dosing	Formulary-dependent; early recovery for active OUD should achieve the target of 16 mg daily (as tolerated) demonstrated in RCT to be associated with best outcomes; low-induction maintenance is guided by patient response; buprenorphine implant for those well-stabilized on 8 mg or lower daily dose
Half-life	37 hours
Metabolism	Hepatic; somewhat affected by cytochrome P450 isoenzymes; fewer drug–drug interactions
Adverse effects	Moderate; opioid class effects (gastrointestinal hypomotility, sweating, sedation, urinary retention, sexual side effects, hypogonadal syndrome, sleep-disordered breathing)
Contraindications	None; caution in co-occurring sedative dependent patients
Pregnancy	Acceptable for OUD in pregnant women, safe for breastfeeding
Diversion potential	High; office-based prevention policies and patient education/engagement required; may transfer to an opioid treatment program setting for supervised dosing
Overdose risk	Low; greatest when not retained in treatment; coprescribing intranasal naloxone rescue kit advised; note that due to buprenorphine's high affinity naloxone requirement for reversal of overdose is often greater

Note. DEA = Drug Enforcement Administration; COWS = Clinical Opiate Withdrawal Scale; RCT = randomized controlled trial.

given too soon after opioid detoxification. Antagonist stabilization will indirectly reduce opioid craving through reduction of psychologically triggered anticipatory craving, since patients are aware that using opioids when they are taking an opioid antagonist will not result in opioid intoxication. This stands in contrast to agonist therapy, where using opioids may result in opioid intoxication, depending on the potency of opioids used.

Beginning a patient on agonist therapy is faster and easier due to rapid relief of opioid craving and withdrawal. Initiating antagonist therapy requires endurance of opioid craving and withdrawal prior to stabilization, and as such poses greater risk for patient dropout during the induction (see the Selecting Antagonist Therapy section in this chapter). Several algorithms to optimize antagonist initiation have been studied (e.g., single-dose buprenorphine

TABLE 25.3

Naltrexone Maintenance in Clinical Treatment of Opioid Use Disorder (OUD): Antagonist at Mu-Opioid Receptor

Not a controlled substance	May be administered by any office-based prescriber; however, extended-release naltrexone (ER-NTX) requires special pharmacy delivery and storage infrastructure
Formulary in United States	Brand and generic tablet, 50 mg, not recommended for OUD maintenance treatment due to poor patient adherence Brand (Vivitrol®) depot solution: ER-NTX, gluteal intramuscular injection, 380 mg lasting 4 weeks
Induction dosing	Oral tablet may be used to test tolerability prior to first dose ER-NTX, initial 25 mg titrating to 50 mg daily following opioid washout (dosing too soon may precipitate opioid withdrawal) Induction with ER-NTX is identical to maintenance, 380 mg IM every 4 weeks
Maintenance dosing	380 mg IM every 4 weeks; oral tablet supplementation may be advisable in those experiencing loss of effect near 3 weeks or undergoing high risk for relapse conditions
Half-life	5–10 days (ER-NTX)
Metabolism	Hepatic; interim assessment of hepatic panel advised for infrequent hepatotoxicity of clinical significance; this is more important in those with medical comorbidity affecting hepatic functioning
Adverse effects	Modest; headache, nausea, insomnia, elevated transaminases, injection site reactions, hypertension, nasopharyngitis
Contraindications	Pregnant or planning pregnancy, foreseeable need for opioid analgesia
Pregnancy	Contraindicated for pregnancy and breastfeeding
Diversion potential	None
Overdose risk	None direct; greatest when not retained in treatment; coprescribing intranasal naloxone rescue kit advised

Note. IM = intramuscular.

plus escalating-dose oral naltrexone; Sullivan et al., 2017); however, these strategies are not yet disseminated in general practice. Beyond medication protocol improvement, there is an urgent need for the development of novel psychosocial strategies to support antagonist induction and distress tolerance during opioid withdrawal syndromes more generally; this is reviewed in the Integration of Pharmacotherapy with Nonpharmacological Approaches section later in this chapter.

Antagonist therapy may be terminated without any adverse discontinuation syndrome. In contrast, agonist therapies are challenging to discontinue, due to the re-emergence of opioid withdrawal as the dose is decreased. Informed consent may summarize that antagonist therapy is difficult to begin but easier to end, whereas agonist therapies are easier to begin but difficult to end. No known duration of treatment has yet been scientifically defined for any of these

medications, but opioid relapse following agonist and antagonist discontinuation is common, and discontinuation requires close monitoring to prevent opioid relapse. All patients should be informed that prolonged treatment reduces opioid tolerance and that relapse following sustained abstinence has elevated risk for fatal overdose.

Supervised injection heroin therapy is an evidence-based agonist approach to treatment-refractory heroin OUD (Strang et al., 2015), which is used in Europe and Canada but is unavailable in the United States. This model provides a safe environment and controlled dosing of safely manufactured heroin that the patient self-injects daily. It requires more intensive monitoring than buprenorphine or methadone treatment, as there is greater risk for seizure and overdose, and it reduces patient use of illicit heroin, with benefits particularly in improved physical health and reduced crime (Metrebian et al.,

TABLE 25.4

Factors to Consider in Selecting Antagonist Versus Agonist Maintenance for Opioid Use Disorder

Patient care variables important to collaborative decision making	Agonist	Antagonist
Ease of induction	easier	challenging
Ease of termination	challenging	easier
Time commitment	greater, especially for methadone	low
Cost to patient	U.S. state-dependent	U.S. state-dependent
Retention in care	higher	lower
Safety	buprenorphine safer than methadone	safe
Diversion	high	none
Overdose risk	buprenorphine safer than methadone	none
Tolerability	acceptable	acceptable
Adolescent	buprenorphine	off-label
Pregnant	methadone gold standard, buprenorphine acceptable	contraindicated
Older adult		unknown
Pain	buprenorphine safer	may pose antagonist conflict in acute care
Alcohol	indicated	FDA-indicated for both, preferred in motivated patients
Human immuno-deficiency virus; hepatitis C virus	buprenorphine safer than methadone more evidence to support good outcomes	less evidence to support good outcomes

Note. FDA = U.S. Food and Drug Administration.

2015). Recent evidence suggests that injection hydromorphone is as effective as injection heroin (Oviedo-Joekes et al., 2016) but may be easier to disseminate due to federal restrictions associated with Schedule I controlled substances (heroin) and prevalent stigma and bias against heroin substitution therapy.

Selecting agonist therapy: Buprenorphine versus methadone. Methadone maintenance remains the most studied treatment for OUD and is still the gold standard of care in terms of efficacy and patient retention in treatment. Methadone is a synthetic opioid agonist with high intrinsic activity (full agonism) at MOR. It also has agonist activity at both kappa and delta opioid receptors (Kristensen, Christensen, & Christrup, 1995) as well as antagonist activity at the ionotropic N-methyl-D-aspartate glutamate receptor (Doi et al., 2016), but the functional significance of these non-mu opioid effects in clinical treatment of OUD remains unknown. It is a Schedule II medication available in oral tablet and liquid dosing formulations and is administered once daily within federally regulated opioid treatment programs rather than in general office-based settings (in contrast to the use of methadone in office-based pain management, which does not require such restrictions in setting and regulatory environment; see Table 25.1).

Buprenorphine has moderate intrinsic activity but very high affinity and slow dissociation from MOR, functioning as a partial agonist (i.e., <50% activation) with dose–response ceiling effects (Cowan, Lewis, & Macfarlane, 1997). Buprenorphine will competitively replace a full agonist and persistently bind to MOR, which also allows it to have functional antagonist properties. The advantage of buprenorphine compared with methadone is its capacity to successfully ameliorate opioid withdrawal and craving while minimizing adverse opioid agonist effects in opioid-tolerant individuals (i.e., those with OUD), particularly sedation, euphoria, and the potential for respiratory depression with intentional or unintentional overdose. This renders buprenorphine a more tolerable and safer therapy than methadone. It is also available in office-based practice by prescribers who have completed federally required training to use it in the treatment of

OUD. Non-mu opioid activity of buprenorphine includes low potency partial agonism at nociceptin receptors, which are thought to be responsible for lower analgesic effects at higher doses, and functional antagonism at delta and kappa opioid receptors, which are still of unclear significance in clinical treatment of OUD (Cami-Kobeci, Polgar, Khroyan, Toll, & Husbands, 2011).

Buprenorphine is a Schedule III medication available in multiple formulations: sublingual tablet or films and buccal film, suitable for daily dosing, and the more recently approved 6-month depot implant and 4-week injectable depot formulations for longer term maintenance dosing (see Table 25.2). Daily dosed regimens are preferentially dispensed as buprenorphine combined with the MOR antagonist naloxone in a 4:1 dosing ratio, to prevent injection misuse of buprenorphine (naloxone is not bioavailable transmucosally but has potent antagonist effects if injected). Buprenorphine–naloxone combined products have equivalent efficacy as buprenorphine mono products but lower abuse liability (Alho, Sinclair, Vuori, & Holopainen, 2007). Situational exceptions to this include dosing in a contained/observed setting, dosing to pregnant women, and dosing for those with documented allergy to naloxone (which is very rare); all of these are cases in which it is more acceptable to weigh the benefit of the buprenorphine mono formulation over the potential risk of abuse liability.

Multiple RCTs reviewing comparisons of buprenorphine and methadone for heroin OUD demonstrate that buprenorphine at fixed doses of 16 mg daily or greater is equivalently effective at reducing opioid use early in treatment as methadone dosing of 85 mg daily or greater. However, it appears that flexibly dosed buprenorphine, which is standard in U.S. community practice and recommended by World Health Organization treatment guidelines for agonist therapy (World Health Organization, 2009), and includes daily dosing of less than 16 mg, may be inferior to higher dose methadone (80 mg daily or greater, representing the U.S. community practice standard) for both opioid abstinence and retention in treatment (Hser et al., 2014; Minozzi, Amato, Bellisario, Ferri, & Davoli, 2013).

Long-term follow-up of patients randomly assigned to methadone versus buprenorphine demonstrated equivalent reductions in mortality and reduced opioid use compared with no treatment; however, those randomized to methadone had greater opioid abstinence and superior treatment retention (Hser et al., 2016).

Selection of buprenorphine versus methadone must balance factors favoring methadone (abstinence efficacy, treatment retention, and daily supervision) with factors favoring buprenorphine (convenience of office-based care, safety, and tolerability), as well as patient preference and access. Both are considered first-line treatments for OUD.

Selecting antagonist therapy: Naltrexone versus buprenorphine. In the United States, only one large RCT ($N = 570$) has evaluated the relative effectiveness of outpatient treatment with buprenorphine + naloxone in sublingual film formulation (BN) versus extended-release naltrexone (ER-NTX; Lee et al., 2017). The results of this study confirmed that BN induction is significantly easier for patients than is ER-NTX, with a 28% dropout rate during induction to ER-NTX versus a 6% dropout rate for BN. Interestingly, one site that avoided the use of opioid detoxification with buprenorphine or methadone and instead utilized a clonidine (nonopioid) taper protocol had the most success with ER-NTX initiation, presumably because the duration of opioid wash-out required prior to ER-NTX induction was briefer, and all opioid withdrawal occurred in a monitored residential setting to protect against relapse. This has important implications for optimizing ER-NTX initiation, as the more common community treatments for opioid detoxification occur in brief stay settings (e.g., 4–7 days) and utilize the long-acting opioids methadone and buprenorphine for detoxification; patients seeking ER-NTX following these protocols typically endure 10 to 14 days opioid withdrawal syndrome as outpatients, with greater risk for opioid access and relapse, before being sufficiently opioid free to safely initiate ER-NTX.

When study analysis was limited to only patients successfully inducted to BN and ER-NTX treatment, outcomes were equally effective for opioid reduction, retention in treatment, opioid craving, and prevention of opioid overdose. Overdose events clustered among those with medication induction failure (9 of 28 overdose events) and occurred with equal frequency for both medication groups during the follow-up study period (10 of 28 in ER-NTX and 9 of 28 in BN), typically after a substantial period off study medication. Adverse events differed only by site reactions (a risk limited to ER-NTX depot formulation). These findings were consistent with a smaller ($N = 165$) outpatient multisite, open-label RCT conducted in Norway that compared flexibly dosed BN (sublingual tablet formulation) to ER-NTX over a 12-week study period (Tanum et al., 2017). Of 143 individuals initiating treatment following detoxification (at least 1 week) in a residential setting, the number of opioid-abstinent days and retention in treatment were equivalent for BN and ER-NTX, but ER-NTX was associated with less heroin use on using days compared with the BN group, lower heroin craving, and a reduction of days using benzodiazepines. Significantly more adverse events occurred with precipitated withdrawal in the ER-NTX group. ER-NTX participants reported greater satisfaction with treatment than did BN participants. Long-term follow-up on this study is ongoing.

Risk management of treatment without agonist or antagonist therapy: The problem of opioid withdrawal, relapse, and overdose.   Despite robust evidence for the superiority of agonist and antagonist treatment of OUD to psychosocial treatment alone, medications continue to be significantly underutilized. Many patients, if receiving any treatment, are completing brief opioid detoxification followed by outpatient treatment without medication for OUD (Hadland et al., 2017). Although medications such as the central alpha-2 adrenergic agonist clonidine or lofexidine are widely prescribed to treat opioid withdrawal syndromes, their efficacy in symptom relief is inferior to opioid agonist treatment and is associated with significantly greater dropout and risk for relapse and overdose (Gowing, Farrell, Ali, & White, 2016; Marsch et al., 2005). Controlled studies with buprenorphine show that for both heroin OUD

(Woody et al., 2008) and prescription opioid OUD (Weiss et al., 2011), rapid return to opioid use following brief stabilization and taper is the majority outcome, even for participants receiving intensive psychosocial treatments and weekly medical appointments allowing multiple medications directed toward symptom relief of opioid withdrawal (i.e., in addition to alpha-2 agonists, medications targeting anxiety, sleep, gastrointestinal distress, and nonopioid pain relievers). Given barriers to medication for OUD and common public bias against medications for OUD affecting patient decision making regarding for "drug-free" treatment, there is an urgent need to develop more effective medical and psychosocial interventions to ameliorate acute opioid withdrawal and to better engage patients in care, as well as to facilitate successful medication taper during long-term recovery. Although extended residential treatment is ideal for drug-free treatment approaches to OUD, it is frequently unavailable and/or unaffordable, and overdose and relapse rates following discharge remain high (Ravndal & Amundsen, 2010; Sannibale et al., 2003). Although psychosocial therapies have not yet been tested for the enhancement of distress tolerance during opioid withdrawal, research on tapering benzodiazepines provides a model for this approach. CBT for benzodiazepine taper has been shown to improve taper success compared with slow taper alone (Otto et al., 2010). This treatment uses interoceptive exposure techniques (i.e., exposure to feared physical sensations) to enhance tolerance of withdrawal symptoms and reduce anxiety symptoms. Application of this approach to OUD has potential to improve the ability to persist through opioid withdrawal by reducing anxious responding to its core physical and affective symptoms.

BEST APPROACHES FOR ASSESSING TREATMENT RESPONSE AND MANAGING SIDE EFFECTS

Treatment response to OUD medication is measured by (a) toxicological confirmation of nonprescribed opioid abstinence and adherence to prescribed opioid therapy (whether analgesic prescription or agonist therapy for OUD); (b) retention in treatment;

(c) patient self-report on OUD behaviors and thoughts/cravings, quality of life, and functioning; (d) objective measures of patient quality of life and functioning, such as functional health measures, employment/school functioning, family status, and legal status; and (e) collateral data (e.g., family reports, clinician reports, service utilization review reports, employer/school/probation reports) regarding clinical outcomes (Chou et al., 2009; Kleber et al., 2007). Special considerations have been developed for assessment of pregnant women treated for OUD, generally following the same principles while adding measures of fetal viability and emphasizing repeal of criminal sanctions that deter prenatal care engagement (Committee Opinion No. 711: Opioid Use and Opioid Use Disorder in Pregnancy, 2017).

Significant research gaps remain regarding the optimal quality measure outcomes for different patient populations (i.e., considering phase of life, sociological determinants of health, and diagnostic comorbidities; Clark et al., 2015); as well as cost-effectiveness measures relating to quality of care, structure of care, and functional and health outcomes associated with different models of care provided (Chou et al., 2016; Mattke, Predmore, Sloss, Wilks, & Watkins, 2018). The absence of such guidance, combined with the absence of integrated/coordinated care centers, results in each treatment center creating local and conflicting policies and procedures for managing issues such as medication nonadherence, relapse to opioid or other substance use, and exacerbation of mental health symptoms or pain during treatment. In this context, many patients end up between services (i.e., too medically or psychiatrically ill for substance use disorder settings and using too many substances for admission to medical or psychiatric services) or discharged from services without viable alternative treatment options available to them. The most pragmatic treatment outcome considered primary for chronic OUD is retaining individuals' treatment engagement in efforts to reduce harms associated with substance use and co-occurring illnesses and to facilitate substance use reduction efforts and supports.

Dosing is fixed for depot formulations of antagonist therapy and buprenorphine, but oral agonist therapies have flexibly tailored dosing ranges aimed at eliminating opioid withdrawal and mitigating craving (see Tables 25.1, 25.2, and 25.3). Dosing of agonist therapy during early stabilization is a predictor of outcome. Methadone maintenance response is dose dependent, with higher dosing (60 mg daily or more) recommended for optimal stabilization (Ling, Wesson, Charuvastra, & Klett, 1996), including among pregnant women with OUD, who also frequently experience increased dosing requirements during third trimester (Wilder, Hosta, & Winhusen, 2017). Similarly, buprenorphine doses are recommended to be at least 16 mg daily during early phases of treatment (Mattick, Breen, Kimber, & Davoli, 2014). There is convergent evidence to suggest that adolescent and adult patients who do not achieve opioid abstinence with buprenorphine within the first 2 to 4 weeks of treatment may need psychosocial treatment intensification in order to achieve a good outcome with buprenorphine (Marcovitz, McHugh, Volpe, Votaw, & Connery, 2016; McDermott et al., 2015; Subramaniam et al., 2011).

The management of adverse effects of treatment is medication specific and formulation specific (see Tables 25.1, 25.2, and 25.3), with methadone maintenance having the largest burden of side effects and drug interactions, and buprenorphine and ER-NTX having a lower burden. Methadone exerts full opioid effects and has greater need for monitoring tolerability and safety. Induction dosing is a time of risk for oversedation and respiratory depression (Bell, Trinh, Butler, Randall, & Rubin, 2009). Once a patient is stabilized, this risk is reduced, but management must continue to assess for medication interactions that would augment methadone blood levels and/or substance use of alcohol and sedatives which may exert synergistic effects on respiratory depression or pulmonary compromise. Hepatic metabolism of methadone is complex and involves multiple cytochrome P450 isoenzymes; potentiation or inhibition of these isoenzymes is the source of most drug interactions with methadone (McCance-Katz, Sullivan, & Nallani, 2010). Changes in mental status should prompt investigation of changes in medications being taken (prescribed and over-the-counter), substance use, or mental health symptom changes. Methadone is dose dependently associated with cardiac QTc prolongation (i.e., the time between ventricular depolarization and complete repolarization is abnormally long), which carries risk of sudden arrhythmia and death, yet baseline QTc assessment has not demonstrated any significance in preventing or predicting QTc prolongation with methadone maintenance (Pani, Trogu, Maremmani, & Pacini, 2013). In contrast, there is no evidence that buprenorphine or naltrexone is associated with QTc prolongation.

Buprenorphine has low intrinsic activity at MOR and is pharmacologically a partial agonist, activating MOR with less than half the potency of full agonists such as methadone. In opioid-tolerant individuals, this results in a "ceiling effect" on both euphoric effects and respiratory depression, significantly improving safety and tolerability. Even in opioid-naïve individuals, intravenous administration is associated with only partial respiratory depressant effects (Dahan, 2006), making it safer for both OUD patients and opioid-naïve individuals exposed to diverted supplies. Opioid class effects are mild in comparison with methadone and drug interactions are fewer (McCance-Katz et al., 2010). Sleep-disordered breathing can occur in both methadone and buprenorphine-maintained patients and may require dosing adjustments (DeVido, Connery, & Hill, 2015).

Due to its high affinity for MOR and partial agonist activity at MOR, buprenorphine will behave as a competitive antagonist if MOR are occupied by full agonist ligands (e.g., morphine, fentanyl, oxycodone, hydrocodone). Therefore, induction with buprenorphine in active OUD patients requires patients to abstain until they are in mild to moderate opioid withdrawal (a score of 8 or greater on the COWS; Wesson & Ling, 2003), to avoid precipitating opioid withdrawal. Transitions from long-acting opioids such as methadone generally require longer abstinence (36 hours) and it is prudent to wait until a COWS threshold of 13 is reached to avoid precipitated withdrawal during induction. Office-based inductions give an initial 2 to 4 mg dose, and within an hour, a patient usually experiences sufficient relief to take the rest of the day's divided doses at home. Stabilization at 16 mg daily maintenance can

be rapidly achieved in most patients within the first 3 days of induction.

ER-NTX is the recommended antagonist therapy for OUD, due to low adherence with oral naltrexone. Oral naltrexone may be used during the induction phase to test tolerability prior to administering the 4-week depot formulation (ER-NTX). Patients need to be opioid-free for at least 7 days to avoid precipitating opioid withdrawal. Oral naltrexone may also be used during maintenance phases of treatment to supplement dosing toward the end of the 4-week period or as needed to manage patients in high-risk situations during the second half of the depot dosing. Common side effects include nausea, headache, and insomnia, and for depot injection site reactions, hypertension and nasopharyngitis. Naltrexone may be associated with hepatotoxicity; baseline and interim hepatic monitoring is advised during treatment. Most patients having mild to moderate elevation of liver enzymes during treatment are asymptomatic and do not warrant treatment discontinuation. Although sporadic reports in the literature have implied that naltrexone, because of MOR antagonism, may cause depressed mood in some patients, controlled studies do not support this observation (Krupitsky et al., 2016), even among patients having co-occurring major depressive disorder (Mysels, Cheng, Nunes, & Sullivan, 2011) or scoring high on scales of depression at baseline (Zaaijer et al., 2015).

MEDICATION MANAGEMENT ISSUES

Following successful initiation of agonist or antagonist therapy, problems with adherence to medication taking and dropout from treatment pose barriers to patient recovery. Controlled clinical trials demonstrate improved treatment retention with both agonist (Mattick et al., 2009; Weiss et al., 2011; Woody et al., 2008) and depot antagonist (Krupitsky et al., 2011) treatments, compared with placebo or no medication.

Community and cohort studies of ER-NTX demonstrate frequent medication discontinuation, particularly within the first 6 months of treatment, if incentives are not paired with the monthly injection appointment (Comer et al., 2006; Jarvis et al.,

2017). This appears to be related to patient under-estimation of relapse risk (Williams et al., 2017), as well as to the ease of discontinuation, which is not subjectively appreciable since there is no ensuing opioid withdrawal. Efforts to support an enhanced ER-NTX delivery platform, while increasing access to ER-NTX, still demonstrate many patients receiving only three or fewer consecutive monthly doses (Cousins, Crèvecoeur-MacPhail, Kim, & Rawson, 2018) and further suggest that patients at greatest risk for medication nonadherence are those who are homeless, injection opioid users, or have co-occurring psychiatric disorders (Cousins et al., 2016).

Head-to-head studies of retention in treatment for agonist therapies favor methadone over buprenorphine for longer treatment retention (Hser et al., 2014; Mattick et al., 2014), including treatment for individuals with HIV (Woody et al., 2014) and pregnant women (Minozzi et al., 2013). However, the flexibility of office-based buprenorphine compared with daily methadone maintenance may be more appealing, and clinicians may leverage this preference to incentivize buprenorphine adherence. Patients who discontinue agonist therapy and do not use illicit opioids will experience the onset of opioid withdrawal syndrome within days, which in nearly all cases will prompt either a return to medication adherence, or alternatively, a relapse to illicit opioid use. The recent development of longer acting formulations of buprenorphine holds promise for improved medication adherence (Rosenthal & Goradia, 2017).

Diversion

Diversion of medication (selling or giving away one's medication) is not a risk with antagonist therapy, given its lack of psychoactive effects, but is a significant public health concern with agonist therapies, which continue to be widely available in illicit supply and commonly shared among opioid-using social networks (Johnson & Richert, 2015). Supervised medication administration is protective but limited by cost and inconvenience for many individuals seeking treatment for OUD, and there is insufficient data to determine whether developing novel systems for agonist medication supervision would in fact decrease medication diversion in a cost-effective

manner (Saulle, Vecchi, & Gowing, 2017). Federally regulated opioid treatment programs employ structured diversion control programs to closely monitor agonist dispensation, allowing take-home doses of liquid methadone only to patients assessed to be clinically stable, motivated in recovery, unlikely to be involved in diversion for profit, and reliable in medication adherence (see Drug Enforcement Agency Diversion Control Division, Section VI, https://www.deadiversion.usdoj.gov/pubs/manuals/pract/section6.htm).

Products containing only buprenorphine have been widely diverted for injection misuse, and thus the development of the combined buprenorphine–naloxone formulation in 2002 provided a successful improvement in diversion prevention compared with office-based buprenorphine treatment (Comer, Sullivan, et al., 2010). This combined product is the standard of care currently utilized in U.S. maintenance therapy for all nonpregnant patients treated for OUD, yet diversion of these products remains problematic (Larance et al., 2014). A newer formulation of buprenorphine, the buprenorphine subdermal implant, a 6-month slow-release rod delivery system surgically placed in the upper arm, is approved by the FDA for maintaining buprenorphine-stabilized patients engaged in recovery treatment (Rosenthal et al., 2013; Rosenthal et al., 2016). Although not yet widely utilized, the implant offers significant diversion reduction potential compared with daily administration of more commonly prescribed oral forms of buprenorphine (e.g., sublingual tablet or film strip, buccal film). Monthly injectable buprenorphine was approved by the FDA on November 30, 2017 and should soon be accessible for treatment of OUD patients who have been stably maintained on an oral formulation for a minimum of 7 days. It is expected that the FDA will soon follow with approval of a weekly subcutaneous depot buprenorphine formulation, and these new depot products promise to improve treatment adherence and diversion problems (Rosenthal & Goradia, 2017; Walsh et al., 2017).

Practice recommendations for safety and diversion prevention include expanding access to treatment, since community surveys of patients in treatment indicate that a substantial number of them reported prior attempts to self-treat with illicit buprenorphine products (Schuman-Olivier et al., 2013; Wright et al., 2016). Additional recommendations include prescribing limited quantities and refills; utilization of prescription monitoring databases to assess prescription filling and renewal, as well as to check controlled substances from other prescribers; implementation of safe storage (a lockbox for buprenorphine or take-home methadone supply) and disposal; preferential prescribing of film strips for those with children in the home (the most childproof of the oral formulations); use of designated pharmacies to fill prescriptions; and use of treatment agreements to prevent diversion. Prescribers may also implement random pill counts and toxicology to confirm buprenorphine adherence.

Overdose

Treatment nonadherence and dropout is associated with both return to opioid use and elevated overdose risk, especially in those who have sustained weeks of opioid abstinence, resulting in loss of opioid tolerance. Evidence that maintenance in agonist therapy prevents overdose death is robust (Sordo et al., 2017), and evidence that ER-NTX therapy prevents overdose is growing (Krupitsky et al., 2013; Lee et al., 2016; Lee et al., 2017). It is recommended that all patients be educated about naloxone antagonist reversal of opioid overdose and that patients and families be provided access to take-home naloxone rescue kits (see the Emerging Trends section in this chapter; see also Fairbairn, Coffin, & Walley, 2017). Optimal practice policy includes repeated patient education about elevated overdose potential following opioid abstinence and obtaining consent to alert emergency contacts if a patient drops out of treatment.

EVALUATION OF PHARMACOLOGICAL APPROACHES ACROSS THE LIFESPAN

Despite high rates of OUD among youth of ages 18 to 25, few controlled clinical trials of OUD pharmacotherapies exist for adolescents (Minozzi, Amato, Bellisario, & Davoli, 2014). Outpatient buprenorphine/naloxone maintenance is the only FDA-approved pharmacotherapy for adolescents aged 16 years and

older, based on favorable outcome, safety, and cost-effectiveness of a single multisite national RCT comparing buprenorphine/naloxone detoxification taper with maintenance treatment (Woody et al., 2008). In the United States, methadone maintenance can be offered to adolescents of ages 16 to 18, but only to those with two prior failed attempts at OUD treatment and only with parental assent; it is therefore rarely used in adolescent OUD. Although ER-NTX antagonist therapy is being empirically used in care of adolescents with OUD (Fishman, 2008), research is sorely needed to assess its efficacy and safety in this cohort. The absence of clinical research in this age cohort has a catastrophic impact on public prevention and treatment: Only 2.4% of U.S. adolescents in substance use treatment for heroin use disorder receive OUD pharmacotherapy, and only 0.4% of U.S. adolescents in substance use treatment for prescription opioid use disorder receive OUD pharmacotherapy (Feder et al., 2017). Even among older youth, a national study of commercial insurance claims assessing whether a prescription for either buprenorphine or naltrexone was filled within 6 months of OUD diagnosis likewise demonstrated disappointingly low rates, with only 22% of those aged 18 to 20 years receiving medication, and females, Hispanic Americans, and African Americans aged 13 to 25 years significantly less likely to receive medication compared with non-Hispanic White males in this age group (Hadland et al., 2017).

Less is known about the efficacy and safety of OUD pharmacotherapies in adults 65 years and older, as no controlled clinical trials have been conducted despite this cohort's prevalence of chronic pain disorders and opioid analgesic use, misuse, substance use disorders, and medical vulnerability to opioid overdose (Le Roux, Tang, & Drexler, 2016; West, Severtson, Green, & Dart, 2015). Clinicians treating older adults are advised to routinely reassess dosing requirements to mitigate aging effects on adverse consequences of agonist maintenance (e.g., fall risk, respiratory and gastrointestinal effects).

In contrast, a large evidence base supports the safety and efficacy of agonist therapies in the treatment of pregnant women with OUD (reviewed in Reddy, Davis, Ren, & Greene, 2017). In utero opioid exposure due to untreated OUD is associated with poor maternal–fetal outcomes, with terato-genic risks including premature birth and stillbirth, low birth weight, oral cleft, ventricular septal and atrial septal defects, and clubfoot (Lind et al., 2017). Agonist maintenance greatly reduces these teratogenic risks and facilitates planning for safe delivery and treatment of *neonatal abstinence syndrome* (NAS; also increasingly referred to as *neonatal opioid withdrawal syndrome* [NOWS] to distinguish it specifically from broader syndromes of neonatal abstinence that may involve exposure to multiple different drugs), which refers to opioid withdrawal occurring in the baby following placental separation (Wurst, Zedler, Joyce, Sasinowski, & Murrelle, 2016; Zedler et al., 2016). A randomized, double-blind comparison of methadone and buprenorphine for pregnant women with OUD found that both treatments were safe and effective for both mother and child outcomes, with no significant differences between these medications (H. E. Jones et al., 2010). Mothers can safely breastfeed on either agonist maintenance, given the minimal transmission in breast milk and the significant positive outcomes of breastfeeding on maternal and child health, including reduced severity of NAS. Polysubstance use during pregnancy is most predictive of NAS severity in infants of buprenorphine-maintained mothers; treatment focus is thus on abstinence from all substances (Jansson et al., 2017).

Sadly, extensive barriers remain that deter pregnant OUD women from seeking appropriate prenatal care, including civil and criminal penalties for drug use during pregnancy (18 states allow criminal charges of child abuse, with consequent termination of all parental rights), the absence of pregnant women-centered treatment in 31 of 50 states, and continuing barriers to access to agonist maintenance across most of the United States. (Krans & Patrick, 2016). As with all other OUD cohorts, rates of psychiatric comorbidity—especially depression, trauma, and anxiety disorders—among pregnant OUD women are high, yet adequate mental health treatment remains largely inaccessible to them. A recent analysis of all deaths during pregnancy or postpartum (not limited to OUD pregnant women) in Philadelphia, PA between 2010 and 2014 demonstrated that 49% were attributable to substance

overdose, domestic violence/homicide, and suicide (Mehta, Bachhuber, Hoffman, & Srinivas, 2016). Given the frequency of recent hospital contact prior to death, these data suggest that more intensive mental health screening and interventions are warranted to support maternal–child safety in general and may be significantly magnified among those identified as having OUD. Collaborative approaches to care, such as mental health services embedded within prenatal care, are feasible and hold promise for improved care for pregnant women with OUD (Mittal & Suzuki, 2017).

CONSIDERATION OF POTENTIAL SEX DIFFERENCES

OUD has historically been more prevalent in men than women. However, as with other substance use disorders, this gap is narrowing, largely due to a roughly equal representation of men and women among those dependent upon prescription opioids (Back, Payne, Simpson, & Brady, 2010). Notably, heroin use is rising twice as quickly in women relative to men (Centers for Disease Control and Prevention, 2015) and the prevalence of prescription opioid overdoses has risen at a higher rate in women relative to men (Centers for Disease Control and Prevention, 2013). Accordingly, OUD in women is a significant and increasing concern.

Several sex differences in OUD have been identified. Women appear to more rapidly escalate from initiation to dependence relative to men (known as a telescoping course of illness; Lewis, Hoffman, & Nixon, 2014) and experience more severe functional consequences (McHugh et al., 2013); women are also more likely to report using opioids to mitigate negative affect (McHugh et al., 2013) and are more likely to be diagnosed with mood or anxiety disorders (Lewis et al., 2014). Animal and human research has identified several sex differences in the effects of opioids; however, these studies— particularly in human models—have yielded equivocal results, and the animal and human models often do not align. For example, some studies report greater opioid analgesia in women (Niesters et al., 2010), whereas others have failed to find a difference (Comer, Cooper, et al., 2010); these findings contrast with evidence for greater opioid analgesia in male rodents (Cicero, Nock, & Meyer, 1996). Research has been more consistent with respect to self-reported adverse opioid side effects. For example, women are more likely than men to report experiencing side effects such as nausea, dizziness, and fatigue (Comer, Cooper, et al., 2010; Fillingim et al., 2005). Several factors complicate the study of sex differences in drug effects, such as ovarian hormones (Harte-Hargrove, Varga-Wesson, Duffy, Milner, & Scharfman, 2015), drug dose, acute versus chronic pain models, and whether the participant is opioid-naïve; therefore, cautious interpretation is recommended.

Pharmacotherapy treatment outcomes appear similar for men and women (McHugh et al., 2013; Smyth, Fagan, & Kernan, 2012; Ziedonis et al., 2009). Induction and dosing procedures are identical for men and women, and only slightly altered for pregnant women. Limitations include the fact that women are underrepresented in OUD clinical trials and sex-specific analyses are often underpowered or not conducted.

INTEGRATION OF PHARMACOTHERAPY WITH NONPHARMACOLOGICAL APPROACHES: BENEFITS AND CHALLENGES

Nonpharmacological approaches to OUD include behavioral therapies, mutual support groups (e.g., Narcotics Anonymous), peer support (e.g., recovery coaching), and case management. These psychosocial therapies are understudied in OUD, and no guidelines exist for matching optimal psychosocial treatment to individual patients. OUD behavioral therapies include drug counseling, structured CBT, and contingency management (CM). CM has the largest effects among behavioral therapies for OUD patients (Dutra et al., 2008), using basic behavioral principles of reinforcement to modify target behaviors. For example, patients can earn an incentive (monetary or other prize) for desired behaviors, such as provision of opioid-negative urine screens. CM has been associated with decreased use of other substances (e.g., cocaine,

nicotine) among those in methadone maintenance therapy (Schottenfeld et al., 2005; Sigmon et al., 2016), as well as improved treatment attendance (Rhodes et al., 2003), and it has been associated with favorable opioid use outcomes, even among those not on OUD pharmacotherapy (Petry & Carroll, 2013).

The addition of counseling to buprenorphine maintenance has not yielded reliable benefits (Weiss et al., 2011) but may improve outcomes among certain high-risk subgroups, such as those with injection drug use and polydrug use (Weiss et al., 2014). However, studies of buprenorphine maintenance often use highly structured and frequent (weekly) medical management conditions, or medical counseling, which may have obscured the benefits of additional behavioral therapies (Carroll & Weiss, 2017). Intensive medication management is unavailable in virtually all primary care settings, and the addition of structured psychosocial treatments may be advisable in this context. Active participation in self-help groups is another key component associated with favorable outcomes in later stages of recovery after discontinuing agonist therapy (Weiss, Griffin, McHugh, & Karakula, 2017).

Several barriers limit the ability to integrate OUD pharmacologic and psychosocial treatments, primarily the cost of staff training and staffing for evidence-based psychosocial treatments. Examples of cost-effective innovations include the Veterans Health Administration expansion of CM services through investment in training and reimbursement (Petry, DePhilippis, Rash, Drapkin, & McKay, 2014) and use of technology to deliver behavioral interventions on demand and outside of office hours (Carroll et al., 2008).

INTEGRATED APPROACHES FOR ADDRESSING COMMON COMORBID DISORDERS

Co-occurring mental health disorders are common among those with OUD. Population-based estimates suggest that more than two thirds of this population will meet criteria for a co-occurring mental health disorder, predominantly anxiety and depressive disorders (Grella et al., 2009); this rate is likely to be even higher among those in treatment settings. Behavioral therapies may be of benefit for these subgroups, and several treatments have shown promise for the treatment of co-occurring mental health and substance use disorders, such as the treatment of bipolar disorder (Weiss et al., 2009) and posttraumatic stress disorder (Mills et al., 2012).

There is a significant research gap in psychopharmacotherapies for those with co-occurring disorders. In the absence of such research, current clinical practice is to prescribe for these individuals according to the evidence-based algorithms and guidelines for both disorders individually, while attempting to minimize the use of controlled substances with abuse liability (Kleber et al., 2007). Colocation of psychiatry and opioid treatment services has demonstrated good outcomes related to improved adherence in mental health care (Brooner et al., 2013).

The management of pain disorders in OUD patients has advanced significantly during the past decade. Principles of treatment include effective functional pain relief; avoidance of opioid relapse; and in the case of opioid analgesia, the prevention of diversion, misuse, and intentional or unintentional overdose (Demidenko et al., 2017; Sen et al., 2016). Patients with OUD are opioid tolerant and will generally require higher dosing of opioid analgesics. Maintenance on OUD agonist therapy is recommended, with pain management added to this for acute and chronic pain syndromes. When possible, nonopioid therapies are preferred, including pharmacotherapies (e.g., nonsteroidal anti-inflammatory medications; medications targeting neuropathic pain such as gabapentin, carbamazepine, and calcium channel blockers; and topical analgesics such as lidocaine patches applied to the region of pain), surgical interventions addressing root causes, exercise/physical therapies, and complementary therapies (e.g., acupuncture, mindfulness-based therapies), as well as supportive mental health interventions targeting distress tolerance, acceptance, and coping skills (see Chapter 19, this volume).

During acute pain syndromes, mild to moderate musculoskeletal and neuropathic pain relief may be obtained by adjusting agonist therapy or transiently adding opioid analgesia. For more severe acute syndromes associated with visceral pain, pain of origin in bony structures, or postoperative recovery, collaboration between agonist therapy prescriber and pain team is optimal, as agonist taper or cessation may be recommended over the duration of treatment with more potent opioid analgesia. Engaging family and other recovery supports to prevent opioid relapse is advisable.

With chronic noncancer pain syndromes, the use of opioid therapy is not recommended for most patients entering care; however, it may be appropriate to continue for those already in a chronic opioid therapy for pain management. Efforts to reduce risks of overdose and other poor outcomes include assessing dose requirements; providing more intensive psychosocial supports to treat other co-occurring disorders or social determinants of health; prescribing longer acting, abuse-deterrent formulations whenever possible (Webster, Markman, Cone, & Niebler, 2017); and coprescribing naloxone reversal antagonist kits to patients and family members (Dowell, Haegerich, & Chou, 2016). In practice, the majority of OUD patients on agonist therapy will not be good candidates for chronic opioid analgesia, and those requiring agonist therapy plus opioid analgesia are best managed with the support of experienced pain management and/or mental health experts in a collaborative care setting.

Pharmacotherapies for treating common medical disorders co-occurring with injection OUD, such as HIV and HCV, are well established as collaborative care models, generally utilizing methadone or buprenorphine maintenance for OUD, although ER-NTX is increasingly utilized in primary care of OUD (Korthuis et al., 2017). An example is the Buprenorphine HIV Evaluation and Support trial (BHIVES), in which localizing OUD care with buprenorphine within treatment centers for HIV-positive patients demonstrated significantly improved buprenorphine induction, retention, and opioid outcomes (Fiellin et al., 2011). Medications used to treat HIV and HCV are safe and effective in patients maintained on either buprenorphine or methadone (Kosloski et al., 2017; Saxon et al.,

2013) but require knowledge of specific drug inter-actions for monitoring safety and dose adjustments (McCance-Katz et al., 2010; Meemken, Hanhoff, Tseng, Christensen, & Gillessen, 2015). Less evidence is available on OUD agonist therapy safety in patients with HIV/HCV coinfection; however, sufficient guidelines exist to recommend specific and time-phased medication treatments and monitoring for drug–drug interactions with agonist therapies (Taylor, Swan, & Matthews, 2013). There is some indication that methadone dosing requirements may be higher in OUD patients with HIV coinfection (Roncero et al., 2017).

EMERGING TRENDS

Naloxone Dissemination

Naloxone is a rapidly-acting opioid antagonist that can effectively reverse opioid intoxication and overdose. It may be effectively administered intra-venously or intraosseously (i.e., into the bone) in hospital and emergency response settings but is also now available in simple-to-use intranasal and intramuscular formulations, which allows it to be effectively deployed in community settings with minimal training requirements. Naloxone prevention of opioid overdose death has been championed since the 1990s and is now considered an essential aspect of opioid overdose prevention strategies in the United States, both for OUD-related drug overdose prevention, as well as for coprescription with chronic opioid analgesic maintenance to prevent potential medication-related overdose (reviewed in Fairbairn et al., 2017). Naloxone education and community dissemination has been associated with significant reductions in OUD-related overdose fatalities, and there is no evidence that its dissemination has contributed negatively to increased illicit opioid use. Training is minimal and community bystanders and trained emergency responders both demonstrate successful implementation (Walley et al., 2013). A growing cause for concern is the increase in illicit fentanyl analogues in opioid and nonopioid drug supplies (particularly in the Northeast, South, and Midwest U.S. regions), whose potency and rapid respiratory depressive effects make naloxone rescue less effective and

more challenging to deliver (multiple administra-tions are required for rescue). Indeed, fentanyl-associated deaths have sharply increased in the United States. since 2014 (O'Donnell, Gladden, & Seth, 2017).

Emergency Department Buprenorphine Induction

The imperative of broad naloxone dissemination for prevention must be coordinated with successful recruitment of patients rescued from fatal opioid overdose into evidence-based treatment for OUD. Unfortunately, current emergency protocols and fragmentation of substance and mental health treatments from medical treatment centers have posed significant barriers to successful treatment recruitment of naloxone-rescued patients. Additionally, naloxone rescue precipitates a robust and aversive opioid withdrawal syndrome, incentivizing patients to discharge abruptly and seek illicit opioid relapse for relief. This ineffective cycling may be repaired by emergency protocols that offer agonist therapy induction immediately to stabilized patients. Evidence has been demonstrated that OUD patients presenting to emergency departments with opioid withdrawal may be successfully induced to buprenorphine maintenance and retained in OUD treatment in primary care with positive outcomes at 30 and 60 days (D'Onofrio et al., 2017) and is currently being further evaluated in a national, multisite clinical trial (see https://clinicaltrials.gov; NCT03023930, Opioid Use Disorder in the Emergency Department: CTN 0069). This model of care has important potential to engage those experiencing postnaloxone rescue, whose best prevention strategy would be engagement in OUD pharmacotherapy and psychosocial treatments. Innovative community program collaborative efforts among law enforcement, hospitals, and substance use treatment centers have made initial progress in reducing repeated overdose rescues and connecting patients with OUD care, and they play a vital community role in raising awareness of solutions to the opioid crisis and access to needed health and social supports (e.g., Project Outreach/PCO Hope in Plymouth County, MA; see https://projectoutreachplymouth.com/).

TOOL KIT OF RESOURCES

Provider Resources: Treatment of Opioid Use Disorder

Substance Abuse and Mental Health Services Agency (SAMHSA): SAMHSA-HRSA Center for Integrated Health Solutions: This free access website provides one-stop references for evidence-based screening tools; shared decision making; motivational interviewing; screening, brief intervention, and referral to treatment; medication-assisted treatment; pain management; health disparities; health indicators; oral health; substance use; suicide prevention; trauma; and intimate partner violence. https://www.integration.samhsa.gov/clinical-practice/

Providers Clinical Support System: This free access website provides evidence-based topical content training on pharmacotherapy and treatment of substance use disorders. It is developed, updated, and maintained by an interdisciplinary consortium of experts in the field and funded by SAMHSA. Its goals are to educate through webinars (including free continuing education credits), office form templates, and discussion groups; to mentor through a national program matching expert mentors with mentees; and to train all licensed professionals for buprenorphine and other prescribing. https://pcssnow.org/

Veteran's Administration/Department of Defense Clinical Practice Guidelines for the Management of Substance Use Disorders: This free access outlines current, evidence-based guidelines to comprehensive substance use disorder treatment developed by experts in the national Veteran's Administration health care services. https://www.healthquality.va.gov/guidelines/mh/sud/

American Association for the Treatment of Opioid Dependence, Inc.: This free access website provides clinician guidelines, training and education, and support tools as well as patient education materials specifically focused on serving those being treated in state and federally regulated Opioid Treatment Programs. http://www.aatod.org/

Boston University Safe and Competent Opioid Prescribing Education (SCOPE of Pain): This free access website outlines a comprehensive core curriculum for pain management and opioid prescribing. It offers training webinars that may be applied to maintenance of certification and also offers institutional and organizational training. https://www.scopeofpain.com/

Suicide Prevention Resource Center: This free access website offers comprehensive suicide prevention materials for all settings (schools, work, clinical, organizational) and provides links to regional suicide prevention resources for clinicians, patients and families. http://www.sprc.org/

Patient Resources: Education

Opioid Overdose Crisis (National Institute on Drug Abuse): This free access website provides an overview of the opioid crisis in laymen's terms and resources for those seeking further information. https://www.drugabuse.gov/drugs-abuse/opioids/opioid-overdose-crisis

Patient Resources: Community Supports

Narcotics Anonymous Mutual Help Groups: This international peer support organization provides free community groups, recovery sponsors, and educational resources for those with opioid use disorder. https://www.na.org/

Nar-Anon Family Groups: This international peer support organization provides free community groups and educational resources for family members of those with opioid use disorder. https://www.nar-anon.org

Self-Management and Recovery Training (SMART Recovery): This peer support organization provides free community groups to those with substance use disorder and their family members, with an emphasis on cognitive and behavioral skills training to stop substance use. http://www.smartrecovery.org/

National Suicide Prevention Lifeline (1-800-273-8255): This free 24/7 hotline provides support to those thinking about suicide or those concerned about another individual who may be thinking about suicide. https://suicidepreventionlifeline.org/

Patient Resources: Opioid Overdose Prevention and Grief Support

Learn to Cope: This peer support group was developed to provide free education and support to family members and friends of those with opioid use disorder, with a focus on opioid overdose prevention and support for those who have lost a loved one to opioid overdose. http://www.learn2cope.org/

Grief Recovery After a Substance Passing: This peer support group was developed to provide free grief support to those who have lost a loved one due to substance-related cause of death. http://grasphelp.org/about-us/

References

Alho, H., Sinclair, D., Vuori, E., & Holopainen, A. (2007). Abuse liability of buprenorphine–naloxone tablets in untreated IV drug users. *Drug and Alcohol Dependence, 88,* 75–78. http://dx.doi.org/10.1016/j.drugalcdep.2006.09.012

*American Psychiatric Association. (2013). *Diagnostic and statistical manual of mental disorders* (5th ed.). Washington, DC: Author.

Back, S. E., Payne, R. L., Simpson, A. N., & Brady, K. T. (2010). Gender and prescription opioids: Findings from the National Survey on Drug Use and Health. *Addictive Behaviors, 35,* 1001–1007. http://dx.doi.org/10.1016/j.addbeh.2010.06.018

Beaudoin, F. L., Merchant, R. C., & Clark, M. A. (2016). Prevalence and detection of prescription opioid misuse and prescription opioid use disorder among emergency department patients 50 years of age and older: Performance of the Prescription Drug Use Questionnaire, Patient Version. *American Journal of Geriatric Psychiatry, 24,* 627–636. http://dx.doi.org/10.1016/j.jagp.2016.03.010

Bell, J., Trinh, L., Butler, B., Randall, D., & Rubin, G. (2009). Comparing retention in treatment and mortality in people after initial entry to methadone and buprenorphine treatment. *Addiction, 104,* 1193–1200. http://dx.doi.org/10.1111/j.1360-0443.2009.02627.x

Blanco, C., Wall, M. M., Okuda, M., Wang, S., Iza, M., & Olfson, M. (2016). Pain as a predictor of opioid use disorder in a nationally representative sample. *American Journal of Psychiatry, 173,* 1189–1195. http://dx.doi.org/10.1176/appi.ajp.2016.15091179

Bodnar, R. J. (2017). Endogenous opiates and behavior: 2015. *Peptides, 88,* 126–188. http://dx.doi.org/10.1016/j.peptides.2016.12.004

Bohnert, K. M., Ilgen, M. A., Louzon, S., McCarthy, J. F., & Katz, I. R. (2017). Substance use disorders and the risk of suicide mortality among men and women in the US Veterans Health Administration. *Addiction, 112,* 1193–1201. http://dx.doi.org/10.1111/add.13774

Brooner, R. K., Kidorf, M. S., King, V. L., Peirce, J., Neufeld, K., Stoller, K., & Kolodner, K. (2013). Managing psychiatric comorbidity within versus outside of methadone treatment settings: A randomized and controlled evaluation. *Addiction, 108,* 1942–1951. http://dx.doi.org/10.1111/add.12269

*Butler, S. F., Fernandez, K., Benoit, C., Budman, S. H., & Jamison, R. N. (2008). Validation of the revised Screener and Opioid Assessment for Patients with Pain (SOAPP-R). *Journal of Pain, 9,* 360–372. http://dx.doi.org/10.1016/j.jpain.2007.11.014

Cami-Kobeci, G., Polgar, W. E., Khroyan, T. V., Toll, L., & Husbands, S. M. (2011). Structural determinants of opioid and NOP receptor activity in derivatives of buprenorphine. *Journal of Medicinal Chemistry, 54,* 6531–6537. http://dx.doi.org/10.1021/jm2003238

Carroll, K. M., Ball, S. A., Martino, S., Nich, C., Babuscio, T. A., Nuro, K. F., . . . Rounsaville, B. J. (2008). Computer-assisted delivery of cognitive-behavioral therapy for addiction: A randomized trial of CBT4CBT. *American Journal of Psychiatry, 165,* 881–888. http://dx.doi.org/10.1176/appi.ajp.2008.07111835

Carroll, K. M., & Weiss, R. D. (2017). The role of behavioral interventions in buprenorphine maintenance treatment: A review. *American Journal of Psychiatry, 174,* 738–747. http://dx.doi.org/10.1176/appi.ajp.2016.16070792

Center for Behavioral Health Statistics and Quality. (2016). *2015 national survey on drug use and health: Detailed tables.* Substance Abuse and Mental Health Services Administration (Ed.). Rockville, MD.

Centers for Disease Control and Prevention. (2013). Prescription painkiller overdoses: A growing epidemic, especially among women. *CDC Vital Signs.* Retrieved September 9, 2017, from https://www.cdc.gov/vitalsigns/prescriptionpainkilleroverdoses/index.html

Centers for Disease Control and Prevention. (2015). Today's heroin epidemic infographics. Retrieved from https://www.cdc.gov/vitalsigns/heroin/infographic.html

Chou, R., Fanciullo, G. J., Fine, P. G., Adler, J. A., Ballantyne, J. C., Davies, P., . . . Miaskowski, C. (2009). Clinical guidelines for the use of chronic opioid therapy in chronic noncancer pain. *Journal of Pain, 10,* 113–130. http://dx.doi.org/10.1016/j.jpain.2008.10.008

Chou, R., Korthuis, P. T., Weimer, M., Bougatsos, C., Blazina, I., Zakher, B., . . . McCarty, D. (2016). *Medication-assisted treatment models of care for opioid use disorder in primary care settings.* Agency for Healthcare Research and Quality: Rockville, MD.

Cicero, T. J., Ellis, M. S., Surratt, H. L., & Kurtz, S. P. (2014). The changing face of heroin use in the United States: A retrospective analysis of the past 50 years. *JAMA Psychiatry, 71,* 821–826. http://dx.doi.org/10.1001/jamapsychiatry.2014.366

Cicero, T. J., Nock, B., & Meyer, E. R. (1996). Gender-related differences in the antinociceptive properties of morphine. *Journal of Pharmacology and Experimental Therapeutics, 279,* 767–773.

Clark, R. E., Baxter, J. D., Aweh, G., O'Connell, E., Fisher, W. H., & Barton, B. A. (2015). Risk factors for relapse and higher costs among Medicaid members with opioid dependence or abuse: Opioid

*Asterisks indicate assessments or resources.

agonists, comorbidities, and treatment history. *Journal of Substance Abuse Treatment, 57*, 75–80. http://dx.doi.org/10.1016/j.jsat.2015.05.001

Comer, S. D., Cooper, Z. D., Kowalczyk, W. J., Sullivan, M. A., Evans, S. M., Bisaga, A. M., & Vosburg, S. K. (2010). Evaluation of potential sex differences in the subjective and analgesic effects of morphine in normal, healthy volunteers. *Psychopharmacology (Berl), 208*, 45–55. http://dx.doi.org/10.1007/s00213-009-1703-4

Comer, S. D., Sullivan, M. A., Vosburg, S. K., Manubay, J., Amass, L., Cooper, Z. D., . . . Kleber, H. D. (2010). Abuse liability of intravenous buprenorphine/naloxone and buprenorphine alone in buprenorphine-maintained intravenous heroin abusers. *Addiction, 105*, 709–718. http://dx.doi.org/10.1111/j.1360-0443.2009.02843.x

Comer, S. D., Sullivan, M. A., Yu, E., Rothenberg, J. L., Kleber, H. D., Kampman, K., . . . O'Brien, C. P. (2006). Injectable, sustained-release naltrexone for the treatment of opioid dependence: A randomized, placebo-controlled trial. *Archives of General Psychiatry, 63*, 210–218. http://dx.doi.org/10.1001/archpsyc.63.2.210

Committee Opinion No. 711. (2017). Opioid use and opioid use disorder in pregnancy. *Obstetrics & Gynecology, 130*, e81–e94. http://dx.doi.org/10.1097/aog.0000000000002235

Compton, W. M., & Volkow, N. D. (2006). Abuse of prescription drugs and the risk of addiction. *Drug and Alcohol Dependence, 83*(Suppl. 1), S4–S7. http://dx.doi.org/10.1016/j.drugalcdep.2005.10.020

Connery, H. S. (2015). Medication-assisted treatment of opioid use disorder: Review of the evidence and future directions. *Harvard Review of Psychiatry, 23*, 63–75. http://dx.doi.org/10.1097/hrp.0000000000000075

Conway, K. P., Compton, W., Stinson, F. S., & Grant, B. F. (2006). Lifetime comorbidity of *DSM–IV* mood and anxiety disorders and specific drug use disorders: Results from the National Epidemiologic Survey on Alcohol and Related Conditions. *Journal of Clinical Psychiatry, 67*, 247–257.

Cousins, S. J., Crèvecoeur-MacPhail, D., Kim, T., & Rawson, R. A. (2018). The Los Angeles County hub-and-provider network for promoting the sustained use of extended-release naltrexone (XR-NTX) in Los Angeles County (2010–2015). *Journal of Substance Abuse Treatment, 85*, 78–83. http://dx.doi.org/10.1016/j.jsat.2017.02.011

Cousins, S. J., Radfar, S. R., Crèvecoeur-MacPhail, D., Ang, A., Darfler, K., & Rawson, R. A. (2016). Predictors of continued use of extended-released naltrexone (XR-NTX) for opioid-dependence: An analysis of heroin and non-heroin opioid users in Los Angeles County. *Journal of Substance Abuse Treatment, 63*, 66–71. http://dx.doi.org/10.1016/j.jsat.2015.12.004

Cowan, A., Lewis, J. W., & Macfarlane, I. R. (1997). Agonist and antagonist properties of buprenorphine, a new antinociceptive agent. *British Journal of Pharmacology, 60*, 537–545.

D'Onofrio, G., Chawarski, M. C., O'Connor, P. G., Pantalon, M. V., Busch, S. H., Owens, P. H., . . . Fiellin, D. A. (2017). Emergency department-initiated buprenorphine for opioid dependence with continuation in primary care: Outcomes during and after intervention. *Journal of General Internal Medicine, 32*, 660–666. http://dx.doi.org/10.1007/s11606-017-3993-2

Dahan, A. (2006). Opioid-induced respiratory effects: New data on buprenorphine. *Palliative Medicine, 20*(Suppl. 1), s3–s8.

Darke, S., Ross, J., Marel, C., Mills, K. L., Slade, T., Burns, L., & Teesson, M. (2015). Patterns and correlates of attempted suicide amongst heroin users: 11-year follow-up of the Australian treatment outcome study cohort. *Psychiatry Research, 227*, 166–170. http://dx.doi.org/10.1016/j.psychres.2015.04.010

Demidenko, M. I., Dobscha, S. K., Morasco, B. J., Meath, T. H. A., Ilgen, M. A., & Lovejoy, T. I. (2017). Suicidal ideation and suicidal self-directed violence following clinician-initiated prescription opioid discontinuation among long-term opioid users. *General Hospital Psychiatry, 47*, 29–35. http://dx.doi.org/10.1016/j.genhosppsych.2017.04.011

DeVido, J., Connery, H., & Hill, K. P. (2015). Sleep-disordered breathing in patients with opioid use disorders in long-term maintenance on buprenorphine-naloxone: A case series. *Journal of Opioid Management, 11*, 363–366. http://dx.doi.org/10.5055/jom.2015.0285

Doi, S., Mori, T., Uzawa, N., Arima, T., Takahashi, T., Uchida, M., . . . Narita, M. (2016). Characterization of methadone as a β-arrestin-biased μ-opioid receptor agonist. *Molecular Pain, 12*. http://dx.doi.org/10.1177/1744806916654146

Dole, V. P., & Nyswander, M. (1965). A medical treatment for diacetylmorphine (heroin) addiction: A clinical trial with methadone hydrochloride. *Journal of the American Medical Association, 193*, 646–650.

Dole, V. P., Robinson, J. W., Orraca, J., Towns, E., Searcy, P., Caine, E. (1969). Methadone treatment of randomly selected criminal addicts. *New England Journal of Medicine, 280*, 1372–1375. http://dx.doi.org/10.1056/NEJM196906192802502

Dowell, D., Haegerich, T. M., & Chou, R. (2016). CDC Guideline for prescribing opioids for chronic pain: United States, 2016. *Recommendations and Reports, 65*, 1–49. http://dx.doi.org/10.15585/mmwr.rr6501e1

Dutra, L., Stathopoulou, G., Basden, S. L., Leyro, T. M., Powers, M. B., & Otto, M. W. (2008). A meta-analytic review of psychosocial interventions for substance use disorders. *American Journal of*

Psychiatry, 165, 179–187. http://dx.doi.org/10.1176/appi.ajp.2007.06111851

Fairbairn, N., Coffin, P. O., & Walley, A. Y. (2017). Naloxone for heroin, prescription opioid, and illicitly made fentanyl overdoses: Challenges and innovations responding to a dynamic epidemic. *International Journal of Drug Policy, 46*, 172–179. http://dx.doi.org/10.1016/j.drugpo.2017.06.005

Feder, K. A., Krawczyk, N., & Saloner, B. (2017). Medication-assisted treatment for adolescents in specialty treatment for opioid use disorder. *Journal of Adolescent Health, 60*, 747–750. http://dx.doi.org/10.1016/j.jadohealth.2016.12.023

Fiellin, D. A., Weiss, L., Botsko, M., Egan, J. E., Altice, F. L., Bazerman, L. B., . . . O'Connor, P. G. (2011). Drug treatment outcomes among HIV-infected opioid-dependent patients receiving buprenorphine/naloxone. *Journal of Acquired Immune Deficiency Syndromes, 56*(Suppl. 1), S33–S38. http://dx.doi.org/10.1097/QAI.0b013e3182097537

Fillingim, R. B., Ness, T. J., Glover, T. L., Campbell, C. M., Hastie, B. A., Price, D. D., & Staud, R. (2005). Morphine responses and experimental pain: Sex differences in side effects and cardiovascular responses but not analgesia. *Journal of Pain, 6*, 116–124. http://dx.doi.org/10.1016/j.jpain.2004.11.005

Finkelman, M. D., Jamison, R. N., Kulich, R. J., Butler, S. F., Jackson, W. C., Smits, N., & Weiner, S. G. (2017). Cross-validation of short forms of the Screener and Opioid Assessment for Patients with Pain-Revised (SOAPP-R). *Drug and Alcohol Dependence, 178*, 94–100. http://dx.doi.org/10.1016/j.drugalcdep.2017.04.016

Fishman, M. (2008). Precipitated withdrawal during maintenance opioid blockade with extended release naltrexone. *Addiction, 103*, 1399–1401. http://dx.doi.org/10.1111/j.1360-0443.2008.02252.x

Fudala, P. J., Bridge, T. P., Herbert, S., Williford, W. O., Chiang, C. N., Jones, K., . . . Tusel, D. (2003). Office-based treatment of opiate addiction with a sublingual-tablet formulation of buprenorphine and naloxone. *New England Journal of Medicine, 349*, 949–958.

George, O., Le Moal, M., & Koob, G. F. (2012). Allostasis and addiction: Role of the dopamine and corticotropin-releasing factor systems. *Physiology & Behavior, 106*, 58–64. http://dx.doi.org/10.1016/j.physbeh.2011.11.004

Gowing, L., Farrell, M., Ali, R., & White, J. M. (2016). Alpha$_2$-adrenergic agonists for the management of opioid withdrawal. *Cochrane Database of Systematic Reviews, 2016*(5), Art. No.: CD002024. http://dx.doi.org/10.1002/14651858.CD002024.pub5

Grella, C. E., Karno, M. P., Warda, U. S., Niv, N., & Moore, A. A. (2009). Gender and comorbidity among individuals with opioid use disorders in the NESARC study. *Addictive Behaviors, 34*, 498–504. http://dx.doi.org/10.1016/j.addbeh.2009.01.002

Griffin, M. L., McDermott, K. A., McHugh, R. K., Fitzmaurice, G. M., Jamison, R. N., & Weiss, R. D. (2016). Longitudinal association between pain severity and subsequent opioid use in prescription opioid dependent patients with chronic pain. *Drug and Alcohol Dependence, 163*, 216–221. http://dx.doi.org/10.1016/j.drugalcdep.2016.04.023

Gryczynski, J., Schwartz, R. P., Mitchell, S. G., O'Grady, K. E., & Ondersma, S. J. (2014). Hair drug testing results and self-reported drug use among primary care patients with moderate-risk illicit drug use. *Drug and Alcohol Dependence, 141*, 44–50. http://dx.doi.org/10.1016/j.drugalcdep.2014.05.001

Hadland, S. E., Wharam, J. F., Schuster, M. A., Zhang, F., Samet, J. H., & Larochelle, M. R. (2017). Trends in receipt of buprenorphine and naltrexone for opioid use disorder among adolescents and young adults, 2001–2014. *JAMA Pediatrics, 171*, 747–755. http://dx.doi.org/10.1001/jamapediatrics.2017.0745

Han, B., Compton, W. M., Blanco, C., Crane, E., Lee, J., & Jones, C. M. (2017). Prescription opioid use, misuse, and use disorders in U.S. adults: 2015 National Survey on Drug Use and Health. *Annals of Internal Medicine, 293–301*. http://dx.doi.org/10.7326/m17-0865

Harte-Hargrove, L. C., Varga-Wesson, A., Duffy, A. M., Milner, T. A., & Scharfman, H. E. (2015). Opioid receptor-dependent sex differences in synaptic plasticity in the hippocampal mossy fiber pathway of the adult rat. *Journal of Neuroscience, 35*, 1723–1738. http://dx.doi.org/10.1523/jneurosci.0820-14.2015

Hilario, E. Y., Griffin, M. L., McHugh, R. K., McDermott, K. A., Connery, H. S., Fitzmaurice, G. M., & Weiss, R. D. (2015). Denial of urinalysis-confirmed opioid use in prescription opioid dependence. *Journal of Substance Abuse Treatment, 48*, 85–90. http://dx.doi.org/10.1016/j.jsat.2014.07.003

Hser, Y. I., Evans, E., Huang, D., Weiss, R., Saxon, A., Carroll, K. M., . . . Ling, W. (2016). Long-term outcomes after randomization to buprenorphine/naloxone versus methadone in a multi-site trial. *Addiction, 111*, 695–705. http://dx.doi.org/10.1111/add.13238

Hser, Y. I., Saxon, A. J., Huang, D., Hasson, A., Thomas, C., Hillhouse, M., . . . Ling, W. (2014). Treatment retention among patients randomized to buprenorphine/naloxone compared to methadone in a multi-site trial. *Addiction, 109*, 79–87. http://dx.doi.org/10.1111/add.12333

Hughes, A., Williams, M. R., Lipari, R. N., Bose, J., Copello, E. A. P., & Kroutil, L. A. (2016). Prescription drug use and misuse in the United States: Results from the 2015 National Survey on Drug Use and Health. *NSDUH Data Review*. Retrieved from https://www.samhsa.gov/data/sites/default/files/NSDUH-FFR2-2015/NSDUH-FFR2-2015.htm

Jaffee, W. B., Trucco, E., Levy, S., & Weiss, R. D. (2007). Is this urine really negative? A systematic review of tampering methods in urine drug screening and testing. *Journal of Substance Abuse Treatment, 33*, 33–42. http://dx.doi.org/10.1016/j.jsat.2006.11.008

Jansson, L. M., Velez, M. L., McConnell, K., Spencer, N., Tuten, M., Jones, H., . . . DiPietro, J. A. (2017). Maternal buprenorphine treatment and infant outcome. *Drug and Alcohol Dependence, 180*, 56–61. http://dx.doi.org/10.1016/j.drugalcdep.2017.08.001

Jarvis, B. P., Holtyn, A. F., DeFulio, A., Dunn, K. E., Everly, J. J., Leoutsakos, J. S., . . . Silverman, K. (2017). Effects of incentives for naltrexone adherence on opiate abstinence in heroin-dependent adults. *Addiction, 112*, 830–837. http://dx.doi.org/10.1111/add.13724

Jensen, K. P. (2016). A review of genome-wide association studies of stimulant and opioid use disorders. *Molecular Neuropsychiatry, 2*, 37–45. http://dx.doi.org/10.1159/000444755

Johnson, B., & Richert, T. (2015). Diversion of methadone and buprenorphine by patients in opioid substitution treatment in Sweden: Prevalence estimates and risk factors. *International Journal of Drug Policy, 26*, 183–190. http://dx.doi.org/10.1016/j.drugpo.2014.10.003.

Jones, C. M. (2013). Heroin use and heroin use risk behaviors among nonmedical users of prescription opioid pain relievers: United States, 2002–2004 and 2008–2010. *Drug and Alcohol Dependence, 132*, 95–100. http://dx.doi.org/10.1016/j.drugalcdep.2013.01.007

Jones, E. B. (2017). Medication-assisted opioid treatment prescribers in federally qualified health centers: Capacity lags in rural areas. *Journal of Rural Health, epub ahead of print.* http://dx.doi.org/10.1111/jrh.12260

Jones, H. E., Kaltenbach, K., Heil, S. H., Stine, S. M., Coyle, M. G., Arria, A. M., . . . Fischer, G. (2010). Neonatal abstinence syndrome after methadone or buprenorphine exposure. *New England Journal of Medicine, 363*, 2320–2331. http://dx.doi.org/10.1056/NEJMoa1005359

Kaye, A. D., Jones, M. R., Kaye, A. M., Ripoll, J. G., Jones, D. E., Galan, V., . . . Manchikanti, L. (2017). Prescription opioid abuse in chronic pain: An updated review of opioid abuse predictors and strategies to curb opioid abuse (Part 2). *Pain Physician, 20*(2S), S111–S133.

Kleber, H. D., Weiss, R. D., Anton, R. F., Jr., George, T. P., Greenfield, S. F., Kosten, T. R., . . . Regier, D. (2007). Treatment of patients with substance use disorders,

second edition. American Psychiatric Association. *American Journal of Psychiatry, 164*(Suppl. 4), 5–123.

Koob, G. F., & Volkow, N. D. (2016). Neurobiology of addiction: A neurocircuitry analysis. *Lancet Psychiatry, 3*, 760–773. http://dx.doi.org/10.1016/s2215-0366(16)00104-8

Korthuis, P. T., McCarty, D., Weimer, M., Bougatsos, C., Blazina, I., Zakher, B., . . . Chou, R. (2017). Primary care-based models for the treatment of opioid use disorder: A scoping review. *Annals of Internal Medicine, 166*, 268–278. http://dx.doi.org/10.7326/m16-2149

Kosloski, M. P., Zhao, W., Asatryan, A., Kort, J., Geoffroy, P., & Liu, W. (2017). No clinically relevant drug-drug interactions between methadone or buprenorphine-naloxone and antiviral combination glecaprevir and pibrentasvir. *Antimicrobial Agents and Chemotherapy, 61*, 1628–1637. http://dx.doi.org/10.1128/aac.00958-17

Krans, E. E., & Patrick, S. W. (2016). Opioid use disorder in pregnancy: Health policy and practice in the midst of an epidemic. *Obstetrics & Gynecology, 128*, 4–10. http://dx.doi.org/10.1097/aog.0000000000001446

Kreek, M. J., Levran, O., Reed, B., Schlussman, S. D., Zhou, Y., & Butelman, E. R. (2012). Opiate addiction and cocaine addiction: Underlying molecular neurobiology and genetics. *Journal of Clinical Investigation, 122*, 3387–3393. http://dx.doi.org/10.1172/jci60390

Kreek, M. J., & Vocci, F. J. (2002). History and current status of opioid maintenance treatments: Blending conference session. *Journal of Substance Abuse Treatment, 23*, 93–105.

Kristensen, K., Christensen, C. B., & Christrup, L. L. (1995). The mu1, mu2, delta, kappa opioid receptor binding profiles of methadone stereoisomers and morphine. *Life Sciences, 56*, L45–L50.

Krupitsky, E., Nunes, E. V., Ling, W., Gastfriend, D. R., Memisoglu, A., & Silverman, B. L. (2013). Injectable extended-release naltrexone (XR-NTX) for opioid dependence: Long-term safety and effectiveness. *Addiction, 108*, 1628–1637. http://dx.doi.org/10.1111/add.12208

Krupitsky, E., Nunes, E. V., Ling, W., Illeperuma, A., Gastfriend, D. R., & Silverman, B. L. (2011). Injectable extended-release naltrexone for opioid dependence: A double-blind, placebo-controlled, multicentre randomised trial. *Lancet, 377*, 1506–1513. http://dx.doi.org/10.1016/s0140-6736(11)60358-9

Krupitsky, E., Zvartau, E., Blokhina, E., Verbitskaya, E., Wahlgren, V., Tsoy-Podosenin, M., . . . Woody, G. (2016). Anhedonia, depression, anxiety, and craving in opiate dependent patients stabilized on oral naltrexone or an extended release naltrexone implant. *American Journal of Drug and Alcohol*

Abuse, 42, 614–620. http://dx.doi.org/10.1080/00952990.2016.1197231

*Kumar, P. C., Cleland, C. M., Gourevitch, M. N., Rotrosen, J., Strauss, S., Russell, L., & McNeely, J. (2016). Accuracy of the Audio Computer Assisted Self Interview version of the Alcohol, Smoking and Substance Involvement Screening Test (ACASI ASSIST) for identifying unhealthy substance use and substance use disorders in primary care patients. *Drug and Alcohol Dependence, 165*, 38–44. http://dx.doi.org/10.1016/j.drugalcdep.2016.05.030

Larance, B., Lintzeris, N., Ali, R., Dietze, P., Mattick, R., Jenkinson, R., . . . Degenhardt, L. (2014). The diversion and injection of a buprenorphine-naloxone soluble film formulation. *Drug and Alcohol Dependence, 136*, 21–27. http://dx.doi.org/10.1016/j.drugalcdep.2013.12.005

Le Roux, C., Tang, Y., & Drexler, K. (2016). Alcohol and opioid use disorder in older adults: Neglected and treatable illnesses. *Current Psychiatry Reports, 18*, 87. http://dx.doi.org/10.1007/s11920-016-0718-x

Lee, J. D., Friedmann, P. D., Kinlock, T. W., Nunes, E. V., Boney, T. Y., Hoskinson, R. A., Jr., . . . O'Brien, C. P. (2016). Extended-release naltrexone to prevent opioid relapse in criminal justice offenders. *New England Journal of Medicine, 374*, 1232–1242. http://dx.doi.org/10.1056/NEJMoa1505409

Lee, J. D., Nunes, E. V., Jr., Novo, P., Bachrach, K., Bailey, G. L., Bhatt, S., . . . Rotrosen, J. (2017). Comparative effectiveness of extended-release naltrexone versus buprenorphine-naloxone for opioid relapse prevention (X:BOT): A multicentre, open-label, randomised controlled trial. *Lancet, 391*(10118), 309–318. http://dx.doi.org/10.1016/S0140-6736(17)32812-X

Lewis, B., Hoffman, L. A., & Nixon, S. J. (2014). Sex differences in drug use among polysubstance users. *Drug and Alcohol Dependence, 145*, 127–133. http://dx.doi.org/10.1016/j.drugalcdep.2014.10.003

Lind, J. N., Interrante, J. D., Ailes, E. C., Gilboa, S. M., Khan, S., Frey, M. T., . . . Broussard, C. S. (2017). Maternal use of opioids during pregnancy and congenital malformations: A systematic review. *Pediatrics, 139*, e20164131. http://dx.doi.org/10.1542/peds.2016-4131

Ling, W. Charuvastra, C., Kaim, S. C., & Klett, C. J. (1976). Methadyl acetate and methadone as maintenance treatments for heroin addicts. A Veterans Administration cooperative study. *Archives of General Psychiatry, 33*, 709–720.

Ling, W., Wesson, D. R., Charuvastra, C., & Klett, C. J. (1996). A controlled trial comparing buprenorphine and methadone maintenance in opioid dependence. *Archives of General Psychiatry, 53*, 401–407.

Maloney, E., Degenhardt, L., Darke, S., Mattick, R. P., & Nelson, E. (2007). Suicidal behaviour and associated risk factors among opioid-dependent individuals: A case-control study. *Addiction, 102*, 1933–1941. http://dx.doi.org/10.1111/j.1360-0443.2007.01971.x

Marcovitz, D. E., McHugh, R. K., Volpe, J., Votaw, V., & Connery, H. S. (2016). Predictors of early dropout in outpatient buprenorphine/naloxone treatment. *American Journal on Addictions, 25*, 472–477. http://dx.doi.org/10.1111/ajad.12414

Marsch, L. A., Bickel, W. K., Badger, G. J., Stothart, M. E., Quesnel, K. J., Stanger, C., & Brooklyn, J. (2005). Comparison of pharmacological treatments for opioid-dependent adolescents: A randomized controlled trial. *Archives of General Psychiatry, 62*, 1157–1164. http://dx.doi.org/10.1001/archpsyc.62.10.1157

Martins, S. S., Sarvet, A., Santaella-Tenorio, J., Saha, T., Grant, B. F., & Hasin, D. S. (2017). Changes in US lifetime heroin use and heroin use disorder: Prevalence from the 2001–2002 to 2012–2013 National Epidemiologic Survey on Alcohol and Related Conditions. *JAMA Psychiatry, 74*, 445–455. http://dx.doi.org/10.1001/jamapsychiatry.2017.0113

Mattick, R. P., Breen, C., Kimber, J., & Davoli, M. (2009). Methadone maintenance therapy versus no opioid replacement therapy for opioid dependence. *Cochrane Database of Systematic Reviews 3*, CD002209. http://dx.doi.org/10.1002/14651858.CD002209.pub2

Mattick, R. P., Breen, C., Kimber, J., & Davoli, M. (2014). Buprenorphine maintenance versus placebo or methadone maintenance for opioid dependence. *Cochrane Database of Systematic Reviews, 2*, CD002207. http://dx.doi.org/10.1002/14651858.CD002207.pub4

Mattke, S., Predmore, Z., Sloss, E., Wilks, A., & Watkins, K. E. (2018). Evidence for misspecification of a nationally used quality measure for substance use treatment. *Journal for Healthcare Quality, 40*, 228–235.

McCance-Katz, E. F., Sullivan, L. E., & Nallani, S. (2010). Drug interactions of clinical importance among the opioids, methadone and buprenorphine, and other frequently prescribed medications: A review. *American Journal on Addictions, 19*, 4–16. http://dx.doi.org/10.1111/j.1521-0391.2009.00005.x

McDermott, K. A., Griffin, M. L., Connery, H. S., Hilario, E. Y., Fiellin, D. A., Fitzmaurice, G. M., & Weiss, R. D. (2015). Initial response as a predictor of 12-week buprenorphine-naloxone treatment response in a prescription opioid-dependent population. *Journal of Clinical Psychiatry, 76*, 189–194. http://dx.doi.org/10.4088/JCP.14m09096

McHugh, R. K., Devito, E. E., Dodd, D., Carroll, K. M., Potter, J. S., Greenfield, S. F., . . . Weiss, R. D. (2013). Gender differences in a clinical trial for prescription opioid dependence. *Journal of Substance Abuse Treatment, 45*, 38–43. http://dx.doi.org/10.1016/j.jsat.2012.12.007

*McNeely, J., Cleland, C. M., Strauss, S. M., Palamar, J. J., Rotrosen, J., & Saitz, R. (2015). Validation of Self-Administered Single-Item Screening Questions (SISQs) for unhealthy alcohol and drug use in primary care patients. *Journal of General Internal Medicine, 30*, 1757–1764. http://dx.doi.org/10.1007/s11606-015-3391-6

Meemken, L., Hanhoff, N., Tseng, A., Christensen, S., & Gillessen, A. (2015). Drug–drug interactions with antiviral agents in people who inject drugs requiring substitution therapy. *Annals of Pharmacotherapy, 49*, 796–807. http://dx.doi.org/10.1177/1060028015581848

Mehta, P. K., Bachhuber, M. A., Hoffman, R., & Srinivas, S. K. (2016). Deaths from unintentional injury, homicide, and suicide during or within 1 year of pregnancy in Philadelphia. *American Journal of Public Health, 106*, 2208–2210. http://dx.doi.org/10.2105/ajph.2016.303473

Metrebian, N., Groshkova, T., Hellier, J., Charles, V., Martin, A., Forzisi, L., . . . Strang, J. (2015). Drug use, health and social outcomes of hard-to-treat heroin addicts receiving supervised injectable opiate treatment: Secondary outcomes from the Randomized Injectable Opioid Treatment Trial (RIOTT). *Addiction, 110*, 479–90. http://dx.doi.org/10.1111/add.12748

Mills, K. L., Teesson, M., Back, S. E., Brady, K. T., Baker, A. L., Hopwood, S., . . . Ewer, P. L. (2012). Integrated exposure-based therapy for co-occurring posttraumatic stress disorder and substance dependence: A randomized controlled trial. *Journal of the American Medical Association, 308*, 690–699. http://dx.doi.org/10.1001/jama.2012.9071

Minozzi, S., Amato, L., Bellisario, C., & Davoli, M. (2014). Maintenance treatments for opiate-dependent adolescents. *Cochrane Database of Systematic Reviews, 6*, CD007210. http://dx.doi.org/10.1002/14651858.CD007210.pub3

Minozzi, S., Amato, L., Bellisario, C., Ferri, M., & Davoli, M. (2013). Maintenance agonist treatments for opiate-dependent pregnant women. *Cochrane Database of Systematic Reviews, 12*, CD006318. http://dx.doi.org/10.1002/14651858.CD006318.pub3

Mittal, L., & Suzuki, J. (2017). Feasibility of collaborative care treatment of opioid use disorders with buprenorphine during pregnancy. *Substance Abuse, 38*, 261–264. http://dx.doi.org/10.1080/08897077.2015.1129525

Mysels, D. J., Cheng, W. Y., Nunes, E. V., & Sullivan, M. A. (2011). The association between naltrexone treatment and symptoms of depression in opioid-dependent patients. *American Journal of Drug and Alcohol Abuse, 37*, 22–26. http://dx.doi.org/10.3109/00952990.2010.540281

Niesters, M., Dahan, A., Kest, B., Zacny, J., Stijnen, T., Aarts, L., & Sarton, E. (2010). Do sex differences exist in opioid analgesia? A systematic review and meta-analysis of human experimental and clinical studies. *Pain, 151*, 61–68. http://dx.doi.org/10.1016/j.pain.2010.06.012

Nunes, E. V., Gordon, M., Friedmann, P. D., Fishman, M. J., Lee, J. D., Chen, D. T., . . . O'Brien, C. P. (2018). Relapse to opioid use disorder after inpatient treatment: Protective effect of injection naltrexone. *Journal of Substance Abuse Treatment, 85*, 49–55. http://dx.doi.org/10.1016/j.jsat.2017.04.016

O'Donnell, J. K., Gladden, R. M., & Seth, P. (2017). Trends in deaths involving heroin and synthetic opioids excluding methadone, and law enforcement drug product reports, by census region—United States, 2006–2015. *Morbidity and Mortality Weekly Report, 66*, 897–903. http://dx.doi.org/10.15585/mmwr.mm6634a2

Otto, M. W., McHugh, R. K., Simon, N. M., Farach, F. J., Worthington, J. J., & Pollack, M. H. (2010). Efficacy of CBT for benzodiazepine discontinuation in patients with panic disorder: Further evaluation. *Behaviour Research and Therapy, 48*, 720–727. http://dx.doi.org/10.1016/j.brat.2010.04.002

Oviedo-Joekes, E., Guh, D., Brissette, S., Marchand, K., MacDonald, S., Lock, K., . . . Schechter, M. T. (2016). Hydromorphone compared with diacetylmorphine for long-term opioid dependence: A randomized clinical trial. *Journal of the American Medical Association Psychiatry, 73*, 447–55. http://dx.doi.org/10.1001/jamapsychiatry.2016.0109

Pani, P. P., Trogu, E., Maremmani, I., & Pacini, M. (2013). QTc interval screening for cardiac risk in methadone treatment of opioid dependence. *Cochrane Database of Systematic Reviews, 6*, CD008939. http://dx.doi.org/10.1002/14651858.CD008939.pub2

Petry, N. M., & Carroll, K. M. (2013). Contingency management is efficacious in opioid-dependent outpatients not maintained on agonist pharmacotherapy. *Psychology of Addictive Behaviors, 27*, 1036–1043. http://dx.doi.org/10.1037/a0032175

Petry, N. M., DePhilippis, D., Rash, C. J., Drapkin, M., & McKay, J. R. (2014). Nationwide dissemination of contingency management: The Veterans Administration initiative. *American Journal on Addictions, 23*, 205–210. http://dx.doi.org/10.1111/j.1521-0391.2014.12092.x

Ravndal, E., & Amundsen, E. J. (2010). Mortality among drug users after discharge from inpatient treatment: An 8-year prospective study. *Drug and Alcohol Dependence, 108*, 65–69. http://dx.doi.org/10.1016/j.drugalcdep.2009.11.008

Reddy, U. M., Davis, J. M., Ren, Z., & Greene, M. F. (2017). Opioid use in pregnancy, neonatal abstinence syndrome, and childhood outcomes: Executive summary of a joint workshop by the Eunice Kennedy Shriver National Institute of Child Health and Human Development, American College of Obstetricians and Gynecologists, American Academy of Pediatrics, Society for Maternal-Fetal Medicine,

Centers for Disease Control and Prevention, and the March of Dimes Foundation. *Obstetrics & Gynecology, 130,* 10–28. http://dx.doi.org/10.1097/aog.0000000000002054

Rhodes, G. L., Saules, K. K., Helmus, T. C., Roll, J., Beshears, R. S., Ledgerwood, D. M., & Schuster, C. R. (2003). Improving on-time counseling attendance in a methadone treatment program: A contingency management approach. *American Journal of Drug and Alcohol Abuse, 29,* 759–773.

Roncero, C., Fuster, D., Palma-Alvarez, R. F., Rodriguez-Cintas, L., Martinez-Luna, N., & Alvarez, F. J. (2017). HIV And HCV infection among opiate-dependent patients and methadone doses: The PROTEUS study. *AIDS Care,* 1–6. http://dx.doi.org/10.1080/09540121.2017.1313384

Rosenthal, R. N., & Goradia, V. V. (2017). Advances in the delivery of buprenorphine for opioid dependence. *Drug Design, Development and Therapy, 11,* 2493–2505. http://dx.doi.org/10.2147/dddt.s72543

Rosenthal, R. N., Ling, W., Casadonte, P., Vocci, F., Bailey, G. L., Kampman, K., . . . Beebe, K. L. (2013). Buprenorphine implants for treatment of opioid dependence: Randomized comparison to placebo and sublingual buprenorphine/naloxone. *Addiction, 108,* 2141–2149. http://dx.doi.org/10.1111/add.12315

Rosenthal, R. N., Lofwall, M. R., Kim, S., Chen, M., Beebe, K. L., & Vocci, F. J. (2016). Effect of buprenorphine implants on illicit opioid use among abstinent adults with opioid dependence treated with sublingual buprenorphine: A randomized clinical trial. *Journal of the American Medical Association, 316,* 282–290. http://dx.doi.org/10.1001/jama.2016.9382

Rudd, R. A., Seth, P., David, F., & Scholl, L. (2016). Increases in drug and opioid-involved overdose deaths: United States, 2010–2015. *Morbidity and Mortality Weekly Report, 65,* 1445–1452. http://dx.doi.org/10.15585/mmwr.mm655051e1

Sannibale, C., Hurkett, P., van den Bossche, E., O'Connor, D., Zador, D., Capus, C., Gregory, K., & McKenzie, M. (2003). Aftercare attendance and post-treatment functioning of severely substance dependent residential treatment clients. *Drug and Alcohol Review, 22,* 181–190. http://dx.doi.org/10.1080/09595230100100624

Saroyan, J. M., Evans, E. A., Segoshi, A., Vosburg, S. K., Miller-Saultz, D., & Sullivan, M. A. (2016). Interviewing and urine drug toxicology screening in a pediatric pain management center: An analysis of analgesic nonadherence and aberrant behaviors in adolescents and young adults. *Clinical Journal of Pain, 32,* 1–6. http://dx.doi.org/10.1097/ajp.0000000000000231

Saulle, R., Vecchi, S., & Gowing, L. (2017). Supervised dosing with a long-acting opioid medication in the management of opioid dependence. *Cochrane Database of Systematic Reviews, 4,* CD011983. http://dx.doi.org/10.1002/14651858.CD011983.pub2

Saxon, A. J., Ling, W., Hillhouse, M., Thomas, C., Hasson, A., Ang, A., . . . Jacobs, P. (2013). Buprenorphine/naloxone and methadone effects on laboratory indices of liver health: A randomized trial. *Drug and Alcohol Dependence, 128,* 71–76. http://dx.doi.org/10.1016/j.drugalcdep.2012.08.002

Schottenfeld, R. S., Chawarski, M. C., Pakes, J. R., Pantalon, M. V., Carroll, K. M., & Kosten, T. R. (2005). Methadone versus buprenorphine with contingency management or performance feedback for cocaine and opioid dependence. *American Journal of Psychiatry, 162,* 340–349. http://dx.doi.org/10.1176/appi.ajp.162.2.340

Schuman-Olivier, Z., Connery, H., Griffin, M. L., Wyatt, S. A., Wartenberg, A. A., Borodovsky, J., . . . Weiss, R. D. (2013). Clinician beliefs and attitudes about buprenorphine/naloxone diversion. *American Journal on Addictions, 22,* 574–580. http://dx.doi.org/10.1111/j.1521-0391.2013.12024.x

Sen, S., Arulkumar, S., Cornett, E. M., Gayle, J. A., Flower, R. R., Fox, C. J., & Kaye, A. D. (2016). New pain management options for the surgical patient on methadone and buprenorphine. *Current Pain and Headache Reports, 20,* 16. http://dx.doi.org/10.1007/s11916-016-0549-9

Sigmon, S. C., Miller, M. E., Meyer, A. C., Saulsgiver, K., Badger, G. J., Heil, S. H., & Higgins, S. T. (2016). Financial incentives to promote extended smoking abstinence in opioid-maintained patients: A randomized trial. *Addiction, 111,* 903–912. http://dx.doi.org/10.1111/add.13264

Smyth, B. P., Fagan, J., & Kernan, K. (2012). Outcome of heroin-dependent adolescents presenting for opiate substitution treatment. *Journal of Substance Abuse Treatment, 42,* 35–44. http://dx.doi.org/10.1016/j.jsat.2011.07.007

Sordo, L., Barrio, G., Bravo, M. J., Indave, B. I., Degenhardt, L., Wiessing, L., . . . Pastor-Barriuso, R. (2017). Mortality risk during and after opioid substitution treatment: Systematic review and meta-analysis of cohort studies. *BMJ, 357,* j1550. http://dx.doi.org/10.1136/bmj.j1550

Strang, J., Groshkova, T., Uchtenhagen, A., van den Brink, W., Haasen, C., Schechter, M. T., . . . Metrebian, N. (2015). Heroin on trial: Systematic review and meta-analysis of randomised trials of diamorphine-prescribing as treatment for refractory heroin addiction. *British Journal of Psychiatry, 207,* 5–14. http://dx.doi.org/10.1192/bjp.bp.114.149195

Subramaniam, G. A., Warden, D., Minhajuddin, A., Fishman, M. J., Stitzer, M. L., Adinoff, B., . . . Woody, G. E. (2011). Predictors of abstinence: National Institute of Drug Abuse multisite buprenorphine/naloxone treatment trial in opioid-dependent youth.

Journal of the American Academy of Child and Adolescent Psychiatry, 50, 1120–1128. http://dx.doi.org/10.1016/j.jaac.2011.07.010

Sullivan, M., Bisaga, A., Pavlicova, M., Choi, C. J., Mishlen, K., Carpenter, K. M., . . . Nunes, E. V. (2017). Long-acting injectable naltrexone induction: A randomized trial of outpatient opioid detoxification with naltrexone versus buprenorphine. *American Journal of Psychiatry, 174,* 459–467. http://dx.doi.org/10.1176/appi.ajp.2016.16050548

Tanum, L., Solli, K. K., Latif, Z., Benth, J. Š., Opheim, A., Sharma-Haase, K., . . . Kunøe, N. (2017). Effectiveness of injectable extended-release naltrexone vs daily buprenorphine-naloxone for opioid dependence: A randomized clinical noninferiority trial. *Journal of the American Medical Association Psychiatry, 74,* 1197–1205. http://dx.doi.org/10.1001/jamapsychiatry.2017.3206

Taylor, L. E., Swan, T., & Matthews, G. V. (2013). Management of hepatitis C virus/HIV coinfection among people who use drugs in the era of direct-acting antiviral-based therapy. *Clinical Infectious Diseases, 57*(Suppl. 2), S118–S124. http://dx.doi.org/10.1093/cid/cit326

Vocci, F. J., Acri, J., & Elkashef, A. (2005). Medication development for addictive disorders: The state of the science. *American Journal of Psychiatry, 162,* 1432–1440. http://dx.doi.org/10.1176/appi.ajp.162.8.1432

Walley, A. Y., Doe-Simkins, M., Quinn, E., Pierce, C., Xuan, Z., & Ozonoff, A. (2013). Opioid overdose prevention with intranasal naloxone among people who take methadone. *Journal of Substance Abuse Treatment, 44,* 241–247. http://dx.doi.org/10.1016/j.jsat.2012.07.004

Walsh, S. L., Comer, S. D., Lofwall, M. R., Vince, B., Levy-Cooperman, N., Kelsh, D., . . . Kim, S. (2017). Effect of buprenorphine weekly depot (CAM2038) and hydromorphone blockade in individuals with opioid use disorder: A randomized clinical trial. *JAMA Psychiatry, 74,* 894–902. http://dx.doi.org/10.1001/jamapsychiatry.2017.1874

Webster, L. R., Markman, J., Cone, E. J., & Niebler, G. (2017). Current and future development of extended-release, abuse-deterrent opioid formulations in the United States. *Postgraduate Medicine, 129,* 102–110. http://dx.doi.org/10.1080/00325481.2017.1268902

Weiss, R. D., Griffin, M. L., Jaffee, W. B., Bender, R. E., Graff, F. S., Gallop, R. J., & Fitzmaurice, G. M. (2009). A "community-friendly" version of integrated group therapy for patients with bipolar disorder and substance dependence: A randomized controlled trial. *Drug and Alcohol Dependence, 104,* 212–219. http://dx.doi.org/10.1016/j.drugalcdep.2009.04.018

Weiss, R. D., Griffin, M. L., McHugh, R. K., & Karakula, S. (2017). *Association between mutual-help groups and abstinence among prescription opioid dependent patients, with and without agonist treatment, during 42-month post-treatment follow-up.* Poster presented at the annual meeting of the College of Problems on Drug Dependence, Montreal, Canada.

Weiss, R. D., Griffin, M. L., Potter, J. S., Dodd, D. R., Dreifuss, J. A., Connery, H. S., & Carroll, K. M. (2014). Who benefits from additional drug counseling among prescription opioid-dependent patients receiving buprenorphine–naloxone and standard medical management? *Drug and Alcohol Dependence, 140,* 118–122. http://dx.doi.org/10.1016/j.drugalcdep.2014.04.005

Weiss, R. D., Potter, J. S., Fiellin, D. A., Byrne, M., Connery, H. S., Dickinson, W., . . . Ling, W. (2011). Adjunctive counseling during brief and extended buprenorphine-naloxone treatment for prescription opioid dependence: A 2-phase randomized controlled trial. *Archives of General Psychiatry, 68,* 1238–1246. http://dx.doi.org/10.1001/archgenpsychiatry.2011.121

*Wesson, D. R., & Ling, W. (2003). The Clinical Opiate Withdrawal Scale (COWS). *Journal of Psychoactive Drugs, 35,* 253–259. http://dx.doi.org/10.1080/02791072.2003.10400007

West, N. A., Severtson, S. G., Green, J. L., & Dart, R. C. (2015). Trends in abuse and misuse of prescription opioids among older adults. *Drug and Alcohol Dependence, 149,* 117–121. http://dx.doi.org/10.1016/j.drugalcdep.2015.01.027

Wilder, C. M., Hosta, D., & Winhusen, T. (2017). Association of methadone dose with substance use and treatment retention in pregnant and postpartum women with opioid use disorder. *Journal of Substance Abuse Treatment, 80,* 33–36. http://dx.doi.org/10.1016/j.jsat.2017.06.005

Williams, A. R., Barbieri, V., Mishlen, K., Levin, F. R., Nunes, E. V., Mariani, J. J., & Bisaga, A. (2017). Long-term follow-up study of community-based patients receiving XR-NTX for opioid use disorders. *American Journal on Addictions, 26,* 319–325. http://dx.doi.org/10.1111/ajad.12527

Witkin, J. M., Statnick, M. A., Rorick-Kehn, L. M., Pintar, J. E., Ansonoff, M., Chen, Y., . . . Ciccocioppo, R. (2014). The biology of nociceptin/orphanin FQ (N/OFQ) related to obesity, stress, anxiety, mood, and drug dependence. *Pharmacology & Therapeutics, 141,* 283–299. http://dx.doi.org/10.1016/j.pharmthera.2013.10.011

Wise, R. A., & Koob, G. F. (2014). The development and maintenance of drug addiction. *Neuropsychopharmacology, 39,* 254–262. http://dx.doi.org/10.1038/npp.2013.261

Woody, G., Bruce, D., Korthuis, P. T., Chhatre, S., Hillhouse, M., Jacobs, P., Ling, W. (2014). HIV risk reduction with buprenorphine-naloxone or methadone: Findings from a randomized trial. *Journal of Acquired Immune Deficiency Syndromes, 66,* 288–293. http://dx.doi.org/10.1097/QAI.0000000000000165

Woody, G. E., Poole, S. A., Subramaniam, G., Dugosh, K., Bogenschutz, M., Abbott, P., . . . Fudala, P. (2008). Extended vs short-term buprenorphine-naloxone for treatment of opioid-addicted youth: A randomized trial. *Journal of the American Medical Association, 300,* 2003–2011. http://dx.doi.org/10.1001/jama.2008.574

World Health Organization. (2009). *Guidelines for the psychosocially assisted pharmacological treatment of opioid dependence.* Geneva, Switzerland: WHO Press.

Wright, N., D'Agnone, O., Krajci, P., Littlewood, R., Alho, H., Reimer, J., . . . Maremmani, I. (2016). Addressing misuse and diversion of opioid substitution medication: Guidance based on systematic evidence review and real-world experience. *Journal of Public Health (Oxf), 38,* e368–e374. http://dx.doi.org/10.1093/pubmed/fdv150

Wu, L. T., Zhu, H., & Swartz, M. S. (2016). Treatment utilization among persons with opioid use disorder in the United States. *Drug and Alcohol Dependence, 169,* 117–127. http://dx.doi.org/10.1016/j.drugalcdep.2016.10.015

Wurst, K. E., Zedler, B. K., Joyce, A. R., Sasinowski, M., & Murrelle, E. L. (2016). A Swedish population-based study of adverse birth outcomes among pregnant women treated with buprenorphine or methadone: Preliminary findings. *Substance Abuse, 10,* 89–97. http://dx.doi.org/10.4137/sart.s38887

*Yudko, E., Lozhkina, O., & Fouts, A. (2007). A comprehensive review of the psychometric properties of the Drug Abuse Screening Test. *Journal of Substance Abuse Treatment, 32,* 189–198. http://dx.doi.org/10.1016/j.jsat.2006.08.002

Zaaijer, E. R., van Dijk, L., de Bruin, K., Goudriaan, A. E., Lammers, L. A., Koeter, M. W., . . . Booij, J. (2015). Effect of extended-release naltrexone on striatal dopamine transporter availability, depression and anhedonia in heroin-dependent patients. *Psychopharmacology (Berl), 232,* 2597–2607. http://dx.doi.org/10.1007/s00213-015-3891-4

Zedler, B. K., Mann, A. L., Kim, M. M., Amick, H. R., Joyce, A. R., Murrelle, E. L., & Jones, H. E. (2016). Buprenorphine compared with methadone to treat pregnant women with opioid use disorder: A systematic review and meta-analysis of safety in the mother, fetus and child. *Addiction, 111,* 2115–2128. http://dx.doi.org/10.1111/add.13462

Ziedonis, D. M., Amass, L., Steinberg, M., Woody, G., Krejci, J., Annon, J. J., . . . Ling, W. (2009). Predictors of outcome for short-term medically supervised opioid withdrawal during a randomized, multicenter trial of buprenorphine–naloxone and clonidine in the NIDA clinical trials network drug and alcohol dependence. *Drug and Alcohol Dependence, 99,* 28–36. http://dx.doi.org/10.1016/j.drugalcdep.2008.06.016

CHAPTER 26

PHARMACOLOGICAL TREATMENT OF SEDATIVE AND ANXIOLYTIC USE DISORDERS

Angela M. Heads, Michael F. Weaver, and Paula Lopez-Gamundi

Sedatives and tranquilizers—including benzodiazepines, selective benzodiazepine receptor subtype agonists, and barbiturates—are widely prescribed for the treatment of anxiety or insomnia by psychiatrists and other physicians. Due to their abuse and misuse potential, sedatives are classified as controlled substances. There are two main patterns of misuse of sedatives and anxiolytics: deliberate abuse because of their euphoric effects or inadvertent misuse in an attempt to self-medicate psychological symptoms. Often, patients who self-medicate were prescribed the medication for the treatment of anxiety or insomnia and began using the drug in ways not authorized by the prescriber (e.g., dose escalation). There are dangerous health consequences associated with abuse and misuse of sedatives.

In this chapter, we provide an overview of the epidemiology of sedative and anxiolytic use disorders and considerations in assessing and diagnosing sedative use disorder. We then discuss pharmacological approaches in the treatment of sedative use disorders, medication management, and management of treatment response and side effects. We provide an overview of lifespan considerations and potential sex differences in the treatment of sedative use disorders and discuss integrated approaches to treatment.

EPIDEMIOLOGY AND PREVALENCE

It is estimated that about 5% of Americans are legally prescribed sedatives or anxiolytics at any given time (National Center for Health Statistics, 2016). Although in most cases, these medications are prescribed and used safely, there is significant abuse and misuse potential. In a national survey, approximately 6.5 million people in the United States aged 12 years or older reported nonmedical use of prescription medications; about 330,000 misused sedatives, and 1.9 million reported misusing tranquilizers in the 30 days prior to the survey (Substance Abuse and Mental Health Services Administration, 2015). Nonmedical use of sedatives and tranquilizers may lead to abuse or dependence (Becker, Fiellin, & Desai, 2007).

Misuse of sedatives and anxiolytics is often an attempt to self-medicate psychological symptoms, such as anxiety. Sedatives also may be abused to induce euphoric effects or to treat the unpleasant effects from the use of illicit stimulants. These self-medication attempts often result in dose escalation, which may lead to dangerous side effects (Weaver, 2015).

Sedatives and anxiolytics are central nervous system depressants. Dose escalation may result in sedative intoxication and associated acute psychological and physical symptoms, including impaired

http://dx.doi.org/10.1037/0000133-026
APA Handbook of Psychopharmacology, S. M. Evans (Editor-in-Chief)

judgment, mood lability, inappropriate behavior, relaxed inhibitions, nystagmus, and slowed motor reflexes (Lewis, 2013; Weaver, 2015). As the dose increases beyond the tolerance level of the consumer, more impairment occurs. Severe overdose can lead to dangerous consequences, such as suppression of the autonomic respiratory drive, weak and rapid pulse, coma, or death (Weaver, 2010).

There is no pharmacological treatment approved by the U.S. Food and Drug Administration (FDA) for sedative use disorder. In cases where there is a need to discontinue sedatives, it is possible that pharmacological approaches can be useful in reducing craving, ameliorating withdrawal symptoms, or treating the underlying anxiety or insomnia. Despite the high prevalence of sedative use and risk for their misuse, there are a limited number of studies exploring pharmacologic interventions in the discontinuation of benzodiazepines and other sedatives.

The conventional approach to managing sedative and anxiolytic use disorders is gradual dose reduction, which often results in significant withdrawal symptoms. Uncomfortable physical and psychological withdrawal symptoms increase the likelihood of patient noncompliance with and eventual discontinuation of dose reduction, which decreases the likelihood of achieving sustained abstinence. This has prompted an interest in exploring pharmacological approaches to discontinuation, with a focus on ameliorating withdrawal symptoms or managing the underlying anxiety or insomnia.

The most commonly explored drugs include anticonvulsants, beta blockers, and antidepressants (Parr, Kavanagh, Cahill, Mitchell, & Young, 2008; Oude Voshaar, Couvée, van Balkom, Mulder, & Zitman, 2006). These approaches have had mixed results. Recently, researchers have demonstrated increased interest in flumazenil, a gamma-aminobutyric acid benzodiazepine receptor antagonist. Flumazenil has been indicated primarily for the reversal of the sedative effects of benzodiazepines, often in the case of suspected overdose (Thomson, Donald, & Lewin, 2006). Preliminary data indicate that flumazenil can reduce benzodiazepine withdrawal sequelae (Hood, Norman, Hince, Melichar, & Hulse, 2014). These pharmacological approaches are discussed in more detail in the next section.

DIAGNOSING SEDATIVE USE DISORDERS

Diagnosis of sedative use disorder relies on criteria outlined in the *Diagnostic and Statistical Manual of Mental Disorders* (fifth edition; *DSM–5*; American Psychiatric Association, 2013). Diagnosis is usually accomplished through semistructured interviews. According to *DSM–5*, diagnosing a sedative use disorder requires clinically significant impairment or distress over a 12-month period. In addition, at least two of 11 other criteria must be met:

- tolerance;
- withdrawal symptoms on dosage reduction or discontinuation;
- cravings;
- using more than planned;
- being unable to quit despite attempts;
- great amount of time spent obtaining the substance or recovering from the effects;
- social, recreational, or occupational activities reduced or given up due to substance use;
- failure to fulfill work, academic, or home obligations;
- persistent social and interpersonal problems due to substance use;
- continued use despite negative physical or psychological consequences; and
- continued use in physically hazardous situations.

Depending on the number of criteria met, a patient will be diagnosed with mild (two–three criteria), moderate (four–five criteria), or severe (six or more criteria) sedative use disorder. The presence of these criteria can be determined during a clinical interview, and there are some available screening tools that may be useful in clinical settings. For example, the Drug Abuse Screening Test is a 10-item questionnaire that screens for problematic drug use (Skinner, 1982). The Substance Use Brief Screen is used to screen for past-year use of illicit drugs (McNeely et al., 2015).

EVIDENCE-BASED PHARMACOLOGICAL TREATMENTS OF SEDATIVE USE DISORDERS

Presently, there are no recommended or approved pharmacological approaches for the treatment of sedative use disorders. Medication-assisted treatments for sedative use disorder typically target reduction of withdrawal symptoms, reduction of psychological craving, or treatment for underlying anxiety or insomnia symptoms (Oude Voshaar et al., 2006; Parr et al., 2008).

The overall consensus is that sedative use disorders should be treated through discontinuation using a gradual dose reduction method, with an ultimate goal of abstinence. The most commonly prescribed sedatives are benzodiazepines (Grohol, 2016). Therefore, the majority of treatment research has been focused on these drugs, with most common approaches including gradual dose reduction alone, gradual dose reduction with the addition of a long half-life benzodiazepine replacement, adjunctive antidepressants (covered more in the section of this chapter on Integrated Approaches for Addressing Common Comorbid Disorders), and non-benzodiazepine anxiolytics or anticonvulsants to treat anxiety and insomnia symptoms (Oude Voshaar et al., 2006; Parr et al., 2008).

Considerations in choosing a pharmacologic treatment include whether the sedative use disorder resulted from long-term prescribed treatment for anxiety or insomnia or whether it resulted from illicit sedative use (Lingford-Hughes, Welch, Nutt, & the British Association for Psychopharmacology, 2004). There is some evidence that high-dose benzodiazepine users may be less likely to achieve and maintain abstinence using a gradual dose reduction approach alone. In a study of a gradual dose treatment for individuals with complicated (defined as high dose, co-occurring alcohol use disorder or co-occurring psychiatric disorder) benzodiazepine dependence, 20% of participants successfully discontinued their benzodiazepine use and another 60% reduced their use by the end of treatment (Vorma, Naukkarinen, Sarna, & Kuoppasalmi, 2002). In the same sample, data collected 6 and 12 months after the end of treatment showed that only 25% of the original participants were abstinent. An examination of patient characteristics in this sample revealed that having lower benzodiazepine doses prior to treatment, having no previous unsuccessful attempts at withdrawal, and having higher life satisfaction predicted abstinence at 12 months following treatment completion (Vorma, Naukkarinen, Sarna, & Kuoppasalmi, 2003). A more complicated pattern of use may have implications for the success of gradual dose reduction. Liebrenz, Boesch, Stohler, and Caflisch (2010) have suggested an agonist replacement approach for high-dose users, long-term users, and individuals with especially problematic patterns of benzodiazepine use. However, no recommendations have been made for a specific medication.

Several factors should be weighed when considering potential pharmacological treatments for sedative use disorders. Despite having similar effects, currently available benzodiazepines have different pharmacodynamics (effect and mechanism by which the effects occur) and pharmacokinetics (onset of action and duration of drug effect). Benzodiazepines enhance the inhibitory effects of gamma-aminobutyric acid (GABA) at the $GABA_A$ receptor complex by binding to specific benzodiazepine receptors (BZ1 & BZ2; Weaver, 2015). This results in the sedative, anxiolytic, muscle relaxant, and anticonvulsant effects of benzodiazepines. Some benzodiazepines (e.g., lorazepam, temazepam) are metabolized by the process of direct conjugation (via glucuronyl transferase), whereas others (e.g., alprazolam, diazepam) are first metabolized by the cytochrome P-450 isozyme 3A4 or 3A5 (Altamura et al., 2013; Weaver, 2015). Several different benzodiazepines are currently prescribed, each with different rates of onset, varying intensities of euphoric effects, and different durations of action. Clinical evidence indicates that benzodiazepines with a faster onset of action and greater euphoric effect are more likely to be abused, and benzodiazepines requiring a prodrug active metabolite mechanism are less likely to be abused (O'Brien, 2005; Poisnel, Dhilly, Le Boisselier, Barre, & Debruyne, 2009). A prodrug initially is inactive in the body but then forms active metabolites; this results in delayed effects, making the drug a less likely choice for intentional abuse. Benzodiazepines with rapid onset and short duration of action include alprazolam and lorazepam, so they are most popular for abuse, along with intermediate-duration benzodiazepines, such as diazepam and chlordiazepoxide; clonazepam has a longer duration of action and less euphoria compared with other benzodiazepines and is not as popular for recreational use. Therefore, Liebrenz et al. (2010) posited that a slow-onset benzodiazepine with a long half-life would be an ideal agonist for substitution.

There is some support for this substitution approach with patients who previously have been unsuccessful in discontinuing benzodiazepines due to rebound anxiety or withdrawal symptoms. Researchers have recommended continued treatment using a relatively long-acting benzodiazepine with these patients (O'Brien, 2005). For example, Weizman, Gelkopf, Melamed, Adelson, and Bleich (2003) compared clonazepam detoxification and clonazepam maintenance treatment in patients in methadone treatment and found that 27.3% of patients in the detoxification group achieved abstinence from benzodiazepines while 78.8% of patients in the maintenance treatment refrained from using benzodiazepines other than the maintenance dose of clonazepam. Survival analysis showed that the maintenance treatment was more successful than the detoxification treatment 12 months later. Additionally, a case report described the use of a maintenance treatment approach with clonazepam on a patient prescribed lormetazepam for social anxiety disorder (Maremmani et al., 2013). The authors described a gradual replacement of lormetazepam with clonazepam, which was eventually reduced to 1 mg per day. The patient did not experience withdrawal symptoms and had improvements in social and cognitive functioning. These studies have promising results. However, the published results from controlled trials comparing outcomes for maintenance versus withdrawal approaches leave clinicians with few treatment alternatives other than supervised withdrawal for patients with sedative use disorder (Zador, 2017).

As previously mentioned, the most widely used approach for managing sedative use disorder is gradual dose reduction. There is no universally recognized schedule for dose reduction. However, it has been suggested that a period of 4 to 8 weeks is suitable for most patients to avoid withdrawal symptoms (Soyka, 2017). Abrupt reduction or cessation of sedatives can result in withdrawal symptoms, including anxiety, agitation, tremor, hyperreflexia, elevated heart rate, sweating, elevated blood pressure, and increased body temperature. More serious symptoms include hallucinations and seizures (American Psychiatric Association, 2013). There is significant variability in the point at which an individual may develop withdrawal symptoms, making it difficult to predict who will have problems. An abrupt cessation of sedatives may result in acute withdrawal symptoms (Weaver, 2015). Conversely, if gradual dose reduction takes place over an extended period of time, this may result in the patient experiencing uncomfortable, albeit milder, withdrawal symptoms over a longer period of time (Oude Voshaar et al., 2006). This will decrease the likelihood that patients will comply with the discontinuation plan (Ashton, 2005). Therefore, a few studies have examined whether an adjunctive pharmacological intervention could facilitate the process by helping to manage symptoms of withdrawal. Table 26.1 shows the primary outcomes from select studies examining the use of various pharmacological agents to manage withdrawal symptoms in patients who are decreasing or discontinuing benzodiazepines.

Although pharmacotherapy may be helpful in the treatment of withdrawal from sedatives, there is no standard protocol (Weaver, 2015). In addition to the longer acting benzodiazepines, medications including beta blockers (e.g., propranolol) and anticonvulsants (e.g., phenobarbital, carbamazepine) have been explored in the management of sedative withdrawal symptoms. Beta blockers have been used to treat tremor and cardiovascular symptoms related to withdrawal from sedatives (Lader, Tylee, & Donoghue, 2009; O'Brien, 2005). Barbiturates such as phenobarbital have been used to treat acute sedative withdrawal syndrome in a variety of clinical settings. Phenobarbital binds to the $GABA_A$ receptor and its half-life is at least twice as long as the longer acting benzodiazepines. It has been found to be effective in the management of sedative withdrawal symptoms (Kawasaki, Jacapraro, & Rastegar, 2012). Other anticonvulsants, such as carbamazepine and gabapentin, have been used for treatment of mild to moderate alcohol withdrawal (Weaver, 2015) and show potential for treating withdrawal from sedatives (Bramness, Sandvik, Engeland, & Skurtveit, 2010). Topiramate also shows some promise for managing withdrawal from benzodiazepines (Cheseaux,

TABLE 26.1

Results of Select Study Outcomes in Treatment of Sedative Use Disorders

Study	Medication tested	Dose	Duration of treatment	Sample	M:F ratio	Primary outcome
Weizman, Gelkopf, Melamed, Adelson, and Bleich, 2003	clonazepam maintenance vs. clonazepam detox	6 mg daily for 2 weeks followed by either a gradual detoxification until no clonazepam was used or a gradual tapering until an individual maintenance dose was achieved	4 to 8 weeks	66 adults in methadone maintenance treatment meeting criteria for benzodiazepine use disorder	not reported	in the detox group, 9/33 (27.3%) were benzodiazepine free after 2 months; in the maintenance group, 26/33 (78.8%) refrained from abusing additional benzodiazepines over the maintenance dose after 2 months
C. H. Ashton, Rawlins, and Tyrer, 1990	buspirone vs. placebo	5 mg three times per day	4 weeks	23 adult chronic benzodiazepine users	6:6 placebo, 3:8 buspirone	at 6 and 12 months after diazepam withdrawal, 11 patients in the placebo group and six in the buspirone group were still abstinent
Cheseaux, Monnat, and Zullino, 2003	topiramate	300 mg first day, 500 mg second day, followed by taper until Day 9	14 days	case study of 1 adult male	n/a	successful taper with withdrawal symptoms including insomnia and nausea during the first days; continued abstinence after 2 months
Lader, Farr, and Morton, 1993	alpidem vs. placebo	usual dose of abused benzodiazepine for Weeks 1 and 2, 25 mg twice daily of placebo with half dose of abused benzodiazepine for Weeks 3 and 4, 50 mg alpidem twice daily or placebo only for Weeks 5 to 6, then half dose of alpidem or placebo followed by discontinuation	8 weeks	25 adults	8:17	alpidem found not effective in benzodiazepine withdrawal: nine of 12 placebo patients withdrew successfully and four of 13 alpidem-treated patients withdrew successfully; increased anxiety symptom levels in alpidem-treated patients
Cantopher, Olivieri, Cleave, and Edwards, 1990	slow withdrawal vs. abrupt withdrawal + propranolol	40 mg three times per day	17 weeks	31 adults	10:6 slow withdrawal, 12:3 abrupt withdrawal	of 16 patients in the slow withdrawal group, 11 successfully withdrew; of the 15 abrupt withdrawal patients, 4 successfully withdrew

Note. n/a = not applicable.

Monnat, & Zullino, 2003; Michopoulos, Douzenis, Christodoulou, & Lykouras, 2006). It acts through inhibition of kainate-activated receptors. This mechanism of action is believed to be responsible for its anticonvulsant effects and may also mitigate withdrawal by reducing activation of noradrenergic neurons in the locus coeruleus (Vgontzas, Kales, & Bixler, 1995). Support of topiramate for the management of sedative withdrawal is lacking; sufficient evidence obtained through controlled trials is needed to determine whether it offers benefits beyond other anticonvulsants (Shinn & Greenfield, 2010).

It is commonly recommended that more serious withdrawal be managed medically using a long-acting sedative, with close medical supervision in either an inpatient or outpatient setting (Weaver, 2015). However, support for this approach is not consistent in the research. A meta-analysis examining the effectiveness of treatment approaches for benzodiazepine discontinuation, which included 14 studies with a total of 927 participants who were treated with a gradual dose reduction plus any adjunctive pharmacological treatment, found no benefit above gradual dose reduction alone (Parr et al., 2008). Despite these results, addiction scientists continue to develop and research new adjunctive pharmacological treatments (see Emerging Trends section of this chapter).

BEST APPROACHES FOR ASSESSING TREATMENT RESPONSE AND MANAGING SIDE EFFECTS

There are several approaches to assessing treatment response for sedative use disorder. The initial evaluation is important for providing a history of substance use, a baseline level of sedative use including quantity and frequency, severity of problems related to substance use, cravings, and triggers for use. Collecting assessment data at follow-up allows clinicians to evaluate the benefit of pharmacotherapy for sedative use disorder. Progress monitoring can provide useful information for diagnosis and treatment planning, facilitate coordination of care among providers, and improve treatment outcomes (Goodman, McKay, & DePhilippis, 2013).

The most common source of information is self-report. Although none are available specific to sedative use disorder, several instruments exist for collection of self-report data related to substance use. For example, the Addiction Severity Assessment Tool (Butler et al., 2005) and the Addiction Severity Index (McLellan et al., 1992) have acceptable psychometric properties available to provide clinicians with information on health problems, daily functioning, relational functioning, and severity of substance use. Additionally, the Severity of Dependence Scale is a brief (5-item) instrument designed to measure the degree of dependence experienced by substance users. The instrument has been validated for use with sedative-using patients (De Las Cuevas, Sanz, De La Fuente, Padilla, & Berenguer, 2000). Timeline followback is a widely used and validated technique for collecting information; it has been used to assess treatment response in a number of behavioral interventions, and in substance use treatment it has been used to assess the quantity and frequency of use (Hjorthøj, Hjorthøj, & Nordentoft, 2012). Timeline followback asks individuals whether they have engaged in a specific behavior over a specified time period. It can be used in an interview format or self-administered on paper or via computer.

Urine drug testing is frequently used in substance use disorders treatment as a way to objectively evaluate compliance with treatment. It is used to verify the presence of prescribed medication and to screen for the presence of other substances, including the sedative for which the patient is receiving treatment. Unexpected or problematic results can be an opportunity to discuss treatment, with a goal of supporting compliance and appropriate behavior (Weaver, 2015). Unfortunately, no individual immunoassay kit can recognize all benzodiazepines (Glover & Allen, 2010). For example, most tests can reliably detect alprazolam and diazepam but often yield false negative results for lorazepam and clonazepam. Confirmatory laboratory testing using gas or liquid chromatography and mass spectroscopy or tandem mass spectroscopy can be requested, usually from an outside laboratory for specific sedative metabolites if there is significant clinical concern. This requires expertise, additional cost, and a longer time to receive results (several days), making it impractical for urgent decision making (Warner & Lorch, 2015).

Medication compliance also can be measured through monitoring of medication refill requests. When medications other than the abused sedative are prescribed to treat the underlying anxiety or insomnia problems, monitoring of medication refills can help the clinician to determine whether the patient is actively taking the medication. This process is facilitated through the Prescription Drug Monitoring Program (PDMP), a statewide electronic database that collects information on medications dispensed. Created for the purpose of promoting the use of medications for legitimate purposes (Morgan, Weaver, Sayeed, & Orr, 2013), a PDMP is now in each state of the United States. If the patient has been switched to another benzodiazepine, the PDMP may help the clinician obtain information on the rate at which the patient is using the medication (Weaver, 2015). This would not, however, account for medications obtained illegally.

Side effects of pharmacological intervention are a concern. Although most medications explored in the treatment of sedative use disorder are well tolerated, the side effects of benzodiazepines include drowsiness, fatigue, and difficulties with concentration. When choosing a longer acting benzodiazepine to aid in discontinuation of the abused sedative, the side-effect profile for that specific drug should be considered. Studies of the use of propranolol in discontinuation of sedatives have not reported adverse events, indicating that it may be a relatively safe option in managing some symptoms of withdrawal from sedatives and anxiolytics. Carbamazepine side effects include sedation, headache, nausea, and cognitive impairment (Schweizer, Rickels, Case, & Greenblatt, 1991). The most commonly reported side effect for phenobarbital and gabapentin was sedation (Crockford, White, & Campbell, 2001; Kawasaki et al., 2012). Flumazenil has been explored in the treatment of benzodiazepine intoxication and withdrawal. According to the results of a recent meta-analysis, flumazenil's most common side effects are anxiety, agitation, nausea, and vomiting (Penninga, Graudal, Ladekarl, & Jürgens, 2016).

MEDICATION MANAGEMENT ISSUES

Monitoring of response is an important component of evaluating the effectiveness of sedative use disorders treatment. In pharmacological treatment, it is widely recognized that its ability to confer benefits is contingent on the patient taking at least the minimum therapeutic dose. The reasons for noncompliance with medications are varied and include cost, side effects, co-occurring psychiatric diagnoses, and lack of external accountability for treatment (Tkacz, Severt, Cacciola, & Ruetsch, 2011).

Tools for medication monitoring include pill counts, electronic pill bottles, and self-report. These indirect measures can be subject to memory lapses or dishonesty on the part of the patient. To circumvent such error, in clinical trials compounds frequently are added to medications, which can be detected in urine under ultraviolet lighting. Riboflavin is the most commonly used compound and has a number of desirable features, including being nontoxic, water soluble, and inexpensive. Although this visual inspection can enhance interrater variability, it can also yield false positive readings (Herron et al., 2013). Although this approach is used in research settings, it is not practical in community treatment settings.

EVALUATION OF PHARMACOLOGICAL APPROACHES ACROSS THE LIFESPAN

There is frequently cited concern about the long-term use of benzodiazepines and *Z-drugs*. Z-drugs are nonbenzodiazepine hypnotics approved for the treatment of insomnia. These medications include zolpidem (Ambien®), zaleplon (Sonata®), and eszopiclone (Lunesta®). Long-term use of benzodiazepines and Z-drugs has been associated with drug dependence, cognitive decline, and injuries due to falls (Cumming & Le Couteur, 2003; Lader, 2011). There is also some evidence that long-term use of benzodiazepines places patients at increased risk for Alzheimer's disease (Lader, 2011; Yaffe & Boustani, 2014). In older populations (65 years and older), there is even greater risk of harm related to prolonged use of benzodiazepines and other sedatives. There are age-related changes in older adults that affect their ability to metabolize benzodiazepines with longer half-lives, which results in accumulation of the drug in the body (Bogunovic & Greenfield, 2004). This may account for sensitivity to the medication, as evidenced by increased sedation, confusion, and unsteadiness. Short-acting benzodiazepines that undergo glucuronidation (the metabolic process whereby substances are combined with glucuronic acid, rendering them water soluble and more easily excreted through urine) are recommended for older adults if discontinuation is not an option (Turnheim, 2003).

Older adults are prescribed sedatives and hypnotics at a higher rate than that for younger adults (Donoghue & Lader, 2010; Paulose-Ram, Safran, Jonas, Gu, & Orwig, 2007). Recently, there has been a trend toward increasing numbers of prescriptions for Z-drugs, whereas prescriptions for benzodiazepines are declining. This is due to the perception among prescribing physicians, primarily general practitioners, that Z-drugs are safer and more effective in older adults (Siriwardena, Qureshi, Gibson, Collier, & Latham, 2006).

In some cases, it may be necessary to discontinue sedatives. As mentioned earlier, gradual dose reduction is the most frequently used method for discontinuing sedatives. Due to a lack of research comparing methods for discontinuation of sedatives and anxiolytics in elderly populations, there are no clear guidelines for how this should take place. Managing common symptoms of withdrawal such as insomnia, anxiety, irritability, and tremor—which occur in about half of patients who discontinue benzodiazepines—should be an important consideration.

Despite the concerns regarding use of sedatives and anxiolytics in older adults, research on discontinuation is sparse. A recent systematic review of the literature examining interventions for discontinuing sedatives and anxiolytics in older adults found only eight articles meeting inclusion criteria: original research evaluating interventions for long-term use of benzodiazepines or Z-drugs that included adults at least 65 years old in the study sample (Reeve et al., 2017). Three of these studies examined pharmacological treatments to aid in the discontinuation of benzodiazepines (see Table 26.2 for a summary).

Garzón, Guerrero, Aramburu, and Guzmán (2009) conducted an 18-week, randomized, placebo-controlled crossover trial to evaluate the effect of melatonin on sleep quality and in the facilitation of the discontinuation of benzodiazepines. The sample consisted of 22 adults (7 men, 15 women) over the age of 65 with a history of insomnia. The participants received melatonin treatment (5 mg/day) for 2 months and 2 months of placebo. Participants were randomly assigned to either receive the treatment condition first followed by the control condition or vice versa. The benzodiazepine discontinuation rate was significantly greater in those receiving melatonin compared with placebo and baseline. The treatment was well tolerated, with no adverse effects of melatonin reported.

Petrovic et al. (1999) demonstrated the feasibility of a 1-week pharmacological replacement therapy prior to benzodiazepine withdrawal in a sample of older adults. This study involved replacing the benzodiazepine with trazodone or lormetazepam for 1 week before complete withdrawal. Successful discontinuation was higher, though not significantly, in the trazodone group than for the lormetazepam group (80% vs. 75%, respectively). There were no significant differences in sleep quality between the two groups and no significant side effects were reported (Petrovic et al., 1999). This study was followed by a randomized placebo-controlled trial that found a significantly higher discontinuation rate in participants assigned to the lormetazepam treatment (80%) versus placebo (50%). Findings also included worse withdrawal symptoms in the placebo group. At 1 year following the study, 46% of participants who discontinued remained abstinent (Petrovic, Pevernagie, Mariman, Van Maele, & Afschrift, 2002). Concern related to prolonged use of sedatives and anxiolytics in older adults and the potential for accidents and injuries due to increased sedation highlight the importance of continued research on the treatment of sedative use disorder in older adults.

Adolescents are another sparsely researched group. Substance use disorders that begin in adolescence are challenging to treat and often lead to later problems. Usual treatment of adolescent substance use disorders involves psychosocial interventions to

TABLE 26.2

Representative Studies Examining Sedative Withdrawal Interventions With Adults Over Age 65

Study	Medication tested	Dose	Duration of treatment	Sample	M:F ratio	Primary outcome
Garzón, Guerrero, Aramburu, and Guzmán, 2009	melatonin	5 mg melatonin substitution for 2 months followed by 2 months of placebo, and vice versa	18 weeks	22 adults with a history of insomnia (mean age 74.7 years)	7:15	64.3% were able to discontinue benzodiazepines during melatonin substitution
Petrovic et al., 1999	trazodone or lormetazepam	50 mg trazodone, 1 mg lormetazepam	6 weeks	56 adults (mean age 80.9 years)	15:41	successful discontinuation was higher in the trazodone group (80.0%) vs. the lormetazepam group (75.0%) but finding was not significant ($p > 0.05$)
Petrovic, Pevernagie, Mariman, Van Maele, and Afschrift, 2002	lormetazepam vs. placebo	1 mg lormetazepam	1 week	40 adults (mean age 81.5 years)	6:14 placebo, 7:13 lormetazepam	discontinuation rate was significantly higher in the lormetazepam group (80.0 vs. 50.0%, $p < 0.05$)

address family and individual problems, along with 12-step programs and in some cases detoxification interventions. Pharmacological interventions are used less often in adolescent populations than in adult populations (Kaplan & Ivanov, 2011). There is limited use of pharmacological interventions for substance use disorders in adolescence, with the main focus being addressing withdrawal symptoms. There are currently no published reports of pharmacotherapy for the treatment of sedative use disorders in adolescents.

CONSIDERATION OF POTENTIAL SEX DIFFERENCES

Research has consistently shown sex differences in the rates of substance use disorders, with men exhibiting higher rates. There are also important sex differences in the course, symptoms, treatment, and consequences of substance use disorders and there is some evidence that problematic use of sedatives is higher in women than in men. The phenomenon of quickly advancing from initiation of substance use to dependence and treatment, known as *telescoping*, occurs in women more often than in men (Greenfield, Back, Lawson, & Brady, 2010; Piazza, Vrbka, & Yeager, 1989). Women in the United States are prescribed benzodiazepines more often than men (Olfson, King, & Schoenbaum, 2015). Further, research has shown that women are more likely to use substances to cope with negative affect and anxiety (Hearon et al., 2011). An examination of a national database revealed that women had higher rates of past-year nonmedical use of sedatives or tranquilizers. This study did not find significant sex associations for abuse or dependence (Becker et al., 2007). Data from the Substance Abuse and Mental Health Services Administration (2017) indicate that women were more likely to report past-year sedative use (8.8% in 2015 and 8.9% in 2016) compared with men (5.9% in 2016 and 5.8% in 2016); however, men and women reported similar levels (between 0.5% and 0.7% in 2015 and 2016) of sedative misuse.

Women seek specialized treatment for substance use disorders less often than men (Brady & Ashley, 2005). When women do seek treatment, it is more likely to be through primary health care or mental health providers (Greenfield et al., 2007). Although it is generally understood that women tend to be prescribed sedatives and anxiolytics at higher rates and may be at risk for misuse, there are no studies examining sex differences in pharmacological approaches to treating sedative use disorder. Oude Voshaar et al. (2006) noted that in a total of 17 different strategies evaluated, the age and sex distribution of the study samples did not match that of the general population and may be indicative of selective recruitment toward younger men. When considering the mechanisms of action for medications used in addiction treatment, it is reasonable to explore how sex differences may affect treatment response.

Sex differences have been described for sedatives and tranquilizers, with studies showing women metabolize some benzodiazepines at different rates than men. There is some evidence that diazepam is metabolized at a faster rate in women (Greenblatt, Allen, Harmatz, & Shader, 1980; Ochs et al., 1981), while the clearance of other benzodiazepines such as lorazepam and oxazepam generally is slower in women (Marazziti et al., 2013). Possible explanations for these differences include cytochrome enzymes CYP3A4 and CYP2C19, which have been found to be more highly expressed in women than men (Franconi, Brunelleschi, Steardo, & Cuomo, 2007). Sex differences in sedative effects of Z-drugs, such as zolpidem, have prompted the FDA to change the recommended dosage of the medication. Studies have indicated that women are more susceptible to daytime drowsiness after taking zolpidem for insomnia because of slower elimination (Kuehn, 2013). Based on these findings, it is possible that women and men may require different doses of benzodiazepines and Z-drugs. Given that treatment of sedative use disorder primarily focuses on tapering, with or without a longer acting medication, or on replacing the abused sedative with another medication to treat insomnia or anxiety, consideration of sex differences is important. Although these studies provide evidence of sex differences related to the pharmacotherapy of medications being explored, there are no published studies explicitly exploring sex differences.

INTEGRATION OF PHARMACOTHERAPY WITH NONPHARMACOLOGICAL APPROACHES: BENEFITS AND CHALLENGES

The treatment of substance use disorders is complex, often necessitating a combination of medical and behavioral interventions. Medication alone does not address the many family, social, occupational, and legal issues that often accompany addiction. Additionally, many individuals with substance use disorders also have co-occurring psychiatric disorders. When psychological and social factors are not addressed, the likelihood of relapse increases.

There are several evidence-based behavioral interventions that are helpful in the treatment of substance use disorders. Psychological interventions can be helpful in treating sedative use disorders by facilitating the initiation of treatment, encouraging abstinence, treating the underlying disorder (anxiety or insomnia), and preventing relapse. The most commonly used psychosocial interventions are motivational interviewing, cognitive behavior therapy (CBT), relapse prevention, and contingency management.

Motivational interviewing (Miller & Rollnick, 2013), which is informed by the transtheoretical model of behavior change (Prochaska & Velicer, 1997), can be used to help motivate the patient to reduce or stop drug use. Motivational interviewing facilitates the patient's movement through the stages of behavioral change identified in the transtheoretical model by encouraging a focus on identifying a specific behavior to be changed, resolving ambivalence about change, creating a plan for change, and strengthening commitment to change (Miller & Rollnick, 2013).

Research has also demonstrated the effectiveness of behavioral approaches using contingency management principles for treatment of substance use disorders. Contingency management involves providing patients with tangible rewards, such as monetary incentives for desired behaviors (e.g., negative urine drug tests, attending therapy sessions). In voucher-based reinforcement therapy, patients with negative urine drug tests receive vouchers they can exchange for goods or services (Higgins et al., 1991). Another contingency management method is the variable magnitude reinforcement procedure, in which participants receive entries for a prize drawing in exchange for desired behaviors, such as negative drug screens and attendance at therapy sessions (Petry, Martin, Cooney, & Kranzler, 2000; Petry, Martin, & Simcic, 2005). This method commonly is known as the *fishbowl*, in reference to the container from which prize slips are drawn. Other contingency management approaches exist and have been used by researchers to promote abstinence from many types of substances, including sedatives (Petry et al., 2017; Prendergast, Podus, Finney, Greenwell, & Roll, 2006).

CBT is widely used in substance use disorders treatment and relapse prevention. CBT helps patients identify life stressors and develop strategies for managing stress by addressing deficits in coping skills, and it encourages patients to be active in identifying high-risk situations for benzodiazepine use. In their Cochrane Review examining the effectiveness of psychosocial interventions in the treatment of benzodiazepine use disorders, Darker, Sweeney, Barry, Farrell, and Donnelly-Swift (2015) found some evidence that CBT combined with dose tapering is more likely to be successful for discontinuing benzodiazepines when compared with tapering alone at up to 3 months posttreatment. These results did not hold at 6 months and later (Darker et al., 2015). Similarly, results of a meta-analysis of 29 studies examining a combination of pharmacotherapy and psychological interventions found that the integration of pharmacotherapy and CBT provided an additive effect when compared with gradual dose reduction alone (Oude Voshaar et al., 2006). In this meta-analysis, two types of interventions were identified: minimal intervention and systematic discontinuation. Minimal intervention refers to giving advice to discontinue the drug in the form of a letter or meeting. Systematic discontinuation comprises treatment programs led by a physician or psychologist. Three studies reviewed in the meta-analysis included minimal intervention (total $n = 601$, mean age = 71 years, M:F ratio 1:5). One study employed systematic discontinuation alone (total $n = 107$, mean age = 62 years, M:F ratio 1:2.6). Five studies used systematic discontinuation with psychotherapy (total *n* = 357, mean age = 56 years, M:F ratio 1:1.4). There were 21 studies examining a combination of systematic discontinuation and pharmacotherapy (total *n* = 1333, mean age = 52 years, M:F ratio 1:1.3). Both minimal intervention and systematic discontinuation were more effective than treatment as usual. Augmentation of systematic discontinuation with imipramine (two studies) was more effective than systematic discontinuation alone. The combination of systematic discontinuation with CBT (two studies) was superior to discontinuation alone (Oude Voshaar et al., 2006). This indicates that CBT along with pharmacotherapy may be helpful during the early phases of recovery.

There is evidence for the additive benefits of contingency management, CBT, and relapse prevention approaches in treatment for other substance use disorders. A meta-analytic review conducted by Dutra et al. (2008) examining the efficacy of psychosocial treatments for substance use disorders found low to moderate effect size estimates for CBT ($d = 0.28$, 95% confidence interval [CI] = 0.06 to 0.51) and relapse prevention ($d = 0.32$, 95% CI = 0.06 to 0.56), and moderately high effect sizes for contingency management alone ($d = 0.58$, 95% CI = 0.25 to 0.90). Although the combination of contingency management and CBT yielded high effect size estimates ($d = 1.02$, 95% CI = −0.05 to 2.09), these estimates were unreliable due to the small sample size ($N = 2$), suggesting that more research should include this treatment combination to further elucidate additive benefits. In addition, these results did not specifically involve studies of treatment of sedative use disorder and only included two studies combining CBT and contingency management. Combining pharmacological and behavioral interventions may be beneficial in improving treatment outcomes for patients with sedative use disorder, but more research is needed in this area.

INTEGRATED APPROACHES FOR ADDRESSING COMMON COMORBID DISORDERS

Sedative use disorders often co-occur with other substance use disorders or psychiatric disorders. The majority of individuals with sedative use disorder were prescribed the medication to treat anxiety or sleep disorders and became dependent due to long-term use (Ashton, 2005). Therefore, it is common to find individuals with a sedative use disorder who also have an underlying anxiety disorder or sleep disorder.

Often, recreational use of sedatives is part of a pattern of polysubstance abuse (Ashton, 2004). Reasons given for recreational use of sedatives include the sense of euphoria achieved from intravenous use or high doses of sedatives, such as benzodiazepines (Ashton, 2005); offsetting the negative effects of another substance, such as cocaine or methamphetamine (McLarnon, Darredeau, Chan, & Barrett, 2014); or increasing the intoxicating effects of another drug. When treating sedative use disorder, it is important to consider whether there is also the need to treat a co-occurring disorder. Alcohol and sedative use disorders commonly co-occur and sedative and tranquilizer users are more likely to engage in hazardous alcohol use or have an alcohol use disorder (McCabe, Cranford, & Boyd, 2006).

Common psychiatric disorders comorbid with sedative use disorder include depression and anxiety. In a study examining benzodiazepine use and abuse in patients dually diagnosed with a psychiatric disorder (schizophrenia, schizoaffective disorder, bipolar disorder) and a substance use disorder (alcohol, cannabis, and/or cocaine use disorder), Brunette, Noordsy, Xie, and Drake (2003) reported that many patients who were prescribed benzodiazepines also met criteria for a sedative use disorder. Although treatment approaches were not clearly described, authors identified sedative use as a further complicating aspect of treatment in this sample and cautioned against the prescribing of sedatives to individuals with co-occurring psychiatric and substance use disorders (Brunette et al., 2003). Similarly, Clark, Xie, and Brunette (2004) found that patients with major depressive disorder and a substance use disorder had higher rates of benzodiazepine use and tended to use benzodiazepines that have a higher abuse potential (e.g., alprazolam). They recommended alternatives to short-acting benzodiazepines, stating that longer acting benzodiazepines (e.g., clonazepam) may offer relief from anxiety symptoms in patients with comorbid anxiety disorders.

Additionally, nonpharmacologic options such as CBT have demonstrated efficacy for treating insomnia and anxiety disorders (Hofmann & Smits, 2008).

Given that there are no approved medications for the treatment of sedative use disorder, one strategy has been to reduce substance use by targeting the psychiatric symptoms. Researchers note that antidepressants may have benefits as an adjunctive therapy in benzodiazepine use disorder (Lader et al., 2009). Because antidepressants downregulate monoaminergic receptors, reduce depression and anxiety levels, and are typically well tolerated by patients, they may be a useful adjunct therapy for benzodiazepine detoxification (Lader, Tylee, & Donoghue, 2009). Of particular interest is paroxetine, a selective serotonin reuptake inhibitor. In one study, patients who were administered paroxetine during an 8-week benzodiazepine taper had significantly higher rates of benzodiazepine discontinuation than those who did not receive paroxetine (Nakao, Takeuchi, Nomura, Teramoto, & Yano, 2006). Although the successful results in discontinuation rates are promising, Nakao et al. (2006) found no significant changes in depression, anxiety, or withdrawal symptoms in patients who received paroxetine.

The tricyclic antidepressant imipramine also has shown promise in facilitating benzodiazepine discontinuation after taper. Rickels et al. (2000) conducted a study with 107 patients with generalized anxiety disorder who had been long-term benzodiazepine users. These patients underwent benzodiazepine taper treatment paired with imipramine, buspirone, or placebo. Those who received imipramine were significantly more likely to achieve abstinence 3 months posttaper than patients who underwent taper treatment with placebo (Rickels et al., 2000). Those who received buspirone were more likely (although not significantly so) to achieve abstinence than those who received placebo. In another study, Rynn et al. (2003) examined imipramine and buspirone as an adjunct to tapering in 40 patients with panic disorder who were discontinuing benzodiazepines. All three treatments resulted in reductions in anxiety and depression symptoms as measured by the Hamilton Anxiety Rating Scale and the Hamilton Depression Rating Scale. There were no significant differences found across treatment conditions in withdrawal symptoms or success in tapering. Imipramine was not effective in mitigating withdrawal symptoms or improving taper outcomes in patients with panic disorder (Rynn et al., 2003).

However, at least one other study did find that the addition of paroxetine was helpful in reducing psychiatric symptoms but added only limited value for benzodiazepine discontinuation. In a double-blind placebo-controlled study, Zitman and Couvée (2001) reported that benzodiazepine-dependent patients with major depressive disorder had reduced rates of anxiety, depression, and insomnia during diazepam tapering when given paroxetine compared with those who received placebo. However, improvement in psychiatric symptoms did not result in greater success in discontinuing benzodiazepines. Thus, preliminary evidence indicates that while paroxetine has beneficial effects for the discontinuation of benzodiazepines in nondepressed patients, it yields limited benefits for depressed patients dependent on sedatives.

Withdrawal symptoms can be particularly acute for patients with underlying anxiety disorders. There is growing support for the treatment of generalized anxiety disorder with the anticonvulsant pregabalin. Pregabalin (sold under the trade name Lyrica®) is a medication used in the treatment of neuropathic pain, seizure disorder, and generalized anxiety disorder. It has been examined as a potentially effective method for ameliorating anxiety symptoms when discontinuing benzodiazepine therapy in patients with generalized anxiety disorder. Pregabalin reduces excitatory activity in stimulated neuronal systems and thus may effectively counteract the inhibitory GABAergic modulation that characterizes benzodiazepine dependence (Hadley, Mandel, & Schweizer, 2012). In a study of 106 adults ages 18 to 65 years (81.1% White, 71.7% women) randomized to receive placebo ($n = 50$) or pregabalin ($n = 56$), Hadley et al. (2012) found that pregabalin was associated with a significantly greater reduction in Hamilton Anxiety Rating Scale scores and Physician Withdrawal Checklist scores compared with placebo. Additionally, of the patients who completed the study, 95% of those receiving pregabalin remained relapse free by the end of the study. Moreover, those in the pregabalin group showed lower rates of somatic and psychic anxiety, less severe withdrawal symptoms during benzodiazepine discontinuation, and better patient and clinician-rated assessments of global improvement by the end of the study than the placebo group. Future research should focus on validating these findings through another randomized, double-blind, placebo-controlled study.

When choosing medications to treat anxiety and sleep disorders in individuals with problematic sedative or anxiolytic use, other recommendations have included gabapentin, beta blockers, selective serotonin reuptake inhibitors or serotonin and norepinephrine reuptake inhibitors for anxiety, trazodone or melatonin for sleep, and antihistamines such as diphenhydramine for anxiety or insomnia (Casher, Gih, & Bess, 2011).

EMERGING TRENDS

Poor outcomes associated with dose tapering regimens have triggered interest in pharmacotherapeutic interventions for the management of sedative withdrawal symptoms, specifically those associated with benzodiazepine use. By pairing the taper dose with certain psychopharmacological agents (e.g., GABA receptor antagonists, antidepressants, and anticonvulsants), one may more effectively reduce the severity of withdrawal symptoms and improve dose tapering outcomes (Podhorna, 2002).

One drug of increasing interest is flumazenil, a GABA$_A$ benzodiazepine receptor antagonist/partial agonist. Flumazenil is primarily used to treat suspected benzodiazepine overdoses and to reverse side effects associated with general anesthesia. Current research indicates that flumazenil infusions also can be paired with tapering to treat benzodiazepine withdrawal symptoms (Hood et al., 2014). In a randomized control experiment, patients given flumazenil infusions paired with oxazepam tapering displayed a significant reduction in benzodiazepine withdrawal symptoms, cravings, and postdetoxification relapse than patients who received tapering alone or were in the placebo group (Gerra, Zaimovic, Giusti, Moi, & Brewer, 2002). When paired with a rapid dose-tapering oxazepam regimen, flumazenil infusions resulted in good management of subjective withdrawal symptoms,

high patient acceptance, and reduced psychological distress over the withdrawal period compared with baseline (Hulse et al., 2013). Flumazenil also seems to be tolerated well with antidepressants. For example, participants who were given flumazenil infusions paired with rapid clonazepam tapering after being stabilized on antidepressants prior to drug discontinuation experienced significantly reduced withdrawal symptoms, high treatment completion, and substantial 6-month abstinence (Quaglio et al., 2012). Flumazenil shows promise as a pharmacotherapeutic agent for the management of sedative withdrawal for both rapid and gradual tapers and for patients on antidepressants.

In addition to reducing the severity of withdrawal symptoms during detoxification, clinicians and researchers are also interested in pharmacotherapeutic interventions that can manage long-term withdrawal symptoms. One promising medication is baclofen, a GABA$_B$ benzodiazepine receptor agonist that has been used in preclinical and clinical studies as an anticraving agent for alcohol (Addolorato & Leggio, 2010). Although significantly more research must be conducted to understand the efficacy and safety of baclofen, a case series indicates that baclofen was effective in the management of craving and withdrawal in patients with benzodiazepine dependence, yielding relatively long abstinence periods that ranged from a minimum of 6 months to the final follow-up time point of 1 year (Shukla, Kandasamy, Kesavan, & Benegal, 2014). Baclofen was also found to be effective in the treatment of withdrawal symptoms for gamma-hydroxybutyrate, a central nervous system depressant whose mechanism of action and drug effects are similar to those of benzodiazepines (Kamal, Loonen, Dijkstra, & De Jong, 2015).

Thus, there is some evidence of potential medication-assisted treatments for sedative use disorder. However, this evidence is relatively weak. Future research is warranted examining whether a medication may be helpful in reducing withdrawal symptoms, decreasing craving, and treating the underlying symptoms of anxiety or insomnia. Further, the debate continues about whether complete discontinuation or reduction in use should be the ultimate goal of pharmacotherapy.

SUMMARY

The discovery of an effective and safe pharmacological intervention for the treatment of sedative use disorder continues to be elusive. There are no medications approved for the treatment of sedative and anxiolytic use disorder. Treating underlying symptoms in individuals with anxiety and sleep disorders is important in the management of sedative use disorder. Currently, the combination of psychosocial interventions and gradual dose reduction, with or without a supporting medication, to treat withdrawal symptoms is the recommended approach, having the most supporting evidence.

Patients with sedative use disorder working toward reducing or discontinuing their sedative use should be provided with information on local treatment resources in the community. In the United States, the American Society of Addiction Medicine and the American Academy of Addiction Psychiatry certify physicians in the treatment of substance use disorders. Other behavioral health providers with experience in treating substance use disorders can be found through the National Association for Alcohol and Drug Abuse Counselors. Additionally, the Substance Abuse and Mental Health Services Administration maintains a treatment-finder guide on its website. The Tool Kit of Resources later in this chapter also includes several other helpful tools and sources of information.

TOOL KIT OF RESOURCES

Sedative Use Disorders

Patient Resources

American Society of Addiction Medicine: http://www.asam.org

American Academy of Addiction Psychiatry: http://www.aaap.org

National Institute on Drug Abuse: Classes of Commonly Misused Prescription Drugs: https://www.drugabuse.gov/publications/research-reports/misuse-prescription-drugs/which-classes-prescription-drugs-are-commonly-misused

*Asterisks indicate assessments or resources.

National Institute on Drug Abuse: Understanding Drug Use and Addiction: https://www.drugabuse.gov/publications/drugfacts/understanding-drug-use-addiction

Smart Recovery Toolbox: http://www.smartrecovery.org/resources/toolchest.htm

Substance Abuse and Mental Health Services Administration (SAMHSA): Behavioral Health Treatment Services Locator: http://findtreatment.samhsa.gov

Weaver, M. F. (2017). *Addiction treatment.* Newburyport, MA: Carlat Publishing.

Provider Resources

American Academy of Addiction Psychiatry: http://www.aaap.org

American Society of Addiction Medicine: http://www.asam.org

Drug Abuse Screening Test (DAST-10): https://cde.drugabuse.gov/instrument/e9053390-ee9c-9140-e040-bb89ad433d69

SAMHSA: Behavioral Health Treatment Services Locator: http://findtreatment.samhsa.gov

Weaver, M. F. (2017). *Addiction treatment.* Newburyport, MA: Carlat Publishing.

Substance Use Brief Screen (SUBS): McNeely, J., Strauss, S. M., Saitz, R., Cleland, C. M., Palamar, J. J., Rotrosen, J., & Gourevitch, M. N. (2015). A brief patient self-administered substance use screening tool for primary care: Two-site validation study of the Substance Use Brief Screen (SUBS). *The American Journal of Medicine, 128*, 784.e9–784.e19. http://dx.doi.org/10.1016/j.amjmed.2015.02.007

References

Addolorato, G., & Leggio, L. (2010). Safety and efficacy of baclofen in the treatment of alcohol-dependent patients. *Current Pharmaceutical Design, 16*, 2113–2117. http://dx.doi.org/10.2174/138161210791516440

Altamura, A. C., Moliterno, D., Paletta, S., Maffini, M., Mauri, M. C., & Bareggi, S. (2013). Understanding the pharmacokinetics of anxiolytic drugs. *Expert Opinion on Drug Metabolism & Toxicology, 9*, 423–440. http://dx.doi.org/10.1517/17425255.2013.759209

American Psychiatric Association. (2013). *Diagnostic and statistical manual of mental disorders* (5th ed.). Washington, DC: Author.

Ashton, C. H., Rawlins, M. D., & Tyrer, S. P. (1990). A double-blind placebo-controlled study of buspirone in diazepam withdrawal in chronic benzodiazepine users. *The British Journal of Psychiatry, 157,* 232–238. http://dx.doi.org/10.1192/bjp.157.2.232

Ashton, H. (2004). Benzodiazepine dependence. In P. Haddad, S. Dursun, & B. Deakin (Eds.), *Adverse syndromes and psychiatric drugs: A clinical guide* (pp. 239–259). Oxford, England: Oxford University Press. http://dx.doi.org/10.1093/med/9780198527480.003.0013

*Ashton, H. (2005). The diagnosis and management of benzodiazepine dependence. *Current Opinion in Psychiatry, 18,* 249–255. http://dx.doi.org/10.1097/01.yco.0000165594.60434.84

Becker, W. C., Fiellin, D. A., & Desai, R. A. (2007). Non-medical use, abuse and dependence on sedatives and tranquilizers among U.S. adults: Psychiatric and socio-demographic correlates. *Drug and Alcohol Dependence, 90,* 280–287. http://dx.doi.org/10.1016/j.drugalcdep.2007.04.009

Bogunovic, O. J., & Greenfield, S. F. (2004). Practical geriatrics: Use of benzodiazepines among elderly patients. *Psychiatric Services, 55,* 233–235. http://dx.doi.org/10.1176/appi.ps.55.3.233

Brady, T. M., & Ashley, O. S. (2005). *Women in substance abuse treatment: Results from the Alcohol and Drug Services Study* (DHHS Publication No. SMA 04-3968, Analytic Series A-26). Rockville, MD: Substance Abuse and Mental Health Services Administration, Office of Applied Studies.

Bramness, J. G., Sandvik, P., Engeland, A., & Skurtveit, S. (2010). Does Pregabalin (Lyrica®) help patients reduce their use of benzodiazepines? A comparison with gabapentin using the Norwegian Prescription Database. *Basic & Clinical Pharmacology & Toxicology, 107,* 883–886.

Brunette, M. F., Noordsy, D. L., Xie, H., & Drake, R. E. (2003). Benzodiazepine use and abuse among patients with severe mental illness and co-occurring substance use disorders. *Psychiatric Services, 54,* 1395–1401. http://dx.doi.org/10.1176/appi.ps.54.10.1395

*Butler, S. F., Budman, S. H., McGee, M. D., Davis, M. S., Cornelli, R., & Morey, L. C. (2005). Addiction Severity Assessment Tool: Development of a self-report measure for clients in substance abuse treatment. *Drug and Alcohol Dependence, 80,* 349–360. http://dx.doi.org/10.1016/j.drugalcdep.2005.05.005

Cantopher, T., Olivieri, S., Cleave, N., & Edwards, J. G. (1990). Chronic benzodiazepine dependence: A comparative study of abrupt withdrawal under propranolol cover versus gradual withdrawal. *The British Journal of Psychiatry, 156,* 406–411. http://dx.doi.org/10.1192/bjp.156.3.406

Casher, M. I., Gih, D., & Bess, J. D. (2011). Benzodiazepines and stimulants for patients with substance use disorders: Careful assessment, close monitoring are

essential when prescribing drugs with abuse potential. *Current Psychiatry, 10,* 58–62, 64–67.

Cheseaux, M., Monnat, M., & Zullino, D. F. (2003). Topiramate in benzodiazepine withdrawal. *Human Psychopharmacology: Clinical and Experimental, 18,* 375–377. http://dx.doi.org/10.1002/hup.497

Clark, R. E., Xie, H., & Brunette, M. F. (2004). Benzodiazepine prescription practices and substance abuse in persons with severe mental illness. *The Journal of Clinical Psychiatry, 65,* 151–155. http://dx.doi.org/10.4088/JCP.v65n0202

Crockford, D., White, W. D., & Campbell, B. (2001). Gabapentin use in benzodiazepine dependence and detoxification. *The Canadian Journal of Psychiatry, 46,* 287–287. http://dx.doi.org/10.1177/070674370104600315

Cumming, R. G., & Le Couteur, D. G. (2003). Benzodiazepines and risk of hip fractures in older people: A review of the evidence. *CNS Drugs, 17,* 825–837. http://dx.doi.org/10.2165/00023210-200317110-00004

Darker, C. D., Sweeney, B. P., Barry, J. M., Farrell, M. F., & Donnelly-Swift, E. (2015). Psychosocial interventions for benzodiazepine harmful use, abuse or dependence. *Cochrane Database of Systematic Reviews,* (5): CD009652.

*De Las Cuevas, C., Sanz, E. J., De La Fuente, J. A., Padilla, J., & Berenguer, J. C. (2000). The Severity of Dependence Scale (SDS) as screening test for benzodiazepine dependence: SDS validation study. *Addiction, 95,* 245–250. http://dx.doi.org/10.1046/j.1360-0443.2000.95224511.x

Donoghue, J., & Lader, M. (2010). Usage of benzodiazepines: A review. *International Journal of Psychiatry in Clinical Practice, 14,* 78–87. http://dx.doi.org/10.3109/13651500903447810

Dutra, L., Stathopoulou, G., Basden, S. L., Leyro, T. M., Powers, M. B., & Otto, M. W. (2008). A meta-analytic review of psychosocial interventions for substance use disorders. *The American Journal of Psychiatry, 165,* 179–187. http://dx.doi.org/10.1176/appi.ajp.2007.06111851

Franconi, F., Brunelleschi, S., Steardo, L., & Cuomo, V. (2007). Gender differences in drug responses. *Pharmacological Research, 55,* 81–95. http://dx.doi.org/10.1016/j.phrs.2006.11.001

Garzón, C., Guerrero, J. M., Aramburu, O., & Guzmán, T. (2009). Effect of melatonin administration on sleep, behavioral disorders and hypnotic drug discontinuation in the elderly: A randomized, double-blind, placebo-controlled study. *Aging Clinical and Experimental Research, 21,* 38–42. http://dx.doi.org/10.1007/BF03324897

Gerra, G., Zaimovic, A., Giusti, F., Moi, G., & Brewer, C. (2002). Intravenous flumazenil versus oxazepam tapering in the treatment of benzodiazepine withdrawal: A randomized, placebo-controlled study. *Addiction Biology, 7,* 385–395. http://dx.doi.org/10.1080/1355621021000005973

Glover, S. J., & Allen, K. R. (2010). Measurement of benzodiazepines in urine by liquid chromatography-tandem mass spectrometry: Confirmation of samples screened by immunoassay. *Annals of Clinical Biochemistry, 47,* 111–117. http://dx.doi.org/10.1258/acb.2009.009172

Goodman, J. D., McKay, J. R., & DePhilippis, D. (2013). Progress monitoring in mental health and addiction treatment: A means of improving care. *Professional Psychology: Research and Practice, 44,* 231–246. http://dx.doi.org/10.1037/a0032605

Greenblatt, D. J., Allen, M. D., Harmatz, J. S., & Shader, R. I. (1980). Diazepam disposition determinants. *Clinical Pharmacology and Therapeutics, 27,* 301–312. http://dx.doi.org/10.1038/clpt.1980.40

Greenfield, S. F., Back, S. E., Lawson, K., & Brady, K. T. (2010). Substance abuse in women. *Psychiatric Clinics of North America, 33,* 339–355. http://dx.doi.org/10.1016/j.psc.2010.01.004

Greenfield, S. F., Brooks, A. J., Gordon, S. M., Green, C. A., Kropp, F., McHugh, R. K., . . . Miele, G. M. (2007). Substance abuse treatment entry, retention, and outcome in women: A review of the literature. *Drug and Alcohol Dependence, 86,* 1–21. http://dx.doi.org/10.1016/j.drugalcdep.2006.05.012

Grohol, J. (2016). Top 25 psychiatric medication prescriptions for 2013. *Psych Central.* Retrieved November 6, 2017, from https://psychcentral.com/lib/top-25-psychiatric-medication-prescriptions-for-2013/

Hadley, S. J., Mandel, F. S., & Schweizer, E. (2012). Switching from long-term benzodiazepine therapy to pregabalin in patients with generalized anxiety disorder: A double-blind, placebo-controlled trial. *Journal of Psychopharmacology, 26,* 461–470. http://dx.doi.org/10.1177/0269881111405360

Hearon, B. A., Calkins, A. W., Halperin, D. M., McHugh, R. K., Murray, H. W., & Otto, M. W. (2011). Anxiety sensitivity and illicit sedative use among opiate-dependent women and men. *The American Journal of Drug and Alcohol Abuse, 37,* 43–47. http://dx.doi.org/10.3109/00952990.2010.535581

Herron, A. J., Mariani, J. J., Pavlicova, M., Parrinello, C. M., Bold, K. W., Levin, F. R., . . . Bisaga, A. (2013). Assessment of riboflavin as a tracer substance: Comparison of a qualitative to a quantitative method of riboflavin measurement. *Drug and Alcohol Dependence, 128,* 77–82. http://dx.doi.org/10.1016/j.drugalcdep.2012.08.007

Higgins, S. T., Delaney, D. D., Budney, A. J., Bickel, W. K., Hughes, J. R., Foerg, F., & Fenwick, J. W. (1991). A behavioral approach to achieving initial cocaine abstinence. *The American Journal of Psychiatry, 148,* 1218–1224. http://dx.doi.org/10.1176/ajp.148.9.1218

Hjorthøj, C. R., Hjorthøj, A. R., & Nordentoft, M. (2012). Validity of timeline follow-back for self-reported use of cannabis and other illicit substances—systematic review and meta-analysis. *Addictive Behaviors, 37,* 225–233. http://dx.doi.org/10.1016/j.addbeh.2011.11.025

Hofmann, S. G., & Smits, J. A. J. (2008). Cognitive-behavioral therapy for adult anxiety disorders: A meta-analysis of randomized placebo-controlled trials. *The Journal of Clinical Psychiatry, 69,* 621–632. http://dx.doi.org/10.4088/JCP.v69n0415

Hood, S. D., Norman, A., Hince, D. A., Melichar, J. K., & Hulse, G. K. (2014). Benzodiazepine dependence and its treatment with low dose flumazenil. *British Journal of Clinical Pharmacology, 77,* 285–294. http://dx.doi.org/10.1111/bcp.12023

Hulse, G., O'Neil, G., Morris, N., Bennett, K., Norman, A., & Hood, S. (2013). Withdrawal and psychological sequelae, and patient satisfaction associated with subcutaneous flumazenil infusion for the management of benzodiazepine withdrawal: A case series. *Journal of Psychopharmacology, 27,* 222–227. http://dx.doi.org/10.1177/0269881112446532

Kamal, R. M., Loonen, A. J. M., Dijkstra, B. A. G., & De Jong, C. A. (2015). Baclofen as relapse prevention in the treatment of gamma-hydroxybutyrate dependence: A case series. *Journal of Clinical Psychopharmacology, 35,* 313–318. http://dx.doi.org/10.1097/JCP.0000000000000315

Kaplan, G., & Ivanov, I. (2011). Pharmacotherapy for substance abuse disorders in adolescence. *Pediatric Clinics of North America, 58,* 243–258, xiii. http://dx.doi.org/10.1016/j.pcl.2010.10.010

Kawasaki, S. S., Jacapraro, J. S., & Rastegar, D. A. (2012). Safety and effectiveness of a fixed-dose phenobarbital protocol for inpatient benzodiazepine detoxification. *Journal of Substance Abuse Treatment, 43,* 331–334. http://dx.doi.org/10.1016/j.jsat.2011.12.011

Kuehn, B. M. (2013). FDA warning: Driving may be impaired the morning following sleeping pill use. *Journal of the American Medical Association, 309,* 645–646. http://dx.doi.org/10.1001/jama.2013.323

Lader, M. (2011). Benzodiazepines revisited—will we ever learn? *Addiction, 106,* 2086–2109. http://dx.doi.org/10.1111/j.1360-0443.2011.03563.x

Lader, M., Farr, I., & Morton, S. (1993). A comparison of alpidem and placebo in relieving benzodiazepine withdrawal symptoms. *International Clinical Psychopharmacology, 8,* 31–36. http://dx.doi.org/10.1097/00004850-199300810-00005

Lader, M., Tylee, A., & Donoghue, J. (2009). Withdrawing benzodiazepines in primary care. *CNS Drugs, 23,* 19–34. http://dx.doi.org/10.2165/0023210-200923010-00002

Lewis, T. F. (2013). *Substance abuse and addiction treatment: Practical application of counseling theory.* London, England: Pearson Higher Education.

Liebrenz, M., Boesch, L., Stohler, R., & Caflisch, C. (2010). Agonist substitution—a treatment alternative for high-dose benzodiazepine-dependent patients? *Addiction, 105,* 1870–1874. http://dx.doi.org/10.1111/j.1360-0443.2010.02933.x

Lingford-Hughes, A. R., Welch, S., Nutt, D. J., & the British Association for Psychopharmacology. (2004). Evidence-based guidelines for the pharmacological management of substance misuse, addiction and comorbidity: Recommendations from the British Association for Psychopharmacology. *Journal of Psychopharmacology, 18,* 293–335. http://dx.doi.org/10.1177/026988110401800321

Marazziti, D., Baroni, S., Picchetti, M., Piccinni, A., Carlini, M., Vatteroni, E., . . . Dell'Osso, L. (2013). Pharmacokinetics and pharmacodynamics of psychotropic drugs: Effect of sex. *CNS Spectrums, 18,* 118–127. http://dx.doi.org/10.1017/S1092852912001010

Maremmani, A. G. I., Rovai, L., Rugani, F., Bacciardi, S., Pacini, M., Dell'osso, L., & Maremmani, I. (2013). Clonazepam as agonist substitution treatment for benzodiazepine dependence: A case report. *Case Reports in Psychiatry, 2013,* 367594. http://dx.doi.org/10.1155/2013/367594

McCabe, S. E., Cranford, J. A., & Boyd, C. J. (2006). The relationship between past-year drinking behaviors and nonmedical use of prescription drugs: Prevalence of co-occurrence in a national sample. *Drug and Alcohol Dependence, 84,* 281–288. http://dx.doi.org/10.1016/j.drugalcdep.2006.03.006

McLarnon, M. E., Darredeau, C., Chan, J., & Barrett, S. P. (2014). Motives for the non-prescribed use of psychiatric medications: Relationships with psychopathology, other substance use and patterns of use. *Journal of Substance Use, 19,* 421–428. http://dx.doi.org/10.3109/14659891.2013.845697

McLellan, A. T., Kushner, H., Metzger, D., Peters, R., Smith, I., Grissom, G., . . . Argeriou, M. (1992). The fifth edition of the Addiction Severity Index. *Journal of Substance Abuse Treatment, 9*(3), 199–213.

*McNeely, J., Strauss, S. M., Saitz, R., Cleland, C. M., Palamar, J. J., Rotrosen, J., & Gourevitch, M. N. (2015). A brief patient self-administered substance use screening tool for primary care: Two-site validation study of the Substance Use Brief Screen (SUBS). *The American Journal of Medicine, 128,* 784.e9–784.e19. http://dx.doi.org/10.1016/j.amjmed.2015.02.007

Michopoulos, I., Douzenis, A., Christodoulou, C., & Lykouras, L. (2006). Topiramate use in alprazolam addiction. *The World Journal of Biological Psychiatry, 7,* 265–267. http://dx.doi.org/10.1080/15622970600671036

Miller, W., & Rollnick, S. (2013). *Applications of motivational interviewing: Motivational interviewing: Helping people change.* New York, NY: Guilford Press.

Morgan, L., Weaver, M., Sayeed, Z., & Orr, R. (2013). The use of prescription monitoring programs to reduce opioid diversion and improve patient safety. *Journal of Pain & Palliative Care Pharmacotherapy, 27,* 4–9. http://dx.doi.org/10.3109/15360288.2012.738288

Nakao, M., Takeuchi, T., Nomura, K., Teramoto, T., & Yano, E. (2006). Clinical application of paroxetine for tapering benzodiazepine use in non-major-depressive outpatients visiting an internal medicine clinic. *Psychiatry and Clinical Neurosciences, 60,* 605–610. http://dx.doi.org/10.1111/j.1440-1819.2006.01565.x

National Center for Health Statistics. (2016). *Health, United States, 2015: With special feature on racial and ethnic health disparities.* Hyattsville, MD: U.S. Department of Health and Human Services, Centers for Disease Control and Prevention.

O'Brien, C. P. (2005). Benzodiazepine use, abuse, and dependence. *The Journal of Clinical Psychiatry, 66*(Suppl. 2), 28–33.

Ochs, H. R., Greenblatt, D. J., Divoll, M., Abernethy, D. R., Feyerabend, H., & Dengler, H. J. (1981). Diazepam kinetics in relation to age and sex. *Pharmacology, 23,* 24–30. http://dx.doi.org/10.1159/000137524

Olfson, M., King, M., & Schoenbaum, M. (2015). Benzodiazepine use in the United States. *JAMA Psychiatry, 72*(2), 136–142. http://dx.doi.org/10.1001/jamapsychiatry.2014.1763

Oude Voshaar, R. C., Couvée, J. E., van Balkom, A. J. L. M., Mulder, P. G. H., & Zitman, F. G. (2006). Strategies for discontinuing long-term benzodiazepine use: Meta-analysis. *The British Journal of Psychiatry, 189,* 213–220. http://dx.doi.org/10.1192/bjp.189.3.213

Parr, J. M., Kavanagh, D. J., Cahill, L., Mitchell, G., & Young, R. (2008). Effectiveness of current treatment approaches for benzodiazepine discontinuation: A meta-analysis. *Addiction, 104,* 13–24. http://dx.doi.org/10.1111/j.1360-0443.2008.02364.x

Paulose-Ram, R., Safran, M. A., Jonas, B. S., Gu, Q., & Orwig, D. (2007). Trends in psychotropic medication use among U.S. adults. *Pharmacoepidemiology and Drug Safety, 16,* 560–570. http://dx.doi.org/10.1002/pds.1367

Penninga, E. I., Graudal, N., Ladekarl, M. B., & Jürgens, G. (2016). Adverse events associated with flumazenil treatment for the management of suspected benzodiazepine intoxication—A systematic review with meta-analyses of randomised trials. *Basic & Clinical Pharmacology & Toxicology, 118,* 37–44. http://dx.doi.org/10.1111/bcpt.12434

Petrovic, M., Pevernagie, D., Mariman, A., Van Maele, G., & Afschrift, M. (2002). Fast withdrawal from benzodiazepines in geriatric inpatients: A randomised double-blind, placebo-controlled trial. *European Journal of Clinical Pharmacology, 57,* 759–764. http://dx.doi.org/10.1007/s00228-001-0387-4

Petrovic, M., Pevernagie, D., Van Den Noortgate, N., Mariman, A., Michielsen, W., & Afschrift, M. (1999). A programme for short-term withdrawal from benzodiazepines in geriatric hospital inpatients: Success rate and effect on subjective sleep quality. *International Journal of Geriatric Psychiatry, 14,* 754–760. http://dx.doi.org/10.1002/(SICI)1099-1166(199909)14:9<754::AID-GPS15>3.0.CO;2-E

Petry, N. M., Alessi, S. M., Olmstead, T. A., Rash, C. J., & Zajac, K. (2017). Contingency management treatment for substance use disorders: How far has it come, and where does it need to go? *Psychology of Addictive Behaviors, 31,* 897–906. http://dx.doi.org/10.1037/adb0000287

Petry, N. M., Martin, B., Cooney, J. L., & Kranzler, H. R. (2000). Give them prizes, and they will come: Contingency management for treatment of alcohol dependence. *Journal of Consulting and Clinical Psychology, 68,* 250–257. http://dx.doi.org/10.1037/0022-006X.68.2.250

Petry, N. M., Martin, B., & Simcic, F., Jr. (2005). Prize reinforcement contingency management for cocaine dependence: Integration with group therapy in a methadone clinic. *Journal of Consulting and Clinical Psychology, 73,* 354–359. http://dx.doi.org/10.1037/0022-006X.73.2.354

Piazza, N. J., Vrbka, J. L., & Yeager, R. D. (1989). Telescoping of alcoholism in women alcoholics. *International Journal of the Addictions, 24,* 19–28. http://dx.doi.org/10.3109/10826088909047272

Podhorna, J. (2002). The experimental pharmacotherapy of benzodiazepine withdrawal. *Current Pharmaceutical Design, 8,* 23–43. http://dx.doi.org/10.2174/1381612023396636

Poisnel, G., Dhilly, M., Le Boisselier, R., Barre, L., & Debruyne, D. (2009). Comparison of five benzodiazepine-receptor agonists on buprenorphine-induced μ-opioid receptor regulation. *Journal of Pharmacological Sciences, 110,* 36–46. http://dx.doi.org/10.1254/jphs.08249FP

Prendergast, M., Podus, D., Finney, J., Greenwell, L., & Roll, J. (2006). Contingency management for treatment of substance use disorders: A meta-analysis. *Addiction, 101*(11), 1546–1560. http://dx.doi.org/10.1111/j.1360-0443.2006.01581.x

Prochaska, J. O., & Velicer, W. F. (1997). The transtheoretical model of health behavior change. *American Journal of Health Promotion, 12,* 38–48. http://dx.doi.org/10.4278/0890-1171-12.1.38

Quaglio, G., Pattaro, C., Gerra, G., Mathewson, S., Verbanck, P., Des Jarlais, D. C., & Lugoboni, F. (2012). High dose benzodiazepine dependence:

Description of 29 patients treated with flumazenil infusion and stabilised with clonazepam. *Psychiatry Research, 198,* 457–462. http://dx.doi.org/10.1016/j.psychres.2012.02.008

Reeve, E., Ong, M., Wu, A., Jansen, J., Petrovic, M., & Gnjidic, D. (2017). A systematic review of interventions to deprescribe benzodiazepines and other hypnotics among older people. *European Journal of Clinical Pharmacology, 73,* 927–935. http://dx.doi.org/10.1007/s00228-017-2257-8

Rickels, K., DeMartinis, N., García-España, F., Greenblatt, D. J., Mandos, L. A., & Rynn, M. (2000). Imipramine and buspirone in treatment of patients with generalized anxiety disorder who are discontinuing long-term benzodiazepine therapy. *The American Journal of Psychiatry, 157,* 1973–1979. http://dx.doi.org/10.1176/appi.ajp.157.12.1973

Rynn, M., García-España, F., Greenblatt, D. J., Mandos, L. A., Schweizer, E., & Rickels, K. (2003). Imipramine and buspirone in patients with panic disorder who are discontinuing long-term benzodiazepine therapy. *Journal of Clinical Psychopharmacology, 23,* 505–508. http://dx.doi.org/10.1097/01.jcp.0000088907.24613.3f

Schweizer, E., Rickels, K., Case, W. G., & Greenblatt, D. J. (1991). Carbamazepine treatment in patients discontinuing long-term benzodiazepine therapy. Effects on withdrawal severity and outcome. *Archives of General Psychiatry, 48,* 448–452. http://dx.doi.org/10.1001/archpsyc.1991.01810290060012

Shinn, A. K., & Greenfield, S. F. (2010). Topiramate in the treatment of substance-related disorders: A critical review of the literature. *The Journal of Clinical Psychiatry, 71,* 634–648. http://dx.doi.org/10.4088/JCP.08r04062gry

Shukla, L., Kandasamy, A., Kesavan, M., & Benegal, V. (2014). Baclofen in the short-term maintenance treatment of benzodiazepine dependence. *Journal of Neurosciences in Rural Practice, 5,* S53–S54. http://dx.doi.org/10.4103/0976-3147.145203

Siriwardena, A. N., Qureshi, Z., Gibson, S., Collier, S., & Latham, M. (2006). GPs' attitudes to benzodiazepine and "Z-drug" prescribing: A barrier to implementation of evidence and guidance on hypnotics. *The British Journal of General Practice, 56*(533), 964–967.

Skinner, H. A. (1982). The drug abuse screening test. *Addictive Behaviors, 7,* 363–371. http://dx.doi.org/10.1016/0306-4603(82)90005-3

*Soyka, M. (2017). Treatment of benzodiazepine dependence. *The New England Journal of Medicine, 376,* 1147–1157. http://dx.doi.org/10.1056/NEJMra1611832

Substance Abuse and Mental Health Services Administration. (2015). *Behavioral health trends in the United States: Results from the 2014 National Survey on Drug Use and*

Health (HHS Publication No. SMA 15-4927, NSDUH Series H-50). Rockville, MD: Author.

Substance Abuse and Mental Health Services Administration. (2017). *Results from the 2016 National Survey on Drug Use and Health: Detailed tables.* Rockville, MD: Author.

Thomson, J. S., Donald, C., & Lewin, K. (2006). Use of flumazenil in benzodiazepine overdose. *Emergency Medicine Journal, 23,* 162–162.

Tkacz, J., Severt, J., Cacciola, J., & Ruetsch, C. (2011). Compliance with buprenorphine medication-assisted treatment and relapse to opioid use. *The American Journal on Addictions, 21,* 55–62. http://dx.doi.org/10.1111/j.1521-0391.2011.00186.x

Turnheim, K. (2003). When drug therapy gets old: Pharmacokinetics and pharmacodynamics in the elderly. *Experimental Gerontology, 38,* 843–853. http://dx.doi.org/10.1016/S0531-5565(03)00133-5

Vgontzas, A. N., Kales, A., & Bixler, E. O. (1995). Benzodiazepine side effects: Role of pharmacokinetics and pharmacodynamics. *Pharmacology, Biochemistry, and Behavior, 51,* 205–223. http://dx.doi.org/10.1159/000139363

Vorma, H., Naukkarinen, H., Sarna, S., & Kuoppasalmi, K. (2002). Treatment of out-patients with complicated benzodiazepine dependence: Comparison of two approaches. *Addiction, 97,* 851–859. http://dx.doi.org/10.1046/j.1360-0443.2002.00129.x

Vorma, H., Naukkarinen, H., Sarna, S., & Kuoppasalmi, K. (2003). Long-term outcome after benzodiazepine withdrawal treatment in subjects with complicated dependence. *Drug and Alcohol Dependence, 70,* 309–314. http://dx.doi.org/10.1016/S0376-8716(03)00014-0

Warner, E. A., & Lorch, E. (2015). Laboratory diagnosis. In A. Herron & T. K. Brennan (Eds.), *The ASAM essentials of addiction medicine* (2nd ed., pp. 127–133). Philadelphia, PA: Lippincott Williams & Wilkins.

Weaver, M. F. (2010). Medical sequelae of addiction. In D. Brizer & R. Castaneda (Eds.), *Clinical Addiction Psychiatry* (pp. 24–36). Cambridge, England: Cambridge University Press.

Weaver, M. F. (2015). Prescription sedative misuse and abuse. *The Yale Journal of Biology and Medicine, 88*(3), 247–256.

Weizman, T., Gelkopf, M., Melamed, Y., Adelson, M., & Bleich, A. (2003). Treatment of benzodiazepine dependence in methadone maintenance treatment patients: A comparison of two therapeutic modalities and the role of psychiatric comorbidity. *Australian and New Zealand Journal of Psychiatry, 37,* 458–463. http://dx.doi.org/10.1046/j.1440-1614.2003.01211.x

Yaffe, K., & Boustani, M. (2014). Benzodiazepines and risk of Alzheimer's disease. *British Medical Journal, 349,* g5312. http://dx.doi.org/10.1136/bmj.g5312

*Zador, D. (2017). Treating benzodiazepine dependence—Abstinence or maintenance? In K. Wolff, J. White, & S. Karch (Eds.), *The Sage handbook of drug & alcohol studies: Biological approaches* (pp. 485–490). Washington, DC: Sage.

Zitman, F. G., & Couvée, J. E. (2001). Chronic benzodiazepine use in general practice patients with depression: An evaluation of controlled treatment and taper-off—Report on behalf of the Dutch Chronic Benzodiazepine Working Group. *The British Journal of Psychiatry, 178,* 317–324. http://dx.doi.org/10.1192/bjp.178.4.317

CHAPTER 27

PHARMACOLOGICAL TREATMENT OF TOBACCO USE DISORDER

David J. Drobes

Human consumption of tobacco dates back to pre-Columbian America, with its earliest uses largely for ceremonial and medicinal purposes. The tobacco plant was introduced to Europe in the early 1500s and quickly spread along shipping routes throughout the world. Gradually, methods for cultivating and ingesting tobacco became more efficient, with mass production (i.e., industrial cigarette rolling machines) and marketing of tobacco cigarettes beginning in the 1920s. All of these developments led to substantially increased usage, with per capita consumption in the United States peaking in the 1950s, when more than half of adult men smoked.

Tobacco use disorder (TUD) is the contemporary diagnostic classification for maladaptive intake of nicotine from tobacco products (American Psychiatric Association, 2013). In this chapter, I review current pharmacological treatments for TUD, as well as assessment and diagnostic conventions and related treatment considerations. Psychologists have been integrally involved with research and application of both pharmacological and nonpharmacological treatments for TUD. The chapter should be informative for psychologists who directly oversee pharmacological treatments for individuals with TUD, and for those who provide primarily nonpharmacological treatment but need to be informed as to available medication approaches. Although cigarette smoking remains the predominant form of tobacco use and is the focus of this chapter, other tobacco

products (e.g., smokeless tobacco, cigars, cigarillos, e-cigarettes) can support addictive behavior and may benefit from similar treatment approaches.

EPIDEMIOLOGY AND PREVALENCE

The smoking rate in the United States and other developed countries has decreased substantially over the past 50 years, with a current rate of approximately 15% among all U.S. adults (Jamal et al., 2016; U.S. Department of Health and Human Services, 2014). Much of this decrease can be attributed to a growing public awareness from the 1960s onward regarding the detrimental health impact of tobacco use, along with evidence concerning the effects of secondhand smoke on the health of nonsmokers. Despite overall downward trends in smoking within the United States, smoking rates vary considerably according to sex (17.5% among men vs. 13.5% among women), race/ethnicity (31.8% among American Indians/Alaska natives vs. 16.5% among non-Hispanic Blacks/Whites vs. 10.7% among Hispanics vs. 9% among Asians), education (from 40% to 4.5%, with lower rates among those with greater education), poverty status (25.3% among those below poverty level vs. 14.3% among those above poverty level), geographic region (from 12.3% to 18.5% according to U.S. census region), and sexual orientation (20.5% among lesbian/gay/bisexual adults vs. 15.3% among straight

http://dx.doi.org/10.1037/0000133-027
APA Handbook of Psychopharmacology, S. M. Evans (Editor-in-Chief)

adults; Jamal et al., 2016). In addition, smoking rates are considerably higher among adults with (35.8%) versus without (14.7%) serious psychological distress (Jamal et al., 2016). Smoking prevalence also differs widely across the world, with the highest per capita consumption rates in Eastern European countries (e.g., Russia, Belarus, Montenegro) and the lowest among certain African and Asian countries (e.g., South Africa, India, Mali; World Health Organization, 2017). Tobacco use remains the top preventable cause of death and disease in the United States; currently, there are approximately 40 million adult smokers, and nearly half a million annual deaths are attributed to tobacco use (U.S. Department of Health and Human Services, 2014).

In the 1960s and 1970s, treatment methods to assist smokers in their quit attempts focused on behavioral and related approaches (e.g., nicotine fading, aversive therapy, coping response training, cigarette substitution, relaxation training, supportive counseling), with programs often combining and delivering these components concurrently or sequentially. Although early behavioral smoking cessation methods were generally efficacious, in the 1980s the field began to emphasize brief interventions, such as those that could be delivered efficiently in busy health care settings. In 1984, in concert with a rapidly developing understanding of the neurophysiology and psychopharmacology of nicotine addiction, the first pharmacological treatment for smoking cessation, nicotine polacrilex gum, was approved by the U.S. Food and Drug Administration (FDA). Initially only available as a prescription medication, nicotine gum was approved in 1996 as an over-the-counter medication. Several additional forms of nicotine replacement therapy (NRT) subsequently were approved, including a nicotine patch (prescription: 1992; over the counter: 1996), a nicotine nasal spray (prescription: 1996), a nicotine inhaler (prescription: 1997), and most recently the nicotine lozenge (over the counter: 2003). In addition to NRT, two nonnicotine pharmacological agents have been approved for smoking cessation in the United States: bupropion hydrochloride (Zyban®) in 1997 and varenicline tartrate (Chantix®) in 2006. A detailed description of these first-line pharmacological treatments is provided later in this chapter, and second-line (non–FDA-approved) pharmacotherapies, such as

clonidine and nortriptyline, are described as well. The *Clinical Practice Guideline for Treating Tobacco Use and Dependence* (Fiore et al., 2008) provides a comprehensive review of both approved and nonapproved pharmacological treatments. Source information for the clinical guideline and other patient and provider materials for smoking cessation are provided at the end of the chapter, in the Tool Kit of Resources.

Nicotine is the primary tobacco constituent that supports the initiation, development, and persistence of smoking addiction. A naturally occurring ligand that closely resembles endogenous acetylcholine, nicotine binds preferentially to nicotinic acetylcholine receptors in brain regions integral to addiction. Most notably, nicotine activates dopaminergic neurons in the ventral tegmental area, which has projections to the nucleus accumbens that are associated with hedonically rewarding and reinforcing effects upon activation. Nicotine serves as a primary reinforcer; for instance, it supports self-administration in both animal and human models (Corrigall, 1992; Henningfield & Goldberg, 1983). In addition, nicotine is a strong secondary reinforcer, such that initially neutral stimuli that become closely associated with nicotine delivery become reinforcers themselves (Caggiula et al., 2001; Palmatier et al., 2007). Those secondary (conditioned) reinforcement properties can be attained by sensory (taste, smell, and feel) aspects of smoking (Rose & Levin, 1991), as well as by a variety of exteroceptive stimuli and interoceptive (e.g., mood) states (Oliver, MacQueen, & Drobes, 2013).

The addictive potential of tobacco products is largely dependent on the speed at which nicotine is delivered to key neural regions following intake, as well as chemical characteristics that support nicotine absorption and bioavailability. In general, nicotine delivered through smoking has the greatest abuse liability, with pharmacologically active doses delivered to the brain within 7 to 10 seconds of inhalation. Indeed, a high percentage (31%) of experimenters with cigarettes transition to regular or daily use (Choi, Pierce, Gilpin, Farkas, & Berry, 1997), with earlier age of first use (i.e., by age 14 years) associated with the highest rates of later tobacco abuse or dependence (e.g., Substance Abuse and Mental Health Services Administration, 2015). In one study, 40% of seventh grade students (ages 12–13 years) who had used tobacco reported at least one symptom of dependence (DiFranza et al., 2002), providing further evidence of the addictive potential of tobacco in cigarette form. In contrast, medicinal NRT products are associated with slower delivery and much less (if any) abuse potential.

DIAGNOSING TOBACCO USE DISORDER

A diagnosis of TUD requires endorsement of at least two of 11 criteria from the *Diagnostic and Statistical Manual of Mental Disorders* (fifth edition; *DSM–5*; American Psychiatric Association, 2013). These criteria are essentially the same as for other substance use disorders, although the relevance to TUD varies across the criteria. Two of the criteria specifically denote physiological dependence (i.e., tolerance and withdrawal), which reflect neuroadaptations that occur with extended exposure to nicotine (e.g., upregulation of nicotinic acetylcholine brain receptors). Tobacco withdrawal has its own set of criteria in the *DSM–5* (American Psychiatric Association, 2013), including seven symptoms (four required for diagnosis) that occur upon abrupt cessation of tobacco use. The other *DSM–5* criteria for TUD generally relate to a lack of control over use and disruption to daily living.

The clinical significance of many of these criteria are subjective, thus requiring clinical expertise in tobacco use to administer assessments and assign a formal diagnosis. The *DSM–5* further specifies that one can exhibit a mild (two or three criteria), moderate (four or five criteria), or severe (six or more criteria) form of the disorder, with some suggestion that clinicians may reserve the term *addiction* for those who exhibit a severe TUD. However, there is no clear evidence that individuals who exhibit six or more criteria are qualitatively different from those who exhibit four or five criteria, placing some doubt on this more restrictive use of the term addiction.

In current practice, few prescribers or recommenders of pharmacotherapy for TUD apply a formal *DSM–5* diagnosis. Rather, most clinicians focus on a persistent pattern of tobacco intake, considering factors such as usage amount (e.g., number of cigarettes per day), length of usage (e.g., years smoking), and reported lack of control over intake (e.g., difficulty in reducing intake or quitting). Fundamentally,

consideration of whether a smoker is addicted to nicotine may be an important step in treatment planning and evaluation, but this does not depend critically on the presence or absence of a *DSM–5* diagnosis. Rather, there are several general definitions of addiction that may be considered in relation to one's tobacco use behavior. According to the National Institute on Drug Abuse, addiction is defined as a chronic, relapsing brain disease characterized by compulsive drug seeking and drug taking, despite their harmful consequences. The Society of Addiction Medicine provides further detail on the neurophysiological aspects and associated behavioral patterns key to addiction. Consideration of the *DSM–5* criteria can be a helpful tool in making a determination of addiction, but it should be noted that a *DSM–5* diagnosis of tobacco use disorder is not equivalent to presence of addiction. For instance, a person conceivably could exhibit a *DSM–5* tobacco use disorder based on the presence of two criteria and yet not be addicted. It should be further noted that a *DSM–5* or addiction diagnosis is not required to benefit from smoking cessation pharmacotherapy. Indeed, several forms of NRT are available over the counter, and tobacco use even at nonaddictive levels can cause serious health problems, further diminishing the necessity of a formal diagnosis prior to medication treatment.

Regardless of whether a formal *DSM–5* diagnosis is met or addiction is present, there are benefits to administering diagnostic and evaluative assessments to smokers. These include the potential to tailor medication treatment according to level of nicotine dependence and other factors (e.g., Lerman et al., 2004), as well as tracking the success of treatment over time. There are many assessment instruments to assist in evaluation, treatment planning, and outcomes assessment for smokers who may be candidates for medication treatment. Some of the most widely used relevant measures for smokers are listed in Table 27.1, including those related to motivation to quit, addiction or dependence, nicotine withdrawal, and urges or cravings to smoke. For instance, the Stage of Change algorithm (Prochaska, DiClemente, & Norcross, 1992), associated with the transtheoretical model of behavior change, places a smoker according to whether he or she is more (action or preparation) or relatively less

TABLE 27.1

Smoking Assessment Measures for Diagnosis, Treatment Planning, and Evaluation

Measure	Items	Scores	Citation
Motivation to quit			
Contemplation Ladder (TP)	1	overall score	Biener and Abrams, 1991
Reasons for quitting (TP)	12	2 subscales	Curry, Wagner, and Grothaus, 1990
Stages of change (TP)	3	overall stage	Prochaska, DiClemente, and Norcross, 1992
Nicotine dependence/tobacco use disorder			
Cigarette Dependence Scale–12 (D)	12	overall score	Etter, Le Houezec, and Perneger, 2003
Cigarette Dependence Scale–5 (D)	5	overall score	Etter, Le Houezec, and Perneger, 2003
Diagnostic and Statistical Manual (DSM–5; D)	11	overall score	American Psychiatric Association, 2013
Fagerström Test for Nicotine Dependence (D)	6	overall score	Heatherton, Kozlowski, Frecker, and Fagerström, 1991
Heaviness of Smoking Index (D)	2	overall score	Heatherton, Kozlowski, Frecker, Rickert, and Robinson, 1989
Hooked on Nicotine Checklist (D)	10	overall score	Wellman et al., 2005
Nicotine Dependence Syndrome Scale (D, TP)	19	5 subscales	Shiffman, Waters, and Hickcox, 2004
Wisconsin Smoking Dependence Motives Scale (D, TP)	68	13 subscales	Piper et al., 2004
Nicotine withdrawal			
Minnesota Withdrawal Scale (TP, E)	13	overall score	Hughes and Hatsukami, 1986
Shiffman–Jarvik Withdrawal Scale (TP, E)	23	5 subscales	Shiffman and Jarvik, 1976
Wisconsin Smoking Withdrawal Scale (TP, E)	28	overall score and 7 subscales	Welsch et al., 1999
Urge/craving			
Questionnaire of Smoking Urges (TP, E)	32	overall score and 2 subscales	Tiffany and Drobes, 1991
Questionnaire of Smoking Urges—Brief (TP, E)	10	overall score and 2 subscales	Cox, Tiffany, and Christen, 2001
Shiffman Craving Scale (TP, E)	4	overall score	Shiffman et al., 2003
Tobacco Craving Questionnaire (TP, E)	47	overall score and 4 subscales	Heishman, Singleton, and Moolchan, 2003

Note. TP = treatment planning; D = diagnosis; E = evaluation. From "Nicotine," by T. H. Brandon, D. J. Drobes, J. W. Ditre, and A. Elibero, in *Pharmacology and Treatment of Substance Abuse: Evidence- and Outcome-Based Perspectives* (p. 270), by L. M. Cohen, F. L. Collins, A. M. Young, D. E. McChargue, T. R. Leffingwell, and K. L. Cook (Eds.), 2009, New York, NY: Routledge. Copyright 2009 by Taylor and Francis Group, LLC. Adapted with permission.

(contemplation, precontemplation) immediately interested in quitting, whereas the Contemplation Ladder (Biener & Abrams, 1991) is an instrument that provides a continuous index of readiness to consider smoking cessation. The most widely used self-report assessment of nicotine addiction is the Fagerström Test for Nicotine Dependence (FTND; Heatherton, Kozlowski, Frecker, & Fagerström, 1991). A subset of two items from the FTND that reliably predicts biomarkers of use and cessation success (i.e., number of cigarettes smoked per day, time to first cigarette of the day) constitutes the Heaviness of Smoking Index (Heatherton, Kozlowski, Frecker, Rickert, & Robinson, 1989). For nicotine withdrawal, several validated indices assess individual symptoms or domains of functioning during periods of smoking abstinence (Hughes & Hatsukami, 1986; Shiffman & Jarvik, 1976; Welsch et al., 1999). Finally, measures of smoking craving can be either brief (e.g., Shiffman et al., 2003) or provide a more detailed assessment (e.g., Tiffany & Drobes, 1991). The Tiffany–Drobes

Questionnaire on Smoking Urges obtains scores for two aspects of craving: those that represent desire and intention to smoke, primarily for pleasurable effects (Factor 1), and those that are more immediate and intense and relate primarily to removal of negative affect or withdrawal (Factor 2).

EVIDENCE-BASED PHARMACOLOGICAL TREATMENTS OF TOBACCO USE DISORDER

Pharmacological approaches for smoking cessation counteract the disruptive effects of nicotine withdrawal during the quitting process, either by directly replacing nicotine or by addressing the neurochemical actions of nicotine in the brain. Nicotine withdrawal is a constellation of subjective emotional, behavioral, and cognitive disturbances experienced by smokers on removal (or reduction) of nicotine after an extended period of use. The *DSM–5* (American Psychiatric Association, 2013) includes seven specific tobacco withdrawal symptoms, which cover a range of emotional, cognitive, and physiological disruptions. Although not listed specifically in the *DSM–5* as a withdrawal symptom, craving also frequently occurs as part of this syndrome. Tobacco withdrawal generally begins within 24 hours of cessation or reduction, peaks at 2 to 3 days, and can last for 2 to 3 weeks or longer (American Psychiatric Association, 2013). It is notable that some withdrawal symptoms (e.g., craving, anger) can onset quite rapidly (within 30 minutes after cessation) among heavy smokers (Hendricks et al., 2006), which may partially explain the high rate of smoking among these individuals. Withdrawal can be a major impediment to successful quitting in the hours and days at the beginning of a cessation attempt.

The *Clinical Practice Guideline for Treating Tobacco Use and Dependence* (Fiore et al., 2008) recommends that all smokers attempting to quit be encouraged to use one or more FDA-approved medications. Each of the first-line agents that are FDA-approved for smoking cessation has been demonstrated to significantly increase rates of long-term smoking abstinence, approximately doubling the rates of successful quitting relative to placebo (Fiore et al., 2008). In this section, I describe each of the approved medication approaches, then discuss general issues related to pharmacotherapy for smokers.

Nicotine Replacement Medications

Nicotine replacement medications are the most common pharmacotherapy for the treatment of TUD, and they have received considerable empirical support. NRT facilitates smoking cessation by partially replacing nicotine in circulation, thereby minimizing withdrawal symptoms. NRT is typically initiated at the onset of a cessation attempt (i.e., the first 8–12 weeks) to coincide with the time period of peak tobacco withdrawal. NRT currently is available in five forms: chewing gum, transdermal patches, intranasal spray, inhaler devices, and lozenges. Each of these products can be considered a form of agonist treatment, though they vary in administration method, daily dose, and delivery duration. Table 27.2 summarizes characteristics of each FDA-approved NRT. At typical doses, NRT delivers one third to one half of the plasma nicotine levels achieved by smoking (Balfour & Fagerström, 1996), though higher doses to achieve more complete replacement levels appear to be associated with decreased smoking in both treatment (e.g., Dale et al., 1995) and nontreatment (e.g., Hatsukami et al., 2007) settings. Of the approved NRT forms, the nicotine nasal spray reaches its peak concentration most rapidly, followed by the gum, lozenge, and oral inhaler, which have similar concentration curves. The nicotine transdermal patch has the slowest onset but provides more consistent blood levels of nicotine over a longer period of time. Consistent with these differences in distribution speed, abuse liability is lowest for the patch and highest for the nasal spray.

Empirical support. A meta-analysis of 117 randomized controlled trials of nicotine replacement for smoking cessation indicated that commercially available forms of NRT significantly improved abstinence rates and increased the odds of quitting approximately 1.6 fold over placebo or no NRT (Stead et al., 2012). Actual 6-month quit rates with a single form of NRT are in the 25% range, with higher quit rates (approximately 36%) with nicotine patch combined with nicotine gum

TABLE 27.2

FDA-Approved Medications for Smoking Cessation

Pharmacotherapy/ availability	Advantages (A)/ disadvantages (D)	Dosing	Duration	Adverse effects	Precautions/ contraindications
Nicotine-based pharmacotherapies					
Nicotine patch[OTC/G] *24-hour patch* (7, 14, 21 mg) *16-hour patch* (5, 10, 15 mg)	A: easy to use (apply once per day), few side effects; D: slow onset, no acute dosing	> 10 cpd: 21 mg/day for 6 wk 14 mg/day for 2 wk 7 mg/day for 2 wk	8–10 wk (varies by patch product and strength)	Local skin reaction (50% mild, 10% causing discontinuation); vivid dreams or insomnia (can occur if worn overnight)	Caution in unstable cardiac disease (e.g., recent heart attack)
Nicotine gum[OTC/G] *regular, mint, orange* (2, 4 mg)	A: flexible dosing, faster onset than patches; D: often used incorrectly	> 20 cpd: 4 mg gum < 20 cpd: 2 mg gum (every 1–2 hr)	Up to 12 wk	Mouth soreness, jaw ache, nausea, hiccups, extra salivation	Acidic food/drink 15 min before or during use decreases absorption
Nicotine nasal spray[Rx] *metered spray* (0.5 mg)	A: flexible dosing, rapid onset; D: side effects, poor compliance	1–2 sprays/hr (up to 5 times/hr or 40 times/day)	3–6 mo (gradually decrease)	Nasal irritation (80%–90%); possible dependence (10%–20%)	Caution with asthma, rhinitis, sinusitis, and nasal polyps
Nicotine oral inhaler[Rx] *10 mg cartridge* (4 mg inhaled vapor)	A: mimics hand–mouth behavior; D: costly, frequent use required	6–16 cartridges/day	Up to 6 mo	Cough; local irritation of mouth and throat (40%), usually mild	Avoid acidic food/drink 15 min before or during use
Nicotine lozenge[OTC] *mint, cherry* (2, 4 mg)	A: flexible dosing, ease of use; D: poor compliance	up to 24 pieces/day at least 8–9 pieces/day initially	Up to 12 wk (6 wk then taper)	Nausea (12%–15%), hiccups, cough, heartburn, insomnia, headache, mouth soreness	Avoid acidic food/drink 15 min before or during use
Nonnicotine pharmacotherapies					
Bupropion SR[Rx/G] *Zyban* (150 mg)	A: ease of use (pill form), can be combined with NRT; D: medical contraindications	Start 1–2 wk before TQD (150 mg/day for 3 days, then 150 mg twice/day)	Up to 12 wk (maintenance up to 6 mo)	Insomnia, dry mouth, nervousness, difficulty concentrating, seizure risk (0.1%)	Caution with history of seizures, eating disorders, significant head trauma
Varenicline[Rx] *Chantix* (0.5, 1 mg)	A: ease of use (pill form), no known drug interactions; D: nausea	Start 1–2 wk before TQD (0.5 mg/day for 3 days, then 0.5 mg twice/day for 4 days, then 1 mg twice/day)	Up to 12 wk (maintenance up to 3 mo)	Nausea (30%), sleep disturbance, constipation, flatulence, vomiting	Adjust dose if kidney function is impaired, safety of use with NRT is unknown

Note. FDA = U.S. Food and Drug Administration; OTC = over the counter; G = generic form available; cpd = cigarettes per day; wk = week; Rx = prescription only; mo = month; SR = sustained release; NRT = nicotine replacement therapy; TQD = target quit date. From "Nicotine," by T. H. Brandon, D. J. Drobes, J. W. Ditre, and A. Elibero, in *Pharmacology and Treatment of Substance Abuse: Evidence- and Outcome-Based Perspectives* (p. 282), by L. M. Cohen, F. L. Collins, A. M. Young, D. E. McChargue, T. R. Leffingwell, and K. L. Cook (Eds.), 2009, New York, NY: Routledge. Copyright 2009 by Taylor and Francis Group, LLC. Adapted with permission.

(Fiore et al., 2008). The improved odds of quitting with NRT are largely independent of therapy duration, the intensity of additional support provided, or the setting in which the NRT is offered. Moreover, nicotine replacement agents do not differ in their effects on withdrawal discomfort, urges to smoke, perceived helpfulness, or rates of abstinence (Hajek et al., 1999). It should be noted, however, that most reviews and meta-analyses only examine treatment outcomes for approximately 6 to 12 months postcessation. A systematic review of the long-term effect of NRT revealed that although the relative efficacy of a single course of NRT remains constant over many years, the extant literature tends to overestimate the lifetime benefit and cost-efficacy by about 30% (Etter & Stapleton, 2006).

Mechanisms of action. There are several mechanisms of action by which NRT medications enhance smoking cessation. First, NRTs reduce the severity of nicotine withdrawal by providing nicotine itself, making it easier for people to tolerate the disruption associated with a quit attempt. Second, NRTs may reduce the rewarding effects of nicotine derived from smoking tobacco by occupying receptors prior to smoking. Finally, NRTs may facilitate the use of coping strategies for dealing with the psychological and behavioral aspects of a TUD (e.g., coping with stress or boredom, craving reduction, managing hunger and weight gain).

Precautions and considerations. Although each form of nicotine replacement is associated with specific precautions, the clinical guidelines (Fiore et al., 2008) recommend that special consideration be given before using NRT with patients who present with acute cardiovascular disease or who may be pregnant. However, there is currently no empirical evidence of increased cardiovascular risk with NRT use, even among high-risk outpatients with cardiac disease (Fiore et al., 2008; Joseph, 1996). Also, there is very limited data on the use of NRT among pregnant women, and the available evidence is mixed (Fiore et al., 2008). In general, most experts agree that the risks associated with continued smoking outweigh those associated with NRT use, but to date no product is FDA-approved for pregnant women.

Bupropion

Bupropion relieves the symptoms of craving and nicotine withdrawal, and it attenuates the weight gain that often occurs after smoking cessation. Currently available in two sustained-release (SR) forms, bupropion initially was marketed as an antidepressant (Wellbutrin®). In 1997, bupropion became the first nonnicotine medication to gain FDA approval for the long-term maintenance of smoking cessation (Zyban®). See Table 27.2 for additional important characteristics of bupropion.

Empirical support. Bupropion has been shown to double quit rates when compared with placebo (Hughes et al., 1999). A meta-analysis of 31 randomized trials of bupropion for smoking cessation revealed that the odds ratio of abstinence at 6 or more months was 1.94 for bupropion SR relative to placebo (Hughes, Stead, & Lancaster, 2007). There is also evidence that bupropion can be effective when offered in a primary care–oriented health care system setting, where a combination of bupropion and minimal or moderate counseling was associated with 12-month quit rates of 23.6% to 33.2% (Swan et al., 2003). Finally, the results of a double-blind, placebo-controlled comparison of bupropion to nicotine transdermal patch indicated that treatment with bupropion alone resulted in significantly greater 1-year rates of smoking cessation (30.3% vs. 16.4%) than did use of the nicotine patch alone (Jorenby et al., 1999). The quit rates were modestly improved (35.5%) when bupropion and the patch were combined. While there is certainly room for improvement in the quit rates achieved with bupropion (as with other smoking cessation pharmacotherapies), these data supported the first nonnicotine-based medication for smoking cessation and offered a distinct alternative to NRT.

Mechanisms of action. Bupropion's exact mechanism of action in tobacco cessation has not been clearly delineated. However, there is evidence that bupropion has a specific effect on neural pathways believed to underlie nicotine addiction (Dwoskin, Rauhut, King-Pospisil, & Bardo, 2006), including the inhibition of neuronal reuptake of dopamine and norepinephrine. There is also evidence that bupropion antagonizes nicotinic receptors in the brain and blocks nicotine's reinforcing effects. The fact that only some antidepressants aid long-term smoking cessation (e.g., bupropion, nortriptyline), whereas others do not (e.g., selective serotonin reuptake inhibitors), suggests that their mechanisms of action may be independent of antidepressant effects (Hughes et al., 2007). Indeed, studies have shown bupropion to be equally efficacious in smokers with or without a history of depression (Hayford et al., 1999).

Precautions and considerations. Treatment with bupropion SR should be initiated while the patient is still smoking, because approximately 1 week of treatment is necessary to achieve steady-state blood levels prior to a cessation attempt. Bupropion is contraindicated, or to be used with caution, among smokers with a history of seizure disorders or a history of factors known to increase the risk of seizures (e.g., bulimia or anorexia nervosa, serious head trauma, alcoholism). There is a risk of about 1 in 1,000 of seizures associated with bupropion use (Hughes et al., 2007). Bupropion SR may be preferable for smokers who favor oral medications or have a history of clinical depression. The safety of bupropion for use in human pregnancy has not been established.

Varenicline

Varenicline (Chantix) is an orally administered partial agonist of α4β2 nicotinic acetylcholine receptors. Varenicline was developed from the naturally occurring alkaloid compound cytisine, a drug derived from the plant *Cytisus Laburnum L.* (Golden Rain). It is the first nonnicotine medication to be developed specifically for use in smoking cessation. Evidence to date suggests that varenicline can increase the odds of successful long-term smoking cessation between two- and threefold when compared with placebo. The main adverse effect of varenicline is mild to moderate nausea. See Table 27.2 for additional important characteristics of varenicline.

Empirical support. A recent meta-analysis of 27 randomized controlled trials of varenicline for smoking cessation revealed that the odds ratio for continuous or sustained abstinence at 6 months or longer was 2.24 for varenicline relative to placebo

(Cahill, Lindson-Hawley, Thomas, Fanshawe, & Lancaster, 2016), with an earlier meta-analysis showing 6-month abstinence rates of 33% (Fiore et al., 2008). Varenicline was also effective at a substandard or variable dose, with an odds ratio of 2.08. Furthermore, varenicline was shown to increase the probability of quitting relative to bupropion by an odds ratio of 1.39 and relative to single-product NRT use by an odds ratio of 1.25. However, based on an earlier review, varenicline was not more effective than combination NRT (Cahill, Stevens, Perera, & Lancaster, 2013). When compared with placebo, varenicline appears to attenuate cravings to smoke, negative affect withdrawal symptoms, and some reinforcing effects of smoking (e.g., Brandon et al., 2011).

Mechanisms of action. Varenicline is a highly selective α4β2 nicotinic receptor partial agonist that stimulates dopamine and simultaneously blocks nicotinic receptors (Foulds, 2006). As a partial agonist, varenicline is hypothesized to alleviate craving and withdrawal symptoms by stimulating and maintaining moderate levels of dopamine in the mesolimbic region of the brain. The antagonist properties of varenicline are hypothesized to reduce nicotine-mediated activation of the dopaminergic system by blocking nicotine binding, thus reducing smoking satisfaction and psychological reward in those who continue to smoke while taking the drug (Brandon et al., 2011; Coe et al., 2005).

Precautions and considerations. The most frequently reported adverse effect of varenicline in clinical trials was dose-dependent nausea, experienced in 30% to 40% of users. These effects generally have been reported as mild to moderate, diminished over time, and were not associated with medication discontinuation. Unlike bupropion and some nicotine-based medications, varenicline does not appear to reduce postcessation weight gain (Jorenby et al., 2006). Although serious adverse events with varenicline were rare in the initial randomized controlled trials, postmarketing observations of neuropsychiatric adverse events (e.g., suicidality, hostility, agitation) led the FDA to mandate a black box warning in 2009. In response, a recently completed multinational randomized clinical trial further examined varenicline safety and efficacy in smokers with and without psychiatric disorders, in comparison with bupropion, nicotine patch, and placebo (Anthenelli et al., 2016). This study did not show a significant increase in neuropsychiatric events associated with either nonnicotine medication (i.e., varenicline or bupropion), in comparison with nicotine patch or placebo. Subsequently, the black box warning was removed from the product insert. In this trial, varenicline was more effective in terms of continuous abstinence from 9 to 12 weeks and 9 to 24 weeks (33.5% and 21.8%, respectively) following treatment, relative to bupropion (22.6% and 16.2%), nicotine patch (23.4% and 15.7%), and placebo (12.5% and 9.4%) conditions. At present, varenicline is not approved for use with pregnant women.

Additional Pharmacotherapy Considerations

Several considerations can guide selection of the most appropriate pharmacotherapy approach to smoking cessation for each individual smoker. These include determining the utility of concurrently using more than one pharmacotherapy, using non–FDA-approved medicines as second-line treatments, and following guidance for choosing among the available pharmacotherapy options. In the following sections I briefly review each of these topics.

Combination pharmacotherapies. Combination NRT involves the use of a long-acting product that delivers relatively constant levels of nicotine (i.e., nicotine patch) in combination with a short-acting product that permits acute nicotine delivery (e.g., nicotine gum or nasal spray). Research indicates that NRT combinations may provide greater efficacy in relieving withdrawal and enabling cessation than monotherapy, with an estimated odds ratio of 1.9 relative to the nicotine patch alone (Fiore et al., 2008). NRT also can be combined with bupropion to achieve greater rates of smoking abstinence than with either treatment alone, with evidence that nicotine patch with bupropion achieves a 6-month abstinence rate of 28.9% (Fiore et al., 2008). However, one review concluded there was insufficient evidence that adding bupropion to NRT provides any additional long-term benefit (Hughes et al., 2007), despite FDA approval for this combination. Some researchers

suggest that bupropion in combination with nicotine patch may be appropriate for patients who have high levels of nicotine dependence, have a history of psychiatric problems, or who have previously failed to quit (Frishman, Mitta, Kupersmith, & Ky, 2006), and this combination has received FDA approval. One study has shown that varenicline combined with nicotine patch was associated with improved cessation rates at end of treatment ($OR = 1.85$) and at 6-month follow-up ($OR = 1.98$), relative to varenicline alone (Koegelenberg et al., 2014). Further research is needed to understand the potential efficacy and safety for this combined medication approach.

Second-line agents. Pharmacologic agents that have not received FDA approval for smoking cessation but are recommended as second-line agents if first-line pharmacotherapies are not effective include clonidine and nortriptyline (Fiore et al., 2008). Clonidine is a centrally acting α_2-adrenergic agonist that reduces sympathetic outflow from the central nervous system and is approved for use as an antihypertensive agent. A recent meta-analysis concluded that clonidine was an effective agent for tobacco cessation, with a pooled odds ratio of 1.63 relative to placebo (Cahill et al., 2013). Nortriptyline, a tricyclic antidepressant, has also demonstrated efficacy for smoking cessation in long-term studies with a 2.03 odds ratio compared with placebo (Cahill et al., 2013). The high incidence of side effects (e.g., sedation and dizziness for clonidine, risk of arrhythmias and postural hypotension for nortriptyline) relegates each to second-line status.

Medication selection. Aside from the ubiquitous recommendation that higher medication doses are appropriate for heavier smokers, the field lacks a clearly validated approach for selecting among the various FDA-approved (and nonapproved) medications for smoking cessation. One study demonstrated superior efficacy for bupropion as compared with nicotine patch or placebo, but no significant improvement when bupropion and patch were combined (Jorenby et al., 1999). Another study (Piper et al., 2009) compared six separate medication conditions: lozenge, patch, bupropion, patch + lozenge, bupropion + lozenge, and placebo. Findings indicated that each active medication condition was superior to placebo without statistical correction for multiple comparisons, but only patch + lozenge was associated with significantly higher abstinence rates at 6 months with statistical correction. A more recent study compared nicotine patch, varenicline, and combined NRT (patch + lozenge) and found that each condition was equally efficacious in producing smoking abstinence at 26 weeks posttreatment (Baker et al., 2016). There is also recent evidence from a large-scale multinational randomized controlled trial that varenicline is associated with higher abstinence rates 9 to 12 weeks following treatment than bupropion and nicotine patch, with both of the latter treatments more effective than placebo (Anthenelli et al., 2016).

Hughes (2013) has provided guidance for choosing among medications, based on existing literature as well as practical considerations. After determining if there are specific precautions for certain medications, Hughes suggests the clinician outline the pros and cons of each noncontraindicated first-line medication and allow the smoker to choose. Prior experience with any of the medications also should be considered. Furthermore, existing guidelines (Fiore et al., 2008) and evidence described previously in this chapter suggest that medication combinations should be recommended. This can include NRT combinations that employ the nicotine patch with a more fast-acting form (e.g., gum, nasal spray), to address both the steady-state replacement of nicotine via the patch and the acute (emergency) treatment of situational urges and cravings via one of the faster-acting forms. Another medication combination that appears be effective involves the nicotine patch together with bupropion (Fiore et al., 2008).

BEST APPROACHES FOR ASSESSING TREATMENT RESPONSE AND MANAGING SIDE EFFECTS

Assessing treatment response for TUD can be relatively straightforward, with positive outcomes characterized by a sustained cessation of tobacco use. Most commonly, self-report is adequate for obtaining this information, and in large-scale studies it has been shown to correlate well with biochemical indices of use. In smaller scale research settings, or

in populations that may have particular incentive or propensity to mislead (e.g., those in medical treatment, pregnant smokers), biochemical confirmation of abstinence is recommended. The most common biochemical index is carbon monoxide (CO), with published guidelines for levels that confirm abstinence (Hughes et al., 2003). A CO level from 8 to 10 parts per million is commonly used as a cutoff to determine abstinence (Benowitz et al., 2002), although a recent analysis indicated that a much lower CO cutoff of 3 has greater specificity for determining abstinence (Cropsey et al., 2014).

It should be noted that CO, although highly sensitive to recent smoking, does not provide a reliable index of abstinence over a longer period of time. CO also varies considerably as a function of baseline levels, as well as activity level and metabolic factors. Alternatively, nicotine and its major metabolite, cotinine, provide direct and reliable indices of abstinence over a more extended period, and for this reason they generally are preferred for confirming abstinence. These biomarkers can be assayed from blood, saliva, or urine; for the latter two, test strips can be conveniently used in clinical settings. An important caveat is that these indices cannot confirm smoking abstinence for someone currently using NRT, as the nicotine from the NRT product will lead to positive test results.

MEDICATION MANAGEMENT ISSUES

As with most medications, those used for treatment of TUD are only effective to the extent that the medication is actually taken. That is, not taking the medication (or enough of it) is likely to be associated with disappointing outcomes. Thus, it is not surprising that medications are much more effective when combined with behavioral approaches. Behavioral treatments may increase adherence to medication regimens, and they may offer support for cessation attempts that increases self-efficacy for quitting, which in turn may encourage proper medication use.

One issue that arises in the context of NRT is whether to continue use of the medication if a slip occurs. When NRTs initially were approved and marketed, users were warned away from continued use once a slip occurred, due to fear of nicotine overdose. This concern has been rebuked, as NRT at recommended doses typically delivers nicotine far below what most smokers have adapted to. As such, the nicotine introduced by a smoking slip will not be enough to have toxic effects, and the benefits of potential cessation from continuing to use the NRT product outweigh this nominal risk. On the other hand, if an individuals has resumed a regular smoking rate (i.e., has relapsed), the safest course is to terminate NRT until a new quit attempt is initiated.

Another consideration is the potential for abuse and dependence with medications for TUD. As discussed previously, each of the NRTs and varenicline are agonist therapies that can be associated with similar reinforcing effects as the original tobacco product. Fortunately, the abuse liability is low for NRT products (e.g., West et al., 2000). Even with extended use (i.e., beyond the recommended acute treatment period), the potential for harmful effects are significantly lower than for cigarettes. Although the typical and recommended NRT course is short term (e.g., 8 weeks), a longer course of medication can be safely recommended and has demonstrated improved efficacy (e.g., Schnoll et al., 2015). It should be noted that after a full recommended course of smoking cessation pharmacotherapy, there should be little expectation of substantially increased withdrawal, craving, or relapse risk upon treatment discontinuation. In contrast, premature pharmacotherapy termination is associated with increased symptoms (e.g., withdrawal, craving) and ultimately treatment failure (e.g., Liberman et al., 2013). Such findings reinforce the importance of complete medication compliance, which may be supported by counseling and contingency management approaches. Finally, there is evidence that extended precessation use of NRT or varenicline is associated with greater abstinence (e.g., Brandon et al., 2018; Hajek, McRobbie, Myers, Stapleton, & Dhanji, 2011; Hawk et al., 2012; Rose, Behm, Westman, & Kukovich, 2006; Rose, Herskovic, Behm, & Westman, 2009). This association can be attributed to antagonist effects of the medication, whereby smoking cigarettes prior to cessation is no longer reinforcing due to receptor occupancy from the medication.

EVALUATION OF PHARMACOLOGICAL APPROACHES ACROSS THE LIFESPAN

Tobacco use among those who ultimately meet criteria for TUD typically begins in early to mid-adolescence. In contrast, the vast majority of randomized clinical trials for smoking cessation medications have been conducted with adult smokers, with very few studies examining pharmacotherapy for adolescent smokers. In one study among teenagers who smoked six or more cigarettes per day, bupropion at a dose of 300 mg/day (but not 150 mg/day) was associated with a significantly higher quit rate (22.6%) than placebo (11.5%) at the end of the 6-week medication period; however, these differences did not persist once medication was discontinued (Muramoto, Leischow, Sherrill, Matthews, & Strayer, 2007). In another study, adolescents who smoked at least 10 cigarettes per day had higher abstinence rates using the nicotine patch during active treatment (18%), relative to nicotine gum (6.5%) or placebo (2.5%), and these significant differences were maintained 3 months after study completion (Moolchan et al., 2005). More generally, a meta-analysis of randomized controlled trials for pharmacotherapy among adolescent smokers found inconsistent efficacy across studies (Kim et al., 2011). Notably, it is not clear for many of these studies if they specifically examined heavier (i.e., addicted) smokers for whom these medications were developed.

On the other end of the lifespan spectrum, many studies examining smoking cessation pharmacotherapy include older adults, and efficacy generally does not appear to be moderated by age. A recent review was not able to ascertain the most effective form of pharmacotherapy for smoking cessation in older adults due to a lack of comparative trials, but it did suggest there is ample evidence that NRT is effective for smoking cessation in this population (Cawkwell, Blaum, & Sherman, 2015). It is notable that the smoking rate is substantially lower among individuals over the age of 65, with part of this decrease due to a higher mortality rate among smokers in this age range (Jamal et al., 2018).

CONSIDERATION OF POTENTIAL SEX DIFFERENCES

Men and women have differed historically in terms of the prevalence of smoking, and research over the past 2 decades has sought to uncover mechanisms that may underlie differential smoking behavior as a function of sex. In this section I briefly review the topic of sex differences in smoking behavior, including the effectiveness of pharmacotherapy for smoking cessation.

Prevalence

The smoking rate as a function of sex has shifted considerably over the past century. Men have smoked at much higher rates than women throughout most of the 20th century, with peak rates for men at exceeding 50% in the 1950s, when smoking rates among women were approximately 25% (Centers for Disease Control and Prevention, 1999). However, given societal trends and aggressive marketing practices of tobacco companies, smoking among women has increased since the 1920s, peaking in the 1960s and 1970s at approximately 30% to 35%, even while rates had begun to decrease among men. The rate for women approached that of men in the 1980s, a pattern that has persisted for the past 30 years. Not surprisingly, as the uptake of smoking among women increased, so did the burden of disease and death associated with smoking behavior, with lung cancer surpassing breast cancer as the leading cause of cancer death among women in 1987 (Ernster, 1994). At present, smoking rates among men and women in the United States are approximately 16.7% and 13.6%, respectively (Jamal et al., 2016).

Pharmacological Treatments

Women are more likely to attempt smoking cessation than men (e.g., Shiffman, Brockwell, Pillitteri, & Gitchell, 2008), although men generally are more successful in their attempts than women over the long term (Smith, Bessette, Weinberger, Sheffer, & McKee, 2016). Perkins (1996) reported that men are more sensitive than women to the reinforcing effects of nicotine, based on laboratory demonstrations that men were more likely to adjust their smoking behavior as a function of nicotine content (see also

Perkins, Donny, & Caggiula, 1999). It was also observed that men are better able to detect differences between doses of nicotine administered via nasal spray (Perkins, 1999; Perkins, Jacobs, Sanders, & Caggiula, 2002). These findings led to the suggestion that men may benefit disproportionately from NRT for smoking cessation. This hypothesis has received some support, including evidence that NRT is less effective in reducing certain withdrawal symptoms among women (Wetter et al., 1999). Overall, this literature has been mixed, with some findings indicating that NRT is as effective for women and others concluding that men benefit more (see Munafò, Bradburn, Bowes, & David, 2004; Perkins & Scott, 2008; Shiffman, Sweeney, & Dresler, 2005).

This remains a controversial issue, with recent calls for NRT clinical trials to more routinely include sex as a variable a priori and to have sufficient statistical power to detect potential sex differences (e.g., Weinberger, Smith, Kaufman, & McKee, 2014). These trials should also seek to examine potential sex differences as a function of parameters such as NRT dose and duration. Furthermore, Weinberger et al. (2014) suggested that researchers consider the role of menstrual cycle phase on NRT effects among women, based on evidence that withdrawal symptoms and cravings appear to be more pronounced during the late luteal (premenstrual) phase (e.g., Allen, Allen, & Pomerleau, 2009; Carpenter, Upadhyaya, LaRowe, Saladin, & Brady, 2006), as well as mixed findings as to whether women are less likely to be successful in quit attempts initiated during this phase (e.g., Franklin & Allen, 2009). Relatedly, given that oral contraceptives may speed the metabolism of nicotine (see Allen, Weinberger, Wetherill, Howe, & McKee, 2017), studies regarding the impact of contraception on cessation outcomes with NRT are needed. Given the complex relationships between hormonal fluctuations and nicotine withdrawal, well-controlled trials are needed to determine if NRT efficacy differs among pre- versus postmenopausal women.

Several studies have examined potential sex differences in the effectiveness of bupropion for smoking cessation. In one analysis of 12 randomized cessation trials, it was found that overall women were less likely to quit successfully, but that bupropion was equally effective for men and women (Scharf & Shiffman, 2004). Similarly, a large-scale, multisite study conducted in France showed men to be more successful overall in quitting with bupropion or placebo, but the effectiveness of bupropion did not differ as a function of sex (Aubin et al., 2004). Overall, it appears that bupropion can be recommended for use equally among men and women smokers. In contrast, despite a number of individual studies not showing a sex difference in treatment outcome with varenicline, a recent meta-analysis indicated that varenicline was more effective for women at short- and immediate-term outcomes (McKee, Smith, Kaufman, Mazure, & Weinberger, 2016). That is, varenicline removed the disparity seen with placebo, whereby men typically have better outcomes than women.

INTEGRATION OF PHARMACOTHERAPY WITH NONPHARMACOLOGICAL APPROACHES: BENEFITS AND CHALLENGES

Medication treatment and behavioral counseling are each beneficial for smoking cessation, yet the highest level of effectiveness is observed when they are combined (Fiore et al., 2008; Stead, Koilpillai, Fanshawe, & Lancaster, 2016). Indeed, quit rates are approximately doubled when medication and behavioral approaches are combined, and a greater number of counseling sessions is associated with higher quit rates when medications are used (Fiore et al., 2008). Behavioral counseling can improve quit rates when using medication by increasing adherence to the medication regimen or by addressing issues that are not targeted by medications. For instance, learning to cope with high-risk (trigger) situations that may be associated with increased urges and cravings to smoke is often the focus of behavioral treatments, whereas NRT does not specifically reduce cue-induced cravings. Conversely, to the extent that medications can decrease withdrawal symptoms and craving during the early stages of a quit attempt, this may increase one's implementation of behavioral strategies. Behavioral support for smoking cessation can range from brief advice to more intensive or specialized counseling,

and it can be delivered through diverse formats (e.g., individual counseling, group counseling, telephone quitlines, self-help materials, smartphone apps, online). Often, the simple technique of setting a target quit date (TQD) can be helpful, for instance by generating motivation to quit and channeling resources and support for quitting, engaging in stimulus control prior to quitting (e.g., removing smoking paraphernalia and other proximal cues for smoking), and developing a repertoire of behavioral skills that can be implemented once the TQD occurs. Interestingly, the timing of a TQD can predict smoking cessation outcomes, in that those who choose a TQD less than a week away are more likely to have quit at the end of treatment and a 6-month follow-up (Zawertailo et al., 2017).

Many specific types or components of behavioral therapies have been examined for smoking cessation, with details that go beyond the scope of this chapter. Some common elements of behavioral problem-solving or skills-training approaches for smoking cessation include (a) identifying internal or external triggers that present an elevated risk for smoking or relapse, (b) developing effective cognitive behavioral skills for coping with high-risk situations, and (c) providing an adequate understanding of the addictive nature of smoking and setting accurate expectations for the quitting process (e.g., cravings and withdrawal symptoms and course). Several detailed guides for behavioral treatment are available (e.g., McEwen, Hajek, McRobbie, & West, 2006; Perkins, Conklin, & Levine, 2008), as well as validated self-help treatments that incorporate effective strategies in the context of smoking cessation or relapse prevention (Brandon et al., 2004).

INTEGRATED APPROACHES FOR ADDRESSING COMMON COMORBID DISORDERS

It is difficult to address treatment for TUD without considering the frequent comorbidity with a range of psychiatric and medical disorders. Not only are individuals with mental health issues far more likely to smoke, they also smoke more cigarettes more often than those without mental illness (e.g., American Psychiatric Association, 2013; Breslau,

1995; Jamal et al., 2016; John, Meyer, Rumpf, & Hapke, 2004; Lasser et al., 2000; Weinberger & George, 2006). Indeed, smokers with mental illness consume 40% of all cigarettes smoked (Substance Abuse and Mental Health Services Administration, 2012). Mental health diagnoses associated with particularly high rates of smoking include mood and anxiety (including posttraumatic stress disorder) disorders, substance use disorders, attention-deficit/ hyperactivity disorder, and schizophrenia. Although there is little recent data concerning smoking rates in persons with specific mental health diagnoses, in 2016 adults who had experienced serious psychological distress were more than twice as likely (35.8% vs. 14.7%) to be current smokers that adults who did not report serious psychological distress (Jamal et al., 2018). In 2006, the smoking rate among persons with schizophrenia was 80%, as compared with the general smoking rate of approximately 20% at that time (e.g., Keltner & Grant, 2006). In 2013, the smoking rate among individuals who experienced a major depressive episode within the past year was 22%, as compared with 13.3 % among those without a past-year major depressive episode (Substance Abuse and Mental Health Services Administration, 2014).

The reasons for high comorbidity between psychiatric conditions and smoking are not well understood. There is considerable overlap between the neurobiological pathways involved in smoking, addiction, and various forms of psychiatric disturbance, and this is an active area of research. Self-medication models suggest that smokers with psychiatric disturbance may be alleviating their cognitive and affective symptoms via smoking (e.g., Evans & Drobes, 2009). It is also possible that these individuals are more susceptible to nicotine withdrawal, which is also consistent with a self-medication hypothesis. To date, there is little evidence to support specialized treatment approaches (pharmacological and/or psychological) for these comorbid populations, yet this is an active area of research. In the meantime, the medications discussed in this chapter generally have been shown to be effective in comorbid populations and should be utilized unless contraindicated.

EMERGING TRENDS

As reviewed in this chapter, a number of pharmacological approaches to treating TUD have demonstrated empirical support. Yet, there remains considerable room for improvement in the short- and long-term success rates for these treatments. Novel nicotine delivery systems under investigation include rapid-release nicotine gum; buccal adhesive nicotine tablets; a pulmonary nicotine inhaler; and nicotine-based straws, lollipops, wafers, and drops (see reviews by Foulds, 2006; Frishman et al., 2006). Also of interest are (a) medications capable of blocking the CYP2A6 enzyme (an enzyme that accounts for individual differences in the rate of nicotine metabolism); (b) agents (e.g., lobeline) that produce pharmacologic effects similar to but weaker than those of nicotine; (c) nicotine vaccines, which are designed to reduce the distribution of nicotine to the brain; and (d) cytisine, a natural alkaloid that operates as a partial agonist of nicotinic acetylcholine receptors (similar to varenicline).

Several current and future trends may amplify the successful treatment of TUD with medications. First, as TUD is a chronic, relapsing disorder, successful cessation often requires repeated quit attempts with multiple methods over time. During this period of rapid change in health care delivery and compensation models, it is critically important for advocates to continue highlighting the chronic nature of TUD and the importance of repeat coverage for smoking cessation. Second, although current medications for TUD have greatly improved cessation rates, there remains an alarmingly high rate of treatment failure and relapse. An improved understanding of nicotinic receptor subtypes that underlie distinct tobacco use phenotypes—including those pertaining to various aspects of nicotine reward and reinforcement, stages along the tobacco use trajectory (i.e., initiation, persistence, relapse), and affective or cognitive disruptions during abstinence—may lead to more targeted pharmacotherapies for TUD (e.g., Brunzell, Stafford, & Dixon, 2015; Mineur, Mose, Blakeman, & Picciotto, 2018).

Third, the recent emergence of e-cigarettes within the U.S. market, though not approved as a smoking cessation treatment in the United States, are anecdotally being used as a cessation strategy by large numbers of smokers. These products may work similarly to existing NRTs but their closer resemblance to smoking may serve as a better substitute for those behaviors. It should be noted that the research and clinical community remains divided over concerns regarding the long-term health impact of these and newer products (e.g., heat-not-burn) and the danger they may bring in terms of normalizing smoking-like behavior on a societal level. Clearly, more research is needed to determine the individual and societal effects of these products, including studies regarding how, when, and for whom these products can lead to smoking cessation. In addition, research and regulatory policy regarding e-cigarettes must recognize a recent disturbing trend in which certain types of e-cigarettes that contain high levels of nicotine with less visible emissions (e.g., JUUL e-cigarette) have become very popular among youth. The challenge for researchers, clinicians, and policymakers is finding the balance between promoting e-cigarettes as a viable treatment option that helps to move smokers away from combustible cigarettes (if supported by accumulating evidence) without increasing nicotine uptake or addiction among youth.

Finally, many online and mobile apps have been validated for smoking cessation in recent years (see Shahab & McEwen, 2009; Taylor et al., 2017). Increasing use of technology (e-health, mobile tracking) may improve utilization of pharmacotherapy for smokers. For instance, new systems that can detect craving or situational triggers for smoking in real-time have the potential to signal timely usage of medications (e.g., nicotine gum, lozenge) or behavioral strategies to avoid smoking.

TOOL KIT OF RESOURCES

Tobacco Use Disorder

Patient Resources

American Cancer Society: https://www.cancer.org/healthy/stay-away-from-tobacco/guide-quitting-smoking

American Heart Association: http://www.heart.org/HEARTORG/HealthyLiving/QuitSmoking/Quit-Smoking_UCM_001085_SubHomePage.jsp

American Lung Association: http://www.lung.org/stop-smoking/i-want-to-quit/how-to-quit-smoking.html

Centers for Disease Control and Prevention: https://www.cdc.gov/tobacco/quit_smoking/how_to_quit/index.htm

National Cancer Institute: https://www.smokefree.gov/

Provider Resources

Society for Research on Nicotine & Tobacco: http://www.srnt.org/

http://www.treatobacco.net: Contains independent, authoritative information on the treatment of tobacco dependence—sponsored by the Society for Research on Nicotine & Tobacco and the Society for the Study of Addiction

Fiore, M., Jaen, C., Baker, T., Bailey, W., Benowitz, N., Curry, S., . . . Wewers, M. E. (2008). *Clinical practice guideline: Treating tobacco use dependence.* Washington, DC: U.S. Department of Health and Human Services, Public Health Service. https://www.ahrq.gov/professionals/clinicians-providers/guidelines-recommendations/tobacco/index.html

McEwen, A., Hajek, P., McRobbie, H., & West, R. (2006). *Manual of smoking cessation: A guide for counsellors and practitioners.* Oxford, England: Blackwell Publishing. http://dx.doi.org/10.1002/9780470757864

References

Allen, A. M., Weinberger, A. H., Wetherill, R. R., Howe, C. L., & McKee, S. A. (2017). Oral contraceptives and cigarette smoking: A review of the literature and future directions. *Nicotine & Tobacco Research, ntx258,* 1–10. http://dx.doi.org/10.1093/ntr/ntx258

Allen, S. S., Allen, A. M., & Pomerleau, C. S. (2009). Influence of phase-related variability in premenstrual symptomatology, mood, smoking withdrawal, and smoking behavior during ad libitum smoking, on smoking cessation outcome. *Addictive Behaviors, 34,* 107–111. http://dx.doi.org/10.1016/j.addbeh.2008.08.009

Anthenelli, R. M., Benowitz, N. L., West, R., St. Aubin, L., McRae, T., Lawrence, D., . . . Evins, A. E. (2016). Neuropsychiatric safety and efficacy of varenicline, bupropion, and nicotine patch in smokers with and without psychiatric disorders (EAGLES): A double-blind, randomised, placebo-controlled clinical trial. *The Lancet, 387,* 2507–2520. http://dx.doi.org/10.1016/S0140-6736(16)30272-0

American Psychiatric Association. (2013). *Diagnostic and statistical manual of mental disorders* (5th ed.). Washington, DC: Author.

*Asterisks indicate assessments or resources.

Aubin, H. J., Lebargy, F., Berlin, I., Bidaut-Mazel, C., Chemali-Hudry, J., & Lagrue, G. (2004). Efficacy of bupropion and predictors of successful outcome in a sample of French smokers: A randomized placebo-controlled trial. *Addiction, 99,* 1206–1218. http://dx.doi.org/10.1111/j.1360-0443.2004.00814.x

Baker, T. B., Piper, M. E., Stein, J. H., Smith, S. S., Bolt, D. M., Fraser, D. L., & Fiore, M. C. (2016). Effects of nicotine patch vs varenicline vs combination nicotine replacement therapy on smoking cessation at 26 weeks: A randomized clinical trial. *JAMA: Journal of the American Medical Association, 315,* 371–379. http://dx.doi.org/10.1001/jama.2015.19284

Balfour, D. J., & Fagerström, K. O. (1996). Pharmacology of nicotine and its therapeutic use in smoking cessation and neurodegenerative disorders. *Pharmacology & Therapeutics, 72,* 51–81. http://dx.doi.org/10.1016/S0163-7258(96)00099-X

Benowitz, N. L., Iii, P. J., Ahijevych, K., Jarvis, M. J., Hall, S., LeHouezec, J., . . . Velicer, W. (2002). Biochemical verification of tobacco use and cessation. *Nicotine & Tobacco Research, 4,* 149–159. http://dx.doi.org/10.1080/14622200210123581

*Biener, L., & Abrams, D. B. (1991). The Contemplation Ladder: Validation of a measure of readiness to consider smoking cessation. *Health Psychology, 10,* 360–365. http://dx.doi.org/10.1037/0278-6133.10.5.360

Brandon, T. H., Drobes, D. J., Ditre, J. W., & Elibero, A. (2009). Nicotine. In L. M. Cohen, F. L. Collins, A. M. Young, D. E. McChargue, T. R. Leffingwell, & K. L. Cook (Eds.), *Pharmacology and Treatment of Substance Abuse: Evidence- and Outcome-Based Perspectives* (pp. 267–293). New York, NY: Routledge.

Brandon, T. H., Drobes, D. J., Unrod, M., Heckman, B. W., Oliver, J. A., Roetzheim, R. C., . . . Small, B. J. (2011). Varenicline effects on craving, cue reactivity, and smoking reward. *Psychopharmacology, 218,* 391–403. http://dx.doi.org/10.1007/s00213-011-2327-z

Brandon, T. H., Meade, C. D., Herzog, T. A., Chirikos, T. N., Webb, M. S., & Cantor, A. B. (2004). Efficacy and cost-effectiveness of a minimal intervention to prevent smoking relapse: Dismantling the effects of amount of content versus contact. *Journal of Consulting and Clinical Psychology, 72,* 797–808. http://dx.doi.org/10.1037/0022-006X.72.5.797

Brandon, T. H., Unrod, M., Drobes, D. J., Sutton, S. K., Hawk, L. W., Simmons, V. N., . . . Cahill, S. P. (2018). Facilitated extinction training to improve pharmacotherapy for smoking cessation: A pilot feasibility trial. *Nicotine & Tobacco Research, 20,* 1189–1197. http://dx.doi.org/10.1093/ntr/ntx203

Breslau, N. (1995). Psychiatric comorbidity of smoking and nicotine dependence. *Behavior Genetics, 25,* 95–101. http://dx.doi.org/10.1007/BF02196920

Brunzell, D. H., Stafford, A. M., & Dixon, C. I. (2015). Nicotinic receptor contributions to smoking: Insights from human studies and animal models. *Current Addiction Reports, 2,* 33–46. http://dx.doi.org/10.1007/s40429-015-0042-2

Caggiula, A. R., Donny, E. C., White, A. R., Chaudhri, N., Booth, S., Gharib, M. A., . . . Sved, A. F. (2001). Cue dependency of nicotine self-administration and smoking. *Pharmacology, Biochemistry and Behavior, 70,* 515–530. http://dx.doi.org/10.1016/S0091-3057(01)00676-1

Cahill, K., Lindson-Hawley, N., Thomas, K. H., Fanshawe, T. R., & Lancaster, T. (2016). Nicotine receptor partial agonists for smoking cessation. *Cochrane Database of Systematic Reviews, 5,* CD006103.

Cahill, K., Stevens, S., Perera, R., & Lancaster, T. (2013). Pharmacological interventions for smoking cessation: An overview and network meta-analysis. *Cochrane Database of Systematic Reviews, 5,* CD009329.

Carpenter, M. J., Upadhyaya, H. P., LaRowe, S. D., Saladin, M. E., & Brady, K. T. (2006). Menstrual cycle phase effects on nicotine withdrawal and cigarette craving: A review. *Nicotine & Tobacco Research, 8,* 627–638. http://dx.doi.org/10.1080/14622200600910793

Cawkwell, P. B., Blaum, C., & Sherman, S. E. (2015). Pharmacological smoking cessation therapies in older adults: A review of the evidence. *Drugs & Aging, 32,* 443–451. http://dx.doi.org/10.1007/s40266-015-0274-9

Centers for Disease Control and Prevention. (1999). Achievements in public health, 1990–1999: Tobacco use—United States, 1900–1999. *Morbidity and Mortality Weekly Report, 48,* 986–993.

Choi, W. S., Pierce, J. P., Gilpin, E. A., Farkas, A. J., & Berry, C. C. (1997). Which adolescent experimenters progress to established smoking in the United States. *American Journal of Preventive Medicine, 13,* 385–391. http://dx.doi.org/10.1016/S0749-3797(18)30159-4

Coe, J. W., Brooks, P. R., Vetelino, M. G., Wirtz, M. C., Arnold, E. P., Huang, J., . . . O'Neill, B. T. (2005). Varenicline: An α4β2 nicotinic receptor partial agonist for smoking cessation. *Journal of Medicinal Chemistry, 48,* 3474–3477. http://dx.doi.org/10.1021/jm050069n

Corrigall, W. A. (1992). A rodent model for nicotine self-administration. *Neuromethods: Animal Models of Drug Addiction, 24,* 315–344.

*Cox, L. S., Tiffany, S. T., & Christen, A. G. (2001). Evaluation of the Brief Questionnaire of Smoking Urges (QSU-brief) in laboratory and clinical settings. *Nicotine & Tobacco Research, 3,* 7–16. http://dx.doi.org/10.1080/14622200020032051

Cropsey, K. L., Trent, L. R., Clark, C. B., Stevens, E. N., Lahti, A. C., & Hendricks, P. S. (2014). How low should you go? Determining the optimal cutoff for exhaled carbon monoxide to confirm smoking abstinence when using cotinine as reference. *Nicotine & Tobacco Research, 16,* 1348–1355. http://dx.doi.org/10.1093/ntr/ntu085

*Curry, S., Wagner, E. H., & Grothaus, L. C. (1990). Intrinsic and extrinsic motivation for smoking cessation. *Journal of Consulting and Clinical Psychology, 58,* 310–316. http://dx.doi.org/10.1037/0022-006X.58.3.310

Dale, L. C., Hurt, R. D., Offord, K. P., Lawson, G. M., Croghan, I. T., & Schroeder, D. R. (1995). High-dose nicotine patch therapy. Percentage of replacement and smoking cessation. *Journal of the American Medical Association, 274,* 1353–1358. http://dx.doi.org/10.1001/jama.1995.03530170033028

DiFranza, J. R., Savageau, J. A., Rigotti, N. A., Fletcher, K., Ockene, J. K., McNeill, A. D., . . . Wood, C. (2002). Development of symptoms of tobacco dependence in youths: 30 month follow up data from the DANDY study. *Tobacco Control, 11,* 228–235. http://dx.doi.org/10.1136/tc.11.3.228

Dwoskin, L. P., Rauhut, A. S., King-Pospisil, K. A., & Bardo, M. T. (2006). Review of the pharmacology and clinical profile of bupropion, an antidepressant and tobacco use cessation agent. *CNS Drug Reviews, 12,* 178–207. http://dx.doi.org/10.1111/j.1527-3458.2006.00178.x

Ernster, V. L. (1994). The epidemiology of lung cancer in women. *Annals of Epidemiology, 4,* 102–110. http://dx.doi.org/10.1016/1047-2797(94)90054-X

*Etter, J. F., Le Houezec, J., & Perneger, T. V. (2003). A self-administered questionnaire to measure dependence on cigarettes: The cigarette dependence scale. *Neuropsychopharmacology, 28,* 359–370. http://dx.doi.org/10.1038/sj.npp.1300030

Etter, J. F., & Stapleton, J. A. (2006). Nicotine replacement therapy for long-term smoking cessation: A meta-analysis. *Tobacco Control, 15,* 280–285. http://dx.doi.org/10.1136/tc.2005.015487

Evans, D. E., & Drobes, D. J. (2009). Nicotine self-medication of cognitive-attentional processing. *Addiction Biology, 14,* 32–42. http://dx.doi.org/10.1111/j.1369-1600.2008.00130.x

Fiore, M., Jaen, C., Baker, T., Bailey, W., Benowitz, N., Curry, S., . . . Wewers, M. E. (2008). *Clinical practice guideline: Treating tobacco use dependence.* Washington, DC: U.S. Department of Health and Human Services, Public Health Service.

Foulds, J. (2006). The neurobiological basis for partial agonist treatment of nicotine dependence: Varenicline. *International Journal of Clinical Practice, 60,* 571–576. http://dx.doi.org/10.1111/j.1368-5031.2006.00955.x

Franklin, T. R., & Allen, S. S. (2009). Influence of menstrual cycle phase on smoking cessation treatment outcome: A hypothesis regarding the discordant findings in the literature. *Addiction, 104,* 1941–1942. http://dx.doi.org/10.1111/j.1360-0443.2009.02758.x

Frishman, W. H., Mitta, W., Kupersmith, A., & Ky, T. (2006). Nicotine and non-nicotine smoking cessation pharmacotherapies. *Cardiology in Review, 14,* 57–73. http://dx.doi.org/10.1097/01.crd.0000172309.06270.25

Hatsukami, D., Mooney, M., Murphy, S., LeSage, M., Babb, D., & Hecht, S. (2007). Effects of high dose transdermal nicotine replacement in cigarette smokers. *Pharmacology, Biochemistry and Behavior, 86,* 132–139. http://dx.doi.org/10.1016/j.pbb.2006.12.017

Hajek, P., McRobbie, H. J., Myers, K. E., Stapleton, J., & Dhanji, A. R. (2011). Use of varenicline for 4 weeks before quitting smoking: Decrease in ad lib smoking and increase in smoking cessation rates. *Archives of Internal Medicine, 171,* 770–777. http://dx.doi.org/10.1001/archinternmed.2011.138

Hajek, P., West, R., Foulds, J., Nilsson, F., Burrows, S., & Meadow, A. (1999). Randomized comparative trial of nicotine polacrilex, a transdermal patch, nasal spray, and an inhaler. *Archives of Internal Medicine, 159,* 2033–2038. http://dx.doi.org/10.1001/archinte.159.17.2033

Hawk, L. W., Jr., Ashare, R. L., Lohnes, S. F., Schlienz, N. J., Rhodes, J. D., Tiffany, S. T., . . . Mahoney, M. C. (2012). The effects of extended pre-quit varenicline treatment on smoking behavior and short-term abstinence: A randomized clinical trial. *Clinical Pharmacology and Therapeutics, 91,* 172–180. http://dx.doi.org/10.1038/clpt.2011.317

Hayford, K. E., Patten, C. A., Rummans, T. A., Schroeder, D. R., Offord, K. P., Croghan, I. T., . . . Hurt, R. D. (1999). Efficacy of bupropion for smoking cessation in smokers with a former history of major depression or alcoholism. *The British Journal of Psychiatry, 174,* 173–178. http://dx.doi.org/10.1192/bjp.174.2.173

*Heatherton, T. F., Kozlowski, L. T., Frecker, R. C., & Fagerström, K. O. (1991). The Fagerström test for nicotine dependence: A revision of the Fagerström tolerance questionnaire. *British Journal of Addiction, 86,* 1119–1127. http://dx.doi.org/10.1111/j.1360-0443.1991.tb01879.x

*Heatherton, T. F., Kozlowski, L. T., Frecker, R. C., Rickert, W., & Robinson, J. (1989). Measuring the heaviness of smoking: Using self-reported time to the first cigarette of the day and number of cigarettes smoked per day. *British Journal of Addiction, 84,* 791–800. http://dx.doi.org/10.1111/j.1360-0443.1989.tb03059.x

*Heishman, S. J., Singleton, E. G., & Moolchan, E. T. (2003). Tobacco Craving Questionnaire: Reliability and validity of a new multifactorial instrument. *Nicotine & Tobacco Research, 5,* 645–654. http://dx.doi.org/10.1080/1462220031000158681

Hendricks, P. S., Ditre, J. W., Drobes, D. J., & Brandon, T. H. (2006). The early time course of smoking withdrawal effects. *Psychopharmacology, 187,* 385–396. http://dx.doi.org/10.1007/s00213-006-0429-9

Henningfield, J. E., & Goldberg, S. R. (1983). Control of behavior by intravenous nicotine injections in human subjects. *Pharmacology, Biochemistry and Behavior, 19,* 1021–1026. http://dx.doi.org/10.1016/0091-3057(83)90409-4

Hughes, J. R. (2013). An updated algorithm for choosing among smoking cessation treatments. *Journal of Substance Abuse Treatment, 45,* 215–221. http://dx.doi.org/10.1016/j.jsat.2013.01.011

Hughes, J. R., Goldstein, M. G., Hurt, R. D., & Shiffman, S. (1999). Recent advances in the pharmacotherapy of smoking. *Journal of the American Medical Association, 281,* 72–76. http://dx.doi.org/10.1001/jama.281.1.72

*Hughes, J. R., & Hatsukami, D. (1986). Signs and symptoms of tobacco withdrawal. *Archives of General Psychiatry, 43,* 289–294. http://dx.doi.org/10.1001/archpsyc.1986.01800030107013

Hughes, J. R., Keely, J. P., Niaura, R. S., Ossip-Klein, D. J., Richmond, R. L., & Swan, G. E. (2003). Measures of abstinence in clinical trials: Issues and recommendations. *Nicotine & Tobacco Research, 5*(1), 13–25.

Hughes, J. R., Stead, L. F., & Lancaster, T. (2007). Antidepressants for smoking cessation. *Cochrane Database of Systematic Reviews, 1,* CD000031.

Jamal, A., King, B. A., Neff, L. J., Whitmill, J., Babb, S. D., & Graffunder, C. M. (2016). Current cigarette smoking among adults—United States, 2005–2015. *Morbidity and Mortality Weekly Report, 65,* 1205–1211. http://dx.doi.org/10.15585/mmwr.mm6544a2

Jamal, A., Phillips, E., Gentzke, A. S., Homa, D. M., Babb, S. D., King, B. A., & Neff, L. J. (2018). Current cigarette smoking among adults—United States, 2016. *Morbidity and Mortality Weekly Report, 67,* 53–59. http://dx.doi.org/10.15585/mmwr.mm6702a1

John, U., Meyer, C., Rumpf, H. J., & Hapke, U. (2004). Smoking, nicotine dependence and psychiatric comorbidity—a population-based study including smoking cessation after three years. *Drug and Alcohol Dependence, 76,* 287–295. http://dx.doi.org/10.1016/j.drugalcdep.2004.06.004

Jorenby, D. E., Hays, J. T., Rigotti, N. A., Azoulay, S., Watsky, E. J., Williams, K. E., . . . Reeves, K. R. (2006). Efficacy of varenicline, an α4β2 nicotinic acetylcholine receptor partial agonist, vs placebo or sustained-release bupropion for smoking cessation: A randomized controlled trial. *Journal of the American Medical Association, 296,* 56–63. http://dx.doi.org/10.1001/jama.296.1.56

Jorenby, D. E., Leischow, S. J., Nides, M. A., Rennard, S. I., Johnston, J. A., Hughes, A. R., . . . Baker, T. B. (1999). A controlled trial of sustained-release bupropion, a nicotine patch, or both for smoking cessation. *The New England Journal of Medicine, 340,* 685–691. http://dx.doi.org/10.1056/NEJM199903043400903

Joseph, A. M. (1996). Nicotine replacement therapy for cardiac patients. *American Journal of Health Behavior, 20*(5), 261–269.

Keltner, N. L., & Grant, J. S. (2006). Smoke, smoke, smoke that cigarette. *Perspectives in Psychiatric Care, 42,* 256–261. http://dx.doi.org/10.1111/j.1744-6163.2006.00085.x

Kim, Y., Myung, S.-K., Jeon, Y.-J., Lee, E.-H., Park, C.-H., Seo, H. G., & Huh, B. Y. (2011). Effectiveness of pharmacologic therapy for smoking cessation in adolescent smokers: Meta-analysis of randomized controlled trials. *American Journal of Health-System Pharmacy, 68,* 219–226. http://dx.doi.org/10.2146/ajhp100296

Koegelenberg, C. F. N., Noor, F., Bateman, E. D., van Zyl-Smit, R. N., Bruning, A., O'Brien, J., . . . Irusen, E. M. (2014). Efficacy of varenicline combined with nicotine replacement therapy vs varenicline alone for smoking cessation: A randomized clinical trial. *JAMA, 312,* 155–161. http://dx.doi.org/10.1001/jama.2014.7195

Lasser, K., Boyd, J. W., Woolhandler, S., Himmelstein, D. U., McCormick, D., & Bor, D. H. (2000). Smoking and mental illness: A population-based prevalence study. *Journal of the American Medical Association, 284,* 2606–2610. http://dx.doi.org/10.1001/jama.284.20.2606

Lerman, C., Kaufmann, V., Rukstalis, M., Patterson, F., Perkins, K., Audrain-McGovern, J., & Benowitz, N. (2004). Individualizing nicotine replacement therapy for the treatment of tobacco dependence: A randomized trial. *Annals of Internal Medicine, 140,* 426–433. http://dx.doi.org/10.7326/0003-4819-140-6-200403160-00009

Liberman, J. N., Lichtenfeld, M. J., Galaznik, A., Mastey, V., Harnett, J., Zou, K. H., . . . Kirchner, H. L. (2013). Adherence to varenicline and associated smoking cessation in a community-based patient setting. *Journal of Managed Care Pharmacy, 19,* 125–131. http://dx.doi.org/10.18553/jmcp.2013.19.2.125

McEwen, A., Hajek, P., McRobbie, H., & West, R. (2006). *Manual of smoking cessation: A guide for counsellors and practitioners.* Oxford, England: Blackwell Publishing. http://dx.doi.org/10.1002/9780470757864

McKee, S. A., Smith, P. H., Kaufman, M., Mazure, C. M., & Weinberger, A. H. (2016). Sex differences in varenicline efficacy for smoking cessation: A meta-analysis. *Nicotine & Tobacco Research, 18,* 1002–1011. http://dx.doi.org/10.1093/ntr/ntv207

Mineur, Y. S., Mose, T. N., Blakeman, S., & Picciotto, M. R. (2018). Hippocampal α7 nicotinic ACh receptors contribute to modulation of depression-like behaviour in C57BL/6J mice. *British Journal of Pharmacology, 175,* 1903–1914. http://dx.doi.org/10.1111/bph.13769

Moolchan, E. T., Robinson, M. L., Ernst, M., Cadet, J. L., Pickworth, W. B., Heishman, S. J., & Schroeder, J. R. (2005). Safety and efficacy of the nicotine patch and gum for the treatment of adolescent tobacco addiction. *Pediatrics, 115,* e407–e414. http://dx.doi.org/10.1542/peds.2004-1894

Munafò, M., Bradburn, M., Bowes, L., & David, S. (2004). Are there sex differences in transdermal nicotine replacement therapy patch efficacy? A meta-analysis. *Nicotine & Tobacco Research, 6,* 769–776. http://dx.doi.org/10.1080/14622200410001696556

Muramoto, M. L., Leischow, S. J., Sherrill, D., Matthews, E., & Strayer, L. J. (2007). Randomized, double-blind, placebo-controlled trial of 2 dosages of sustained-release bupropion for adolescent smoking cessation. *Archives of Pediatric & Adolescent Medicine, 161,* 1068–1074. http://dx.doi.org/10.1001/archpedi.161.11.1068

Oliver, J. A., MacQueen, D. A., & Drobes, D. J. (2013). Deprivation, craving and affect: Intersecting constructs in addiction. In P. Miller (Ed.), *Comprehensive addictive behaviors and disorders: Vol. 1. Principles of addiction* (pp. 395–403). San Diego, CA: Elsevier. http://dx.doi.org/10.1016/B978-0-12-398336-7.00041-3

Palmatier, M. I., Liu, X., Matteson, G. L., Donny, E. C., Caggiula, A. R., & Sved, A. F. (2007). Conditioned reinforcement in rats established with self-administered nicotine and enhanced by noncontingent nicotine. *Psychopharmacology, 195,* 235–243. http://dx.doi.org/10.1007/s00213-007-0897-6

Perkins, K. A. (1996). Sex differences in nicotine versus nonnicotine reinforcement as determinants of tobacco smoking. *Experimental and Clinical Psychopharmacology, 4,* 166–177. http://dx.doi.org/10.1037/1064-1297.4.2.166

Perkins, K. A. (1999). Nicotine discrimination in men and women. *Pharmacology, Biochemistry, and Behavior, 64,* 295–299.

Perkins, K. A., Conklin, C. A., & Levine, M. D. (2008). *Cognitive-behavioral therapy for smoking cessation: A practical guidebook to the most effective treatments.* New York, NY: Routledge.

Perkins, K. A., Donny, E., & Caggiula, A. R. (1999). Sex differences in nicotine effects and self-administration: Review of human and animal evidence. *Nicotine & Tobacco Research, 1,* 301–315. http://dx.doi.org/10.1080/14622299050011431

Perkins, K. A., Jacobs, L., Sanders, M., & Caggiula, A. R. (2002). Sex differences in the subjective and reinforcing effects of cigarette nicotine dose. *Psychopharmacology, 163,* 194–201. http://dx.doi.org/10.1007/s00213-002-1168-1

Perkins, K. A., & Scott, J. (2008). Sex differences in long-term smoking cessation rates due to nicotine patch. *Nicotine & Tobacco Research, 10,* 1245–1250. http://dx.doi.org/10.1080/14622200802097506

*Piper, M. E., Piasecki, T. M., Federman, E. B., Bolt, D. M., Smith, S. S., Fiore, M. C., & Baker, T. B. (2004). A multiple motives approach to tobacco dependence: The Wisconsin Inventory of Smoking Dependence Motives (WISDM-68). *Journal of Consulting and Clinical Psychology, 72,* 139–154. http://dx.doi.org/10.1037/0022-006X.72.2.139

Piper, M. E., Smith, S. S., Schlam, T. R., Fiore, M. C., Jorenby, D. E., Fraser, D., & Baker, T. B. (2009). A randomized placebo-controlled clinical trial of 5 smoking cessation pharmacotherapies. *Archives of General Psychiatry, 66,* 1253–1262. http://dx.doi.org/10.1001/archgenpsychiatry.2009.142

*Prochaska, J. O., DiClemente, C. C., & Norcross, J. C. (1992). In search of how people change: Applications to addictive behaviors. *American Psychologist, 47,* 1102–1114. http://dx.doi.org/10.1037/0003-066X.47.9.1102

Rose, J. E., Behm, F. M., Westman, E. C., & Kukovich, P. (2006). Precessation treatment with nicotine skin patch facilitates smoking cessation. *Nicotine & Tobacco Research, 8,* 89–101. http://dx.doi.org/10.1080/14622200500431866

Rose, J. E., Herskovic, J. E., Behm, F. M., & Westman, E. C. (2009). Precessation treatment with nicotine patch significantly increases abstinence rates relative to conventional treatment. *Nicotine & Tobacco Research, 11,* 1067–1075. http://dx.doi.org/10.1093/ntr/ntp103

Rose, J. E., & Levin, E. D. (1991). Inter-relationships between conditioned and primary reinforcement in the maintenance of cigarette smoking. *British Journal of Addiction, 86,* 605–609. http://dx.doi.org/10.1111/j.1360-0443.1991.tb01816.x

Scharf, D., & Shiffman, S. (2004). Are there gender differences in smoking cessation, with and without bupropion? Pooled- and meta-analyses of clinical trials of bupropion SR. *Addiction, 99*, 1462–1469. http://dx.doi.org/10.1111/j.1360-0443.2004.00845.x

Schnoll, R. A., Goelz, P. M., Veluz-Wilkins, A., Blazekovic, S., Powers, L., Leone, F. T., . . . Hitsman, B. (2015). Long-term nicotine replacement therapy: A randomized clinical trial. *JAMA Internal Medicine, 175*, 504–511.

Shahab, L., & McEwen, A. (2009). Online support for smoking cessation: A systematic review of the literature. *Addiction, 104*, 1792–1804. http://dx.doi.org/10.1111/j.1360-0443.2009.02710.x

Shiffman, S., Brockwell, S. E., Pillitteri, J. L., & Gitchell, J. G. (2008). Use of smoking-cessation treatments in the United States. *American Journal of Preventive Medicine, 34*, 102–111. http://dx.doi.org/10.1016/j.amepre.2007.09.033

*Shiffman, S., Shadel, W. G., Niaura, R., Khayrallah, M. A., Jorenby, D. E., Ryan, C. F., & Ferguson, C. L. (2003). Efficacy of acute administration of nicotine gum in relief of cue-provoked cigarette craving. *Psychopharmacology, 166*, 343–350. http://dx.doi.org/10.1007/s00213-002-1338-1

Shiffman, S., Sweeney, C. T., & Dresler, C. M. (2005). Nicotine patch and lozenge are effective for women. *Nicotine & Tobacco Research, 7*, 119–127. http://dx.doi.org/10.1080/14622200412331328439

*Shiffman, S., Waters, A., & Hickcox, M. (2004). The Nicotine Dependence Syndrome Scale: A multi-dimensional measure of nicotine dependence. *Nicotine & Tobacco Research, 6*, 327–348. http://dx.doi.org/10.1080/1462220042000202481

*Shiffman, S. M., & Jarvik, M. E. (1976). Smoking withdrawal symptoms in two weeks of abstinence. *Psychopharmacology, 50*, 35–39. http://dx.doi.org/10.1007/BF00634151

Smith, P. H., Bessette, A. J., Weinberger, A. H., Sheffer, C. E., & McKee, S. A. (2016). Sex/gender differences in smoking cessation: A review. *Preventive Medicine, 92*, 135–140. http://dx.doi.org/10.1016/j.ypmed.2016.07.013

Stead, L. F., Koilpillai, P., Fanshawe, T. R., & Lancaster, T. (2016). Combined pharmacotherapy and behavioural interventions for smoking cessation. *Cochrane Database of Systematic Reviews, 3*, CD008286.

Stead, L. F., Perera, R., Bullen, C., Mant, D., Hartmann-Boyce, J., Cahill, K., & Lancaster, T. (2012). Nicotine replacement therapy for smoking cessation. *Cochrane Database of Systematic Reviews, 11*, CD000146.

Substance Abuse and Mental Health Services Administration. (2012). *Results from the 2011 National Survey on Drug Use and Health: Mental health findings* (HHS Publication No. SMA 12-4725). Rockville, MD: Author.

Substance Abuse and Mental Health Services Administration. (2014). *Results from the 2013 National Survey on Drug Use and Health: Summary of national findings* (HHS Publication No. SMA 14-4863). Rockville, MD: Author.

Substance Abuse and Mental Health Services Administration. (2015). *Behavioral health trends in the United States: Results from the 2014 National Survey on Drug Use and Health* (HHS Publication No. SMA 15-4927). Retrieved from http://www.samhsa.gov/data/

Swan, G. E., McAfee, T., Curry, S. J., Jack, L. M., Javitz, H., Dacey, S., & Bergman, K. (2003). Effectiveness of bupropion sustained release for smoking cessation in a health care setting: A randomized trial. *Archives of Internal Medicine, 163*, 2337–2344. http://dx.doi.org/10.1001/archinte.163.19.2337

Taylor, G. M. J., Dalili, M. N., Semwal, M., Civljak, M., Sheikh, A., & Car, J. (2017). Internet-based interventions for smoking cessation. *Cochrane Database of Systematic Reviews, 9*(9), CD007078.

*Tiffany, S. T., & Drobes, D. J. (1991). The development and initial validation of a questionnaire on smoking urges. *British Journal of Addiction, 86*, 1467–1476. http://dx.doi.org/10.1111/j.1360-0443.1991.tb01732.x

U.S. Department of Health and Human Services. (2014). *The health consequences of smoking—50 years of progress: A report of the Surgeon General.* Atlanta, GA: Centers for Disease Control and Prevention, National Center for Chronic Disease Prevention and Health Promotion, Office on Smoking and Health.

Weinberger, A. H., & George, T. P. (2006, January). Comorbid tobacco dependence and psychiatric disorders. *Psychiatric Times, 25*. Retrieved from http://www.psychiatrictimes.com/bipolar-disorder/comorbid-tobacco-dependence-and-psychiatric-disorders

Weinberger, A. H., Smith, P. H., Kaufman, M., & McKee, S. A. (2014). Consideration of sex in clinical trials of transdermal nicotine patch: A systematic review. *Experimental and Clinical Psychopharmacology, 22*, 373–383. http://dx.doi.org/10.1037/a0037692

*Wellman, R. J., DiFranza, J. R., Savageau, J. A., Godiwala, S., Friedman, K., & Hazelton, J. (2005). Measuring adults' loss of autonomy over nicotine use: The Hooked on Nicotine Checklist. *Nicotine & Tobacco Research, 7*, 157–161. http://dx.doi.org/10.1080/14622200412331328394

*Welsch, S. K., Smith, S. S., Wetter, D. W., Jorenby, D. E., Fiore, M. C., & Baker, T. B. (1999). Development and validation of the Wisconsin Smoking Withdrawal Scale. *Experimental and Clinical Psychopharmacology, 7*, 354–361. http://dx.doi.org/10.1037/1064-1297.7.4.354

West, R., Hajek, P., Foulds, J., Nilsson, F., May, S., & Meadows, A. (2000). A comparison of the abuse liability and dependence potential of nicotine patch, gum, spray and inhaler. *Psychopharmacology, 149,* 198–202. http://dx.doi.org/10.1007/s002130000382

Wetter, D. W., Kenford, S. L., Smith, S. S., Fiore, M. C., Jorenby, D. E., & Baker, T. B. (1999). Gender differences in smoking cessation. *Journal of Consulting and Clinical Psychology, 67,* 555–562. http://dx.doi.org/10.1037/0022-006X.67.4.555

World Health Organization. (2017). *WHO report on the global tobacco epidemic, 2017: Monitoring tobacco use and prevention policies.* Geneva, Switzerland: Author.

Zawertailo, L., Ragusila, A., Voci, S., Ivanova, A., Baliunas, D., & Selby, P. (2017). Target quit date timing as a predictor of smoking cessation outcomes. *Psychology of Addictive Behaviors, 31,* 655–663. http://dx.doi.org/10.1037/adb0000301

CHAPTER 28

PHARMACOLOGICAL TREATMENT OF BEHAVIORAL ADDICTIONS

*Meredith K. Ginley, Kristyn Zajac, Carla J. Rash,
and Nancy M. Petry*

Certain substance use disorders, such as nicotine, opioid, and alcohol use disorders, have efficacious pharmacotherapies (National Institute on Drug Abuse, 2014). Medications for these disorders largely target neurotransmitter systems affected by the substance of abuse. Behavioral addictions, in contrast, do not involve ingestion of any substance, and their neurophysiology remains elusive. To date, the U.S. Food and Drug Administration (FDA) has not approved any medication to treat a behavioral addiction. However, initial experimental trials of medications for gambling disorder and other putative behavioral addictions have been conducted. In this chapter, we review research on pharmacotherapy for gambling disorder, Internet gaming disorder, and Internet addiction. We also briefly discuss treatments for other potential behavioral addictions (e.g., shopping, eating), although much less data exist on these conditions.

EPIDEMIOLOGY AND PREVALENCE

Debate remains around the evidence for and classification of behavioral addictions. The American Psychiatric Association's Substance Use and Related Disorders Work Group included gambling disorder under the Substance-Related and Addictive Disorder classification in the fifth edition of the *Diagnostic and Statistical Manual of Mental Disorders* (*DSM–5*; American Psychiatric Association, 2013). The work group recommended Internet gaming disorder, a pattern of excessive gaming behavior that results in clinical impairment, as a condition requiring further study in the research appendix of the *DSM–5*. Another condition that has received substantial attention is Internet addiction, which refers to a range of activities that can occur in excess on the Internet, from social network use to shopping and beyond. Internet addiction is not included in the *DSM–5*.

Estimates of the past-year prevalence of gambling disorder range from 0.1% (Bonke & Borregaard, 2006) to 0.7% (Ferris & Wynne, 2001) among studies using nationally representative samples and *DSM*-based criteria. Past-year prevalence rates for Internet gaming disorder obtained from large samples range from 0.3% (Wittek et al., 2016) to 4.9% (Desai, Krishnan-Sarin, Cavallo, & Potenza, 2010). The wide interval in prevalence for this disorder may be due in part to the use of different assessment instruments and criteria across studies. Rates are even more variable for Internet addiction. In studies using large nationally representative samples, prevalence rates for Internet addiction range from 0.6% (Kim et al., 2016) to 22.2% (Ahmadi, 2014). A lack of clear consensus on symptoms or symptom

Dr. Nancy Petry passed away on July 18, 2018. She contributed to all aspects of preparing this chapter for publication. We feel fortunate for all her contributions to the field of behavioral addictions and for her mentorship.

http://dx.doi.org/10.1037/0000133-028
APA Handbook of Psychopharmacology, S. M. Evans (Editor-in-Chief)

thresholds for Internet addiction and a wide range of assessment instruments hinders conclusive prevalence estimates.

From a historical perspective, researchers have been conducting randomized pharmacological treatment studies for gambling disorder for approximately 15 years, although results are far from conclusive. Pharmacological studies for Internet gaming disorder are quite new, with the first randomized trials published in 2012. No large randomized pharmacotherapy trials for Internet addiction have been published to date. Unclear prevalence estimates, symptomology, and illness classifications likely have influenced the timing and rate of initiation of randomized pharmacotherapy trials.

DIAGNOSING BEHAVIORAL ADDICTIONS

Systematic and evidence-based assessments of gambling disorder and Internet gaming disorder are currently available. Standardized criteria for assessment of Internet addiction have not yet been established.

Gambling Disorder

The *DSM–5* gambling disorder diagnostic criteria include (a) excessive thinking about gambling, (b) betting in increasing amounts, (c) being unable to stop or reduce gambling, (d) experiencing withdrawal symptoms when not able to gamble (e.g., craving, irritability, restlessness), (e) gambling to escape negative feelings or situations, (f) gambling more money or for longer periods of time in an attempt to regain past losses, (g) relying on others to cover monetary losses from gambling, (h) lying or covering up gambling, or (i) losing important opportunities or relationships because of gambling. Endorsement of four or more of the nine diagnostic criteria within the past year indicates gambling disorder. In addition, the gambling behavior must not be better explained by a manic episode.

Several self-report assessments of gambling disorder criteria exist. The South Oaks Gambling Screen (SOGS; Lesieur & Blume, 1987) is a widely used self-report screening measure based on *DSM–III–R* criteria and was initially developed for use in treatment-seeking samples. The SOGS generates higher prevalence rates than several other regularly used assessments (Stinchfield, 2002). Other commonly used measures include the Canadian Problem Gambling Index to assess gambling habits and patterns of play (CPGI; Ferris & Wynne, 2001), and a 9-item subset of the scale that focuses on problem severity (referred to as the Problem Gambling Severity Index; PGSI). The CPGI and PGSI are more conservative than the SOGS and are designed to capture gambling-related problems in the general population. However, these measures assess a range of gambling behaviors and associated problems rather than *DSM* criteria (Currie, Hodgins, & Casey, 2013).

Two structured clinical interviews, the National Opinion Research Center Screen DSM–IV Screen for Gambling Problems (NODS; Gerstein et al., 1999) and the Diagnostic Interview for Gambling Severity (DIGS; Winters, Specker, & Stinchfield, 1996), have evidence of validity and reliability (Gerstein et al., 1999; Hodgins, 2004; Stinchfield, Govoni, & Frisch, 2007; Weinstock, Whelan, Meyers, & McCausland, 2007; Wickwire, Burke, Brown, Parker, & May, 2008). Both are based on *DSM–IV* criteria, with the NODS intended to capture gambling-related symptoms in the general population and the DIGS designed for treatment-seeking samples. The NODS can be rescored to capture *DSM–5* gambling disorder diagnosis without reducing internal consistency, and this approach may improve classification accuracy (Petry, Blanco, Stinchfield, & Volberg, 2013).

Internet Gaming Disorder

Internet gaming disorder criteria listed for further study in the *DSM–5* include (a) excessive thinking about gaming, (b) being unable to stop or reduce gaming, (c) loss of interest in other activities, (d) experiencing withdrawal symptoms when not able to game (e.g., restlessness, irritability, difficulty sleeping), (e) gaming to escape negative feelings or situations, (f) needing to game for longer periods of time or needing new equipment or games to get the same enjoyment from gaming, (g) lying or covering up gaming, (h) continued gaming despite problems, or (i) losing important opportunities or relationships because of gaming. The *DSM–5* suggests endorsement of at least five of the nine criteria within the past year, but cautions that these criteria and the cutoff for diagnosis need additional study.

Brief self-report screening instruments for Internet gaming disorder based on *DSM–5* criteria are internally valid: The Video Game Dependency Scale (VGDS; Rehbein, Kliem, Baier, Mößle, & Petry, 2015), the Internet Gaming Disorder-20 Test (IGD-20; Pontes, Király, Demetrovics, & Griffiths, 2014), and the Internet Gaming Disorder Scale (IGD; Lemmens, Valkenburg, & Gentile, 2015) all have some support for their concurrent validity. Two structured clinical interviews based on *DSM–5* criteria for Internet gaming disorder, the Structured Clinical Interview for Internet Gaming Disorder (SCI-IGD; Koo, Han, Park, & Kwon, 2017) and the Diagnostic Criteria of Internet Addiction for College Students (DC-IA-C; Ko et al., 2014), have adequate sensitivity and specificity for classification status. Despite the availability of valid brief self-report screening instruments and structured clinical interviews, many studies rely on various measures of symptom and frequency assessment with little consensus on a standard of measurement.

Internet Addiction

Criteria for Internet addiction are not defined by the *DSM–5* or any other formal consensus. Reflecting the variations in operationalization, studies have used as many as 45 different measures to capture a range of symptoms and constructs related to Internet addiction (Laconi, Rodgers, & Chabrol, 2014). The most frequently used screening measure is the Internet Addiction Test (IAT; Young, 1998a), a 20-item measure modeled after *DSM–IV* substance use dependence and pathological gambling diagnostic criteria. Despite frequent use of the IAT, evaluations reveal mixed findings on its reliability and factor structure validity (Laconi et al., 2014). Although many versions of Internet addiction measures are readily available, determination of the best assessment approach is challenging in the absence of a consensus on diagnostic criteria or defining features.

EVIDENCE-BASED PHARMACOLOGICAL TREATMENTS OF BEHAVIORAL ADDICTIONS

Pharmacological treatments have been evaluated preliminarily for gambling disorder, and to a lesser extent for Internet gaming disorder and Internet addiction.

Neurobiology and Neurochemical Mechanisms

To date, pharmacological trials for behavioral addictions have focused on two medication classes: opioid antagonists and antidepressants.

Opioid antagonists. The reward deficiency theory posits that addictions, including behavioral addictions, stem from genetic variations that lead to a reduction in dopamine receptors in the brain. Decreased dopamine sensitivity in brain regions responsible for excitement and reward lead individuals to seek novel and high-sensation rewards, such as drugs, alcohol, and behaviors like gambling, video gaming, or Internet use, to increase dopamine levels (Blum et al., 1996; Comings & Blum, 2000). Medications that act on the brain regions involved in reward (e.g., opioid antagonists) are successfully used to treat some substance use disorders (Rösner et al., 2010; Veilleux, Colvin, Anderson, York, & Heinz, 2010). Less is known about their effectiveness for treating gambling disorder and other putative behavioral addictions.

Antidepressants. Reduced serotonin function has been linked to increased impulsivity and greater aggression in both animals (Robbins & Dalley, 2017) and humans (Neufang et al., 2016). Drugs that target the serotonergic system are hypothesized to reduce behavioral impulsivity (Grant et al., 2003). Selective serotonin reuptake inhibitors are primarily used to treat depression and anxiety disorders, as well as obsessive-compulsive disorder and attention-deficit/hyperactivity disorder (ADHD), and they may act through increasing the sensitization of dopamine-like receptors in addition to their effects on serotonin (Willner, Hale, & Argyropoulos, 2005).

Treatment of Internet gaming disorder has involved the use of the norepinephrine–dopamine reuptake inhibitor bupropion. This medication is primarily an antidepressant, with additional use in smoking cessation treatment for individuals with or without comorbid depression (Torrens, Fonseca, Mateu, & Farré, 2005). Bupropion acts through increasing extracellular concentrations of both dopamine and norepinephrine, and it may block both peripheral and central nicotine effects (Slemmer, Martin, & Damaj, 2000). Bupropion as a pharmacological treatment option for substance use disorders other than nicotine has had limited success (e.g., cocaine use disorder, Margolin et al., 1995; methamphetamine use disorder, Elkashef et al., 2008).

To identify studies of pharmacological treatments for this chapter, we first specified the scope and limits of our review. Inclusion criteria were that studies (a) use a randomized controlled trial design for a pharmacological treatment targeting gambling disorder, Internet gaming disorder, or Internet addiction; (b) have at least 25 participants per group, a sample size threshold recommended for detecting stable effects (Chambless & Hollon, 1998); (c) have a placebo or no treatment control group; and (d) measure severity of problems, symptoms, or the behavior (either in time or money spent).

We conducted database searches in June 2017 and included all studies published before that date. Studies were excluded if they (a) focused on prevention rather than treatment or (b) were not available in English.

Gambling Disorder

Six placebo-controlled randomized clinical trials of pharmacological treatments for gambling disorder met our criteria (see Table 28.1). Four of these trials evaluated opioid antagonists, and two evaluated selective serotonin reuptake inhibitors. Nearly all trials found no significant treatment effects on symptoms of gambling disorder. In a study of adults with a primary diagnosis of gambling disorder, Grant and colleagues (2006) found that the opioid antagonist nalmefene improved gambling-related symptoms and general clinical impressions compared with placebo. This trial randomized participants to three different nalmefene dosage levels (25, 50, or 100 mg/day) or a placebo control group. The 50 mg/day dosage is commonly used in alcohol treatment (Berg, Pettinati, & Volpicelli, 1996; Morris, Hopwood, Whelan, Gardiner, & Drummond, 2001; Volpicelli et al., 1997). Overall placebo response was high, with 34% of patients classified as responders. Nonetheless, the lowest medication dose condition (25 mg/day) and standard dose condition (50 mg/day) significantly reduced gambling-related symptoms relative to the placebo condition, as measured by the Yale-Brown Obsessive Compulsive Scale Modified for Pathological Gambling (PG-YBOCS;

Pallanti, DeCaria, Grant, Urpe, & Hollander, 2005). However, only the lowest dosage condition significantly improved clinicians' ratings of patients' overall functioning, as measured by the Clinical Global Impression Scale (CGI; Guy, 1976). The highest dose (100 mg/day) yielded no additional therapeutic benefit (Grant et al., 2006) beyond the placebo response.

However, three other studies of opioid antagonists (nalmefene or naltrexone) in adult samples with gambling disorder found no significant benefit in terms of gambling-related symptom reduction or clinician ratings of patient functioning (Grant, Odlaug, Potenza, Hollander, & Kim, 2010; Kovanen et al., 2016; Toneatto, Brands, & Selby, 2009). These trials included a range of medication dosages. Two (Grant et al., 2010; Kovanen et al., 2016) used similar doses as the Grant et al. (2006) study. In the study by Grant and colleagues (2010), 60% of individuals in the placebo group were classified as responders, compared with 47% of those receiving 20 mg/day and 56% of those assigned to 40 mg/day of nalmefene. In the Kovanen et al. (2016) trial, participants were instructed to take naltrexone as needed when experiencing gambling-related urges or cravings, rather than prescribing a daily dose. On average, participants took the naltrexone no more than three times per week. By the end of the treatment period, participants in the placebo group were only taking the medication about two times a week and participants in the naltrexone group only one time per week. Participants in all groups reported a significant reduction in symptoms, with participants in the placebo group having similar rates of symptom reduction compared with those in the active conditions. Participants in the third opioid antagonist trial (Toneatto et al., 2009) had both gambling and alcohol use problems. Daily doses of naltrexone were increased over the course of the trial if self-reports indicated that the medication dosage was not helping to reduce alcohol use. Participants reached a mean medication dosage of 100 mg/day ($SD = 59.4$) of naltrexone. At the 12-month follow-up, a 50% reduction in money spent on gambling was found for both the active treatment and placebo control groups (Toneatto et al., 2009). In all three studies, opioid antagonists reduced gambling-related symptoms at rates similar to placebo controls. Overall, no studies

TABLE 28.1

Evidence-Based Pharmacological Treatments for Behavioral Addictions

First author, year	Treatment	n	Duration (weeks)	Male (%)	Completed treatment (%)	Primary outcome variable(s)	Significant results relative to control or other conditions
Gambling disorder							
Grant, 2003	Placebo	40	16	75	60	PG-YBOCS, CGI	No differences
	Paroxetine (10–60 mg/day)	36	44	58			
Saiz-Ruiz, 2005	Placebo	33	24	90	58	CCPGQ, CGI	No differences
	Sertraline (M = 95 mg/day)	33		90	55		
Grant, 2006	Placebo	51	16	67	47	PG-YBOCS, CGI	Benefits of nalmefene (25 mg/day) and nalmefene (50 mg/day) vs. placebo on PG-YBOCS; benefits of nalmefene (25 mg/day) vs. placebo on CGI
	Nalmefene (25 mg/day)	52		54	37		
	Nalmefene (50 mg/day)	52		56	29		
	Nalmefene (100 mg/day)	52		50	29		
Grant, 2010	Placebo	74	16	58	62	PG-YBOCS, CGI	No differences
	Nalmefene (20 mg/day)	77		(overall)	57		
	Nalmefene (40 mg/day)	82		44			
Toneatto, 2009	Placebo	25	11	93	76	$, Days	No differences
	Naltrexone (25–250 mg/day)	27		(overall)	70		
Kovanen, 2016	Placebo	51	20	59	73	$, Days, PG-YBOCS	No differences
	Naltrexone (50 mg/day)	50		74	64		
Internet gaming disorder							
Han, 2012	Placebo + education	28	8	100	86	Weekly gaming (hr); YIAS	Benefits of bupropion on reductions in gaming time and YIAS vs. placebo
	Bupropion + education	29		100	89		
Song, 2016	No treatment control	33	6	100	Not reported	YIAS, CGI	Benefits of bupropion and escitalopram vs. placebo; benefit of bupropion vs. escitalopram
	Bupropion	44		100			
	Escitalopram	42		100			
Internet addiction							
Dell'Osso, 2008	Placebo	7	9	71	88	Nonessential Internet use (hr/wk);	No differences
	Escitalopram	7		(overall)	77	Obsessive-compulsive Internet use (IC-IUD-YBOCS)	

Note. PG-YBOCS = Yale-Brown Obsessive-Compulsive Scale for Pathological Gambling; CGI = Clinical Global Impression Scale; CCPGQ = Criteria for Control of Pathological Gambling Questionnaire; $ = gambling-related expenditures; Days = frequency of days with gambling behavior; hr = hours; YIAS = Young Internet Addiction Scale; wk = week; IC-IUD-YBOCS = impulsive-compulsive Internet usage disorder Yale-Brown Obsessive Compulsive Scale.

support the use of naltrexone at the higher dose (i.e., 100 mg/day), and support for its efficacy at lower dosages is mixed at best (Grant et al., 2006, 2010).

The other studies (Grant et al., 2003; Saiz-Ruiz et al., 2005) evaluated the antidepressants paroxetine and sertraline in samples of adults with gambling disorder and found no posttreatment differences in gambling disorder symptoms or clinician ratings of patient functioning between medications and placebo. Sixty-seven percent of paroxetine treatment completers were classified as responders compared with 63% of those treated with placebo (Grant et al., 2003). Similarly, 74% of the sertraline-treated completers were classified as responders compared with 72% of those treated with placebo (Saiz-Ruiz et al., 2005).

Internet Gaming Disorder

Two randomized trials of pharmacological treatments for Internet gaming disorder met inclusion criteria for this review (Han & Renshaw, 2012; Song et al., 2016; see Table 28.1). These trials evaluated selective serotonin reuptake inhibitor and norepinephrine–dopamine reuptake inhibitor class antidepressant medications in male samples. In a sample of adolescents and young adults with comorbid Internet gaming disorder and major depressive disorder, the antidepressant bupropion plus an educational intervention resulted in significant reductions in time spent gaming and Internet gaming disorder symptoms compared with placebo plus an educational intervention (Han & Renshaw, 2012). Reductions in symptoms were maintained at 4-week follow-up in both the medication and placebo groups. Improvements in symptoms of Internet gaming disorder and depression were significantly correlated across both conditions (Han & Renshaw, 2012). Because the sample had comorbid depression, the efficacy of bupropion for individuals with Internet gaming disorder with no other psychiatric disorders remains unclear. It is possible that bupropion reduced depression symptoms, which in turn indirectly improved gaming symptoms. Thus, these results are not necessarily generalizable to individuals with Internet gaming disorder who do not have comorbid depression.

Song and colleagues (2016) randomly assigned adolescent and young adult participants to one of two medication groups: bupropion or the anti-depressant escitalopram. Participants who declined further treatment (i.e., agreed to study assessments but elected not to take any medication) were not randomized. These participants were instead followed over time as a no-treatment comparison group. Both bupropion and escitalopram reduced symptoms of Internet gaming disorder compared with the no-treatment group. Participants receiving bupropion had a significantly greater reduction in clinician-rated symptom severity and larger improvements in overall functioning as measured by the CGI (Guy, 1976) than those receiving escitalopram. Important differences between the medication groups relative to the control group, particularly the unwillingness of participants in the control condition to be randomized to a medication condition, could have influenced the findings. In addition, because this study did not include a placebo control to rule out potential expectancy effects, it is difficult to draw conclusions about the efficacy of either medication.

Internet Addiction

No pharmacological treatments for Internet addiction met inclusion criteria. One randomized trial of escitalopram for Internet addiction was identified (Dell'Osso et al., 2008), but it included only seven adult participants per condition. Hours spent on nonessential Internet use and symptoms of obsessive and compulsive Internet use did not differ between escitalopram and placebo conditions, with a significant decrease in both hours per week of Internet use and Internet addiction symptoms compared with baseline in both conditions.

Overall, we did not find evidence that any class of medication is efficacious for treating behavioral addictions. The neurobiological regions or neurochemical processes responsible for behavioral addictions remain unclear. It is possible that the prefrontal cortex and striatum are desensitized to reward in individuals with behavioral addictions compared with controls (Weng et al., 2013; Yuan et al., 2013; Zois et al., 2017). However, neither targeting dopamine, as suggested by the reward deficiency theory, nor serotonin via antidepressants appears to be sufficient for creating behavior change, at least not in the studies conducted to date.

BEST APPROACHES FOR ASSESSING TREATMENT RESPONSE AND MANAGING SIDE EFFECTS

Valid self-report and structured clinical interview assessments based on diagnostic criteria are commonly used for determining inclusion into pharmacotherapy treatment trials (see earlier section of this chapter on Diagnosing Behavioral Addictions); however, the most commonly used assessment of treatment response across all pharmacological treatment studies for behavioral addictions was the CGI (Guy, 1976), a measure of clinician-reported symptom severity. A trained clinician completes the CGI subjective report of symptom severity improvement after a patient initiates pharmacotherapy. Per the assessment instructions, the rater judges the severity of each patient in the context of the rater's experience with the symptom severity of the patient population under study. Ratings of improvement can range from 1 (*very much improved*) to 7 (*very much worse*). Patients rated 1 or 2 are generally considered treatment responders (Guy, 1976).

Measures tied to symptom severity for specific behavioral or putative behavioral addictions have also been used to assess treatment response. For the assessment of gambling disorder symptom severity, the PG-YBOCS is a 10-item measure that captures severity of thoughts, urges, and behaviors related to gambling (Pallanti et al., 2005). The PG-YBOCS has validity and reliability in treatment-seeking samples as well as good sensitivity to change in gambling symptom severity (Pallanti et al., 2005). For Internet gaming disorder, the Young Internet Addiction Scale (YIAS; Young, 1998b), a self-report measure modeled after *DSM–IV* criteria for pathological gambling, has been used in pharmacological studies (Han & Renshaw, 2012; Park, Lee, Sohn, & Han, 2016; Song et al., 2016). However, instead of measuring symptoms specific to Internet gaming disorder, the YIAS measures symptoms associated with Internet overuse more generally and not exclusively for gaming.

Management of side effects from medications to treat behavioral addictions have been handled on a medication-by-medication and trial-by-trial basis, with very limited information provided about side effects in trials for Internet gaming disorder. In trials reporting medication side effects, antidepressants were generally found to be well tolerated, with low dropout rates due to side effects (Dell'Osso et al., 2008; Grant et al., 2003; Saiz-Ruiz et al., 2005). Most side effects from opioid antagonists were found to be mild to moderate (Kovanen et al., 2016, Toneatto et al., 2009). The two studies that reported dropout rates by nalmefene medication dosage (Grant et al., 2006, 2010) reported that higher dosages corresponded with higher percentages of dropouts due to side effects. The most commonly reported side effects were nausea, insomnia, and dizziness (Grant et al., 2006). Current side effect management recommendations for pharmacological treatment of behavioral addictions do not exist, and any future recommendations should first consider evidence for the efficacy of the therapeutic invention.

MEDICATION MANAGEMENT ISSUES

As with many chronic conditions (McLellan, Lewis, O'Brien, & Kleber, 2000), dropout rates in addictions treatment often reach or exceed 50% (Dutra et al., 2008; Stahler, Mennis, & DuCette, 2016), leaving many individuals without a full treatment dose. The mean dropout rates in pharmacotherapy trials for gambling disorder ranged from 27% (Toneatto et al., 2009) to 65% (Grant et al., 2006) across the six studies included in this review. These dropout rates are similar to those from a large nalmefene trial in patients with alcohol use disorder (38% in nalmefene-treated patients; Gual et al., 2013). Dropout rates in the treatment of Internet gaming disorder and Internet addiction, when reported, were lower than dropout rates for gambling disorder treatment. However, conclusions about differences in dropout rates across populations cannot be made due to differences in samples (e.g., age, comorbidity) and study designs.

EVALUATION OF PHARMACOLOGICAL APPROACHES ACROSS THE LIFESPAN

Gambling disorder rates are highest among individuals in their 20s and 30s (Welte, Barnes, Tidwell, & Hoffman, 2011), but treatment-seeking samples tend to be older, with a mean age of 42 years (Granero et al., 2014). The majority of systematic studies of pharmacotherapy approaches for gambling disorder have focused on participants in their mid-40s (Grant et al., 2003, 2006, 2010; Kovanen et al., 2016), capturing the population most likely to be seeking treatment for gambling disorder (Granero et al., 2014).

Internet gaming disorder is primarily a problem of adolescence and young adulthood (Haagsma, Pieterse, & Peters, 2012; Mentzoni et al., 2011). The randomized pharmacotherapy trials for Internet gaming disorder have focused on adolescents and young adults in their late teens to early 20s (Han & Renshaw, 2012; Park et al., 2016; Song et al., 2016). This age range is also consistent with the age range of individuals most afflicted by this problem.

In a large sample of individuals aged 18 to 65 years assessed for Internet addition, younger age was associated with higher rates of problematic use (Kim et al., 2016). In the only known pharmacological study of Internet addiction (Dell'Osso et al., 2008), the participants were in their late 30s on average. Future studies of pharmacological approaches for behavioral addictions across the lifespan thus may enhance their relevance by targeting the age cohorts most affected by these conditions.

CONSIDERATION OF POTENTIAL SEX DIFFERENCES

Gambling disorder is more prevalent in males than females (Petry, Stinson, & Grant, 2005), and males also have an earlier age of onset (Grant & Kim, 2002). Women may be more likely to progress quickly to becoming symptomatic and to seek treatment sooner after symptoms manifest, although this pattern is not consistent in all samples (Grant, Chamberlain, Schreiber, & Odlaug, 2012; Grant & Kim, 2002). Gambling preferences also vary by sex, with women more likely to gamble primarily on slot machines, and men reporting higher frequencies of betting on cards, sports, and animals (Grant & Kim, 2002). In their meta-analysis of pharmacological treatment trials for pathological gambling, Pallesen and colleagues (2007) found that studies with a greater proportion of male participants had smaller treatment effect sizes. It is possible the improved treatment outcomes for female gamblers are due to

genetic or physiological differences or the nature and course of symptoms.

Similarly, males, particularly adolescent males, are significantly more likely to develop Internet gaming disorder than females (Festl, Scharkow, & Quandt, 2013; Wittek et al., 2016). Pharmacological treatment studies have primarily focused on male samples, with little to no data available on females' responses to pharmacotherapy.

Internet addiction may be equally prevalent in males and females (Durkee et al., 2012), although similar to gambling disorder, the expression may differ by sex. Females are significantly more likely to overuse social networking websites (Andreassen & Pallesen, 2014; Dufour et al., 2016), whereas males tend to use online games and sexual sites excessively (Dufour et al., 2016). As with Internet gaming disorder, the literature is too limited to point to trends in sex differences in pharmacological treatment response.

INTEGRATION OF PHARMACOTHERAPY WITH NONPHARMACOLOGICAL APPROACHES: BENEFITS AND CHALLENGES

According to reviews of psychotherapy for gambling disorder, cognitive behavior therapy (CBT) has the most evidence of efficacy for reduction of gambling-related symptoms (Oei, Raylu, & Casey, 2010; Pallesen, Mitsem, Kvale, Johnsen, & Molde, 2005; Petry et al., 2006; Petry, Ginley, & Rash, 2017; Toneatto & Ladoceur, 2003). CBT for gambling disorder typically focuses on the identification of internal and external cues for gambling, exploring cognitive distortions related to gambling (e.g., beliefs about luck, illusions of control), developing and practicing alternative responses when faced with cues and triggers, and exploring alternatives to gambling (see Petry, 2005). Long-term therapy or inpatient treatment is likely unnecessary for patients without additional complications, such as comorbid psychiatric or substance use disorders (Toneatto & Ladoceur, 2003). Further, for individuals who are not seeking treatment or are experiencing lower severity symptoms, brief motivational or feedback interventions have some support (Larimer et al.,

2012; Martens, Arterberry, Takamatsu, Masters, & Dude, 2015; Neighbors et al., 2015; Petry, Rash, & Alessi, 2016; Petry, Weinstock, Ledgerwood, & Morasco, 2008).

Randomized psychotherapy trials for Internet gaming disorder and Internet addiction are limited. Our recent review of the treatment literature (Zajac, Ginley, Chang, & Petry, 2017), along with other reviews for Internet gaming disorder and Internet addiction (King & Delfabbro, 2014; Kuss & Lopez-Fernandez, 2016; Przepiorka, Blachnio, Miziak, & Czuczwar, 2014; Winkler, Dörsing, Rief, Shen, & Glombiewski, 2013), found that all treatments for these behavioral addictions are currently considered "experimental" per the Chambless et al. (1998) criteria for treatment efficacy. This classification means there have not been sufficient well-controlled studies that show the superiority of a treatment compared with a wait-list control or another treatment. The majority of studies identified focused on CBT and family therapy; however, few found any evidence of differential symptom reduction, and many were limited by methodological design issues and lack of standardized measurement of outcomes. Approaches that integrate pharmacotherapy and psychotherapy for behavioral addictions have not received enough research attention to warrant any recommendations.

INTEGRATED APPROACHES FOR ADDRESSING COMMON COMORBID DISORDERS

Estimates of comorbidity between gambling disorder and substance use disorders have been as high as 76% in a nationally representative sample (Kessler et al., 2008), and the severity of gambling symptoms corresponds with increased severity of substance use problems. Nicotine use disorder is most common, with rates around 60% (Kessler et al., 2008; Lorains, Cowlishaw, & Thomas, 2011). Rates of comorbid alcohol use disorder are estimated at 28%, followed by rates for an illicit drug use disorder (17%; Lorains et al., 2011). Additionally, comorbidity of gambling disorders with mood (38%) and anxiety disorders (37%) is common (Lorains et al., 2011). Medications that address a specific comorbidity—

bipolar disorders—may reduce both gambling- and mania-related symptoms (Hollander, Pallanti, Allen, Sood, & Baldini Rossi, 2005). However, research on pharmacotherapy approaches for other conditions commonly comorbid with gambling disorder is limited. CBT targeting problem gambling has shown some success in reducing symptoms beyond the gambling disorder itself (e.g., depressive symptomology; Carlbring & Smit, 2008; Petry et al., 2006). Additionally, in a sample of substance use disorder treatment patients who screened positive for gambling-related problems, individuals randomly assigned to a CBT intervention that included motivational interviewing had significant reductions in money wagered and gambling symptoms compared with patients randomly assigned to a brief advice control. This significant between-condition effect remained over a 2-year follow-up (Petry et al., 2016).

Comorbidity is common between Internet gaming disorder and depression (Desai et al., 2010; Gentile et al., 2011; van Rooij, Schoenmakers, Vermulst, van den Eijnden, & van de Mheen, 2011), anxiety (Gentile et al., 2011; van Rooij et al., 2014), and ADHD (Choo et al., 2010; Gentile et al., 2011; Walther, Morgenstern, & Hanewinkel, 2012). Internet gaming disorder has also been linked to cigarette smoking and other substance use disorders (Desai et al., 2010; van Rooij et al., 2014; Walther et al., 2012). Pharmacological studies of Internet gaming disorder have focused on the treatment of comorbid major depressive disorder and comorbid ADHD. For individuals with comorbid major depressive disorder, treatment with antidepressants may reduce gaming time, Internet gaming disorder symptoms, and depression (Han & Renshaw, 2012). A study of adolescents with comorbid Internet gaming disorder and ADHD compared two medications typically prescribed for ADHD: a norepinephrine reuptake inhibitor (atomoxetine) and a central nervous system stimulant (methylphenidate). Both medications reduced gaming-related symptoms and impulsivity. However, this trial did not include a placebo control group, limiting interpretation of findings (Park et al., 2016). Efforts made in pharmacological treatment studies to include populations with common comorbid conditions are beneficial for understanding the treatment of co-occurring symptomology.

Carli and colleagues (2013) found 20 studies that evaluated comorbidity between Internet addiction and other mental health conditions, including ADHD, major depressive disorder, anxiety disorders, and obsessive-compulsive disorders. As with gambling disorder and Internet gaming disorder, comorbidity between Internet addiction and alcohol use disorders are common (Ko et al., 2008; Yen, Ko, Yen, Chen, & Chen, 2009). However, we did not identify any treatment trials of pharmacotherapies or integrated approaches for the treatment of Internet addiction and comorbid conditions.

EMERGING TRENDS

Few randomized clinical trials on pharmacological treatments for behavioral addictions, particularly for Internet gaming disorder and Internet addiction, are available, perhaps due to how recently these conditions have been described. Gambling disorder is the only behavioral addiction included in the Substance Use and Other Addictive Behaviors section of the *DSM–5*. Internet gaming disorder is listed as a condition needing further study. Internet addiction remains unclassified.

Standardized assessment measures based on *DSM–5* criteria for behavioral addictions are limited. Currently, only gambling disorder has valid interviews and assessment measures of symptoms. With Internet gaming disorder, consistent measurement of symptoms is now possible with the *DSM–5* criteria. However, different interpretations and operationalizations of the criteria exist (Petry et al., 2014). Consensus agreement on the symptoms of Internet addiction should precede the development and validation of assessment measures. Additionally, future research should focus on studies that capture or rule out the specific and lasting adverse impacts from Internet overuse not better accounted for by another mental health condition or addictive disorder.

Initial operationalization exists for several other potential behavioral addictions, including shopping, exercise, sex, eating, and tanning. Like Internet addiction, the literature on these conditions has a range of established criteria and assessment measures, and few, if any, systematically evaluated pharmacological or psychotherapeutic interventions (Petry & O'Brien,

2013; Starcevic & Khazaal, 2017). Prevalence rates for these conditions are not yet established. Several of them may represent permutations of existing mental health conditions. For example, sex addiction may have more symptom overlap with sexual dysfunction disorders than behavioral addictions. Eating addiction may better align with eating disorder–related diagnoses than behavioral addictions. Shopping addiction may be more closely related to obsessive-compulsive disorder or hoarding disorder than behavioral addictions. Treatment recommendations for these behavioral patterns will likely correspond with the interventions for the mental health condition with which these symptoms most closely align.

In conclusion, no pharmacological treatment for any behavioral addiction is approved by the FDA or has demonstrated efficacy in more than one placebo-controlled randomized trial. However, psychosocial interventions for gambling disorder do have support, with CBT providing the most consistently favorable outcomes (see Tool Kit of Resources). An emerging trend in the area of gambling disorder treatment is a focus on brief, Internet-based psychotherapy delivery to increase treatment accessibility and acceptability (Casey et al., 2017; Toneatto, 2016). For the treatment of Internet gaming disorder and Internet addiction, no pharmacological treatment is efficacious, nor is sufficient evidence available regarding psychosocial interventions for these conditions. The development of valid measures for Internet gaming disorder and a consensus about the symptoms of Internet addiction will enhance future research on pharmacological and psychotherapeutic treatments for these conditions.

TOOL KIT OF RESOURCES

Behavioral Addictions

Patient Resources

National Council on Problem Gambling: http://www.ncpgambling.org/

Petry, N. M. (2019). *Pause and reset: A parent's guide to preventing and overcoming problems with gaming.* New York, NY: Oxford University Press.

ReSTART: Residential Treatment for Problematic Use: https://netaddictionrecovery.com

Your First Step to Change: http://s96539219.onlinehome.us/toolkits/FirstStepSite/main.htm

Provider Resources

Kuss, D. J., & Lopez-Fernandez, O. (2016). Internet addiction and problematic Internet use: A systematic review of clinical research. *World Journal of Psychiatry, 22,* 143–176.

Petry, N. M. (2005). *Pathological gambling: Etiology, comorbidity, and treatment.* Washington, DC: American Psychological Association.

Petry, N. M., Ginley, M. K., & Rash, C. J. (2017). A systematic review of treatments for problem gambling. *Psychology of Addictive Behaviors, 31,* 951–961.

Petry, N. M., Rehbein, F., Gentile, D. A., Lemmens, J. S., Rumpf, H. J., Mößle, T., . . . Auriacombe, M. (2014). An international consensus for assessing Internet gaming disorder using the new *DSM–5* approach. *Addiction, 109,* 1399–1406.

Przepiorka, A. M., Blachnio, A., Miziak, B., & Czuzcwar, S. J. (2014). Clinical approaches to treatment of Internet addiction. *Pharmacological Reviews, 66,* 187–191.

Zajac, K., Ginley, M. K., Chang, R., & Petry, N. M. (2017). Treatments for Internet gaming disorder and Internet addiction: A systematic review. *Psychology of Addictive Behaviors, 31,* 979–994.

References

Ahmadi, K. (2014). Internet addiction among Iranian adolescents: A nationwide study. *Acta Medica Iranica, 52,* 467–472.

American Psychiatric Association. (2013). *Diagnostic and statistical manual of mental disorders* (5th ed.). Washington, DC: Author.

Andreassen, C. S., & Pallesen, S. (2014). Social network site addiction: An overview. *Current Pharmaceutical Design, 20,* 4053–4061. http://dx.doi.org/10.2174/13816128113199990616

Berg, B. J., Pettinati, H. M., & Volpicelli, J. R. (1996). A risk-benefit assessment of naltrexone in the treatment of alcohol dependence. *Drug Safety, 15,* 274–282. http://dx.doi.org/10.2165/00002018-199615040-00005

Blum, K., Sheridan, P. J., Wood, R. C., Braverman, E. R., Chen, T. J., Cull, J. G., & Comings, D. E. (1996). The D$_2$ dopamine receptor gene as a determinant of reward deficiency syndrome. *Journal of the Royal Society of Medicine, 89,* 396–400. http://dx.doi.org/10.1177/014107689608900711

Bonke, J., & Borregaard, K. (2006). *The prevalence and heterogeneity of at-risk and pathological gamblers: The Danish case.* Copenhagen, Denmark: The Danish National Institute of Social Research.

Carlbring, P., & Smit, F. (2008). Randomized trial of Internet-delivered self-help with telephone support for pathological gamblers. *Journal of Consulting and Clinical Psychology, 76,* 1090–1094. http://dx.doi.org/10.1037/a0013603

Carli, V., Durkee, T., Wasserman, D., Hadlaczky, G., Despalins, R., Kramarz, E., . . . Kaess, M. (2013). The association between pathological Internet use and comorbid psychopathology: A systematic review. *Psychopathology, 46,* 1–13. http://dx.doi.org/10.1159/000337971

Casey, L. M., Oei, T. P. S., Raylu, N., Horrigan, K., Day, J., Ireland, M., & Clough, B. A. (2017). Internet-based delivery of cognitive behaviour therapy compared to monitoring, feedback and support for problem gambling: A randomised controlled trial. *Journal of Gambling Studies, 33,* 993–1010. http://dx.doi.org/10.1007/s10899-016-9666-y

Chambless, D. L., Baker, M. J., Baucom, D. H., Beutler, L. E., Calhoun, K. S., Crits-Christoph, P., & Woody, S. R. (1998). Update on empirically validated therapies, II. *The Clinical Psychologist, 51*(1), 3–16.

Chambless, D. L., & Hollon, S. D. (1998). Defining empirically supported therapies. *Journal of Consulting and Clinical Psychology, 66,* 7–18. http://dx.doi.org/10.1037/0022-006X.66.1.7

Choo, H., Gentile, D. A., Sim, T., Li, D., Khoo, A., & Liau, A. K. (2010). Pathological video-gaming among Singaporean youth. *Annals of the Academy of Medicine, Singapore, 39,* 822–829.

Comings, D. E., & Blum, K. (2000). Reward deficiency syndrome: Genetic aspects of behavioral disorders. *Progress in Brain Research, 126,* 325–341. http://dx.doi.org/10.1016/S0079-6123(00)26022-6

Currie, S. R., Hodgins, D. C., & Casey, D. M. (2013). Validity of the Problem Gambling Severity Index interpretive categories. *Journal of Gambling Studies, 29,* 311–327. http://dx.doi.org/10.1007/s10899-012-9300-6

Dell'Osso, B., Hadley, S., Allen, A., Baker, B., Chaplin, W. F., & Hollander, E. (2008). Escitalopram in the treatment of impulsive-compulsive Internet usage disorder: An open-label trial followed by a double-blind discontinuation phase. *The Journal of Clinical Psychiatry, 69,* 452–456. http://dx.doi.org/10.4088/JCP.v69n0316

*Asterisks indicate assessments or resources.

Ginley et al.

Desai, R. A., Krishnan-Sarin, S., Cavallo, D., & Potenza, M. N. (2010). Video-gaming among high school students: Health correlates, gender differences, and problematic gaming. *Pediatrics, 126*, e1414–e1424. http://dx.doi.org/10.1542/peds.2009-2706

Dufour, M., Brunelle, N., Tremblay, J., Leclerc, D., Cousineau, M. M., Khazaal, Y., . . . Berbiche, D. (2016). Gender differences in Internet use and Internet problems among Quebec high school students. *The Canadian Journal of Psychiatry, 61*, 663–668. http://dx.doi.org/10.1177/0706743716640755

Durkee, T., Kaess, M., Carli, V., Parzer, P., Wasserman, C., Floderus, B., . . . Wasserman, D. (2012). Prevalence of pathological Internet use among adolescents in Europe: Demographic and social factors. *Addiction, 107*, 2210–2222. http://dx.doi.org/10.1111/j.1360-0443.2012.03946.x

Dutra, L., Stathopoulou, G., Basden, S. L., Leyro, T. M., Powers, M. B., & Otto, M. W. (2008). A meta-analytic review of psychosocial interventions for substance use disorders. *The American Journal of Psychiatry, 165*, 179–187. http://dx.doi.org/10.1176/appi.ajp.2007.06111851

Elkashef, A. M., Rawson, R. A., Anderson, A. L., Li, S. H., Holmes, T., Smith, E. V., . . . Weis, D. (2008). Bupropion for the treatment of methamphetamine dependence. *Neuropsychopharmacology, 33*, 1162–1170. http://dx.doi.org/10.1038/sj.npp.1301481

Ferris, J. A., & Wynne, H. J. (2001). *The Canadian Problem Gambling Index*. Ottawa, ON: Canadian Centre on Substance Abuse.

Festl, R., Scharkow, M., & Quandt, T. (2013). Problematic computer game use among adolescents, younger and older adults. *Addiction, 108*, 592–599. http://dx.doi.org/10.1111/add.12016

Gentile, D. A., Choo, H., Liau, A., Sim, T., Li, D., Fung, D., & Khoo, A. (2011). Pathological video game use among youths: A two-year longitudinal study. *Pediatrics, 127*, e319–e329. http://dx.doi.org/10.1542/peds.2010-1353

Gerstein, D., Volberg, R. A., Toce, M. T., Harwood, H., Johnson, R. A., Buie, T., & Hill, M. A. (1999). *Gambling Impact and Behavior Study: Report to the National Gambling Impact Study commission*. Chicago, IL: National Opinion Research Center.

Granero, R., Penelo, E., Stinchfield, R., Fernandez-Aranda, F., Savvidou, L. G., Fröberg, F., . . . Jiménez-Murcia, S. (2014). Is pathological gambling moderated by age? *Journal of Gambling Studies, 30*, 475–492.

Grant, J. E., Chamberlain, S. R., Schreiber, L. R., & Odlaug, B. L. (2012). Gender-related clinical and neurocognitive differences in individuals seeking treatment for pathological gambling. *Journal of Psychiatric Research, 46*, 1206–1211. http://dx.doi.org/10.1016/j.jpsychires.2012.05.013

Grant, J. E., & Kim, S. W. (2002). Gender differences in pathological gamblers seeking medication treatment. *Comprehensive Psychiatry, 43*, 56–62. http://dx.doi.org/10.1053/comp.2002.29857

Grant, J. E., Kim, S. W., Potenza, M. N., Blanco, C., Ibanez, A., Stevens, L., . . . Zaninelli, R. (2003). Paroxetine treatment of pathological gambling: A multi-centre randomized controlled trial. *International Clinical Psychopharmacology, 18*, 243–249. http://dx.doi.org/10.1097/00004850-200307000-00007

Grant, J. E., Odlaug, B. L., Potenza, M. N., Hollander, E., & Kim, S. W. (2010). Nalmefene in the treatment of pathological gambling: Multicentre, double-blind, placebo-controlled study. *The British Journal of Psychiatry, 197*, 330–331. http://dx.doi.org/10.1192/bjp.bp.110.078105

Grant, J. E., Potenza, M. N., Hollander, E., Cunningham-Williams, R., Nurminen, T., Smits, G., & Kallio, A. (2006). Multicenter investigation of the opioid antagonist nalmefene in the treatment of pathological gambling. *The American Journal of Psychiatry, 163*, 303–312. http://dx.doi.org/10.1176/appi.ajp.163.2.303

Gual, A., He, Y., Torup, L., van den Brink, W., Mann, K., & the ESENSE 2 Study Group. (2013). A randomised, double-blind, placebo-controlled, efficacy study of nalmefene, as-needed use, in patients with alcohol dependence. *European Neuropsychopharmacology, 23*, 1432–1442. http://dx.doi.org/10.1016/j.euroneuro.2013.02.006

Guy, W. (1976). *ECDEU assessment manual for psychopharmacology*. Rockville, MD: US Department of Health, and Welfare.

Haagsma, M. C., Pieterse, M. E., & Peters, O. (2012). The prevalence of problematic video gamers in the Netherlands. *Cyberpsychology, Behavior, and Social Networking, 15*, 162–168. http://dx.doi.org/10.1089/cyber.2011.0248

Han, D. H., & Renshaw, P. F. (2012). Bupropion in the treatment of problematic online game play in patients with major depressive disorder. *Journal of Psychopharmacology, 26*, 689–696. http://dx.doi.org/10.1177/0269881111400647

Hodgins, D. C. (2004). Using the NORC DSM Screen for Gambling Problems as an outcome measure for pathological gambling: Psychometric evaluation. *Addictive Behaviors, 29*, 1685–1690. http://dx.doi.org/10.1016/j.addbeh.2004.03.017

Hollander, E., Pallanti, S., Allen, A., Sood, E., & Baldini Rossi, N. (2005). Does sustained-release lithium reduce impulsive gambling and affective instability versus placebo in pathological gamblers with bipolar spectrum disorders? *The American Journal of Psychiatry, 162*, 137–145. http://dx.doi.org/10.1176/appi.ajp.162.1.137

Kessler, R. C., Hwang, I., LaBrie, R., Petukhova, M., Sampson, N. A., Winters, K. C., & Shaffer, H. J.

(2008). *DSM–IV* pathological gambling in the National Comorbidity Survey Replication. *Psychological Medicine, 38,* 1351–1360. http://dx.doi.org/10.1017/S0033291708002900

Kim, B. S., Chang, S. M., Park, J. E., Seong, S. J., Won, S. H., & Cho, M. J. (2016). Prevalence, correlates, psychiatric comorbidities, and suicidality in a community population with problematic Internet use. *Psychiatry Research, 244,* 249–256. http://dx.doi.org/10.1016/j.psychres.2016.07.009

King, D. L., & Delfabbro, P. H. (2014). Internet gaming disorder treatment: A review of definitions of diagnosis and treatment outcome. *Journal of Clinical Psychology, 70,* 942–955. http://dx.doi.org/10.1002/jclp.22097

Ko, C. H., Yen, J. Y., Chen, S. H., Wang, P. W., Chen, C. S., & Yen, C. F. (2014). Evaluation of the diagnostic criteria of Internet gaming disorder in the *DSM–5* among young adults in Taiwan. *Journal of Psychiatric Research, 53,* 103–110. http://dx.doi.org/10.1016/j.jpsychires.2014.02.008

Ko, C. H., Yen, J. Y., Yen, C. F., Chen, C. S., Weng, C. C., & Chen, C. C. (2008). The association between Internet addiction and problematic alcohol use in adolescents: The problem behavior model. *CyberPsychology & Behavior, 11,* 571–576. http://dx.doi.org/10.1089/cpb.2007.0199

Koo, H. J., Han, D. H., Park, S. Y., & Kwon, J. H. (2017). The Structured Clinical Interview for DSM–5 Internet gaming disorder: Development and validation for diagnosing IGD in adolescents. *Psychiatry Investigation, 14,* 21–29. http://dx.doi.org/10.4306/pi.2017.14.1.21

Kovanen, L., Basnet, S., Castrén, S., Pankakoski, M., Saarikoski, S. T., Partonen, T., . . . Lahti, T. (2016). A randomised, double-blind, placebo-controlled trial of as-needed naltrexone in the treatment of pathological gambling. *European Addiction Research, 22,* 70–79. http://dx.doi.org/10.1159/000435876

*Kuss, D. J., & Lopez-Fernandez, O. (2016). Internet addiction and problematic Internet use: A systematic review of clinical research. *World Journal of Psychiatry, 6,* 143–176. http://dx.doi.org/10.5498/wjp.v6.i1.143

Laconi, S., Rodgers, R. F., & Chabrol, H. (2014). The measurement of Internet addiction: A critical review of existing scales and their psychometric properties. *Computers in Human Behavior, 41,* 190–202. http://dx.doi.org/10.1016/j.chb.2014.09.026

Larimer, M. E., Neighbors, C., Lostutter, T. W., Whiteside, U., Cronce, J. M., Kaysen, D., & Walker, D. D. (2012). Brief motivational feedback and cognitive behavioral interventions for prevention of disordered gambling: A randomized clinical trial. *Addiction, 107,* 1148–1158. http://dx.doi.org/10.1111/j.1360-0443.2011.03776.x

Lemmens, J. S., Valkenburg, P. M., & Gentile, D. A. (2015). The Internet Gaming Disorder Scale. *Psychological Assessment, 27,* 567–582. http://dx.doi.org/10.1037/pas0000062

Lesieur, H. R., & Blume, S. B. (1987). The South Oaks Gambling Screen (SOGS): A new instrument for the identification of pathological gamblers. *The American Journal of Psychiatry, 144,* 1184–1188. http://dx.doi.org/10.1176/ajp.144.9.1184

Lorains, F. K., Cowlishaw, S., & Thomas, S. A. (2011). Prevalence of comorbid disorders in problem and pathological gambling: Systematic review and meta-analysis of population surveys. *Addiction, 106,* 490–498. http://dx.doi.org/10.1111/j.1360-0443.2010.03300.x

Margolin, A., Kosten, T. R., Avants, S. K., Wilkins, J., Ling, W., Beckson, M., . . . Bridge, P. (1995). A multicenter trial of bupropion for cocaine dependence in methadone-maintained patients. *Drug and Alcohol Dependence, 40,* 125–131. http://dx.doi.org/10.1016/0376-8716(95)01198-6

Martens, M. P., Arterberry, B. J., Takamatsu, S. K., Masters, J., & Dude, K. (2015). The efficacy of a personalized feedback-only intervention for at-risk college gamblers. *Journal of Consulting and Clinical Psychology, 83,* 494–499. http://dx.doi.org/10.1037/a0038843

McLellan, A. T., Lewis, D. C., O'Brien, C. P., & Kleber, H. D. (2000). Drug dependence, a chronic medical illness: Implications for treatment, insurance, and outcomes evaluation. *Journal of the American Medical Association, 284,* 1689–1695. http://dx.doi.org/10.1001/jama.284.13.1689

Mentzoni, R. A., Brunborg, G. S., Molde, H., Myrseth, H., Skouverøe, K. J., Hetland, J., & Pallesen, S. (2011). Problematic video game use: Estimated prevalence and associations with mental and physical health. *Cyberpsychology, Behavior, and Social Networking, 14,* 591–596. http://dx.doi.org/10.1089/cyber.2010.0260

Morris, P. L., Hopwood, M., Whelan, G., Gardiner, J., & Drummond, E. (2001). Naltrexone for alcohol dependence: A randomized controlled trial. *Addiction, 96,* 1565–1573. http://dx.doi.org/10.1046/j.1360-0443.2001.961115654.x

National Institute on Drug Abuse. (2014). *Addiction medications.* Retrieved from https://www.drugabuse.gov/publications/principles-adolescent-substance-use-disorder-treatment-research-based-guide/evidence-based-approaches-to-treating-adolescent-substance-use-disorders/addiction-medications

Neighbors, C., Rodriguez, L. M., Rinker, D. V., Gonzales, R. G., Agana, M., Tackett, J. L., & Foster, D. W. (2015). Efficacy of personalized normative feedback as a brief intervention for college student gambling: A randomized controlled trial. *Journal of Consulting and Clinical*

Psychology, 83, 500–511. http://dx.doi.org/10.1037/a0039125

Neufang, S., Akhrif, A., Herrmann, C. G., Drepper, C., Homola, G. A., Nowak, J., . . . Romanos, M. (2016). Serotonergic modulation of "waiting impulsivity" is mediated by the impulsivity phenotype in humans. *Translational Psychiatry, 6,* e940. http://dx.doi.org/10.1038/tp.2016.210

Oei, T. P., Raylu, N., & Casey, L. M. (2010). Effectiveness of group and individual formats of a combined motivational interviewing and cognitive behavioral treatment program for problem gambling: A randomized controlled trial. *Behavioural and Cognitive Psychotherapy, 38,* 233–238. http://dx.doi.org/10.1017/S1352465809990701

Pallesen, S., Mitsem, M., Kvale, G., Johnsen, B. H., & Molde, H. (2005). Outcome of psychological treatments of pathological gambling: A review and meta-analysis. *Addiction, 100,* 1412–1422. http://dx.doi.org/10.1111/j.1360-0443.2005.01204.x

Pallesen, S., Molde, H., Arnestad, H. M., Laberg, J. C., Skutle, A., Iversen, E., . . . Holsten, F. (2007). Outcome of pharmacological treatments of pathological gambling: A review and meta-analysis. *Journal of Clinical Psychopharmacology, 27,* 357–364. http://dx.doi.org/10.1097/jcp.013e3180dcc304d

Pallanti, S., DeCaria, C. M., Grant, J. E., Urpe, M., & Hollander, E. (2005). Reliability and validity of the pathological gambling adaptation of the Yale-Brown Obsessive-Compulsive Scale (PG-YBOCS). *Journal of Gambling Studies, 21,* 431–443. http://dx.doi.org/10.1007/s10899-005-5557-3

Park, J. H., Lee, Y. S., Sohn, J. H., & Han, D. H. (2016). Effectiveness of atomoxetine and methylphenidate for problematic online gaming in adolescents with attention deficit hyperactivity disorder. *Human Psychopharmacology: Clinical and Experimental, 31,* 427–432. http://dx.doi.org/10.1002/hup.2559

Petry, N. M. (2005). *Pathological gambling: Etiology, comorbidity, and treatment.* Washington, DC: American Psychological Association. http://dx.doi.org/10.1037/10894-000

Petry, N. M., Ammerman, Y., Bohl, J., Doersch, A., Gay, H., Kadden, R., . . . Steinberg, K. (2006). Cognitive-behavioral therapy for pathological gamblers. *Journal of Consulting and Clinical Psychology, 74,* 555–567. http://dx.doi.org/10.1037/0022-006X.74.3.555

Petry, N. M., Blanco, C., Stinchfield, R., & Volberg, R. (2013). An empirical evaluation of proposed changes for gambling diagnosis in the *DSM–5. Addiction, 108,* 575–581. http://dx.doi.org/10.1111/j.1360-0443.2012.04087.x

*Petry, N. M., Ginley, M. K., & Rash, C. J. (2017). A systematic review of treatments for problem gambling.

Psychology of Addictive Behaviors, 31, 951–961. http://dx.doi.org/10.1037/adb0000290

Petry, N. M., & O'Brien, C. P. (2013). Internet gaming disorder and the *DSM–5. Addiction, 108,* 1186–1187. http://dx.doi.org/10.1111/add.12162

Petry, N. M., Rash, C. J., & Alessi, S. M. (2016). A randomized controlled trial of brief interventions for problem gambling in substance abuse treatment patients. *Journal of Consulting and Clinical Psychology, 84,* 874–886. http://dx.doi.org/10.1037/ccp0000127

*Petry, N. M., Rehbein, F., Gentile, D. A., Lemmens, J. S., Rumpf, H. J., Mößle, T., . . . O'Brien, C. P. (2014). An international consensus for assessing Internet gaming disorder using the new *DSM–5* approach. *Addiction, 109,* 1399–1406. http://dx.doi.org/10.1111/add.12457

Petry, N. M., Stinson, F. S., & Grant, B. F. (2005). Comorbidity of *DSM–IV* pathological gambling and other psychiatric disorders: Results from the National Epidemiologic Survey on Alcohol and Related Conditions. *The Journal of Clinical Psychiatry, 66,* 564–574. http://dx.doi.org/10.4088/JCP.v66n0504

Petry, N. M., Weinstock, J., Ledgerwood, D. M., & Morasco, B. (2008). A randomized trial of brief interventions for problem and pathological gamblers. *Journal of Consulting and Clinical Psychology, 76,* 318–328. http://dx.doi.org/10.1037/0022-006X.76.2.318

Pontes, H. M., Király, O., Demetrovics, Z., & Griffiths, M. D. (2014). The conceptualisation and measurement of *DSM–5* Internet gaming disorder: The development of the IGD-20 Test. *PLoS ONE, 9*(10), e110137. http://dx.doi.org/10.1371/journal.pone.0110137

*Przepiorka, A. M., Blachnio, A., Miziak, B., & Czuczwar, S. J. (2014). Clinical approaches to treatment of Internet addiction. *Pharmacological Reviews, 66,* 187–191. http://dx.doi.org/10.1016/j.pharep.2013.10.001

Rehbein, F., Kliem, S., Baier, D., Mößle, T., & Petry, N. M. (2015). Systematic validation of Internet gaming disorder criteria needs to start somewhere: A reply to Kardefelt-Winther. *Addiction, 110,* 1360–1362. http://dx.doi.org/10.1111/add.12995

Robbins, T. W., & Dalley, J. W. (2017). Impulsivity, risky choice, and impulse control disorders: Animal models. In J.-C. Dreher & L. Tremblay (Eds.), *Decision neuroscience: An integrative perspective* (pp. 81–93). London, England: Academic Press. http://dx.doi.org/10.1016/B978-0-12-805308-9.00007-5

Rösner, S., Hackl-Herrwerth, A., Leucht, S., Vecchi, S., Srisurapanont, M., & Soyka, M. (2010). Opioid antagonists for alcohol dependence. *The Cochrane Library.* Available from: http://www.thehealthwell.info/node/70211 http://dx.doi.org/10.1002/14651858.CD001867.pub3

Saiz-Ruiz, J., Blanco, C., Ibáñez, A., Masramon, X., Gómez, M. M., Madrigal, M., & Díez, T. (2005). Sertraline treatment of pathological gambling: A pilot study. *The Journal of Clinical Psychiatry, 66*, 28–33. http://dx.doi.org/10.4088/JCP.v66n0104

Slemmer, J. E., Martin, B. R., & Damaj, M. I. (2000). Bupropion is a nicotinic antagonist. *The Journal of Pharmacology and Experimental Therapeutics, 295*, 321–327.

Song, J., Park, J. H., Han, D. H., Roh, S., Son, J. H., Choi, T. Y., . . . Lee, Y. S. (2016). Comparative study of the effects of bupropion and escitalopram on Internet gaming disorder. *Psychiatry and Clinical Neurosciences, 70*, 527–535. http://dx.doi.org/10.1111/pcn.12429

Stahler, G. J., Mennis, J., & DuCette, J. P. (2016). Residential and outpatient treatment completion for substance use disorders in the U.S.: Moderation analysis by demographics and drug of choice. *Addictive Behaviors, 58*, 129–135. http://dx.doi.org/10.1016/j.addbeh.2016.02.030

Starcevic, V., & Khazaal, Y. (2017). Relationships between behavioural addictions and psychiatric disorders: What is known and what is yet to be learned? *Frontiers in Psychiatry, 8*, 53. http://dx.doi.org/10.3389/fpsyt.2017.00053

Stinchfield, R. (2002). Reliability, validity, and classification accuracy of the South Oaks Gambling Screen (SOGS). *Addictive Behaviors, 27*, 1–19. http://dx.doi.org/10.1016/S0306-4603(00)00158-1

Stinchfield, R., Govoni, R., & Frisch, G. R. (2007). A review of screening and assessment instruments for problem and pathological gambling. In G. Smith, D. C. Hodgins, & R. Williams (Eds.), *Research and measurement issues in gambling studies* (pp. 179–213). New York, NY: Academic Press.

Toneatto, T. (2016). Single-session interventions for problem gambling may be as effective as longer treatments: Results of a randomized control trial. *Addictive Behaviors, 52*, 58–65. http://dx.doi.org/10.1016/j.addbeh.2015.08.006

Toneatto, T., Brands, B., & Selby, P. (2009). A randomized, double-blind, placebo-controlled trial of naltrexone in the treatment of concurrent alcohol use disorder and pathological gambling. *The American Journal on Addictions, 18*, 219–225. http://dx.doi.org/10.1080/10550490902787007

Toneatto, T., & Ladoceur, R. (2003). Treatment of pathological gambling: A critical review of the literature. *Psychology of Addictive Behaviors, 17*, 284–292. http://dx.doi.org/10.1037/0893-164X.17.4.284

Torrens, M., Fonseca, F., Mateu, G., & Farré, M. (2005). Efficacy of antidepressants in substance use disorders with and without comorbid depression. A systematic review and meta-analysis. *Drug and Alcohol Dependence, 78*, 1–22. http://dx.doi.org/10.1016/j.drugalcdep.2004.09.004

van Rooij, A. J., Kuss, D. J., Griffiths, M. D., Shorter, G. W., Schoenmakers, M. T., & van de Mheen, D. (2014). The (co-)occurrence of problematic video gaming, substance use, and psychosocial problems in adolescents. *Journal of Behavioral Addictions, 3*, 157–165. http://dx.doi.org/10.1556/JBA.3.2014.013

van Rooij, A. J., Schoenmakers, T. M., Vermulst, A. A., van den Eijnden, R. J., & van de Mheen, D. (2011). Online video game addiction: Identification of addicted adolescent gamers. *Addiction, 106*, 205–212. http://dx.doi.org/10.1111/j.1360-0443.2010.03104.x

Veilleux, J. C., Colvin, P. J., Anderson, J., York, C., & Heinz, A. J. (2010). A review of opioid dependence treatment: Pharmacological and psychosocial interventions to treat opioid addiction. *Clinical Psychology Review, 30*, 155–166. http://dx.doi.org/10.1016/j.cpr.2009.10.006

Volpicelli, J. R., Rhines, K. C., Rhines, J. S., Volpicelli, L. A., Alterman, A. I., & O'Brien, C. P. (1997). Naltrexone and alcohol dependence. Role of subject compliance. *Archives of General Psychiatry, 54*, 737–742. http://dx.doi.org/10.1001/archpsyc.1997.01830200071010

Walther, B., Morgenstern, M., & Hanewinkel, R. (2012). Co-occurrence of addictive behaviours: Personality factors related to substance use, gambling and computer gaming. *European Addiction Research, 18*, 167–174. http://dx.doi.org/10.1159/000335662

Weinstock, J., Whelan, J. P., Meyers, A. W., & McCausland, C. (2007). The performance of two pathological gambling screens in college students. *Assessment, 14*, 399–407. http://dx.doi.org/10.1177/1073191107305273

Weiser, E. B. (2000). Gender differences in Internet use patterns and Internet application preferences: A two-sample comparison. *CyberPsychology & Behavior, 3*, 167–178. http://dx.doi.org/10.1089/109493100316012

Welte, J. W., Barnes, G. M., Tidwell, M. C. O., & Hoffman, J. H. (2011). Gambling and problem gambling across the lifespan. *Journal of Gambling Studies, 27*, 49–61. http://dx.doi.org/10.1007/s10899-010-9195-z

Weng, C. B., Qian, R. B., Fu, X. M., Lin, B., Han, X. P., Niu, C. S., & Wang, Y. H. (2013). Gray matter and white matter abnormalities in online game addiction. *European Journal of Radiology, 82*, 1308–1312. http://dx.doi.org/10.1016/j.ejrad.2013.01.031

Wickwire, E. M., Jr., Burke, R. S., Brown, S. A., Parker, J. D., & May, R. K. (2008). Psychometric evaluation of the National Opinion Research Center DSM–IV Screen for Gambling Problems (NODS). *The American Journal on Addictions, 17*, 392–395. http://dx.doi.org/10.1080/10550490802268934

Willner, P., Hale, A. S., & Argyropoulos, S. (2005). Dopaminergic mechanism of antidepressant action in depressed patients. *Journal of Affective Disorders, 86*, 37–45. http://dx.doi.org/10.1016/j.jad.2004.12.010

Winkler, A., Dörsing, B., Rief, W., Shen, Y., & Glombiewski, J. A. (2013). Treatment of Internet addiction: A meta-analysis. *Clinical Psychology Review, 33*, 317–329. http://dx.doi.org/10.1016/j.cpr.2012.12.005

Winters, K. C., Specker, S., & Stinchfield, R. D. (1996). *Diagnostic Interview for Gambling Severity (DIGS)*. Minneapolis, MN: University of Minnesota Medical School.

Wittek, C. T., Finserås, T. R., Pallesen, S., Mentzoni, R. A., Hanss, D., Griffiths, M. D., & Molde, H. (2016). Prevalence and predictors of video game addiction: A study based on a national representative sample of gamers. *International Journal of Mental Health and Addiction, 14*, 672–686. http://dx.doi.org/10.1007/s11469-015-9592-8

Yen, J. Y., Ko, C. H., Yen, C. F., Chen, C. S., & Chen, C. C. (2009). The association between harmful alcohol use and Internet addiction among college students: Comparison of personality. *Psychiatry and Clinical Neurosciences, 63*, 218–224. http://dx.doi.org/10.1111/j.1440-1819.2009.01943.x

Young, K. S. (1998a). *Caught in the net: How to recognize signs of Internet addiction and a winning strategy for recovery*. New York, NY: John Wiley & Sons.

Young, K. S. (1998b). Internet addiction: The emergence of a new clinical disorder. *CyberPsychology & Behavior, 1*, 237–244. http://dx.doi.org/10.1089/cpb.1998.1.237

Yuan, K., Cheng, P., Dong, T., Bi, Y., Xing, L., Yu, D., . . . Tian, J. (2013). Cortical thickness abnormalities in late adolescence with online gaming addiction. *PLoS One, 8*, e53055. http://dx.doi.org/10.1371/journal.pone.0053055

*Zajac, K., Ginley, M. K., Chang, R., & Petry, N. M. (2017). Treatments for Internet gaming disorder and Internet addiction: A systematic review. *Psychology of Addictive Behaviors, 31*, 979–994. http://dx.doi.org/10.1037/adb0000315

Zois, E., Kiefer, F., Lemenager, T., Vollstädt-Klein, S., Mann, K., & Fauth-Bühler, M. (2017). Frontal cortex gray matter volume alterations in pathological gambling occur independently from substance use disorder. *Addiction Biology, 22*, 864–872. http://dx.doi.org/10.1111/adb.12368

PSYCHOPHARMACOLOGY IN CONTEXT: ISSUES PERTANING TO PROFESSIONAL TRAINING, POLICY, AND INDUSTRY

PROFESSIONAL PSYCHOLOGY IN THE CONTEXT OF PSYCHOPHARMACOLOGY: ETHICAL ISSUES, EDUCATION, AND TRAINING

Lynette A. Pujol and Bret A. Moore

Approximately 18% of Americans aged 18 or older (43.7 million adults) experienced a mental health disorder in the past year (Lipari, Van Horn, Hughes, & Williams, 2017). An estimated 9.8 million people (4% of the U.S. adult population) had a serious mental illness in the past year, which is defined as any mental, behavioral, or emotional disorder that substantially interferes with or limits one or more major life activities (Substance Abuse and Mental Health Services Administration, Center for Behavioral Health Statistics and Quality, 2015). The same percentage of adults admits serious thoughts of suicide (Substance Abuse and Mental Health Services Administration, Center for Behavioral Health Statistics and Quality, 2015). Mental health disorders are also prevalent in American youth; one in five aged 13 to 18 experiences a severe mental health disorder during their lifetime (Merikangas et al., 2010). Additionally, suicide is the third leading cause of death among persons aged 10 to 14, and the second cause of death among persons ages 15 to 34 (Centers for Disease Control and Prevention, 2013).

GROWTH IN THE USE OF PSYCHOTROPICS

Treatment for psychiatric conditions, especially the use of psychopharmacologic agents, has grown in recent years in the United States. Approximately one of six adults took a psychiatric drug at least once in 2013, with twofold to threefold increases considering race/ethnicity, age, and sex (Moore & Mattison, 2017). Three psychiatric diagnostic groups are among the top 20 diagnostic categories in primary care settings (i.e., psychoses, excluding major depressive disorder; attention-deficit/hyperactivity disorder; and anxiety states), and antidepressants are the third most prescribed drug class (Hing, Rui, & Palso, 2013). Psychotropic medication use is also common among children and adolescents in the United States. Seven and one-half percent (7.5%) of children and adolescents ages 6 to 17 received medications for behavioral or emotional difficulties in 2011 to 2012 (Howie, Pastor, & Lukacs, 2014). Psychotropic medication prescriptions for non-institutionalized adolescents increased by fivefold for any psychotropic medication, and were up to

Disclaimer: The view(s) expressed herein are those of the author(s) and do not reflect the official policy or position of U.S. Army Regional Health Command—Central, the U.S. Army Medical Department, the U.S. Army Office of the Surgeon General, the U.S. Department of the Army and Department of Defense, or the U.S. government.

http://dx.doi.org/10.1037/0000133-029
APA Handbook of Psychopharmacology, S. M. Evans (Editor-in-Chief)

28 times higher for girls for treatment for ADHD from 1988 to 2010 (Howie et al., 2014).

Given these statistics of the prevalence of both psychiatric disorders and psychotropic medication use, it is not surprising that clinical psychologists frequently find themselves in the middle of psychopharmacologic treatment concerns. Often consulted first when a patient experiences a problem, psychologists are in a position to judge whether a patient's symptoms necessitate a referral for a medication consultation, making them primary referral sources for prescribers. Patients generally see psychologists more frequently than prescribing providers and therefore may hear about efficacy or side-effects before prescribing providers. Further, some psychologists have training and experience to consult with physicians (i.e., recommend medications) and/or have actual prescriptive authority. In fact, prescriptive authority for psychologists appears to have received new wind, with several states passing recent laws. Psychologists debate the appropriate level of knowledge of psychopharmacologic treatments needed for the general practitioner, consultant, and/or prescriber, but it is clear that "no" or "a little" knowledge is not adequate for competent practice in any role.

ETHICS AND TRAINING IN PSYCHOLOGY

Quality training and ethical practice have always been a focus in the profession of psychology. It is no surprise, then, that the prescriptive authority for psychologists (RxP) movement engenders questions regarding appropriate training and ethical practice. In fact, training and ethical issues in RxP are foci for opponents of prescriptive authority both within and outside the profession of psychology. Ethical considerations were discussed early on in the literature (Buelow & Chafetz, 1996), and later expanded to the present form. This chapter contains information on the evolution of ethical guidelines in psychopharmacology.

As growth in the use of psychotropic medications ensues, questions regarding ethical and competent practice emerge. What should all psychologists know about psychotropic medications to best serve their patients? What ethical principles exist or are needed regarding prescriptive authority? What type of training is necessary and sufficient for psychologists involved in providing education to patients, consulting, and prescribing? While the answers to some of these questions continue to be debated, the current ethical and training guidelines regarding psychopharmacology are reviewed in this chapter. In spite of considerable progress in the areas of ethics and training, challenges and decisions for the future remain. A few of these future challenges will be discussed at the end of the chapter.

PROFESSIONAL ETHICS

Ethical guides can be aspirational or prescriptive, general or specific, or best practices for certain conditions or areas of practice. The American Psychological Association (APA) uses different terminology to distinguish between various guides for behavior; therefore, it is important to understand the terminology used by APA.

Principles and Code of Conduct
The APA's *Ethical Principles of Psychologists and Code of Conduct* (2017b) describes aspects of ethical practice for psychologists. The Preamble and General Principles sections are aspirational, detailing higher-level principles to be used when considering ethical questions. Readers will be familiar with the principles of beneficence and nonmaleficence, fidelity and responsibility, integrity, justice, and respect for people's rights and dignity (APA, 2017b). Consistent with the general aspirational principles, but more specific to practice is the Code of Conduct, which specifies the expected behavior of psychologists in a wide range of practice situations. Violations of the code of conduct are enforceable and include a variety of sanctions, to include reporting to state and federal agencies.

Standards, Clinical Practice Guidelines, and Professional Practice Guidelines
In addition to aspirational principles and an ethics code, APA has approved standards and guidelines. Like the ethics code, standards are mandatory and enforceable. Standards set forth criteria for conduct, performance, services, or products in psychology

(https://www.apa.org/about/policy/approved-guidelines.aspx). Examples of standards relevant to psychopharmacology practice are the *Designation Criteria for Education and Training Programs in Preparation for Prescriptive Authority* (APA, 2009a) and the *Recommended Postdoctoral Education and Training Program in Psychopharmacology for Prescriptive Authority* (APA, 2009b).

Clinical practice guidelines (CPGs), also called treatment guidelines, are research-based recommendations that are considered best practice for the treatment of certain disorders. APA has not traditionally produced CPGs, although they are moving in this direction by appointing a task force designed to oversee the production of CPGs and by publishing a recent CPG for posttraumatic stress disorder (PTSD) in adults (Clinical Practice Guideline for the Treatment of PTSD in Adults; APA, 2017a).

Professional practice guidelines are different than clinical practice guidelines because they are directed at general conduct in a specific domain, though not for a certain disorder. These guidelines are aspirational, not exhaustive or applicable to every clinical encounter, and are intended to inspire the highest level of professional practice (McGrath & Rom-Rymer, 2010). APA has produced professional practice guidelines that address practice with certain populations (e.g., persons with disabilities) or in specific areas of practice (e.g., telepsychology).

STATE LAW AND INSTITUTIONAL FORMULARIES

Prescribing psychologists must also comply with state law. Some state laws limit categories of drugs that can be prescribed by psychologists and/or populations to whom medications may be prescribed. For example, Illinois does not allow psychologists to prescribe benzodiazepine Schedule III controlled substances or to patients who are younger than 17 years of age or older than 65 years of age (see the Tool Kit of Resources in this chapter for links to information about state laws). Institutions (e.g., hospitals) also have formularies instituted by a Pharmacy and Therapeutics Committee or similar forum. Psychologists seeking to prescribe in these institutions will need to understand the process of approval for the institution and comply.

CURRENT ETHICAL GUIDELINES FOR PSYCHOLOGISTS INVOLVED IN PHARMACOLOGICAL ISSUES

The current APA *Practice Guidelines Regarding Psychologists' Involvement in Pharmacological Issues* (2011) evolved from increasing interest and progress in the prescriptive authority movement. Early suggestions for adding ethical standards for the developing prescription privileges movement were made by Buelow and Chafetz (1996). Using a term they previously coined for prescribing psychologists, "pharmacopsychologist," they describe seven additional ethical considerations in assessment, treatment, and evaluation. These guidelines emphasize the provision of high-quality clinical pharmacopsychology practice, to include assessment, diagnosis, conceptualization, treatment planning, treatment, treatment evaluation, and reassessment. Most of the guidelines highlight integrative practice and the priority of psychotherapy when possible and warranted by the condition. Guidelines call for special attention to and accurate referral of medically ill patients, avoidance of polypharmacy, longitudinal measurement of outcomes of psychotherapy and pharmacotherapy, adverse side effect monitoring, and evaluation of the cost–benefit ratio of prescribing (Buelow & Chafetz, 1996).

Other suggestions about ethics and training came from an article about professional issues in pharmacotherapy (McGrath et al., 2004). These authors focus on the need to create a psychological model of prescribing consistent with maintaining psychotherapy as a primary activity versus migrating to a prescriber-only model characterized by brief medication encounters. In a psychological model, the patient is considered the decision maker and the psychologist serves as the consultant to the patient regarding various treatment options. This collaborative approach involves exploration of the meaning of medications in treatment from the perspective of the psychologist as well as the patient. Additionally, McGrath et al. (2004) urge psychologists to be aware and critical of the role of pharmaceutical companies in participation in research, research publications, marketing, and clinical decision making (see also Chapter 31, this volume).

A growing recognition of the need to address ethics in a more formal way for those involved in pharmacological practice was made by early proponents of RxP. Led by Beth Rom-Rymer, then president of APA's Division 55 (American Society for the Advancement of Pharmacotherapy), a task force was organized to formalize expected ethical behavior related to pharmacotherapy (APA, 2011). Because the field was emerging, aspirational practice guidelines were created as opposed to an enforceable code. Like other professional practice guidelines published by APA, the guidelines are not meant to apply to psychologists who have no involvement in the practice of pharmacotherapy. The *Practice Guidelines Regarding Psychologists' Involvement in Pharmacological Issues* (APA, 2011) delineates a continuum of involvement in pharmacotherapy. Given the continued growth of the use of psychopharmacologic drugs, one might contend that every psychologist involved in patient care needs to be familiar with the end of the continuum that describes psychologists who provide information to patients, but do not have a role in assisting the medical prescriber or patient in choosing a medication. These roles are also subject to various state laws, some of which prohibit a discussion of medication by some psychologists (e.g., those employed by schools).

The three levels specified by the *Practice Guidelines Regarding Psychologists' Involvement in Pharmacological Issues* (APA, 2011) are providing information, collaborating, and prescribing. Seventeen guidelines are given in five categories, including general, education, assessment, intervention and consultation, and relationships. Using a step analogy (Smyer et al., 1993), providing information is the first step, while collaborating and prescribing are successive steps. The hierarchal step model connotes increased training and responsibility as involvement with pharmacologic agents increases. For those who wish to avoid a hierarchal presentation, these three activities can also be conceptualized as three points along a continuum or three concentric circles. Psychologists who prescribe medications are expected to consider all 17 guidelines, while those who do not prescribe are expected to consider only those guidelines related to the pharmacotherapeutic activities they perform.

A full listing of the seventeen guidelines is contained in Table 29.1. A brief overview of the three activities will be delineated here.

Psychologists involved in any of the three activities regarding pharmacotherapy (i.e., providing information, collaborating, or prescribing) are encouraged to objectively consider their competence prior to engaging in any activity related to psychotropic medication and to seek consultation as needed (Guideline 1; APA, 2011). Those involved in pharmacotherapy are to identify an appropriate level of knowledge for the activity in which they engage and the populations they serve, then seek education to attain and maintain that level of knowledge (Guideline 4; APA, 2011), to include the potential adverse effects of psychotropic medications (Guideline 5; APA, 2011). In addition to knowing about medications, psychologists involved in pharmacotherapy understand their views have the potential to affect their patients, and therefore, evaluate their own feelings and attitudes regarding the use of medication for psychological disorders (Guideline 2; APA, 2011). Similarly, patients have feelings and attitudes about the use of medication that may affect adherence, and discussion of these feelings is potentially beneficial (Guideline 9; APA, 2011). Creating a therapeutic relationship that allows for the comfortable exploration of issues surrounding medication use is encouraged (Guideline 10; APA, 2011). Finally, psychologists involved in any level of pharmacotherapeutic activity maintain appropriate relationships with providers of biological interventions (Guideline 17; APA, 2011).

Guidelines relevant for psychologists involved in collaborating and prescribing are added to the next step. In these roles, sensitivity to individual differences from a biological perspective, as well as from psychosocial and interpersonal perspectives, may be relevant to recommending or prescribing medications (Guideline 3; APA, 2011). Broad categories of individual differences include developmental stage, age, aging, education, sex and gender, language, health status, and cultural and ethnic factors (Guideline 3; APA, 2011). For example, drugs may have differential effects due to racial/ethnic genetic polymorphisms, individual variation in metabolism, or reduced organ function due to aging and/or medical comorbidities. Additionally, a patient's socioeconomic

TABLE 29.1

Practice Guidelines for Psychologists' Involvement in Pharmacological Issues

Guideline	Relevant activities		
	Providing information[a]	Collaborating	Prescribing
General			
Guideline 1. Psychologists are encouraged to consider objectively the scope of their competence in pharmacotherapy and to seek consultation as appropriate before offering recommendations about psychotropic medications.	X	X	X
Guideline 2. Psychologists are urged to evaluate their own feelings and attitudes about the role of medication in the treatment of psychological disorders, as these feelings and attitudes can potentially affect communications with patients.	X	X	X
Guideline 3. Psychologists involved in prescribing or collaborating are sensitive to the developmental, age and aging, educational, sex and gender, language, health status, and cultural/ethnicity factors that can moderate the interpersonal and biological aspects of pharmacotherapy relevant to the populations they serve.		X	X
Education			
Guideline 4. Psychologists are urged to identify a level of knowledge concerning pharmacotherapy for the treatment of psychological disorders that is appropriate to the populations they serve and the type of practice they wish to establish, and to engage in educational experiences as appropriate to achieve and maintain that level of knowledge.	X	X	X
Guideline 5. Psychologists strive to be sensitive to the potential for adverse effects associated with the psychotropic medications used by their patients.	X	X	X
Guideline 6. Psychologists involved in prescribing or collaborating are encouraged to familiarize themselves with the technological resources that can enhance decision-making during the course of treatment.		X	X
Assessment			
Guideline 7. Psychologists with prescriptive authority strive to familiarize themselves with key procedures for monitoring the physical and psychological sequelae of the medications used to treat psychological disorders, including laboratory examinations and overt signs of adverse or unintended effects.			X
Guideline 8. Psychologists with prescriptive authority regularly strive to monitor the physiological status of the patients they treat with medication, particularly when there is a physical condition that might complicate the response to psychotropic medication or predispose a patient to experience an adverse reaction.			X
Guideline 9. Psychologists are encouraged to explore issues surrounding patient adherence and feelings about medication.	X	X	X

(*continues*)

TABLE 29.1

Practice Guidelines for Psychologists' Involvement in Pharmacological Issues (*Continued*)

	Relevant activities		
Guideline	Providing information[a]	Collaborating	Prescribing
Intervention and Consultation			
Guideline 10. Psychologists are urged to develop a relationship that will allow the populations they serve to feel comfortable exploring issues surrounding medication use.	X	X	X
Guideline 11. To the extent deemed appropriate, psychologists involved in prescribing or collaboration adopt a biopsychosocial approach to case formulation that considers both psychosocial and biological factors.		X	X
Guideline 12. The psychologist with prescriptive authority is encouraged to use an expanded informed consent process to incorporate additional issues specific to prescribing.			X
Guideline 13. When making decisions about the use of psychological treatments, pharmacotherapy, or their combination, the psychologist with prescriptive authority considers the best interests of the patient, current research, and when appropriate, the needs of the community.			X
Guideline 14. Psychologists involved in prescribing or collaborating strive to be sensitive to the subtle influences of effective marketing on professional behavior and the potential for bias in information in their clinical decisions about the use of medications.		X	X
Guideline 15. Psychologists with prescriptive authority are encouraged to use interactions with the patient surrounding the act of prescribing to learn more about the patient's characteristic patterns of interpersonal behavior.			X
Relationships			
Guideline 16. Psychologists with prescriptive authority are sensitive to maintaining appropriate relationships with other providers of psychological services.			X
Guideline 17. Psychologists are urged to maintain appropriate relationships with providers of biological interventions.	X	X	X

Note. Adapted from "Practice Guidelines Regarding Psychologists' Involvement in Pharmacological Issues" by American Psychological Association Division 55 (American Society for the Advancement of Pharmacotherapy) Task Force on Practice Guidelines, 2011, *American Psychologist, 66*, pp. 838–839. Copyright 2011 by the American Psychological Association.
[a]This is the term adopted in the guidelines document to refer to instances in which the psychologist plays no role in the decision-making process. It parallels the discussion in the educational literature on Level 1.

status may be a factor in compliance due to an inability to afford a prescribed drug on a regular basis. Psychologists who collaborate or prescribe are encouraged to be aware of technological resources that provide information that can enhance the decision-making process (Guideline 6; APA, 2011). Additionally, individuals recommending medications and prescribing are encouraged to be sensitive to the subtle influences of pharmaceutical market-

ing on their clinical decision making (Guideline 14; APA, 2011).

The third step or level contains additional guidelines relevant for prescribers of psychotropic medications. Psychologists with prescriptive authority must know physical and laboratory procedures for monitoring both the physical and psychological effects of medications, to include adverse and unintended effects (Guideline 7; APA, 2011).

Regular monitoring is especially important for patients with physical conditions that could complicate treatment, which might include a response to treatment or a predisposition to an adverse reaction (Guideline 8; APA, 2011). Because prescribing involves additional considerations for patients, an expanded consent form is recommended (Guideline 12; APA, 2011). Guideline 12 comes with 16 elements of an expanded informed consent, to include a description of the medication, why the medication is prescribed, the availability of other treatment options compared with the recommended medication, how the medication is to be taken, potential benefits and risks, expected consequences of abrupt discontinuation, and the role of medication and psychotherapy in the treatment plan, among other elements. Prescribing psychologists are encouraged to take into account the best interests of the patient, current research, and at times, the community, when considering decisions about pharmacotherapy, psychotherapy, or a combination as treatment (Guideline 13; APA, 2011). Consistent with McGrath et al. (2004), psychologists with prescriptive authority are urged to learn about the patient's patterns of interpersonal behavior through interactions that surround the act of prescribing (Guideline 15; APA, 2011). Finally, prescribers maintain appropriate relationships with providers of psychological services (Guideline 16) in addition to appropriate relationships with providers of biological interventions (Guideline 17; APA, 2011).

No discussion of ethics in psychopharmacology would be complete without mentioning the influence of pharmaceutical companies on psychologists at all levels of psychopharmacologic involvement. With global sales projected to be $1.12 trillion by 2022 ("Global pharma market," 2016), pharmaceutical companies have immense cultural and economic power. In 2016, the United States held approximately 45% of the global pharmaceutical market, valued at approximately $445 billion (Statista, 2016). Decisions of pharmaceutical companies affect psychologists in a variety of ways, from choosing which drugs to develop to the design, implementation, and analysis of clinical trials, publications, and the marketing and sales of drugs (see Chapter 31, this volume, for a full review).

They have become known for wielding power and influence over prescribers in subtle ways (e.g., providing free educational lunches and collegial "friendship") and overt ways (e.g., paying large sums of money for promoting a product or consulting).

Cosgrove and Moore (2010) provide a summary of some the ways pharmaceutical companies affect decisions to prescribe. These authors offer several suggestions for practitioners to avoid ethical dilemmas when considering the impact of pharmaceutical companies on day-to-day practice. In a prescribing therapeutic relationship, especially when treatment recommendations could lead to adverse effects for the patient, the importance of an ongoing and forthright informed consent process in the context of a good therapeutic alliance is critical (Cosgrove & Bursztajn, 2010). Cosgrove and Moore (2010) propose several actions to improve informed consent and prescribing practice, which include a healthy skepticism of pharmaceutical literature and studies, even when published in highly esteemed academic journals, an in-depth knowledge of marketing strategies—especially those used for "me too" drugs (i.e., drugs that are structurally similar to already known compounds or have the same mechanism of action)—and familiarity with statistical and methodological flaws common in clinical trials and research sponsored by pharmaceutical companies. Continuing education sponsored by industry should also be assumed to be biased toward the product produced by the sponsor. Although pharmaceutical companies and professional societies have taken some positive steps to minimize bias, the profit motive remains, and the steps forward primarily target the most egregious practices (e.g., luxury weekend trips to exotic locales for prescribers). Psychologists will do well to utilize the Cochrane Central Register of Controlled Trials and other repositories of research information that rate research bias and report on comparisons between industry-sponsored and non–industry-sponsored research (Cosgrove & Moore, 2010). Additionally, intentionally seeking information and continuing education from organizations that do not accept funding from pharmaceutical companies is warranted in today's industry-dominated climate (Cosgrove & Moore, 2010).

EDUCATION AND TRAINING IN PSYCHOPHARMACOLOGY

The American Psychological Association Recommended Postdoctoral Education and Training Program in Psychopharmacology for Prescriptive Authority (APA, 2009b) contains current standards for training. In addition to holding a doctorate degree, psychologists must also have a current state license as a psychologist and practice as a health service provider where defined by state law or APA. Central to the recommendations is a competency-based model that focuses on the integration of knowledge and skills and requires an evaluation demonstrating mastery. In addition to didactic instruction, case-based learning methods and skills-based demonstrations are required throughout the curriculum. Eight didactic core content areas are delineated: basic science (e.g., anatomy and physiology, biochemistry); neurosciences; physical assessment and laboratory exams; clinical medicine and pathophysiology; clinical and research pharmacology and psychopharmacology; clinical pharmacotherapeutics; research; and professional, ethical, and legal issues. Although course hours are determined by the institutions offering training, a minimum of 400 didactic contact hours are required. Supervised clinical experience must be sufficient to achieve competency and be approved by the training director of the program. The standards recommend a capstone evaluation that involves a review of the portfolio of supervised experience and application of knowledge, skills, and attitudes in response to unrehearsed clinical situations that range in difficulty (APA, 2009b).

Over the years, a number of educational institutions have offered programs for training in psychopharmacology. Currently, Alliant International University, Fairleigh Dickinson University, New Mexico State University, and the Chicago School of Professional Psychology offer a master's degree in clinical psychopharmacology. These institutions differ slightly in the format of training. For example, faculty at Alliant International University deliver didactic content in all-day weekend real-time lectures once per month, while faculty at Fairleigh Dickinson University deliver didactic content through asynchronous online lectures that can be accessed at any time and weekly real-time online discussions with faculty. Additionally, most programs have some requirement for in-person attendance for learning physical examination and/or other program content. The Chicago School of Professional Psychology's new psychopharmacology program is specifically tailored to psychologists who want prescriptive authority in Illinois. Although there are differences in all RxP laws, Illinois law requires more coursework than other states thus far.

PRESCRIPTIVE AUTHORITY LAWS

Five states have passed RxP legislation as of this writing. New Mexico passed the first state law in 2002, and Louisiana passed a law in 2004. More recent laws have been passed in Illinois (2015), Iowa (2016), and Idaho (2017). Additionally, prescriptive authority is granted to appropriately trained psychologists in Guam, the U.S. Public Health Service, the Indian Health Service, and the U.S. military. See Chapter 1, this volume, for a full discussion of the history of prescriptive authority legislation and current issues involving legislation.

ISSUES IN ETHICS, EDUCATION, AND TRAINING

An important aspect of the ethical guidelines for psychopharmacology is the maintenance of a primary identification as a psychologist. Early articles on ethics called a psychologist's method of practice the "psychological" or "psychobiological model" to differentiate it from the medical model (McGrath & Rom-Rymer, 2010). The clear intent of the ethical guidelines is for psychologists to retain a psychological "home base," even when equipped to provide psychopharmacologic information to patients, consultation to physicians, and/or to prescribe medications. Inherent in the maintenance of the psychological role is a biopsychosocial evaluation and treatment approach. For some psychologists, retaining a primary identity as a psychologist, whether advising the patient, consulting, or prescribing, means that pharmacologic information or intervention is one more tool, albeit a potentially powerful one, in the array of possible interventions. For those with prescriptive authority, the presumed goal of obtaining additional skills is the ability to deliver evidence-based treatment incorporating psychopharmacology, psychotherapy, and/or combined treatment, a practice sometimes referred to as *integrative*. Although some hold integrative practice to be the gold standard for RxP, little true integrative research has been performed. Studies that involve head-to-head comparisons of drugs are limited, with fewer studies still including one or more treatment groups involving an evidenced-based psychotherapy. There are some notable exceptions, such as the Treatment for Adolescents with Depression Study (TADS; March et al., 2007). In the TADS study, funded by the National Institute of Mental Health, adolescents with depression were randomized to one of four treatments: fluoxetine, placebo with clinical management, cognitive behavior therapy (CBT) alone, or a combination of fluoxetine and CBT. Results revealed that combination treatment was the safest and most effective treatment for adolescents with depression (March et al., 2007). What was remarkable about this study was the inclusion of medication alone, CBT alone, and a combination of medication and CBT, in addition to the placebo arms and the real-world representativeness of the sample.

Cultural competency is critical to psychological practice and in psychopharmacology. Polymorphisms of cytochrome P450 enzymes vary in different racial or ethnic populations and may affect the metabolism of medications. Ethical guidelines in pharmacotherapy also indicate the need for awareness of cultural factors concerning the use of medications. The *Diagnostic and Statistical Manual of Mental Disorders* (American Psychiatric Association, 2013) provides an Outline for Cultural Formulation and an associated Cultural Formulation Interview that involves questions regarding the cultural identity of the individual, cultural conceptualizations of distress, psychosocial stressors and cultural features of vulnerability and resilience, and the cultural features of the relationship between the individual and the clinician (pp. 750–759). Cultural differences are often not readily apparent to a clinician. For example, a psychiatric diagnosis and/or treatment with

medication could affect the ability to deploy of an active duty military member. American advertising, oriented toward turning to medicine as a cure, may or may not be consistent with the cultural beliefs of a devout Buddhist who immigrated to America. Moreover, the superiority of complementary and alternative medicine as a cure of the cause of the illness and/or for symptoms of illness may be prominent in certain cultures. Making a cultural formulation of patients for whom psychiatric medication is being considered will ultimately affect the therapeutic relationship and outcome of treatment in a positive manner.

Another issue in ethics and training is how or to what extent psychologists with prescriptive authority can or will be distinguished from other prescribing practitioners. For example, institutional economic pressures, rural practice, and/or a personal preference for psychopharmacologic involvement may push some prescribers to practice more akin to the medical model than an integrated psychological model. Little evidence on how prescribers with prescriptive authority actually practice is available to date. A recent survey of prescribing psychologists uses indirect evidence and concludes that even though more patients were seen by prescribers for medication alone than therapy alone, they were not biased towards using medications versus psychosocial interventions (Linda & McGrath, 2017). Since there are a wide variety of approaches to prescribing medications, the distinction between how different professionals practice may be more ideological than based on real-world practice; that is, not all psychiatrists and nurse practitioners have short medication management visits, and some practice a biopsychosocial approach. Nevertheless, psychologists with prescriptive authority are urged to consider their approach carefully based on their training and experience, the practice setting, and current ethical guidelines.

When applied to the consulting role, knowledge and skills in psychopharmacology are considered by some authors to be beneficial to collaboration with physicians and mental health professionals and superior to a prescribing practice (Robiner, Tumlin, & Tompkins, 2013). The Canadian Psychological Association agrees, endorsing a collaborative model as the "optimal standard" (p. 27) for psychologists (Canadian Psychological Association Task Force on Prescriptive Authority for Psychologists in Canada, 2010). The definition of collaboration and educational requirements presumed to be adequate for information giving and consultation are lacking. In practice, the consultation–liaison model is one in which a patient is evaluated and formal consultation ensues, generally to a requesting physician. Opponents of prescriptive authority endorse consultative practice, but do not always appreciate that the consultant has just as much need to know the pharmacodynamics, pharmacokinetics, individual differences, and medical comorbidities as prescribers, although they may assume less liability than prescribers. Ethical guidelines call for a consideration of the level of training needed in a particular area of practice and the obligation of the psychologist to pursue the required amount of education (APA, 2011, Guideline 4). Psychologists indicate that they collaborate regularly with a wide variety of medical professionals, according to APA Center for Workforce Studies (APA, 2015, Figure 5a). Other surveys show that providing information about medications is the subject of conversation in these consultations (Meyers, 2006; Robiner et al., 2013). Psychologists are frequently in the position of referring patients for a medication consultation. As psychologists become more integrated into primary care and medical settings, relationships with medical providers develop and consultation about the appropriateness of medication for a particular patient may be discussed. In the past, psychologists have not been in a position to recommend particular medications. However, with appropriate training, formal consultation or prescribing in settings in which prescribing is allowed may be beneficial for the primary care provider or other medical professional. Therefore, special attention to the type of training needed to perform such consultation is advised.

The training received by RxP providers is likely the most debated topic among psychologists as well as other providers (i.e., physicians, psychiatrists, psychiatric nurse practitioners). For psychologists opposed to prescriptive authority, points of contention regarding training are primarily related to

beliefs that psychotherapy will be lost as a focus of psychology (e.g., Mojtabai & Olfson, 2008), as well as concerns about the comprehensiveness and cost of training (Robiner et al., 2013). Much of the debate involves the perceived inadequacy of RxP training when compared with that of other prescribing professionals. Robiner et al. (2013) point out that psychologists with prescriptive authority have the least undergraduate training in sciences (e.g., chemistry, organic chemistry, microbiology) that are generally a prerequisite for entry into programs that lead to prescriptive authority (e.g., medical school, optometry, podiatry, nursing, and physician's assistant training), and that a reduced number of advanced courses are required in RxP training programs. They argue that current guidelines require fewer hours and less practical experience than required for the first psychologists in the U.S. Department of Defense Psychopharmacology Demonstration Project (PDP; Sammons & Brown, 1997). Specifically, trainees in the PDP received more biochemistry and basic science preparation than required by the current didactic guidelines, as well as more intensive clinical requirements following didactic training (Robiner et al., 2013).

Proponents of prescriptive authority counter opponents with the argument that prescribing psychologists are better trained to treat persons with emotional and behavioral disorders than a variety of other professionals with prescriptive authority (e.g., nurses, physicians), that an entire medical school curriculum is not needed to prescribe psychotropics, and that the safety record for prescribing psychologists thus far has been good (Muse & McGrath, 2010). These authors contend that psychologists receive much more training in some areas (e.g., research, psychosocial interventions) than other providers of mental health services (Muse & McGrath, 2010). In a recent study, Linda and McGrath (2017) surveyed prescribing psychologists and medical colleagues who worked with them. These authors found "an overwhelmingly favorable evaluation" (p. 44) of prescribing psychologists by medical colleagues with whom they work. Medical colleagues valued the RxP's own practice, in addition to seeing the prescribing psychologist as a source of information (Linda & McGrath, 2017).

FUTURE ISSUES IN ETHICS, EDUCATION, AND TRAINING

What is the future of the ethical guidelines? As more psychologists obtain training to provide information, consultation, or prescriptions, there may be a need for codification of the current aspirational guidelines. Previous research in ethics has shown that in general, human beings are very poor evaluators of their own competence, seeing themselves as "better than average" most of the time (Johnson, Barnett, Elman, Forrest, & Kaslow, 2012). The current ethical guidelines urge psychologists to identify the knowledge needed given their patient population and type of involvement with psychopharmacologic practice, to attain that knowledge, and to maintain it (APA, 2011). Medical knowledge expands at a fast pace, necessitating continual commitment to update information. Given that humans are poor judges of their own performance, tending to allow themselves the benefit of the doubt, some codification of the aspirational guidelines will likely be necessary in the future, not only to draw distinct lines between ideal and unacceptable practice, but as a protection to consumers.

As more psychologists perceive a need to be more knowledgeable about psychotropic medications, the future of education and training may include recommendations for an increased emphasis on science prerequisite courses in the predoctoral work or during doctoral training. Some authors propose moving psychopharmacologic training to the doctoral years as an alternative to the postdoctoral years in order to reduce the cost and time of training, to attract more applicants interested in a biopsychosocial orientation, and to increase the number of people interested in prescriptive authority legislative initiatives (e.g., Fagan, Ax, Liss, Resnick, & Moody, 2007; Resnick, Ax, Fagan, & Nussbaum, 2012). Although debate regarding how psychologists should incorporate psychopharmacology into

practice will likely continue, it is clear that increases in psychopharmacologic knowledge and skills are necessary for all psychologists.

TOOL KIT OF RESOURCES

Psychopharmacology Training Programs Offering the Master's Degree in Clinical Psychopharmacology

Alliant International University: https://www.alliant.edu

Chicago School of Professional Psychology: https://www.thechicagoschool.edu

Fairleigh Dickinson University: http://www.fdu.edu

New Mexico State University: https://www.nmsu.edu

Information on State Laws

Idaho Board of Psychologist Examiners: https://legislature.idaho.gov/statutesrules/idstat/title54/t54ch23/sect54-2317/

Iowa Board of Psychology: https://www.legis.iowa.gov/docs/publications/lgi/86/attachments/ssb1093.html

Illinois Board of Psychological Examiners: http://www.ilga.gov/legislation/ilcs/ilcs3.asp?ActID=1294&ChapterID=24

New Mexico Board of Psychological Examiners: http://www.ilga.gov/legislation/ilcs/ilcs3.asp?ActID=1294&ChapterID=24

Louisiana State Board of Medical Examiners: http://www.lsbme.la.gov

References

American Psychiatric Association. (2013). *Diagnostic and statistical manual of mental disorders* (5th ed.). Washington, DC: Author.

American Psychological Association. (2009a). *American Psychological Association designation criteria for education and training programs in preparation for prescriptive authority*. Washington, DC: Author. Retrieved from http://www.apa.org/education/grad/rxp-designation-criteria.pdf

American Psychological Association. (2009b). *Recommended postdoctoral education and training program in psychopharmacology for prescriptive authority*. Washington, DC: Author. Retrieved from https://www.apa.org/about/policy/rxp-model-curriculum.pdf

*Asterisks indicate assessments or resources.

American Psychological Association. (2017a). *Clinical practice guideline for the treatment of posttraumatic stress disorder (PTSD) in adults*. Washington, DC: Guideline Development Panel for the Treatment of PTSD in Adults. Retrieved from http://www.apa.org/about/offices/directorates/guidelines/clinical-practice.aspx

American Psychological Association. (2017b). *Ethical principles of psychologists and code of conduct* (2002, Amended June 1, 2010 and January 1, 2017). Retrieved from http://www.apa.org/ethics/code/index.aspx

American Psychological Association, Center for Workforce Studies. (2015). *2015 APA survey of psychology health service providers*. Washington, DC: Author. Retrieved from https://www.apa.org/workforce/publications/15-health-service-providers/figure5a.pdf

*American Psychological Association Division 55 (American Society for the Advancement of Pharmacotherapy) Task Force on Practice Guidelines. (2011). Practice guidelines regarding psychologists' involvement in pharmacological issues. *American Psychologist, 66*, 835–849. http://dx.doi.org/10.1037/a0025890

Buelow, G. D., & Chafetz, M. D. (1996). Proposed ethical practice guidelines for clinical pharmaco-psychology: Sharpening a new focus in psychology. *Professional Psychology: Research and Practice, 27*, 53–58. http://dx.doi.org/10.1037/0735-7028.27.1.53

Canadian Psychological Association Task Force on Prescriptive Authority for Psychologists in Canada. (2010). *Report to the Canadian Psychological Association Board of Directors*. Retrieved from http://www.cpa.ca/docs/File/Task_Forces/CPA_RxPTaskForce_FinalReport_Dec2010_RevJ17.pdf

Centers for Disease Control and Prevention (CDC). (2013). Web-based Injury Statistics Query and Reporting System (WISQARS) [Online]. Atlanta, GA: CDC National Center for Injury Prevention and Control. Retrieved from https://www.cdc.gov/injury/wisqars/pdf/leading_causes_of_death_by_age_group_2013-a.pdf

Cosgrove, L., & Bursztajn, H. J. (2010). Strengthening conflict-of-interest policies in medicine. *Journal of Evaluation in Clinical Practice, 16*, 21–24. http://dx.doi.org/10.1111/j.1365-2753.2009.01106.x

*Cosgrove, L., & Moore, B. A. (2010). Professional, legal, ethical and interprofessional issues in clinical psychopharmacology. In M. Muse & B. A. Moore (Eds.), *Handbook of Clinical Psychopharmacology for Psychologists* (pp. 457–481). Hoboken, NJ: Wiley.

Fagan, T. J., Ax, R. K., Liss, M., Resnick, R. J., & Moody, S. (2007). Prescriptive authority and preference for training. *Professional Psychology: Research and Practice, 38*, 104–111. http://dx.doi.org/10.1037/0735-7028.38.1.104

Global pharma market will reach 1.12 trillion in 2022. (2016, September 18). Retrieved from http://pharmaceuticalcommerce.com/business-and-finance/global-pharma-market-will-reach-1-12-trillion-2022

Hing, E., Rui, P., & Palso, K. (2013). National Ambulatory Medical Care Survey: 2013 State and National Summary Tables. Atlanta, GA: Centers for Disease Control and Prevention National Center for Health Statistics. Retrieved from http://www.cdc.gov/nchs/ahcd/ahcd_products.htm

Howie, L. D., Pastor, P. N., & Lukacs, S. L. (2014, April). Use of medication prescribed for emotional or behavioral difficulties among children aged 6–17 years in the United States, 2011–2012. *NCHS Data Brief, 148*, 1–8.

Johnson, W. B., Barnett, J. E., Elman, N. S., Forrest, L., & Kaslow, N. J. (2012). The competent community: Toward a vital reformulation of professional ethics. *American Psychologist, 67*, 557–569. http://dx.doi.org/10.1037/a0027206

*Linda, W. P., & McGrath, R. E. (2017). The current status of prescribing psychologists: Practice patterns and medical professional evaluations. *Professional Psychology: Research and Practice, 48*, 38–45. http://dx.doi.org/10.1037/pro0000118

Lipari, R. N., Van Horn, S., Hughes, A., & Williams, M. (2017). *State and substate estimates of any mental illness from the 2012–2014 National Surveys on Drug Use and Health. The CBHSQ Report: July 20, 2017*. Rockville, MD: Center for Behavioral Health Statistics and Quality, Substance Abuse and Mental Health Services Administration; https://www.samhsa.gov/data/sites/default/files/report_3189/ShortReport-3189.html

March, J. S., Silva, S., Petrycki, S., Curry, J., Wells, K., Fairbank, J., . . . Severe, J. (2007). The Treatment for Adolescents With Depression Study (TADS): Long-term effectiveness and safety outcomes. *Archives of General Psychiatry, 64*, 1132–1143. http://dx.doi.org/10.1001/archpsyc.64.10.1132

*McGrath, R. E., & Rom-Rymer, B. (2010). Ethical considerations in pharmacotherapy for psychologists. In R. E. McGrath & B. A. Moore (Eds.), *Pharmacotherapy for psychologists: Prescribing and collaborative roles* (pp. 89–104). Washington, DC: American Psychological Association. http://dx.doi.org/10.1037/12167-005

McGrath, R. E., Wiggins, J. G., Sammons, M. T., Levant, R. F., Brown, A., & Stock, W. (2004). Professional issues in pharmacotherapy for psychologists. *Professional Psychology: Research and Practice, 35*, 158–163. http://dx.doi.org/10.1037/0735-7028.35.2.158

Merikangas, K. R., He, J. P., Burstein, M., Swanson, S. A., Avenevoli, S., Cui, L., . . . Swendsen, J. (2010). Lifetime prevalence of mental disorders in U.S. adolescents: Results from the National Comorbidity

Survey Replication—Adolescent Supplement (NCS-A). *Journal of the American Academy of Child & Adolescent Psychiatry, 49*, 980–989. http://dx.doi.org/10.1016/j.jaac.2010.05.017

Meyers, L. (2006). Psychologists and psychotropic medication. *Monitor on Psychology, 37*, 46. http://www.apa.org/monitor/jun06/psychotropic.aspx

Mojtabai, R., & Olfson, M. (2008). National trends in psychotherapy by office-based psychiatrists. *Archives of General Psychiatry, 65*, 962–970. http://dx.doi.org/10.1001/archpsyc.65.8.962

Moore, T. J., & Mattison, D. R. (2017). Adult utilization of psychiatric drugs and differences by sex, age, and race. *JAMA Internal Medicine, 177*, 274–275. http://dx.doi.org/10.1001/jamainternmed.2016.7507

Muse, M., & McGrath, R. E. (2010). Making the case for prescriptive authority. In R. E. McGrath & B. A. Moore (Eds.), *Pharmacotherapy for psychologists: Prescribing and collaborative roles* (pp. 9–27). Washington, DC: American Psychological Association. http://dx.doi.org/10.1037/12167-001

Resnick, R. J., Ax, R. K., Fagan, T. J., & Nussbaum, D. (2012). Predoctoral prescriptive authority curricula: A training option. *Journal of Clinical Psychology, 68*, 246–262. http://dx.doi.org/10.1002/jclp.20828

Robiner, W. N., Tumlin, T. R., & Tompkins, T. L. (2013). Psychologists and medications in the era of inter-professional care: Collaboration is less problematic and costly than prescribing. *Clinical Psychology: Science and Practice, 20*, 489–507. http://dx.doi.org/10.1111/cpsp.12054

Sammons, M. T., & Brown, A. B. (1997). The Department of Defense Psychopharmacology Demonstration Project: An evolving program for postdoctoral education in psychology. *Professional Psychology: Research and Practice, 28*, 107–112. http://dx.doi.org/10.1037/0735-7028.28.2.107

Smyer, M. A., Balster, R. L., Egli, D., Johnson, D. L., Kilbey, M. M., Leith, N. J., & Puente, A. E. (1993). Summary of the Report of the Ad Hoc Task Force on Psychopharmacology of the American Psychological Association. *Professional Psychology: Research and Practice, 24*, 394–403. http://dx.doi.org/10.1037/0735-7028.24.4.394

Statista: The Statistics Portal. (2016). *U.S. Pharmaceutical Industry—Statistics and Facts*. Retrieved from https://www.statista.com/topics/1719/pharmaceutical-industry

Substance Abuse and Mental Health Services Administration, Center for Behavioral Health Statistics and Quality. (2015). *Behavioral health trends in the United States: Results from the 2014 National Survey on Drug Use and Health* (HHS Publication No. SMA 15-4927, NSDUH Series H-50). Retrieved from https://www.samhsa.gov/data/sites/default/files/NSDUH-FRR1-2014/NSDUH-FRR1-2014.pdf

PSYCHOLOGISTS AND INTEGRATED BEHAVIORAL HEALTH CARE WITHIN THE FRAMEWORK OF PSYCHOPHARMACOLOGY

Ana J. Bridges

According to national epidemiological studies, approximately 15% of children, 20% to 40% of adolescents, and 20% to 25% of adults have experienced sufficiently elevated clinical symptoms to meet full criteria for a psychiatric disorder in the past year (Center for Behavioral Health Statistics and Quality, 2016; Kessler, Chiu, Demler, & Walters, 2005; Kessler et al., 2012). The most common disorders youth experience are anxiety disorders (25%), behavior disorders (16%), and mood disorders (10%; Kessler et al., 2012). In adults, anxiety disorders (18%), mood disorders (10%), and impulse control disorders (9%) are most common (Kessler et al., 2005). While a significant proportion of the population will experience symptoms consistent with a diagnosable psychiatric disorder, relatively few individuals seek help. For instance, Wang et al. (2005) found that only 36% of adults with a psychiatric disorder seek care from a health care provider. Instead, most people prefer to manage problems on their own or seek assistance from informal sources of care (Mojtabai et al., 2011). When it does occur, care is most often sought from medical providers rather than specialty mental health providers (Wang et al., 2005). This has resulted in Kessler and Stafford (2008) asserting that primary care is the de facto mental health system.

Not surprisingly, given where people with mental health problems prefer to seek care, primary care providers, rather than psychiatrists or specialty mental health care providers, prescribe most psychotropic medications that patients receive (Mark, Levit, & Buck, 2009). However, primary care providers often lack proper training in the diagnosis and treatment of common psychiatric problems. For example, according to one meta-analysis of 41 studies, general practitioners fail to recognize approximately 52% of patients with major depression (Mitchell, Vaze, & Rao, 2009) and many self-report low confidence in their ability to manage psychiatric concerns in their patients (Loeb, Bayliss, Binswanger, Candrian, & deGruy, 2012).

MODELS OF INTEGRATED BEHAVIORAL HEALTH CARE

Integrated behavioral health care broadly refers to any medical system (from primary care clinics to specialty care clinics and hospitals) that includes a behavioral health specialist as part of the medical health care team (Byrd, O'Donohue, & Cummings, 2005). Psychologists have been part of many secondary and tertiary health care systems for some time (e.g., psychologists integrated into oncology units in hospitals). In fact, by the late 1800s there was already a movement to place mental health facilities inside medical hospitals and, in 1902, the first psychiatric ward of a hospital opened (Holland, 2002). However, integration into primary care settings is much more recent. The first mention of integrating mental health and physical health into primary care

http://dx.doi.org/10.1037/0000133-030
APA Handbook of Psychopharmacology, S. M. Evans (Editor-in-Chief)

clinics occurred in 1967, long after psychologists had already been part of other health care systems (Kazak, Nash, Hiroto, & Kaslow, 2017). However, at that time integration was being done in an ad hoc manner by a few isolated organizations or professionals who each developed their own language for describing what they were doing (Peek, 2013). Since then, especially due to the passage of the Patient Protection and Affordable Care Act (ACA; Public Law No: 111–148) on March 23, 2010, efforts to create a common nomenclature and to develop practice guidelines have flourished.

For the purposes of this chapter, I focus on primary care as the setting in which integration takes place. In order for a primary care setting to be integrated, the care must result from "a practice team of primary care and behavioral health clinicians, working together with patients and families, using a systematic and cost-effective approach to provide patient-centered care for a defined population. This care may address mental health and substance abuse conditions, health behaviors (including their contribution to chronic medical illnesses), life stressors and crises, stress-related physical symptoms, and ineffective patterns of health care utilization" (Peek & the National Integration Academy Council, 2013, p. 15). The behavioral health specialist is often, but not always, a mental health professional such as a psychologist, licensed clinical social worker, or licensed counselor (Robinson & Reiter, 2016).

There are many different ways medical systems can be integrated, and systems can be classified by degree of integration (Doherty, McDaniel, & Baird, 1996; see also Table 30.1). At a relatively low level of integration, the behavioral health specialist has separate space from the medical providers, maintains separate patient medical records, and provides services after a formal referral from a medical provider. At the highest level of integration, sometimes called the *primary care behavioral health model of integrated care* (Robinson & Reiter, 2016), behavioral health specialists use shared space with the medical provider; document in the same patient medical record; and consult on a frequent, informal, and ongoing basis. In fact, in primary care behavioral health, the behavioral health specialist is seen as a primary care provider "extender"—meaning that the primary

care provider is able to expand her services for her patients by including this team member.

Integrated care systems may also differ in the patients they serve (from a well-defined set of patients, such as those with clinical depression, to any patient with a set of psychiatric symptoms or behaviors that are interfering with the patient's health) and the frequency and length of sessions (for instance, from weekly 1-hour meetings to monthly 20-minute meetings). To illustrate, Unützer et al. (2002) developed a collaborative care system to treat depression in elderly primary care patients. The health care team, including the primary care providers, nurses, case managers, psychologists, and a consulting psychiatrist, used a stepped-care approach that began with screening for depression, psychoeducation, care management, medication, and psychotherapy (with each component added as needed, depending on how the patient responded). This model used a targeted group of patients (older adults who screened positive for depression), a set of targeted interventions (including problem-solving therapy and behavioral activation), and telephonic follow-ups for 1 year. A rather different model of integrated care was described by Robinson and Reiter (2016), who provided a "day in the life" of a behavioral health specialist in a primary care behavioral health setting. The hypothetical behavioral health specialist in their example begins her day by participating in a primary care team "huddle" wherein scheduled patients are reviewed, then bounces from seeing a 37-year-old female with medically unexplained symptoms (30-minute session focused on assessment and mindfulness skills) to seeing a 2-year-old boy to screen for autism. The day includes scheduled sessions and "warm hand-offs" (i.e., same-day visits with people identified by the primary care provider as requiring the involvement of a behavioral health specialist for their care), some administration time, and even a patient group. Many of these patients will not require a scheduled follow-up visit.

Despite these differences, all integrated care systems share some common features. The focus is on whole-person care provided by a team of health professionals, rather than fragmented care that occurs in professional siloes (Byrd et al., 2005).

TABLE 30.1

Levels of Medical and Behavioral Health Care Integration

	Coordinated services
Location:	Medical and behavioral health care providers are in separate facilities.
Clinical services:	Services are provided according to separate professional practice standards, with separate medical records, practice guidelines, and minimal sharing of treatment plans across providers.
Patient experience:	Patient physical and behavioral health needs are treated as separate issues.
Referrals:	Referrals are formal and patient is responsible for navigating separate organizations/practice sites.
	Colocated services
Location:	Medical and behavioral health care providers are in the same facility but may be in separate wings or offices.
Clinical services:	Services may be provided with some coordination (e.g., sharing scheduling or office staff, same screening procedures, some sharing of treatment plans), but typically behavioral and medical records are kept separate.
Patient experience:	Patient physical and behavioral health needs are treated in close proximity but remain largely independent.
Referrals:	Referrals are internal and more frequent than in the coordinated services model.
	Integrated services
Location:	Medical and behavioral health care providers are in the same space in the same facility, with offices or exam rooms shared between medical and behavioral health providers.
Clinical services:	Services are fully integrated. Medical and behavioral health providers meet as a team to develop collaborative treatment plans. Medical and behavioral health records are kept together, in the same patient chart.
Patient experience:	Patient's behavioral and physical health care needs are treated simultaneously by members of the team. The clinic is a "one-stop shop" for the patient.
Referrals:	Referrals and provider consultations are informal, frequent, and seamless. No additional paperwork or consent forms are required.

Note. Adapted from *Review and Proposed Standard Framework for Levels of Integrated Healthcare* (pp. 10–13), by B. Heath, P. Wise Romero, and K. A. Reynolds, 2013, Washington, DC: SAMHSA-HRSA Center for Integrated Health Solutions; https://www.integration.samhsa.gov/integrated-care-models/A_Standard_Framework_for_Levels_of_Integrated_Healthcare.pdf. In the public domain.

The purpose is to better manage patient health concerns and reduce barriers to accessing care (Blount, 1998). There is an emphasis on continual evaluation and quality improvement (Peek, 2013) and a focus on population health (Robinson & Reiter, 2016). Population health is defined as "the health outcomes of a group of individuals, including the distribution of such outcomes within the group" (Kindig & Stoddart, 2003, p. 381). In contrast to individual health care, in which the goal is to maximize the health outcomes of an individual person, integrated health care is focused on maximizing the health outcomes of a group of people. This means attending to not only the efficacy of a treatment approach

or intervention but also to the percentage of the population who can receive that treatment. This dual focus on efficacy and reach is called *treatment impact* (Abrams et al., 1996).

PSYCHOPHARMACOLOGY AND THE BEHAVIORAL HEALTH SPECIALIST

The primary role of the behavioral health specialist in the primary care team, regardless of the degree of integration, is to provide direct patient care. Depending on the position, model, and behavioral health specialists' training, the role may also include program evaluation, development of patient care algorithms, and administration, as well as (of course) consultation with primary care providers and other members of the health care team (Robinson & Reiter, 2016).

However, one important role behavioral health specialists often find that they need to navigate when they are part of the primary care team is that of consultant to medical providers regarding psychopharmacological interventions for patients with psychiatric disorders. This is a particularly challenging role for most behavioral health specialists, who may lack formal training in psychopharmacology. Although in a handful of states and in some special settings, psychologists with additional training may in fact obtain prescriptive authority (American Psychological Association, 2017; see Chapter 29, this volume, for more details), this is outside the scope of practice for most psychologists and other behavioral health specialists.

Tension may arise because the primary care provider will often seek the expertise of a behavioral health specialist regarding medications to augment treatment, but the behavioral health specialist's role must remain within the scope of his or her professional practice (American Psychological Association Division 55 Task Force on Practice Guidelines, 2011). For instance, without proper training and certification, most psychologists and social workers should not provide primary care providers with recommendations regarding specific medications or therapeutic doses for prescriptions. So, what are the activities that behavioral health specialists may engage in while remaining within their scope of practice? In the following sections, I review a few. Additional resources are provided at the end of this chapter (in the Tool Kit of Resources).

Psychodiagnostics

One critical role a behavioral health specialist may provide to the patient that can inform psychopharmacological interventions is to conduct a psychiatric evaluation of the patient. The depth or scope of such an evaluation depends on the model of integrated care that the behavioral health specialist operates within (see Table 30.1); in a more colocated model, a traditional comprehensive assessment is possible, but in a primary care behavioral health

model, diagnostic interviewing should remain brief (under 30 minutes). In either case, psychodiagnostic assessments of patients should rely on standardized measures that are normed on people like the patient and that have good psychometric properties (e.g., reliability and validity for diagnostic purposes). Examples of instruments and websites for assessment resources are provided in the Tool Kit of Resources at the end of this chapter. For instance, the Mini International Neuropsychiatric Interview (MINI; Sheehan et al., 1998) assesses over a dozen of the most common psychiatric disorders and can be administered in approximately 15 minutes. There are versions for both adult and pediatric patients. The newest version (MINI 7.0.2) has been recently updated to reflect *Diagnostic and Statistical Manual of Mental Disorders, 5th Edition* (*DSM–5*; American Psychiatric Association, 2013) criteria. In some cases, the entire measure need not be administered; the behavioral health specialist may select only certain modules or sections in order to focus on a particular likely set of diagnoses the patient may carry. Behavioral health specialists may instead opt to administer more targeted measures to assist with clinical diagnostics, such as the Patient Health Questionnaire (PHQ-9; Kroenke, Spitzer, & Williams, 2001) to assess for depression or the Generalized Anxiety Disorders 7-item scale (Spitzer, Kroenke, Williams, & Löwe, 2006) to assess anxiety. The new *DSM–5* website includes several disorder-specific measures for both adults and children.

Consultation

Perhaps following a diagnostic assessment or clinical interview with the patient, or perhaps through direct interaction with the primary care provider, the behavioral health specialist may serve an important consultation role regarding the appropriateness of pharmacological treatment for a patient. While, as noted previously, specific recommendations about medications and doses are typically outside the scope of practice for most behavioral health specialists, there are other consultation activities that may be helpful. For instance, the behavioral health specialist may provide research evidence to the primary care provider about whether medication is an evidence-based approach to treating people with a particular disorder. Sources of that evidence are best obtained through systematic reviews such as those published by Cochrane (https://www.cochrane.org/) or through reputable organizations, such as the World Health Organization (see, for example, http://www.who.int/mental_health/management/psychotropic/en/) or the National Institutes of Health (https://www.nimh.nih.gov/health/topics/mental-health-medications/index.shtml), but meta-analyses or single randomized controlled trials may also be helpful.

Web-based informatics are also available to assist behavioral health specialists in consulting with prescribing providers about pharmacological interventions for patients. For instance, behavioral health specialists can learn to search for answers to clinical care questions by using the PICO format. The PICO acronym refers to (P) patient, problem, or population; (I) intervention; (C) comparison, control, or comparator, and (O) outcome (Spring, 2007). One database that can be helpful when searching for the latest health care informatics is the Trip database (https://www.tripdatabase.com/#pico). Here, you can enter in clinical questions in the PICO format to quickly access evidence. For instance, you can ask whether in (P) patients with social anxiety disorder, does (I) medication augment (C) cognitive behavior therapy to (O) reduce symptoms? The results are even organized by type of article (e.g., ongoing clinical trials, primary research, controlled trials, evidence-based synopses, or systematic reviews), corresponding with increasingly strong levels of research evidence. These can be particularly helpful resources to suggest to medical providers if questions about the relative benefits of one versus another type of treatment are part of the consultation question.

Psychoeducation

Many times patients can be confused about prescriptions. A behavioral health specialist can help prescribing medical providers free up their time by taking on the role of communicating with patients regarding their prescriptions—the purpose of the medication, dosing instructions, possible side effects, and so forth (American Psychological Association Division 55 Task Force on Practice Guidelines, 2011). Of course, behavioral health

specialists should ensure that they possess accurate information and understand the specific instructions that the prescribing provider wants to convey to the patient. In fact, knowledge of psychotropic medications is one of the core competencies articulated by numerous scholars for primary care behavioral health providers (e.g., McDaniel et al., 2014; Robinson & Reiter, 2016; Strosahl, 2005; see also the Tool Kit of Resources).

Monitoring

Another method of helping to free up the medical provider's time by assisting with patient care is for the medical provider to stagger patient follow-up visits so that they alternate between the medical provider and the behavioral health specialist (Robinson & Reiter, 2016). The patient, for instance, can be scheduled to follow up with the behavioral health specialist 2 weeks after beginning a new psychotropic medication. At this follow-up visit, the behavioral health specialist can inquire about the patient's well-being, see if there were any concerns or side effects, and complement medical treatment with targeted behavioral interventions, if appropriate. This staggered schedule of follow-up visits allows the health care team to monitor potentially serious complications on a more frequent basis while a patient adjusts to a medication change, often at a lower cost to the patient and a reduced burden to the primary care physician, which is particularly important given the possibility that some medications, such as selective serotonin reuptake inhibitors, may result in increases in suicidality in patients (especially adolescents; Barbui, Esposito, & Cipriani, 2009).

Intervention

In most cases, a combination of pharmacological and psychotherapeutic interventions is ideal to treat disorders. For instance, research syntheses suggest that adding psychotherapy to pharmacotherapy results in significant improvements in depression symptoms and lower premature termination of treatment compared with pharmacotherapy alone (Cuijpers, Dekker, Hollon, & Andersson, 2009; Pampallona, Bollini, Tibaldi, Kupelnick, & Munizza, 2004). In addition, patients on the whole express a preference for psychological treatments over pharmacological treatments for psychiatric concerns (McHugh, Whitton, Peckham, Welge, & Otto, 2013). It is therefore beneficial for behavioral health specialists to see their role as providing intervention to patients to address whatever psychiatric concerns may be present, even if medications are being prescribed for the same concern. Evidence-based interventions can be adapted for the type of integrated care facility in which the behavioral health specialist works, but some useful resources for identifying possible interventions to be utilized or adapted include websites (such as the American Psychological Association's Society of Clinical Psychology website at https://www.div12.org/psychological-treatments and the SAMHSA/HRSA Center for Integrated Care Solutions website at https://www.integration.samhsa.gov/), books (such as Gatchel & Oordt, 2003; Hunter, Goodie, Oordt, & Dobmeyer, 2009; O'Donohue, Byrd, Cummings, & Henderson, 2006; Robinson & Reiter, 2016), and journal issues (such as volume 21, issue 3 of *Cognitive and Behavioral Practice*, 2014, or volume 35, issue 2 of *Families, Systems, & Health*, 2017). The Society of Clinical Psychology has amassed a list of empirically supported treatments for various psychiatric disorders. The website includes descriptions about the treatments and information for further training or clinical resources. Although nearly all of these treatments were developed to be delivered in traditional care settings and therefore tend to require 12+ sessions, many of the principles of change can be adapted for delivery in primary care settings. Hunter et al. (2009) described how common behavioral and cognitive intervention strategies can be adapted from specialty care to the rapid pace of primary care (that is, to be delivered in one to four 30-minute sessions). They focus on interventions that patients can practice outside of session, so that the time the behavioral health specialist spends with a patient can be more focused on instruction, encouragement, correction, and monitoring. Recently, academic journals have begun publishing papers that provide "mini-manuals" or "how to" guides for treating specific behavioral health concerns, including insomnia (Goodie & Hunter, 2014), suicidality (Bryan, Corso, & Macalanda, 2014), and even posttraumatic stress disorder (Cigrang et al., 2017).

Medication Adherence

An important role a behavioral health specialist may play in assisting with pharmacological interventions for primary care patients is to assist with medication nonadherence. A large proportion of patients do not adhere to prescription instructions (Olfson, Marcus, Tedeschi, & Wan, 2006). Common reasons patients report difficulties with medication adherence include lack of financial resources to purchase required medications, undesirable side effects, and a sense that medication is either ineffective or no longer required (American Psychological Association Division 55 Task Force on Practice Guidelines, 2011). One task psychologists can take on to support pharmacotherapy is to recognize and assist patients who show some ambivalence or barriers to adhering to medication recommendations.

Interventions to increase adherence to medication regimens have been developed. For instance, Rollnick, Mason, and Butler (1999) suggested that interventions focus on understanding the reasons why patients may not be adhering to a recommended medical regimen, with the behavioral health specialist being as nonjudgmental and collaborative as possible, and then flexibly working with patients to identify these barriers, enhance patient self-efficacy, and negotiate adherence treatment goals. This approach relies heavily on motivational enhancement. Systematic reviews of interventions related to increasing adherence to pharmacotherapy for depression in primary care patients concluded that psychoeducation is insufficient to enhance adherence, but multifaceted and collaborative care interventions that included a mental health care specialist as part of the primary care team are sufficient (Chong, Aslani, & Chen, 2011; Vergouwen, Bakker, Katon, Verheij, & Koerselman, 2003). Levensky (2005) described brief strategies that are appropriate for primary care behavioral health practitioners to use to increase medication adherence in patients. Strategies include assessing readiness to use medications, providing psychoeducation about the nature of the condition for which medication is being prescribed and about the medication itself, increasing skills that the patient may need to adhere properly to the recommended regimen (e.g., memory aids, problem-solving skills, self-monitoring), and enhancing motivation.

If cost is a barrier to medication adherence, the behavioral health specialist can work with a patient case manager to see whether there are resources available to assist with prescription costs. Many pharmaceutical companies provide samples to providers that can be used to help a patient for a brief period of time. Prescription assistance programs, such as the Partnership for Prescription Assistance (https://www.pparx.org/), can also be explored. Some are run by pharmaceutical companies, while others are run by states or nonprofit organizations. Some have eligibility requirements, such as limiting assistance to people with specific health conditions or individuals who are receiving government-funded health care. A behavioral health specialist or case manager can assist patients with completing eligibility paperwork to receive such services.

Communication/Liaison

Sometimes patients will reveal concerns about their prescribed medications to their behavioral health specialist, but do not feel comfortable addressing those concerns directly with their primary care provider. In other cases, the patient does not reveal any concerns, but the behavioral health specialist notes that the patient appears not to be improving or even to be worsening. In each of these cases, the behavioral health specialist can communicate the concerns with the primary care provider so she can make adjustments, as needed. Behavioral health specialists can also work with patients to increase their communication skills so that patients can more effectively advocate for their own needs.

SUMMARY AND FUTURE DIRECTIONS

Primary care has been and likely will continue to be the most frequent setting wherein patients suffering from psychiatric difficulties seek care. The embedding of mental health professionals into the primary care team is therefore beneficial to better identify and treat such patients. However, challenges remain. The pipeline of psychologists trained in integrated care practice is growing but remains behind the demand for professionals who can fill such positions

(American Psychological Association, 2016; Hall et al., 2015). Many psychologists trained in traditional techniques of psychotherapy struggle to limit assessments and interventions to the 15 to 30 minutes required for most integrated primary care practices, at least initially (Robinson & Reiter, 2016). There is a general lack of providers with experience in integrated care (both medical and behavioral) who can model best practices for new trainees, and organizations are finding that they must commit extra time and resources to adequate training (Hall et al., 2015). Furthermore, funding for integrated care is challenging; traditional medical and behavioral health providers use separate billing codes, and many insurance providers will not allow for the billing of two services for the same condition in the same day (Robinson & Reiter, 2016). Although integrated care practices are considered "one-stop shops" for primary care patients (e.g., Hetrick et al., 2017), a well-functioning primary care practice relies on a robust network of community partners—outside providers who can serve as referral sources for patients with serious mental illness or those in need of longer term psychotherapy and more complex pharmacological treatment. As the American Psychological Association's (2016) resolution indicates, there are clear efforts underway to address each of these major barriers and challenges.

The behavioral health specialists who take on these roles within health care teams often face requests to assist with pharmacological treatment of patients. Although specific recommendations regarding medications and dosage are beyond the scope of professional practice for most behavioral health specialists, there are many supportive roles they can take on. Assisting prescribing medical providers by conducting psychodiagnostic assessments, monitoring medication effects, providing adjunct therapeutic interventions, addressing medication nonadherence, and enhancing communication between the patient and primary care provider are all well within the expertise of a behavioral health specialist. Primary care providers express high satisfaction with behavioral health specialists who can assist them with managing patients (Funderburk, Fielder, DeMartini, & Flynn, 2012; Torrence et al.,

2014). As long as each member of the team is aware and respectful of their roles and responsibilities, integrated behavioral health care teams function well to assist patients with psychiatric concerns that may require medication.

TOOL KIT OF RESOURCES

Assessment Instruments Appropriate for Integrated Behavioral Health Care Practice

Mini International Neuropsychiatric Interview: www.harmresearch.org/index.php/mini-international-neuropsychiatric-interview-mini/

Substance Abuse and Mental Health Services Administration–Health Resources Services Administration Center for Integrated Health Care Solutions: https://www.integration.samhsa.gov/clinical-practice/screening-tools

Patient Health Questionnaire-9 and Generalized Anxiety Disorders 7: https://www.phqscreeners.com

DSM–5 Online Assessment Measures: https://www.psychiatry.org/psychiatrists/practice/dsm/educational-resources/assessment-measures#Disorder

Consultation/Informatics Resources

Cochrane systematic reviews: https://www.cochrane.org

World Health Organization: www.who.int/mental_health/en/

National Institutes of Health: https://www.nimh.nih.gov/health/topics/index.shtml

Trip database: https://www.tripdatabase.com#pico

General Resources

Substance Abuse and Mental Health Services Administration–Health Resources Services Administration Center for Integrated Health Care Solutions: https://www.integration.samhsa.gov/

Agency for Healthcare Research and Quality: https://integrationacademy.ahrq.gov

Patient-Centered Primary Care Collaborative: https://www.pcpcc.org

Integrated Behavioral Health Partners: www.ibhpartners.org

Behavioral Health Consultant Core Competencies: https://neupsykey.com/behavioral-health-consultant-core-competencies/

*Asterisks indicate assessments or resources.

Behavioral Consultation and Primary Care: A Guide to Integrating Services: https://www.behavioralconsultationandprimarycare.com/

References

Abrams, D. B., Orleans, C. T., Niaura, R. S., Goldstein, M. G., Prochaska, J. O., & Velicer, W. (1996). Integrating individual and public health perspectives for treatment of tobacco dependence under managed health care: A combined stepped-care and matching model. *Annals of Behavioral Medicine, 18*, 290–304. http://dx.doi.org/10.1007/BF02895291

American Psychiatric Association. (2013). *Diagnostic and statistical manual of mental Disorders, 5th edition.* Washington, DC: Author.

American Psychological Association. (2016). *Resolution of psychologists in integrated primary care and specialty health settings.* Retrieved from http://www.apa.org/about/policy/integrated-primary-care.aspx

American Psychological Association. (2017). *Idaho becomes fifth state to allow psychologists to prescribe medications.* Retrieved from www.apa.org/news/press/releases/2017/04/idaho-psychologists-medications.aspx

American Psychological Association Division 55 (American Society for the Advancement of Pharmacotherapy) Task Force on Practice Guidelines. (2011). Practice guidelines regarding psychologists' involvement in pharmacological issues. *American Psychologist, 66*, 835–849. http://dx.doi.org/10.1037/a0025890

Barbui, C., Esposito, E., & Cipriani, A. (2009). Selective serotonin reuptake inhibitors and risk of suicide: A systematic review of observational studies. *Canadian Medical Association Journal, 180*, 291–297. http://dx.doi.org/10.1503/cmaj.081514

Blount, A. (1998). Introduction to integrated primary care. In A. Blount (Ed.), *Integrated primary care: The future of medical and mental health collaboration* (pp. 1–43). New York, NY: W. W. Norton & Co.

Bryan, C. J., Corso, K. A., & Macalanda, J. (2014). An evidence-based approach to managing suicidal patients in the patient-centered medical home. *Cognitive and Behavioral Practice, 21*, 269–281. http://dx.doi.org/10.1016/j.cbpra.2014.04.006

Byrd, M. R., O'Donohue, W. T., & Cummings, N. A. (2005). The case for integrated care: Coordinating behavioral health care with primary care medicine. In W. T. O'Donohue, M. R. Byrd, N. A. Cummings, & D. A. Henderson (Eds.), *Behavioral integrative care: Treatments that work in the primary care setting* (pp. 1–14). New York, NY: Brunner Routledge.

Center for Behavioral Health Statistics and Quality. (2016). *2015 National Survey on Drug Use and Health:*

Detailed tables. Rockville, MD: Substance Abuse and Mental Health Services Administration.

Cigrang, J. A., Rauch, S. A., Mintz, J., Brundige, A. R., Mitchell, J. A., Najera, E., . . . Peterson, A. L., & the STRONG STAR Consortium. (2017). Moving effective treatment for posttraumatic stress disorder to primary care: A randomized controlled trial with active duty military. *Families, Systems, & Health, 35,* 450–462. http://dx.doi.org/10.1037/fsh0000315

Chong, W. W., Aslani, P., & Chen, T. F. (2011). Effectiveness of interventions to improve antidepressant medication adherence: A systematic review. *International Journal of Clinical Practice, 65,* 954–975. http://dx.doi.org/10.1111/j.1742-1241.2011.02746.x

Cuijpers, P., Dekker, J., Hollon, S. D., & Andersson, G. (2009). Adding psychotherapy to pharmacotherapy in the treatment of depressive disorders in adults: A meta-analysis. *The Journal of Clinical Psychiatry, 70,* 1219–1229. http://dx.doi.org/10.4088/JCP.09r05021

Doherty, W. J., McDaniel, S. H., & Baird, M. A. (1996). Five levels of primary care/behavioral healthcare collaboration. *Behavioral Healthcare Tomorrow, 5,* 25–27.

Funderburk, J. S., Fielder, R. L., DeMartini, K. S., & Flynn, C. A. (2012). Integrating behavioral health services into a university health center: Patient and provider satisfaction. *Families, Systems, & Health, 30,* 130–140. http://dx.doi.org/10.1037/a0028378

Gatchel, R. J., & Oordt, M. S. (2003). *Clinical health psychology and primary care: Practical advice and clinical guidance for successful collaboration.* Washington, DC: American Psychological Association. http://dx.doi.org/10.1037/10592-000

Goodie, J. L., & Hunter, C. L. (2014). Practical guidance for targeting insomnia in primary care settings. *Cognitive and Behavioral Practice, 21,* 261–268. http://dx.doi.org/10.1016/j.cbpra.2014.01.001

Hall, J., Cohen, D. J., Davis, M., Gunn, R., Blount, A., Pollack, D. A., . . . Miller, B. F. (2015). Preparing the workforce for behavioral health and primary care integration. *Journal of the American Board of Family Medicine, 28*(Suppl. 1), S41–S51. http://dx.doi.org/10.3122/jabfm.2015.S1.150054

Heath, B., Wise Romero, P., & Reynolds, K. A. (2013). Review and proposed standard framework for levels of integrated healthcare. Washington, DC: SAMHSA-HRSA Center for Integrated Health Solutions. Retrieved from https://www.integration.samhsa.gov/integrated-care-models/A_Standard_Framework_for_Levels_of_Integrated_Healthcare.pdf

Hetrick, S. E., Bailey, A. P., Smith, K. E., Malla, A., Mathias, S., Singh, S. P., . . . McGorry, P. D. (2017). Integrated (one-stop shop) youth health care: Best available evidence and future directions. *The Medical Journal of Australia, 207,* S5–S18. http://dx.doi.org/10.5694/mja17.00694

Holland, J. C. (2002). History of psycho-oncology: Overcoming attitudinal and conceptual barriers. *Psychosomatic Medicine, 64,* 206–221. http://dx.doi.org/10.1097/00006842-200203000-00004

Hunter, C. L., Goodie, J. L., Oordt, M. S., & Dobmeyer, A. C. (2009). *Integrated behavioral health in primary care: Step-by-step guidance for assessment and intervention.* Washington, DC: American Psychological Association. http://dx.doi.org/10.1037/11871-000

Kazak, A. E., Nash, J. M., Hiroto, K., & Kaslow, N. J. (2017). Psychologists in patient-centered medical homes (PCMHs): Roles, evidence, opportunities, and challenges. *American Psychologist, 72,* 1–12. http://dx.doi.org/10.1037/a0040382

Kessler, R., & Stafford, D. (2008). Primary care is the de facto mental health system. In R. Kessler & D. Stafford (Eds.), *Collaborative medicine case studies* (pp. 9–21). New York, NY: Springer. http://dx.doi.org/10.1007/978-0-387-76894-6_2

Kessler, R. C., Avenevoli, S., Costello, E. J., Georgiades, K., Green, J. G., Gruber, M. J., . . . Merikangas, K. R. (2012). Prevalence, persistence, and sociodemographic correlates of *DSM–IV* disorders in the National Comorbidity Survey Replication Adolescent Supplement. *Archives of General Psychiatry, 69,* 372–380. http://dx.doi.org/10.1001/archgenpsychiatry.2011.160

Kessler, R. C., Chiu, W. T., Demler, O., & Walters, E. E. (2005). Prevalence, severity, and comorbidity of 12-month *DSM–IV* disorders in the National Comorbidity Survey Replication. *Archives of General Psychiatry, 62,* 617–627. http://dx.doi.org/10.1001/archpsyc.62.6.617

Kindig, D., & Stoddart, G. (2003). What is population health? *American Journal of Public Health, 93,* 380–383. http://dx.doi.org/10.2105/AJPH.93.3.380

*Kroenke, K., Spitzer, R. L., & Williams, J. B. W. (2001). The PHQ-9: Validity of a brief depression severity measure. *Journal of General Internal Medicine, 16,* 606–613. http://dx.doi.org/10.1046/j.1525-1497.2001.016009606.x

Levensky, E. R. (2005). Increasing medication adherence in chronic illnesses: Guidelines for behavioral healthcare clinicians working in primary care settings. In W. T. O'Donohue, M. R. Byrd, N. A. Cummings, & D. A. Henderson (Eds.), *Behavioral integrative care: Treatments that work in the primary care setting* (pp. 347–366). New York, NY: Brunner Routledge.

Loeb, D. F., Bayliss, E. A., Binswanger, I. A., Candrian, C., & deGruy, F. V. (2012). Primary care physician perceptions on caring for complex patients with medical and mental illness. *Journal of General Internal Medicine, 27,* 945–952. http://dx.doi.org/10.1007/s11606-012-2005-9

Mark, T. L., Levit, K. R., & Buck, J. A. (2009). Datapoints: Psychotropic drug prescriptions by medical specialty.

Psychiatric Services, 60, 1167. http://dx.doi.org/10.1176/ps.2009.60.9.1167

McDaniel, S. H., Grus, C. L., Cubic, B. A., Hunter, C. L., Kearney, L. K., Schuman, C. C., . . . Johnson, S. B. (2014). Competencies for psychology practice in primary care. *American Psychologist, 69,* 409–429. http://dx.doi.org/10.1037/a0036072

McHugh, R. K., Whitton, S. W., Peckham, A. D., Welge, J. A., & Otto, M. W. (2013). Patient preference for psychological vs pharmacologic treatment of psychiatric disorders: A meta-analytic review. *The Journal of Clinical Psychiatry, 74,* 595–602. http://dx.doi.org/10.4088/JCP.12r07757

Mitchell, A. J., Vaze, A., & Rao, S. (2009). Clinical diagnosis of depression in primary care: A meta-analysis. *The Lancet, 374,* 609–619. http://dx.doi.org/10.1016/S0140-6736(09)60879-5

Mojtabai, R., Olfson, M., Sampson, N. A., Jin, R., Druss, B., Wang, P. S., . . . Kessler, R. C. (2011). Barriers to mental health treatment: Results from the National Comorbidity Survey Replication. *Psychological Medicine, 41,* 1751–1761. http://dx.doi.org/10.1017/S0033291710002291

O'Donohue, W. T., Byrd, M. R., Cummings, N. A., & Henderson, D. A. (2006). *Behavioral integrative care: Treatments that work in the primary care setting.* New York, NY: Brunner Routledge.

Olfson, M., Marcus, S. C., Tedeschi, M., & Wan, G. J. (2006). Continuity of antidepressant treatment for adults with depression in the United States. *The American Journal of Psychiatry, 163,* 101–108. http://dx.doi.org/10.1176/appi.ajp.163.1.101

Pampallona, S., Bollini, P., Tibaldi, G., Kupelnick, B., & Munizza, C. (2004). Combined pharmacotherapy and psychological treatment for depression: A systematic review. *Archives of General Psychiatry, 61,* 714–719. http://dx.doi.org/10.1001/archpsyc.61.7.714

Peek, C. J. (2013). Integrated behavioral health and primary care: A common language. In M. R. Talen & A. Burke Valeras (Eds.), *Integrated behavioral health in primary care: Evaluating the evidence, identifying the essentials* (pp. 9–31). New York, NY: Springer. http://dx.doi.org/10.1007/978-1-4614-6889-9_2

Peek, C. J. and the National Integration Academy Council. (2013). Lexicon for behavioral health and primary care integration: Concepts and definitions developed by expert consensus. *AHRQ Publication No.13-IP001-EF,* 15. Rockville, MD: Agency for Healthcare Research and Quality. Available at: http://integrationacademy.ahrq.gov/sites/default/files/Lexicon.pdf.

Robinson, P. J., & Reiter, J. T. (2016). *Behavioral consultation and primary care: A guide to integrating services* (2nd ed.). New York, NY: Springer. http://dx.doi.org/10.1007/978-3-319-13954-8

Rollnick, S., Mason, P., & Butler, C. (1999). *Health behavior change: A guide for practitioners.* Philadelphia, PA: Churchill Livingstone.

*Sheehan, D. V., Lecrubier, Y., Sheehan, K. H., Amorim, P., Janavs, J., Weiller, E., . . . Dunbar, G. C. (1998). The Mini-International Neuropsychiatric Interview (M.I.N.I.): The development and validation of a structured diagnostic psychiatric interview for *DSM–IV* and ICD–10. *The Journal of Clinical Psychiatry, 59*(Suppl. 20), 22–33.

*Spitzer, R. L., Kroenke, K., Williams, J. B. W., & Löwe, B. (2006). A brief measure for assessing generalized anxiety disorder: The GAD-7. *Archives of Internal Medicine, 166,* 1092–1097. http://dx.doi.org/10.1001/archinte.166.10.1092

Spring, B. (2007). Evidence-based practice in clinical psychology: What it is, why it matters; what you need to know. *Journal of Clinical Psychology, 63,* 611–631. http://dx.doi.org/10.1002/jclp.20373

Strosahl, K. D. (2005). Training behavioral health and primary care providers for integrated care: A core competencies approach. In W. T. O'Donohue, M. R. Byrd, N. A. Cummings, & D. A. Henderson (Eds.), *Behavioral integrative care: Treatments that work in the primary care setting* (pp. 15–52). New York, NY: Brunner Routledge.

Torrence, N. D., Mueller, A. E., Ilem, A. A., Renn, B. N., DeSantis, B., & Segal, D. L. (2014). Medical provider attitudes about behavioral health consultants in integrated primary care: A preliminary study. *Families, Systems, & Health, 32,* 426–432. http://dx.doi.org/10.1037/fsh0000078

Unützer, J., Katon, W., Callahan, C. M., Williams, J. W., Jr., Hunkeler, E., Harpole, L., . . . Langston, C., & the IMPACT Investigators (2002). Collaborative care management of late-life depression in the primary care setting: A randomized controlled trial. *JAMA: Journal of the American Medical Association, 288,* 2836–2845. http://dx.doi.org/10.1001/jama.288.22.2836

Vergouwen, A. C. M., Bakker, A., Katon, W. J., Verheij, T. J., & Koerselman, F. (2003). Improving adherence to antidepressants: A systematic review of interventions. *The Journal of Clinical Psychiatry, 64,* 1415–1420. http://dx.doi.org/10.4088/JCP.v64n1203

Wang, P. S., Lane, M., Olfson, M., Pincus, H. A., Wells, K. B., & Kessler, R. C. (2005). Twelve-month use of mental health services in the United States: Results from the National Comorbidity Survey Replication. *Archives of General Psychiatry, 62,* 629–640. http://dx.doi.org/10.1001/archpsyc.62.6.629

THE ROLE OF THE PHARMACEUTICAL INDUSTRY IN THE TREATMENT OF MENTAL HEALTH DISORDERS

Bethea A. Kleykamp and Jack E. Henningfield

The pharmaceutical industry's role as an innovator of drug treatments for mental health disorders began in the middle of the 20th century with the development of chlorpromazine (i.e., Largactil®, Thorazine®) by the French pharmaceutical company Rhône-Poulenc (Ban, 2001, 2006, 2007; López-Muñoz, Álamo, & García-García, 2011). At the time, chlorpromazine was determined to be more effective for managing psychotic symptoms (e.g., delusions, hallucinations) compared with existing alternatives, such as morphine. As a result, chlorpromazine was approved as a prescription drug and used by psychiatric facilities across the world to manage patient health and behavior. Historians have noted that the commercial success of chlorpromazine stimulated the development of other psychotropic drugs and contributed to the role of the pharmaceutical industry in treating mental health disorders (Ban, 2007). Another key contributor to the commercialization of medications was the growing endorsement of the biomedical model of mental health disorders, or the theory that brain diseases involve chemical imbalances that can be corrected with drugs (Deacon, 2013; more history can be found in Chapter 1, this volume.)

While the 1900s held much promise for the role of the pharmaceutical industry in mental health, there has been a growing concern that there is a diminishing pipeline of approved medications for mental health disorders (Berk, 2012; Fibiger, 2012; Hyman, 2012; O'Brien, Thomas, Hodgkin, Levit, & Mark, 2014). This slowing of medication development is thought to be associated with various factors, such as failure of animal trials to translate well into human trials, undesirable side effect profiles, and the inherent complexity of the human brain (DiMasi, Grabowski, & Hansen, 2016; O'Brien et al., 2014). Another key contributor to lagging drug development is the challenging regulatory environment involved in gaining approval for the marketing and distribution of such medications (O'Brien et al., 2014). As represented in Figure 31.1, regulatory authorities such as the U.S. Food and Drug Administration (FDA) require that companies conduct multiple phases of preclinical and human testing prior to submitting new drug applications (NDAs; O'Brien et al., 2014). Other regulatory authorities have similar requirements, such as the European Medicines Agency. As reflected in the figure, the

Dr. Henningfield works for the consulting firm PinneyAssociates. PinneyAssociates consults with pharmaceutical companies that market a wide variety of prescription and over-the-counter medications, including prescription opioids and stimulants. In addition, PinneyAssociates has provided services for Reynolds American, Inc. on tobacco harm minimization and noncombustible tobacco products. RAI was recently acquired by British American Tobacco. Dr. Henningfield has worked with a variety of organizations, including the National Institutes of Health (NIH)/National Institute on Drug Abuse (NIDA), U.S. Food and Drug Administration (FDA), World Health Organization, and the U.S. Surgeon General's Office across the last 4 decades. Dr. Kleykamp was previously employed by PinneyAssociates and currently works as a research associate professor at the University of Rochester School of Medicine and Dentistry where she is also the communications director for the Analgesic, Anesthetic, and Addiction Clinical Trial Translations, Innovations, Opportunities, and Networks (ACTTION) public–private partnership, which has received research contracts, grants, or other revenue from FDA, multiple pharmaceutical and device companies, and other sources. She previously completed predoctoral and postdoctoral fellowships supported by the NIH/NIDA, and has worked for the health care technology assessment company Hayes, Inc. All of these past and present affiliations have the potential to influence the content of this chapter, although all efforts have been made to limit their impact, including having no support or oversight of the writing of the chapter by any clients served by PinneyAssociates.

http://dx.doi.org/10.1037/0000133-031
APA Handbook of Psychopharmacology, S. M. Evans (Editor-in-Chief)
Copyright © 2019 by the American Psychological Association. All rights reserved.

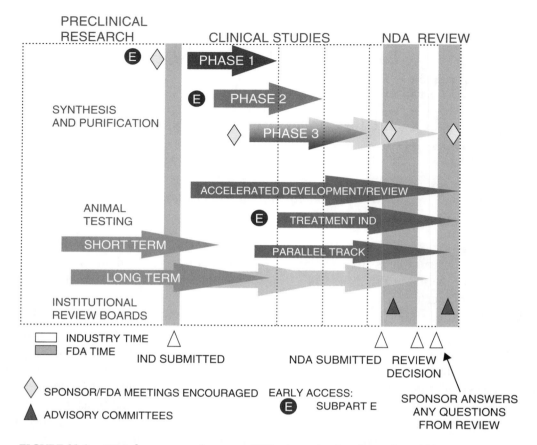

FIGURE 31.1. FDA drug approval process. IND = investigational new drug; NDA = new drug application. From *New Drug Development and Review Process*, by U.S. Food and Drug Administration, 2016, Silver Spring, MD: Author; https://www.fda.gov/Drugs/ DevelopmentApprovalProcess/SmallBusinessAssistance/ucm053131.htm. In the public domain.

clinical evaluation component of an NDA includes three premarketing phases and sometimes a fourth phase that includes postmarketing surveillance (i.e., the monitoring of drug safety after a medication has been marketed and distributed to the public). Some estimates suggest that final approval of an NDA can take upwards of 10 years and 2.5 billion dollars to achieve, highlighting the enormous investment necessary for bringing new drugs to market (DiMasi, Grabowski, and Hansen, 2016).

An additional, but very important, consideration for drug development related to mental health is the FDA requirement that any drug with central nervous system (CNS) activity be considered for abuse potential (U.S. Food and Drug Administration Center for Drug Evaluation and Research, 2017). Abuse potential is defined as the likelihood that the

drug could be abused or used for nontherapeutic reasons such as to achieve a desired psychological or physiological effect. Abuse potential studies, which can include nonclinical and clinical studies, are critical in determining if the drug should be regulated or placed in one of five distinct categories or schedules depending on the drug's acceptable medical use and the drug's abuse or dependency potential. All in all, the extensive process of CNS drug development and potential need for abuse potential evaluations make the successful development and approval of such medications quite challenging. A consequence of these regulatory and economic burdens includes a low number of NDA approvals, with an average of only 26 FDA approvals per year since 2003 for all drugs, including those related to mental health (Moses et al., 2015).

Drug pricing concerns are also very important considerations related to pharmaceutical investment in drug development. The issue is a growing concern in the United States, as reflected by a congressional hearing addressing the drug supply chain that took place on December 13, 2017, among the members of the Committee on Energy and Commerce and the Subcommittee on Health (Examining the Drug Supply Chain, 2017). Such concerns are, at least in part, related to increasing costs of biomedical research investments, with one estimate suggesting that between 1995 and 2005 costs increased from 43% to 369% across multiple therapeutic areas, with a 101% inflation-adjusted increase for neuroscience research (e.g., neurological disorders, mental health, substance abuse; Dorsey et al., 2009). Unfortunately, such investments have not been matched by federal funding, with one study finding that industry-funded registered trials in the www.ClinicalTrials.gov registry increased by 43% between 2006 and 2013, while trials funded by the National Institutes of Health (NIH) decreased by 24% during the same time period (Ehrhardt, Appel, & Meinert, 2015). As noted later in the chapter, other considerations influencing drug pricing include drug market exclusivity and patent rights, as well as the influence of various stakeholders, including insurance companies, the hospital industry, and pharmacy benefits managers (companies that negotiate drug price discounts for insurers and employers). These legitimate and growing concerns around drug pricing highlight the key role that the pharmaceutical industry plays and likely will continue to play in generating research and treatments for mental health disorders in the 21st century (Dorsey et al., 2009; Ehrhardt et al., 2015).

EXAMPLES OF MENTAL HEALTH DISORDERS ADDRESSED BY PHARMACEUTICAL COMPANY RESEARCH AND NEW DRUG DEVELOPMENT

The following sections examine four commonly diagnosed mental health disorders that have been impacted by the pharmaceutical industry. The disorders discussed are: attention-deficit/hyperactivity disorder, anxiety disorders, pain and pain-related disorders, and tobacco dependence.

Attention-Deficit/Hyperactivity Disorder

Attention-deficit/hyperactivity disorder (ADHD; see also Chapter 16, this volume), previously identified as attention deficit disorder or hyperkinetic reaction of childhood, is a brain disorder marked by an ongoing pattern of inattention and/or hyperactivity–impulsivity that interferes with functioning or development (National Institute of Mental Health, 2016). The diagnosis of ADHD among children and adults has increased considerably in recent years (Collins & Cleary, 2016; Nyarko et al., 2017). Similarly, the prescribing of ADHD medications has increased on a global level, albeit with much variability across countries and regions of the world (Scheffler, Hinshaw, Modrek, & Levine, 2007). The most widely prescribed ADHD medications are stimulants, including methylphenidate and amphetamine (Catalá-López et al., 2017). However, the more recent development and approval of nonstimulant medications such as atomoxetine (Strattera®) have altered prescribing patterns, as has the availability of generic, more affordable forms of ADHD medications (Budur, Mathews, Adetunji, Mathews, & Mahmud, 2005; U.S. Food and Drug Administration, 2017). Recent estimates suggest that there are 18 ADHD medicines under development by the pharmaceutical industry (Pharmaceutical Research and Manufacturers of America, 2017).

While increased diagnosis and prescribing practices are ideally reflective of better treatment options for patients diagnosed with ADHD, there can be unintended consequences, including increased misuse and diversion of stimulant medications (Kaye & Darke, 2012). The misuse of prescription stimulants (taking stimulants without a valid prescription or use other than as prescribed) has become a serious problem in the United States and abroad, especially on college campuses (Franke et al., 2011; McCabe, West, Teter, & Boyd, 2014; Weyandt et al., 2016). Risk factors thought to contribute to misuse include ease of drug access, academic failure/low educational attainment in middle and high school, previous substance use, and adverse childhood experiences (Ford, Sacra, & Yohros, 2017; Forster, Gower, Borowsky, & McMorris, 2017; Nargiso, Ballard, & Skeer, 2015). In addition, misuse of stimulants for purposes of cognitive enhancement is a continuing concern; for example, among college students studying for exams (Turner et al., 2003; Munro, Weyandt, Marraccini, & Oster, 2017; Sussman, Pentz, Spruijt-Metz, & Miller, 2006; Weyandt et al., 2013). These concerns highlight the fact that misuse of prescription stimulants, as well as their beneficial effects as therapeutic interventions, must be weighed so as to best support the patient while mitigating unintentional risks.

Anxiety Disorders

Anxiety disorders are one of the most commonly diagnosed mental health conditions; 18.1% of American adults (42 million) are estimated to be living with an anxiety disorder (National Alliance on Mental Illness, 2017; readers are also referred to Chapter 9, this volume, for further discussion). Generally, selective serotonin reuptake inhibitors and selective serotonin norepinephrine reuptake inhibitors are first-line treatments for anxiety (Bystritsky, Khalsa, Cameron, & Schiffman, 2013; Thibaut, 2017). While anxiety medications such as benzodiazepines were historically first-line treatments, concerns regarding their detrimental effects on cognition and potential for abuse has limited their use over time (Bystritsky et al., 2013; Thibaut, 2017). Such concerns are even more salient for older adult patients, who might be particularly susceptible to the cognitive- and behavior-impairing effects of such drugs due to metabolic differences or cognitive aging (Hilmer et al., 2007; Woolcott et al., 2009; Markota, Rummans, Bostwick, & Lapid, 2016).

An evolving area of research and development related to anxiety is the possibility that medicines previously thought to have no therapeutic benefit, such as "club drugs" (e.g., MDMA, ecstasy) or psychedelics (e.g., psilocybin), may provide long-term relief from anxiety-related disorders (Griffiths et al., 2016; Johnson & Griffiths, 2017; Oehen, Traber, Widmer, & Schnyder, 2013; Sessa, 2017; Sessa & Nutt, 2015). The role that pharmaceutical companies will play in the development of such medicines is unclear. The development and marketing of such novel substances could benefit from the existing infrastructure associated with the pharmaceutical industry. In contrast, however, psychedelics also carry social and political stigma that might not align with industry goals (Gautam & Pan, 2016; Kneller, 2010; Ku, 2015).

Overall, while there have been advances in the pharmacological treatment of anxiety through improved safety and tolerability of such medications, there has been little improvement in efficacy (Farach et al., 2012). For many patients, pharmacological treatments do not lead to sustained remission of anxiety (Bandelow et al., 2015). Part of the challenge in helping these patients relates to the pervasive nature of anxiety and the lack of specific biomarkers associated with its diagnosis (Bandelow et al., 2017). The incredible impact of anxiety on society will no doubt prompt the pharmaceutical industry to continue its efforts on developing efficacious treatments, perhaps with a focus on medications that target specific subtypes of serotonergic receptors more precisely than existing medications (Farach et al., 2012).

Pain and Pain-Related Disorders

The development of medicines for the treatment of pain is among the most important and challenging task faced by pharmaceutical companies in the 21st century. Pain is represented by a complex set of medical disorders with diverse types, etiologies, and treatment modalities (Institute of Medicine, 2011; Merskey & Bogduk, 1994; readers are also referred to Chapter 19, this volume, for a more in-depth discussion of this topic). In the United States, the economic consequences of pain are also enormous, with an estimated annual societal cost of $560 to $635 billion (Gaskin & Richard, 2012) and total costs related to prescription medications estimated to be $17.8 billion annually for adult patients with nonmalignant chronic pain (noncancerous pain for 3 months or longer, or pain persisting beyond the time of expected healing; Rasu et al., 2014). The development and marketing of pain medications is complicated and risky, due in part to the very nature of pain being a subjective experience that is not necessarily associated with known tissue damage (Institute of Medicine, 2011; Merskey & Bogduk, 1994). For example, a medicine such as morphine that is generally recognized as effective for treating pain due to burns, cancer, and/or injury may be of little benefit for pain associated with a condition such as fibromyalgia. Further, morphine might be less effective for certain dental- and joint-related pain compared with drugs with no abuse potential, such as over-the-counter nonsteroidal anti-inflammatory drugs (NSAIDs; e.g., ibuprofen; Institute of Medicine, 2011). The subjective component of pain complicates diagnosis, treatment, and evaluation of treatments, but it does not lessen the devastatingly debilitating and sometimes suicide-provoking nature of pain. In fact, the World Health Organization recognizes the treatment of pain as a human right, and several international treaties deem the withholding of pain treatment as a human rights violation that can be considered "torture" and/or "cruel, inhuman, and degrading" (Lohman, Schleifer, & Amon, 2010; World Health Organization, 2007).

As has been seen in news headlines in recent years, opioid analgesic medications meant to treat pain can have serious societal side effects, including increased morbidity and mortality as exemplified by the officially designated opioid crisis in the United States (Katz, 2017). At the time of this writing, the United States is witnessing daily media and professional publication of accounts of inappropriate opioid prescribing that have contributed to an epidemic of opioid overdose deaths that in 2016 exceeded 90 per day nationwide (Gostin, Hodge, Jr, & Noe, 2017; Katz, 2017; Scholten & Henningfield, 2016; Volkow & Collins, 2017). In response to such concerns, the FDA has required risk management programs and intensive postmarketing surveillance, including prescription drug monitoring, to more quickly and accurately detect problems (Dart, 2009; Dasgupta & Schnoll, 2009). The FDA has also incentivized the development of less abusable analgesic products by the pharmaceutical industry, including abuse deterrent formulations (Cone, Buchhalter, Henningfield, & Schnoll, 2014). Future efforts to offset the risks associated with prescription opioid abuse and dependence include expanded access to treatment on demand and medication-assisted therapies for opioid addiction (Volkow & Collins, 2017). The challenge to the pharmaceutical industry is working with diverse sectors of society, government, and professional organizations, including representatives of people with pain, to do their best to develop and market the most effective and safest possible medications.

Substance Use: Tobacco Use

Smoked tobacco continues to be the leading cause of death and disease in the United States and other parts of the world, making the treatment of tobacco dependence an important public health goal within and outside of the pharmaceutical industry (Carter et al., 2015). Since 1984, the following smoking cessation pharmacotherapies have been developed by the pharmaceutical industry and approved for use by the FDA: nicotine gum, nicotine patches, nicotine lozenges, nicotine nasal spray, bupropion, nicotine inhalers, varenicline, and combination nicotine replacement therapy (NRT; Harmey, Griffin, & Kenny, 2012; see also Chapter 27, this volume). In addition, nicotine gum, patches, and lozenges were approved for over-the-counter availability between 1996 and 2002, allowing for greater access among smokers trying to quit tobacco use (Shiffman & Sweeney, 2008). The most recent non-NRT medication to be approved for smoking cessation in the United States was varenicline in 2006. Thus, it has been more than a decade since a novel, innovative FDA-approved medication was developed by the pharmaceutical industry.

This lull in medication development related to smoking cessation has prompted the Society for Research on Nicotine and Tobacco and the American Psychological Association to petition the FDA and the U.S. Department of Health and Human Services to encourage smoking cessation medication development by industry (Association for the Treatment of Tobacco Use and Dependence and Society for Research on Nicotine and Tobacco, 2009; Foulds et al., 2009). In addition to these policy efforts, researchers are exploring novel medications, devices, and combination treatments aimed at smoking cessation. For example, a recent study found beneficial effects of an FDA-approved drug for weight management, lorcaserin, on smoking cessation combined with counseling in a randomized, placebo-controlled trial of adult smokers (Shanahan, Rose, Glicklich, Stubbe, & Sanchez-Kam, 2017). In addition, controversial interventions such as electronic cigarettes (vaporized nicotine devices), as well the psychedelic drug psilocybin (mentioned above as a novel treatment for anxiety), have been examined in controlled trials with cessation as a key endpoint (Hartmann-Boyce et al., 2016; Johnson, Garcia-Romeu, & Griffiths, 2017). E-cigarettes have been quite divisive in the field of public health, especially in the United States, with continuing debate regarding whether these products help or hinder smoking cessation efforts (Kalkhoran & Glantz, 2016; Glasser et al., 2017; Kozlowski, 2017). The pharmaceutical industry does not currently manufacture or distribute e-cigarettes and it is not clear what role they would play, if any, in the future of e-cigarettes as a cessation product.

ADDITIONAL CONSIDERATIONS

The intersection of the pharmaceutical industry with the management of mental health disorders raises unique issues that deserve consideration. These issues including the role of regulatory science in managing the development and approval of medications, the positive and negative impacts of the advertising and marketing associated with pharmaceutical products, and the ethical considerations that arise when for-profit entities are involved in the treatment of mental health disorders.

Regulatory Science

Regulatory science is a distinct scientific discipline with "independent goals and measures not found in either the basic or applied sciences" (Ashley, Backinger, van Bemmel, & Neveleff, 2014; Uchiyama, 1995, p. 186). Regulatory science is important for ensuring that drugs under development will be appropriately evaluated so that they can be regulated and approved using the most rigorous available evidence. Programs for regulatory scientists include the Tobacco Regulatory Science Program, an FDA Center for Tobacco Products (CTP)/NIH collaboration that awards funding to tobacco-related research centers to create Tobacco Centers of Regulatory Science (National Institutes of Health, 2013). This program provides for a mix of research that serves FDA's regulatory needs while advancing the state of the science in areas such as pharmaceutical development and scientific training. Similarly, the FDA

Center for Drug Evaluation and Research, which is separate from the CTP, has a Division of Applied Regulatory Science located in the Office of Clinical Pharmacology (Rouse et al., 2017). This division is unique in that it performs applied research and review across the translational research spectrum, including in vitro and in vivo laboratory research, in silico computational modeling and informatics, and integrated clinical research covering clinical pharmacology, experimental medicine, and postmarket analyses, all of which can inform drug development. In addition to federal programs, many academic institutions offer degrees in the study of regulatory science (e.g., University of Maryland School of Pharmacy, University of Southern California School of Pharmacy).

Pharmaceutical Advertising and Marketing

Historically, the marketing practices of pharmaceutical companies (including advertising) were primarily controlled by the Federal Trade Commission (FTC). However, this changed in 1962 in the wake of the thalidomide disaster, during which the Federal Food, Drug, and Cosmetic Act was amended and the FDA, not the FTC, was granted authority over prescription drugs and advertising (Donohue, 2006). Over time, the advertising practices of industry have moved from being focused on physicians and health care providers (e.g., calls or visits to offices by representatives of the pharmaceutical industry) to direct-to-consumer advertising (Donohue, 2006). While direct-to-consumer advertising has benefits, such as promoting patient involvement in health care, including mental health care (Becker, 2015), it also has the potential of under communicating risks for particular treatments or contributing to physicians feeling pressured to prescribe a drug that a patient mentions during a visit.

Additional changes that have impacted pharmaceutical advertising and marketing include increased Internet advertising via social media and mobile devices (Donohue, 2006; Donohue, Cevasco, & Rosenthal, 2007; Mackey, 2016; Sullivan, Aikin, Chung-Davies, & Wade, 2016) as well as increased promotion of off-label prescribing (i.e., prescribing a medication outside the terms of its regulatory approval; Sharma et al., 2016). The potential for unforeseen risks associated with off-label promotion and prescribing has prompted concerns regarding the ethics of such practices (Painter et al., 2017; Sharma et al., 2016). In a recent case, Pfizer agreed to pay $2.3 billion related to the promotion of off-label use of four drugs—Geodon® (antipsychotic), Bextra® (anti-inflammatory), Zyvox® (antibiotic), and Lyrica® (antiepileptic)—which contributed to increased prescribing and related false claims to the U.S. government's Medicare and Medicaid programs (Tanne, 2009). Legal ramifications and regulatory control over advertising and marketing by the pharmaceutical industry continues to evolve, and will likely be a key issue impacting the net positive or negative effects of pharmaceutical medications on mental health in the 21st century.

Ethical Concerns and Conflicts of Interest

Part of the shift to direct-to-consumer advertising has led to increased scrutiny of face-to-face interactions between the representatives from industry and physicians (Fickweiler, Fickweiler, & Urbach, 2017; Wazana, 2000). For example, such interactions and resulting conflicts of interest may prompt some clinicians to overstate the efficacy of particular psychiatric drugs or be more likely to prescribe particular brand-name medications over others, as has been suggested for the antidepressant medication, Pristiq® (desvenlafaxine; DeJong et al., 2016; MacKenzie & Rogers, 2015). Efforts have been made to control such conflicts of interest, including a report from the Institute of Medicine (IOM; 2009) titled *Conflict of Interest in Medical Research, Education, and Practice* (Institute of Medicine Committee on Conflict of Interest in Medical Research Education and Practice, 2009). The report was prompted by concerns regarding the growing role of industry in funding research and medical education, and the potential bias that such funding can introduce to the care of patients. The report addressed how professionals working in science and health care should navigate relationships with industry, including the receipt of funding or gifts. In addition to the IOM report, the federal Physician Payments Sunshine Act of 2010 was passed, which requires pharmaceutical and medical device companies to publicly report payments to physicians and teaching hospitals,

further increasing the transparency of such relationships (Agrawal, Brennan, & Budetti, 2013). Of note is that while the Sunshine Act is meant to increase transparency of payments from the pharmaceutical industry, it does not necessarily prohibit such payments.

In addition to the above concerns, there are ethical considerations related to the pharmaceutical industry funding of academic research. For example, peer-reviewed publications or testimony provided by panel members with industry affiliations or disclosures have been suggested to be biased in favor of the pharmaceutical industry (Bekelman et al., 2003; Cosgrove & Krimsky, 2012; Ebrahim et al., 2016; Etter, Burri, & Stapleton, 2007; Lundh, Lexchin, Mintzes, Schroll, & Bero, 2017). This includes concerns that industry-sponsored trials of nicotine replacement therapy are more likely to produce statistically significant results and larger odds ratios compared with trials that are not industry sponsored (Etter et al., 2007).

However, it should also be noted that there can also be potential benefits associated with pharmaceutical involvement in science. For example, a marketing campaign associated with the approval of nicotine gum and patches for over-the-counter sales has been noted as an important positive health intervention for smokers in a Centers for Disease Control and Prevention *Morbidity and Mortality Weekly Report*, given that this effort removed barriers to obtaining smoking cessation (Burton et al., 1997). In this case, the increased availability and promotion of effective treatments for tobacco dependence, specifically nicotine gum and patches, not only served the needs of a pharmaceutical company to increase sales of products, but increased the number of smokers seeking out medications that can improve their chances of stopping smoking and thus promoted health (Shiffman et al., 1997). Thus, despite the challenges associated with financial conflicts of interest, it is important to point out that there are ways to work ethically and collaboratively across industry, government, and university sectors (Lehmann et al., 2012). The most important strategy for maintaining scientific integrity in such complicated relationships is to promote full disclosure and complete transparency around potential competing interests and financial reimbursements (Smith, 1998). Such disclosures are essential for supporting ethical conduct of research, while ideally allowing for private sector entities such as the pharmaceutical industry to fully contribute to innovation, economic development, and public health goals.

CONCLUSIONS AND FUTURE DIRECTIONS

As noted throughout this chapter, the pharmaceutical industry plays an important role in the treatment of mental health disorders (additional information can also be located in the Tool Kit of Resources). Such companies must navigate the enormous cost and time investment necessary to bring drugs to market that can help patients live happier and healthier lives (Morgan, Grootendorst, Lexchin, Cunningham, & Greyson, 2011). The pharmaceutical industry continues to evolve, which ideally will help to improve its ability to generate safe and effective treatments. For example, pharmaceutical companies have shifted away from concentrating drug development inside companies towards outsourcing early-stage research and development to smaller pharma and biotech companies (Morgan, Lopert, & Greyson, 2008). These changes reflect the idea that innovation is most possible in smaller companies given the risks involved with innovative work, which was not the case in previous decades (O'Brien et al., 2014). Thus, the historical business model for pharmaceutical companies appears to be shifting, and this transition is likely to impact drug development and the role of the industry in treating mental health disorders in the 21st century.

Despite these shifts in business practices, there continues to be the promise of new, efficacious pharmacological treatments, as discussed throughout the chapter with respect to mental health disorders such as ADHD, pain, anxiety, and tobacco dependence. Other areas of innovation that are likely to impact the pharmaceutical industry include the use of neuroimaging outcomes in the drug development process (Smucny, Wylie, & Tregellas, 2014; Tregellas, 2014) and the use of genetic data in guiding the prescribing of medications and precision medicine (Bousman et al., 2017; Daly, 2017; Pérez et al., 2017; Peterson et al., 2017; Rosenblat, Lee, & McIntyre, 2017). Further, as noted previously in this chapter, unconventional pharmacological therapeutics such as ketamine for treatment-resistant depression (DeWilde, Levitch, Murrough, Mathew, & Iosifescu, 2015) and psychedelics (e.g., psilocybin) for anxiety or depression (Johnson & Griffiths, 2017; Thomas, Malcolm, & Lastra, 2017) offer promising new directions for mental health treatments. Lastly, combination products that include drugs and devices are likely to be a key development in addressing mental health disorders in the 21st century (Bayarri, 2015). For example, in late 2017 the FDA approved the combination of the medication Abilify® (aripiprazole; indicated for treating schizophrenia, bipolar disorder, and depression) with an ingestible sensor embedded in the medication to assist patients and providers in tracking medication adherence. This technological development is extremely important given that the full benefit of effective medications is only achieved if patients are willing and able to adhere to prescribed treatment regimens (De las Cuevas & de Leon, 2017; Osterberg & Blaschke, 2005). Adherence to pharmacological treatments can be particularly challenging for individuals with mental health disorders (Cramer & Rosenheck, 1998). Likewise, research continues to support the idea that for many psychotropic medications, combined treatment with behavioral interventions and/or psychotherapy are better than pharmacological treatments alone (Cuijpers, Dekker, Hollon, & Andersson, 2009; Fiore & the Clinical Practice Guideline Treating Tobacco Use and Dependence 2008 Update Panel, Liaisons, and Staff, 2008).

As noted in this chapter, there are complex and unique challenges associated with the involvement of the pharmaceutical industry in developing and marketing products that society hopes and expects will serve to treat disease. The pharmaceutical industry is by definition commercial, thus making it essential that laws and regulatory policy ensure that incentives, standards, and oversight of such an industry are kept in check with the ultimate goal of serving society. Achieving the right balance in this effort through the interplay of commercial interests, regulation, and policy may be as challenging as carrying out the scientific effort required for drug development. A key example of this challenge is growing concern over the high cost of prescription drugs in the United States, with per capita spending in 2013 more than double ($858) than that of the average of 19 other industrialized nations ($400; Kesselheim, Avorn, & Sarpatwari, 2016). A primary driver of such high drug prices is the ability for pharmaceutical companies to have market exclusivity on brand name drugs after FDA approval, as well as the granting of patents. Further compounding the issue is the limited negotiating power of payers(in part because of coverage requirements imposed on government-funded drug benefits), and physician prescribing choices when comparable alternatives are available at different costs. Strategies to rectify the imbalances among all these factors contributing to drug pricing will be a key issue in U.S. health care reform in coming decades.

Despite these challenges and drawbacks, the private sector has an important role in serving the greater public good and the health of society. Such a role is reflected in the historic comments made by public health leader and former Surgeon General Dr. C. Everett Koop, in his address, "Health and Health Care for the 21st Century: For All the People" (Koop, 2006): "I urge health professionals and their professional organizations, foundations, and the private sector to support efforts that look at the 21st century from beginning to end as an opportunity for better health for all" (p. 2092). Dr. Koop's words offer an important reminder that all stakeholders involved in influencing health, including those with commercial interests such as the pharmaceutical industry, should keep human health and well-being the primary focus of their work.

TOOL KIT OF RESOURCES

The Pharmaceutical Industry and Treatments for Mental Health Disorders

U.S. Food and Drug Administration Resources

Drug Guidance Documents: https://www.fda.gov/Drugs/GuidanceComplianceRegulatoryInformation/Guidances/default.htm

Drug Development and Approval Information: https://www.fda.gov/Drugs/DevelopmentApprovalProcess/; https://www.accessdata.fda.gov/scripts/cder/daf/index.cfm

Drug Recalls: https://www.fda.gov/Drugs/DrugSafety/DrugRecalls/default.htm

*Asterisks indicate assessments or resources.

Safety Information and Adverse Event Reporting Program (FDA MedWatch): https://www.fda.gov/Safety/MedWatch/default.htm

International Organizations

World Health Organization and International Controls: http://www.who.int/medicines/access/controlled-substances/en/

World Health Organization Model Lists of Essential Medicines: http://www.who.int/medicines/publications/essentialmedicines/en/

Searchable Database for European Medicines Agency Approved Medicines: http://www.ema.europa.eu/ema/index.jsp?curl=pages/includes/medicines/medicines_landing_page.jsp&mid=

European Medicines Agency Marketing Authorisation: http://www.ema.europa.eu/ema/index.jsp?curl=pages/regulation/general/general_content_001595.jsp&mid=WC0b01ac0580b18a3d

European Medicines Agency Guideline on Non-Clinical Investigation of the Dependence Potential of Medicinal Products: http://www.ema.europa.eu/ema/index.jsp?curl=pages/regulation/general/general_content_000989.jsp&mid=WC0b01ac058002956f

Industry-Sponsored Resources

The Pharmaceutical Research and Manufacturers of America: https://www.phrma.org/

The Coalition to Prevent ADHD Medication Misuse: http://www.cpamm.org/

More Than My Diagnosis: http://www.morethanmydiagnosis.com/

Other Federal Resources

National Institute of Mental Health: Mental Health Medications: https://www.nimh.nih.gov/health/topics/mental-health-medications/index.shtml

DailyMed: https://dailymed.nlm.nih.gov/dailymed/

References

*Agrawal, S., Brennan, N., & Budetti, P. (2013). The Sunshine Act—effects on physicians. *The New England Journal of Medicine, 368,* 2054–2057. http://dx.doi.org/10.1056/NEJMp1303523

Ashley, D. L., Backinger, C. L., van Bemmel, D. M., & Neveleff, D. J. (2014). Tobacco regulatory science: Research to inform regulatory action at the Food and Drug Administration's Center for Tobacco Products.

Nicotine & Tobacco Research, 16, 1045–1049.
http://dx.doi.org/10.1093/ntr/ntu038

Association for the Treatment of Tobacco Use and
Dependence (ATTUD) and Society for Research
on Nicotine and Tobacco (SRNT). (2009). *Petition
pursuant to Title 21, Chapter 9, Subchapter V, Part A
of the Federal Food, Drug, and Cosmetic Act and
21 CFR 10.30* Retrieved from https://c.ymcdn.com/
sites/srnt.site-ym.com/resource/resmgr/About_SRNT/
Positions/2009/Citizens%E2%80%99_Petition_
re-_NRT_L.pdf

Ban, T. A. (2001). Pharmacotherapy of mental illness—
a historical analysis. *Progress in Neuro-Psychopharmacology & Biological Psychiatry, 25,* 709–727.
http://dx.doi.org/10.1016/S0278-5846(01)00160-9

Ban, T. A. (2006). The role of serendipity in drug discovery.
Dialogues in Clinical Neuroscience, 8(3), 335–344.

Ban, T. A. (2007). Fifty years chlorpromazine: A historical
perspective. *Neuropsychiatric Disease and Treatment,
3*(4), 495–500.

Bandelow, B., Michaelis, S., & Wedekind, D. (2017).
Treatment of anxiety disorders. *Dialogues in Clinical
Neuroscience, 19*(2), 93–107.

Bandelow, B., Reitt, M., Röver, C., Michaelis, S., Görlich, Y.,
& Wedekind, D. (2015). Efficacy of treatments for
anxiety disorders: A meta-analysis. *International
Clinical Psychopharmacology, 30,* 183–192. http://
dx.doi.org/10.1097/YIC.0000000000000078

Bayarri, L. (2015). Drug-device combination products:
Regulatory landscape and market growth. *Drugs
of Today, 51,* 505–513. http://dx.doi.org/10.1358/
dot.2015.51.8.2376223

*Becker, S. J. (2015). Direct-to-consumer marketing: A
complementary approach to traditional dissemination
and implementation efforts for mental health and
substance abuse interventions. *Clinical Psychology:
Science and Practice, 22,* 85–100. http://dx.doi.org/
10.1111/cpsp.12086

Bekelman, J. E., Li, Y., & Gross, C. P. (2003). Scope and
impact of financial conflicts of interest in biomedical
research: A systematic review. *JAMA, 289,* 454–465.
http://dx.doi.org/10.1001/jama.289.4.454

Berk, M. (2012). Pathways to new drug discovery in neuropsychiatry. *BMC Medicine, 10,* 151. http://dx.doi.org/
10.1186/1741-7015-10-151

Bousman, C. A., Forbes, M., Jayaram, M., Eyre, H.,
Reynolds, C. F., Berk, M., . . . Ng, C. (2017). Antidepressant prescribing in the precision medicine
era: A prescriber's primer on pharmacogenetic tools.
BMC Psychiatry, 17, 60. http://dx.doi.org/10.1186/
s12888-017-1230-5

Budur, K., Mathews, M., Adetunji, B., Mathews, M., &
Mahmud, J. (2005). Non-stimulant treatment for

attention deficit hyperactivity disorder. *Psychiatry,
2*(7), 44–48.

Burton, S., Kemper, K., Baxter, T., Shiffman, S., Gitchell, J.,
Currence, C., & the Centers for Disease Control and
Prevention. (1997). Impact of promotion of the Great
American Smokeout and availability of over-the-
counter nicotine medications, 1996. *Morbidity and
Mortality Weekly Report, 46*(37), 867–871.

Bystritsky, A., Khalsa, S. S., Cameron, M. E., & Schiffman, J.
(2013). Current diagnosis and treatment of anxiety
disorders. *P&T, 38*(1), 30–57.

Carter, B. D., Abnet, C. C., Feskanich, D., Freedman, N. D.,
Hartge, P., Lewis, C. E., . . . Jacobs, E. J. (2015).
Smoking and mortality—beyond established causes.
The New England Journal of Medicine, 372, 631–640.
http://dx.doi.org/10.1056/NEJMsa1407211

Catalá-López, F., Hutton, B., Núñez-Beltrán, A., Page, M. J.,
Ridao, M., Macías Saint-Gerons, D., . . . Moher, D.
(2017). The pharmacological and non-pharmaco-
logical treatment of attention deficit hyperactivity
disorder in children and adolescents: A systematic
review with network meta-analyses of randomised
trials. *PLoS One, 12,* e0180355. http://dx.doi.org/
10.1371/journal.pone.0180355

Collins, K. P., & Cleary, S. D. (2016). Racial and ethnic
disparities in parent-reported diagnosis of ADHD:
National Survey of Children's Health (2003, 2007,
and 2011). *The Journal of Clinical Psychiatry, 77,*
52–59. http://dx.doi.org/10.4088/JCP.14m09364

Cone, E., Buchhalter, A., Henningfield, J., & Schnoll, S.
(2014). The new science of abuse-deterrence
assessment of pharmaceutical products; FDA proposed guidance and category 1 laboratory studies.
Pharmaceutica Analytica Acta, 5(9), 317.

Cosgrove, L., & Krimsky, S. (2012). A comparison of
DSM–IV and *DSM–5* panel members' financial associations with industry: A pernicious problem persists.
PLoS Medicine, 9, e1001190. http://dx.doi.org/
10.1371/journal.pmed.1001190

Cramer, J. A., & Rosenheck, R. (1998). Compliance with
medication regimens for mental and physical disorders.
Psychiatric Services, 49, 196–201. http://dx.doi.org/
10.1176/ps.49.2.196

Cuijpers, P., Dekker, J., Hollon, S. D., & Andersson, G.
(2009). Adding psychotherapy to pharmacotherapy
in the treatment of depressive disorders in adults:
A meta-analysis. *The Journal of Clinical Psychiatry, 70,*
1219–1229. http://dx.doi.org/10.4088/JCP.09r05021

Daly, A. K. (2017). Pharmacogenetics: A general review on
progress to date. *British Medical Bulletin, 124,* 65–79.

Dart, R. C. (2009). Monitoring risk: Post marketing
surveillance and signal detection. *Drug and Alcohol
Dependence, 105*(Suppl. 1), S26–S32. http://dx.doi.org/
10.1016/j.drugalcdep.2009.08.011

Dasgupta, N., & Schnoll, S. H. (2009). Signal detection in post-marketing surveillance for controlled substances. *Drug and Alcohol Dependence, 105*(Suppl. 1), S33–S41. http://dx.doi.org/10.1016/j.drugalcdep.2009.05.019

De las Cuevas, C., & de Leon, J. (2017). Reviving research on medication attitudes for improving pharmaco-therapy: Focusing on adherence. *Psychotherapy and Psychosomatics, 86*, 73–79. http://dx.doi.org/10.1159/000450830

Deacon, B. J. (2013). The biomedical model of mental disorder: A critical analysis of its validity, utility, and effects on psychotherapy research. *Clinical Psychology Review, 33*, 846–861. http://dx.doi.org/10.1016/j.cpr.2012.09.007

DeJong, C., Aguilar, T., Tseng, C. W., Lin, G. A., Boscardin, W. J., & Dudley, R. A. (2016). Pharma-ceutical industry–sponsored meals and physician prescribing patterns for Medicare beneficiaries. *JAMA Internal Medicine, 176*, 1114–1122. http://dx.doi.org/10.1001/jamainternmed.2016.2765

DeWilde, K. E., Levitch, C. F., Murrough, J. W., Mathew, S. J., & Iosifescu, D. V. (2015). The promise of ketamine for treatment-resistant depression: Current evidence and future directions. *Annals of the New York Academy of Sciences, 1345*, 47–58. http://dx.doi.org/10.1111/nyas.12646

DiMasi, J. A., Grabowski, H. G., & Hansen, R. W. (2016). Innovation in the pharmaceutical industry: New estimates of R&D costs. *Journal of Health Economics, 47*(Suppl. C), 20–33. http://dx.doi.org/10.1016/j.jhealeco.2016.01.012

Donohue, J. (2006). A history of drug advertising: The evolving roles of consumers and consumer protection. *Milbank Quarterly, 84*, 659–699. http://dx.doi.org/10.1111/j.1468-0009.2006.00464.x

Donohue, J. M., Cevasco, M., & Rosenthal, M. B. (2007). A decade of direct-to-consumer advertising of prescrip-tion drugs. *The New England Journal of Medicine, 357*, 673–681. http://dx.doi.org/10.1056/NEJMsa070502

Dorsey, E. R., Thompson, J. P., Carrasco, M., de Roulet, J., Vitticore, P., Nicholson, S., . . . Moses, H., III. (2009). Financing of U.S. biomedical research and new drug approvals across therapeutic areas. *PLoS One, 4*, e7015. http://dx.doi.org/10.1371/journal.pone.0007015

Ebrahim, S., Bance, S., Athale, A., Malachowski, C., & Ioannidis, J. P. (2016). Meta-analyses with industry involvement are massively published and report no caveats for antidepressants. *Journal of Clinical Epidemiology, 70*, 155–163. http://dx.doi.org/10.1016/j.jclinepi.2015.08.021

Ehrhardt, S., Appel, L. J., & Meinert, C. L. (2015). Trends in National Institutes of Health funding for clinical trials registered in clinicaltrials.gov.

JAMA, 314, 2566–2567. http://dx.doi.org/10.1001/jama.2015.12206

Etter, J. F., Burri, M., & Stapleton, J. (2007). The impact of pharmaceutical company funding on results of randomized trials of nicotine replacement therapy for smoking cessation: A meta-analysis. *Addiction, 102*, 815–822. http://dx.doi.org/10.1111/j.1360-0443.2007.01822.x

Examining the Drug Supply Chain: Committee on Energy and Commerce, Subcommittee on Health, House of Representatives, 115th Congress. (2017). Retrieved from https://energycommerce.house.gov/hearings/examining-drug-supply-chain/

Farach, F. J., Pruitt, L. D., Jun, J. J., Jerud, A. B., Zoellner, L. A., & Roy-Byrne, P. P. (2012). Pharmacological treatment of anxiety disorders: Current treatments and future directions. *Journal of Anxiety Disorders, 26*, 833–843. http://dx.doi.org/10.1016/j.janxdis.2012.07.009

Fibiger, H. C. (2012). Psychiatry, the pharmaceutical industry, and the road to better therapeutics. *Schizophrenia Bulletin, 38*, 649–650. http://dx.doi.org/10.1093/schbul/sbs073

*Fickweiler, F., Fickweiler, W., & Urbach, E. (2017). Interactions between physicians and the pharma-ceutical industry generally and sales representatives specifically and their association with physicians' attitudes and prescribing habits: A systematic review. *BMJ Open, 7*, e016408. http://dx.doi.org/10.1136/bmjopen-2017-016408

Fiore, M. C., & the Clinical Practice Guideline Treating Tobacco Use and Dependence 2008 Update Panel, Liaisons, and Staff. (2008). A clinical practice guideline for treating tobacco use and dependence: 2008 update: A U.S. Public Health Service report. *American Journal of Preventive Medicine, 35*, 158–176. http://dx.doi.org/10.1016/j.amepre.2008.04.009

Ford, J. A., Sacra, S. A., & Yohros, A. (2017). Neighbor-hood characteristics and prescription drug misuse among adolescents: The importance of social dis-organization and social capital. *International Journal on Drug Policy, 46*, 47–53. http://dx.doi.org/10.1016/j.drugpo.2017.05.001

Forster, M., Gower, A. L., Borowsky, I. W., & McMorris, B. J. (2017). Associations between adverse childhood experiences, student-teacher relationships, and non-medical use of prescription medications among adolescents. *Addictive Behaviors, 68*, 30–34. http://dx.doi.org/10.1016/j.addbeh.2017.01.004

Foulds, J., Hughes, J., Hyland, A., Le Houezec, J., McNeill, A., Melvin, C., . . . Zeller, M. (2009). *Barriers to use of FDA-approved smoking cessation medications: Implications for policy action.* Madison, WI: Society for Research on Nicotine and Tobacco.

Retrieved from https://c.ymcdn.com/sites/srnt.site-ym.com/resource/resmgr/About_SRNT/Positions/2009/Barriers_to_Use_of_FDA-Appro.pdf

Franke, A. G., Bonertz, C., Christmann, M., Huss, M., Fellgiebel, A., Hildt, E., & Lieb, K. (2011). Non-medical use of prescription stimulants and illicit use of stimulants for cognitive enhancement in pupils and students in Germany. *Pharmacopsychiatry, 44,* 60–66. http://dx.doi.org/10.1055/s-0030-1268417

Gaskin, D. J., & Richard, P. (2012). The economic costs of pain in the United States. *The Journal of Pain, 13*(8), 715–724. http://dx.doi.org/10.1016/j.jpain.2012.03.009

*Gautam, A., & Pan, X. (2016). The changing model of big pharma: Impact of key trends. *Drug Discovery Today, 21,* 379–384. http://dx.doi.org/10.1016/j.drudis.2015.10.002

Glasser, A. M., Collins, L., Pearson, J. L., Abudayyeh, H., Niaura, R. S., Abrams, D. B., & Villanti, A. C. (2017). Overview of electronic nicotine delivery systems: A systematic review. *American Journal of Preventive Medicine, 52,* e33–e66. http://dx.doi.org/10.1016/j.amepre.2016.10.036

Gostin, L. O., Hodge, J. G., Jr., & Noe, S. A. (2017). Reframing the opioid epidemic as a national emergency. *JAMA, 318,* 1539–1540. http://dx.doi.org/10.1001/jama.2017.13358

Griffiths, R. R., Johnson, M. W., Carducci, M. A., Umbricht, A., Richards, W. A., Richards, B. D., . . . Klinedinst, M. A. (2016). Psilocybin produces substantial and sustained decreases in depression and anxiety in patients with life-threatening cancer: A randomized double-blind trial. *Journal of Psychopharmacology, 30,* 1181–1197. http://dx.doi.org/10.1177/0269881116675513

Harmey, D., Griffin, P. R., & Kenny, P. J. (2012). Development of novel pharmacotherapeutics for tobacco dependence: Progress and future directions. *Nicotine & Tobacco Research, 14,* 1300–1318. http://dx.doi.org/10.1093/ntr/nts201

Hartmann-Boyce, J., McRobbie, H., Bullen, C., Begh, R., Stead, L. F., & Hajek, P. (2016). Electronic cigarettes for smoking cessation. *The Cochrane Database of Systematic Reviews, 9,* CD010216.

Hilmer, S. N., Mager, D. E., Simonsick, E. M., Cao, Y., Ling, S. M., Windham, B. G., . . . Abernethy, D. R. (2007). A drug burden index to define the functional burden of medications in older people. *Archives of Internal Medicine, 167,* 781–787. http://dx.doi.org/10.1001/archinte.167.8.781

Hyman, S. E. (2012). Revolution stalled. *Science Translational Medicine, 4*(155), 155cm11. http://dx.doi.org/10.1126/scitranslmed.3003142

Institute of Medicine. (2011). *Relieving pain in America: A blueprint for transforming prevention, care, education, and research.* Washington, DC: National Academies Press.

Institute of Medicine Committee on Conflict of Interest in Medical Research Education and Practice. (2009). *Conflict of interest in medical research, education, and practice.* Washington, DC: National Academies Press.

Johnson, M. W., Garcia-Romeu, A., & Griffiths, R. R. (2017). Long-term follow-up of psilocybin-facilitated smoking cessation. *The American Journal of Drug and Alcohol Abuse, 43,* 55–60. http://dx.doi.org/10.3109/00952990.2016.1170135

Johnson, M. W., & Griffiths, R. R. (2017). Potential therapeutic effects of psilocybin. *Neurotherapeutics, 14,* 734–740. http://dx.doi.org/10.1007/s13311-017-0542-y

Kalkhoran, S., & Glantz, S. A. (2016). E-cigarettes and smoking cessation in real-world and clinical settings: A systematic review and meta-analysis. *The Lancet Respiratory Medicine, 4,* 116–128. http://dx.doi.org/10.1016/S2213-2600(15)00521-4

Katz, J. (2017). Drug deaths in America are rising faster than ever. *The New York Times.* Retrieved from https://www.nytimes.com/interactive/2017/06/05/upshot/opioid-epidemic-drug-overdose-deaths-are-rising-faster-than-ever.html

Kaye, S., & Darke, S. (2012). The diversion and misuse of pharmaceutical stimulants: What do we know and why should we care? *Addiction, 107,* 467–477. http://dx.doi.org/10.1111/j.1360-0443.2011.03720.x

Kesselheim, A. S., Avorn, J., & Sarpatwari, A. (2016). The high cost of prescription drugs in the United States: Origins and prospects for reform. *JAMA, 316,* 858–871. http://dx.doi.org/10.1001/jama.2016.11237

Kneller, R. (2010). The importance of new companies for drug discovery: Origins of a decade of new drugs. *Nature Reviews. Drug Discovery, 9,* 867–882. http://dx.doi.org/10.1038/nrd3251

Koop, C. E. (2006). Health and health care for the 21st century: For all the people. *American Journal of Public Health, 96,* 2090–2092. http://dx.doi.org/10.2105/AJPH.2006.098962

Kozlowski, L. T. (2017). Minors, moral psychology, and the harm reduction debate: The case of tobacco and nicotine. *Journal of Health Politics, Policy and Law, 42,* 1099–1112. http://dx.doi.org/10.1215/03616878-4193642

*Ku, M. S. (2015). Recent trends in specialty pharma business model. *Journal of Food and Drug Analysis, 23,* 595–608. http://dx.doi.org/10.1016/j.jfda.2015.04.008

Lehmann, L. S., Kaufman, D. J., Sharp, R. R., Moreno, T. A., Mountain, J. L., Roberts, J. S., & Green, R. C. (2012). Navigating a research partnership between academia and industry to assess the impact of personalized genetic testing. *Genetics in Medicine, 14,* 268–273. http://dx.doi.org/10.1038/gim.2011.59

Lohman, D., Schleifer, R., & Amon, J. J. (2010). Access to pain treatment as a human right. *BMC Medicine, 8,* 8–8. http://dx.doi.org/10.1186/1741-7015-8-8

López-Muñoz, F., Álamo, C., & García-García, P. (2011). The discovery of chlordiazepoxide and the clinical introduction of benzodiazepines: Half a century of anxiolytic drugs. *Journal of Anxiety Disorders, 25,* 554–562. http://dx.doi.org/10.1016/j.janxdis.2011.01.002

*Lundh, A., Lexchin, J., Mintzes, B., Schroll, J. B., & Bero, L. (2017). Industry sponsorship and research outcome. *Cochrane Database of Systematic Reviews, 2017,* MR000033. http://dx.doi.org/10.1002/14651858.MR000033.pub3

MacKenzie, R., & Rogers, W. (2015). Potential conflict of interest and bias in the RACGP's Smoking Cessation Guidelines: Are GPs provided with the best advice on smoking cessation for their patients? *Public Health Ethics, 8,* 319–331. http://dx.doi.org/10.1093/phe/phv010

*Mackey, T. K. (2016). Digital direct-to-consumer advertising: A perfect storm of rapid evolution and stagnant regulation comment on "Trouble spots in online direct-to-consumer prescription drug promotion: A content analysis of FDA warning letters." *International Journal of Health Policy and Management, 5,* 271–274. http://dx.doi.org/10.15171/ijhpm.2016.11

Markota, M., Rummans, T. A., Bostwick, J. M., & Lapid, M. I. (2016, November). Benzodiazepine use in older adults: Dangers, management, and alternative therapies. *Mayo Clinic Proceedings, 91,* 1632–1639. http://dx.doi.org/10.1016/j.mayocp.2016.07.024

McCabe, S. E., West, B. T., Teter, C. J., & Boyd, C. J. (2014). Trends in medical use, diversion, and non-medical use of prescription medications among college students from 2003 to 2013: Connecting the dots. *Addictive Behaviors, 39,* 1176–1182. http://dx.doi.org/10.1016/j.addbeh.2014.03.008

Merskey, H., & Bogduk, N. (1994). *Classification of chronic pain, IASP Task Force on Taxonomy.* Seattle, WA: International Association for the Study of Pain Press. Retrieved from http://www.iasp-pain.org

Morgan, S., Grootendorst, P., Lexchin, J., Cunningham, C., & Greyson, D. (2011). The cost of drug development: A systematic review. *Health Policy, 100,* 4–17. http://dx.doi.org/10.1016/j.healthpol.2010.12.002

Morgan, S., Lopert, R., & Greyson, D. (2008). Toward a definition of pharmaceutical innovation. *Open Medicine, 2*(1), e4–e7.

Moses, H., III, Matheson, D. H., Cairns-Smith, S., George, B. P., Palisch, C., & Dorsey, E. R. (2015). The anatomy of medical research: US and international comparisons. *JAMA, 313,* 174–189. http://dx.doi.org/10.1001/jama.2014.15939

Munro, B. A., Weyandt, L. L., Marraccini, M. E., & Oster, D. R. (2017). The relationship between nonmedical use of prescription stimulants, executive functioning and academic outcomes. *Addictive Behaviors, 65,* 250–257. http://dx.doi.org/10.1016/j.addbeh.2016.08.023

Nargiso, J. E., Ballard, E. L., & Skeer, M. R. (2015). A systematic review of risk and protective factors associated with nonmedical use of prescription drugs among youth in the United States: A social ecological perspective. *Journal of Studies on Alcohol and Drugs, 76,* 5–20. http://dx.doi.org/10.15288/jsad.2015.76.5

National Alliance on Mental Illness. (2017). *Mental health facts in America.* Retrieved from https://www.nami.org/NAMI/media/NAMI-Media/Infographics/GeneralMHFacts.pdf

National Institute of Mental Health. (2016). *Attention deficit hyperactivity disorder* [Press release]. Retrieved from https://www.nimh.nih.gov/health/topics/attention-deficit-hyperactivity-disorder-adhd/index.shtml

National Institutes of Health. (2013). *FDA and NIH create first-of-kind Tobacco Centers of Regulatory Science.* Retrieved from https://www.nih.gov/news-events/news-releases/fda-nih-create-first-kind-tobacco-centers-regulatory-science

Nyarko, K. A., Grosse, S. D., Danielson, M. L., Holbrook, J. R., Visser, S. N., & Shapira, S. K. (2017). Treated prevalence of attention-deficit/hyperactivity disorder increased from 2009 to 2015 among school-aged children and adolescents in the United States. *Journal of Child and Adolescent Psychopharmacology, 27,* 731–734. http://dx.doi.org/10.1089/cap.2016.0196

O'Brien, P. L., Thomas, C. P., Hodgkin, D., Levit, K. R., & Mark, T. L. (2014). The diminished pipeline for medications to treat mental health and substance use disorders. *Psychiatric Services, 65,* 1433–1438. http://dx.doi.org/10.1176/appi.ps.201400044

Oehen, P., Traber, R., Widmer, V., & Schnyder, U. (2013). A randomized, controlled pilot study of MDMA (± 3,4-Methylenedioxymethamphetamine)-assisted psychotherapy for treatment of resistant, chronic post-traumatic stress disorder (PTSD). *Journal of Psychopharmacology, 27,* 40–52. http://dx.doi.org/10.1177/0269881112464827

Osterberg, L., & Blaschke, T. (2005). Adherence to medication. *The New England Journal of Medicine, 353,* 487–497. http://dx.doi.org/10.1056/NEJMra050100

Painter, J. T., Owen, R., Henderson, K. L., Bauer, M. S., Mittal, D., & Hudson, T. J. (2017). Analysis of the appropriateness of off-label antipsychotic use for mental health indications in a veteran population. *Pharmacotherapy, 37,* 438–446. http://dx.doi.org/10.1002/phar.1910

Pérez, V., Salavert, A., Espadaler, J., Tuson, M., Saiz-Ruiz, J., Sáez-Navarro, C., . . . Menchón, J. M., & the AB-GEN Collaborative Group. (2017). Efficacy of prospective pharmacogenetic testing in the treatment of major depressive disorder: Results of a randomized, double-blind clinical trial. *BMC Psychiatry, 17*, 250. http://dx.doi.org/10.1186/s12888-017-1412-1

Peterson, K., Dieperink, E., Anderson, J., Boundy, E., Ferguson, L., & Helfand, M. (2017). Rapid evidence review of the comparative effectiveness, harms, and cost-effectiveness of pharmacogenomics-guided antidepressant treatment versus usual care for major depressive disorder. *Psychopharmacology, 234*, 1649–1661. http://dx.doi.org/10.1007/s00213-017-4622-9

Pharmaceutical Research and Manufacturers of America. (2017). *Medicines in Development 2017: Mental Illness*. Retrieved from http://phrma-docs.phrma.org/files/dmfile/MentalIllness_MIDReport_2017.pdf

Rasu, R. S., Vouthy, K., Crowl, A. N., Stegeman, A. E., Fikru, B., Bawa, W. A., & Knell, M. E. (2014). Cost of pain medication to treat adult patients with non-malignant chronic pain in the United States. *Journal of Managed Care & Specialty Pharmacy, 20*, 921–928. http://dx.doi.org/10.18553/jmcp.2014.20.9.921

Rosenblat, J. D., Lee, Y., & McIntyre, R. S. (2017). Does pharmacogenomic testing improve clinical outcomes for major depressive disorder? A systematic review of clinical trials and cost-effectiveness studies. *The Journal of Clinical Psychiatry, 78*, 720–729. http://dx.doi.org/10.4088/JCP.15r10583

Rouse, R., Kruhlak, N., Weaver, J., Burkhart, K., Patel, V., & Strauss, D. G. (2017). Translating new science into the drug review process: The US FDA's Division of Applied Regulatory Science. *Therapeutic Innovation & Regulatory Science, 52*, 244–255. http://dx.doi.org/10.1177%2F2168479017720249.

Scheffler, R. M., Hinshaw, S. P., Modrek, S., & Levine, P. (2007). The global market for ADHD medications. *Health Affairs, 26*, 450–457. http://dx.doi.org/10.1377/hlthaff.26.2.450

Scholten, W., & Henningfield, J. E. (2016). Negative outcomes of unbalanced opioid policy supported by clinicians, politicians, and the media. *Journal of Pain & Palliative Care Pharmacotherapy, 30*, 4–12. http://dx.doi.org/10.3109/15360288.2015.1136368

Sessa, B. (2017). MDMA and PTSD treatment: "PTSD: From novel pathophysiology to innovative therapeutics." *Neuroscience Letters, 649*, 176–180. http://dx.doi.org/10.1016/j.neulet.2016.07.004

Sessa, B., & Nutt, D. (2015). Making a medicine out of MDMA. *The British Journal of Psychiatry, 206*, 4–6. http://dx.doi.org/10.1192/bjp.bp.114.152751

Shanahan, W. R., Rose, J. E., Glicklich, A., Stubbe, S., & Sanchez-Kam, M. (2017). Lorcaserin for smoking cessation and associated weight gain: A randomized 12-week clinical trial. *Nicotine & Tobacco Research, 19*(8), 944–951.

Sharma, A. N., Arango, C., Coghill, D., Gringras, P., Nutt, D. J., Pratt, P., . . . Hollis, C. (2016). BAP Position Statement: Off-label prescribing of psychotropic medication to children and adolescents. *Journal of Psychopharmacology, 30*, 416–421. http://dx.doi.org/10.1177/0269881116636107

Shiffman, S., Gitchell, J., Pinney, J. M., Burton, S. L., Kemper, K. E., & Lara, E. A. (1997). Public health benefit of over-the-counter nicotine medications. *Tobacco Control, 6*, 306–310. http://dx.doi.org/10.1136/tc.6.4.306

Shiffman, S., & Sweeney, C. T. (2008). Ten years after the Rx-to-OTC switch of nicotine replacement therapy: What have we learned about the benefits and risks of non-prescription availability? *Health Policy, 86*, 17–26. http://dx.doi.org/10.1016/j.healthpol.2007.08.006

Smith, R. (1998). Beyond conflict of interest. Transparency is the key. *BMJ, 317*, 291–292. http://dx.doi.org/10.1136/bmj.317.7154.291

Smucny, J., Wylie, K. P., & Tregellas, J. R. (2014). Functional magnetic resonance imaging of intrinsic brain networks for translational drug discovery. *Trends in Pharmacological Sciences, 35*, 397–403. http://dx.doi.org/10.1016/j.tips.2014.05.001

Sullivan, H. W., Aikin, K. J., Chung-Davies, E., & Wade, M. (2016). Prescription Drug promotion from 2001–2014: Data from the U.S. Food and Drug Administration. *PLoS One, 11*, e0155035. http://dx.doi.org/10.1371/journal.pone.0155035

Sussman, S., Pentz, M. A., Spruijt-Metz, D., & Miller, T. (2006). Misuse of "study drugs": Prevalence, consequences, and implications for policy. *Substance Abuse Treatment, Prevention, and Policy, 1*, 15. http://dx.doi.org/10.1186/1747-597X-1-15

Tanne, J. H. (2009). Pfizer agrees to pay record fine for promotion of off-label use of four drugs. *BMJ, 339*, b3657. http://dx.doi.org/10.1136/bmj.b3657

Thibaut, F. (2017). Anxiety disorders: A review of current literature. *Dialogues in Clinical Neuroscience, 19*(2), 87–88.

Thomas, K., Malcolm, B., & Lastra, D. (2017). Psilocybin-assisted therapy: A review of a novel treatment for psychiatric disorders. *Journal of Psychoactive Drugs, 49*, 446–455. http://dx.doi.org/10.1080/02791072.2017.1320734

Tregellas, J. R. (2014). Neuroimaging biomarkers for early drug development in schizophrenia. *Biological Psychiatry, 76*, 111–119. http://dx.doi.org/10.1016/j.biopsych.2013.08.025

Turner, D. C., Robbins, T. W., Clark, L., Aron, A. R., Dowson, J., & Sahakian, B. J. (2003). Cognitive enhancing effects of modafinil in healthy volunteers. *Psychopharmacology, 165,* 260–269. http://dx.doi.org/10.1007/s00213-002-1250-8

Uchiyama, M. (1995). Regulatory science. *PDA Journal of Pharmaceutical Science and Technology, 49*(4), 185–187.

U.S. Food and Drug Administration. (2016). *New drug development and review process.* Retrieved from https://www.fda.gov/Drugs/DevelopmentApprovalProcess/SmallBusinessAssistance/ucm053131.htm

U.S. Food and Drug Administration. (2017). *FDA approves first generic Strattera for the treatment of ADHD* [Press release]. Retrieved from https://www.fda.gov/NewsEvents/Newsroom/PressAnnouncements/ucm561096.htm

U.S. Food and Drug Administration Center for Drug Evaluation and Research. (2017). *Assessment of abuse potential of drugs: Guidance for industry.* Silver Spring, MD: Author. Retrieved from https://www.fda.gov/downloads/drugs/guidancecomplianceregulatoryinformation/guidances/ucm198650.pdf

Volkow, N. D., & Collins, F. S. (2017). The role of science in addressing the opioid crisis. *The New England Journal of Medicine, 377,* 391–394. http://dx.doi.org/10.1056/NEJMsr1706626

Wazana, A. (2000). Physicians and the pharmaceutical industry: Is a gift ever just a gift? *JAMA, 283,* 373–380. http://dx.doi.org/10.1001/jama.283.3.373

Weyandt, L. L., Marraccini, M. E., Gudmundsdottir, B. G., Zavras, B. M., Turcotte, K. D., Munro, B. A., & Amoroso, A. J. (2013). Misuse of prescription stimulants among college students: A review of the literature and implications for morphological and cognitive effects on brain functioning. *Experimental and Clinical Psychopharmacology, 21,* 385–407. http://dx.doi.org/10.1037/a0034013

Weyandt, L. L., Oster, D. R., Marraccini, M. E., Gudmundsdottir, B. G., Munro, B. A., Rathkey, E. S., & McCallum, A. (2016). Prescription stimulant medication misuse: Where are we and where do we go from here? *Experimental and Clinical Psychopharmacology, 24,* 400–414. http://dx.doi.org/10.1037/pha0000093

Woolcott, J. C., Richardson, K. J., Wiens, M. O., Patel, B., Marin, J., Khan, K. M., & Marra, C. A. (2009). Meta-analysis of the impact of 9 medication classes on falls in elderly persons. *Archives of Internal Medicine, 169,* 1952–1960. http://dx.doi.org/10.1001/archinternmed.2009.357

World Health Organization. (2007). *Access to controlled medications programme framework* (WHO/PSM/QSM/2007.2). Retrieved from http://www.who.int/medicines/areas/quality_safety/Framework_ACMP_withcover.pdf?ua=

CHAPTER 32

NONPHARMACOLOGICAL NEUROTHERAPEUTICS: PRINCIPLES AND METHODS OF BRAIN STIMULATION THERAPY

Marc L. Copersino

It may seem unusual to include a chapter devoted to nonpharmacological approaches in a psychopharmacology handbook. However, brain function relies on a highly interdependent system of electrical and biochemical mechanisms that can be modulated pharmacologically through psychoactive drugs as well as nonpharmacologically through electrical stimulation of the brain. It is, therefore, worthwhile to explore and contrast nonpharmacological approaches that are used to activate and inhibit basic brain cell and regional function for the treatment of neuropsychiatric disorders. In this chapter, I provide an introduction to the general principles and concepts associated with brain stimulation, then discuss common brain stimulation strategies and device types, including a review of their clinical applications (and supporting evidence from clinical trials) and risks, mechanisms of action, and examples of use in basic and translational research.

For reasons addressed at greater length later in this chapter, brain stimulation therapies traditionally have been used when pharmacological treatment options have been unsuccessful or cannot be tolerated, or to provide a reversible alternative to ablative psychosurgery (i.e., brain lesioning). While brain stimulation therapies continue to be used under these circumstances, the accelerating pace of innovation in the neurosciences has greatly improved our understanding of the effects of electrical stimulation on the brain, which is contributing to its greater acceptability and clinical accessibility.

WHAT IS THERAPEUTIC BRAIN STIMULATION?

In addition to pharmacotherapy, brain stimulation constitutes a second class of medical therapeutics for the treatment of neuropsychiatric disorders. Brain stimulation therapy is defined here as the use of medical devices to effectuate electrical stimulation of the central nervous system via focally applied electrodes or an electromagnetic pulse in order to achieve different therapeutic effects for a variety of psychiatric and neurological conditions. The list of conditions that brain stimulation is used to treat continues to grow but most notably includes epilepsy, pain, and mood and movement disorders, as well as other emerging clinical applications.

The therapeutic use of electrical stimulation appears to have originated in ancient Rome when electrogenic fish were used to treat headaches (see Higgins & George, 2009). Although the practitioners of that time were not aware of bioelectricity, they were aware that this practice produced analgesia. Despite this long history, the mechanisms of action associated with various brain stimulation therapies remain under debate. It is important, however, to distinguish therapeutic mechanisms of action

http://dx.doi.org/10.1037/0000133-032
APA Handbook of Psychopharmacology, S. M. Evans (Editor-in-Chief)
Copyright © 2019 by the American Psychological Association. All rights reserved.

(i.e., what produces the therapeutic effect) from the effects of stimulation on the brain.

The functional unit of the brain is the neuron, which receives and transmits electrochemical signals. In a historic series of papers, Alan L. Hodgkin and Andrew F. Huxley at the Physiological Laboratory at the University of Cambridge described and quantified the flow of electric current through the surface membrane of a neuron (i.e., the Hodgkin–Huxley Model; see Catterall, Raman, Robinson, Sejnowski, & Paulsen, 2012). The neuron holds a small amount of electrical voltage (similar to a battery) due to positively and negatively charged ions (e.g., potassium, sodium, chloride, calcium) that polarize the membrane by forming gradients along the inside and outside of the cell. The net balance of these ions produces a *resting voltage* (also called a *membrane* or *resting potential*) of approximately −0.07 volts, which provides the potential energy for intracellular signal transfer and postsynaptic neurotransmission. Neurons are called "electrically excitable cells" because stimulus-driven changes to cross-membrane ion concentration (e.g., from an electrical field) can trigger ionic depolarization (i.e., change the membrane potential from negative to positive), thereby carrying an electrical impulse, or potential, across the axon to the nerve terminal. Thus, electrical stimulation of the brain triggers the intracellular electrical activity responsible for

synaptic signal transmission that, similar to the pharmacological actions of drugs, modulates neural excitatory and inhibitory processes in adjacent neurons (see Chapter 2, this handbook, for more detail on these concepts).

Brain stimulation therapies do not, however, stimulate neurons in isolation but rather in assemblages forming electrically excitable tissue. There are several variables associated with stimulation of nervous tissue that are described as fundamental to understanding how various stimulation methods and parameters affect the brain (Brocker & Grill, 2013; Higgins & George, 2009; Peterchev et al., 2012; Ranck, 1975; see Table 32.1 for a summary of the general parameters associated with electrical stimulation of the brain). As discussed in greater detail in the section of this chapter on Types of Brain Stimulation Therapies, the first variable involves the parameters of the device used to effectuate electrical stimulation. All brain stimulation devices either use electrodes to apply an electrical current or a magnetic coil to induce an electrical current. The flow of electricity through a coil (or wire) produces a magnetic field, the strength of which can be controlled by the amount of current applied to the coil. A change in the magnetic field (e.g., by turning the power source on and off) induces a magnetic pulse outside the head that activates the neural tissue beneath the skull.

TABLE 32.1

General Stimulation Parameters Associated With Electrical Stimulation of the Brain

Parameter	Examples	Affects
Device characteristics	Composition, size, placement, and electrical properties of the stimulating electrodes or coil	Spatial distribution of the electrical field
Qualities of the electrical current delivered or induced	Waveform (shape), frequency (waves per second), amplitude (wave height), pulse width, directionality (direct or alternating current), repetition frequency	Temporal characteristics of the electrical field
Pulse-delivery protocol and session characteristics	Within-session characteristics (number and duration of pulses and the time interval between pulses) Between-session characteristics (total number of sessions and the time interval between them)	Amount and duration of exposure
Properties of the neural tissue	Electrical conductivity and permittivity	Efficiency or attenuation of source activity

Peterchev and colleagues (2012) refer to device characteristics—such as the composition, size, placement, and electrical properties of the stimulating electrodes or coil—as parameters modulating the spatial distribution of the electrical field. For example, different electrode and coil configurations on human head models have been used to evaluate and compare the electrical field stimulation strength and focality of various stimulation paradigms (Lee, Lisanby, Laine, & Peterchev, 2014). For a review of methodological considerations in the selection of brain stimulation devices involving one or more transcranial electrodes, see Guleyupoglu, Schestatsky, Edwards, Fregni, and Bikson (2013).

The second set of variables associated with how electrical stimulation affects the brain involves the qualities of the electrical current delivered or induced. The parameters of an electrical current applied to electrodes or a coil include its waveform (shape), frequency (waves per second), amplitude (wave height), pulse width, directionality (direct or alternating current), and repetition frequency. Peterchev et al. (2012) refer to these variables as those affecting the "temporal characteristics of the electromagnetic field" (p. 437).

A related, but qualitatively different, third set of variables that similarly pertain to how the electrical current is delivered or induced involve the pulse-delivery protocol and other session characteristics. These parameters include within-session (number and duration of pulses and the time interval between pulses) and between-session characteristics (total number of sessions and the time interval between them).

The fourth set of variables associated with how electrical stimulation affects the brain involves the properties of the neural tissue to which it is delivered, including its electrical and dielectric (or "insulating") properties. This concerns the electrical conductivity of the biological material—in other words, how easily it enables electricity to pass through—and its electrical permittivity—or how well it transmits electricity. Although neural tissue is a good conductor of electricity, the skull has low electrical conductivity. As a result, electrical stimulation of the brain via transcranial electrodes requires sufficient intensity to overcome source activity attenuation at the skull and

stimulate the brain tissue underneath. Because both tissue and bone have good magnetic permeability, however, there is no notable source activity attenuation at the skull when brain stimulation methods are used in which an electromagnetic pulse is delivered via a coil (Scharfetter, Casañas, & Rosell, 2003).

STIMULATION PARAMETERS AND THERAPEUTIC DOSE

Traditionally, the concept of *dose* in brain stimulation therapies has been relative rather than fixed; in other words, it has been based on individual response measures. For example, the proper "dose" of electroconvulsive therapy is the individual's seizure threshold (i.e., the amount necessary to induce a seizure), or the proper dose of transcranial magnetic therapy is the individual's motor threshold (i.e., the amount necessary to induce a finger twitch). Thus, the dose that works for one person may be different than that for another. One notable limitation of relative dosing is that measuring a threshold in itself exposes the participant to some quantity of stimulation, the effects of which are unknown.

Because of increasingly better understanding of the effects of electrical stimulation on the brain, there is a growing interest in developing dosing protocols with greater scientific rigor that can be fully described and replicated (Peterchev et al., 2012). Despite these advances, one of the biggest challenges associated with the use of brain stimulation therapies remains establishing standardized dosing regimens that approximate what exists for pharmacotherapy.

While there may be some differences of opinion regarding fixed (mg) versus weight-adjusted (mg/kg) medication dosing regimens, best-practice approaches recognize that each regimen has its merits under different circumstances (Pan, Zhu, Chen, Xia, & Zhou, 2016). In contrast, in brain stimulation therapies, there is no equivalent to standardized dose or dose-correction algorithms based on an individual characteristic. One of the challenges associated with establishing standardized dosing is the large number of stimulation parameters, including properties of the stimulating electrodes or coil, qualities of the electrical current applied to the electrodes or coil, pulse duration and the interval between pulse sequences, and the total number of brain stimulation sessions and the interval between them. Correspondingly, there are an exponentially larger number of possible stimulation parameter combinations.

Peterchev and colleagues (Peterchev et al., 2012; Peterchev, Rosa, Deng, Prudic, & Lisanby, 2010) have sought to limit the stimulus parameters in defining dose to only those externally applied and controlled, rather than including any physiologic or behavioral response to stimulation. Accordingly, *fixed dosing* (also referred to as *response-independent* or *open-loop dosing*) paradigms control stimulation parameters via preprogrammed protocols that do not vary across individuals. The principle benefits of fixed dosing are that it enables standardization, replication, and between-group comparison.

There is, however, a large amount of interindividual variability in response to brain stimulation, some of which may be attributed to subject characteristics (e.g., anatomical differences), but for others, characteristics of responders versus nonresponders have not been clearly differentiated (Kim et al., 2014; López-Alonso, Cheeran, Río-Rodríguez, & Fernández-del-Olmo, 2014). The biggest limitation of fixed dosing, therefore, is its inability to automatically adjust to individual differences affecting brain stimulation outcome. To address the limitations of fixed-dosing paradigms, *adaptive*, or *closed-loop*, *dosing* paradigms present a new approach that enables real-time changes to stimulation parameters based on clinical response (F. T. Sun & Morrell, 2014). Although similar to the individualized dosing of the past (i.e., establishing dose based on individual motor or seizure threshold), the closed-loop paradigm is different in that it represents real-time adaptive dosing based on biological feedback. While this approach is promising, several challenges to developing effective closed-loop neurostimulation systems remain, including insufficient biological markers for the prediction and assessment of brain stimulation treatment response and the limited availability of clinical sensor technology.

Applying knowledge about the effects of electrical stimulation on the brain continues to enhance understanding of dosing in the context of brain stimulation therapy. Similarly, examining the clinical outcomes associated with varying modifiable stimulation parameters contributes to a growing knowledge base regarding therapeutic mechanisms of action. However, due to the large variation of brain stimulation types, there are important distinctions between mechanisms of action across different types of therapies. Further discussion of mechanism of action, therefore, requires a more in-depth examination of specific brain stimulation types.

TYPES OF BRAIN STIMULATION THERAPIES

The variety of brain stimulation methods and techniques is quite large and continues to grow. As is true for drugs, medical devices are federally regulated by the U.S. Food and Drug Administration (FDA) to provide a reasonable assurance of their safety and effectiveness. The FDA categorizes medical devices as Class I, II, or III, based on their safety risk and corresponding degree of regulatory control—with Class I representing low risk (e.g., bandages, gauze), Class II moderate risk (e.g., wheelchairs, syringes), and Class III high risk (e.g., pacemakers, heart valves, implantable neurostimulators; for more information, see https://www.fda.gov/MedicalDevices/ResourcesforYou/Consumers/ucm142523.htm). Brain stimulation devices comprise only a small fraction of the medical devices regulated by the FDA, and they generally are categorized as neurostimulatory (e.g., implantable deep brain and vagus nerve stimulation systems) or neurotherapeutic (e.g., noninvasive electromagnetic and transcutaneous or cranial electrotherapies). However, these categories are primarily intended to guide the FDA's Office of Device Evaluation in making review group assignments (i.e., matching regulatory review of new devices to the committee best qualified to perform the review) and are not intended to be comprehensive. Device classifications are identified (by number) in Title 21 and Chapter I of the *Code of Federal Regulations*, which is the part of the federal rules and regulations dedicated to the FDA and the Department of Health and Human Services. A link to the FDA Medical Device Database is among the resources provided in the Tool Kit of Resources at the end of this chapter.

The sections that follow provide a summary of the most common brain stimulation therapies for the treatment of psychological disorders, including electroconvulsive therapy, magnetic seizure therapy, transcranial magnetic stimulation, deep brain stimulation, and vagus nerve stimulation. Each section first addresses historical perspectives, then describes proposed mechanisms of action, medical conditions for which use of these devices currently is approved by the FDA, emerging clinical applications, and research applications. Individual sections also identify several important and recurring themes across brain stimulation therapies. A summary of clinical indications and other investigational uses of brain stimulation therapies appears in Table 32.2.

Electroconvulsive Therapy

Electroconvulsive therapy (ECT) is a noninvasive form of brain stimulation in which brief, intense electrical current is applied to the patient's head via electrodes to induce a major motor seizure. The use of therapeutically induced seizure was pioneered in the early 1930s by Hungarian neurophysiologist

Ladislas Meduna, who considered the motionlessness of catatonic schizophrenia and the uncontrollable muscle movement of epilepsy to be diametrically opposite expressions of the same underlying processes (Fink, 1985). Initially, therapeutic seizures were induced chemically, first using intramuscular camphor and subsequently pentylenetetrazol injection (Gazdag, Bitter, Ungvari, Baran, & Fink, 2009). Electrical induction of seizure using ECT was invented by Italian neuropathologist and psychiatrist Ugo Cerletti as a safer alternative to the chemical induction of seizure; by the 1940s it was in common use as a principal treatment for severe mental illness, most notably depression (cf. Shorter, 1997).

Despite having unmatched efficacy in the treatment of depression, as well as the existence of personal testimonies by high profile advocates (Dukakis & Tye, 2007), ECT remains controversial principally

TABLE 32.2

Brain Stimulation Devices With Accompanying FDA-Approved Clinical and Investigational Uses

Device	Approved for	Investigational use only
Electroconvulsive therapy	Bipolar disorder Depression	Catatonia Mania Schizophrenia Schizoaffective disorder
Magnetic seizure therapy	—	Bipolar depression Depression Treatment-resistant schizophrenia
Transcranial magnetic stimulation	Bipolar depression Depression Headache	Obsessive-compulsive disorder Pain Parkinson's disease Posttraumatic stress disorder Schizophrenia Stroke Substance use disorders
Deep brain stimulation	Epilepsy Movement disorder/dystonia Parkinsonian symptoms Treatment-resistant depression Treatment resistant obsessive-compulsive disorder	Dystonia Obsessive-compulsive disorder Tourette's disorder
Vagus nerve stimulation	Epilepsy Headache (noninvasive vagus nerve stimulation only) Treatment-resistant depression	Parkinson's disease Stroke

Note. FDA = U.S. Food and Drug Administration.

because of its association with the stigma of "shock treatment." In other words, common perceptions about modern ECT are influenced by its reputation, which in large part has been shaped by popular media (Sienaert, 2016) as a painful and dangerous procedure used as a means to subdue or control patients. However, ECT as practiced today is quite unlike ECT of the past. In modern practice, ECT patients are given muscle relaxants to avoid injuries from the strong muscle contractions and general anesthesia to avoid pain. It is also typically administered on an outpatient basis.

Proposed mechanisms of action. Although ECT is the oldest method of brain stimulation that is still in use today, there is no general consensus regarding its mechanism of action. However, the crucial component of the depression-relieving effect of ECT appears to be seizure activity, as opposed to the other effects of electrical stimulation (Cronholm & Ottosson, 1996).

Clinical indications. The FDA approval of ECT in the *Code of Federal Regulations* (FDA Electroconvulsive Therapy Device Rule, 2018) is fairly broad in that it is approved for the treatment of "severe psychiatric disturbances (e.g., severe depression)." The strongest evidence of its treatment efficacy is for unipolar and bipolar depression (Dierckx, Heijnen, van den Broek, & Birkenhäger, 2012). There is also evidence for the efficacy of ECT in the treatment of bipolar mania (Medda, Toni, & Perugi, 2014) and of schizophrenia and schizoaffective disorder (Weiner & Reti, 2017). To date, ECT is regarded as the biological "gold standard" in depression treatment efficacy in that no clinical trial has identified an active comparator (drug or device) that is superior to ECT in short-term outcome. Unlike typical antidepressant medications (e.g., monoamine oxidase inhibitors, selective serotonin reuptake inhibitors, tricyclic antidepressants), ECT is among the treatments for depression that promote rapid mood enhancement. Nonetheless, ECT typically is reserved for intractable depression as a method of last resort because of ongoing controversy surrounding brain stimulation stigma and perception of safety.

Risks. Although safer than in the past, even modern ECT retains the risk of cognitive side effects. The most notable cognitive side effect of ECT appears to be retrograde amnesia for autobiographical memory (Coleman et al., 1996; Sackeim et al., 1993), which can be minimized by altering stimulation parameters such as electrode placement (Sackeim et al., 2007). Although the degree to which modern ECT retains risks of cognitive side effects remains controversial, there has been a significant reduction in apprehension and stigma associated with ECT. This greater acceptability is reflected in efforts to reclassify ECT from being a high-risk to a moderate-risk device (McDonald, Weiner, Fochtmann, & McCall, 2016). Specifically, the FDA released a draft document for public comment, based on the recommendations of an FDA advisory panel, that proposed the reclassification of ECT devices from Class III to Class II for use in treating severe unipolar or bipolar depression in adults who are treatment-resistant or who require a rapid response due to the severity of their psychiatric or medical condition (Neurological Devices; Reclassification of Electroconvulsive Therapy Devices, 2015). The most notable change resulting from such reclassification would be an increase in ECT availability to consumers.

Research applications. Research using ECT is predominantly aimed toward gaining a better understanding of its mechanisms of action and examining ways to make it safer and more effective. One line of research uses brain imaging methods to examine biological markers of ECT success. Studies using electroencephalograms (EEGs) to examine the electrophysiological correlates of therapeutic efficacy and cognitive side effects have been conducted for nearly as long as ECT has been in existence (see Krystal et al., 2000, for review). Recent reviews of functional neuroimaging studies of ECT—including EEG (Farzan, Boutros, Blumberger, & Daskalakis, 2014; Fosse & Read, 2013), single-photon emission computed tomography, and positron emission tomography (Fosse & Read, 2013)—have identified patterns of frontal and temporal deactivation that may contribute to its therapeutic mechanism of action in complex ways, including the activation of the hypothalamic–pituitary–adrenal axis and dopamine systems.

Structural imaging studies of ECT have identified regional gray matter volume increases in the medial temporal lobes (Ota et al., 2015) and limbic region (Thomann et al., 2017), particularly ipsilateral to (i.e., on the same side of the body as) the stimulation side (Bouckaert et al., 2016), as well as modulations of resting state neural coupling (Thomann et al., 2017). These regional changes in gray matter volume suggest that a neurotrophic (i.e., promotion of nerve tissue growth) effect of ECT could play a role in its therapeutic effect (Ota et al., 2015). In addition to biomarkers identified via brain imaging studies, neurochemical biomarkers of ECT effectiveness have also been identified, including tissue-plasminogen activator (Hoirisch-Clapauch, Mezzasalma, & Nardi, 2014), an enzyme that helps dissolve blood clots and promote brain plasticity, and neurogranin (Kranaster, Blennow, Zetterberg, & Sartorius, 2017), a dendritic protein associated with synaptic plasticity.

Although the identification of biomarkers may facilitate adaptive dosing approaches in the future, ECT dosing is studied more directly by examining the clinical effects of manipulating stimulation parameters. Although the crucial component of the depression-relieving effect of ECT appears to be seizure activity (Cronholm & Ottosson, 1996), researchers have found markedly different effectiveness and minimization of adverse cognitive effects based on the adjustment of stimulation parameters (Peterchev et al., 2010; Sackeim et al., 2007).

Research focusing on the manipulation of stimulation parameters has enabled the development of new methods of administering ECT that reduce adverse cognitive effects and increase effectiveness. For example, such new methods as ultrabrief-pulse right unilateral ECT (Gálvez, Hadzi-Pavlovic, Waite, & Loo, 2017), individualized low-amplitude seizure therapy (Peterchev, Krystal, Rosa, & Lisanby, 2015; Radman & Lisanby, 2017), and focal electrically administered seizure therapy (Sahlem et al., 2016) have shown improvements over traditional ECT.

Magnetic Seizure Therapy

In an effort to duplicate the clinical efficacy of ECT but further minimize its potential adverse cognitive consequences, magnetic seizure therapy (MST) was developed as a new seizure-induction technique (Lisanby, Luber, Schlaepfer, & Sackeim, 2003; Y. Sun et al., 2016). Unlike ECT, which uses electrodes to apply an electrical current, MST uses a transcranial magnetic stimulator (discussed in greater detail in the section of this chapter on Transcranial Magnetic Stimulation) to induce an electrical current beneath the surface of the skull. Because the electromagnetic pulse passes through the skull, it requires a lower electrical field strength than does ECT to generate sufficient current in the brain to activate neurons.

Proposed mechanisms of action.   As with ECT, the induction of seizure activity is regarded to be the mechanism of therapeutic action for MST.

Clinical indications.   There is research evidence for the efficacy and safety of MST in treating unipolar and bipolar depression (Cretaz, Brunoni, & Lafer, 2015) and, in a pilot study, treatment-resistant schizophrenia (Tang et al., 2018). Although MST does not currently have FDA approval for the treatment of any condition, at least one randomized clinical trial of its efficacy and safety is underway (University of Texas Southwestern Medical Center, 2018).

Risks.   The risks associated with MST appear to be minimal. In comparison with ECT, the seizures induced via MST are of shorter duration and require a shorter recovery period. MST also has greater focality of activation and avoids stimulation of brain structures thought to be associated with the adverse cognitive effects of ECT (Deng, Lisanby, & Peterchev, 2011; McClintock, Tirmizi, Chansard, & Husain, 2011).

Research applications.   There is not a large body of research using MST. However, similar to ECT, there is evidence that efficacy can be further enhanced through the adjustment of stimulation parameters (Lee, Lisanby, Laine, & Peterchev, 2016; Lee et al., 2014).

Transcranial Magnetic Stimulation

A transcranial magnetic stimulator is a noninvasive device that activates neural tissue below the skull through electromagnetic induction. The device includes a power source that delivers pulses of electric current to a coil placed on the head, thus generating an electromagnetic field outside of the head that induces an electrical field inside of the head. Although the device is similar to what is used in MST, transcranial magnetic stimulation (TMS) is a therapeutic technique that activates spatially discrete regions of the cerebral cortex using a lower frequency electrical field than MST, and it is not intended to induce a seizure.

Because a static magnetic field does not induce an electric field, the TMS device delivers a single magnetic pulse of brief duration. However, the frequency and type of magnetic pulse delivered are modifiable, resulting in multiple stimulus-delivery approaches, including single-pulse TMS, in which individual pulses are typically administered no more than once every few seconds; paired-pulse TMS, in which pairs of stimuli are administered separated by intervals of usually no more than 0.02 seconds; and repetitive-pulse TMS (rTMS), in which "trains" of pulses are administered. The effect of applying combinations of repeated- and paired-pulse TMS on cortical excitability also have been examined in clinical research settings (Khedr, Gilio, & Rothwell, 2004). When used clinically, rTMS pulses may be applied in the range of hundreds or thousands over the course of a single 1-hour session. For more detailed reviews of standard nomenclature and basic principles of TMS see, Huang et al. (2009) and Rossi, Hallett, Rossini, and Pascual-Leone (2009).

Proposed mechanisms of action. The delivery of TMS decreases or increases cortical excitability depending on the stimulation parameters applied to the neural tissue. When TMS is delivered repeatedly at frequencies below 1 Hz (called *low-frequency* or *slow rTMS*), it is believed to promote the long-term depression, or inhibition, of adjacent neuronal activity. In contrast, when delivered at frequencies above 1 Hz (called *high-frequency* or *fast rTMS*), it is believed to promote long-term potentiation, or excitation, of adjacent neurons. As an extension, the therapeutic effect of TMS is hypothesized to manifest as long-term depression or long-term potentiation of sufficiently lengthy duration to achieve synaptic plasticity (Hoogendam, Ramakers, & Di Lazzaro, 2010). Beyond this general description, the therapeutic mechanism of action of TMS remains a subject of debate but is generally regarded to depend on the method of TMS used and the clinical condition or disorder being targeted.

As with other forms of brain stimulation, hypotheses regarding mechanism of action are inferred from research examining the clinical effects of manipulating stimulation parameters and identifying the biomarkers associated with positive outcomes. Positive outcomes associated with TMS for the treatment of depression have primarily been observed when high-frequency rTMS is applied to the dorsolateral prefrontal cortex. This makes theoretical sense given the role of the dorsolateral prefrontal cortex in modulating affective and cognitive control mechanisms, as well as the state of hypofrontality identified in depression and other psychiatric disorders. For more information about TMS mechanisms of action, see Dubin (2017) and Hoogendam et al. (2010).

Clinical indications. In 2008, the FDA approved the use of rTMS to deliver repetitive pulsed magnetic fields to induce neural action potentials in the prefrontal cortex to treat symptoms of major depressive disorder in patients who have not benefited from at least one antidepressant medication and currently are not on any antidepressant therapy (FDA Repetitive Transcranial Magnetic Stimulation System Rule, 2018). Traditional TMS and rTMS have an effective depth penetration of about 1 to 1.5 cm beneath the surface of the skull. Via traditional methods, direct cortical activation is accompanied by secondary activation of deeper brain structures, the mechanisms of which are not well understood. In 2013, on the basis of being determined "substantially equivalent" to traditional TMS, the FDA approved a method of deep TMS (dTMS) that uses a coil designed to activate neural tissue up to 6 cm below the surface of the skull. Despite improvements resulting from new coil configurations (Wei, Li, Lu, Wang, & Yi, 2017), decreased focality and a dearth of accompanying safety data limit the clinical utility of dTMS.

Current best-practice guidelines for use of TMS therapy in the treatment of unipolar depression recommend delivery of traditional rTMS to the left prefrontal cortex for a minimum of 4 and a maximum of 6 weeks (Perera et al., 2016). Though generally well tolerated, early use of TMS was criticized for its questionable efficacy in the treatment of depression. However, its efficacy and safety have improved significantly over time. Meta-reviews of meta-analytic studies with rTMS for the treatment of depression generally show it to be effective and safe in the treatment of medication-refractory depression (Dell'Osso et al., 2011; Janicak & Dokucu, 2015). Results of these meta-reviews indicate that despite there being heterogeneous effect sizes across meta-analyses, the effect sizes for TMS efficacy in treating depression are at least comparable to those of antidepressant medications, even though studies included only treatment-resistant or treatment-intolerant patients. However, further studies are needed to optimize dosing and stimulation parameters, to describe the durability of treatment response, and to identify prognostic markers.

In 2014, the FDA granted approval for the use of TMS to deliver brief duration, rapidly alternating magnetic fields (i.e., pulsed magnetic fields) in the treatment of migraine headache (FDA Transcranial Magnetic Stimulator for Headache Rule, 2018). There is evidence for the clinical effectiveness of both single- and repetitive-pulse TMS as a treatment for acute migraine with or without aura, as well as some evidence for its use as a preventative treatment for migraine headache (Lipton & Pearlman, 2010; Schwedt & Vargas, 2015).

The use of TMS for the treatment of various other disorders also has been examined. Based on a meta-analysis of its efficacy across psychiatric disorders, rTMS has been recommended for depression, for auditory verbal hallucinations, and possibly for negative symptoms associated with schizophrenia (Slotema, Blom, Hoek, & Sommer, 2010). The conclusion drawn from a review of the Cochrane Schizophrenia Group Trials Register (Dougall, Maayan, Soares-Weiser, McDermott, & McIntosh, 2015) is that TMS for the reduction of psychotic symptoms associated with schizophrenia is inconclusive, though some evidence suggests temporoparietal TMS may improve auditory hallucinations and positive symptoms of schizophrenia. There is also evidence that rTMS is helpful for acute and maintenance treatment for catatonic schizophrenia in individuals for whom pharmacological interventions have been unsuccessful or who have safety concerns with ECT (Stip, Blain-Juste, Farmer, Fournier-Gosselin, & Lespérance, 2018). Furthermore, there is emerging evidence for the efficacy of rTMS in the treatment of

Parkinson's disease (Moisello et al., 2015), obsessive-compulsive disorder (Rehn, Eslick, & Brakoulias, 2018), posttraumatic stress disorder (Kozel et al., 2018), and substance use disorders (Makani, Pradhan, Shah, & Parikh, 2017).

Risks. Generally, TMS is a well-tolerated treatment. Although side effects such as headache and local pain at the site of stimulation are common, they are generally mild in severity (Taylor, Galvez, & Loo, 2018). Severe adverse effects, such as inadvertent seizure induction, mania, or hearing impairment, are rare but possible with standard TMS (Taylor et al., 2018). A comprehensive review of TMS safety considerations is included in the consensus statement from the International Workshop on the Present and Future of TMS: Safety and Ethical Guidelines (Rossi et al., 2009).

Research applications. Similar to other brain stimulation therapies, one area of research using TMS is aimed at improving and broadening its clinical efficacy. The examination of modifiable stimulation parameters in TMS has led to many variations in technique, including theta-burst stimulation, which is intended to mimic the theta rhythm firing patterns in EEG signals (TBS; Chung, Hoy, & Fitzgerald, 2015); intermittent theta-burst stimulation (Bulteau et al., 2017); H-coil induction of deep brain structures, or deep-brain TMS (Bersani et al., 2013); cerebellar transcranial magnetic stimulation (Hardwick, Lesage, & Miall, 2014); and EEG-alpha-wave-frequency synchronized TMS (Leuchter et al., 2015). Also similar to other brain stimulation therapies, imaging techniques have been used to examine biomarkers of therapeutic effectiveness, which in turn has improved knowledge regarding mechanism of action (Dubin, 2017).

Deep Brain Stimulation

Deep brain stimulation (DBS) is an invasive method of brain stimulation requiring neurosurgery. During the surgery, electrodes are implanted in specific brain regions. The electrodes are connected via wires under the skin to a battery-powered stimulator called an *implantable pulse generator*, which controls the amount of current delivered to the electrodes. The device settings and stimulation levels are adjusted noninvasively using a programming device. Unlike deep-brain TMS, effective depth of penetration is irrelevant because the electrical current is delivered through the wires directly to the electrodes implanted in the brain.

The use of DBS grew out of ablative neurosurgery (i.e., brain lesioning) for movement disorders, a common practice during the mid-20th century. Prior to the development of alternative therapies, irreversible lesioning of brain areas was the only treatment for movement disorders, such as Parkinson's disease and essential tremor (Obeso et al., 1997). Despite the success of the medication levodopa for the treatment of Parkinson's disease, dyskinesia associated with long-term levodopa therapy remains a common side effect. Stereotaxic surgery has greatly improved neurosurgical precision and has led to the need for smaller resections than performed in the past. Despite this, ablative neurosurgery remains controversial due to its association with other irreversible psychosurgeries, notably frontal lobotomy and the memory of its widespread and irresponsible use.

It was serendipitously discovered by Benabid et al. (1993) that electrical stimulation of discrete brain regions at frequencies higher than 60 Hz during the mapping phase of neurosurgery suppressed Parkinsonian tremor. Since then, DBS not only has been used as a reversible alternative to ablative psychosurgery but also as an adjunct to levodopa therapy.

Proposed mechanisms of action. Although DBS commonly is regarded as "virtual lesioning" of the brain, its specific mechanisms of action remain a subject of debate. Several review papers have proposed mechanisms of action for DBS, including one by McIntyre, Savasta, Kerkerian-Le Goff, and Vitek (2004) that presented four hypothesized mechanisms: "depolarization blockade, synaptic inhibition, synaptic depression, and stimulation-induced modulation of pathological network activity" (p. 1239). Montgomery and Gale (2008) reviewed possible therapeutic mechanisms of DBS action and described the challenges inherent to proposing mechanisms of action in complex dynamical systems. Finally, Udupa and Chen (2015) identified different aspects of DBS mechanisms of action according to the modality of

investigation, the disease under study, the stimulation target, and the animal model used in the investigation.

Clinical indications. The FDA provided initial approval for DBS in 1997 for the treatment of motor symptoms associated with movement disorders. The specific use indication for DBS is what determines the placement of the stimulating electrodes. For example, bilateral stimulation of the internal globus pallidus or the subthalamic nucleus is indicated for adjunctive therapy in reducing symptoms of advanced, levodopa-responsive Parkinson's disease that are not adequately controlled with medication (see Bronstein et al., 2011, for an expert consensus on best practices for the use of DBS to treat Parkinson's disease). For the treatment of epilepsy, DBS is approved for stimulation at the seizure foci in the brain. However, FDA approvals for use of DBS in the treatment of Parkinsonian tremor and essential tremor do not specify a particular target region. Nor are locations specified in DBS for the treatment of dystonia, for which the FDA granted a humanitarian device exemption that waives some regulatory requirements in order to provide patients with access to a medical device that otherwise would be unavailable to them.

In addition to treating movement disorders, DBS has been used as an alternative to ablative neurosurgery for the treatment of psychiatric disorders, and it has been granted a humanitarian device exemption for the treatment of obsessive-compulsive disorder (see Chapter 11, this handbook, for information on the pharmacological treatment of obsessive-compulsive disorder). Specifically, DBS is indicated for bilateral stimulation of the anterior limb of the internal capsule—adjunctive to medications and as an alternative to anterior capsulotomy (i.e., lesioning the anterior limb of the internal capsule)—for treatment of chronic, severe, treatment-resistant obsessive-compulsive disorder in adults who have not responded positively to at least three selective serotonin reuptake inhibitors. There is some evidence for the efficacy of DBS in the treatment of other conditions as well, including thalamic DBS for Tourette's disorder (Issac, Chandra, & Nagaraju, 2016), DBS of the nucleus accumbens for the treatment of addiction (Müller et al., 2013), DBS of the hypothalamus or nucleus accumbens for obesity (Bétry, Thobois, Laville, & Disse, 2018), DBS of the subcallosal cingulate gyrus for treatment-resistant depression (Kennedy et al., 2011), and DBS of the medial forebrain bundle in an animal model of depression (Thiele, Furlanetti, Pfeiffer, Coenen, & Döbrössy, 2018).

Risks.   The risks associated with DBS are primarily surgery related, including the possibility of bleeding, stroke, infection, and (in rare cases) death. Long-term mortality analysis of patients with Parkinson's disease who were treated with DBS revealed survival rates of 99% and 94% at 3 and 5 years, respectively, with death usually occurring due to vascular events or infection (Rocha et al., 2014). However, movement disorders induced by DBS also have been reported (Baizabal-Carvallo & Jankovic, 2016).

Research applications.   As is true for other brain stimulation technologies, a better understanding of stimulation parameters in DBS helps enhance knowledge about concepts such as dose and mechanisms of action. Because DBS is surgical, neurostimulation is delivered outside of clinical settings and parameters pertaining to within- and between-session characteristics thus are not applicable. There is, however, substantial variability in DBS based on device characteristics, such as electrode placement and geometry, as well as other variables pertaining to anatomical targeting and properties of the delivered current that alter the electric field and can control neural activation. For example, examination of the clinical differences between voltage-limited and constant-current delivery of electrical charge have identified superiority of the latter because it controls for increasing electrode impedance over time after implantation (Bronstein et al., 2015). See Kuncel and Grill (2004) for an overview of DBS stimulation parameters, and Hariz (2014) for a review of how variation in stimulus parameters is contributing to the development of new DBS techniques. See also Lempka, Howell, Gunalan, Machado, and McIntyre (2018) for characterization of the stimulus waveforms generated by implantable pulse generators that can alter the efficacy and utility of DBS.

In comparison with noninvasive technologies, there have been greater advances in the use of adaptive, or closed-loop, dosing paradigms in implantable forms of brain stimulation, including DBS. The study and application of adaptive DBS has been particularly fruitful in part because it already makes use of sensor technology (e.g., to monitor intracranial EEG in DBS for epilepsy). For example, in a nonhuman primate study, adaptive DBS that made real-time changes to stimulation parameters in response to primary motor cortex activity had greater benefits in alleviating Parkinsonian motor symptoms than did response-independent stimulation (Rosin et al., 2011). Beudel and Brown (2016) reviewed other potential feedback signals in adaptive DBS for Parkinson's disease. There also has been progress in developing an adaptive DBS system for the treatment of Tourette's disorder via a safety and proof-of-concept study that used flexible programming settings as a first step toward personalized, responsive brain stimulation (Okun et al., 2013).

Similar to other brain stimulation technologies, biological markers of DBS success have been examined using brain imaging methods. For example, studies have identified network connectivity changes associated with both rapid-onset (Choi, Riva-Posse, Gross, & Mayberg, 2015) and longer term (van Hartevelt et al., 2014) effects of DBS.

Vagus Nerve Stimulation

The vagus nerve is the 10th and longest of the 12 pairs of cranial nerve bundles emanating from the brain, and it carries information to and from the organ systems of the body (e.g., heart, lungs, stomach, intestines). Part of the autonomic nervous system, it plays an important role in modulating involuntary body functions, including heart rhythm and digestion. Its connection between the organ systems and the brain creates complex mind–body functional relationships that are not well understood (e.g., psychosomatic illness, wellness approaches to mental health) and that continue to be studied.

Similar to DBS, vagus nerve stimulation (VNS) is an invasive method of neurostimulation that requires surgery. In VNS, however, electrodes are not implanted in the brain but rather wrapped around the vagus nerve—usually but not exclusively on the left side to avoid cardiac complications. As in DBS, the electrodes are connected to wires that run under the skin and connect to a battery-powered stimulator, which controls the amount of current delivered to the electrodes. The device settings and stimulation levels are similarly adjusted noninvasively using a programming device.

Proposed mechanisms of action. The mechanisms of action for VNS in the treatment of epilepsy and depression are not entirely understood. With regard to epilepsy, there is evidence to suggest that the locus coeruleus and dorsal raphe nucleus play a mediating role, as indicated through their release of antiepileptic neuromodulators when activated by VNS and the abolishment of VNS-induced seizure suppression when these areas are lesioned (Krahl & Clark, 2012). With respect to depression, there is evidence that, similar to the pharmacologic effects of antidepressant medication, VNS affects neurotransmission of norepinephrine, serotonin, gamma-aminobutyric acid, and glutamate (Ben-Menachem et al., 1994; Krahl & Clark, 2012). Because the efficacy of VNS in both epilepsy (R. George et al., 1994) and depression (Aaronson et al., 2017) improves over time, there appears to be neural plasticity–associated changes related to processes that researchers have yet to explain.

Clinical indications. Animal studies have established the ability of VNS to synchronize the electrical activity of the brain (Bailey & Bremer, 1938), but it was American neuroscientist Jake Zabara who first demonstrated in an animal model that VNS not only could stop seizures during acute stimulation but also have lasting effects beyond the duration of neuro-stimulation (cf. Higgins & George, 2009). Subsequent clinical trials demonstrated efficacy of VNS in the reduction of seizures in humans (Ben-Menachem et al., 1994), an effect that also persists over time (R. George et al., 1994), such that VNS was approved by the FDA for the treatment of epilepsy in 1997. As a point of clarification regarding terminology, the FDA refers to the VNS device as an "implanted autonomic nerve stimulator." Furthermore, VNS should not be confused with noninvasive, transcutaneous VNS, referred to by the FDA simply as noninvasive VNS, which is VNS delivered via a handheld portable device for the treatment of headache.

The observation that some patients treated with VNS for epilepsy also reported incidental improvements in mood has led to studies examining the mood-enhancing properties of VNS. In July 2005, the FDA approved VNS as an adjunctive, or augmentive, treatment for severe, recurrent unipolar and bipolar depression. Specifically, VNS is indicated for the adjunctive long-term treatment of chronic or recurrent depression in adults who have not had an adequate response to four or more antidepressant treatments. Because its mood-enhancing effects take longer to appear in comparison with other treatments for depression (including ECT), VNS cannot be considered a treatment for acute treatment-resistant depression. Similar to its efficacy in the treatment of epilepsy, VNS for depression also appears to improve, or have a cumulative effect, over time. Studies identifying VNS-enhanced memory consolidation suggest its possible application in the treatment of Alzheimer's disease and other types of dementias. See M. S. George et al. (2002) for a discussion of potential VNS utility in the treatment of other neuropsychiatric disorders, including anxiety, obesity, and chronic pain.

Risks. Similar to DBS, the risks associated with VNS are primarily surgery related, including the possibility of bleeding, stroke, infection, and (in rare cases) death. The complications and safety associated with 247 VNS implantations over 25 years at a single center were examined (Révész, Rydenhag, & Ben-Menachem, 2016). Complications occurred in 2% of patients and were most commonly postoperative hematoma, infection, and vocal cord palsy. Other studies suggest VNS may contribute to sleep-related breathing disorders in adults with epilepsy. There is normally a high rate of sudden unexpected death in epilepsy, and it is unclear if VNS can help reduce epilepsy-related mortality rates.

Research applications. Research examining biomarkers associated with positive clinical outcomes also has contributed to hypotheses about VNS mechanisms of action. For example, a body of research examining changes in EEG synchronization between VNS responders and nonresponders provides evidence for EEG desynchronization as an important mechanism of antiepileptic action.

Research using other brain imaging techniques has identified differences between VNS responders and nonresponders in functional network reorganization (Fraschini et al., 2014); regional cerebral blood flow changes in the thalamus and limbic system (Vonck et al., 2008), including the amygdala and hippocampus (Van Laere, Vonck, Boon, Versijpt, & Dierckx, 2002); and hippocampal gray matter volume changes (Perini et al., 2017).

Other research has examined the clinical effects of manipulating stimulation parameters in order to guide optimized dosing parameters. For example, research identifying interactive effects of pulse width and intensity on both plasticity- and memory-enhancing effects of VNS may help guide dosing considerations to optimize VNS efficacy (Loerwald, Borland, Rennaker, Hays, & Kilgard, 2018).

EMERGING TRENDS

Neuroscientific advances have fueled a rapid growth in knowledge and technology innovations pertaining to brain stimulation methods and clinical applications. Although there have been advances across brain stimulation methods, the use of TMS in research is considerably broader than for other brain stimulation technologies, given its enormous applicability for probing neurocognitive functioning in alert individuals. For example, TMS has been used as a diagnostic tool to probe specific cortical circuits in neurological diseases, including dementia (Cantone et al., 2014) and corticobasal ganglia degeneration syndromes (Issac, Chandra, & Nagaraju, 2016). It also is used extensively as a tool for examining cognitive processing in a variety of contexts, including language mapping of Broca's region (Sakreida et al., 2018) and mapping of other brain–cognition relationships, as well as to study the effects of drugs on TMS-evoked electromyographic responses (pharmaco-TMS-EMG; Ziemann, 2004; Ziemann et al., 2015).

In addition to TMS, there are emerging clinical uses of other brain imaging technologies as well. For example, a growing body of research is examining the utility of interventional radiology methods in DBS, including diffusion tensor imaging (Coenen et al., 2014; Kovanlikaya, Heier, & Kaplitt, 2014) and other advanced magnetic resonance imaging methods (Lucas-Neto et al., 2015; Nagahama et al., 2015), to optimize DBS surgery by helping to clarify the selection of anatomical targets. Another example of technological innovation involves the use of adaptive, or closed-loop, dosing paradigms in implantable forms of brain stimulation. Although the use of biological sensor technology is not new in DBS, a small but growing area of research is also examining potential physiological feedback monitoring systems for adaptive VNS dosing paradigms (e.g., extracellular pH monitoring for use in closed-loop VNS for the treatment of obesity; Cork et al., 2018).

SUMMARY

Brain stimulation therapy involves the use of medical devices that effectuate electrical stimulation of the central nervous system to achieve therapeutic effects. Electrical stimulation of the brain triggers the intracellular electrical activity responsible for synaptic signal transmission, which—similar to the pharmacological actions of drugs—modulates neural excitatory and inhibitory processes in adjacent neurons. Manipulation of stimulation parameters (e.g., characteristics of the stimulation device and electrical current) affects stimulation dosage. The most common brain stimulation therapies for the treatment of psychological disorders include ECT, MST, TMS, DBS, and VNS. To varying degrees for different therapies, our ability to explain the interrelation of stimulation parameters, therapeutic dose, and mechanism of action remains limited. However, the accelerating pace of innovation in the neurosciences assures continued growth in knowledge and methods pertaining to brain stimulation therapies.

TOOL KIT OF RESOURCES

Brain Stimulation Therapy

General Patient Information

American Psychiatric Association: What Is Electroconvulsive Therapy (ECT)?: https://www.psychiatry.org/patients-families/ect

American Psychological Association. (2009). A pacemaker for your brain? Electric brain stimulation may give hope to people with unremitting depression.

Monitor on Psychology, 40, 36. Retrieved from http://www.apa.org/monitor/2009/03/pacemaker.aspx

National Alliance on Mental Illness: ECT, TMS, and Other Brain Stimulation Therapies: https://www.nami.org/Learn-More/Treatment/ECT,-TMS-and-Other-Brain-Stimulation-Therapies

National Institute of Mental Health: Brain Stimulation Therapies (vagus nerve stimulation, repetitive transcranial magnetic stimulation, magnetic seizure therapy, and deep brain stimulation): https://www.nimh.nih.gov/health/topics/brain-stimulation-therapies/brain-stimulation-therapies.shtml

National Institute of Neurological Disorders and Stroke: Deep Brain Stimulation for Parkinson's Disease: https://www.ninds.nih.gov/Disorders/All-Disorders/Parkinsons-Disease-Information-Page

National Library of Medicine: MedlinePlus Medical Encyclopedia: Deep Brain Stimulation: https://medlineplus.gov/ency/article/007453.htm

National Library of Medicine: MedlinePlus Medical Encyclopedia: Electroconvulsive Therapy: https://medlineplus.gov/ency/article/007474.htm

National Parkinson Foundation: Parkinson's Disease—Guide to Deep Brain Stimulation Therapy: http://www.parkinson.org/sites/default/files/Guide_to_DBS_Stimulation_Therapy.pdf

Nuland, S. (2001, February). *Sherwin Nuland: How electroshock therapy changed me* [Video file]. Retrieved from https://www.ted.com/talks/sherwin_nuland_on_electroshock_therapy?language=en

Review Documents for Professionals

The Clinical TMS Society: Recommendations for TMS Therapy for Major Depressive Disorder: Perera, T., George, M. S., Grammer, G., Janicak, P. G., Pascual-Leone, A., & Wirecki, T. S. (2016). The Clinical TMS Society consensus review and treatment recommendations for TMS therapy for major depressive disorder. *Brain Stimulation, 9*, 336–346. http://dx.doi.org/10.1016/j.brs.2016.03.010

Safety of TMS Consensus Group: Consensus Statement From the International Workshop on Present and Future of TMS—Safety and Ethical Guidelines, Siena, Italy, March 7–9, 2008: Rossi, S., Hallett, M., Rossini, P. M., & Pascual-Leone, A. (2009). Safety, ethical considerations, and application guidelines for the use of transcranial magnetic stimulation in clinical practice and research. *Clinical Neurophysiology, 120*, 2008–2039. http://dx.doi.org/10.1016/j.clinph.2009.08.016

The World Federation of Societies of Biological Psychiatry: WFSBP Guidelines on Brain Stimulation Treatments in Psychiatry: Schlaepfer, T. E., George, M. S., Mayberg, H., & WFSBP Task Force on Brain Stimulation. (2010). WFSBP guidelines on brain stimulation treatments in psychiatry. *World Journal of Biological Psychiatry, 11*, 2–18. http://dx.doi.org/10.3109/15622970903170835

Professional Conference and Training Opportunities

Duke University Medical Center: Course in Transcranial Magnetic Stimulation: https://psychiatry.duke.edu/transcranial-magnetic-stimulation-course

International Brain Stimulation Conference: Organized by Elsevier and sponsored by and integrated with the journal *Brain Stimulation*: https://www.elsevier.com/events/conferences/international-brain-stimulation-conference

The Medical University of South Carolina: Department of Psychiatry and Behavioral Sciences, Brain Stimulation Lab, Brain Stimulation Intensive Courses (Transcranial Magnetic Stimulation Intensive Course and Electroconvulsive Therapy Intensive Course): https://education.musc.edu/colleges/medicine/departments/psychiatry/divisions-and-programs/divisions/bsl/about/course

Databases

ClinicalTrials.gov: Privately and publicly funded clinical studies of brain stimulation that are open for subject recruitment: https://clinicaltrials.gov/ct2/results?term=Brain+Stimulation+Therapies&recr=Open

Food and Drug Administration: Medical Device Database—a list of all medical devices with their associated classifications, product codes, premarket review organizations, and other regulatory information: https://www.accessdata.fda.gov/scripts/cdrh/cfdocs/cfPCD/classification.cfm

References

Aaronson, S. T., Sears, P., Ruvuna, F., Bunker, M., Conway, C. R., Dougherty, D. D., . . . Zajecka, J. M. (2017). A 5-year observational study of patients with treatment-resistant depression treated with vagus nerve stimulation or treatment as usual: Comparison of response, remission, and suicidality. *The American Journal of Psychiatry, 174*, 640–648. http://dx.doi.org/10.1176/appi.ajp.2017.16010034

*Asterisks indicate assessments or resources.

Bailey, P., & Bremer, F. (1938). A sensory cortical representation of the vagus nerve. *Journal of Neurophysiology, 1*, 405–412. http://dx.doi.org/10.1152/jn.1938.1.5.405

Baizabal-Carvallo, J. F., & Jankovic, J. (2016). Movement disorders induced by deep brain stimulation. *Parkinsonism & Related Disorders, 25*, 1–9. http://dx.doi.org/10.1016/j.parkreldis.2016.01.014

Benabid, A. L., Pollak, P., Seigneuret, E., Hoffmann, D., Gay, E., & Perret, J. (1993). Chronic VIM thalamic stimulation in Parkinson's disease, essential tremor and extra-pyramidal dyskinesias. *Acta Neurochirurgica. Supplementum, 58*, 39–44.

Ben-Menachem, E., Mañon-Espaillat, R., Ristanovic, R., Wilder, B. J., Stefan, H., Mirza, W., . . . First International Vagus Nerve Stimulation Study Group. (1994). Vagus nerve stimulation for treatment of partial seizures: 1. A controlled study of effect on seizures. *Epilepsia, 35*, 616–626. http://dx.doi.org/10.1111/j.1528-1157.1994.tb02482.x

*Bersani, F. S., Minichino, A., Enticott, P. G., Mazzarini, L., Khan, N., Antonacci, G., . . . Biondi, M. (2013). Deep transcranial magnetic stimulation as a treatment for psychiatric disorders: A comprehensive review. *European Psychiatry, 28*, 30–39. http://dx.doi.org/10.1016/j.eurpsy.2012.02.006

Bétry, C., Thobois, S., Laville, M., & Disse, E. (2018). Deep brain stimulation as a therapeutic option for obesity: A critical review. *Obesity Research & Clinical Practice, 12*, 260–269. http://dx.doi.org/10.1016/j.orcp.2018.02.004

Beudel, M., & Brown, P. (2016). Adaptive deep brain stimulation in Parkinson's disease. *Parkinsonism & Related Disorders, 22*(Suppl. 1), S123–S126. http://dx.doi.org/10.1016/j.parkreldis.2015.09.028

Bouckaert, F., De Winter, F.-L., Emsell, L., Dols, A., Rhebergen, D., Wampers, M., . . . Vandenbulcke, M. (2016). Grey matter volume increase following electroconvulsive therapy in patients with late life depression: A longitudinal MRI study. *Journal of Psychiatry & Neuroscience?, 41*, 105–114. http://dx.doi.org/10.1503/jpn.140322

Brocker, D. T., & Grill, W. M. (2013). Principles of electrical stimulation of neural tissue. *Handbook of Clinical Neurology, 116*, 3–18. http://dx.doi.org/10.1016/B978-0-444-53497-2.00001-2

Bronstein, J. M., Tagliati, M., Alterman, R. L., Lozano, A. M., Volkmann, J., Stefani, A., . . . DeLong, M. R. (2011). Deep brain stimulation for Parkinson disease: An expert consensus and review of key issues. *Archives of Neurology, 68*, 165. http://dx.doi.org/10.1001/archneurol.2010.260

Bronstein, J. M., Tagliati, M., McIntyre, C., Chen, R., Cheung, T., Hargreaves, E. L., . . . Okun, M. S. (2015). The rationale driving the evolution of deep brain stimulation to constant-current devices. *Neuromodulation, 18*, 85–88, 89. http://dx.doi.org/10.1111/ner.12227

Bulteau, S., Sébille, V., Fayet, G., Thomas-Ollivier, V., Deschamps, T., Bonnin-Rivalland, A., . . . Sauvaget, A. (2017). Efficacy of intermittent theta burst stimulation (iTBS) and 10-Hz high-frequency repetitive transcranial magnetic stimulation (rTMS) in treatment-resistant unipolar depression: Study protocol for a randomised controlled trial. *Trials, 18*, 17. http://dx.doi.org/10.1186/s13063-016-1764-8

Cantone, M., Di Pino, G., Capone, F., Piombo, M., Chiarello, D., Cheeran, B., . . . Di Lazzaro, V. (2014). The contribution of transcranial magnetic stimulation in the diagnosis and in the management of dementia. *Clinical Neurophysiology, 125*, 1509–1532. http://dx.doi.org/10.1016/j.clinph.2014.04.010

Catterall, W. A., Raman, I. M., Robinson, H. P. C., Sejnowski, T. J., & Paulsen, O. (2012). The Hodgkin-Huxley heritage: From channels to circuits. *The Journal of Neuroscience, 32*, 14064–14073. http://dx.doi.org/10.1523/JNEUROSCI.3403-12.2012

Choi, K. S., Riva-Posse, P., Gross, R. E., & Mayberg, H. S. (2015). Mapping the "depression switch" during intraoperative testing of subcallosal cingulate deep brain stimulation. *JAMA Neurology, 72*, 1252–1260. http://dx.doi.org/10.1001/jamaneurol.2015.2564

Chung, S. W., Hoy, K. E., & Fitzgerald, P. B. (2015). Theta-burst stimulation: A new form of TMS treatment for depression? *Depression and Anxiety, 32*, 182–192. http://dx.doi.org/10.1002/da.22335

Coenen, V. A., Allert, N., Paus, S., Kronenbürger, M., Urbach, H., & Mädler, B. (2014). Modulation of the cerebello-thalamo-cortical network in thalamic deep brain stimulation for tremor: A diffusion tensor imaging study. *Neurosurgery, 75*, 657–670. http://dx.doi.org/10.1227/NEU.0000000000000540

Coleman, E. A., Sackeim, H. A., Prudic, J., Devanand, D. P., McElhiney, M. C., & Moody, B. J. (1996). Subjective memory complaints prior to and following electroconvulsive therapy. *Biological Psychiatry, 39*, 346–356. http://dx.doi.org/10.1016/0006-3223(95)00185-9

Cork, S. C., Eftekhar, A., Mirza, K. B., Zuliani, C., Nikolic, K., Gardiner, J. V., . . . Toumazou, C. (2018). Extracellular pH monitoring for use in closed-loop vagus nerve stimulation. *Journal of Neural Engineering, 15*, 016001. http://dx.doi.org/10.1088/1741-2552/aa8239

Cretaz, E., Brunoni, A. R., & Lafer, B. (2015). Magnetic seizure therapy for unipolar and bipolar depression: A systematic review. *Neural Plasticity, 2015*, 521398. http://dx.doi.org/10.1155/2015/521398

Cronholm, B., & Ottosson, J. O. (1996). Experimental studies of the therapeutic action of electroconvulsive therapy in endogenous depression. The role of the electrical stimulation and of the seizure studied by variation of stimulus intensity and modification by lidocaine of seizure discharge. *Convulsive Therapy, 12*(3), 172–194.

Dell'Osso, B., Camuri, G., Castellano, F., Vecchi, V., Benedetti, M., Bortolussi, S., & Altamura, A. C. (2011). Meta-review of metanalytic studies with repetitive transcranial magnetic stimulation (rTMS) for the treatment of major depression. *Clinical Practice and Epidemiology in Mental Health, 7,* 167–177. http://dx.doi.org/10.2174/1745017901107010167

Deng, Z.-D., Lisanby, S. H., & Peterchev, A. V. (2011). Electric field strength and focality in electroconvulsive therapy and magnetic seizure therapy: A finite element simulation study. *Journal of Neural Engineering, 8,* 016007. http://dx.doi.org/10.1088/1741-2560/8/1/016007

Dierckx, B., Heijnen, W. T., van den Broek, W. W., & Birkenhäger, T. K. (2012). Efficacy of electroconvulsive therapy in bipolar versus unipolar major depression: A meta-analysis. *Bipolar Disorders, 14,* 146–150. http://dx.doi.org/10.1111/j.1399-5618.2012.00997.x

Dougall, N., Maayan, N., Soares-Weiser, K., McDermott, L. M., & McIntosh, A. (2015). Transcranial magnetic stimulation (TMS) for schizophrenia. *Cochrane Database of Systematic Reviews,* (8): CD006081.

Dubin, M. (2017). Imaging TMS: Antidepressant mechanisms and treatment optimization. *International Review of Psychiatry, 29,* 89–97. http://dx.doi.org/10.1080/09540261.2017.1283297

Dukakis, K., & Tye, L. (2007). *Shock: The healing power of electroconvulsive therapy.* New York, NY: Penguin Group.

Farzan, F., Boutros, N. N., Blumberger, D. M., & Daskalakis, Z. J. (2014). What does the electroencephalogram tell us about the mechanisms of action of ECT in major depressive disorders? *The Journal of ECT, 30,* 98–106. http://dx.doi.org/10.1097/YCT.0000000000000144

FDA Electroconvulsive Therapy Device Rule, 21 C.F.R. § 882.5940 (2018).

FDA Repetitive Transcranial Magnetic Stimulation System Rule, 21 C.F.R. § 882.5805 (2018).

FDA Transcranial Magnetic Stimulator for Headache Rule, 21 C.F.R. § 882.5808 (2018).

Fink, M. (1985). Historical article: Autobiography of L. J. Meduna. *Convulsive Therapy, 1*(1), 43–57.

Fosse, R., & Read, J. (2013). Electroconvulsive treatment: Hypotheses about mechanisms of action. *Frontiers in Psychiatry, 4,* 94. http://dx.doi.org/10.3389/fpsyt.2013.00094

Fraschini, M., Demuru, M., Puligheddu, M., Floridia, S., Polizzi, L., Maleci, A., . . . Marrosu, F. (2014). The

re-organization of functional brain networks in pharmaco-resistant epileptic patients who respond to VNS. *Neuroscience Letters, 580,* 153–157. http://dx.doi.org/10.1016/j.neulet.2014.08.010

Gálvez, V., Hadzi-Pavlovic, D., Waite, S., & Loo, C. K. (2017). Seizure threshold increases can be predicted by EEG quality in right unilateral ultrabrief ECT. *European Archives of Psychiatry and Clinical Neuroscience, 267,* 795–801. http://dx.doi.org/10.1007/s00406-017-0777-y

Gazdag, G., Bitter, I., Ungvari, G. S., Baran, B., & Fink, M. (2009). László Meduna's pilot studies with camphor inductions of seizures: The first 11 patients. *The Journal of ECT, 25,* 3–11. http://dx.doi.org/10.1097/YCT.0b013e31819359fc

George, M. S., Nahas, Z., Bohning, D. E., Kozel, F. A., Anderson, B., Chae, J.-H., . . . Mu, C. (2002). Vagus nerve stimulation therapy: A research update. *Neurology, 59,* S56–S61. http://dx.doi.org/10.1212/WNL.59.6_suppl_4.S56

George, R., Salinsky, M., Kuzniecky, R., Rosenfeld, W., Bergen, D., Tarver, W. B., Wernicke, J. F., & the First International Vagus Nerve Stimulation Study Group. (1994). Vagus nerve stimulation for treatment of partial seizures: 3. Long-term follow-up on first 67 patients exiting a controlled study. *Epilepsia, 35,* 637–643. http://dx.doi.org/10.1111/j.1528-1157.1994.tb02484.x

*Guleyupoglu, B., Schestatsky, P., Edwards, D., Fregni, F., & Bikson, M. (2013). Classification of methods in transcranial electrical stimulation (tES) and evolving strategy from historical approaches to contemporary innovations. *Journal of Neuroscience Methods, 219,* 297–311. http://dx.doi.org/10.1016/j.jneumeth.2013.07.016

Hardwick, R. M., Lesage, E., & Miall, R. C. (2014). Cerebellar transcranial magnetic stimulation: The role of coil geometry and tissue depth. *Brain Stimulation, 7,* 643–649. http://dx.doi.org/10.1016/j.brs.2014.04.009

Hariz, M. (2014). Deep brain stimulation: New techniques. *Parkinsonism & Related Disorders, 20*(Suppl. 1), S192–S196. http://dx.doi.org/10.1016/S1353-8020(13)70045-2

Higgins, E. S., & George, M. S. (2009). *Brain stimulation therapies for clinicians.* Washington, DC: American Psychiatric Association.

Hoirisch-Clapauch, S., Mezzasalma, M. A. U., & Nardi, A. E. (2014). Pivotal role of tissue plasminogen activator in the mechanism of action of electroconvulsive therapy. *Journal of Psychopharmacology, 28,* 99–105. http://dx.doi.org/10.1177/0269881113507639

Hoogendam, J. M., Ramakers, G. M. J., & Di Lazzaro, V. (2010). Physiology of repetitive transcranial magnetic stimulation of the human brain. *Brain*

Stimulation, 3, 95–118. http://dx.doi.org/10.1016/j.brs.2009.10.005

Huang, Y.-Z., Sommer, M., Thickbroom, G., Hamada, M., Pascual-Leonne, A., Paulus, W., . . . Ugawa, Y. (2009). Consensus: New methodologies for brain stimulation. *Brain Stimulation, 2,* 2–13. http://dx.doi.org/10.1016/j.brs.2008.09.007

Issac, T. G., Chandra, S. R., & Nagaraju, B. C. (2016). Transcranial magnetic stimulation (TMS) as a tool for early diagnosis and prognostication in cortico-basal ganglia degeneration (CBD) syndromes: Review of literature and case report. *Indian Journal of Psychological Medicine, 38,* 81–83. http://dx.doi.org/10.4103/0253-7176.175133

Janicak, P. G., & Dokucu, M. E. (2015). Transcranial magnetic stimulation for the treatment of major depression. *Neuropsychiatric Disease and Treatment, 11,* 1549–1560. http://dx.doi.org/10.2147/NDT.S67477

Kennedy, S. H., Giacobbe, P., Rizvi, S. J., Placenza, F. M., Nishikawa, Y., Mayberg, H. S., & Lozano, A. M. (2011). Deep brain stimulation for treatment-resistant depression: Follow-up after 3 to 6 years. *The American Journal of Psychiatry, 168,* 502–510. http://dx.doi.org/10.1176/appi.ajp.2010.10081187

Khedr, E. M., Gilio, F., & Rothwell, J. (2004). Effects of low frequency and low intensity repetitive paired pulse stimulation of the primary motor cortex. *Clinical Neurophysiology, 115,* 1259–1263. http://dx.doi.org/10.1016/j.clinph.2003.08.025

Kim, J.-H., Kim, D.-W., Chang, W. H., Kim, Y.-H., Kim, K., & Im, C.-H. (2014). Inconsistent outcomes of transcranial direct current stimulation may originate from anatomical differences among individuals: Electric field simulation using individual MRI data. *Neuroscience Letters, 564,* 6–10. http://dx.doi.org/10.1016/j.neulet.2014.01.054

Kovanlikaya, I., Heier, L., & Kaplitt, M. (2014). Treatment of chronic pain: Diffusion tensor imaging identification of the ventroposterolateral nucleus confirmed with successful deep brain stimulation. *Stereotactic and Functional Neurosurgery, 92,* 365–371. http://dx.doi.org/10.1159/000366002

Kozel, F. A., Motes, M. A., Didehbani, N., DeLaRosa, B., Bass, C., Schraufnagel, C. D., . . . Hart, J., Jr. (2018). Repetitive TMS to augment cognitive processing therapy in combat veterans of recent conflicts with PTSD: A randomized clinical trial. *Journal of Affective Disorders, 229,* 506–514. http://dx.doi.org/10.1016/j.jad.2017.12.046

Krahl, S. E., & Clark, K. B. (2012). Vagus nerve stimulation for epilepsy: A review of central mechanisms. *Surgical Neurology International, 3*(Suppl. 4), 255–259. http://dx.doi.org/10.4103/2152-7806.103015

Kranaster, L., Blennow, K., Zetterberg, H., & Sartorius, A. (2017). Electroconvulsive therapy does not alter the synaptic protein neurogranin in the cerebrospinal fluid of patients with major depression. *Journal of Neural Transmission, 124,* 1641–1645. http://dx.doi.org/10.1007/s00702-017-1802-z

Krystal, A. D., West, M., Prado, R., Greenside, H., Zoldi, S., & Weiner, R. D. (2000). EEG effects of ECT: Implications for rTMS. *Depression and Anxiety, 12,* 157–165. http://dx.doi.org/10.1002/1520-6394(2000)12:3<157::AID-DA7>3.0.CO;2-R

Kuncel, A. M., & Grill, W. M. (2004). Selection of stimulus parameters for deep brain stimulation. *Clinical Neurophysiology, 115,* 2431–2441. http://dx.doi.org/10.1016/j.clinph.2004.05.031

Lee, W. H., Lisanby, S. H., Laine, A. F., & Peterchev, A. V. (2014). Stimulation strength and focality of electroconvulsive therapy and magnetic seizure therapy in a realistic head model. *Proceedings of the 36th Annual International Conference of the IEEE Engineering in Medicine and Biology Society,* 410–413. http://dx.doi.org/10.1109/EMBC.2014.6943615

Lee, W. H., Lisanby, S. H., Laine, A. F., & Peterchev, A. V. (2016). Comparison of electric field strength and spatial distribution of electroconvulsive therapy and magnetic seizure therapy in a realistic human head model. *European Psychiatry, 36,* 55–64. http://dx.doi.org/10.1016/j.eurpsy.2016.03.003

Lempka, S. F., Howell, B., Gunalan, K., Machado, A. G., & McIntyre, C. C. (2018). Characterization of the stimulus waveforms generated by implantable pulse generators for deep brain stimulation. *Clinical Neurophysiology, 129,* 731–742. http://dx.doi.org/10.1016/j.clinph.2018.01.015

Leuchter, A. F., Cook, I. A., Feifel, D., Goethe, J. W., Husain, M., Carpenter, L. L., . . . George, M. S. (2015). Efficacy and safety of low-field synchronized transcranial magnetic stimulation (sTMS) for treatment of major depression. *Brain Stimulation, 8,* 787–794. http://dx.doi.org/10.1016/j.brs.2015.05.005

Lipton, R. B., & Pearlman, S. H. (2010). Transcranial magnetic simulation in the treatment of migraine. *Neurotherapeutics, 7,* 204–212. http://dx.doi.org/10.1016/j.nurt.2010.03.002

Lisanby, S. H., Luber, B., Schlaepfer, T. E., & Sackeim, H. A. (2003). Safety and feasibility of magnetic seizure therapy (MST) in major depression: Randomized within-subject comparison with electroconvulsive therapy. *Neuropsychopharmacology, 28,* 1852–1865. http://dx.doi.org/10.1038/sj.npp.1300229

Loerwald, K. W., Borland, M. S., Rennaker, R. L., II, Hays, S. A., & Kilgard, M. P. (2018). The interaction of pulse width and current intensity on the extent of cortical plasticity evoked by vagus nerve stimulation. *Brain Stimulation, 11,* 271–277. http://dx.doi.org/10.1016/j.brs.2017.11.007

López-Alonso, V., Cheeran, B., Río-Rodríguez, D., & Fernández-del-Olmo, M. (2014). Inter-individual variability in response to non-invasive brain stimulation paradigms. *Brain Stimulation, 7,* 372–380. http://dx.doi.org/10.1016/j.brs.2014.02.004

*Lucas-Neto, L., Reimão, S., Oliveira, E., Rainha-Campos, A., Sousa, J., Nunes, R. G., . . . Campos, J. G. (2015). Advanced MR imaging of the human nucleus accumbens—Additional guiding tool for deep brain stimulation. *Neuromodulation, 18,* 341–348. http://dx.doi.org/10.1111/ner.12289

Makani, R., Pradhan, B., Shah, U., & Parikh, T. (2017). Role of repetitive transcranial magnetic stimulation (rTMS) in treatment of addiction and related disorders: A systematic review. *Current Drug Abuse Reviews, 10,* 31–43. http://dx.doi.org/10.2174/1874473710666171129225914

*McClintock, S. M., Tirmizi, O., Chansard, M., & Husain, M. M. (2011). A systematic review of the neurocognitive effects of magnetic seizure therapy. *International Review of Psychiatry, 23,* 413–423. http://dx.doi.org/10.3109/09540261.2011.623687

McDonald, W. M., Weiner, R. D., Fochtmann, L. J., & McCall, W. V. (2016). The FDA and ECT. *The Journal of ECT, 32,* 75–77. http://dx.doi.org/10.1097/YCT.0000000000000326

McIntyre, C. C., Savasta, M., Kerkerian-Le Goff, L., & Vitek, J. L. (2004). Uncovering the mechanism(s) of action of deep brain stimulation: Activation, inhibition, or both. *Clinical Neurophysiology, 115,* 1239–1248. http://dx.doi.org/10.1016/j.clinph.2003.12.024

Medda, P., Toni, C., & Perugi, G. (2014). The mood-stabilizing effects of electroconvulsive therapy. *The Journal of ECT, 30,* 275–282. http://dx.doi.org/10.1097/YCT.0000000000000160

Moisello, C., Blanco, D., Fontanesi, C., Lin, J., Biagioni, M., Kumar, P., . . . Ghilardi, M. F., & the Sensory Motor Integration Lab (SMILab). (2015). TMS enhances retention of a motor skill in Parkinson's disease. *Brain Stimulation, 8,* 224–230. http://dx.doi.org/10.1016/j.brs.2014.11.005

*Montgomery, E. B. J., Jr., & Gale, J. T. (2008). Mechanisms of action of deep brain stimulation(DBS). *Neuroscience and Biobehavioral Reviews, 32,* 388–407. http://dx.doi.org/10.1016/j.neubiorev.2007.06.003

Müller, U. J., Voges, J., Steiner, J., Galazky, I., Heinze, H.-J., Möller, M., . . . Kuhn, J. (2013). Deep brain stimulation of the nucleus accumbens for the treatment of addiction. *Annals of the New York Academy of Sciences, 1282,* 119–128. http://dx.doi.org/10.1111/j.1749-6632.2012.06834.x

Nagahama, H., Suzuki, K., Shonai, T., Aratani, K., Sakurai, Y., Nakamura, M., & Sakata, M. (2015). Comparison of magnetic resonance imaging sequences for depicting the subthalamic nucleus for deep brain stimulation. *Radiological Physics and Technology, 8,* 30–35. http://dx.doi.org/10.1007/s12194-014-0283-0

Neurological Devices; Reclassification of Electroconvulsive Therapy Devices, 80 Fed. Reg. 81223 (proposed December 29, 2015) (to be codified at 21 C.F.R. pt. 882).

Obeso, J. A., Rodríguez, M. C., Gorospe, A., Guridi, J., Alvarez, L., & Macias, R. (1997). Surgical treatment of Parkinson's disease. *Bailliere's Clinical Neurology, 6*(1), 125–145.

Okun, M. S., Foote, K. D., Wu, S. S., Ward, H. E., Bowers, D., Rodriguez, R. L., . . . Sanchez, J. C. (2013). A trial of scheduled deep brain stimulation for Tourette syndrome: Moving away from continuous deep brain stimulation paradigms. *JAMA Neurology, 70,* 85–94. http://dx.doi.org/10.1001/jamaneurol.2013.580

Ota, M., Noda, T., Sato, N., Okazaki, M., Ishikawa, M., Hattori, K., . . . Kunugi, H. (2015). Effect of electroconvulsive therapy on gray matter volume in major depressive disorder. *Journal of Affective Disorders, 186,* 186–191. http://dx.doi.org/10.1016/j.jad.2015.06.051

Pan, S.-D., Zhu, L.-L., Chen, M., Xia, P., & Zhou, Q. (2016). Weight-based dosing in medication use: What should we know? *Patient Preference and Adherence, 10,* 549–560.

Perera, T., George, M. S., Grammer, G., Janicak, P. G., Pascual-Leone, A., & Wirecki, T. S. (2016). The Clinical TMS Society consensus review and treatment recommendations for TMS therapy for major depressive disorder. *Brain Stimulation, 9,* 336–346. http://dx.doi.org/10.1016/j.brs.2016.03.010

Perini, G. I., Toffanin, T., Pigato, G., Ferri, G., Follador, H., Zonta, F., . . . D'Avella, D. (2017). Hippocampal gray volumes increase in treatment-resistant depression responding to vagus nerve stimulation. *The Journal of ECT, 33,* 160–166. http://dx.doi.org/10.1097/YCT.0000000000000424

Peterchev, A. V., Krystal, A. D., Rosa, M. A., & Lisanby, S. H. (2015). Individualized low-amplitude seizure therapy: Minimizing current for electroconvulsive therapy and magnetic seizure therapy. *Neuropsychopharmacology, 40,* 2076–2084. http://dx.doi.org/10.1038/npp.2015.122

Peterchev, A. V., Rosa, M. A., Deng, Z.-D., Prudic, J., & Lisanby, S. H. (2010). Electroconvulsive therapy stimulus parameters: Rethinking dosage. *The Journal of ECT, 26,* 159–174. http://dx.doi.org/10.1097/YCT.0b013e3181e48165

Peterchev, A. V., Wagner, T. A., Miranda, P. C., Nitsche, M. A., Paulus, W., Lisanby, S. H., . . . Bikson, M. (2012). Fundamentals of transcranial electric and magnetic stimulation dose: Definition, selection, and reporting practices. *Brain Stimulation, 5,* 435–453. http://dx.doi.org/10.1016/j.brs.2011.10.001

Radman, T., & Lisanby, S. H. (2017). New directions in the rational design of electrical and magnetic seizure therapies: Individualized low amplitude seizure therapy (iLAST) and magnetic seizure therapy (MST). *International Review of Psychiatry, 29*, 63–78. http://dx.doi.org/10.1080/09540261.2017.1304898

Ranck, J. B. J., Jr. (1975). Which elements are excited in electrical stimulation of mammalian central nervous system: A review. *Brain Research, 98*, 417–440. http://dx.doi.org/10.1016/0006-8993(75)90364-9

Rehn, S., Eslick, G. D., & Brakoulias, V. (2018). A meta-analysis of the effectiveness of different cortical targets used in repetitive transcranial magnetic stimulation (rTMS) for the treatment of obsessive-compulsive disorder (OCD). *Psychiatric Quarterly, 89*, 645–665. http://dx.doi.org/10.1007/s11126-018-9566-7

Révész, D., Rydenhag, B., & Ben-Menachem, E. (2016). Complications and safety of vagus nerve stimulation: 25 years of experience at a single center. *Journal of Neurosurgery. Pediatrics, 18*, 97–104. http://dx.doi.org/10.3171/2016.1.PEDS15534

Rocha, S., Monteiro, A., Linhares, P., Chamadoira, C., Basto, M. A., Reis, C., . . . Vaz, R. (2014). Long-term mortality analysis in Parkinson's disease treated with deep brain stimulation. *Parkinson's Disease, 2014*, 717041. http://dx.doi.org/10.1155/2014/717041

Rosin, B., Slovik, M., Mitelman, R., Rivlin-Etzion, M., Haber, S. N., Israel, Z., . . . Bergman, H. (2011). Closed-loop deep brain stimulation is superior in ameliorating parkinsonism. *Neuron, 72*, 370–384. http://dx.doi.org/10.1016/j.neuron.2011.08.023

Rossi, S., Hallett, M., Rossini, P. M., & Pascual-Leone, A. (2009). Safety, ethical considerations, and application guidelines for the use of transcranial magnetic stimulation in clinical practice and research. *Clinical Neurophysiology, 120*, 2008–2039. http://dx.doi.org/10.1016/j.clinph.2009.08.016

Sackeim, H. A., Prudic, J., Devanand, D. P., Kiersky, J. E., Fitzsimons, L., Moody, B. J., . . . Settembrino, J. M. (1993). Effects of stimulus intensity and electrode placement on the efficacy and cognitive effects of electroconvulsive therapy. *The New England Journal of Medicine, 328*, 839–846. http://dx.doi.org/10.1056/NEJM199303253281204

Sackeim, H. A., Prudic, J., Fuller, R., Keilp, J., Lavori, P. W., & Olfson, M. (2007). The cognitive effects of electroconvulsive therapy in community settings. *Neuropsychopharmacology, 32*, 244–254. http://dx.doi.org/10.1038/sj.npp.1301180

Sahlem, G. L., Short, E. B., Kerns, S., Snipes, J., DeVries, W., Fox, J. B., . . . Sackeim, H. A. (2016). Expanded safety and efficacy data for a new method of performing electroconvulsive therapy: Focal electrically administered seizure therapy. *The Journal of ECT, 32*, 197–203. http://dx.doi.org/10.1097/YCT.0000000000000328

Sakreida, K., Lange, I., Willmes, K., Heim, S., Binkofski, F., Clusmann, H., & Neuloh, G. (2018). High-resolution language mapping of Broca's region with transcranial magnetic stimulation. *Brain Structure & Function, 223*(3), 1297–1312.

Scharfetter, H., Casañas, R., & Rosell, J. (2003). Biological tissue characterization by magnetic induction spectroscopy (MIS): Requirements and limitations. *IEEE Transactions on Biomedical Engineering, 50*, 870–880. http://dx.doi.org/10.1109/TBME.2003.813533

Schwedt, T. J., & Vargas, B. (2015). Neurostimulation for treatment of migraine and cluster headache. *Pain Medicine, 16*(9), 1827–1834. http://dx.doi.org/10.1111/pme.12792

Shorter, E. (1997). *A history of psychiatry: From the era of the asylum to the age of Prozac.* New York, NY: Wiley.

Sienaert, P. (2016). Based on a true story? The portrayal of ECT in international movies and television programs. *Brain Stimulation, 9*, 882–891. http://dx.doi.org/10.1016/j.brs.2016.07.005

*Slotema, C. W., Blom, J. D., Hoek, H. W., & Sommer, I. E. C. (2010). Should we expand the toolbox of psychiatric treatment methods to include repetitive transcranial magnetic stimulation (rTMS)? A meta-analysis of the efficacy of rTMS in psychiatric disorders. *The Journal of Clinical Psychiatry, 71*, 873–884. http://dx.doi.org/10.4088/JCP.08m04872gre

Stip, E., Blain-Juste, M.-E., Farmer, O., Fournier-Gosselin, M.-P., & Lespérance, P. (2018). Catatonia with schizophrenia: From ECT to rTMS. *L'Encéphale, 44*, 183–187. http://dx.doi.org/10.1016/j.encep.2017.09.008

Sun, F. T., & Morrell, M. J. (2014). Closed-loop neurostimulation: The clinical experience. *Neurotherapeutics, 11*, 553–563. http://dx.doi.org/10.1007/s13311-014-0280-3

Sun, Y., Farzan, F., Mulsant, B. H., Rajji, T. K., Fitzgerald, P. B., Barr, M. S., . . . Daskalakis, Z. J. (2016). Indicators for remission of suicidal ideation following magnetic seizure therapy in patients with treatment-resistant depression. *JAMA Psychiatry, 73*, 337–345. http://dx.doi.org/10.1001/jamapsychiatry.2015.3097

Tang, V. M., Blumberger, D. M., McClintock, S. M., Kaster, T. S., Rajji, T. K., Downar, J., . . . Daskalakis, Z. J. (2018). Magnetic seizure therapy in treatment-resistant schizophrenia: A pilot study. *Frontiers in Psychiatry, 8*, 310. http://dx.doi.org/10.3389/fpsyt.2017.00310

*Taylor, R., Galvez, V., & Loo, C. (2018). Transcranial magnetic stimulation (TMS) safety: A practical guide for psychiatrists. *Australasian Psychiatry, 26*, 189–192. http://dx.doi.org/10.1177/1039856217748249

Thiele, S., Furlanetti, L., Pfeiffer, L.-M., Coenen, V. A., & Döbrössy, M. D. (2018). The effects of bilateral, continuous, and chronic deep brain stimulation of the medial forebrain bundle in a rodent model of depression. *Experimental Neurology, 303*, 153–161. http://dx.doi.org/10.1016/j.expneurol.2018.02.002

Thomann, P. A., Wolf, R. C., Nolte, H. M., Hirjak, D., Hofer, S., Seidl, U., . . . Wüstenberg, T. (2017). Neuromodulation in response to electroconvulsive therapy in schizophrenia and major depression. *Brain Stimulation, 10,* 637–644. http://dx.doi.org/10.1016/j.brs.2017.01.578

Udupa, K., & Chen, R. (2015). The mechanisms of action of deep brain stimulation and ideas for the future development. *Progress in Neurobiology, 133,* 27–49. http://dx.doi.org/10.1016/j.pneurobio.2015.08.001

University of Texas Southwestern Medical Center. (2018). *Confirmatory efficacy and safety trial of magnetic seizure therapy for depression* (CREST-MST) (Clinicaltrials.gov Identifier NCT03191058). Retrieved from https://clinicaltrials.gov/ct2/show/NCT03191058

van Hartevelt, T. J., Cabral, J., Deco, G., Møller, A., Green, A. L., Aziz, T. Z., & Kringelbach, M. L. (2014). Neural plasticity in human brain connectivity: The effects of long term deep brain stimulation of the subthalamic nucleus in Parkinson's disease. *PLoS One, 9,* e86496. http://dx.doi.org/10.1371/journal.pone.0086496

Van Laere, K., Vonck, K., Boon, P., Versijpt, J., & Dierckx, R. (2002). Perfusion SPECT changes after acute and chronic vagus nerve stimulation in relation to prestimulus condition and long-term clinical efficacy. *Journal of Nuclear Medicine, 43,* 733–744.

Vonck, K., De Herdt, V., Bosman, T., Dedeurwaerdere, S., Van Laere, K., & Boon, P. (2008). Thalamic and limbic involvement in the mechanism of action of vagus nerve stimulation, a SPECT study. *Seizure, 17,* 699–706. http://dx.doi.org/10.1016/j.seizure.2008.05.001

Wei, X., Li, Y., Lu, M., Wang, J., & Yi, G. (2017). Comprehensive survey on improved focality and penetration depth of transcranial magnetic stimulation employing multi-coil arrays. *International Journal of Environmental Research and Public Health, 14,* 1388. http://dx.doi.org/10.3390/ijerph14111388

*Weiner, R. D., & Reti, I. M. (2017). Key updates in the clinical application of electroconvulsive therapy. *International Review of Psychiatry, 29,* 54–62. http://dx.doi.org/10.1080/09540261.2017.1309362

Ziemann, U. (2004). TMS and drugs. *Clinical Neurophysiology, 115,* 1717–1729. http://dx.doi.org/10.1016/j.clinph.2004.03.006

Ziemann, U., Reis, J., Schwenkreis, P., Rosanova, M., Strafella, A., Badawy, R., & Müller-Dahlhaus, F. (2015). TMS and drugs revisited 2014. *Clinical Neurophysiology, 126,* 1847–1868. http://dx.doi.org/10.1016/j.clinph.2014.08.028

CHAPTER 33

FUTURE DIRECTIONS IN THEORY, RESEARCH, PRACTICE, AND POLICY

Patrick H. DeLeon, Fernanda P. De Oliveira,
and Antonio E. Puente

Over the past decade, our nation's health care system has undergone an unprecedented transformation. Historically, the system relied on providing individually and medically-oriented acute care services that were expected to be reimbursed on a fee-for-service basis. With the rapidly changing landscape, we are now evolving towards a system that strives to objectively measure the quality of health care being provided, rather than the volume of services rendered—and one that will give priority to enhancing prevention, wellness, and population-based initiatives. This will, of necessity as a consequence of the measurement of performance, include attention to the psychosocial-cultural-economic gradient of quality care—which historically has been under-appreciated and therefore underfunded.

The steady advances occurring within the technology and communications fields and their direct applicability to health care has been critical in this evolution. Each of the core health professions (i.e., nursing, medicine, pharmacy, and psychology) has significantly grown in terms of absolute numbers of practitioners, while simultaneously expanding the knowledge base provided within their professional training. Not surprisingly, this has resulted in increased interest in expanding their respective scopes of clinical practice and obtaining a seat at the table in developing health policies that directly impact them and their patients. The health care system of the future will be based on interprofessional (i.e., interdisciplinary) teams of providers, functioning within "closed systems" of care, who demonstrate respect for their colleagues' professional competence and contributions (DeLeon, Sells, Cassidy, Waters, & Kasper, 2015). Integrated care and systematic attention to evidence-based practice will become the norm. No longer will health care be considered the exclusive purview of any one discipline, especially just of medicine; instead, the goal will be to facilitate patients acting as educated consumers, assuming responsibility for their own health status.

One important development in this paradigm shift has been prescriptive authority for psychologists (RxP). Whether or not one ultimately decides to pursue obtaining this clinical privilege, it is important for clinicians, educators, and scientists to understand the societal and clinical context within which the appropriate utilization of psychotropic medications may be expected to significantly enhance the overall quality and reduce the costs of care being provided (Burns, DeLeon, Chemtob, Welch, & Samuels, 1988; Fox et al., 2009). Without question, the catalyst for the RxP quest was the U.S. Department of Defense (DoD) Psychopharmacology Demonstration Project

The views expressed are those of the authors and do not reflect the official policy or position of the Uniformed Services University, the U.S. Department of Defense, or the U.S. government.

The authors appreciate the editorial assistance of Jazmin Rios, graduate student in psychology at the University of North Carolina Wilmington.

http://dx.doi.org/10.1037/0000133-033
APA Handbook of Psychopharmacology, S. M. Evans (Editor-in-Chief)

(PDP), sponsored by U.S. Senator Daniel K. Inouye (D-HI) during congressional deliberations on the Fiscal Year 1989 Appropriations Bill (which became Public Law No. 100-463). At that time, the conferees directed the DoD to establish a "demonstration pilot training project under which military psychologists may be trained and authorized to issue appropriate psychotropic medications under certain circumstances" (DeLeon, Fox, & Graham, 1991, p. 34). From the very beginning, the underlying vision for this proposal was to improve the overall quality of mental health care throughout the nation and not merely within the military community. Accordingly, in many ways, this visionary initiative might reasonably be considered as fostering a clinical, research, and social justice agenda.

WHY THE U.S. DEPARTMENT OF DEFENSE?

Over the years, the DoD has had an impressive history of developing a wide range of innovative health initiatives: for example, the training and utilization of medical corpsmen (medics) for front line, naval, and remote operations; expanded utilization of dentists, nurse practitioners. and physician assistants as primary care providers; and the development of extraordinary life-saving trauma procedures, medications, and specialized equipment. DoD scientists and clinicians have been on the cutting edge of developing visionary telehealth and electronic medical record systems that have allowed for the provision of necessary care over long distances in austere and often extremely hostile environments, as well as designing population-based prevention and public health initiatives. In the rehabilitation arena, as one example, the DoD has been the catalyst for integrating the increasingly sophisticated expertise of the diverse fields of engineering, computer science, and a wide range of health care professions to address the complex needs of wounded warriors, both physical and emotional.

ESTABLISHING AN INTRIGUING POLICY AGENDA

From a health policy perspective, the well-established legal basis underlying the federal supremacy doctrine frees the DoD's leadership from being constrained by historic state scope of practice restrictions (e.g., the portability of state licensure of federal health care personnel). Further, given the magnitude of the DoD's overall budget and the global/international and humanitarian nature of its underlying mission, the resources required to be responsive to congressional interests and presidential administration proposals definitely exist. This has included the development of cutting-edge evidence-based protocols for effectively addressing the needs of those afflicted with the signature war wounds of posttraumatic stress disorder (PTSD) and traumatic brain injuries (TBI). As described elsewhere in this handbook, the DoD ultimately did take the challenge of training psychologists to utilize psychotropic medications seriously and responsibly. In retrospect, perhaps the most significant long-term contribution of the PDP was to clearly demonstrate to psychologists that those in the profession could, in fact, be trained to safely and cost-effectively utilize psychotropic medications clinically in a reasonable and effective fashion. In so doing, the PDP provided an exciting vision of the future for the next generation of psychologists.

It is correct that some psychologists, for example those who have been active in the American Psychological Association's (APA's) Division 28 (Psychopharmacology and Substance Abuse)—which was established in 1967—have long been active in this arena. Whereas the division's primary role entails research, the PDP soon became a catalyst for encouraging collaborative discussions among colleagues who primarily identified themselves as clinicians *or* as educators. Further, given the intense legislative opposition that organized psychiatry generated in response to subsequent state and federal efforts to expand psychology's scope of clinical practice to include psychopharmacology, prescriptive authority per se soon matured into becoming a significant and highly visual health policy agenda within the APA and state association governances. And from the beginning of those deliberations, a small but highly vocal element of the association expressed concern that by obtaining the legal right to utilize drugs therapeutically, psychology would lose its fundamental identity in behavioral science.

On the other hand, others appreciated and became genuinely excited by the vision expressed by the APA Ad Hoc Task Force on Psychopharmacology, established by the Council of Representatives in 1990 and chaired by Michael Smyer, which reported

> The Task Force emphasizes the importance of developing a subspecialty of psychology with comprehensive knowledge and experience in psychopharmacology. Practitioners with combined training in psychopharmacology and psychosocial treatments can reasonably be viewed as a new form of health care professional, expected to bring to health care delivery the best of both psychological and pharmacological knowledge. The contributions of this new form of psychopharmacological intervention have the potential to dramatically improve patient care and make important new advances in treatment. (Smyer et al., 1993, p. 402)

Those serving on the Task Force, which included 2017 APA President Antonio Puente, could further foresee numerous areas of potentially exciting research opportunities for psychology, and especially for those colleagues with an interprofessional orientation. The Task Force included researchers, practitioners, and a psychiatrist, Fuller Torey. The fundamental assumption behind the Task Force was that an insufficient number of people had the opportunity to receive appropriate psychopharmacotherapy. This was especially true in rural and poor urban settings, as well as for a large percentage of ethnic and racial minorities. To compound the situation, socioeconomic issues and lack of accessibility to psychiatrists limited the potential impact of using this type of intervention, especially concomitant with psychotherapy.

One of the underlying principles behind the Task Force's consideration of how to integrate prescription authority into the psychological workforce was the importance of introducing biological concepts to the training for professional education. Specifically, the group believed that early introduction, as early as high school and definitely at the undergraduate

level, to biological and pharmacological concepts was critical to subsequent foundational understanding of psychopharmacological interventions. Three levels of education and training were introduced for all practicing psychologists (detailed information on these levels can be found in Chapter 1, this volume). The first was rudimentary understanding of the use and limitations of psychopharmacological intervention. The second was a midlevel but more in-depth understanding, including specific application of and interaction between psychoactive medicines and mental disorders—for example, examining what types of medications might have the best impact on specific types of depression. Finally, the third level is what today is called prescriptive authority, which entails both classroom and didactic training. Whereas the third level has gained strong support, the first two have not substantially been integrated into current professional education. Hence, in the future, the field might want to focus on the first two steps, so a more comprehensive understanding of all forms of interventions can be gained by all professionals.

THE UNPRECEDENTED TRANSFORMATION OF HEALTH CARE

During the past decade a number of fundamental changes have been occurring in our nation's health care environment, many of which have been reflected in various provisions of President Obama's landmark Patient Protection and Affordable Care Act (ACA; 2010). Perhaps the most significant of these has been the increasing impact of the continuous advances in the computer/technology fields and their direct application to the delivery of, and research programs addressing, quality health care. Health care reimbursement has shifted from fee for the activity to fee for performance. Hence, the focus is now fast becoming reimbursement for empirically derived and supported results, which, has changed the very definition of quality care to cost-effective clinical outcomes focused on patient-relevant improvements.

Historically, it has taken nearly two decades for scientific developments—for example, by scientists at the National Institutes of Health (NIH)—to have a direct impact on the actual delivery of clinical care.

Today, that estimate has been dramatically reduced and new focus areas for research have evolved, including exploring the importance of the psycho-social-behavioral determinants of care, utilizing and disseminating comparative clinical effectiveness research, and the use of apps for real-time patient monitoring and clinical interventions. For instance, the ACA established the Patient-Centered Outcomes Research Institute (PCORI) in 2010 to provide patients with the ability to make better-informed data-based health decisions by funding and disseminating comparative clinical effectiveness research focused on patient-relevant outcomes. Each of these developments has acknowledged that the individual patient is in charge of his or her own health destiny. They have also fostered a serious appreciation for the societal benefits of taking a broader (i.e., public health-oriented) look at the limitations and constraints of our current approach to delivering health care, including historical scope-of-practice licensure limitations. Focus also has been placed on the importance of integrating different kinds of interventions, such as psychotherapy and psychopharmacotherapy.

Numerous studies over the years have consistently confirmed that clinicians who rely on the use of psychotropic medications, rather than on equally or more effective behavioral and psychosocial interventions, are simply not providing true quality care. Perhaps most striking is the fact that less than 20% of psychotropic medications are actually prescribed by psychiatrists, with internists and family practitioners having higher utilization rates (Olfson, Blanco, Wang, Laje, & Correll, 2014). Studies have shown that primary care providers consistently utilize less than effective dosage levels, and perhaps most importantly, underdiagnose mental health issues (Vermani, Marcus, & Katzman, 2011). These findings clearly underscore the critical importance of mental/behavioral health training and its relevance to providing comprehensive quality health care. Further, when one closely studies various sub-populations, such as women, the elderly, children, and people of color, the over-reliance upon psychotropic medications by the general medical system, especially to address behavioral issues, becomes even more pronounced. This is particularly relevant

in addressing the issues of hyperactive children, as well as depression, which have increasingly become major concerns of primary care providers.

Those involved in pursuing legislation to authorize the use of medications by appropriately trained psychologists and other nonphysician health care providers are well aware of organized medicine's frequent reliance on the emotional "public health hazard" argument (i.e., that nonmedical practitioners will affirmatively harm their patients if allowed to utilize these "dangerous medications"). It is this particular argument that was presented by the American Psychiatric Association when the Current Procedural Terminology (CPT) medical code 90863 for psychopharmacological management was presented at the 2013 meeting of the American Medical Association CPT Panel (of which Puente was a member at the time). Using empirically derived support, the APA successfully disputed psychiatry's challenge of allowing the use of this historical code by prescribing psychologists. Further, the field of medicine's historical avoidance of insisting on holding their own members to objective data-based standards and protocols of prescribing calls into question the validity of their underlying assumptions. As we have suggested, the advent of technology and additional scientific discoveries are making it increasingly possible to determine across populations and across diagnoses which prescribing protocols would objectively appear to be most beneficial and cost-effective for individual patients.

We would foresee that one important aspect of this evolution will be the systematic reliance on the expertise of clinical pharmacists, who as a profession are becoming increasingly engaged within the mental health arena and who, without question, have considerable knowledge regarding the impact of medications on patients. We would suggest, for example, that those ultimately responsible for paying for the clinical care being provided and/or those responsible for establishing facility and system quality of care guidelines will soon require regular reviews of the ongoing therapeutic effects of specific medication orders (e.g., examining how long an individual patient should remain on a particular dosage, and whether this approach is resulting in objectively measured positive clinical change, perhaps as determined via monitoring by appropriate apps). Some of those who are now senior clinical pharmacists began their careers when it was deemed unethical to discuss the clinical impact of medications with patients. This reflected the fact that in the mid-20th century, placebos were still often used and the mind-set was that patients did not need to know the names of the medications or the reasons they were prescribed. It would be an understatement to note that this approach is significantly different from today's emphasis on fostering professional collaboration with patients who are to be considered educated consumers of health care. The landscape is definitely changing.

Another transformative change has involved shifting demographics, both within the United States and outside. In the United States, an increasing demand has been attending to this changing face of America. Outside of the United States, the importance of migration and the rapidly shifting cultural landscape calls for a greater appreciation and understanding of cultural diversity. Using the United States as an illustration, increasing evidence has mounted showing that underserved groups (e.g., those in lower socioeconomic levels and ethnic minorities) experience higher rates of chronic diseases, especially mental health problems, that are highly associated with lifestyle choices and psychological status (HHS, 1999). As a consequence, the emergence of combined interventions, behavioral and pharmaceutical, increases the likelihood that these individuals will respond to these types of treatments, and, in turn, the entire health care landscape would be considerably affected positively, both in terms of effectiveness and reduced cost. Unfortunately, the alternative is to continue to rely upon primary health care providers who are demonstratively not trained in the nuances of mental health care nor of psychotropic medications (e.g., Geraghty, Franks, & Kravitz, 2007).

By bringing psychology's extensive expertise in the psychosocial-cultural-behavioral arena into this equation, we are confident that the nation's overall quality of care will be dramatically improved. United States Air Force Lt. Col. Elaine Foster (retired) was one of the first graduates of the PDP. She noted,

The expertise we bring to bear as psychologists is most critical because even a pill will only work within a contextual framework. Trust is key to any therapeutic relationship. Otherwise, when the side effects hit, most people will follow their instinct to stop taking the offending agent. It comes down to the art of instilling hope within the framework of explaining the science. Once a person can place a challenging experience into a context, they are much more willing to continue working collaboratively. This is how I optimize medication effects by combining my training as a psychologist with my knowledge of psychopharmacology. (personal communication, January 1, 2018)

PSYCHOLOGY'S ROLE AS A HEALTH CARE PROFESSION

From a public policy frame of reference, it is important to appreciate that for many of the profession's senior leaders, the notion that psychology might be a bona fide health care profession is a new, if not alien, concept. Most would agree that the profession of psychology evolved from the military and societal needs of World War II, and that mental health per se was at that time viewed as distinct from general health care, which was primarily focused on providing acute care services. The community mental health center movement grew out of the era of President John F. Kennedy, and the community health center initiative began in the Great Society era of President Lyndon Johnson. Almost everyone—at the policy, individual patient, and clinical level—viewed these as two separate entities with almost no overlap (McGuire, 1990; Phares & Trull, 1997; Uhlaner, 1967).

Clinicians and educational training systems specializing in mental health had their own distinct sources of reimbursement and financial support—and often dramatically different levels of societal acceptance (as exemplified by the prolonged and intense legislative efforts to obtain mental health parity). Psychology educational systems were usually within colleges of philosophy or social sciences, rather than within university health profession institutions, and were infrequently associated with schools of public health or schools of law. Interprofessional collaboration and integrated mental health care were rarely considered, though some psychologists succeeded by being employed in university medical centers, particularly within departments of psychiatry. Recent discussions surrounding interprofessional education have stressed the importance of beginning this process in professional students' earliest stages of study, prior to when limiting stereotypes are formed. Psychologists should recognize that, in fact, it was only in 2001, during the APA presidential term of the late Norine Johnson, that the APA bylaws were modified by the membership to expressly recognize psychology's potential contributions to our nation's health care system. This was further delineated by others, including Puente (2011), who asserted that the idea of psychology as involving only mental health was outdated, inappropriate, and did not meet the demands of modern health care. Mental health should and will continue to be central to the profession of psychology. However, the addition of other areas, such as prescription authority, which is now formally APA policy, helps expand the impact of psychological science and the profession into a more vibrant, economical, and impactful health care system.

Looking into the future, one should also appreciate the policy significance of the fact that during the period from President Richard Nixon to President Barack Obama, when health care reform was becoming an increasingly important societal and thus political priority, organized psychology was primarily focused on protecting its independent private practice orientation and was generally in opposition to developing national standards (i.e., protocols) of care or having its clinical practice scientifically evaluated (Chambless & Ollendick, 2001). For many, psychotherapy was considered an "art" rather than a "science," with the human relationship developed being more clinically significant than exploring potentially quantifiable techniques (e.g., Addis & Krasnow, 2000; Fonagy, 1999; Smith, 1995). The growing movement within traditional physical health care toward prepaid capitation and organized systems of care (i.e., health maintenance

organizations [HMOs], managed care, and the ACA's accountable care organizations), was adamantly opposed—often by employing a slightly modified version of the emotional "public health hazard" argument proffered by psychiatry. Further, one could reasonably suggest that it was fundamentally mental health practitioners who, by urging special privacy treatment for patient records, were actively continuing the unfortunate stigma surrounding receiving mental health care. The growing movement toward value-based and holistic care was simply not foreseen.

Further, the integration of psychology into all health care, not just mental health care, provides an additional legislative agenda to require that psychologists be considered in the definition of *physician* according to Medicare and the Centers for Medicaid and Medicare Services (CMS). Currently, of the 13 doctorate-level health care providers, including medicine and dentistry, psychologists are the only ones not considered physicians by those organizations. This is critical in that the system reimburses 52% of the health care dollar for cognitive work, which can only be done by "physicians." As a reminder, 42% is provided for "technical" and noncognitive work, which is essentially how psychologists have been reimbursed historically. The introduction of prescription authority is one further and significant step in destroying this artificial boundary for psychologists. From a public policy perspective, every substantive modification in the status quo often results in further unanticipated policy agendas (Garrison, DeLeon, & Smedley, 2017).

EVOLVING TRAINING MODELS— INCLUDING INTERPROFESSIONAL COLLABORATION

When the APA Council of Representatives began considering the issue of RxP in 1990, a conscious decision was made to conceptualize this as a postdoctoral initiative in order to generate broad-based support from the membership. As described elsewhere in this handbook (see Chapter 29, this volume), the governance proceeded to establish reasonable guidelines for identifying appropriate training models and model legislation for identifying which individual practitioners should be deemed competent to prescribe. It was essentially up to individual state legislatures and psychology licensing boards to ultimately determine the specifics of this evolving practice. In 2017, those involved in pursuing this agenda determined that it would be timely to revisit the original standards and training assumptions. For example, recently there has been increasing momentum to allow students interested in pursuing this clinical expertise to begin their relevant studies at the graduate level, and even for some to begin their studies at the undergraduate level. Proponents for this modification often reference the ever-increasing scientific knowledge base, stressing the intimate relationship between genetics, physiology, and various mental and emotional states.

A persistent criticism of the prescriptive authority movement, one which is especially raised by physicians testifying before state legislatures in opposition to proposed legislation authorizing appropriately trained psychologists to prescribe, concerns the training received by psychologists at the undergraduate and graduate level; namely, that psychologists do not receive sufficient training oriented toward preparing to prescribe. However, with the APA Ad Hoc Task Force on Psychopharmacology training recommendations from 1992, this artificial limitation is no longer viable nor correct. At the heart of this argument is the presumption that only medical schools can adequately train prescribers, and that the curriculum necessary to ensure adequate training in psychotropics cannot be taught and learned outside of a doctoral-level medical program. Again, from a public policy vantage point, this argument was essentially tried, unsuccessfully, in organized medicine's efforts to restrict advanced practice nurses, optometrists, podiatrists, and clinical pharmacists from obtaining prescriptive authority. Under varying conditions, these other nonphysician health care providers have been increasingly able to practice to the full scope of their training, and where objective evidence is available, they have demonstrated equivalent positive outcomes. As their numbers of graduates continue to grow and as they continue to be actively involved in the legislative process at both the federal and state level, they will increasingly shape the role of, and society's expectations for, primary care providers—including their

very definition—far beyond that envisioned by the field of medicine per se.

Looking beyond individual provider-focused care, in 2015 the Institute of Medicine (IOM) released its report on the impact of interprofessional education:

> Patients are integral members of the care team, not solely patients to be treated, and the team is recognized as comprising a variety of health professionals. This changed thinking is the culmination of many social, economic, and technological factors that are transforming the world and forcing the fields of both health care and education to rethink long-established organizational models. . . . Widespread adoption of a model of interprofessional education across the learning continuum is urgently needed. An ideal model would retain the tenets of professional identity formation while providing robust opportunities for interprofessional education and collaborative care. Such a model also would differentiate between learning outcomes per se and the individual, population, and system outcomes that provide the ultimate rationale for ongoing investment in health professions education. (IOM, 2015, pp. xv–xvi)

This visionary evolution towards direct patient involvement in shaping their own health care undoubtedly reflects the increasing advanced educational level of the nation's population.

While the curriculum of postdoctoral training programs in psychopharmacology ensures knowledge of anatomy, physiology, pathophysiology, and other core medical coursework deemed to be essential to understanding the etiology and treatment of mental disorders, many undergraduate and graduate programs in psychology are admittedly lacking in the fundamental coursework for assessing and treating physical conditions. Accordingly, one logical next step in the development of the psychopharmacology educational track for psychologists will be to cultivate greater visibility and opportunities in undergraduate and graduate programs. As young potential mental health providers and researchers review their career options, few who see the value of becoming a prescriber or are intrigued by the scientific complexity surrounding medications may appreciate the opportunity to do so within the field of psychology. Although it is difficult to predict with any certainty why one career path is ultimately chosen, some of the best candidates for this specialty may be lost to other disciplines, such as psychiatric nursing, neuroscience, or psychiatry. Similarly, many early career psychologists who actually do explore available training opportunities in psychopharmacology may shy away out of a belief that they did not receive the necessary foundational knowledge in chemistry, biology, and other core sciences at earlier stages of their education. Accordingly, a necessary part of this evolution should be to strategically increase the specialty's visibility among students, and especially to offer opportunities for readily accessible professional development in early career stages.

THE UNPRECEDENTED IMPACT OF TECHNOLOGY

With increasingly sophisticated and more affordable technology becoming readily available, there has been a growing utilization of simulation laboratory experiences within the health professions and especially within nursing. For example, at the Uniformed Services University, nursing, medicine, and psychology faculty regularly utilize paid actors as patients who role play various mental health symptoms, such as having anxiety attacks, depression, psychosis, and dysfunctional family dynamics. Mental health doctor of nursing practice and clinical psychology graduate students have the opportunity to conduct joint case conferences, including discussions regarding the potential appropriate use of psychotropic medications, for the various scenarios presented by these patient-actors. With the increasing call for interprofessional training by the National Academy of Medicine (NAM)—formerly the Institute of Medicine—as well as by the APA and the national associations of every major health profession, we would expect to eventually see regular

interprofessional seminars focusing on the appropriate use of medications versus behavioral or other therapeutic approaches throughout psychology's graduate school training programs.

On April 27, 2004, President George W. Bush noted,

> The way I like to kind of try to describe health care is, on the research side, we're the best. We're coming up with more innovative ways to save lives and to treat patients. Except when you think about the provider's side, we're kind of still in the buggy era. . . . And there's a lot of talk about productivity gains in our society, and that's because companies and industries have properly used information technology. . . . And yet the health care industry hasn't touched it, except for certain areas. And one area that has is the Veterans Administration [VA]. (Bush, 2004, pp. 698–699)

Later that day, the President signed Executive Order 13335—Incentives for the Use of Health Information Technology and Establishing the Position of the National Health Information Technology Coordinator.

Since then, the VA and DoD have invested heavily, both economically and at the highest administrative policy level, in developing integrated electronic patient records and the ready use of telehealth (including telepharmacy and telemental health). Not surprisingly, the private sector has been increasingly following the federal government's lead, reflected by the steady enactment of legislation mandating the reimbursement of clinical services provided via telehealth.

As we have suggested earlier, substantive change is often an evolutionary process, with each modification gradually leading to another, often unanticipated, change. In the case of telehealth, the issue of licensure mobility soon became a major consideration for patients, practitioners, licensing boards, insurance companies, and those committed to developing comprehensive health policies. The underlying policy issue readily becomes: "Why should geographical location per se determine provider competence?" If an individual psychologist is deemed qualified by appropriate administrative authorities to provide psychotherapy and to prescribe psychotropics in one jurisdiction, should that provider not be considered qualified to utilize those same clinical skills in another jurisdiction? In our judgment, psychology is fortunate that the Association of State and Provincial Psychology Boards (ASPPB) has recently begun to address this important issue by establishing the Psychology Interjurisdictional Compact (PSYPACT), which is a joint initiative with APA and the APA Insurance Trust. This visionary concept proposes an "e-passport" which would allow the provision of psychological services by qualified licensed psychologists via electronic means across jurisdictional boundaries, without additional licensure, in the jurisdiction in which the client was physically present when receiving those services. For many, this approach would seem very similar, if not identical, to possessing a driver's license; that is, one's driver's license allows one to travel across state lines.

From this perspective, it is important to appreciate that over the past several decades advanced practice nurses, physician assistants, and clinical pharmacists have successfully expanded their state and federal scopes of practice to become increasingly recognized as autonomous health professionals with full prescriptive authority. Not surprisingly, this movement has often been actively opposed by corresponding medical specialty societies. Further, one can only speculate how long it will take for those vested in technology (i.e., experts in developing increasingly sophisticated platforms and apps) to offer psychology students who are on clinical internships the capability of exploring which medications might be best suited for any particular patient/client with whom they are working. Similarly, one should also expect the development of virtual centers of psychopharmacological excellence, perhaps fostered jointly by schools of pharmacy and professional psychology, to become available online, thereby functionally removing historical geographical barriers to professional training.

It is also important to appreciate that these changes are not occurring randomly or in a larger policy vacuum. The senior author (DeLeon) recently had the opportunity to serve on the U.S.

Health Resources and Services Administration (HRSA) Advisory Committee on Interdisciplinary, Community-Based Linkages (ACICBL). The committee's *16th Annual Report to the Secretary of Health and Human Services and the U.S. Congress* addressed the growing importance of clinical training sites for the nation:

> Enrollment in virtually all health professions is growing, while changes in the health care system are leading to consolidation of hospitals and a decline in traditional training sites. To expand the number of sites, schools and programs must begin to look to smaller, non-traditional sites such as community-based clinics. However, such sites often lack the resources needed to accept students and provide a broad range of clinical experiences. . . . The recommendations provided in this 16th report of the Advisory Committee for Interdisciplinary, Community-Based Linkages (ACICBL) are intended to address the challenges facing health professions schools in developing new clinical training sites, assisting students in accessing rural or other distant clinical sites, and providing incentives and support to increase the number and promote the quality of preceptors. (Advisory Committee on Interdisciplinary, Community-Based Linkages, 2017, p. 6)

In light of these projected challenges, psychology's training programs will undoubtedly, over time, develop cooperative agreements with major organized systems of health care, including our nation's federally qualified community health centers, the Federal Bureau of Prisons, and especially the VA, which currently is the largest employer of psychologists in the nation. Again, the ACA has provided impressive resources for establishing organized systems of care; for example, patient-centered medical homes (an important initiative without express reference to psychology). A significant proportion of the beneficiaries of each of these systems has a long history of, and continues to possess, a very pressing need for quality psychological services, including in some cases, the appropriate utilization of psychotropic medications. Psychology can make a significant difference in the ability of these systems to fulfill their underlying societal mission. We would further suggest that it will be necessary for the educational leadership of APA to conduct a substantive, long-term-oriented policy discussion surrounding the appropriateness and necessity of telesupervision versus in person supervision, especially in rural and remote areas. Again, as the nation's health care and educational environments evolve, it is necessary to constantly reassess earlier fundamental assumptions.

Doctoral psychology programs located within or closely associated with medical and/or nursing schools may intuitively seem to be particularly well suited to providing additional training for students interested in psychopharmacology. However, our experiences to date strongly suggest that fundamental change is often surprisingly difficult, especially for those who feel that they or their profession may be adversely impacted, notwithstanding any expected societal benefits. Accordingly, we would expect that it would take truly visionary and strong-minded leadership for any school of medicine or nursing to actively engage in this training, even if individual faculty members have a sincere interest and possess the necessary didactic and clinical expertise required. From a more optimistic frame of reference, at the core of psychology's prescriptive authority movement is recognition of the necessity of interprofessional collaboration, a value these programs are increasingly likely to share. Through greater investment in interprofessional academic coursework, they could provide students with the foundational training in psychopharmacology that will be necessary for working on interprofessional health care teams, whether individual students are actually interested in pursuing additional psychopharmacology training or not. It is also our expectation that those psychology students who wish to pursue prescriptive authority will gravitate towards programs that value strong academic training in psychopharmacology and the interprofessional nature of this work—and in which highly creative and visionary faculty are often found.

As the HRSA 16th *Annual Report* strongly suggests, a critical component of health professions training for all disciplines is the internship or residency experience. For those interested in pursuing psychopharmacology education, internship-level opportunities can provide trainees with invaluable exposure to clinical psychopharmacology. Internship experiences within organized health care systems, such as those within state or federal sites, will consider offering rotations in clinical psychopharmacology; for example, by arranging for the possibility of shadowing a prescribing psychologist, psychiatric nurse, psychiatrist, or other relevant prescribing provider. At a minimum, those responsible for the administration of APA-accredited internships should facilitate the development of regular seminars specifically focusing on the potential use of psychotropic medications (pros and cons) for their facility's patient populations. These seminars could be offered for those with an interest in pursuing postdoctoral training, or more generally to increase the interprofessional competence of all trainees. Following the lead of the DoD, we would expect the field of psychology to pursue the natural progression of increased training opportunities by establishing formal postdoctoral fellowships in clinical psychopharmacology within both the public and private sector, as described elsewhere in this handbook (see Chapter 29, this volume).

Another natural progression in the establishment of formal postdoctoral fellowships is the development of subspecialty tracks within clinical psychopharmacology as envisioned by the APA Task Force. Psychologists with training in neuropsychology, clinical health psychology, child psychology, geriatric psychology, and addictions psychology will benefit from programs that offer concentrations aimed at developing their competency to prescribe within their specific subspecialties. This will not only ensure the continued commitment to build on psychologists' traditional competencies, but also advance the goal of integrating prescribing psychologists into primary care, neurorehabilitation, and long-term care settings, among others. Furthermore, as the VA has demonstrated with its postdoctoral initiatives, these will provide excellent research opportunities for interested scientists.

Whether psychologists with specialized training in neuropsychology and clinical health psychology should push for expanded prescription privileges relevant to their practice (i.e., beyond psychotropics) remains a controversial topic, even among proponents of prescriptive authority. Clinical health psychologists, for example, regularly provide treatment in smoking cessation, obesity, sleep disorders, and diabetes management. Prescribing health psychologists have the unique advantage of extensive training in the psychobiosocial model, making them well suited to integrate behavior change and medication management in the treatment of these conditions. With proper training and experience, we believe that they could safely and effectively administer non-steroidal anti-inflammatory drugs, nicotine patches, nonbenzodiazepine hypnotics, and other commonly administered medications in the treatment of physical diseases with strong behavioral and psychological components. Should the treatment provided by prescribing psychologists be expanded to include commonly prescribed medications, such as acetylcholinesterase inhibitors for Alzheimer's disease or dopamine-receptor agonists for Parkinson's disease, for example? Considering the high level of understanding of specific disease process by specialists like neuropsychologists, this seems a likely next step in the evolution of expanding the scope of practice and potential impact for patients.

THE CONTINUING CRITICAL IMPORTANCE OF VISIONARY LEADERSHIP WITHIN THE AMERICAN PSYCHOLOGICAL ASSOCIATION

In August, 1995, the APA Council of Representatives formally endorsed prescriptive authority for appropriately trained psychologists and called for the development of model legislation and a model training curriculum. Since then, APA has solidified this foundation, establishing a national examination for clinicians and a rigorous designation process for training programs. Currently, the training for prescribing psychologists occurs at the postdoctoral level in the form of a master's in clinical psychopharmacology or certificate program. Only three APA-designated training programs currently actively exist (i.e.,

Alliant International University, Fairleigh Dickinson University, and New Mexico State University); with the Chicago School of Professional Psychology not currently APA-designated, and with the University of Hawaii at Hilo having been designated but now focusing on developing a viable and sustainable student enrollment. We further understand that several developing programs are in the process of also pursuing APA designation. Without question, as more states pass legislation authorizing prescription privileges for psychologists, the need for additional training programs will increase dramatically.

From the beginning, those most involved in shaping the agenda for psychology's psychopharmacology professional quest sincerely believed that developing a critical mass of well trained and qualified providers was the necessary first step. In our judgment, the time has arrived for organized psychology to focus on systematically developing both the concrete financial incentives and the clinical opportunities necessary for providing these specialized services. Over our years of involvement in the public policy process, we have learned that it is absolutely necessary to possess both a broadly defined long-term vision and the dedication and persistence required to implement concrete, short-term steps towards one's ultimate goal (DeLeon & Kazdin, 2010). One of the most significant positive clinical consequences of RxP will be that the profession has finally obtained the legal authority (i.e., legal standing) to clinically question, modify, or terminate ongoing medication orders.

There is little question that for the leadership of APA, from the Council of Representatives to the Board of Directors, increasing the scope of practice of psychologists is in the mission and vision. The question of how best to do so, basing training and practice on sound professional education, standards, and scientific information, is critical. One of the interesting challenges being addressed in 2018 by the APA is the role and scope of the master's degree. The possible integration of what has occurred with the existing master's program in psychopharmacology and the further evolution of the role of a master's degree in psychology should be considered. Competency-based training and competency-based provision of care is the future for all health professions.

THE EXAMPLE OF NURSING HOME QUALITY OF CARE

Providing necessary and quality care to our nation's senior citizens represents just one graphic example of where appropriately trained prescribing psychologists can make a substantial difference to society:

> Consider it America's *other* prescription drug epidemic. For decades, experts have warned that older Americans are taking too many unnecessary drugs, often prescribed by multiple doctors, for dubious or unknown reasons. Researchers estimate that 25 percent of people ages 65 to 69 take at least five prescription drugs to treat chronic conditions, a figure that jumps to nearly 46 percent for those between 70 and 79. Doctors say it is not uncommon to encounter patients taking more than 20 drugs to treat acid reflux, heart disease, depression or insomnia or other disorders. Unlike the overuse of opioid painkillers, the polypharmacy problem has attracted little attention, even though its hazards are well documented. (Boodman, 2017, pp. E1, E4)

In 2015, the U.S. Government Accountability Office (GAO) released its report *Antipsychotic Drug Use*. The GAO noted that

> Concerns have been raised about the use of antipsychotic drugs to address the behavioral symptoms of [dementia], primarily due to the FDA [U.S. Food and Drug Administration]'s boxed warning that these drugs may cause an increased risk of death when used by older adults with dementia and the drugs are not approved for this use. (U.S. Government Accountability Office, 2015, "GAO Highlights")

Focusing on older adults residing in nursing homes, the GAO found that about one third of those with dementia who spent more than 100 days in a nursing home were prescribed an antipsychotic; in stark contrast, only approximately 14% of those living outside of a nursing home with similar diagnoses were prescribed an antipsychotic. Individuals who were diagnosed with one of the FDA-approved conditions for antipsychotic drugs—schizophrenia and bipolar disorder—were excluded from the study, as were those with Tourette syndrome and Huntington's disease, for which antipsychotics are recognized as an acceptable treatment. Among other concerns, antipsychotic medications have been found to cause falls, which are particularly dangerous for the elderly.

Currently dementia affects almost 15% of older adults in the United States, and is responsible for an annual cost of between $157 billion and $215 billion for caring for these individuals. It is estimated that dementia costs will more than double by 2040 due to the aging of the American population. In conducting their review, the GAO further noted that

> Clinical guidelines consistently suggest the use of antipsychotic drugs for the treatment of the behavioral symptoms of dementia only when other, non-pharmacological attempts to ameliorate the behaviors have failed, and the individuals pose a threat to themselves or to others. (U.S. Government Accountability Office, 2015, p. 8)

The nation's nursing homes are closely regulated by authorities in the federal government (for example, under the Medicare and Medicaid Conditions for Participation) and also at the state level, where they are required to be licensed. Over the years, various congressional committees have conducted numerous public hearings on the quality (or lack thereof) of care being provided to residents of nursing homes, often emphasizing that there is a clear governmental responsibility for providing necessary protections for these vulnerable citizens. Those genuinely interested in pursuing psychology's prescriptive authority agenda could clearly develop a comprehensive legal and regulatory strategy at the federal and state level for formally recognizing (and ultimately reimbursing) psychology's unique clinical skills, especially in collaboration with colleagues in the clinical pharmacy and advanced practice nursing communities. In conjunction, additional focus is needed on both state and federal reimbursement practices, for without economic backing the future of prescriptive authority would be challenged. Just like allied mental health practitioners with terminal master's degrees (e.g., physician assistants), psychologists with appropriate training should be adequately reimbursed.

EXCITING RESEARCH HORIZONS

The majority of psychopharmacological research today is conducted by psychiatrists in academic settings. As more psychologists become trained in psychopharmacology, however, a natural shift in this dynamic should follow. Psychologists' extensive training in the scientific method makes them particularly well suited to take more of a leadership role in this research, and the same holds true for pharmacotherapy research. Further, psychologists' training in the scientist–practitioner model prepares them to be ideally adept in translational research efforts in psychopharmacology (and some would argue, pharmacology and medicine more broadly). Research on geriatric depression, for example, struggles with the question of significantly higher variability in psychopharmacological treatment response. Approximately 25% of geriatric patients are treatment resistant, while many others are at significantly increased risk of relapse (Knöchel et al., 2015). Several psychosocial and medical factors associated with increased vulnerability to poor treatment response have been identified, such as age of onset, stress, anxiety, bereavement, stroke, and interferon-induced depression. However, the neurobiological substrates that differentiate psychopharmacological treatment response remain largely unknown. Similarly, approximately 25% to 40% of cancer patients develop depressive and anxiety symptoms following diagnosis, although this estimate is likely to be a significant underrepresentation (Smith, 2015). Despite increasing recognition of the emotional distress and treatment-related cognitive difficulties associated with a cancer diagnosis, formal diagnostic evaluations by mental health experts are still frequently lacking in oncology settings.

Psychologists with specialized training in psychopharmacology are ideally equipped to assist in these efforts, given their in-depth knowledge of both subject matters and their ability to bridge the divide between these lines of investigation. Additionally, this same logic suggests that psychologists are able to provide interprofessional research teams with unique insights into the translation of findings to clinical recommendations. Despite our confidence in the shift to increased representation of psychologists in psychopharmacological research, it remains critical that psychologists become more aggressive in efforts to secure research grants for clinical trials of new and current psychotropics (and trials of combined psychotherapy and pharmacology), engage in the scientific discussion through submissions to major journals of related disciplines, and advocate for the critical role psychologists' expertise can play in this field. Some of our colleagues have been successful in these efforts by working within university departments of psychiatry, and finding employment in medical centers can increase opportunities for interprofessional collaborations. Notably, psychologists' greater involvement in psychopharmacology research can serve as an exponential catalyst to establishing psychology's role in this area; as current psychologists in academic settings become ingrained in drug trial research, so will a new generation of psychologists, as more and more opportunities emerge for graduate- and undergraduate-level drug research.

AN EXCITING FUTURE

In conclusion, the delivery of quality health care in our nation is undergoing unprecedented change. Team-based integrated care emphasizing the psychosocial-cultural-economic gradient of quality care will soon become the norm, with reimbursement strategies following. Patients and providers of all disciplines will need to become increasingly attuned to the intimate relationship between the physiological, behavioral, and emotional determinants of health. The historical Cartesian dualism—the view that mind and body are essentially separate entities—will be replaced by exciting advances in scientific knowledge. Substantive knowledge of the effects (short term and long term) of pharmacological agents and their interactions with other proposed interventions will be especially important to clinicians, educators, and researchers specializing in the emotional (i.e., mental health) aspects of health care. Finally, we would further suggest that the profession of psychology and society as a whole would be well served by such a timely and critical integration of psychotherapeutic and psychopharmacologic competencies—one that would, in our judgment, represent the best of former APA President George Miller's call for "giving psychology away."

References

Addis, M. E., & Krasnow, A. D. (2000). A national survey of practicing psychologists' attitudes toward psychotherapy treatment manuals. *Journal of Consulting and Clinical Psychology*, 68(2), 331.

Advisory Committee on Interdisciplinary, Community-Based Linkages. (2017). *Enhancing community-based clinical training sites: Challenges and opportunities—Sixteenth annual report to the Secretary of the U.S. Department of Health and Human Services and to Congress.* Washington, DC: Author.

Boodman, S. G. (2017, December 12). The other big drug problem: Seniors taking too many pills. *The Washington Post*, pp. E1, E4.

Burns, S. M., DeLeon, P. H., Chemtob, C. M., Welch, B. L., & Samuels, R. M. (1988). Psychotropic medication: A new technique for psychology? *Psychotherapy: Theory, Research, Practice, & Training*, 25, 508–515. http://dx.doi.org/10.1037/h0085376

Bush, G. W. (2004). Remarks in a discussion on the benefits of health care information technology in Baltimore, Maryland (April 27, 2004). *Weekly Compilation of Presidential Documents*, 40(18), 697–702.

Chambless, D. L., & Ollendick, T. H. (2001). Empirically supported psychological interventions: Controversies and evidence. *Annual Review of Psychology*, 52(1), 685–716.

DeLeon, P. H., Fox, R. E., & Graham, S. R. (1991). Prescription privileges. Psychology's next frontier? *American Psychologist*, 46, 384–393. http://dx.doi.org/10.1037/0003-066X.46.4.384

DeLeon, P. H., & Kazdin, A. E. (2010). Public policy: Extending psychology's contributions to national priorities. *Rehabilitation Psychology*, 55, 311–319. http://dx.doi.org/10.1037/a0020450

*DeLeon, P. H., Sells, J. R., Cassidy, O., Waters, A. J., & Kasper, C. E. (2015). Health policy: Timely and interdisciplinary. *Training and Education in Professional Psychology*, 9, 121–127. http://dx.doi.org/10.1037/tep0000077

Fonagy, P. (1999). Achieving evidence-based psychotherapy practice: A psychodynamic perspective on the general acceptance of treatment manuals. *Clinical Psychology: Science and Practice*, 6(4), 442–444.

Fox, R. E., DeLeon, P. H., Newman, R., Sammons, M. T., Dunivin, D. L., & Baker, D. C. (2009). Prescriptive authority and psychology: A status report. *American Psychologist*, 64, 257–268. http://dx.doi.org/10.1037/a0015938

*Garrison, E. G., DeLeon, P. H., & Smedley, B. D. (2017). Psychology, public policy, and advocacy: Past, present, and future. *American Psychologist*, 72, 737–752. http://dx.doi.org/10.1037/amp0000209

Geraghty, E. M., Franks, P., & Kravitz, R. L. (2007). Primary care visit length, quality, and satisfaction for standardized patients with depression. *Journal of General Internal Medicine*, 22(12), 1641–1647.

*Institute of Medicine (IOM). (2015). *Measuring the impact of interprofessional education on collaborative practice and patient outcomes.* Washington, DC: The National Academies Press.

Knöchel, C., Alves, G., Friedrichs, B., Schneider, B., Schmidt-Rechau, A., Wenzler, S., . . . Oertel-Knöchel, V. (2015). Treatment-resistant late-life depression: Challenges and perspectives. *Current Neuropharmacology*, 13, 577–591. http://dx.doi.org/10.2174/1570159X1305151013200032

McGuire, F. L. (1990). *Psychology aweigh! A history of clinical psychology in the United States Navy, 1900–1988.* Washington, DC: American Psychological Association.

Olfson, M., Blanco, C., Wang, S., Laje, G., & Correll, C. U. (2014). National trends in the mental health care of children, adolescents, and adults by office-based physicians. *JAMA Psychiatry*, 71, 81–90. http://dx.doi.org/10.1001/jamapsychiatry.2013.3074

Patient Protection and Affordable Care Act (P.L. 111-148), 42 U.S.C. § 18001 et seq. (2010).

Phares, E. J., & Trull, T. J. (1997). *Clinical psychology: Concepts, methods, and profession* (5th ed.). Pacific Grove, CA: Brooks/Cole.

Puente, A. E. (2011). Psychology as a health care profession. *American Psychologist*, 66(8), 781–792. http://dx.doi.org/10.1037/a0025033

Smith, E. W. L. (1995). A passionate, rational response to the "manualization" of psychotherapy. *Psychotherapy Bulletin*, 30(2), 36–40.

Smith, H. R. (2015). Depression in cancer patients: Pathogenesis, implications and treatment (Review).

*Asterisks indicate assessments or resources.

Oncology Letters, 9, 1509–1514. http://dx.doi.org/10.3892/ol.2015.2944

Smyer, M. A., Balster, R. L., Egli, D., Johnson, D. L., Kilbey, M. M., Leith, N. J., & Puente, A. E. (1993). Summary of the report of the ad hoc task force on psychopharmacology of the American Psychological Association. *Professional Psychology: Research and Practice, 24*, 394–403. http://dx.doi.org/10.1037/0735-7028.24.4.394

Uhlaner, J. E. (1967, September). *Chronology of military psychology in the Army.* Paper presented at the meeting of the 1967 Annual Convention of the American Psychological Association, Washington, DC.

U.S. Department of Health and Human Services (HHS). (1999). *Mental health: A report of the Surgeon General.* Rockville, MD: Department of Health and Human Services, Substance Abuse and Mental Health Services Administration, Center for Mental Health Services, National Institutes of Health, National Institute of Mental Health.

U.S. Government Accountability Office (GAO). (2015). *Antipsychotic drug use: HHS has initiatives to reduce use among older adults in nursing homes, but should expand efforts to other settings* (GAO-15-211). Washington, DC: Author.

Vermani, M., Marcus, M., & Katzman, M. A. (2011). Rates of detection of mood and anxiety disorders in primary care: A descriptive, cross-sectional study. *The Primary Care Companion for CNS Disorders, 13*(2), e1–e10.

Index

Dimensional Obsessive-Compulsive Scale
(DOCS), 251
DiPerna, J. C., 352
Direct-to-consumer advertising (DTCA),
7, 122
Disabilities, learning, 363–364
DISCO (Diagnostic Interview for Social
and Communication Disorders),
377
Discontinuation, of sedative/anxiolytic
use disorder, 591
Discontinuation syndrome, 204
Disruptive behavior disorder, 461
Distribution, in psychopharmacology,
51–53
Disulfiram, 482–487, 493–494, 544
Divalproex, 170, 173–174, 285, 382,
514, 519
Diversion, of medication, 573–574
DMS [DMTS] (Delayed Matching to
Sample), 69, 399
DOCS (Dimensional Obsessive-
Compulsive Scale), 251
Doctoral psychology programs, 718.
See also Education, for psychologists
DoD. *See* U.S. Department of Defense
Donepezil plus choline, 404
Donnelly-Swift, E., 599
Dopamine (DA), 26, 170, 219, 534, 547
Dopidines, 413
Dosing
in elderly, 55–56
fixed, 692
intermittent, 145
open-loop, 692
in pregnancy, 55
response-independent, 692
Doxepin, 313–314, 317
Drake, R. E., 600
Dronabinol, 516–517
DRSP (Daily Record of Severity of
Problems), 143
Drug(s)
actions on brain, 36
development of, 64–71, 673, 675–678
dosing of. *See* Dosing
efficacy of, 117, 118–121. *See also*
Efficacy
experimental, 63
factors affecting response to, 62–63
instrumental vs. recreational use of, 42
interactions of, 55–56
medication vs., 42–43
misuse of, 545
pricing of, 675

repeated effects of, 63
route of exposure to, 49
safety/lethality of, 49–51
sensitization to, 47
as term, 44
Drug Attitudinal Inventory, 46
Drug-seeking, in animal laboratory
research, 71–72
Drug testing, 490–491, 542–543, 594
Drug trials, clinical, 110–115, 125–126
*DSM. See Diagnostic and Statistical Manual
of Mental Disorders*
DTCA (direct-to-consumer advertising),
7, 122
Duloxetine, 198, 428, 430
Dutra, L., 600
Dye industry, and psychopharmacology
development, 5
Dysfunction, sexual, 225

Earle, J. F., 385
Eating addiction, 640
Eating Disorder Diagnostic Scale (EDDS),
330
Eating Disorder Examination (EDE),
329–330
Eating Disorder Examination
Questionnaire (EDE-Q), 330
Eating disorders, 327–338
about, 327–328
with BPD, 461
in clinical laboratory research, 95
comorbid disorders with, 337–338
diagnosing, 329–330
emerging trends in, 338
epidemiology/prevalence of, 328–329
evidence-based pharmacotherapy for,
330–334
historical treatments of, 329
nonpharmacological approaches to,
336–337
resources for, 338
sex differences with, 336
treatment management with, 334–336
E-cigarettes, 622–623
Eckman, T. A., 230
Ecological momentary assessment (EMA),
98
Ecological validity, 96–97
ECS (cannabinoid receptor system), 511
ECT. *See* Electroconvulsive therapy
EDDS (Eating Disorder Diagnostic Scale),
330
EDE (Eating Disorder Examination),
329–330

EDE-Q (Eating Disorder Examination
Questionnaire), 330
Edinburgh Postnatal Depression Scale
(EPDS), 144, 147
Education, for psychologists, 656, 659.
See also Training
Edwards, J. G., 593
Effective dose value, 46
Efficacy
of BD treatment, 169–170, 175,
179–180
defined, 6
SGAs vs. FGAs, 220–221, 228
of SSRIs, 144
Eight-arm radial arm maze (RAM), 69
Elderly. *See also* Older adulthood
antipsychotics use in, 228
anxiety disorders in, 205
AUD in, 492–493
benzodiazepines/Z-drugs used in,
595–596
BPD in, 459
dosing in, 55–56, 409
eating disorders in, 335
neurocognitive disorders in, 410–411
and off-label prescribing, 125
pain management in, 435–436
PTSD in, 292
sleep–wake disorders in, 316–317
TUD in, 619
Electrical stimulation. *See* Brain
stimulation therapy
Electroconvulsive therapy (ECT), 151–
152, 184–185, 691, 693–696
Elkashef, A., 535, 540, 542, 547
EMA (ecological momentary assessment),
98
Emergency medicine, 43, 578–579
Emmelkamp, P. M., 361
Emotions, expressed, 230
Endocannabinoids, 26
Endogenous opioid peptides, 26
EPDS (Edinburgh Postnatal Depression
Scale), 144, 147
Epidemiology
alcohol use disorder, 481–482
anxiety disorders, 195–196
attention-deficit/hyperactivity
disorder, 347–349
autism spectrum disorder, 373–374
behavioral addictions, 631–632
bipolar disorder, 165–166
borderline personality disorder,
451–452
cannabis use disorder, 507–509